IMAGING
CHILDREN

SECOND EDITION

To our spouses – our best friends – Austin, Anne, Irene and Rosanna, and our families.

Thank you for your forbearance and love.

This book is also dedicated to our parents, who are our mentors, and, above all, to children everywhere.

IMAGING

CHILDREN

SECOND EDITION   VOLUME 2

Edited by

Helen Carty FRCR FRCPI FRCP FRCPCH FFRRCSI (Hon)
Professor of Paediatric Radiology
Alder Hey Hospital Royal Liverpool Children's NHS Trust and The University of Liverpool
Liverpool
UK

Francis Brunelle MD
Professor and Chairman of Pediatric Radiology
Department of Radiology
Hôpital des Enfants Malades
Paris
France

David A Stringer BSc MBBS FRCR FRCPC
Clinical Professor of Radiology
Clinical Director and Senior Consultant
National University Hospital;
Head of Diagnostic Imaging
KK Women's and Children's Hospital
Singapore

Simon Ching-Shun Kao MBBS DMRD FRCR FACR
Professor of Radiology
University of Iowa College of Medicine
Staff Radiologist, Children's Hospital of Iowa
Iowa City, IA
USA

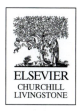

ELSEVIER
CHURCHILL
LIVINGSTONE

EDINBURGH   LONDON   NEW YORK   OXFORD   PHILADELPHIA   ST LOUIS   SYDNEY   TORONTO   2005

ELSEVIER
CHURCHILL
LIVINGSTONE

An imprint of Elsevier Ltd

First edition 1994
Second edition 2005

ISBN 0 4330 7039 3

British Library Cataloguing in Publication Data
A catalogue record for this book is available from the British Library

Library of Congress Cataloging in Publication Data
A catalog record for this book is available from the Library of Congress

Notice
Medical knowledge is constantly changing. Standard safety precautions must be followed, but as new research and clinical experience broaden our knowledge, changes in treatment and drug therapy may become necessary or appropriate. Readers are advised to check the most current product information provided by the manufacturer of each drug to be administered to verify the recommended dose, the method and duration of administration, and contraindications. It is the responsibility of the practitioner, relying on experience and knowledge of the patient, to determine dosages and the best treatment for each individual patient. Neither the Publisher nor the contributors assume any liability for any injury and/or damage to persons or property arising from this publication.
The Publisher

Printed in China
Last digit is the print number: 9 8 7 6 5 4 3 2 1

Working together to grow
libraries in developing countries

www.elsevier.com | www.bookaid.org | www.sabre.org

ELSEVIER   BOOK AID International   Sabre Foundation

Commissioning Editor: *Michael Houston, Alan Ross*
Project Development Manager: *Sheila Black*
Project Manager: *Cheryl Brant*
Illustration Manager: *Mick Ruddy*
Design Manager: *Andy Chapman*
Illustrator: *Robin Dean*

Contents

Contributors

Laurence J Abernethy MRCP FRCR
Consultant Paediatric Radiologist
Department of Radiology
Alder Hey Hospital Royal Liverpool Children's
NHS Trust
Liverpool
UK

Judith E Adams MBBS DMRD FRCR FRCP
Chair, Diagnostic Radiology;
Clinical Academic Group Leader, Imaging
Science & Biomedical Engineering;
Honorary Consultant Radiologist
University of Manchester
Manchester
UK

Hussein Aref MB BCh MSc(Rad)
Assistant Lecturer in Radiology
Department of Radiology
Faculty of Medicine
Alexandria University
Alexandria
Egypt

Eric Arnaud MD
Consultant in Craniofacial Surgery
Department of Pediatric Neurosurgery –
Craniofacial Unit
Hôpital des Enfants Malades
Paris
France

Paul S Babyn MDCM FRCP(C)
Associate Professor of Medical Imaging
Department of Radiology
The Hospital for Sick Children
Toronto, Ontario
Canada

Teresa Berrocal Frutos MD PhD
Pediatric Radiologist
Department of Radiology
Pediatric Radiology Section
University Hospital La Paz
Madrid
Spain

Larissa T Bilaniuk MD FACR
Professor of Radiology
University of Pennsylvania School of Medicine;
Staff Neuroradiologist
Department of Radiology
Children's Hospital of Philadelphia
Philadelphia, PA
USA

Johan G Blickman MD PhD FACR
Professor of Radiology and Pediatrics
Chairman, Department of Radiology
University Medical Centre Nijmegen
Nijmegen
Netherlands

Nigel J Broderick BMedSci BMBS
MRCP(UK) FRCR
Consultant in Radiology
Radiology Department
Nottingham City Hospital
Nottingham
UK

Francis Brunelle MD
Professor and Chairman of Pediatric
Radiology
Department of Radiology
Hôpital des Enfants Malades
Paris
France

Nathalie Capon Degardin MD
Assistant Professor
Department of Pediatric Neurosurgery –
Craniofacial Unit
Hôpital des Enfants Malades
Paris
France

Rita C Carneiro MD
Consultant Radiologist
Department of Radiology
Hospital De Dona Estefânia
Lisbon
Portugal;
Department of Radiology
UNC Hospitals
Chapel Hill, NC
USA

Helen Carty FRCR FRCPI FRCP FRCPCH
FFRRCSI (Hon)
Professor of Paediatric Radiology
Alder Hey Hospital Royal Liverpool Children's
NHS Trust and University of Liverpool
Liverpool
UK

Amparo Castellote MD
Chief of Pediatric MR
Department of Pediatric Radiology
Vall d'Hebron Hospitals
Barcelona
Spain

Gillian Cattell DCR MSc
Advanced Ultrasound Practitioner
Radiology Department
Birmingham Women's Healthcare Trust
Birmingham
UK

Peter G Chait MBBCh FFRAD(D)SA
FRCR(UK) FRCP(C) DABR
Associate Professor of Radiology
University of Toronto
Department of Diagnostic Imaging
The Hospital for Sick Children
Toronto, Ontario
Canada

Valérie Chigot MD
Assistant Professor of Radiology
Department of Radiology
Hôpital des Enfants Malades
Paris
France

W K 'Kling' Chong BMedSci MD MRCP
FRCR
Consultant Paediatric Neuroradiologist
Department of Radiology
Great Ormond Street Hospital for Children
London
UK

Jeanne S Chow MD
Radiologist
Department of Radiology
Children's Hospital Boston
Boston, MA
USA

Elisabeth A M Cornelissen MD PhD
Pediatric Nephrologist
Department of Pediatric Nephrology
University Medical Centre Nijmegen
Nijmegen
The Netherlands

Cinzia Crawley MBBCh BAO FRCR BSc
(Hons)
Consultant Radiologist
Department of Radiology
Alder Hey Hospital Royal Liverpool Children's
NHS Trust
Liverpool
UK

Philippe Demaerel MD, PhD
Professor of Radiology, Consultant
Neuroradiologist
Department of Radiology
University Hospital KU Leuven
Leuven
Belgium

Veronica Donoghue FRCR FFR RCSI
Consultant Paediatric Radiologist
Radiology Department
Children's University Hospital
Dublin
Ireland

Andrew W Duncan MBBS DMRD FFR FRCR
FRCPCh
Consultant Paediatric Radiologist
Department of Paediatric Radiology
Bristol Royal Hospital for Children;
Senior Lecturer in Paediatric Radiology
University of Bristol
Bristol
UK

Ranjana Dwarkanath MBBS DMRD
Specialist Registrar in Radiology
Department of Radiology
Alder Hey Hospital Royal Liverpool Children's
NHS Trust
Liverpool
UK

Goya Enríquez MD
Head of Pediatric Ultrasound
Department of Pediatric Radiology
Vall d'Hebron Hospitals
Barcelona
Spain

Mónica Epelman MD
Clinical Fellow in Pediatric Radiology
Department of Diagnostic Imaging
Hospital for Sick Children and University of
Toronto
Toronto, Ontario
Canada

Judy A Estroff MD
Co-director of Fetal Imaging
Department of Radiology
Children's Hospital Boston
Boston, MA
USA

Wouter F J Feitz MD PhD FEBU
Pediatric Urologist
Pediatric Urology Center
Department of Urology
University Medical Center Nijmegen
Nijmegen
The Netherlands

Olof Flodmark MD PhD FRCPC
Senior Consulting Paediatric Neuroradiologist
& Associate Professor of Neuroradiology
Department of Neuroradiology & MR
Research Center
Karolinska Hospital
Stockholm
Sweden

Lynn A Fordham MD
Associate Professor of Radiology
Section Chief of Pediatric Imaging
Department of Radiology
University of North Carolina School of
Medicine
Chapel Hill, NC
USA

Richard Fotter MD
Professor of Radiology and Chairman
Department of Radiology
Division of Pediatric Radiology
Medical University Graz
Graz
Austria

Donald P Frush MD
Associate Professor of Radiology
Chief, Division of Pediatric Radiology
McGovern Davison Children's Health Center
Department of Radiology
Duke Medical Center
Durham, NC
USA

Ingmar Gaßner MD
Senior Consultant
Section of Pediatric Radiology
Department of Pediatrics
University of Innsbruck Medical School
Innsbruck
Austria

Theresa E Geley MD
Resident
Section of Pediatric Radiology
Department of Pediatrics
University of Innsbruck Medical School
Innsbruck
Austria

Tal Geva MD FACC
Associate Professor of Pediatrics (Radiology)
Harvard Medical School;
Senior Associate, Cardiology
Department of Cardiology
Children's Hospital Boston
Boston, MA
USA

Nadine Girard MD
Professor of Radiology
Université de la Méditerranée;
Department of Radiology
Hôpital Nord
Marseille
France

Dan Greitz MD PhD
Senior Consulting Neuroradiologist
Department of Neuroradiology & MR
Research Center
Karolinska Hospital
Stockholm
Sweden

Christine M Hall FRCR
Professor of Paediatric Radiology
Department of Radiology
Great Ormond Street Hospital for Children
London
UK

Katharine E Halliday MBChB FRCS FRCR
Consultant Paediatric Radiologist
Department of Radiology
Queen's Medical Centre
Nottingham
UK

Walter Huda PhD
Professor of Radiology
Department of Radiology
SUNY Upstate Medical University
Syracuse, NY
USA

Fiorenza Ianzini PhD
Research Scientist
Department of Radiology;
Adjunct Associate Professor
Departments of Radiation, Oncology &
Biomedical Engineering
University of Iowa
Iowa City, IA
USA

Devon Jacobson
Undergraduate BSc Hons (Biology)
University of Western Ontario
London, Ontario;
Research Student
Department of Image Guided Therapy
The Hospital for Sick Children
Toronto, Ontario
Canada

Douglas Jamieson MBChB FFRAD(D)SA
MMED FRCPC
Clinical Associate Professor
Department of Radiology
BC Children's Hospital
Vancouver, British Columbia
Canada

Karl Johnson MRCP FRCR
Consultant Paediatric Radiologist
Radiology Department
Birmingham Children's Hospital
Birmingham
UK

Simon Ching-Shun Kao MBBS DMRD
FRCR FACR
Professor of Radiology
University of Iowa College of Medicine
Staff Radiologist, Children's Hospital of Iowa
Iowa City, IA
USA

In-One Kim MD
Professor of Radiology
Department of Radiology
Seoul National University Hospital and
Seoul National University College of Medicine
Seoul
Korea

Torvid Kiserud MD PhD
Professor of Obstetrics and Gynecology
Division of Obstetrics & Gynecology
Institute of Clinical Medicine
University of Bergen
Bergen
Norway

Denise Kitchiner MD FRCP FRCPCH
Consultant Paediatric Cardiologist
Alder Hey Hospital Royal Liverpool Children's
NHS Trust
Liverpool
UK

Gillian Klafkowski MBChB BSc Hons DMRD
FRCR
Consultant Paediatric Radiologist
Department of Radiology
Warrington District General Hospital
Warrington
UK

Osnat Konen-Cohen MD
Fellow, Diagnostic Imaging
Department of Diagnostic Imaging
The Hospital for Sick Children
Toronto, Ontario
Canada

Sambasiva R Kottamasu MD
Clinical Professor of Radiology
Department of Radiology
Wayne State University School of Medicine;
Radiologist
Covenant Medical Center
Saginaw, MI
USA

Steven J Kraus MD MS
Associate Professor of Radiology & Pediatrics
Department of Radiology
Cincinnati Children's Hospital Medical Center
and University of Cincinnati College of
Medicine
Cincinnati, OH
USA

Ganesh Krishnamurthy MD DNB
Fellow
Department of Diagnostic Imaging
KK Women's and Children's Hospital
Singapore

Elisabeth Lajeunie-Renier (deceased) PhD
Biologist
Department of Clinical Genetics
Hôpital des Enfants Malades
Paris
France

Gabriel B H Lau MBChB FRANZCR
Consultant Radiologist
Department of Diagnostic Imaging
National University Hospital
Singapore

Olivier Levrier MD
Consultant Neuroradiologist
Department of Neuroradiology
CHU Timone
Marseille
France

Franz Lindbichler MD
Senior Registrar
Department of Radiology
Division of Pediatric Radiology
University Hospital Graz
Graz
Austria

Gillian Long MB MRCP DCH DRCOG FRCR
Med FRANZCR
Deputy Director of Radiology
Medical Imaging Department
Mater Children's Hospital
Brisbane
Australia

Javier Lucaya MD
Director
Division of Diagnostic Imaging
Vall d'Hebron Hospitals and
Autonomous University of Barcelona
Barcelona
Spain

Mark T Madsen PhD FAAPM FACR
Professor of Radiology
Department of Radiology
University of Iowa
Iowa City, IA
USA

Kieran McHugh MB FRCR FRCPI
Consultant Paediatric Radiologist
Radiology Department
Great Ormond Street Hospital for Children
London
UK

Josephine M McHugo MBBS FRCR FRCP
FRCPCH
Consultant Radiologist, Head of Specialty and
Honorary Senior Lecturer
Radiology Department
Birmingham Women's Hospital
Birmingham
UK

Maeve McPhillips MBBCh BAO FRCR
Consultant Paediatric Radiologist
Department of Radiology
Royal Hospital for Sick Children
Edinburgh
UK

Benoît Michel MD
Clinical Fellow
Department of Oral and Maxillofacial Surgery
Hôpital des Enfants Malades
Paris
France

Zulf Mughal MBChB FRCP FRCPCH DCH
Consultant Paediatrician & Honorary Senior
Lecturer in Child Health
Department of Paediatrics
Saint Mary's Hospital for Women and Children
Manchester
UK

Helen R Nadel MD FRCPC
Associate Professor of Radiology, University of
British Columbia;
Pediatric Radiologist and Nuclear Medicine
Physician, Head, Division of Nuclear Medicine
Department of Radiology
British Columbia Children's Hospital
Vancouver, British Columbia
Canada

Oscar M Navarro MD
Assistant Professor
University of Toronto;
Department of Diagnostic Imaging
The Hospital for Sick Children
Toronto, Ontario
Canada

Amaka Offiah BSc MBBS MRCP FRCR
Consultant, Academic Radiology
Radiology Department
Great Ormond Street Hospital for Children
London
UK

Øystein E Olsen PhD
Consultant Paediatric Radiologist
Radiology Department
Great Ormond Street Hospital for Children
London
UK

Kamaldine Oudjhane MD MSc
Associate Professor of Radiology
University of Toronto;
Head, Abdomen Imaging
Department of Diagnostic Imaging
The Hospital for Sick Children
Toronto, Ontario
Canada

Catherine M Owens BSc MBBS MRCP
FRCR
Consultant Paediatric Radiologist
Department of Radiology
Great Ormond Street Hospital for Children
London
UK

Frederica Papadopoulou MD
Assistant Professor of Radiology
Department of Radiology
University of Ioannina Medical School
Ioannina
Greece

Danièle Pariente MD
Chief of Pediatric Radiology
Department of Pediatric Radiology
Hôpital Bicêtre
Le Kremlin-Bicêtre
France

Zoltán Patay MD PhD
Head, Section of Neuroradiology
Department of Radiology
King Faisal Specialist Hospital and Research
Centre
Riyadh
Kingdom of Saudi Arabia

Anne Paterson MB BS MRCP FRCR FFR
RCSI
Consultant Paediatric Radiologist
Radiology Department
Royal Belfast Hospital for Sick Children
Belfast
UK

Martin Payne BDS FDSRCPS DDRRCR
Consultant in Dental & Maxillofacial Radiology
and Assessment and Casualty
The Charles Clifford Dental Hospital
Sheffield
UK

David W Pilling MB DCH FRCR FRCPCH
Consultant Paediatric Radiologist
Department of Radiology
Alder Hey Hospital Royal Liverpool Children's
NHS Trust
Liverpool
UK

Elizabeth L Pilling BM BCh MRCPCH
Specialist Registrar Paediatrics
Sheffield Children's Hospital
Sheffield
UK

Stefan Puig MD
Associate Professor
Department of Radiology
Medical University Vienna
Vienna
Austria

Maria T Raissaki MD PhD
Lecturer in Radiology
Department of Radiology
University Hospital of Iraklion
University of Crete
Iraklion
Crete
Greece

Charles Raybaud MD
Professor of Neuroradiology
Department of Neuroradiology
CHU Timone
Marseille
France

Dominique Renier MD
Pediatric Neurosurgeon
Department of Pediatric Neurosurgery
Hôpital des Enfants Malades
Paris
France

Michael Riccabona MD
Professor of Pediatrics and Radiology
Pediatric Radiologist
Department of Radiology
Division of Pediatric Radiology
University Hospital Graz
Graz
Austria

Karen Rosendahl MD PhD
Professor of Paediatric Radiology
Radiology Section
Institute of Surgery
University of Bergen
Bergen
Norway

Andrea Rossi MD
Staff Neuroradiologist
Department of Pediatric Neuroradiology
G. Gaslini Children's Research Hospital
Genoa
Italy

Dawn E Saunders MD MRCP FRCR
Consultant Neuroradiologist
Department of Radiology
Great Ormond Street Hospital for Children
London
UK

Erich Sorantin MD
Professor of Radiology
Department of Radiology
Medical University Graz
Graz
Austria

Alan Sprigg MB ChB DCH DRCOG DMRD
FRCR FRCPCH
Consultant Paediatric Radiologist
Radiology Department
Sheffield Children's Hospital
Sheffield
UK

David A Stringer BSc MB BS FRCR FRCPC
Clinical Professor of Radiology
Clinical Director and Senior Consultant
National University Hospital;
Head of Diagnostic Imaging
KK Women's and Children's Hospital
Singapore

Peter J Strouse MD
Associate Professor of Radiology
Section of Pediatric Radiology
C.S. Mott Children's Hospital
Ann Arbor, MI
USA

Louise E Sweeney MB BCh BAO DCH
DMRD FRCR
Consultant Paediatric Radiologist
Department of Radiology
Royal Belfast Hospital for Sick Children
Belfast
UK

Lawrence Tan Thuan Heng MB BS FRCR
FHKAM (Radiology) FAMS(Radiology) FHKCR
MHA
Chief of Service
Department of Radiology
Hong Kong Baptist Hospital
Kowloon
Hong Kong
China

E L Harvey J Teo MBBS FRCR
Deputy Head of Department, Consultant in
Radiology
Department of Diagnostic Imaging
KK Women's and Children's Hospital
Singapore

Paolo Tortori-Donati MD
Head, Department of Pediatric Neuroradiology
G. Gaslini's Children's Research Hospital
Genoa
Italy

Joanna Turner MB MRCP FRCR
Consultant Radiologist
Department of Radiology
Ulster Hospital
Belfast
UK

Eilish L Twomey MB BCh BAO
Consultant Paediatric Radiologist
Radiology Department
The Children's University Hospital
Dublin
Ireland

Kate A Ward BSc PhD
Research Associate
Imaging Science & Biomedical Engineering
University of Manchester
Manchester
UK

Ulrich V Willi MD
Professor of Paediatric Radiology
Department of Radiology
University Children's Hospital
Zürich
Switzerland

Alex Mun-Ching Wong MD
Neuroradiologist
Department of Diagnostic Radiology
Chang Gung Memorial Hospital
Taoyuan
Taiwan
China

Neville B Wright DMRD FRCR
Consultant Paediatric Radiologist
Department of Radiology
Royal Manchester & Booth Hall Children's
Hospital
Manchester
UK

Robert A Zimmerman MD
Chief of Neuroradiology and MRI
Vice-Chairman of Radiology
Children's Hospital of Philadelphia;
Professor of Radiology & Radiology in
Neurosurgery,
University of Pennsylvania School of Medicine
Department of Radiology
Children's Hospital of Philadelphia
Philadelphia, PA
USA

Foreword

The chief editor Helen Carty's countryman, Oscar Wilde, is supposed to have said: "*I have a very simple taste, only the best is good enough*". For my simple tastes, Professor Carty has made the second edition of *Imaging Children* into a very good textbook. There is thus truth in the saying "*if you want something done – ask a busy person*". I also find, paraphrasing, that "*you can always rely on this editorial team to do the right thing – as soon as they have exhausted all other possibilities*". The partly new group of editors, Brunelle, Carty, Kao and Stringer, have improved most of the chapters in different ways. Most are completely rewritten and there is much new material, reflecting the continued growth and expansion of paediatric radiology.

The second edition is the result of the combined effort of both the editors and around a hundred excellent contributors. It is obvious that the "exclusive European" approach of the first edition has been changed into an international one, "*many contributors, separated only by a common language*". The clinical aspects of paediatric radiology are also enhanced in places by the inclusion of overviews from other specialities to give a background to the imaging.

As my short foreword pointed out in the first edition, paediatric radiology is a challenging and stimulating subject with the rapid development of new radiological modalities and techniques. The editors and authors have, however, been able to master these challenges and produce an excellent textbook that covers the requirements of both the general radiologist with limited exposure to imaging children and the radiologist in the specialised paediatric radiology department.

This is a very well structured textbook of paediatric radiology, richly illustrated with pertinent cases of high quality. Again I would like to congratulate the new team of editors and authors on a job well done and a successful joint effort. The old lady wrote on the envelope of the fiery love letter that she found in her mailbox on putting it into the correct mailbox: "*Incorrectly delivered, accidentally opened, thoroughly enjoyed*". This, on the contrary, was correctly delivered, deliberately opened, but still thoroughly enjoyed!

Hans G Ringertz
Stanford, CA, USA

Acknowledgements

The first edition of *Imaging Children* would not have happened without the editorship of Drs Brian Kendall and Don Shaw. Both are now retired, but their contribution to paediatric radiology continues today. We record our gratitude to them for all they have done and their support for this new edition.

We acknowledge the help of our paediatric colleagues and friends across the world who so willingly gave their time and experience in helping us to achieve this second edition.

We also wish to record our gratitude to our secretaries and assistants – in particular, Dorothy Turner from Alder Hey, the senior editorial assistant. Their good humour and efficiency is much appreciated.

Preface

Masterminding the first edition of a major book is a mammoth task. This second edition has proved no less challenging. Radiology, technology and knowledge have moved on in quantum leaps in the intervening 10 years. Yet, old truths remain and facts known in the 1930s are still true and pertinent today. This second edition of *Imaging Children* embraces the new and the old. It is a complete re-write, with many more authors, including radiologists from the Far East and North America. This reflects the enhanced communication and globalisation of our specialty – Paediatric Radiology.

We dedicate this book to children – everywhere. They, as we stated previously, are not "small adults". Their diseases are different and they deserve this recognition. It is impossible for all children's radiology to be carried out by specialists. We hope this text will assist radiologists for whom children's radiology is a part time activity. We also hope that *Imaging Children* will be helpful to paediatricians who, in many places, have to be their own radiologist. We have been mindful when writing it that our specialty is not technical, though we use technology, but is clinical and that we as radiologists are part of the multidisciplinary team who care for children.

We hope you enjoy it.

HC, FB, DAS, SC-SK

SECTION 8

VASCULAR SYSTEM AND SOFT TISSUE DISORDERS

Vascular System and Soft Tissue Disorders

Laurence J Abernethy, Gillian Klafkowski

IMAGING MODALITIES FOR EVALUATION OF SOFT TISSUE MASSES

PROJECTIONAL RADIOGRAPHY

Conventional radiography plays only a small part in the diagnosis and classification of soft tissue lesions but is important when there are clinical signs of bone or joint involvement. The presence of a large soft tissue haemangioma or vascular malformation may cause growth disturbance in adjacent long bones (Figure 8.1). Vascular malformations may primarily involve skeletal structures. Aneurysmal bone cysts are essentially intraosseous vascular malformations, manifesting as expansile, lytic lesions, usually in the metaphyses of long bones and the posterior elements of vertebrae. Multiple intraosseous venous and lymphatic malformations occur in Gorham–Stout syndrome, which is also known as diffuse skeletal haemangiomatosis or vanishing bone disease; radiographs of this condition typically show progressive osteolysis, pathological fractures, phleboliths and limb shortening.

Projectional radiography may show phleboliths and calcification within soft tissue vascular malformations (Figure 8.2). Vascular calcification may also be visible in idiopathic infantile arterial calcification and progeria. Other causes of soft tissue calcification include connective tissue disorders such as dermatomyositis, haematoma, burns, prolonged immobilization, fat necrosis and iatrogenic extravasation of infusions containing calcium salts. In tropical countries, parasite infestation may produce characteristic patterns of soft tissue calcification. Calcified regional lymph nodes may be visible following tuberculosis (TB) infection or bacille Calmette–Guerin (BCG) immunization.

Radiographic techniques for dimensionally accurate leg length measurement are important in the follow-up of vascular malformations associated with limb hypertrophy, such as Klippel–Trenaunay syndrome.

ULTRASOUND AND COLOUR FLOW IMAGING

Ultrasound (US) is ideally suited to the examination of superficial soft tissue lesions in children. Ultrasound examination is painless and non-invasive and with patience useful images can be obtained even with a restless child. The plane of imaging is infinitely variable and can be adapted to the anatomical location of the lesion for optimal visualization. Colour Doppler is uniquely valuable in providing an instantaneous, real-time assessment of blood flow. Pulsed Doppler US permits spectral analysis of arterial and venous flow and measurement of flow velocities.

The value of ultrasound is limited in the assessment of deep lesions in some anatomical locations. The field of view may not be sufficient to demonstrate the whole of the lesion. Ultrasound cannot penetrate bone and air and so may fail to demonstrate the deep extension of lesions around skeletal structures, in the thorax or in the vicinity of the airway or gastrointestinal tract.

COMPUTED TOMOGRAPHY

Computed tomography (CT) with intravenous contrast enhancement has been used for the assessment of soft tissue haemangiomas. CT involves significant exposure to ionizing radiation, lacks the multiplanar imaging capability of magnetic resonance imaging (MRI) and offers less intrinsic soft tissue contrast, making it less useful in determining tissue and blood flow characteristics. CT has some advantages in the demonstration of calcification and skeletal or visceral involvement but, in general, MRI and US are preferable to CT in the assessment of vascular lesions.

MAGNETIC RESONANCE IMAGING (MRI)

MRI allows non-invasive imaging of soft tissue masses and vascular lesions with no exposure to ionizing radiation. A high level of intrinsic contrast, the capacity for multiplanar imaging and intrinsic sensitivity to high-velocity blood flow make MRI particularly valuable for imaging vascular malformations. MRI optimally demonstrates the anatomical relationships between vascular structures and adjacent organs, nerves, tendons and muscles. MRI does not offer the same capability for real time imaging that ultrasound can provide; imaging times are relatively long and as the images are easily degraded by movement artifact, younger children may require sedation or general anaesthesia. However, MRI is not constrained by the same limitations as ultrasound; the presence of bone, dense calcification and air do not interfere with MR

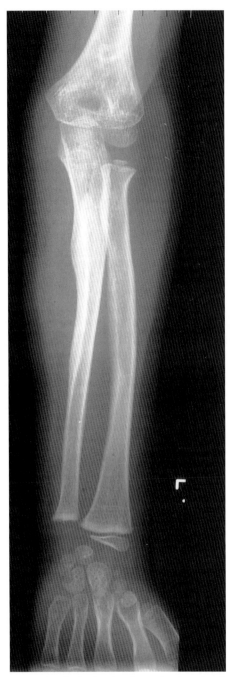

Figure 8.1 Projectional radiographs show bowing and thickening of the shaft of the ulna adjacent to a vascular malformation.

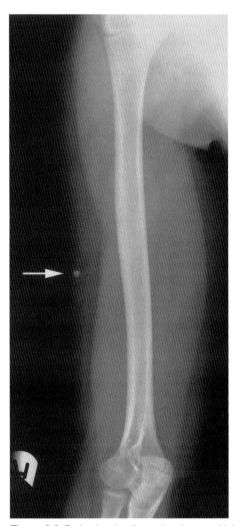

Figure 8.2 Projectional radiographs show a phlebolith within a venous malformation in the upper arm (arrow).

may also cause signal voids on all sequences. Fast flow is visible as flow-related hyperintensity on gradient-echo images.

VENOGRAPHY AND ARTERIOGRAPHY

Invasive, painful diagnostic procedures and exposure to ionizing radiation are avoided whenever possible in the investigation of children but contrast venography and conventional catheter arteriography still have an important role, particularly in preoperative assessment and as a precursor to interventional procedures such as sclerotherapy and embolization of vascular malformations.

Ascending venography involves intravenous injection of radioopaque contrast, usually into a superficial vein on the hand or foot, followed by fluoroscopy and radiographic exposures. This is the optimal technique for demonstrating the patency and anatomical connections of the deep venous systems of the extremities. In patients with venous malformations, ascending venography is often supplemented by direct contrast injection into the lesion to

images. Indeed, in many cases, MRI and ultrasound with colour flow imaging are complementary.

Slow-flow venous malformations can be consistently distinguished from high-flow arteriovenous malformations and arteriovenous fistulae on the basis of MRI findings. Slow-flow venous malformations show predominantly high signal intensity on long TR/TE spin echo sequences, whereas high-flow arteriovenous malformations and fistulae typically contain signal voids caused by time-of-flight effect and turbulence related dephasing. Caution must be exercised, however, because phleboliths and calcification

demonstrate its size, extent and venous drainage pathways. In favourable situations, this may be followed by therapeutic sclerotherapy with injection of agents such as sodium tetradecyl sulphate (STD), ethanolamine oleate or dehydrated ethanol.

Conventional catheter arteriography requires percutaneous arterial puncture and catheter insertion, usually into the femoral artery. Arteriograms are obtained by contrast injection following selective catheterization of the required vessels. Digital subtraction arteriography (DSA) allows optimal visualization of arterial anatomy. In selected cases, arteriography may be followed by embolization therapy using coils, occluding balloons, particulate material, polyvinyl alcohol foam or polymerizing liquid glue.

VASCULAR TUMOURS AND MALFORMATIONS

PROLIFERATIVE HAEMANGIOMAS

Proliferative haemangiomas are benign vascular tumours, which usually appear shortly after birth, although some cutaneous manifestations may be visible at birth in up to 40%. They undergo a proliferative phase of rapid growth, becoming raised, bulky, compressible lesions with a characteristic strawberry-red colour. Following a few weeks of proliferation and growth, they typically enter a phase of stabilization lasting for several months, followed by a phase of involution. In some cases, proliferation is biphasic; the second phase of growth may cause great parental concern if a confident prediction of complete regression has been given. The rate of regression is variable; 50% enter the phase of involution by 5 years of age and 90% by the age of 9 years. The prognosis for cosmetic outcome is not universally favourable; even after involution; some residual abnormality is present in 20–40% of cases, ranging from mild telangiectasia, hyperpigmentation, or hypopigmentation, to persisting fibrofatty masses.

Proliferative haemangiomas occur more frequently in girls than in boys; there is a significant association with prematurity. Systemic haemangiomatosis is a rare condition in which multiple cutaneous and visceral haemangiomas occur. The aetiology of proliferative haemangiomas is not well understood; possible aetiological factors include the persistence of fetal or placental angioblastic tissue, the occurrence of a somatic mutational event or a local increase in angiogenic peptides. The mechanism of involution appears to involve the activation of mast cells, which express interferon and transforming growth factor.

Although eventual stabilization and involution can be expected, proliferative haemangiomas may cause significant symptoms. Ulceration, bleeding and secondary infection occur in 5%, particularly in perioral and anogenital lesions. There is a special category of lesions at dangerous sites, particularly those close to the eye and airway, where rapid proliferation may have disastrous consequences. In the young infant, permanent visual impairment may occur if the eye is occluded for longer than 1 week; a large proliferative haemangioma on the eyelid, therefore, requires urgent investigation and treatment. Similarly, lesions involving the oropharynx, larynx or trachea may rapidly progress to cause airway obstruction and require prompt intervention.

Medical management of symptomatic or dangerous proliferative haemangiomas involves the use of high doses of steroids. If steroid therapy is ineffective, alpha-interferon or chemotherapy with vincristine may be used. Direct steroid injection is used for rapid control of orbital lesions. Laser therapy has proved valuable for cutaneous and airway lesions. If none of these is effective, surgical excision may be necessary, although surgery is avoided wherever possible because of the risks of haemorrhage and long-term scarring.

Imaging is not usually necessary for typical cutaneous proliferative haemangiomas, but it can be very valuable in determining the extent of particularly large lesions and those at dangerous sites. The differential diagnosis of a superficial soft tissue mass in an infant includes infantile fibrosarcoma, rhabdomyosarcoma, neurofibroma, nasal glioma and vascular malformation. If the nature of the lesion is not clinically certain, ultrasound and colour flow imaging may be helpful in showing a typical appearance of a well-defined, solid, echogenic mass, which is intensely hypervascular. In difficult cases, high vessel density and high peak arterial Doppler shift can help to distinguish haemangiomas from other vascular soft tissue masses such as arteriovenous malformations and vascular malignant tumours. Vessel density in excess of 5 per square centimetre and peak arterial Doppler shift greater than 2 kHz, taken together, are highly specific and give a positive predictive value of 97% for the diagnosis of a proliferative haemangioma.

MRI of haemangiomas in the proliferative phase typically shows a lobulated, solid mass with intermediate signal on T1-weighted images and high signal intensity on T2-weighted images (Figure 8.3). Flow voids may be visible within feeding arteries and draining veins. There is intense, uniform enhancement following intravenous gadolinium. In the involuting phase, appearances are more varied and heterogeneous, as the lesions contain varying amounts of fibrous tissue, fat, blood breakdown products and calcification. The appearances are not specific, and so lesions that show progressive enlargement and atypical clinical or imaging features require biopsy.

KASABACH–MERRITT SYNDROME (KMS)

KMS is the association of a severe, life-threatening consumptive coagulopathy with a soft tissue haemangioma, usually occurring in early infancy. The characteristic features are an enlarging soft tissue mass with development of a severe systemic bleeding disorder and marked reduction in platelet count, which may be impossible to correct by platelet transfusion. There may also be evidence of consumption of fibrinogen and other coagulation factors. KMS should not be confused with the low-grade consumptive coagulopathy sometimes seen in children with proliferative haemangiomas and venous malformations. The underlying lesion in infants with KMS is not a typical proliferative haemangioma; recent histological studies suggest that the underlying lesion in KMS is a quite different type of vascular tumour with a pathological resemblance to either a tufted angioma or kaposiform haemangioendothelioma. KMS is a medical emergency that requires treatment with platelet support; systemic steroid therapy, alpha interferon or vincristine therapy may be effective but, in some

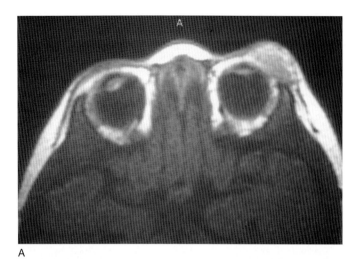

A

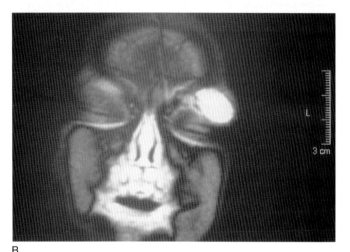

B

Figure 8.3 Proliferative haemangioma of the left upper eyelid. (A) Axial T1-weighted MR image. (B) Coronal fat-suppressed T2-weighted MR image.

cases, embolization of the lesion is necessary to control platelet consumption (Figure 8.4).

ARTERIOVENOUS MALFORMATIONS

Arteriovenous malformations (AVM) consist of a network of abnormal vascular channels comprising both feeding arteries and draining veins. Clinically, high-flow vascular malformations present as a soft tissue mass with cutaneous discolouration, locally increased temperature and palpable arterial pulsation. AVM tend to be present at birth and grow in parallel with the growth of the child, although some lesions manifest unpredictable, aggressive growth, sometimes precipitated by trauma, infection, surgery, puberty or pregnancy. Tissue ischaemia and venous hypertension may cause severe local pain, particularly on exercise. Skin ulceration and uncontrollable haemorrhage may occur and large lesions may result in high-output cardiac failure.

Ultrasound is helpful in confirming the vascular nature of the lesion and demonstrating high-velocity flow within it. MRI provides optimal definition of the overall size of the lesion and its relationship to deep structures. Multiple flow voids are typically present, indicating rapid or turbulent blood flow. Areas of high-signal intensity on T1-weighted images may represent areas of haemorrhage, intravascular thrombosis or flow-related enhancement. MR angiography may be helpful to demonstrate feeding arteries and draining veins but catheter angiography provides optimal definition of the vascular anatomy.

Arteriovenous malformations may be difficult to distinguish from malignant vascular tumours such as rhabdomyosarcoma, soft tissue sarcoma, angiosarcoma and haemangiopericytoma. Helpful signs of an AVM on MRI include the presence of fat within the lesion, muscle atrophy and absence of surrounding oedema. However, aggressive, enlarging lesions may require surgical biopsy. Lesions that appear to be vascular at the periphery but solid at the centre require particular caution.

AVM can often be managed by simple, conservative measures to control symptoms but large and aggressive lesions are difficult and dangerous to treat. In selected cases, embolization or combined embolization and surgery are used. Multiple procedures may be necessary to gain adequate control and treatment must be planned carefully so that future management is not compromised; in particular, proximal occlusion of feeding vessels should be avoided, as this simply stimulates collateral formation, which may cause the lesion to enlarge and also makes subsequent embolization more difficult. Embolization or sclerotherapy should be targeted at the nidus of the lesion, either by superselective arterial catheterization or by a direct percutaneous approach (Figure 8.5).

VENOUS MALFORMATIONS

Venous malformations are very variable; some affected children have diffuse malformations involving both deep and superficial systems, whereas others have localized or segmental abnormalities. Localized, superficial lesions have characteristic clinical features; they are bluish in colour and there is no local increase in skin temperature. They are easily compressible and typically increase in size on Valsalva manoeuvre. They may present with pain due to thrombosis from local trauma. However, deeper lesions are impossible to assess fully on clinical criteria alone and are often much more extensive than initially expected. Grey-scale ultrasound reveals the vascular spaces as hypoechoic structures. Varicosities, stenoses, complex interconnecting channels and venous lakes are typical. Colour flow imaging shows slow, turbulent flow within dilated, compressible vascular spaces.

On MRI, venous malformations have a characteristic serpentine pattern with internal striations and septations and associated muscle atrophy (Figure 8.6). Fibrofatty septations between endothelium-lined vascular spaces produce signal intensity higher than muscle on both T1- and T2-weighted sequences. Orientation along the long axis of the limb, multifocal involvement and absence of enlarged feeding arteries or draining veins are characteristic (Figure 8.7).

Recognition of venous malformations is important in young patients presenting with superficial varicose veins, as conventional surgical treatment is often ineffective and may be harmful. Treatment is difficult but percutaneous sclerotherapy is helpful for

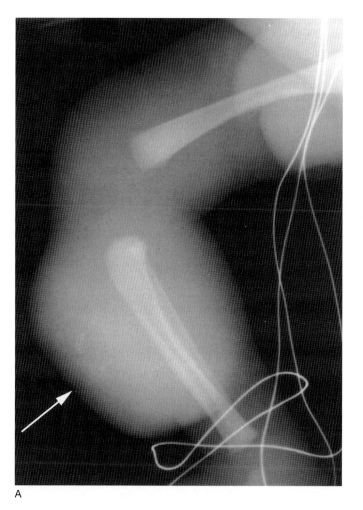

A

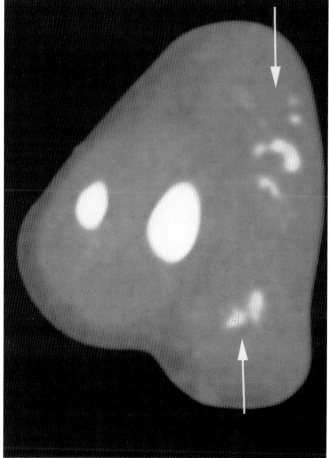

B

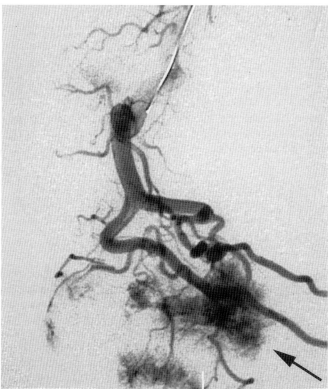

C

Figure 8.4 Kasabach–Merritt syndrome. A newborn baby with a soft tissue haemangioma on the right leg associated with a severe consumptive coagulopathy. (A) Projectional radiographs and (B) CT show a large soft tissue mass containing focal areas of calcification (arrows). (C) Digital subtraction arteriography shows that the tumour is intensely vascular (arrow) with massive enlargement of the feeding vessels.

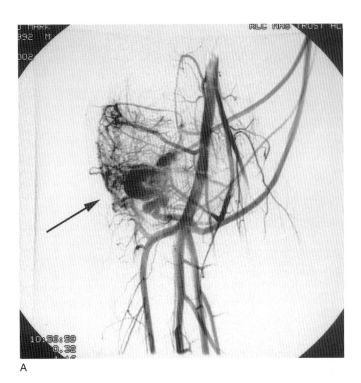

A

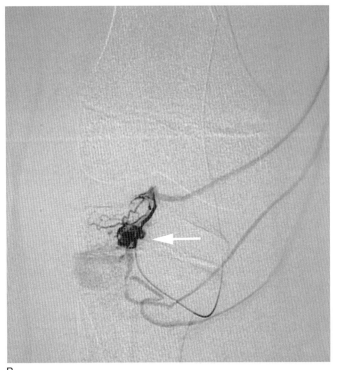

B

Figure 8.5 Arteriovenous malformation adjacent to the right knee. (A) Digital subtraction arteriography shows enlargement of the feeding vessels with early filling of draining veins. (B) Super-selective arteriography of the nidus of the lesion prior to embolization (arrow).

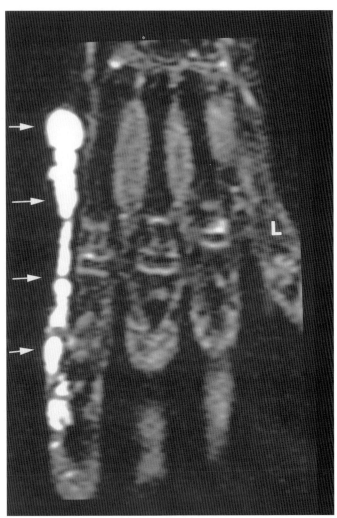

Figure 8.6 Venous malformation affecting the index finger. A T2-weighted MR image shows multiple dilated vascular spaces oriented along the long axis of the finger (arrows), separated by segmental stenoses.

ways. The result of surgical treatment of venous malformations is often disappointing; following incomplete resection, the residual malformation may become aggressive and symptomatic.

CUTANEOUS VENULAR MALFORMATIONS (PORT WINE STAINS)

Venular malformations are usually purely cutaneous lesions, which may have distressing cosmetic effects but are otherwise asymptomatic. Treatment is usually by laser therapy to reduce skin discolouration. However, there may occasionally be associated deep vascular malformations or other developmental abnormalities. Cutaneous facial lesions may be associated with Sturge–Weber syndrome. Midline dorsal lesions over the spine may indicate underlying spinal dysraphism or spinal AVM. Ultrasound and

localized lesions. Direct contrast injection venography (Figure 8.7C) is the essential precursor to sclerotherapy; it is the optimal technique for assessing the size and extent of localized venous malformations and for demonstrating the venous drainage path-

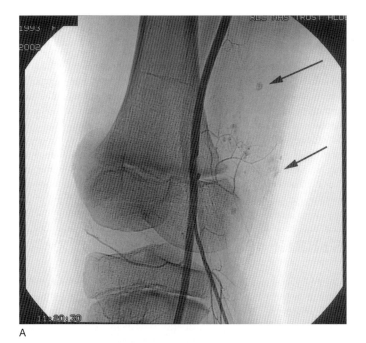

A

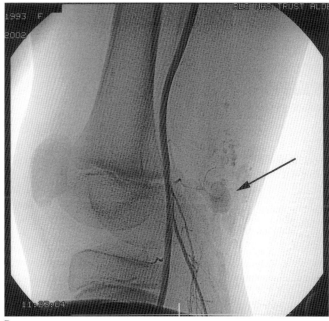

B

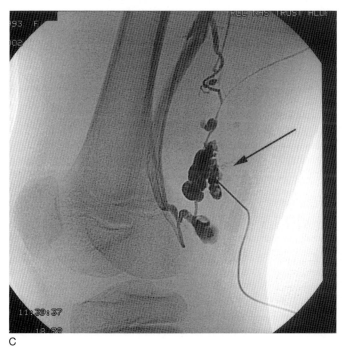

C

Figure 8.7 Venous malformation. (A and B) Arteriography shows slow filling of abnormally dilated venous spaces, which contain phleboliths (arrows). (A) The early phase shows no arterial component, arteriovenous shunting or enlargement of feeding vessels. Phleboliths are visible (arrows). (B) At a later stage, slow filling of the abnormally dilated venous spaces becomes visible (arrow). (C) Direct percutaneous venography reveals dilated venous spaces (arrow) with slow filling of draining veins.

colour flow imaging are useful screening procedures to exclude the presence of an underlying abnormality.

FURTHER READING

Abernethy LJ. Classification and imaging of vascular malformations in children. European Radiology 2003; 13:2483–2497.

Dubois J, Patriquin HB, Garel L, Powell J, Filiatrault D, David M, Grignon A. Soft tissue hemangiomas in infants and children: diagnosis using Doppler sonography. American Journal of Roentgenology 1998; 171:247–252.

Konez O, Burrows PE. Magnetic resonance of vascular anomalies. Magnetic Resonance Imaging Clinics of North America 2002; 10:363–388.

Mulliken JB, Glowacki J. Hemangiomas and vascular malformations in infants and children: a classification based on endothelial characteristics. Plastic Reconstructive Surgery 1982; 69:412–420.

Paltiel HJ, Burrows PE, Kozakewich HP, Zurakowski D, Mulliken JB. Soft tissue vascular anomalies: utility of US for diagnosis. Radiology 2000; 214:747–754.

Yakes WF, Rossi P, Odink H. Arteriovenous malformation management. Cardiovascular and Interventional Radiology 1996; 19:65–71.

SYNDROMAL VASCULAR MALFORMATIONS

KLIPPEL–TRENAUNAY SYNDROME (KTS)

KTS is characterized by a low-flow combined vascular malformation, including venous and lymphatic components in association with a cutaneous venular lesion, which usually has a sharply demarcated, geographical distribution over the affected area. There is typically overgrowth of the affected limb but this is not invariable. Absence of significant arteriovenous shunting distinguishes this condition from Parkes–Weber syndrome but if arteriography is performed it may show multiple small arteriovenous fistulas. Most cases are unilateral and affect the lower limb but the condition is sometimes bilateral, and may affect the upper limb, pelvis, abdomen and thorax.

Projectional radiography is important for demonstration of bone hypertrophy and the accurate measurement of leg length discrepancy. Ultrasound can demonstrate the venous malformation, and is particularly helpful in assessing the patency and valvular competence of the deep venous system and whether there are incompetent perforating veins. MRI can accurately demonstrate soft tissue hypertrophy and the full extent of the underlying venous malformation. When KTS involves the lower limb, there is frequently a large aberrant lateral vein, which may be associated with persistence of the sciatic vein and enlarged suprapubic veins draining to the internal iliac vein. Non-invasive imaging with ultrasound and MRI may adequately demonstrate these anomalies in the majority of cases, which are treated conservatively, but optimal demonstration is achieved by contrast venography. Contrast venography should be performed in patients who are potential candidates for surgery, which may involve excision and stripping of varicose veins or deep venous reconstruction. Ascending venography is performed to evaluate obstruction or hyperplasia of the deep venous system and direct injection into varicosities is performed to delineate the route of drainage. Catheter arteriography is rarely necessary unless there are clinical or imaging features to suggest the presence of arteriovenous shunting.

PARKES–WEBER SYNDROME (PWS)

PWS is distinguished from KTS by the presence of high-flow vascular malformation in association with cutaneous venular malformation and limb hypertrophy. Large lesions may cause high output cardiac failure. The high-flow nature of the vascular malformation may be clinically evident from the presence of hyperthermia, thrill and bruit but Doppler ultrasound is particularly helpful in demonstrating dilated veins with rapid, arterialized flow; complex arteriovenous malformations or simple arteriovenous fistulas may be demonstrated. Full assessment requires catheter arteriography, particularly if embolization therapy is considered to control cardiac failure.

PROTEUS SYNDROME

Proteus syndrome is a congenital hamartomatous disorder characterized by limb overgrowth in association with vascular anomalies, neurocutaneous tumours, hyperkeratosis of the palms and soles, and hyperpigmentation. The condition is asymmetrical. Macrodactyly of the hands and feet and bilateral genu valgum are characteristic; there may also be kyphosis and scoliosis secondary to vertebral dysplasia. The vascular anomalies may include lymphatic, venous and arteriovenous malformations. Ultrasound and MRI are useful in determining the nature of soft tissue masses and evaluating vascular malformations.

STURGE–WEBER SYNDROME (SWS)

Sturge-Weber syndrome (SWS) consists of a facial venular malformation (port wine stain) in the cutaneous area supplied by the V1 division of the trigeminal nerve, associated with a leptomeningeal vascular malformation. The intracranial vascular anomaly characteristically causes seizures and focal neurological deficits (Figure 8.8). CT is optimal for showing the characteristic gyriform calcification over the surface of the affected cerebral hemisphere, most commonly in the temporal and occipital regions. MRI is less sensitive for calcification but can elegantly demonstrate prominence of the cortical sulci with pial vascular enhancement in the affected areas. There may also be abnormal draining veins and enlargement of the choroid plexus within the affected hemisphere. However, no abnormality may be detected by brain imaging in early infancy. Ocular involvement may result in glaucoma. Facial venular malformations involving the V2 and V3 distributions of the trigeminal nerve are usually not associated with intracranial pathology.

MAFFUCCI SYNDROME

Maffucci syndrome is the association between multiple enchondromas and soft tissue venous malformations. Projectional radiography typically shows multiple lytic bone lesions with abnormal bone modelling and growth disturbance, in association with soft tissue swellings that often contain phleboliths. Symptomatic or enlarging lesions require investigation as the bone lesions may undergo malignant transformation to chondrosarcoma.

BLUE RUBBER BLEB NAEVUS SYNDROME

Blue rubber bleb naevus syndrome is a familial condition in which there is progressive development of multiple cutaneous, musculoskeletal and gastrointestinal venous malformations. Venous malformations within the gastrointestinal tract are difficult to demonstrate; they may cause chronic blood loss and intermittent small bowel obstruction due to intussusception.

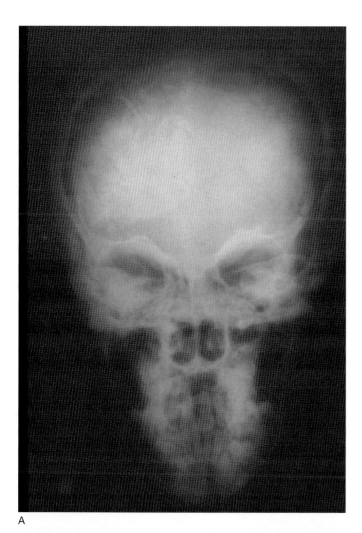

A

B

Figure 8.8 (A) Skull x-ray of a teenager showing extensive calcification of the right cerebral hemisphere typical of Sturge–Weber syndrome. (B) Non-enhanced CT scan of a different child showing typical serpiginous cortical calcification.

HEREDITARY HAEMORRHAGIC TELANGIECTASIA (OSLER–WEBER–RENDU SYNDROME)

Hereditary haemorrhagic telangiectasia (Osler–Weber–Rendu) syndrome is an autosomal dominant condition in which multiple arteriovenous malformations develop in skin, mucosa, lung and brain. Nasal lesions may cause severe, recurrent epistaxis. Pulmonary arteriovenous malformations may cause significant shunting, resulting in cyanosis and finger clubbing; cerebral infarction and abscess may occur because of paradoxical embolism. Chest radiography may reveal round or lobulated masses with draining veins visible as linear extensions to the hilum; contrast enhanced CT is the optimal non-invasive method of assessing the size and number of lesions. Pulmonary arteriography is often combined with coil embolization of feeding vessels for symptomatic lesions.

FURTHER READING

Gloviczki P, Stanson AW, Stickler GB et al. Klippel–Trenaunay syndrome: the risks and benefits of vascular interventions. Surgery 1991; 110:469–479.
Oranje AP. Blue rubber bleb nevus syndrome. Pediatric Dermatology 1986; 3:304–310.
Vaughn R, Selinger A, Howell C et al. Proteus syndrome: diagnosis and surgical management. Journal of Pediatric Surgery 1993; 28:5–10.

LYMPHATIC MALFORMATIONS AND LYMPHOEDEMA

MACROCYSTIC AND MICROCYSTIC LYMPHATIC MALFORMATIONS

Lymphatic malformations (LM) consist of fluid-filled cystic spaces, which originate from lymphatic vessels that fail to develop normal communication with draining vessels. The lesions may be unilocular or multilocular and there is a wide variation in the size of the individual cysts. Microcystic LM (previously known as lymphangioma) consist of multiple tiny cysts within a solid matrix; macrocystic LM (cystic hygroma) may be very large and exert significant mass effect on adjacent structures. Individual cysts typically contain straw-coloured, protein-rich fluid. Haemorrhage or infection may cause rapid enlargement.

LM may occur at any anatomical location except in the central nervous system but about 80% occur in the neck, axilla and mediastinum. Cervical lymphatic malformations are associated with trisomy syndromes, Turner syndrome, Noonan syndrome and fetal alcohol syndrome. Soft tissue LM may be associated with overgrowth of adjacent skeletal structures, particularly in the craniofacial region; histology of resected bone specimens reveals a high incidence of intraosseous LM.

Ultrasound in macrocystic LM characteristically reveals large, thin walled, fluid-filled cystic spaces, which may contain internal septations. If there has been recent haemorrhage or infection,

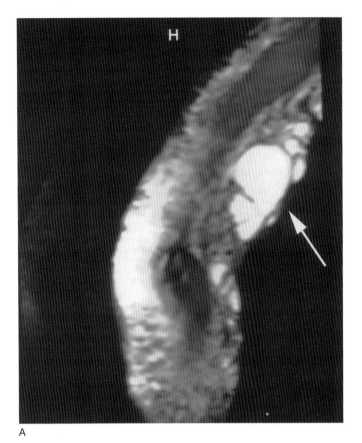

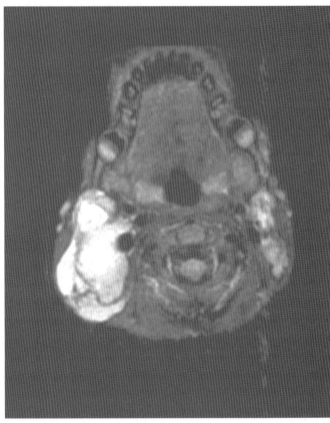

A

B

Figure 8.9 Macrocystic lymphatic malformation. (A) T2-weighted MR image shows multiple thin-walled, fluid-filled cysts (arrow). (B) Typical neck 'cystic hygroma'.

mobile echogenic debris may be visible. The cysts may be mobile but are usually not compressible. Colour Doppler typically shows only sparse blood vessels around the walls of the cysts. Microcystic LM are shown to consist of multiple tiny cysts, sometimes at the limit of ultrasound resolution, within a densely echogenic solid matrix. Grey-scale ultrasound appearances may be similar to those of a proliferative haemangioma but colour Doppler shows that a microcystic LM is largely avascular.

MRI is the optimal modality for assessing the deep extension of LM in areas that are not accessible to ultrasound; for example, a macrocystic LM in the posterior triangle of the neck may show an unexpected extension deep to the carotid and jugular vessels, into the retropharyngeal region and upper mediastinum. Signal characteristics of the fluid within macrocystic LM are variable. Typically, the contents of uncomplicated lesions are hypointense on T1-weighted images and hyperintense on T2-weighted images (Figure 8.9) but following haemorrhage or infection fluid–fluid levels may be visible, with the separate layers showing different signal characteristics. Following intravenous gadolinium, there may be rim and septal enhancement. Microcystic LM appear as diffusely infiltrative solid masses, usually with intermediate signal on T1-weighted images and high signal intensity on T2-weighted images. Lymphoedema may be visible in the adjacent subcutaneous fat. There is usually no enhancement following intravenous gadolinium. Direct contrast injection with very fine needles, usually performed as a preliminary to sclerotherapy, reveals dilated lymphatic spaces with no communication with normal lymphatics (Figure 8.10).

Venolymphatic malformations (VLM) are a common form of combined vascular malformation, containing both venous and cystic lymphatic elements, often in association with a cutaneous venular malformation (port wine stain). Recurrent haemorrhage into a predominantly lymphatic malformation suggests the presence of a venous component. Colour Doppler ultrasound is helpful in demonstrating blood flow within the venous elements.

FURTHER READING

Carpenter CT, Pitcher JD Jr, Davis BJ et al. Cystic hygroma of the arm: a case report and review of the literature. Skeletal Radiology 1996; 25:201–204.

Kathary N, Bulas DI, Newman KD, Schonberg RL. MRI imaging of fetal neck masses with airway compromise: utility in delivery planning. Pediatric Radiology 2001; 31:727–731.

PRIMARY LYMPHOEDEMA

Primary lymphoedema usually affects the lower limbs but may occasionally involve the perineum, upper limbs and face. There is a biphasic pattern of incidence; primary lymphoedema may be present at birth (Milroy's disease) or may develop at the onset of

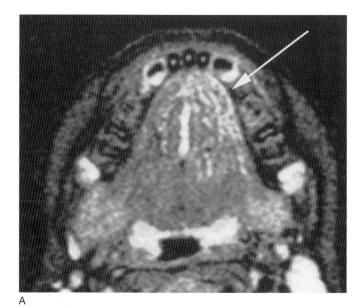

A

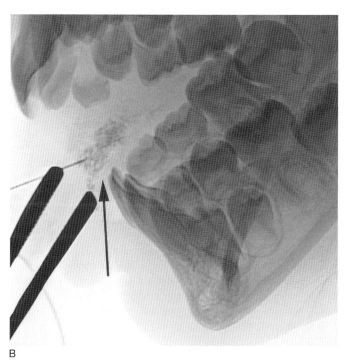

B

Figure 8.10 Microcystic lymphatic malformation of the tongue. (A) T2-weighted axial MR image and (B) direct injection of water soluble contrast with a 28-gauge needle reveal dilated lymphatic spaces (arrow).

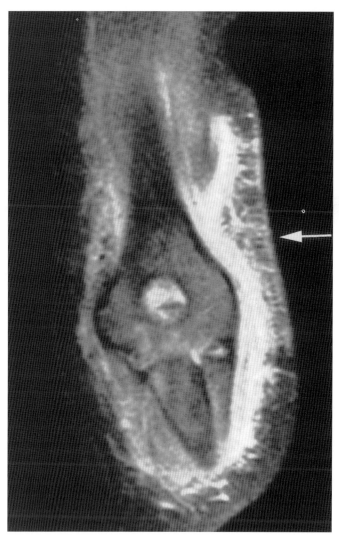

Figure 8.11 Primary lymphoedema of the arm. Heavily T2-weighted MR with fat suppression (MR lymphangiography) reveals a fine network of dilated lymphatics within the superficial soft tissues adjacent to the elbow (arrow).

puberty (lymphoedema praecox). The diagnosis is usually clinical but imaging may be helpful to confirm the diagnosis and to exclude the presence of an underlying vascular malformation. Diffuse soft tissue oedema is present within the affected area; MRI demonstrates a characteristic reticular pattern of fluid accumulation within a network of septal spaces. Heavily T2-weighted MR sequences with fat suppression ('MR lymphangiography') provide optimal demonstration of stationary or slowly moving fluid (Figure 8.11). Lymphography or isotope lymphography have been used to confirm the diagnosis of lymphatic hypoplasia but are rarely necessary in cases with typical clinical features. Lymphatic hyperplasia may be familial and is associated with distichiasis and cardiac anomalies. Ectatic lymphatic channels may leak lymph. Retroperitoneal lymphatic ectasia may cause vaginal discharge.

FURTHER READING

Laor T, Hoffer FA, Burrows PE, Kozakewich HPW. MR lymphangiography in infants, children and young adults. American Journal of Roentgenology 1998; 171:1111–1117.

GORHAM–STOUT SYNDROME OR VANISHING BONE DISEASE

This condition, in which there is a focal area of lymphangiomatosis or other vascular proliferation leading to bone destruction, is

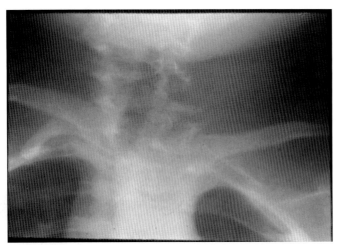

Figure 8.12 Anteroposterior (AP) view of cervical spine showing the typical 'rotting tooth' appearance of vanishing bone disease.

exceedingly rare in childhood. The typical radiological appearances are areas of osteolysis with irregular ends, often referred to as a 'rotting tooth' appearance (Figure 8.12). The lysis most commonly affects the shoulder and pelvic girdles. The course of the disease is variable, ranging from arrest with replacement of the vascular channels by fibrous material to a relentless course culminating in death. On MRI, there is high signal on T2, reflecting the fluid content.

FURTHER READING

Aviv RI, McKugh K, Hunt J. Angiomatosis of bone and soft tissue: a spectrum of disease from diffuse lymphangiomatosis to vanishing bone disease in young patients. Clinical Radiology 2001; 56:184–190.
Dominguez R, Washowich TL. Gorham's disease or vanishing bone disease: plain film, CT and MRI findings of two cases. Pediatric Radiology 1994; 24:316–318.

BENIGN FATTY TUMOURS

LIPOMA

Lipomas rarely occur in children and are composed of mature adipose tissue that is unavailable for systemic metabolism. They are most commonly found on the posterior trunk, upper neck and proximal extremities. Deep lipomas that can rarely be multiple are found in the retroperitoneum, chest wall and hands and feet. Although these soft lesions are usually slow growing they can occasionally enlarge rapidly and cause concern about malignant change. Histologically, the lobulated, thinly encapsulated mass consists of uniform adipocytes with occasional fibrous connective tissue septations.

On plain radiographs it is possible to discern a usually oval mass that is isodense to adjacent subcutaneous fat (Figure 8.13). There may be associated cortical thickening of adjacent bone.

A well-defined and homogeneous lesion with a negative Hounsfield attenuation (-90–120) is seen on CT. MRI will show a lesion that is isointense to fat and therefore hyperintense on T1-weighted sequences and the lesion may be characterized using a fat suppression sequence such as a short T1 inversion recovery sequence (Figure 8.14). Low signal septations may be seen but there is absence of any surrounding oedema.

LIPOBLASTOMA AND LIPOBLASTOMATOSIS

Lipoblastoma and lipoblastomatosis are rare mesenchymal benign tumours of embryonal white fat, the former being a localized well-circumscribed lesion and the latter being the multicentric type that infiltrates the subcutis and adjacent muscles. Males are affected 2–3 times more commonly. These benign tumours usually present in the first 2–3 years of life but may be present at birth. Histologically, they consist of uni- or multivacuolated lipoblasts in between spindle cells suspended in a myxoid stroma. Clinically, they present as painless masses mainly located in the extremities but other sites include the trunk, head, retroperitoneum, perineum and mediastinum. Radiographically, there is a diffuse increase in the radiolucent tissue of part of a limb and affected muscle bundles are both surrounded and separated by fat. With MRI lipoblastoma is mainly high signal on both T1-weighted and T2-weighted sequences but it may also be hypointense to subcutaneous fat on T1-weighted images as immature lipoblasts have a lower signal intensity. MRI is useful with both lipoblastomas and lipoblastomatosis in demonstrating precise anatomical delineation essential for radical excision as this is the treatment of choice.

DIFFUSE LIPOMATOSIS

Diffuse lipomatosis usually has an onset in the first 2 years of life. It is an extremely rare infiltrating overgrowth of mature adipose tissue involving large proportions of an extremity or the trunk. Muscle is diffusely involved and there is often associated osseous hypertrophy and therefore plain radiographs are of importance in suggesting the diagnosis (Figure 8.15). The differential diagnosis from lesions that may diffusely affect a limb and may have associated bone overgrowth and fatty components such as vascular malformations and haemangiomatosis is aided by the use of gadolinium-enhanced MRI.

STEROID LIPOMATOSIS

This diffuse proliferation of fat is due to prolonged endogenous or exogenous adrenocortical hormone stimulation. In Cushing's syndrome, truncal obesity predominates with muscle atrophy and associated osteopenia and osteonecrosis. When steroid levels are normalized the lipomatosis resolves.

NEURAL FIBROLIPOMA (MACRODYSTOPHIA LIPOMATOSA)

This is a rare condition in which there is a sausage-shaped fusiform enlargement of a nerve by fibrofatty tissue (Figure 8.16). It

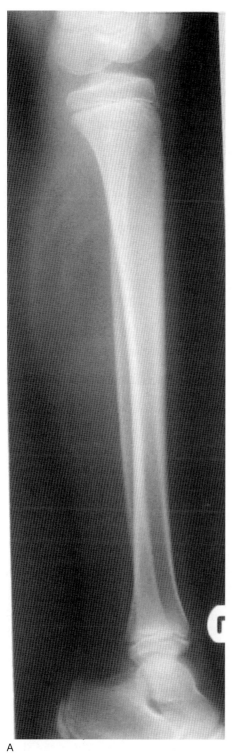

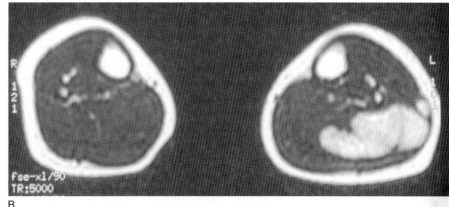

Figure 8.13 (A) Lateral radiograph of the calf. (B) T2-weighted axial sequence of a calf lipoma. Note the radiolucency on the x-ray.

presents as a painful, soft, slowly enlarging mass with signs of a compressive neuropathy. Males are more frequently affected and the lesion is usually found on the hand, wrist or forearm. The median nerve is most commonly affected. In contradistinction to neuromas and neurofibromas there is neural atrophy.

Approximately one-third to two-thirds of cases are associated with macrodactyly.

The lesions have a cable-like appearance on US with bands that are of alternating hyper- and hypoechogenicity. On MRI, the lesions are seen as serpiginous or linear signal voids surrounded by hyperintense fat.

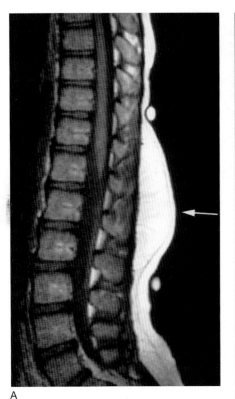 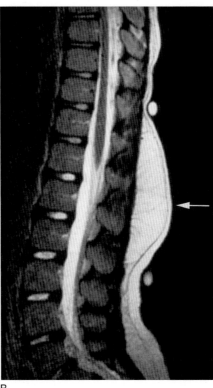 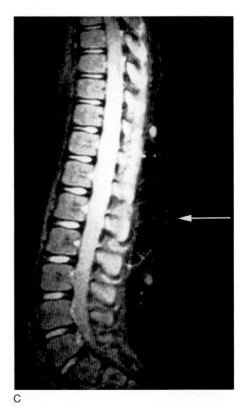

A   B   C

Figure 8.14 Lipoma overlying the lumbar spine. Sagittal MR images: (A) T1-weighted, (B) T2-weighted and (C) T2-weighted with fat suppression. The lesion (arrow) shows high signal intensity on both T1-weighted and T2-weighted images but the high signal disappears with fat suppression, except in the fibrous septations. There is no extension into the spinal canal and the spinal cord is normal.

FIBROMATOSIS

Fibroma and fibromatosis are terms used for tumours that are mainly composed of fibroblasts. Although they appear histologically benign, some behave aggressively and may be locally invasive, with a tendency to recur following local excision. Some may present with multifocal tumours but true metastases do not occur. In some types, spontaneous regression is typical.

BENIGN STERNOMASTOID TUMOUR OF INFANCY (FIBROMATOSIS COLLI)

Benign sternomastoid tumour of infancy is characterized by diffuse or focal enlargement of the sternomastoid muscle, typically first recognized a few weeks after birth and often associated with a history of birth trauma. Shortening of the muscle may cause torticollis, sometimes with secondary facial asymmetry and plagiocephaly. Spontaneous resolution usually occurs over a period of 4–8 months and may be helped by physiotherapy; a minority of cases require surgery for persisting torticollis. Ultrasound typically shows a well-defined mass within the belly of the muscle, which may be isoechoic or slightly hypoechoic (Figure 8.17); CT and MRI show the mass to be homogeneous with similar characteristics to normal muscle.

CONGENITAL GENERALIZED FIBROMATOSIS

Congenital generalized fibromatosis, also known as infantile myofibromatosis, is a deep form of fibromatosis. Solitary and multicentric forms occur with equal frequency. Most cases present in early infancy, with males being affected more often. Microscopically, the lesions consist of spindle cells with features of both fibroblasts and smooth muscle cells. Prognosis is better in the solitary form without visceral involvement and indeed lesions may undergo spontaneous regression. However, the prognosis is less favourable in patients with visceral involvement of organ systems such as bone, soft tissue, skeletal muscle or involvement of organs such as the lung and liver (Figure 8.18). Cutaneous nodules may be commonly found on the head, neck and trunk, may resemble haemangiomas and are often firm. Bone lesions are frequently found in the metaphyses, are eccentric, geographical and may have a sclerotic rim. The differential diagnosis of these osseous lesions includes Langerhans' cell histiocytosis, osteomyelitis and metastatic neuroblastoma. CT may show increased density of the soft tissue lesions compared to the adjacent muscle both with and without intravenous contrast administration and foci of calcification may be seen. MRI is particularly of value in demonstrating the extent of involvement; signal characteristics are variable but lesions with a high content of collagen typically show low signal intensity on both T1- and T2-weighted images.

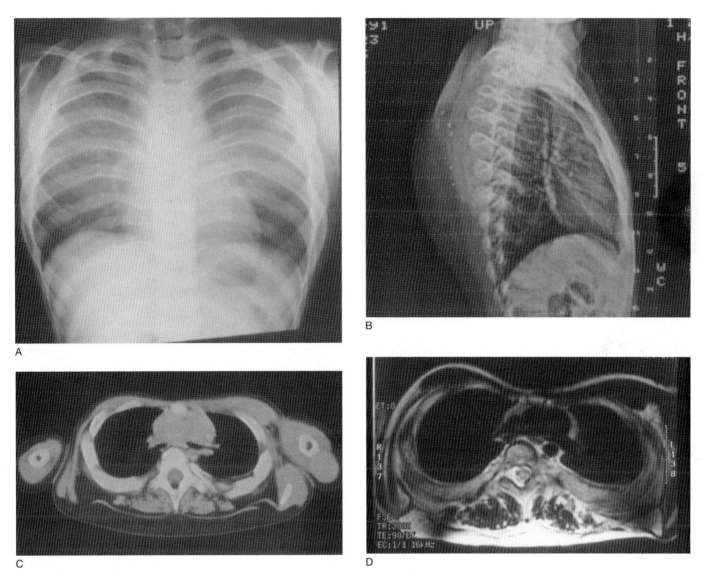

Figure 8.15 (A) Chest x-ray. (B) Lateral scout film of CT scan. (C) Axial lower thoracic slice. (D) Axial T2-weighted MR scan. Girl with diffuse lipomatosis. The CT and MRI have been done following surgery, hence the opacities. Note, massive expansion of posterior ribs, normal anterior ribs and posterior subcutaneous fat, also infiltrating the paravertebral muscles.

INFANTILE (DESMOID-TYPE) FIBROMATOSIS

Infantile fibromatosis is a benign but sometimes locally aggressive tumour, which typically occurs between birth and 5 years of age, arising as a solitary mass in skeletal muscle or the adjacent soft tissues (Figure 8.19). The lesion often grows along nerve sheaths or vascular bundles and may produce periosteal reaction but rarely causes lytic bone lesions. Sites of predilection are the anterior abdominal wall, paravertebral and gluteal muscles, shoulder and upper arm, and head and neck. Surgery provides the best chance of cure if excision can be complete but local recurrence is common after incomplete excision. Imaging is therefore most important in preoperative staging and postoperative follow-up.

Ultrasound typically shows a homogeneous, echogenic, solid mass with poorly defined margins. On CT, infantile fibromatosis shows non-specific appearances of a solid, homogeneous enhancing mass. MRI is the optimal modality for staging the extent of the disease and demonstrating postoperative recurrence; because of high collagen content, lesions typically show low signal intensity on both T1- and T2-weighted sequences (Figure 8.20), although some lesions with relatively less collagen may show high signal intensity on T2-weighted images.

CALCIFYING APONEUROTIC FIBROMA

Also known as juvenile aponeurotic fibroma, this rare form of fibromatosis usually presents during the first two decades of life as an asymptomatic, slowly growing soft tissue mass in the palms of the hand or the soles of the feet. The lesion is found twice as frequently in males. In the hand, the lesions arise from the deep palmar fascia. Plain x-ray may demonstrate a soft tissue mass with fine calcification and sometimes adjacent bone scalloping and therefore the differential diagnosis of these appearances includes

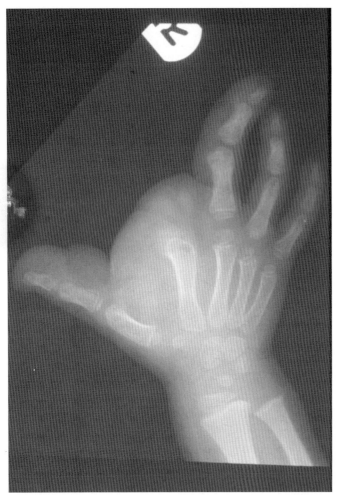

Figure 8.16 View of right hand showing typical increase in the soft tissues and macrodactyly of the middle finger. The index finger had been amputated.

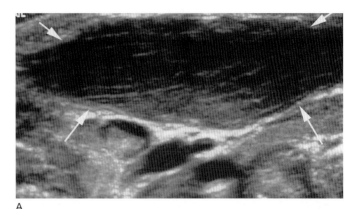

A

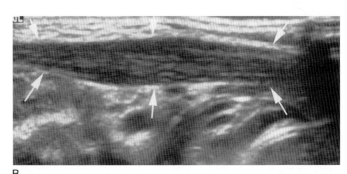

B

Figure 8.17 Benign sternomastoid tumour of infancy. (A) Ultrasound shows a well-defined mass within the belly of the sternomastoid muscle (arrows), which is less echogenic than the normal contralateral muscle (B).

synovial sarcoma and calcifying chondroma. Treatment is by surgical resection but there is a high rate of local recurrence.

NODULAR FASCIITIS

Nodular fasciitis consists of reactive myofibroblastic proliferative lesions found in the subcutaneous tissues, fascia and skeletal muscle, the former site being the most common. These lesions have a large histological variability but can be classified into myxoid, cellular and fibrous. In infants and children, these benign lesions are most commonly found in the head and neck region, although they can occur at any site. The usual history is that of a rapidly growing mass that usually measures less than 3 cm in diameter and has only been noticed for a couple of weeks. Uncommon variants include intravascular, cranial, ossifying and proliferative fasciitis. Cranial fasciitis involves both the scalp and the underlying skull. Erosion of the outer table and an epidural small soft tissue mass may be seen on CT. The fibrous nature of the lesion on MRI may be suggested by the low signal on T1- and T2-weighted images. Recent work regarding the correlation of MRI appearances and the histopathology of nodular fasciitis suggests

that the myxoid subtype may have a characteristic MRI appearance; isointense to muscle on T1-weighted sequences, with homogeneous enhancement following intravenous gadolinium, and high signal intensity on T2-weighted images.

PLEXIFORM NEUROFIBROMA

Plexiform neurofibroma is a peripheral nerve sheath tumour that is typically associated with neurofibromatosis type 1 (Figure 8.21). The tumour produces diffuse enlargement and distortion of nerve trunks; it is histologically benign but may be locally aggressive. MRI scans usually show that the tumours are slightly hyperintense to muscle on T1-weighted images and very hyperintense on T2-weighted images, sometimes with central areas of hypointensity producing a target-like appearance in cross-section (Figure 8.22). Malignant transformation may occur and is accompanied by severe pain.

FURTHER READING

Castellote A, Vazquez E, Vera J et al. Cervicothoracic lesions in infants and children. Radiographics 1999; 19:583–600.

Chung CJ, Armfield KB, Mukherji SK, Fordham LA, Krause WL. Cervical neurofibromas in children with NF-1. Pediatric Radiology 1999; 29:353–356.

Dilley AV, Patel DL, Hicks MJ, Brandt ML. 2001 Lipoblastoma: pathophysiology and surgical management. Journal of Pediatric Surgery 2001; 36:229–231.

Eich GF, Hoeffel J-C, Tschappeler H, Gassner I, Willi UV. Fibrous tumours in children: imaging features of a heterogeneous group of disorders. Paediatric Radiology 1998; 28:500–509.

Gupta SK, Sharma OP, Sharma SV, Sood B, Gupta S. Macrodystrophia lipomatosa: radiographic observations. British Journal of Radiology 1992; 65:769–773.

Kingston CA, Owens CM, Jeanes A, Malone M. Imaging of desmoid fibromatosis in pediatric patients. American Journal of Roentgenology 2002; 178:191–199.

Reister T, Nordshus T, Borthne A et al. Lipoblastoma:MRI appearances of a rare paediatric soft tissue tumour. Pediatric Radiology 1999; 29:542–545.

Robbin MR, Murphey MD, Temple HT, Kransdorf MJ, Choi JJ. Imaging of musculoskeletal fibromatosis. Radiographics 2001; 21:585–600.

GRANULOMA ANNULARE

This is a condition of unknown aetiology. Clinically, this presents as a soft tissue mass, most commonly over the extensor surface of the tibia. The mass is due to a necrobiotic granuloma. It is hypoechoic relative to subcutaneous fat on ultrasound, has low signal on T1 and a low to slightly increased signal on T2 (Figure 8.23). The margins may be poorly defined.

FURTHER READING

Chung S, Frush DP, Prose NH et al. Subcutaneous granuloma annulare: MR imaging features in six children and literature review. Radiology 1999; 210:845–849.

Vandevenne JE, Colpaert CG, De-Schepper AM. Subcutaneous granuloma annulare: MR imaging and literature review. European Radiology 1998; 8:1363–1365.

BENIGN MUSCLE TUMOURS

These include rhabdomyomas. Fetal rhabdomyoma is a rare benign tumour of male children under the age of 3, affecting the neck. A leiomyoma is a benign tumour of smooth muscle. It presents as a well-defined soft tissue mass, with imaging characteristics of muscle density. It is well circumscribed. Pilomatrixoma is a benign

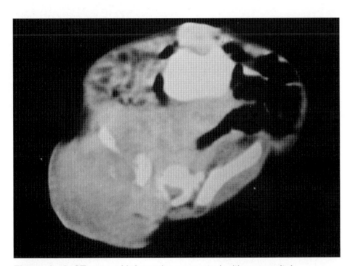

Figure 8.18 CT scan of infant who presented with congenital fibromatosis. Note, huge soft tissue mass infiltrating the pelvis and displacing the abdominal organs.

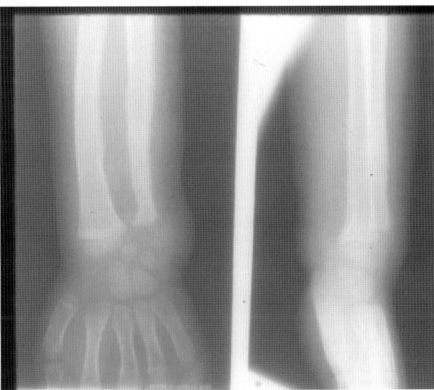

A   B

Figure 8.19 (A) AP and (B) lateral view of forearm of a boy with diffuse fibromatosis. Note soft tissue thickening and bony abnormalities due to the external compression.

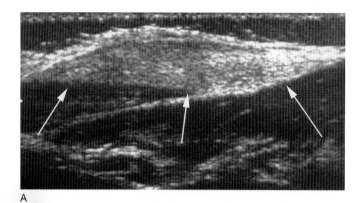

A

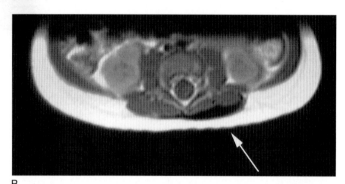

B

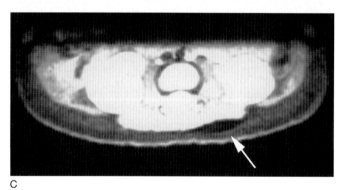

C

Figure 8.20 Infantile fibromatosis affecting the paravertebral muscles. (A) Ultrasound shows a plaque-like echogenic mass (arrows). (B) T1-weighted and (C) T2-weighted MRI scans: the lesion shows low signal intensity on both sequences (arrows).

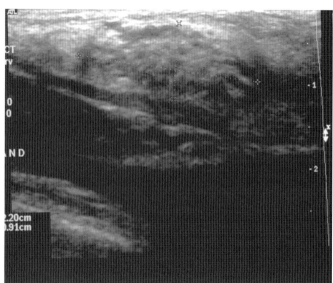

Figure 8.21 Ultrasound of peripheral nerve neurofibroma, which presented as a lump in the hand.

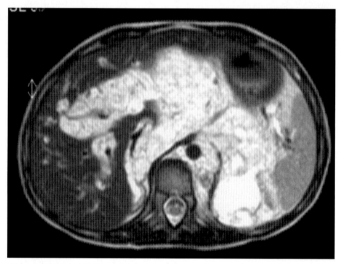

Figure 8.22 Axial T2-weighted sequence of an abdomen MRI showing massive plexiform neurofibroma encasing the vessels.

granuloma surrounding an ingrowing hair follicle. It is located in the subcutaneous tissues. It is a well-circumscribed solid mass whose nature is suggested by location but requires excisional biopsy for confirmation.

SOFT TISSUE SARCOMAS

Palpable soft tissue masses that have developed spontaneously or are apparently associated with a recent episode of trauma pose a major diagnostic challenge. Although the majority of these lesions will prove innocent, some resolving spontaneously, the possibility of a soft tissue sarcoma should always have a place in the list of differential diagnosis. Imaging is of only limited value in the differentiation of benign and malignant masses. The presence or absence of a clearly defined margin is of no diagnostic value; many soft tissue malignancies are well defined because of the presence of a pseudocapsule and ill-defined lesions are frequently caused by benign inflammatory processes such as infection and myositis ossificans. When suspicion is aroused by a non-resolving soft tissue mass, early referral to a specialist paediatric oncology centre is of paramount importance.

RHABDOMYOSARCOMA

The most common soft tissue sarcoma of childhood is rhabdomyosarcoma (RMS), accounting for approximately two-thirds

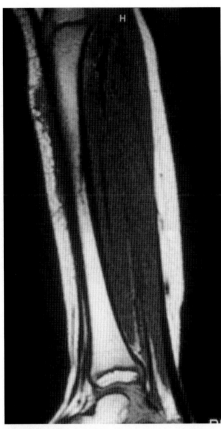

Figure 8.23 T1-weighted image in sagittal plane. Note the low signal soft tissue lesion in the pretibial region.

of all sarcomas in children and 7–8% of malignant solid tumours in childhood. The age incidence of RMS is biphasic, with peaks at 1–4 years and 15–19 years. Histologically, there are two major types of RMS: embryonal (about 75% of RMS cases) and alveolar (10–20%), which tend to occur at different body sites and present in different age groups. Botryoid rhabdomyosarcomas occur in the genital tracts. Embryonal and botryoid tumours have a better prognosis than alveolar lesions. The incidence of embryonal RMS is highest among younger children (0–4 years), while the alveolar RMS presents throughout childhood.

RMS is a highly malignant tumour and is thought to arise from primitive mesenchymal cells committed to develop into striated muscle . RMS can therefore arise virtually anywhere in the body, including sites where healthy striated muscle would not normally be found. Signs and symptoms at presentation will depend on the site of the primary tumour, whether there is extension into contiguous organs and, in some cases, the presence of metastatic disease. There are three main locations of presentation: the head and neck, the genitourinary tract and the limbs. RMS can present very indolently with non-specific and minimal signs and symptoms.

Genetic factors may play an important part in some cases of RMS. An increase in both central nervous system anomalies and genitourinary abnormalities similar to those associated with Wilms' tumour is recognized. Other associations are with Gorlin syndrome, fetal alcohol syndrome, neurofibromatosis and Li–Fraumeni (or family cancer) syndrome.

Ultrasound of peripheral RMS typically shows a solid mass that is less echogenic than normal muscle; colour Doppler often shows intense vascularity. CT and MRI show a solid mass that shows marked enhancement on scans following intravenous contrast. On MRI, the tumour is often isointense with normal muscle on T1-weighted images but hyperintense on T2-weighted images (Figure 8.24).

Metastases may occur to lung, pleura, liver, bone and regional lymph nodes. Radioisotope bone scans and CT of the chest are indicated for staging.

SYNOVIAL SARCOMA

Synovial sarcoma is a malignant soft tissue tumour that originates from primitive mesenchymal cells. It typically occurs in the soft tissues of the arms or legs, often closely related to tendons and bursae but not usually within joints. The tumour typically forms a well-defined, lobulated mass with a pseudocapsule, within which there is often calcification, cystic change and haemorrhage (Figure 8.25).

OTHER SOFT TISSUE SARCOMAS

Other soft tissue sarcomas that may occur in childhood include fibrosarcoma, malignant fibrous histiocytoma, haemangiopericytoma, angiosarcoma and leiomyosarcoma, and rely on biopsy for accurate diagnosis. All tend to show similar imaging features. Haemangiopericytoma and angiosarcoma, in particular, may be intensely vascular (Figure 8.26), and may on occasion be mistaken for vascular malformations. The diagnosis of any soft tissue mass that shows progressive enlargement must be kept under review and a histological diagnosis should be sought if there are any clinical signs to suggest malignancy. Staging and biopsy procedures are best performed in specialist paediatric oncology centres, as an inappropriately performed biopsy may compromise definitive surgery.

FURTHER READING

Bisset GS. MR imaging of soft-tissue masses in children. Magnetic Resonance Imaging Clinics of North America 1996; 4:697–719.

KAPOSI'S SARCOMA

Kaposi's sarcoma, which is an AIDS-related tumour, is rare in affected children, with the exception of African children who may develop a fulminant form (Figure 8.27). This is associated with lymphadenopathy. The prognosis is very poor. Regional metastases are to lymph nodes and distant to the lung.

FURTHER READING

Haller JO. AIDS-related malignancies in pediatrics. Radiology Clinics of North America 1997; 35:1517–1538.

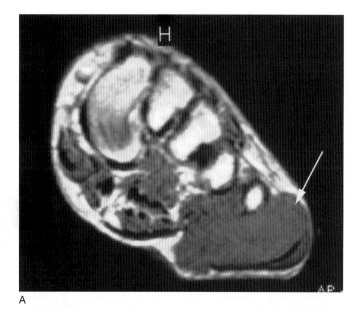

A

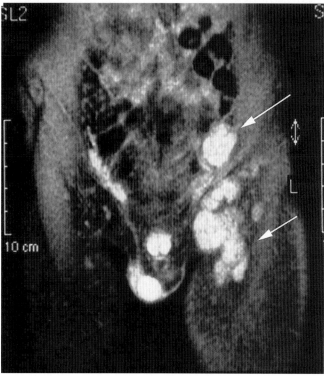

C

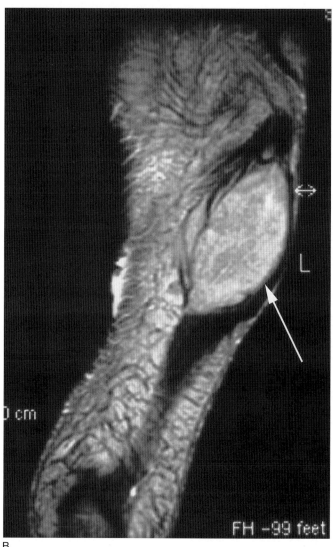

B

Figure 8.24 Rhabdomyosarcoma. MRI scans. (A) Coronal T1-weighted and (B) axial T2-weighted scans of the left foot show a well-defined, fusiform mass on the lateral aspect of the fifth metatarsal (arrows). The tumour shows similar signal characteristics to normal muscle on the T1-weighted image but is hyperintense on the T2-weighted image. Fat-suppressed T2-weighted image of the pelvis (C) shows massive inguinal, iliac and para-aortic lymphadenopathy (arrows).

DISORDERS OF MUSCLE

FIBRODYSPLASIA (MYOSITIS) OSSIFICANS PROGRESSIVA

Progressive myositis ossificans is a hereditary autosomal dominant disorder with variable penetrance having an equal sex distribution. The majority of patients present by 2 years of age with this condition where there is progressive ossification of tendons, muscles and ligaments with associated congenital osseous abnormalities. It initially involves the neck, shoulders and upper extremities with eventual involvement of the chest, abdomen and lower extremities. Progression results in joint ankylosis. Trauma may precipitate exacerbations and surgery at any site may cause acceleration of the ossification. Fractures of the ossified lesions may occur. Skeletal anomalies evident on plain radiographs may occur before the ectopic calcification and include bilateral hallux microdactyly (Figure 8.28) with or without phalangeal synostosis with hallux valgus. Less frequently, microdactyly of the thumbs occurs. Other

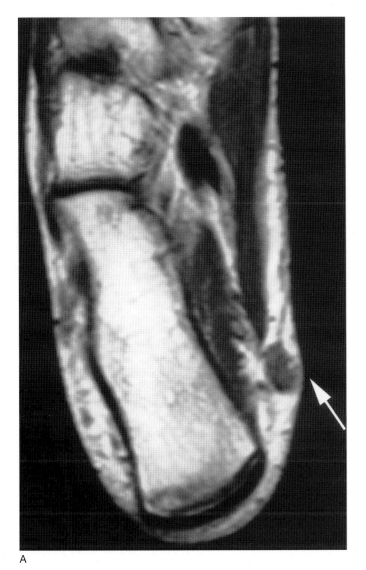

A

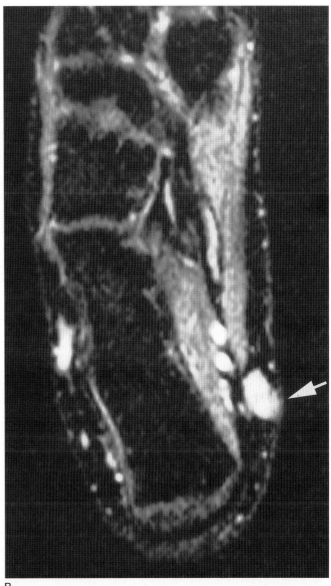

B

Figure 8.25 Synovial sarcoma. MRI scans of the right foot. Axial T1-weighted (A) and T2-weighted (B) images show a small well-defined tumour within the subcutaneous fat on the medial side of the calcaneum (arrows). The tumour shows low signal intensity on T1-weighted images and high signal intensity on T2-weighted images but there are no specific features to indicate its malignant nature.

osseous abnormalities include acetabular dysplasia, narrowed vertebral bodies in the AP diameter and vertebral fusion. On CT, early swelling of the muscular fascial planes is followed by ossification. Affected areas demonstrate uptake of technetium-labelled phosphate (MDP). The prognosis of the disease is poor with a fatal outcome usually within 10–15 years. The major differential diagnosis includes idiopathic calcinosis universalis; however, in the latter, the linear calcification occurs in the extremities as opposed to the predominantly axial distribution of myositis.

FURTHER READING

Kaplan FS, Strear CM, Zasloff MA. Radiographic and scintigraphic features of modelling and remodelling in the heterotopic skeleton of patients who have fibrodysplasia ossificans progressiva. Clinical Orthopaedics and Related Research 1994; 304:238–247.

MYOSITIS OSSIFICANS

Myositis ossificans is a benign and self-limiting condition in which an ossifying soft tissue mass develops, most commonly in muscle but also occasionally in tendons and subcutaneous fat. Approximately 75% of cases have a history of direct trauma but it can occur as a result of burns (sometimes in areas remote from the site of thermal injury) and central or peripheral nervous system disease, and some cases are apparently spontaneous. Myositis ossificans is most commonly seen in athletic male adolescent patients and is rare under the age of 10 years. The lesion usually affects the large muscles of the limbs, in particular, the anterior compartments of the upper arm and leg.

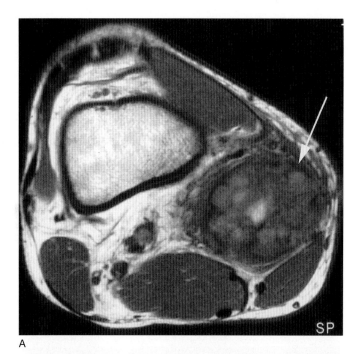

A

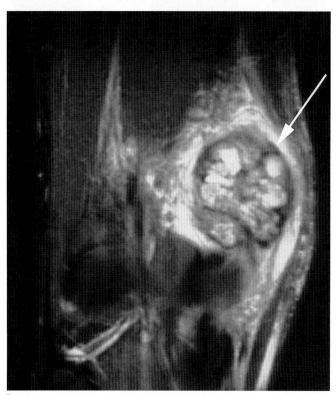

B

Figure 8.26 Angiosarcoma: MRI scans. Axial T1-weighted (A) and coronal fat-suppressed T2-weighted (B) images show a large complex mass with internal haemorrhage and marked surrounding oedema in the medial hamstring muscles adjacent to the distal femur (arrows).

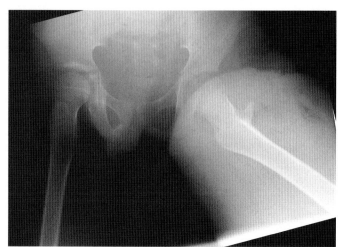

Figure 8.27 Radiograph of Kaposi sarcoma. Note large soft tissue mass with some reactive new bone and gas gangrene.

The typical clinical presentation is the development of a warm and painful soft tissue mass within 2 weeks of an episode of trauma. Projectional radiographs may be normal initially; the earliest radiographic change is a non-specific soft tissue mass. This is followed over the next few weeks by the appearance of amorphous calcific densities within the mass and sometimes periosteal reaction or attachment to the adjacent bone (Figure 8.29). This may simulate an early parosteal osteogenic sarcoma. As the lesion matures or ossifies it tends to do so from the periphery to the centre and there is usually a radiolucent zone separating it from the adjacent bone. CT optimally demonstrates the typical pattern of ossification. These features help to distinguish myositis ossificans from parosteal osteogenic sarcoma but caution is necessary and biopsy is required for lesions that show atypical features. Radiologically, a zoning pattern of peripheral maturation is the most important indicator that the lesion is benign; at 6–8 weeks, a lacy pattern of new bone with a sharp peripheral cortex is formed. Subsequently, the central non-calcified region may enlarge, leaving a residual rim of calcification. After several months, the mass reduces in size and may resolve completely or leave a residual densely ossified mass.

On MRI, in the early phase of the lesion it appears inhomogeneous and hyperintense to fat on T2-weighted sequences and isointense to muscle on T1-weighted sequences and demonstrates contrast enhancement (Figure 8.30). It progressively becomes hyperintense on T2-weighted sequences and can due to oedema display a peritumoral halo of increased signal. Extensive muscle oedema is typical of myositis ossificans and is not usually seen in soft tissue sarcomas, although it may be prominent in soft tissue abscess and haematoma. With maturation, myositis ossificans becomes better defined with an inhomogeneous signal similar to fat due to fat between the bone trabeculae of the lesion.

Technetium 99m diphosphonate bone scans are highly sensitive in the detection of myositis ossificans, demonstrating increased uptake of activity within the damaged area of muscle due to the presence of calcium salts. In the early stages, the vascular and blood pool phases of the scan show most abnormality; the static bone scan may show only a minor increase in uptake. In later stages, once true soft tissue ossification has developed, the static bone scan shows intense uptake. However, the bone scan appear-

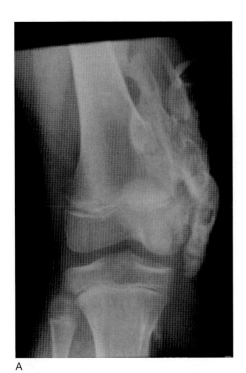

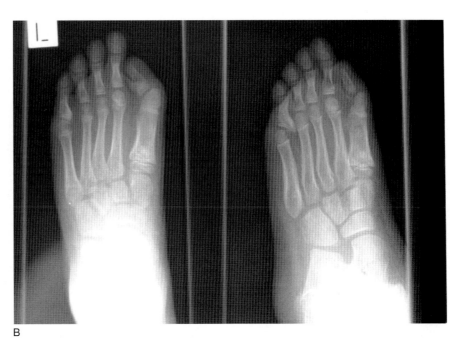

Figure 8.28 Fibrous dysplasia ossificans progressiva. (A) Knee radiograph. (B) Foot radiograph. Note the small hypoplastic big toe and the massive ossification in the muscles surrounding the knee.

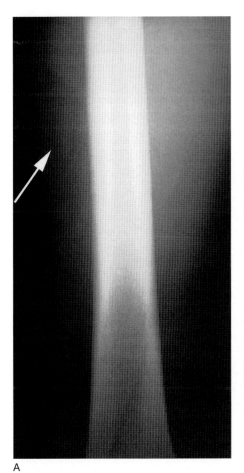

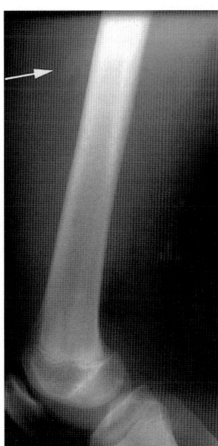

Figure 8.29 Myositis ossificans (early phase). (A) AP and (B) lateral radiographs show soft tissue swelling and subtle calcification adjacent to the shaft of the femur (arrows).

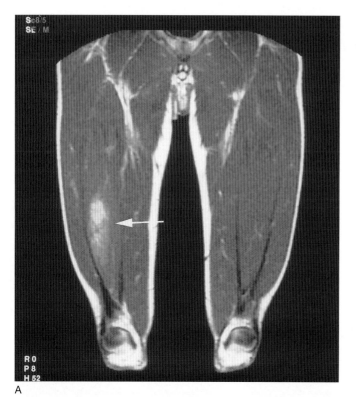

A

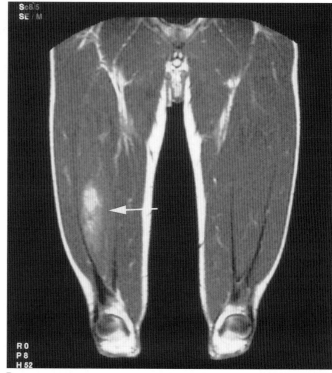

B

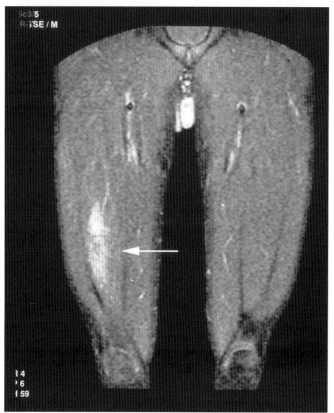

C

Figure 8.30 Myositis ossificans (early phase). MRI scans. Coronal T1-weighted images before (A) and after (B) intravenous gadolinium, and coronal fat-suppressed T2-weighted image (C) show soft tissue swelling in the quadriceps muscles. Unenhanced T1-weighted images (A) show subtle hyperintensity surrounding a central area of low intensity (arrow); following intravenous gadolinium (B), there is intense enhancement (arrow). The lesion shows high signal intensity on fat-suppressed T2-weighted images (C).

ances are non-specific and musculoskeletal infection and tumours may show identical appearances, although serial bone scans showing reduced uptake with maturation may sometimes be helpful.

Ectopic bone formation may develop in neurologically impaired children in transplanted muscles or post-trauma. These sheets of ectopic bone may fracture and cause pain.

FURTHER READING

Parikh, J, Hyare H, Saifuddin A. The imaging features of post-traumatic myositis ossificans, with emphasis on MRI. Clinical Radiology 2002; 57:1058–1066.

TUMORAL CALCINOSIS

Tumoral calcinosis is a rare condition in which large calcified masses develop within the soft tissues (Figure 8.31) in close proximity to large joints. It usually occurs during the first two decades of life with an equal predilection for both sexes. It is most common in people of Afro-Caribbean origin. The disorder is thought to be due to a disorder of phosphate metabolism, as serum calcium levels are normal but the serum phosphate level is raised. Calcified periarticular soft tissue masses of up to 20 cm in size are most commonly found adjacent to the hips, elbows and shoulders but almost never the knees. CT may reveal fluid–fluid levels within the lesions. There is a high rate of local recurrence following surgical resection.

FURTHER READING

Martinez S. Tumoral calcinosis: 12 years later. Seminars in Musculoskeletal Radiology 2002; 6:331–340.

TRAUMA

MUSCLE HAEMATOMA

Most children who present with muscle tears do so from overt trauma – either from direct injury or by sustaining a tear during sporting activity. In these cases, the diagnosis is easy. Frequent sites are the thigh (Figure 8.32), leg and anterior abdominal wall muscles. Other causes of muscle haematomas are haemophilia and rupture of an occult vascular malformation. Plain films are usually non-diagnostic. There may be an increase in the size of the muscle. The ultrasound characteristics of a haematoma depend on the stage of imaging. It is initially echogenic, then of mixed echogenicity with striae and debris, and as the clot retracts it becomes hypoechoic. These features are mirrored on MRI. Bright signal on T1, if the haemorrhage is fresh, then heterogeneous. They are less intense than muscle by about 48 h. They are of high signal on T2. MRI need only be done if the diagnosis is uncertain on ultrasound.

Chronic muscle tears, due to unrecognized trauma, may present as a worrying soft tissue mass. The imaging characteristics usually suggest the diagnosis.

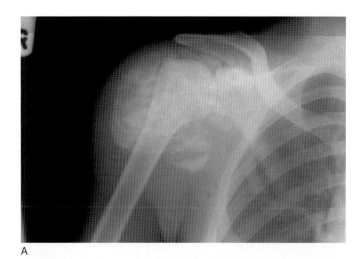

A

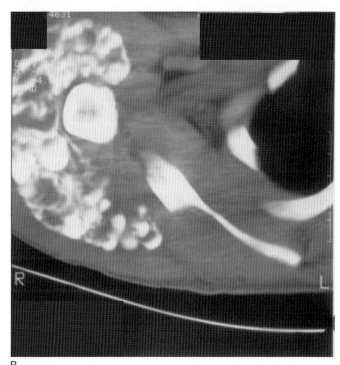

B

Figure 8.31 (A) Shoulder radiograph and (B) CT of an adolescent with tumoral calcinosis.

FURTHER READING

Sanches-Marquez A, Gil-Garcia M, Valls C et al. Sports-related muscle injuries of the lower extremity: MR imaging appearances. European Radiology 1999; 9:1088–1093.

SUBUNGUAL HAEMATOMA

This appears as a lucent lesion in the soft tissues under the nail bed (Figure 8.33).

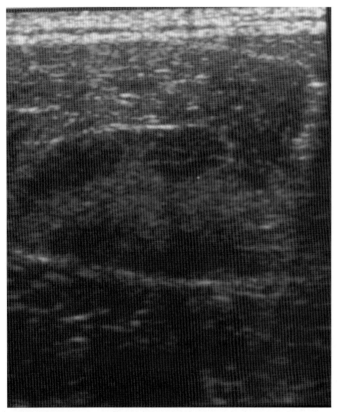

Figure 8.32 Ultrasound of large haematoma in the adductor muscles.

Table 8.1 Soft tissue calcification

Vascular – AVM and phleboliths
Haematoma
Renal osteodystrophy
Hyperparathyroidism
Tumoral calcinosis
Drip extravasation
Helminth infection
Scleroderma
Calcinosis universalis
BCG
Ehlers–Danlos syndrome
Tumour

SOFT TISSUE CALCIFICATION

Calcification within the soft tissues has many causes (Table 8.1). The discovery of calcification on an x-ray has to be related to the clinical history. The location and pattern of it can help, e.g. lesions in the finger pulp are likely in scleroderma, linear opacities at drip sites or typical phleboliths in venous malformations. Individual disorders are described in the relevant chapters.

FAT NECROSIS

Subcutaneous fat necrosis is occasionally seen in young infants. The lesion occurs in brown fat. It may be discovered as an

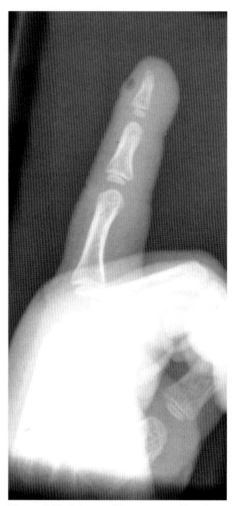

Figure 8.33 Subungual haematoma. Note lucency under the nail.

incidental finding on x-ray or present clinically with indurated subcutaneous tissue, particularly in the buttocks, thighs and cheeks. There is a known association with induced hypothermia for cardiac surgery (Figure 8.34). It resolves spontaneously over some months. This condition is different to sclerema neonatorum in which there is diffuse thickening of subcutaneous tissues described in premature and debilitated infants. In older children who sustain bruising to the fat, necrosis may present clinically as induration. On MRI, this appears as a linear area of very low density on all sequences.

DRIP EXTRAVASATION

Extravasation of intravenous fluids into the soft tissues may cause local necrosis with calcification. By definition this occurs at drip sites (Figure 8.35). The calcification is amorphous and mainly linear as it lies in tissue planes. There is often some thickening of the subcutaneous tissues. Skin sloughing is a consequence.

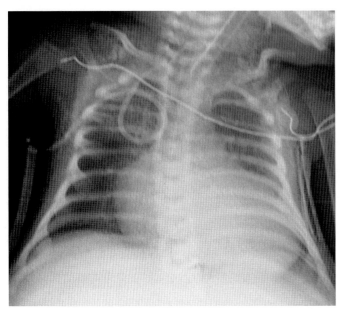

Figure 8.34 Chest radiograph of an infant who had recent cardiac surgery. Note extensive soft tissue calcification around shoulder and in the chest wall due to fat necrosis.

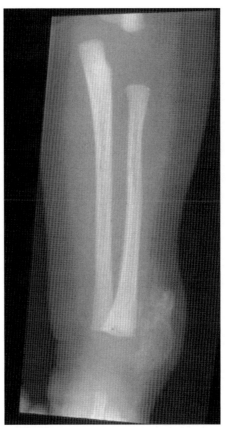

Figure 8.35 Calcification in the soft tissue due to drip extravasation.

PARATHYROID AND RENAL DISEASE

Soft tissue calcification in children with renal osteodystrophy and secondary hyperparathyroidism is much less frequently seen since the advent of modern management of renal failure. The calcification occurs in hydroxyapatite crystals. While it may be visceral, the main radiological abnormalities are peripheral. Arterial calcification is rare in children. The typical distribution of the calcified plaque is periarticular. The plaque may induce surrounding inflammation, become painful and ulcerate through the skin surface. Calcification in parathyroid disorders is described in Chapter 6.5.

EHLERS–DANLOS SYNDROME

This is a group of connective tissues characterized by abnormal collagen synthesis, leading to joint laxity, skin hyperelasticity and fragility. Fragile blood vessels may lead to bleeding. There are 10 different described varieties. There is male predominance. Radiographic findings include subcutaneous calcification, mainly over the exterior surfaces of arms and legs (Figure 8.36). Ectopic bone formation may occur around the hip. Joint effusion, haemarthrosis, subluxation and dislocation are frequent. There is an increased incidence of scoliosis, kyphosis, diaphragmatic hernia and early osteoarthritis. There is also an increased incidence of aortic aneurysm and dissection. Other clinical and radiographic features include arachnodactyly, uniphalangeal thumbs, club feet, radioulnar synostosis, supernumerary teeth and a double ossification centre for the calcaneus and a short proximal phalanx for the little finger.

PSEUDOXANTHOMA ELASTICUM

This is a rare inherited disorder in which there is degeneration of elastic tissue. Radiological manifestations are vascular calcification, and periarticular and subcutaneous calcification. Complications include aortic disease, AV malformation, cardiomyopathy and myocardial infarction, and fibrous metaplasm of the long bones.

FURTHER READING

Taybi H, Lachman RS. Radiology of syndromes, metabolic disorders, and skeletal dysplasias, 3rd edn. Chicago: Year Book Medical Publishers Inc.; 1990.

FOREIGN BODY

Foreign body (FB) puncture wounds in the hands and feet are a frequent occurrence. Wood, glass and metal fragments are the main penetrating substances. Radiographs are taken in two projections, attempting to project the FB away from the bone, with the site of the puncture marked to identify the fragment and its depth; this may need to be repeated following removal to ensure that it is complete, as retained FBs may be the source of granulomas or infection. Wood splinters are almost always non-opaque. Visualization of a glass splinter depends on its composition and location relative

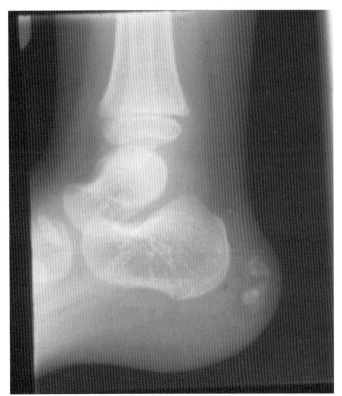

Figure 8.36 Lateral view of calcaneus in a child with Ehlers–Danlos syndrome. Note soft tissue calcification.

to bony structures and its projection, i.e. seen in profile or en face. High-resolution ultrasound is excellent at visualizing non-opaque lesions (Figure 8.37). Most cause an acoustic shadow. Ultrasound should be the first imaging procedure of unexplained lumps, especially on the feet, as the wounding incident is often forgotten. CT is helpful, especially in facial wounds. At MRI, glass and wood produce signal voids, surrounded by inflammatory reaction. Foreign bodies that penetrate the soft tissues and enter the underlying bone may result in an implantation dermoid.

INFANTILE ARTERIAL CALCIFICATION

This is a very rare disease of unknown origin, characterized by intimal calcification in the aorta and its main branches. Clinically, children may present with congestive heart failure, respiratory distress and gastrointestinal symptoms, e.g. vomiting, and ileus. There may be joint stiffness, swelling and fever. Radiologically, subtle calcification may be seen on x-ray but is easily seen on CT. The vessel walls are strongly echogenic at ultrasound.

FURTHER READING

Vera J, Lucaya J, Garcia-Conesa JA, Aso C, Balaguer A. Idiopathic infantile arterial calcification: unusual features. Pediatric Radiology 1990; 20:585–587.

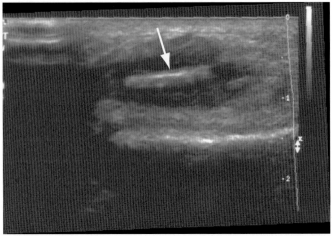

A

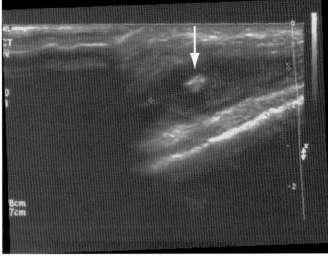

B

Figure 8.37 (A) Longitudinal and (B) transverse ultrasound of foot showing a splinter of glass with surrounding granuloma. This was not visible on x-ray.

VENOUS THROMBOSIS

Occasionally, calcification may develop in thrombosis in veins associated with central lines. Idiopathic venous thrombosis may develop in the inferior vena cava (IVC) without necessarily involving the renal vein. It may be found on x-ray or ultrasound performed for some other reason.

FURTHER READING

Kassner EG, Baumstark A, Kinkhabwala MN, Ablow RC, Haller JO. Calcified thrombus in inferior vena cava in infants and children. Pediatric Radiology 1976; 4:167–171.

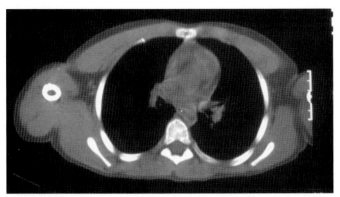

Figure 8.38 CT scan of a boy of 14 who presented with unilateral muscle enlargement over the right scapula. Note hypertrophy of the muscles. Biopsy showed normal muscles.

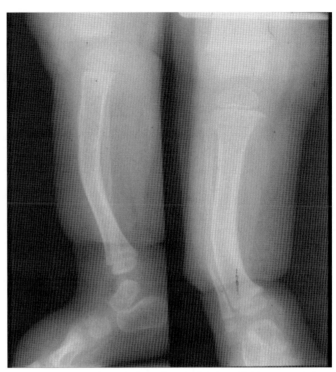

Figure 8.39 Amniotic constriction band over the calf. Note constriction band around the lower calf. There is, in addition, tibial and fibular bowing.

HEMIHYPERTROPHY

There is overgrowth of one side of the body, often presenting clinically in the lower limb, though careful examination shows that this affects all tissues and structures including organs on the ipsilateral side. There is increase in tissue bulk and in limb length. There may be dentition anomalies. The cause is unknown. Hemihypertrophy differs from local gigantism. Congenital hemihypertrophy has a known association with Wilms' tumour, hepatoblastoma, adrenal carcinoma, renal cystic disease and medullary sponge kidneys. Hemihypertrophy may be recognized at birth but more commonly is recognized during infancy.

Beckwith–Wiedemann syndrome, in which organomegaly is the dominant feature, may also be associated with hemihypertrophy.

Radiological assessment should include leg length measurement, bone age monitoring and renal ultrasound. There is no agreed interval at which this surveillance should be done. Most units do it at 3–6 monthly intervals.

FURTHER READING

Taybi H, Lachman RS. Radiology of syndromes, metabolic disorders, and skeletal dysplasias, 3rd edn. Chicago: Year Book Medical Publishers Inc.; 1990.

HEMIATROPHY

This condition, in which one half of the body, including all tissues, is smaller than the other, is also sometimes called hemihypotrophy. It may be difficult to decide whether one side is small and the other normal or that one side is pathologically large and the other normal. Normal organ measurement helps to distinguish between the two conditions. There is no increased risk of malignancy with hemiatrophy. Most hemiatrophy states are associated with neurological deficits, e.g. hemiplegia. It also occurs in Russel–Silver dwarfism.

MUSCULAR DYSTROPHY

The clinical and pathological criteria for this group of neuromuscular disorders are a primary progressive myopathy, a dearth of muscle fibres and replacement by fat, with loss of muscle bulk. These conditions are genetically inherited. The severity ranges from a rapidly progressive course from birth to slowly progressive disease with loss of muscle bulk, scoliosis and respiratory embarrassment.

Duchenne muscular dystrophy is the most frequent inherited neuromuscular disorder. It occurs in males and is an x-linked recessive disorder. It is sometimes referred to as pseudohypertrophic muscular dystrophy, as initially there is an apparent increase in muscle bulk due to the fatty infiltration. Clinically, there is often thigh wasting with apparent calf enlargement. The lower limbs and shoulder girdle are initially affected but with progression the children develop scoliosis, which may be rapid. There is a long 'C' shaped curve. Cardiomyopathy coexists. Death is usual between 18 and 30 years of age. The diagnosis is clinical but the fatty infiltration is well seen on MRI.

Becker muscular dystrophy is similar to Duchenne but has a slower course. Imaging features are similar. Myotonic muscular dystrophy is autosomal dominant in inheritance and affects striated and smooth muscle.

In the 'congenital muscular dystrophies', there are often brain abnormalities in addition to the muscle weakness. These include white matter changes, pachygyria and cerebellar hypoplasia.

MUSCLE HYPERTROPHY

Overuse of muscle groups due to conditioning or habitual tics may result in hypertrophy of an individual muscle or a muscle group and present as a puzzling soft tissue mass. The imaging characteristics are those of muscle (Figure 8.38).

AMNIOTIC CONSTRICTION BAND

In utero, minor placental disruption may lead to the development of amniotic bands, which may cause limb deformities. These range from soft tissue constricting bands to amputation of digits or part of a limb. The anomaly may be demonstrated by antenatal sonography. The radiographic appearance depends on the underlying deformity. Soft tissue constriction without bony abnormality may be visible (Figure 8.39). Amputations are self evident. Craniofacial defects caused by such bands are imaged by CT.

ACKNOWLEDGEMENTS

The structure and contents of this chapter are based upon Chapter 9 in the 1st edition of *Imaging Children*, written by Dr G. Sebag and Dr J. Dubois. We are grateful to Dr H. McDowell for her expert advice on soft tissue sarcomas and to Dr P. Rowlands for advising on the investigation and management of vascular malformations.

SECTION 9

THE HEART

The Heart

Denise Kitchiner, Cinzia Crawley, Tal Geva

GENERAL IMAGING, RADIOLOGY AND ULTRASOUND

Denise Kitchiner, Cinzia Crawley

INCIDENCE OF CARDIOVASCULAR DISEASE

Congenital heart disease occurs in 8 per 1000 live births. Ten lesions account for over 80% of congenital heart disease. They can be divided into three haemodynamic groups (Table 9.1). More than one lesion may coexist. A wide variety of rare or complex conditions make up the remainder. Approximately 80% of infants born with congenital heart disease are likely to reach adulthood. The incidence of congenital heart disease in young adults is 5 per 1000 and rising steadily. Most enjoy good health but many require life-long expert follow-up. Acquired heart disease is rare in children. In developing countries, rheumatic heart disease remains at least as common as congenital heart disease.

AETIOLOGY OF CONGENITAL HEART DISEASE

Congenital heart disease is usually sporadic, with genetic and environmental factors having some influence. There are a wide range of chromosomal or genetic abnormalities, and other associations (Table 9.2). The risk of congenital heart disease increases to 2% in a subsequent pregnancy. There is a tendency for a similar anomaly to recur, although the severity may vary. If two previous children are affected, the risk rises to 6–8%, and offspring of a father with congenital heart disease have a similar risk. If the mother is affected the risk is up to 15%, depending on the lesion. Environmental factors include maternal diabetes, phenylketonuria or rubella, and drugs such as alcohol, lithium or phenytoin.

CARDIAC MORPHOLOGY AND SEQUENTIAL ANALYSIS

ORIENTATION OF HEART

The normal heart lies obliquely in the mediastinum with the right-sided chambers positioned anterior to the left-sided chambers, the right ventricle being the most anterior chamber. The ventricles are positioned slightly inferior and to the left of the atria. The most posterior chamber is the left atrium. The left ventricle is the larger of the two ventricles, it forms the apex of the heart, typically positioned on the left side of the chest. The aortic valve arises inferior, behind and to the right of the pulmonary valve. It is situated centrally within the mediastinum.

The term dextrocardia is confusing. When describing the position of the heart in the chest, both the predominant side of the chest in which the heart lies and the position of the apex should be ascertained; it is important to realize that they do not always correspond. A heart that lies mainly in the right side of the chest may have a left-sided apex. The apex is determined by the orientation of the ventricles as well as by their relative sizes. In a hypoplastic left heart with a relatively small left ventricle the apex will be formed by the right ventricle.

CARDIAC MORPHOLOGY

In congenital heart disease, the position and number of chambers and their connections can become very complex. As a result it has become necessary to define individual chambers as well as terms to define their relationship to each other. Emphasis will be placed on the European model, which differs slightly from that used in North America.

The chambers can be identified by transthoracic echocardiography using the landmarks described below. Some of the features identifying individual chambers can also be appreciated on angiographic studies.

MORPHOLOGICAL RIGHT ATRIUM

The morphological right atrium typically receives the inferior and superior vena cavae. The opening of the former is bounded inferiorly by the eustachian valve. This is a very useful structure in identifying the right atrium on echocardiography. The right atrium also receives the coronary sinus, which after passing along the left atrioventricular groove empties into the right atrium near the orifice of the inferior vena cava. The orifice of the coronary sinus is partially surrounded by the thebesian valve. The internal surface of the right atrium is made up of a smooth posterior part receiving both vena cavae and a rough anterior portion consisting of multiple pectinate muscles. The two surfaces are divided by a ridge of muscle called the crista terminalis. The most constant feature to distinguish the morphological right atrium is the atrial appendage, which is broad and triangular in shape with a rough surface due to the pectinate muscles (Figure 9.1). It arises from the upper aspect of the rough anterior surface in close proximity to the ascending aorta and partially covering the right atrioventricular groove and associated right coronary artery.

MORPHOLOGICAL LEFT ATRIUM

This is the most posterior chamber, typically receiving the pulmonary veins. Similar to the morphological right atrium, the atrial appendage, which is classically fingerlike, is the most constant feature (Figure 9.2). It is closely related to the main pulmonary artery and covers the left atrioventricular groove and part of the circumflex coronary artery. The main body of the left atrium is smooth walled.

MORPHOLOGICAL RIGHT VENTRICLE

Due to the rightward bowing of the ventricular septum the right ventricle is crescent shaped. It is divided into inlet, apical trabecular and outlet portions. The inlet portion lies to the right and inferiorly and is associated with the tricuspid valve. The outlet portion lies superiorly and to the left. The outlet portion or infundibulum is smooth walled and muscular and in a normal heart separates the tricuspid and pulmonary valves. The apical component contains coarse trabeculations, which are most easily identified on angiographic studies (Figure 9.3).

Table 9.1 Incidence of common congenital cardiac lesions

	Condition	Incidence
Left-to-right shunt	Ventricular septal defect	36%
	Atrial septal defect	5%
	Patent arterial duct	9%
	Atrioventricular septal defect	4%
Obstructive lesions	Pulmonary stenosis	9%
	Aortic stenosis	5%
	Coarctation	5%
	Hypoplastic left heart syndrome	4%
Cyanotic lesions	Transposition of the great arteries	4%
	Tetralogy of Fallot	4%

Table 9.2 Congenital disorders associated with cardiac lesions

	Chromosome abnormality	% with heart disease	Commonest cardiovascular abnormalities
Chromosome disorders			
Down	Trisomy 21	50	AVSD, VSD, ASD, Tetralogy of Fallot
Edward	Trisomy 18	90	VSD, ASD, PDA, valve disease
Patau	Trisomy 13	80	PDA, VSD, ASD,
Turner	XO	15	Coarct, AS, PS
Associations			
Cleft lip and palate		25	VSD, PDA, TGA, Tetralogy of Fallot
Diaphragmatic hernia		25	Tetralogy of Fallot
Lung agenesis		20	PDA, VSD, Tetralogy of Fallot, Anomalous pulmonary venous drainage
Omphalocele		20	Tetralogy of Fallot, ASD
Intestinal atresia		10	VSD
Unilateral renal agenesis		17	VSD
Tracheoesophageal fistula		10	VSD, Tetralogy of Fallot
CHARGE association		70	Tetralogy of Fallot, DORV, ASD, VSD, PDA, Coarctation, AVSD
VACTRL association		10	VSD, ASD, Tetralogy of Fallot
Asymmetrical crying facies		44	VSD
Autosomal Dominant			
Beckwith–Wiedemann	11	15+	HCM, ASD, VSD, Tetralogy of Fallot, PDA
DiGeorge	22q11	75	Interrupted aortic arch, Tetralogy of Fallot, Common arterial trunk
Goldenhar		15	Tetralogy of Fallot, VSD
Holt–Oram	12q24.1	100	ASD, VSD, PDA
Tuberose sclerosis	9q34	30+	Rhabdomyomas
Noonan	12q22		PS with dysplastic PV, PDA, HCM
Williams	7q11.2	50–80	Supravalvar AS, stenosis affecting cerebral and renal arteries
Familial SVAS			SVAS
Autosomal recessive			
Smith–Lemli–Opitz	7q32.1	20–100	VSD, PDA, ASD, Tetralogy of Fallot
Thrombocytopenia absent radius		33	ASD, Tetralogy of Fallot

Adapted from Forfar and Arneil's. Textbook of paediatrics, 6th edn. Table 19.6. © Elsevier Ltd 2003.
Note this list is not inclusive: AS, aortic stenosis; AVSD, atrioventricular septal defect; DORV, double outlet right ventricle; HCM, hypertrophic cardiomyopathy; VSD, ventricular septal defect; ASD, atrial septal defect; Coarctation, aortic coarctation; PDA, patent arterial duct; PS, pulmonary stenosis; SVAS, supra valviaortic stenosis; TGA, transposition of the great arteries.

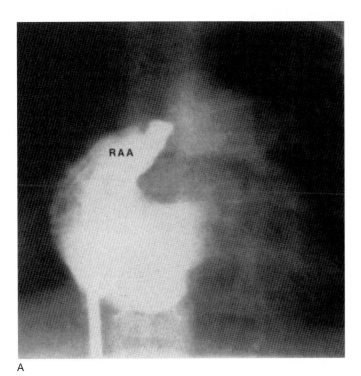
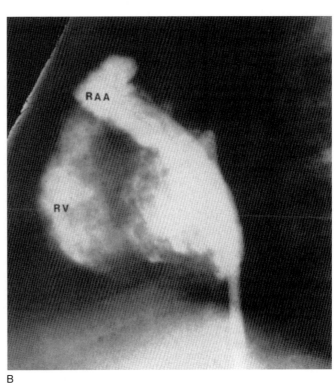

A   B

1Figure 9.1 Normal right atrial angiogram (A) anteroposterior (AP) and (B) lateral views. The catheter is in the inferior vena cava (IVC). Note the broad-based right atrial appendage. RV, right ventricle.

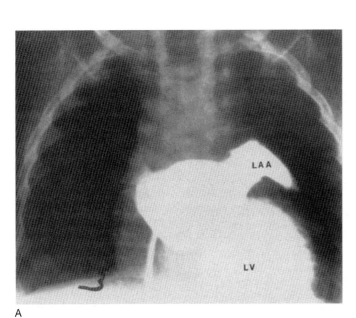
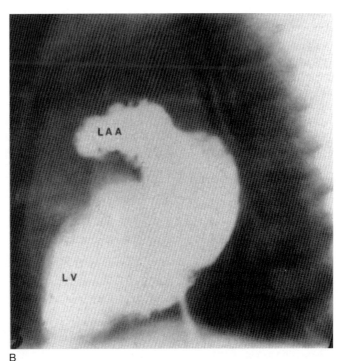

A   B

Figure 9.2 Normal left atrial angiogram. (A) AP and (B) lateral views. The catheter passes from the IVC into left atrium and through the foramen ovale into the left atrium. LAA, left atrial appendage; LV, left ventricle.

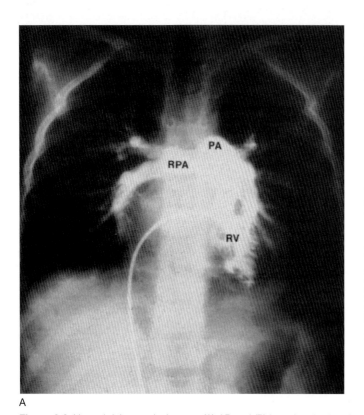
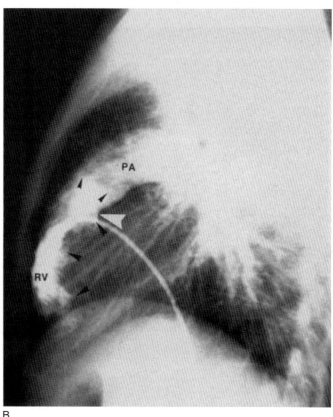

A   B

Figure 9.3 Normal right ventriculogram. (A) AP and (B) lateral projection. Note that in (B) inlet and outlet valves (black arrowheads) are separated by the muscular conus (white arrowhead). RV, right ventricle; PA, main pulmonary artery; RPA, right pulmonary artery.

The tricuspid valve is shaped like a reversed D in short axis view, consisting of the septal leaflet (straight part of the D), anterior leaflet (top right part of reversed D) and posterior or inferior leaflet (inferior right part of reversed D). The tricuspid valve always attaches to the morphological right ventricle, so that its correct identification on echocardiography will also help assess ventricular morphology. The classical features enabling correct identification of the tricuspid valve are the septal attachments of the tendinous cords of the septal leaflet. The tricuspid valve is displaced in a more apical direction than the mitral valve on the four-chamber view. Exceptions to the latter finding are in partial atrioventricular septal defects (AVSD) and double inlet right ventricle.

MORPHOLOGICAL LEFT VENTRICLE

The left ventricle also has inlet, outlet and apical portions. The apical part contains fine trabeculations (Figure 9.4). There is fibrous continuity of the mitral and aortic valves in a normal heart. The mitral valve is circular or elliptical depending on the phase of the cardiac cycle. It consists of anterior and posterior leaflets. There is no septal attachment of the tendinous cords or leaflet. The mitral valve only attaches to the papillary muscles. The anterior leaflet forms part of the outflow tract. Since the atrioventricular valves follow the ventricle, the correct identification on echocardiography of the mitral valve allows confirmation of the position of the morphological left ventricle.

SEQUENTIAL ANALYSIS

Once each chamber and the great vessels have been recognized, then the arrangements of the atria should be described. This should be followed by atrioventricular and ventriculoarterial connections.

The atria can have four different arrangements. 'Situs solitus' is the expected finding in a normal heart with the morphological right atrium on the right and the morphological left atrium on the left side of the body. 'Situs inversus' is the opposite with the morphological right atrium on the left and the morphological left atrium on the right side of the body. The latter may be associated with reverse arrangement of the abdominal organs, i.e. the stomach and spleen are right sided and the liver is mainly left sided (Figure 9.5).

'Isomerism' describes the situation when two right atria or two left atria are present, i.e. right or left isomerism, respectively. When isomerism is present there is variable positioning of the abdominal organs. Usually in left isomerism, there are multiple spleens and azygos continuation of the inferior vena cava (IVC; Figure 9.6). In right isomerism, the spleen is absent. The liver may be midline (Figure 9.7).

When considering connections, the morphological right atrium may be connected to a morphological right ventricle and left atrium to left ventricle, i.e. concordant, or the morphological right atrium may be connected to the morphological left ventricle and morphological left atrium to the morphological right ventricle, i.e. discordant. When the atria are isomeric then this nomenclature cannot be used and the connections are 'ambiguous'.

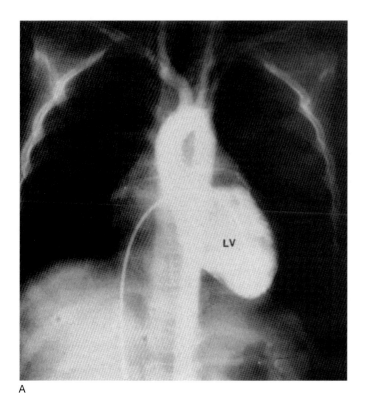

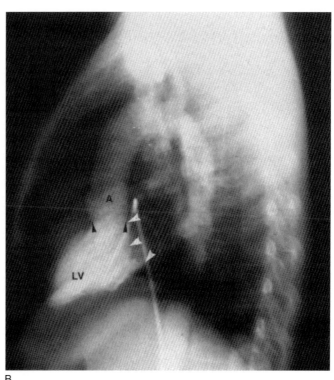

A   B

Figure 9.4 Normal left ventriculogram. (A) AP and (B) lateral projections. Note that the inlet and outlet valves (arrowheads) are in continuity with one another. LV, left ventricle; A, ascending aorta.

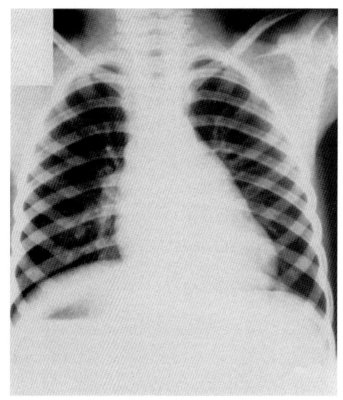

Figure 9.5 Abdominal situs inversus with isolated lavocardia. Note the stomach bubble is on the right.

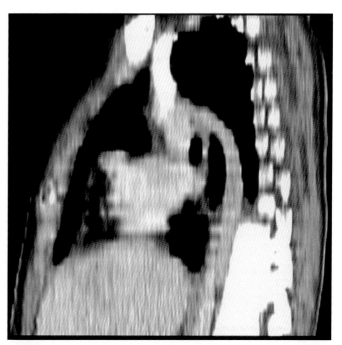

Figure 9.6 Sagittal reconstruction. CT image demonstrates absence of the normal IVC entering the atrium. The azygos vein ascends to join the superior vena cava (SVC) posteriorly. Classical findings of azygos continuation of the IVC.

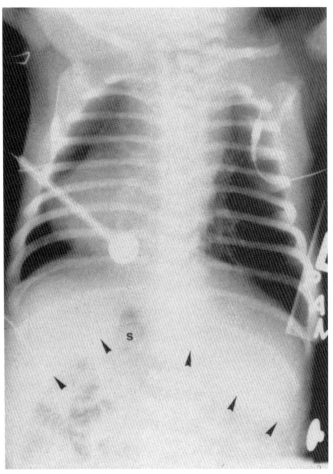

Figure 9.7 Right isomerism. The liver (arrowheads) lies symmetrically across the midline. The stomach (s) is to the right of the midline. The cardiac apex is on the right.

The ventriculoarterial relationship should also be described as concordant or discordant, if possible.

FURTHER READING

Burn J, Brennan P, Little J et al. Recurrence risks in offspring of adults with major heart defects: results from first cohort of British collaborative study. Lancet 1998; 351:311–316.
Hoffman JIE. Incidence, mortality and natural history. In: Anderson RH, Baker EJ, Macartney FJ et al. (eds). Pediatric cardiology, 2nd edn. Edinburgh: Churchill Livingstone; 2002:111–139.
Samanek M, Voriskova M. Congenital heart disease among 818,5569 children born between 1980 and 1990 and their 15 year survival: a prospective Bohemia survival study. Pediatric Cardiology 1999; 20:411–417.
Wren C, O'Sullivan JJ. Survival with congenital heart disease and need for follow-up in adult life. Heart 2001; 85:438–443.

METHODS OF INVESTIGATION

THE CHEST RADIOGRAPH

In older texts, the classical appearances of a chest radiograph were illustrated as the diagnosis of heart disease was in part based on these. With modern early diagnosis and treatment, often antenatal, these patterns are no longer used. The classical patterns will be briefly described here for completeness as in some parts of the world, early diagnosis and treatment are still rare.

The primary diagnostic tool of cardiac disease is by echocardiography. Nonetheless, the radiologist must still be able to identify that there is underlying cardiac disease on the radiograph and must be able to analyze and identify situs, cardiomegaly, pulmonary oedema, pulmonary plethora and oligaemia, and the normal vascular contours. The roles of the radiologist today are to distinguish cardiac from respiratory causes of disease, to monitor position of tubes and lines, and advise and perform cross-sectional imaging.

In many textbooks, the typical appearance of enlargement of individual chambers is described in detail; however, suspected chamber enlargement is now confirmed on ultrasound.

ANALYSIS OF CHEST RADIOGRAPH

TECHNICAL CONSIDERATIONS

A correctly inspired and exposed radiograph is essential in assessing cardiac size. Low lung volumes can erroneously make the heart appear enlarged as well as create the impression of air space opacification simulating pulmonary oedema. The anterior ends of six ribs should be visible above the diaphragm in a correctly inspired film. Tracheal buckling to the right is accentuated in expiration. Over- or underexposure will produce a dark or light film, respectively, leading to difficulty in assessing the pulmonary vascularity. Rotation of the patient alters mediastinal structures, which may appear falsely prominent or difficult to see. Symmetry of the anterior ribs confirms that the film is straight.

TRACHEA

The position of the trachea as well as its contour should be carefully assessed, though this is not always possible in a neonate. Displacement or compression suggests the presence of a mediastinal mass or vascular ring (Figure 9.8). A right aortic arch gives the appearance of an upper right mediastinal mass with indentation of the right side of the trachea (Figure 9.9). A vascular ring due to a double aortic arch may result in indentation of both sides of the trachea on the anteroposterior (AP) view. This is difficult to appreciate in the neonate and young infant but loss of the tracheal air column or narrowing may be seen. The branching pattern of the main bronchi may give clues to the presence of isomerism with bilateral left main bronchi in left isomerism and vice versa in right isomerism, the left main bronchus being longer than the right.

MEDIASTINUM

Abnormally positioned vessels can contribute to mediastinal widening. These include the cervical aortic arch, described later under vascular rings, the right aortic arch and the vertical vein in total anomalous pulmonary venous return and a persistent left superior vena cava (Figure 9.10). In the latter, there may be left upper mediastinal widening due to the left superior vena cava (SVC), which typically drains into the coronary sinus and hence into the right atrium (Figure 9.11).

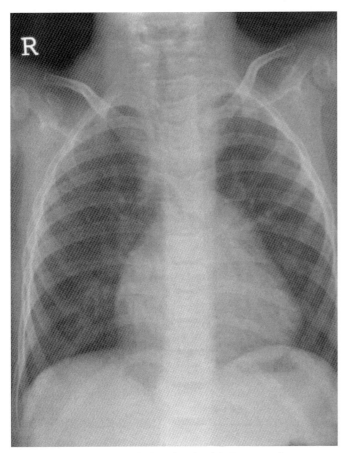

Figure 9.8 The trachea is displaced to the right by a superior mediastinal mass confirmed to be a large jugular varix.

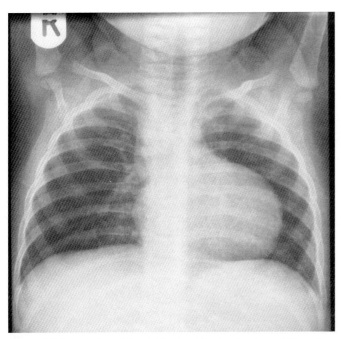

Figure 9.9 Indentation of the right side of the trachea by a right aortic arch.

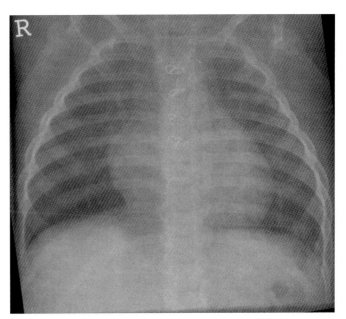

Figure 9.10 Left upper mediastinal widening by a left SVC.

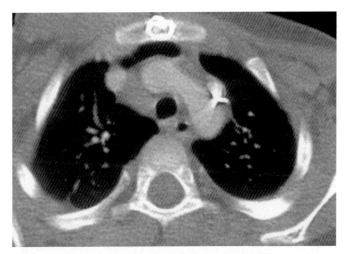

Figure 9.11 Contrast-enhanced CT displaying the left SVC coursing along the left side of the aortic arch.

ABDOMINAL ORGANS

When isomerism or heterotaxy are present then the stomach may be left sided with a midline liver. Bilateral horizontal fissures may be identified in right isomerism with bilateral trilobed lungs.

PULMONARY ARTERY

The position and size of the main and branch pulmonary arteries should be assessed. In general, in untreated right ventricular outflow obstructive lesions the main pulmonary artery is small or not visible, e.g. tetralogy of Fallot or pulmonary atresia and ventricular septal defect. In transposition of the great arteries, the main pulmonary artery may be difficult to appreciate because it often lies behind and in a directly anteroposterior alignment with the aorta. The main pulmonary artery may be enlarged in pulmonary stenosis, atrial septal defect and pulmonary hypertension. In Fallot's tetralogy with absent pulmonary valve, the branch pulmonary arteries can be massive. As a general rule, the right descending pulmonary artery is normally the same size as the trachea. With absence of a right or left pulmonary artery, marked mediastinal shift will be seen to the side of the absent vessel. If a main branch pulmonary artery is hypoplastic then lung hypoplasia occurs with a smaller lung on the involved side as well as mediastinal shift to that side. Confirmation with other imaging studies, e.g. CT or MRI, is usually necessary.

PULMONARY VASCULARITY

Pulmonary vascularity can be described as to be increased, decreased, normal or asymmetrical. Detection of changes is dependent on a good-quality, well-inspired film.

Increased pulmonary blood flow is due to passive congestion when there is pulmonary venous congestion resulting from obstruction along the left side of the heart or due to left-sided failure. Initially, there is a characteristic haziness of the lungs with indistinctness of the vessels (Figure 9.12). Often pleural fluid is present. Frank pulmonary oedema and air space opacification may then develop. On the other hand, active congestion is seen with a left-to-right shunt, e.g. a ventricular septal defect (VSD) or patent ductus curteriosus (PDA). The central and peripheral pulmonary vessels are enlarged. The peripheral vessels may extend into the outer third of the lung. The vessel margins are crisp, unlike in pulmonary venous congestion (Figure 9.13).

Reduced pulmonary blood flow, classically described in tetralogy of Fallot, can be seen in any cause of right-sided obstruction including hypoplastic right heart, Ebstein's anomaly and unilateral absent pulmonary artery (Figure 9.14). Asymmetry in blood flow is often found in Fallot's tetralogy with asymmetrical peripheral pulmonary stenosis. The left lung often has relatively decreased blood flow. Also, in postoperative patients, particularly following a Blalock–Taussig shunt or Glenn procedure (cavopulmonary),

pulmonary blood flows preferentially to the side of the shunt (Figure 9.15). The pattern in pulmonary hypertension is different again and is described below under left-to-right shunts.

AORTA

A right-sided aortic arch indents the trachea on the right (Figure 9.9). There is absence of the normal left aortic knuckle. The

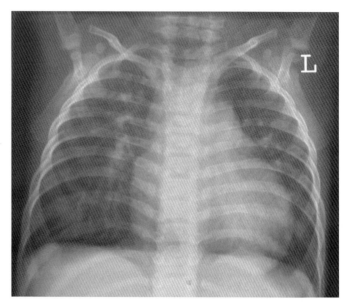

Figure 9.13 Enlarged heart and pulmonary plethora due to a VSD.

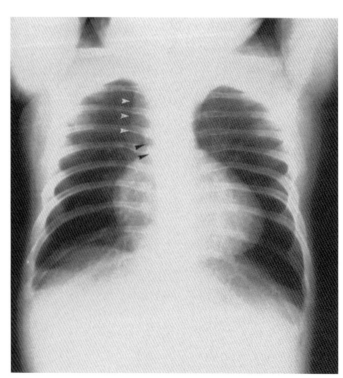

Figure 9.14 Pulmonary oligaemia. The pulmonary trunk and peripheral vessels are small. The aortic arch (black arrowheads) is right sided, displacing the SVC (white arrowheads) laterally. This patient had tetralogy of Fallot.

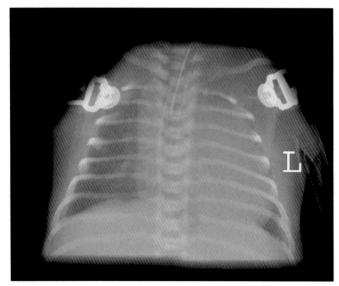

Figure 9.12 Neonate with an enlarged heart and hazy opacification of both lungs due to hypoplastic left heart causing pulmonary oedema.

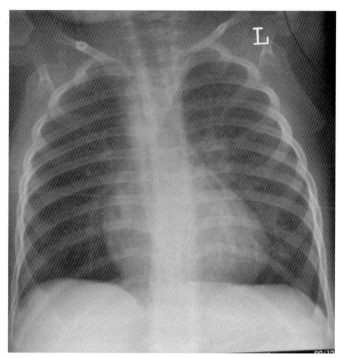

Figure 9.15 Relatively increased vascularity in the left lung due to a left-sided Blalock–Taussig shunt.

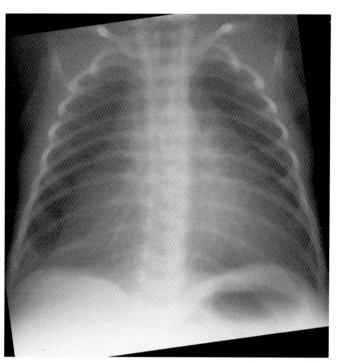

Figure 9.16 Middle mediastinal mass due to a pericardial teratoma giving the false impression of massive cardiomegaly.

ascending aorta is normally barely visible on a normal chest radiograph in a young child. When prominent it is usually due to aortic stenosis, aortic incompetence, coarctation of the aorta, or in Marfan syndrome is due to dilation of the ascending aorta. In coarctation, rib notching is not seen in young children and classical signs (reversed 3 sign, dilated ascending aorta) of coarctation can be very subtle on the chest radiograph. These really only develop in untreated coarctation.

HEART SIZE

The size of the heart and the position and size of the great vessels can be very difficult to assess in the neonate and young infant due to the presence of the thymus and variable degrees of inspiration. Massive cardiomegaly should be differentiated from a mediastinal tumour (Figure 9.16). This is obviously rapidly achieved by echo but change in heart size is often a useful sign. It must be noted that a normal heart size does not exclude underlying cardiac or great vessel pathology. In the older child, cardiomegaly is easier to recognize. Absolute ratios are of limited value but as a rule of thumb, the maximum transverse diameter of the heart should be no more than 60% of the transverse diameter of the chest in young children up to the age of 4. After that it assumes the more normal adult ratio of 50% of the thoracic diameter.

LUNG AERATION

Asymmetry in lung aeration may be due to associated tracheo- or bronchomalacia often found with extrinsic compression of the airways by abnormal vessels. Obstructive emphysema or atelecta-

sis may result. Pulmonary hypoplasia and a smaller volume lung occurs with a hypoplastic pulmonary artery. Generalized hyperinflation is also described in children with respiratory distress due to underlying congenital heart disease and is not necessarily due to proven lung pathology.

The classical radiographs will be described in the relevant section below.

SCIMITAR

This describes the classical radiographic finding of a scimitar or curved linear shadow (which simulates a turkish sword) coursing along the right side of the chest sometimes behind the heart (Figure 9.17). It is due to an anomalous pulmonary vein, which often enters the right atrium or IVC. In so doing, a left-to-right shunt occurs. The chest radiograph is classical. Often there is an associated small right lung with mediastinal shift to the right and volume loss of the right lung. The patient may be asymptomatic if the shunt is small. Dynamic enhanced computed tomography (CT) or magnetic resonance imaging (MRI) are useful in defining the abnormalities (Figure 9.18).

POSTOPERATIVE CHEST RADIOGRAPH

The chest radiograph is particularly useful in the immediate postoperative period whilst the patient is being ventilated in intensive care. In particular, the position of tubes and lines should be carefully followed and evaluated. It is preferable to report radiographs in conjunction with the Intensivist who often adds valuable clinical information. A logical and methodical approach allows the radiologist to assess the often myriad of tubes and lines. External

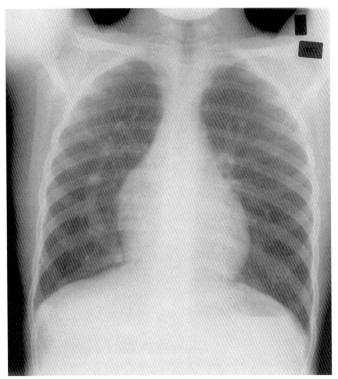

Figure 9.17 Classical scimitar coursing along the right lower chest due to partial anomalous pulmonary venous return.

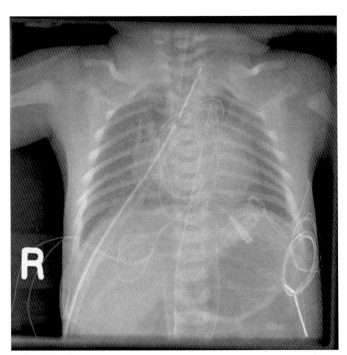

Figure 9.19 CXR immediately postcardiac surgery demonstrates the typical myriad of tubes and lines. Two atrial and two ventricular external pacemaker wires identified by the knot overlying the abdomen. A right atrial pressure catheter is slightly more radiopaque; the external end lies above the stomach. The tip of the nasogastric tube extends into the duodenum.

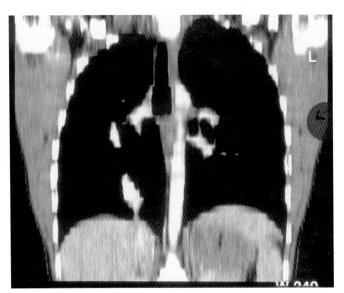

Figure 9.18 Coronal reconstruction from a contrast-enhanced CT demonstrates the partial pulmonary venous return, which drained into the intrahepatic IVC.

pacing wires can be recognized from the double knot on the external portion of the wire. Pressure catheters tend to be slightly more opaque than the pacing wires and will usually be positioned in either atria or the main pulmonary artery (Figure 9.19). Occasionally, they are inadvertently retained requiring subsequent removal. Central lines may enter the chest from the abdominal vessels or via a transhepatic route. Axillary, subclavian or internal jugular veins can be used as vascular access of central lines. The tips

should preferably lie in the superior vena cava. A left-sided SVC may result in inadvertent placement of a line into the coronary sinus and subsequently into the right atrium. Often, the surgeon places a mediastinal drain and a single chest tube in each hemithorax. In some cases, the chest is left open. This should not be mistaken for a pneumothorax or pneumomediastinum (Figure 9.20). Subtle pneumothoraces may be seen as increased clarity of the heart border or hemidiaphragm. A pneumopericardium is not unusual post cardiac surgery, however a large collection may need to be drained as it can cause pericardial tamponade (Figure 9.21).

Postoperative pleural fluid may be related to pulmonary oedema, a postoperative chylothorax resulting from trauma to the thoracic duct or a complication of central venous or arterial line insertion with a resultant haemothorax (Figure 9.22). Occasionally, the phrenic nerve is injured at surgery and diaphragmatic paralysis may only become evident on extubating the patient.

The chest radiograph is invaluable in assessing the position of occlusion devices, e.g. atrial septal defect (ASD) or PDA coils, as well as the position of vascular stents usually in the branch pulmonary arteries. Pulmonary conduits may calcify or be opaque immediately postoperatively. Delayed complications include aneurysmal dilation of a pulmonary patch and a calcified seroma related to a Blalock–Taussig shunt (Figure 9.23).

ECHOCARDIOGRAPHY

The ultrasound examination of the heart is the most important diagnostic technique in congenital heart disease. Cross-

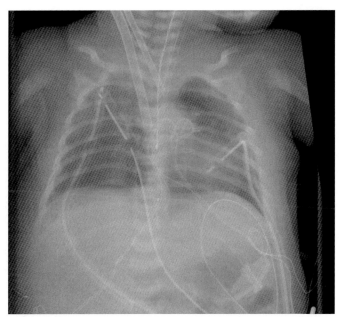

Figure 9.20 Postoperative CXR with the mediastinum still open. The air around the heart is due to this.

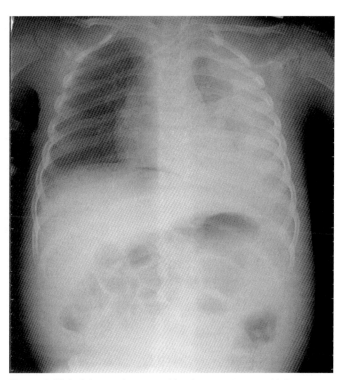

Figure 9.22 Left haemothorax resulting from an attempted left subclavian artery puncture. Pneumoperitoneum due to peritoneal dialysis. Left subclavian venous line in situ.

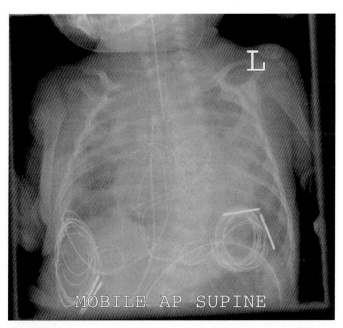

Figure 9.21 Air around the heart due to a postoperative pneumopericardium.

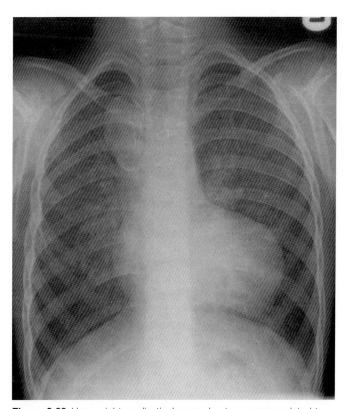

Figure 9.23 Upper right mediastinal mass due to a seroma related to a Blalock–Taussig shunt.

sectional echocardiography provides a two-dimensional view of the structure of the heart. By scanning in various planes, the anatomy and relationship of the heart chambers and great vessels can be defined. Doppler echocardiography provides information on cardiac haemodynamics, including assessment of pressure gradients across stenoses and septal defects. Assessment of left ventricular function is performed using single beam ultrasound ('M-mode' echocardiography).

CROSS-SECTIONAL (TWO-DIMENSIONAL) ECHOCARDIOGRAPHY

The heart is scanned in the parasternal, apical, subcostal and suprasternal views. In infants, there are larger echo windows (without air from the lungs between the probe and the heart) making imaging easier and better definition is achieved by using a higher frequency (8–12 MHz) ultrasound because of the faster heart rate. The higher frequency results in reduced tissue penetration and a frequency of 2–5 MHz is needed for larger children.

The long-axis view is obtained from the left parasternal edge, usually in the fourth intercostal space (Figure 9.24). It allows visualization of the left ventricle, part of the right ventricle, the interventricular septum, left atrium, and aortic and mitral valves.

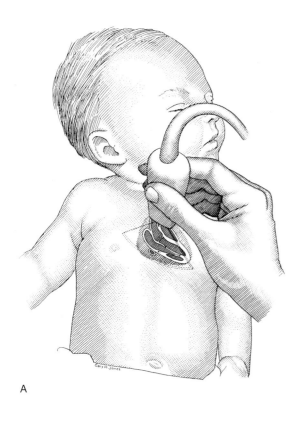

A

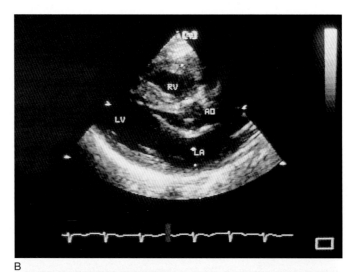

B

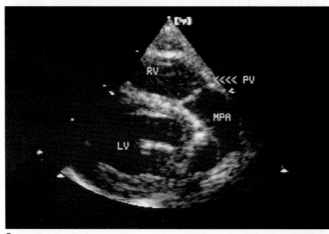

C

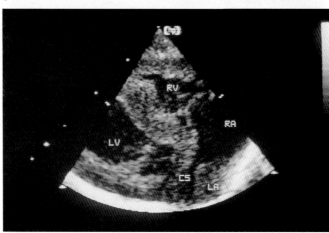

D

Figure 9.24 (A) Diagram showing the position of the transducer and orientation of scanning plane to provide a parasternal long-axis image of the heart. (B) Echocardiogram showing a standard parasternal long-axis image of the heart, ideal for demonstrating the left heart. The mitral valve is widely open in this diastolic frame. Ao, aorta; LV, left ventricle; RV, right ventricle. (C) Tilting towards the left shoulder reveals a long-axis view of the main pulmonary artery (MPA) and pulmonary valve (PV). (D) Tilting to the right, away from the left shoulder, reveals the tricuspid valve between the right atrium (RA) and right ventricle (RV). The coronary sinus (CS) is seen draining into the right atrium. LA, left atrium. (Reproduced with permission from Skinner J, Alverson D, Hunter S (eds). Echocardiography for the neonatologist. Edinburgh: Churchill Livingstone; 2000:43.)

The short-axis view is obtained by rotating the transducer through 90 degrees clockwise from the long axis view (Figure 9.25). The aortic valve is in a central position (Figure 9.25D) with the right ventricular outflow tract anteriorly, bifurcating into the left and right pulmonary arteries. The atria and interatrial septum lie posterior to the aorta.

Angling down towards the apex of the left ventricle brings the mitral valve structures into view, gaping like a 'fish mouth' as the leaflets open and close (Figure 9.25C). Tilting further towards the apex shows the anterolateral and posteromedial papillary muscles (Figure 9.25B).

The four-chamber view is obtained by placing the transducer over the apex or by scanning from the subcostal position (Figure 9.26B and 9.27B). It shows the ventricles, atria, and the interatrial and interventricular septums. The tricuspid valve is attached to the septum closer to the cardiac apex than the mitral valve (Figure

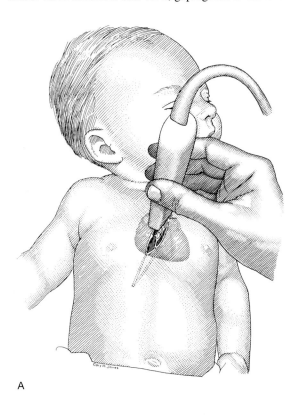

A

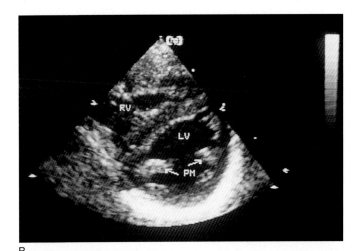

B

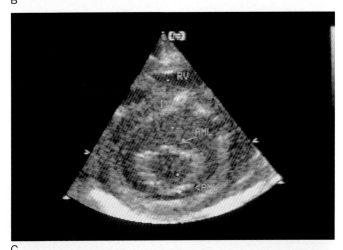

C

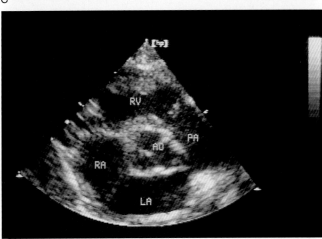

D

Figure 9.25 (A) Diagram showing the position of the transducer and orientation of the scanning plane to provide a parasternal short-axis image of the heart at the aortic valve level. (B) Parasternal short-axis echocardiograph at the level of the papillary muscles (towards the apex of the left ventricle). (C) Tilting away from the apex (towards the right shoulder) brings this view of the mitral valve. AML, anterior mitral valve leaflet; PML, posterior mitral valve leaflet. (D) Further tilt shows this cut at the aortic valve (as in (A)). Note here how three aortic valve leaflets are seen, and how the right heart wraps around the aorta. Tilting the probe further still away from the apex demonstrates the pulmonary artery bifurcation. (Reproduced with permission from Skinner J, Alverson D, Hunter S (eds). Echocardiography for the Neonatologist. Edinburgh: Churchill Livingstone; 2000:44.)

9.27B). Since a tricuspid valve is always associated with a right ventricle, and a mitral valve with the left, this offsetting is used to differentiate the ventricles in complex cases.

The atrial septum is best examined from the subcostal view (Figure 9.27B). Because of the complex shape of the interventricular septum, the search for ventricular septal defects needs to include all the available views. There is also a tiny component of the septal wall, the membranous septum, closely related to the tricuspid and aortic valves. It has atrioventricular and interventricular portions separated by the attachment of the septal leaflet of the tricuspid valve. With posterior tilt of the probe in the four-chamber view, the pulmonary veins can be seen entering the back of the left atrium. The coronary sinus runs in the atrioventricular groove behind the left atrium and opens into the right atrium.

The suprasternal view (Figure 9.28) demonstrates the arch of the aorta, which supplies the brachiocephalic (innominate) artery and the left common carotid artery as it runs superiorly for a short distance before passing backwards and to the left, where it gives rise to the left subclavian artery. Aortic coarctation most commonly appears just after this point.

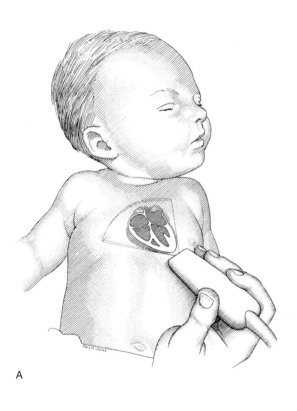

A

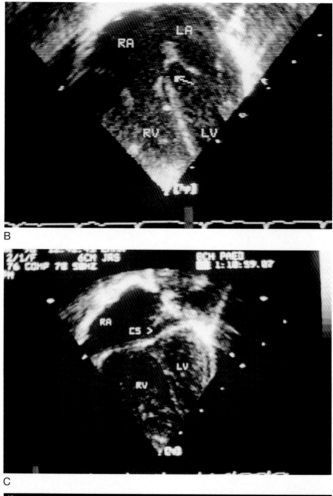

B

C

D

Figure 9.26 (A) Diagram showing the position of the transducer and orientation of scanning plane to provide an apical four-chamber view of the heart. (B) Apical four-chamber echocardiogram. Note that the screen has been inverted. The arrow indicates the lower position of the tricuspid valve as it arises from the septum. This region between the two atrioventricular valves is known as the atrioventricular septum, dividing the left ventricle from the right atrium. (C) Apical view of the heart with the probe angled posteriorly to bring the coronary sinus (CS) into view (not to be confused with a low atrial septal defect!). (D) Apical view of the heart with the probe angled anteriorly and rotated to the right bringing the left ventricular outflow tract and aortic valve into view – this is an apical long axis image. (Reproduced with permission from Skinner J, Alverson D, Hunter S (eds). Echocardiography for the neonatologist. Edinburgh: Churchill Livingstone; 2000:45.)

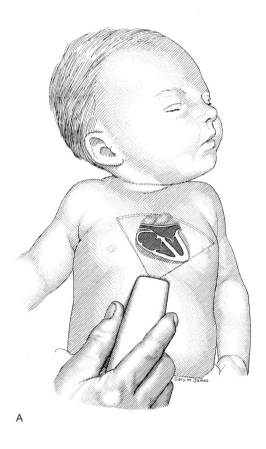

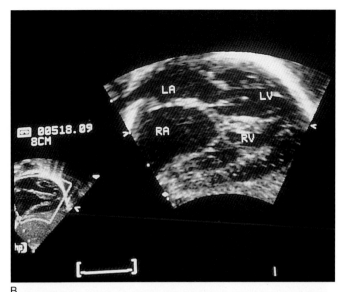

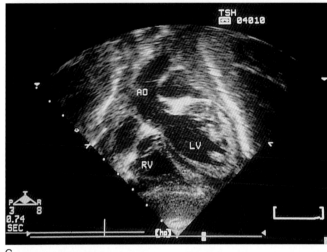

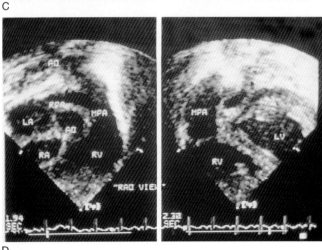

Figure 9.27 (A) Diagram showing the position of the transducer and orientation of the scanning plane to provide a subcostal four-chamber image of the heart. (B) Subcostal four-chamber image demonstrating the four chambers. This is an ideal view to see atrial septal defects. (C) Tilting the probe anteriorly brings the ascending aorta into view. (D) Left: rotating anticlockwise brings the right ventricular outflow tract and pulmonary arteries into view (subcostal short-axis or 'RAO' (right anterior oblique) view). MPA, main pulmonary artery; RPA, right pulmonary artery. Right: rotating clockwise shows the interventricular septum and another view of the right ventricular outflow tract. These views are especially useful in tetralogy of Fallot to assess obstruction of the right ventricular outflow tract. (Reproduced with permission from Skinner J, Alverson D, Hunter S (eds). Echocardiography for the neonatologist. Edinburgh: Churchill Livingstone; 2000:46.)

DOPPLER ECHOCARDIOGRAPHY

This allows the detection of blood flow within the heart and great vessels. There are three modes of Doppler ultrasound: pulsed-wave, continuous wave and colour Doppler. These are complementary, each measuring blood flow velocities in different ways.

PULSED-WAVE DOPPLER ULTRASOUND

This allows accurate sampling of small volumes at precise locations within the heart, provided the velocity is not high. High velocities are measured with continuous wave Doppler.

CONTINUOUS WAVE DOPPLER ULTRASOUND

This allows accurate measurement of high velocities along its path. As it receives signals from all along its course, high velocities coming from a valve or vessel further away or closer must not be confused with the area being imaged.

COLOUR DOPPLER ULTRASOUND

This combines pulsed Doppler and two-dimensional scans, superimposing the Doppler information on the two-dimensional image and colour coding the speed and direction. For example, red and yellow are slow and fast towards the probe, respectively, and

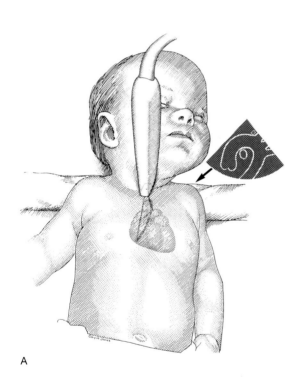

A

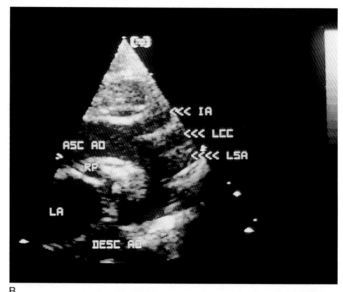

B

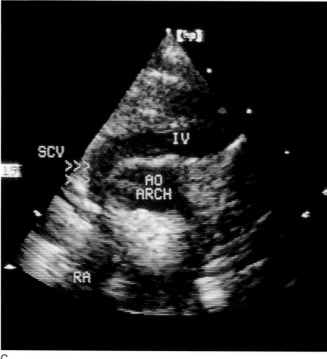

C

Figure 9.28 (A) Diagram showing the position of the transducer and orientation of the scanning plane required to obtain views of the aortic arch with a conventional left-sided aorta. Note that a roll has been placed behind the shoulders to extend the neck. (B) Image of the aortic arch and branches obtained from the suprasternal window. IA, innominate artery (or right brachiocephalic artery); LCC, left common carotid artery; LSA, left subclavian artery. Arch interruptions and coarctations are best viewed like this. (C) With a transverse scanning plane, the innominate vein (IV) drains to the superior caval vein (SCV). (Reproduced with permission from Skinner J, Alverson D, Hunter S (eds). Echocardiography for the neonatologist. Edinburgh: Churchill Livingstone; 2000:47.)

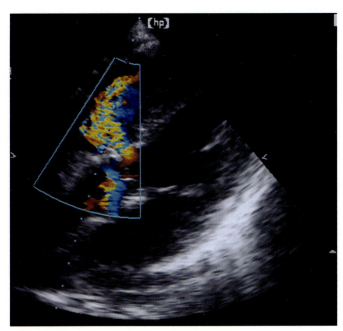

Figure 9.29 Echocardiogram showing VSD.

blue and green are slow and fast away from the probe. Areas of turbulence and high velocity are shown by a mosaic pattern of these colours. This technique is especially useful in detecting ventricular septal defects (VSD), valvar or arterial stenosis, or regurgitation (Figure 9.29).

DETERMINATION OF PRESSURE GRADIENT

The simplified Bernoulli equation is used to estimate pressure drop across a stenosis, a shunt such as a ventricular septal defect, or a regurgitant valve. The peak velocity is measured with continuous wave Doppler and the instantaneous gradient calculated from the formula:

$$4V^2 = P_1 - P_2$$

Where $(P_1 - P_2)$ is the pressure drop across the obstruction (mmHg) and V is the peak velocity (m/s). The Doppler beam must be in line with the flow to avoid underestimation of the peak velocity.

Valvar stenosis

Cardiac catheterization is no longer needed to monitor pressure gradients across valves. The Doppler gradient is not exactly the same as the catheterization gradient and is consistently higher than that measured at catheterization. This is because the Doppler gradient is the maximal instantaneous pressure gradient (the greatest pressure difference before and after the valve at any instant in the cardiac cycle). The catheter gradients reflect the peak to peak gradient (the difference between the highest pressure before and after the stenosis, i.e. not recorded simultaneously). Nevertheless, Doppler gradients are an effective non-invasive method of monitoring changes in valve stenosis.

Pulmonary arterial (PA) pressure

Pulmonary arterial pressure is calculated from the pressure drop between the right ventricle (RV) and the right atrium (RA) by measuring peak velocity of tricuspid regurgitation (TR):

RV systolic pressure = $4 \times$ TR jet velocity^2 + RA pressure

Right ventricular systolic pressure approximates to pulmonary arterial systolic pressure (if the pulmonary valve is not stenotic), and right atrial pressure varies little and can usually be assumed to be 5 or 10 mmHg. The technique is useful, because of the high incidence of trivial or mild tricuspid regurgitation in children with congenital heart diseases and in the normal population. Pulmonary artery pressure can similarly be estimated by measuring the peak velocity across a ventricular septal defect (if there is no pulmonary stenosis), or across an arterial duct.

Assessment of valvar regurgitation

Colour Doppler demonstrates valvar regurgitation but the assessment is subjective and not accurately quantifiable. Trivial valvar regurgitation of all but the aortic valve is seen in normal subjects. Severe atrioventricular valve regurgitation causes dilatation of the respective atrium. Severe aortic or pulmonary valve regurgitation causes dilation of the ventricle.

Assessment of ventricular function

Left ventricle: The most reproducible technique employs M-mode echocardiography to measure the fractional shortening (FS) or percentage reduction of the left ventricular (LV) diameter in systole:

$$FS(\%) = \frac{\text{LV diastolic dimension} - \text{LV systolic dimension}}{\text{LV diastolic dimension}} \times 100$$

The normal value lies between 28% and 44% and is reduced with poor myocardial function, and increased with volume overload, such as a left-to-right shunt through a ventricular septal defect or arterial duct. The measurements are made just beyond the tips of the mitral valve, from the parasternal position. Measurements of septal and posterior wall thickness in diastole assess ventricular hypertrophy (Figure 9.30).

Right ventricle: This has a complex shape and subjective visual assessment from cross-sectional images provides the best assessment of function.

FURTHER READING

Ho SY, McCarthy KP, Josen M, Rigby ML. Anatomic-echocardiographic correlates: an introduction to normal and congenitally malformed hearts. Heart 2001; 86(Suppl II):ii3–ii11.

Skinner J, Alverson D, Hunter S. Echocardiography for the Neonatologist. Edinburgh: Churchill Livingstone; 2000.

Tworetzky W, McElhinney DB, Brook MM et al. Echocardiographic diagnosis alone for the complete repair of major congenital heart defects. Journal of the American College of Cardiology 1999; 33:228–233.

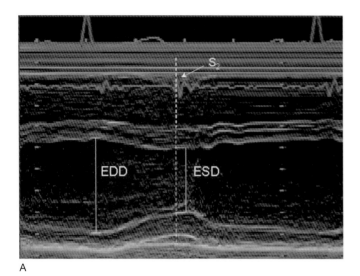

A

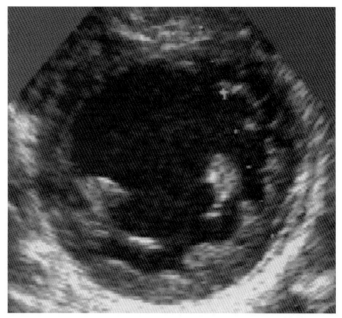

B

Figure 9.30 The M-mode images across the short axis of the left ventricle (A) with the cross-sectional image (B) showing the position from which the M-mode is derived. Fractional shortening is calculated as end diastolic diameter (EDD) – end systolic diameter (ESD) divided by end diastolic diameter x 100. (From Forfar and Arneil's Textbook of paediatrics 6th edn. © Elsevier Ltd 2003.)

CARDIAC COMPUTED TOMOGRAPHY

Spiral CT of the chest using 16-slice scanners and dynamic enhancement with intravenous contrast is increasingly being used to identify the anatomy both pre- and postoperatively in children with congenital heart disease. Reconstructions can be obtained in any plane and viewed with cine loop. The main and both the right and left pulmonary arteries can be assessed for presence, size, position, stenosis and intraluminal filling defects. Patency of vascular stents and wall calcification can be evaluated. The position and size of the aorta can be demonstrated. Coarctation of the aorta is best demonstrated by sagittal oblique reconstructions of the aortic arch and descending aorta. CT is useful in assessing vascular rings and the relationship to the adjacent airways, particularly if access to MRI is limited. Information on anomalous pulmonary venous return and associated abnormalities of the lungs and upper abdominal viscera can be obtained with a single study. The new generation multislice CT scanners with faster imaging, cardiac gating and improved resolution are increasingly being used in place of invasive angiography. Dynamic contrast-enhanced CT may be required to show the relationship of the great vessels to the chest wall prior to repeat surgery. Postoperative complications such as stitch decussation or sternal osteomyelitis are easily assessed with contrast enhancement or, on occasion, CT sinography. The radiation burden to the patient must always be balanced against the utility of the information obtained.

FURTHER READING

Gilkeson RC, Ciancibello L, Zahka K. Pictorial essay. Multidetector CT evaluation of congenital heart disease in pediatric and adult patients. American Journal of Roentgenology 2003; 180:973–980.

Goo HW, Park IS, Ko JK et al. CT of congenital heart disease: normal anatomy and typical pathologic conditions. Radiographics 2003; 23:S147–165.

Kaemmerer H, Stern H, Fratz S et al. Imaging in adults with congenital cardiac disease (ACCD). Thoracic Cardiovascular Surgery 2000; 48:328–335.

Kawano T, Ishii M, Takagi J et al. Three-dimensional helical computed tomographic angiography in neonates and infants with complex congenital heart disease. American Heart Journal 2000; 139:654–660.

CARDIAC MAGNETIC RESONANCE IMAGING

The use of magnetic resonance imaging in evaluating morphology and function in congenital heart disease is advancing at a rapid rate. It is discussed below in 'MRI and Functional Imaging of the Heart'.

CARDIAC CATHETERIZATION

Echocardiography allows the diagnosis and management of most children with heart disease. Cardiac catheterization provides information on pulmonary vascular disease and accurate shunt calculations. Angiography remains superior to echocardiography for coronary and distal pulmonary artery imaging, and is helpful in infants with complex arterial or venous abnormalities. It is usually performed under general anaesthesia. The percutaneous femoral approach is the most frequent, although axillary, brachial or internal jugular routes are occasionally used. In the first few days of life, an atrial septostomy can be performed through the umbilical vein before the venous duct closes.

CALCULATION OF THE LEFT-TO-RIGHT SHUNT

A rise in oxygen saturation of 5% or more between the systemic veins and pulmonary artery indicates a significant left-to-right shunt. Pulmonary to systemic flow ratio (Qp:Qs) is calculated from the oxygen saturations in the aorta (Ao), pulmonary artery (PA), left atrium (LA) and the mixed venous saturation (MV) from the formula:

$$QP:QS = \frac{Ao - MV}{LA - PA}$$

A shunt ratio of less than 1.5:1 is insignificant and one that is more than 1.8:1 is likely to require intervention.

CALCULATION OF PRESSURE GRADIENTS

Pressures are recorded in all chambers and great vessels and peak systolic gradients determined.

CALCULATION OF PULMONARY VASCULAR RESISTANCE

The mean pressure in the atria and great arteries is required for estimation of pulmonary and systemic vascular resistance, which are indexed for body surface area. Pulmonary vascular resistance determines the operability of a child with a left-to-right shunt. Administration of a pulmonary vasodilator such as 100% oxygen or nitric oxide during the catheter procedure identifies whether or not a high resistance is fixed.

ANGIOGRAPHY

This is performed by the injection of radiological contrast into chambers or vessels. Angiography is now less important for the definition of intracardiac defects but remains necessary for abnormalities of the great arteries or veins, in particular the anatomy of abnormal pulmonary or coronary arteries (Figures 9.31 and 9.32).

COMPLICATIONS

These include haemorrhage, femoral artery occlusion, arrhythmia, embolism and cardiac perforation with tamponade. General anaesthetic and angiography carries a high risk in patients with pulmonary hypertension.

INTERVENTIONAL CATHETERIZATION

The majority of paediatric cardiac catheterization includes an interventional procedure. Many complex interventions require radiological and ultrasound (usually transoesophageal) imaging

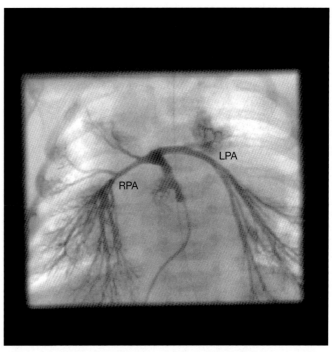

Figure 9.31 Pulmonary angiogram in the main pulmonary artery (MPA) showing small left (LPA) and right pulmonary arteries (RPA).

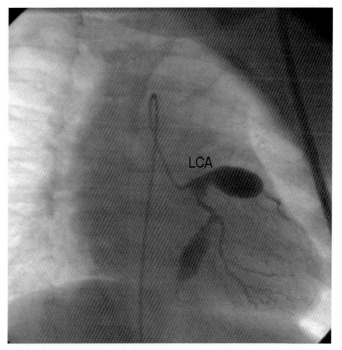

Figure 9.32 Left coronary arteriogram showing an aneurysm of the main left and anterior descending coronary arteries in a child with Kawasaki disease. LCA, left coronary artery. (Reproduced with permission from Forfar and Arneil's. Textbook of paediatrics, 6th edn. © Elsevier Ltd 2003.)

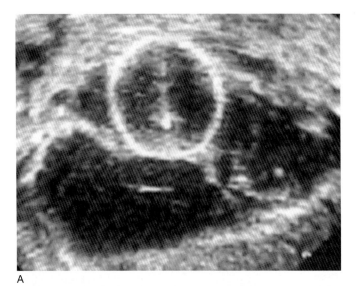

A

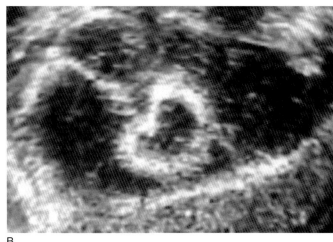

B

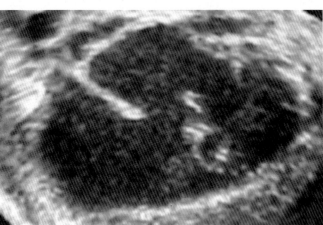

C

Figure 9.33 Balloon atrial septostomy using echocardiographic imaging. A balloon septostomy catheter is advanced from the umbilical or femoral vein into the right atrium and across into the left atrium (A). The balloon is inflated in the left atrium and pulled across the atrial septum (B). (C) The atrial septal defect created is identified with the asterisk. LA, left atrium; RA, right atrium. (Reproduced with permission from Forfar and Arneil's. Textbook of paediatrics, 6th edn. © Elsevier Ltd 2003.)

and are performed by interventional cardiologists. Balloon atrial septostomy (Figure 9.33) was the first reported paediatric interventional catheter procedure. It is still carried out in infants with inadequate cardiac mixing, as in transposition of the great arteries, using either ultrasound or radiographic imaging.

Balloon valvuloplasty is the treatment of choice for pulmonary valve stenosis (Figure 9.34). It is safe and effective (unless the valve is severely dysplastic) and can be performed at any age. Aortic balloon valvuloplasty is an alternative to surgery, unless there is significant regurgitation (Figure 9.35). The results are comparable but both are palliative, and progression occurs. Balloon dilatation is not effective in the treatment of neonatal coarctation and there is a debate regarding its use in infants and young children who have not had previous surgery. Balloon dilatation is the treatment of choice for most residual or recurrent coarctation following surgery (Figure 9.36). Balloon dilatation has also been used for patients with a wide variety of vessel narrowing. In older children and adolescents, balloon-expandable metallic stents may provide more effective and longer-lasting relief of stenoses. There are concerns regarding the use of stents in young children, as growth will not occur. Radiofrequency energy can be used to ablate arrhythmic substrates and to perforate occluded valves, allowing subsequent balloon dilatation, as in the treatment of valvar pulmonary atresia (Figure 9.37).

Closure of the persistent arterial duct with a coil or device is now the procedure of choice for children weighing over 5 kg. Closure of more than 50% of atrial septal defects is possible with one of a variety of devices. Most large ventricular septal defects still require surgical closure, but transcatheter devices are available for muscular defects that are difficult to close surgically. A wide variety of devices are used to occlude collateral vessels and fistulas. Prolonged and multiple procedures raise the issue of radiation dosage.

FURTHER READING

Berger F, Vogel M, Alexi-Meskishvili V et al. Comparison of results and complications of surgical and Amplatzer device closure of atrial septal defects. Journal of Thoracic and Cardiovascular Surgery 1999; 118:674–678.

Bilkis AA, Alwi M, Hasri S et al. The Amplatzer duct occluder: experience in 209 patients. Journal of the American College of Cardiology 2001; 37:258–261.

Pihkala J, Nykanen D, Freedom RM, Benson LN. Interventional cardiac catheterisation. Pediatric Clinics of North America 1999; 46:441–464.

Qureshi SA. Catheterisation and angiography. In: Anderson RH, Baker EJ, Macartney FJ et al. (eds). Pediatric cardiology, 2nd edn. Edinburgh: Churchill Livingstone; 2002:459–511.

Wilkinson JL. Haemodynamic calculations in the catheter laboratory. Heart 2001; 85:113–120.

NUCLEAR STUDIES

The role of nuclear medicine studies in children's heart disease has greatly diminished with the increasing sophistication of echocardiography, CT and MRI. As in adults, myocardial performance imaging with stress testing is useful for myocardial ischaemia in those children with congenital anomaly of the coronary arteries. The most frequently used radiopharmaceutical for this is technetium-labelled sestamibi. The effective dose is 5 mSv (Administration of Radioactive Substances Advisory Committee, December 1998).

First-pass studies using technetium 99m (Tc 99m) DTPA to demonstrate the presence and measurement of shunt size are less frequently performed.

Pulmonary perfusion scintography is requested to demonstrate regional pulmonary blood flow following surgery in which the pulmonary vessels are reconstructed or used as conduits during surgical repair of complex congenital heart disease.

Communication with the department of nuclear medicine is essential to identify the correct site for injection as during surgery the pulmonary arteries may be used as venous conduits and the blood flow becomes diverted systematically.

Suspected pulmonary thromboembolism is still often investigated by V/Q scanning.

FETAL ECHOCARDIOGRAPHY

The routine 20-week anomaly scan examines the heart in the four-chamber view. A normal examination includes identifying the

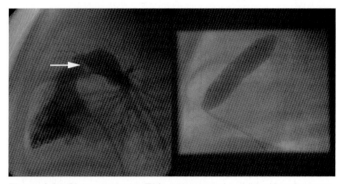

Figure 9.34 Right ventricular (RV) angiogram of a child with pulmonary valve stenosis showing a thickened pulmonary valve (PV) and poststenotic dilatation of the main pulmonary artery (MPA). The balloon catheter is inflated across the valve resulting in relief of the stenosis. (Reproduced with permission from Forfar and Arneil's. Textbook of paediatrics, 6th edn. © Elsevier Ltd 2003.)

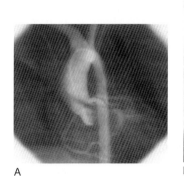
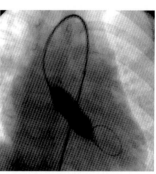

A   B

Figure 9.35 (A) Aortogram showing the narrow jet of negative contrast entering the ascending aorta. There is poststenotic dilatation of the ascending aorta. (B) the balloon is inflated across the aortic valve.

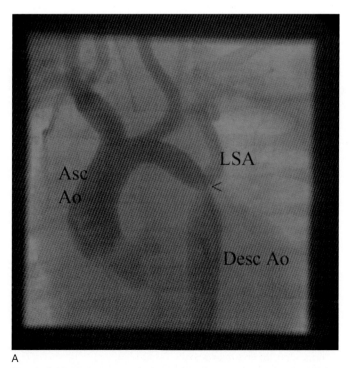
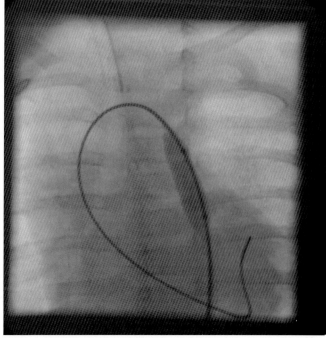

A   B

Figure 9.36 (A) Aortogram (Ao) showing discrete coarctation (arrow) just distal to the origin of the left subclavian artery (LSA). (B) The balloon catheter is positioned across the coarctation and the balloon inflated to stretch the narrowed area.

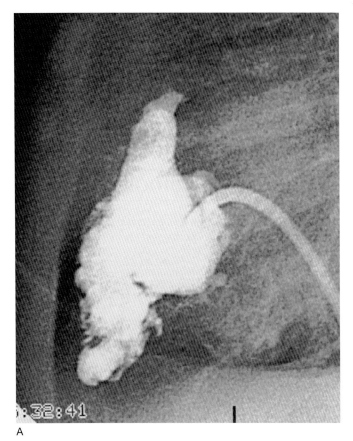

A

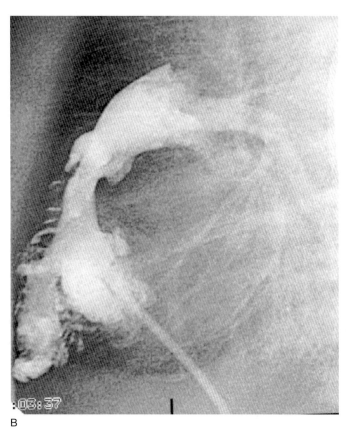

B

Figure 9.37 Right ventricular (RV) angiogram showing pulmonary atresia with an obstruction of the right ventricular outflow tract (A). Following radiofrequency perforation and balloon dilatation, there is flow through the pulmonary valve and into the pulmonary arteries (B). PV, pulmonary valve. (Reproduced with permission from Forfar and Arneil's. Textbook of paediatrics, 6th edn. © Elsevier Ltd 2003.)

cardiac apex to the left, a cardiothoracic ratio of less than 50%, two atria and two ventricles of equal size, and normal atrioventricular valves with the tricuspid valve inserted a little lower in the interventricular septum than the mitral valve. This view should identify fetuses with a hypoplastic left or right ventricle and those with a complete atrioventricular septal defect (Figure 9.38). It will also show marked right atrial dilatation of severe tricuspid regurgitation associated with Ebstein's anomaly of the tricuspid valve and cardiomyopathy. Abnormalities of the great vessels and outlet ventricular septal defects are not seen in the four-chamber view. Lesions such as tetralogy of Fallot, pulmonary atresia with ventricular septal defect, truncus arteriosus, transposition of the great arteries, double outlet right ventricle and some ventricular septal defects will only be detected on more detailed 'five-chamber or outlet views' where the ventricular septum below the great vessels and the ventriculoarterial connections are also identified. Colour Doppler can also detect turbulence in great vessels indicating stenosis, or regurgitation through atrioventricular valves. In some conditions, such as aortic or pulmonary stenosis and coarctation of the aorta, a discrepancy in chamber or great vessel size increases with advancing gestation. Other conditions such as atrial septal defect and patent ductus arteriosus only become apparent postnatally as these features are normal in the fetus. Total anomalous pulmonary venous drainage is difficult to detect antenatally as less than 10% of the circulation passes through the lungs. Thus, there is reduced flow in the pulmonary veins before birth. Even with detailed

cardiac screening performed by an experienced fetal echocardiographer, small septal defects and minor valve abnormalities are frequently outside the resolution and limits of detection of the ultrasound equipment. Antenatal ultrasonographic diagnosis of significant congenital heart disease is now possible in around 50% of cases, although in the UK this figure is rarely achieved.

WHO SHOULD BE REVIEWED BY A SPECIALIST FETAL ECHOCARDIOGRAPHER?

Maternal and familial:

- Mother, partner or previous child with congenital heart disease or congenital complete heart block
- Parental consanguinity
- Mother or partner with 22q11 deletion
- Maternal insulin-dependent diabetes
- Mother taking drugs such as lithium, anticonvulsants or alcohol.

Fetal:

- Multiple fetal pregnancy (monochorionic)
- Increased fetal nuchal translucency (>3.5 mm)
- Other congenital abnormality, e.g. exomphalos, congenital diaphragmatic hernia, tracheoesophageal fistula, bowel obstruction, cleft lip and palate
- Chromosomal abnormality

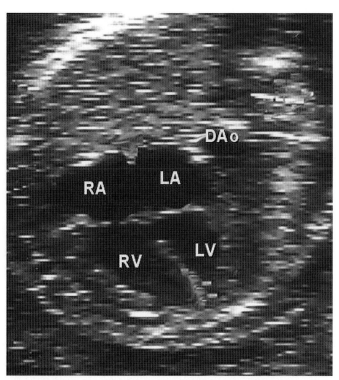

Figure 9.38 Four-chamber view of a fetal heart showing complete atrioventricular septal defect. The left and right components of the atrioventricular valves are at the same level. There is a ventricular septal defect and a primum atrial septal defect. LA, left atrium; LV, left ventricle; RA, right atrium; RV, right ventricle. (Reproduced with permission from Forfar and Arneil's. Textbook of paediatrics, 6th edn. © Elsevier Ltd 2003.)

- Cardiac anomaly detected on routine ultrasound scan, i.e. abnormal four-chamber view
- Fetal cardiac arrhythmia.

The incidence of congenital heart disease in many of these conditions is low and the main benefit is parental reassurance, although repeated scanning may be required for some progressive conditions. An abnormal four-chamber view on the routine 20-week scan is the most likely to result in a diagnosis of congenital heart disease. Extracardiac malformations and chromosomal abnormalities may adversely affect the cardiac outlook.

The main reason for detecting cardiac disease antenatally is still to provide parental choice. Fetal diagnosis gives the family the option of termination or continuation of an affected pregnancy. Antenatal diagnosis of congenital heart disease permits timely and appropriate postnatal management and avoids haemodynamic deterioration and acidosis in duct-dependent lesions. However, there is little evidence that antenatal diagnosis significantly improves survival. Analysis is complicated by the fact that the more severe end of the spectrum of congenital heart disease is diagnosed antenatally.

FURTHER READING

Andrews R, Tulloh R, Sharland G et al. Outcome of staged reconstructive surgery for hypoplastic left heart syndrome following antenatal diagnosis. Heart 2001; 85:474–477.

Bull C. Current and potential future impact of fetal diagnosis on prevalence and spectrum of serious congenital heart disease at term in the UK. Lancet 1999; 354:1242–1247.

Friedman AH, Copel JA, Kleinman CS. Fetal echocardiography and fetal cardiology: indications, diagnosis and management. Seminars in Perinatology 1993; 17:76–88.

Gardiner HM. Fetal echocardiography: 20 years of progress. Heart 2001; 86(Suppl II):ii12–ii22.

Kovalchin JP, Lewin MB, Bezold LI et al. Harmonic imaging in fetal echocardiography. Journal of the American Society of Echocardiography 2001; 14:1025–1029.

Sharland G. Changing impact of fetal diagnosis of congenital heart disease. Archives of Diseases in Childhood 1997; 77:F1–F3.

MRI AND FUNCTIONAL IMAGING OF THE HEART

Tal Geva

Magnetic resonance imaging has evolved from an esoteric test in congenital heart disease (CHD) imaging into a mainstream diagnostic modality whose clinical utility is increasing rapidly. Echocardiography, the established primary non-invasive imaging tool in paediatric cardiology, is capable of providing comprehensive anatomical and haemodynamic information in many patients with congenital and acquired heart disease, is portable, easily accessible and relatively inexpensive. Cardiac catheterization, previously the 'gold standard' for diagnosis of CHD, has evolved into a predominantly interventional and therapeutic modality. Both echocardiography and cardiac catheterization, however, have significant limitations. For example, image quality with echocardiography is often degraded by poor acoustic windows in patients who have undergone cardiac surgery. Cardiac catheterization is invasive, expensive, associated with radiation exposure and carries risks of morbidity and mortality. MRI overcomes many of these limitations and is capable of providing additional unique diagnostic information.

Widespread realization of this potential, however, has been slow until the last few years, during which the field has seen dramatic progress in both technical capabilities and clinical applications. Major advances in hardware design, new pulse sequences and faster image reconstruction techniques now allow rapid high-resolution imaging of complex cardiovascular anatomy in three-dimensional space, quantitative assessment of ventricular dimensions and function, assessment of myocardial function, perfusion and viability, quantification of blood flow rate, tissue characterization, and imaging of non-cardiac structures such as the trachea, bronchi and chest wall. This chapter reviews the clinical applications of MRI in congenital and acquired paediatric heart disease.

CARDIAC MRI TECHNIQUES

CARDIAC AND RESPIRATORY GATING

The heart and central blood vessels are in relatively rapid motion compared to other body structures. There are two principal approaches to obtain clear images of cardiovascular structures. First, images are acquired within an extremely short time period so that motion is 'frozen' (as in real-time MR fluoroscopy). Second, image acquisition is synchronized with the cardiac cycle. Imaging may be synchronized or 'gated' with a pulse oxymetry trace (so-called 'peripheral gating') or, more optimally, with a high-quality electrocardiogram (ECG) signal. Because images are constructed over multiple cardiac cycles, respiratory motion can degrade image quality. The most straightforward approach to minimizing respiratory artifacts is to have the patient hold their breath during image acquisition. Although this solution is often quite effective, it cannot be used in patients who are too young or ill to cooperate. In such cases, respiratory motion compensation can be achieved by synchronizing image data acquisition to the respiratory as well as the cardiac cycle. Respiratory motion can be tracked by either a bellows device placed around the torso or by MRI navigator echoes that concurrently image the position of the diaphragm or heart. The principal limitation of respiratory gating is that it substantially prolongs scan time since image data is only accepted during a portion of the respiratory cycle. A final strategy to minimize respiratory motion artifacts is to acquire multiple images at the same location and average them, thereby minimizing variations due to respiration. As with respiratory triggering, the disadvantage of this approach is increased scan time.

This discussion highlights the need for faster high-quality MRI techniques that will obviate the need for cardiac gating and respiratory motion compensation. Recent advances in gradient coil performance and parallel acquisition methods have achieved this goal and are becoming widely available. Real-time MRI at 30 frames/s is now possible on commercially available clinical scanners albeit at the expense of spatial resolution. However, given the rapid progress in MRI technology, it is conceivable that the goal of obviating the need for ECG and respiratory gating may be achieved shortly after publication of this book.

ANATOMICAL IMAGING AND TISSUE CHARACTERISTICS

Spin echo pulse sequences are usually used to produce images in which flowing blood has low signal intensity and appears dark ('black-blood' imaging). Other tissues appear as varying shades of grey. Though cardiac-gated spin echo sequences produce only one image per location and thus provide only static anatomical information, their advantages include high spatial resolution, excellent blood-myocardium contrast and decreased artifact from metallic biomedical implants (e.g. sternal wires, stents, prosthetic valves). Spin echo sequences are also easily modified to alter tissue contrast and characterize abnormal structures. Their clinical uses include evaluation for arrhythmogenic right ventricular cardiomyopathy, cardiac tumours, constrictive pericardial disease, vessel wall abnormalities and thoracic masses (Figure 9.39). Conventional spin echo sequences are hampered by relatively long scan times (several minutes, depending on the number of phase encoding steps, heart rate and number of signal averages). More recently, fast spin echo sequences have been developed that allow one location to be imaged rapidly enough for the patient to breath-hold (10–15 seconds). A double inversion preparatory pulse is usually applied to suppress the blood signal, and an additional inversion pulse may by applied to suppress signal from fat.

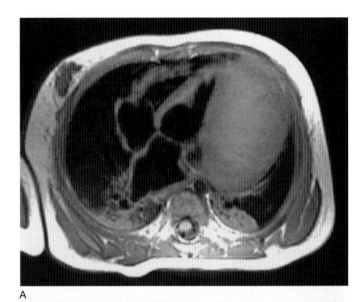

A

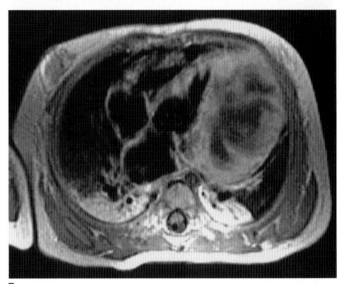

B

Figure 9.39 Axial plane ECG-triggered proton density-weighted fast spin echo with double inversion recovery sequence in a 6-month-old infant with a large left ventricular fibroma. (A) Pre-gadolinium image. (B) Post-gadolinium image showing enhancement of the uninvolved myocardium as well as the myocardium surrounding the hypoperfused tumour's core.

CINE MRI

Cardiac-gated gradient echo sequences can be used to produce multiple images over the cardiac cycle in each anatomical location. These images can then be displayed in a cine loop format to demonstrate the motion of the heart and vasculature over the cardiac cycle. On such cine MR images, flowing blood produces a bright signal, and the myocardium and vessel wall are relatively dark ('bright-blood' imaging). Using a segmented *k*-space technique, cine MRI scan times are reduced so that a single location can be imaged with good temporal and spatial resolution in 5–15 s, thereby permitting breath-hold scanning (Figure 9.40A).

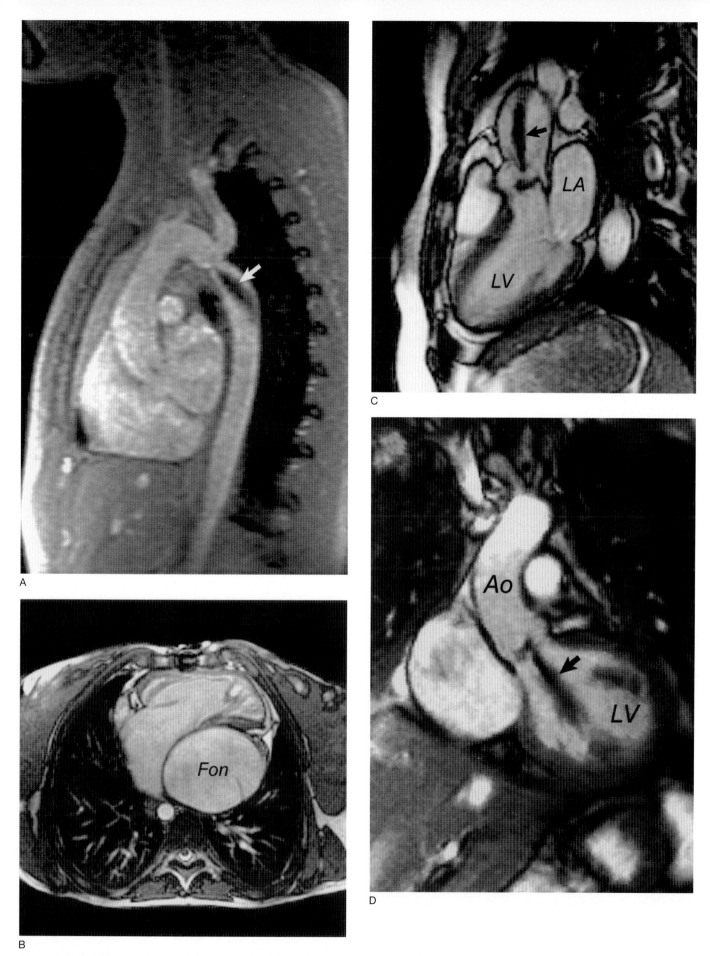

Figure 9.40 Clinical applications of gradient echo cine MRI. (A) ECG-triggered breath-hold segmented *k*-space fast spoiled gradient echo multiphase sequence in a patient with severe coarctation of the aorta. The relatively long echo time allows for clear depiction of the dephasing jet in systole (arrow) indicating high-velocity turbulent flow. (B) Axial plane ECG-triggered steady-state free precession multiphase sequence in a patient with heterotaxy syndrome and single ventricle who is status post Fontan operation. Note the left-sided Fontan pathway (Fon) as well as the clear depiction of intracardiac anatomy. (C) Systolic turbulent jet (arrow) in a patient with aortic valve stenosis. (D) Diastolic turbulent jet (arrow) in a patient with aortic valve regurgitation. Ao, aorta; LA, left atrium; LV, left ventricle.

Steady-state free precession cine MRI sequence is faster and has improved blood–myocardial contrast compared with traditional gradient echo cine sequences (Figure 9.40B). Cine MRI is used to delineate cardiovascular anatomy and assess ventricular function. It is helpful for evaluating the systemic and pulmonary veins, atrial and ventricular septum, intracardiac baffles and pathways (e.g. following Fontan, Mustard, Senning, or Rastelli procedures), ventricular outflow tracts, ventricular-arterial conduits, pulmonary arteries and the aorta. It is also useful in identifying stenotic and regurgitant jets which appear as dark signal voids (Figure 9.40C and D). Myocardial tagging is a modification of cine MRI that allows for a sophisticated analysis of regional myocardial function. Using a preparatory radiofrequency pulse, saturation bands or 'tags' that appear as dark lines on the image are applied to the myocardium at end-diastole (Figure 9.41). By analyzing the movement and deformation of these tags over the cardiac cycle, regional myocardial strain can be quantified.

BLOOD FLOW ANALYSIS

An ECG-gated velocity encoded cine MRI (VEC MRI) sequence, a type of gradient echo sequence, can be used to measure blood flow velocity and quantify blood flow rate. The VEC MRI technique is based on the principle that the signal from hydrogen nuclei (such as those in blood) flowing through specially designed magnetic field gradients accumulates a predictable phase shift that is proportional to its velocity. Multiple phase images are constructed across the cardiac cycle in which the signal amplitude (intensity) of the voxel is proportional to mean flow velocity within that voxel. Using specialized software, regions of interest around a

vessel are defined and the flow rate is automatically calculated (Figure 9.42). VEC MRI flow calculations have been shown by *in vitro* and *in vivo* studies to be accurate and reproducible. When flow encoding is performed in three orthogonal directions, multidimensional flow imaging and shear stress calculation can be accomplished. Development of real-time velocity encoded sequences is in progress with a potential utility analogous to colour Doppler in echocardiography.

MR ANGIOGRAPHY

Another approach for improving the contrast between vascular and non-vascular structures is to intravenously administer a T1-shortening contrast agent, typically a gadolinium chelate (0.2–0.3 mmol/kg injected through an intravenous cannula at a rate of 1.5–3 ml/s), resulting in a bright signal on T1-weighted sequences. This method of angiography is less prone to flow-related artifacts than other MRI techniques and has a short acquisition time. Contrast-enhanced MR angiography (MRA) is usually performed without cardiac gating using a three-dimensional fast-gradient echo acquisition lasting 10–25 s of breath-holding. The time delay between contrast administration and image acquisition determines the vascular territory illustrated, and several serial acquisitions can be performed. The entire procedure takes only a few minutes to perform and yields a high-contrast and high-resolution three-dimensional data set depicting all or part of the thorax (Figure 9.43). Recently developed parallel processing techniques and improved sequence design allow the acquisition time to be shortened to 3–5 s, thus opening the door to time-resolved three-dimensional MRA. The three-dimensional data set can be navigated on

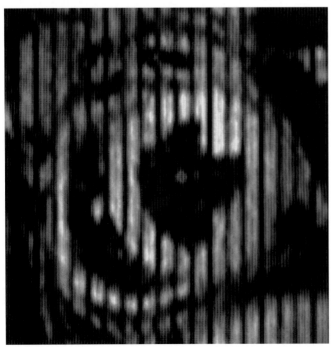

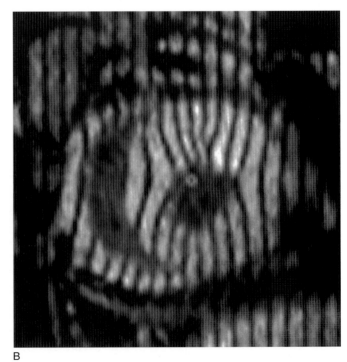

A   B

Figure 9.41 Myocardial tagging. (A) Diastolic frame showing the undistorted tags before the onset of systole; (B) systolic frame showing distortion of the myocardial tags due to cardiac motion. Notice the undistorted tags on the chest wall and liver.

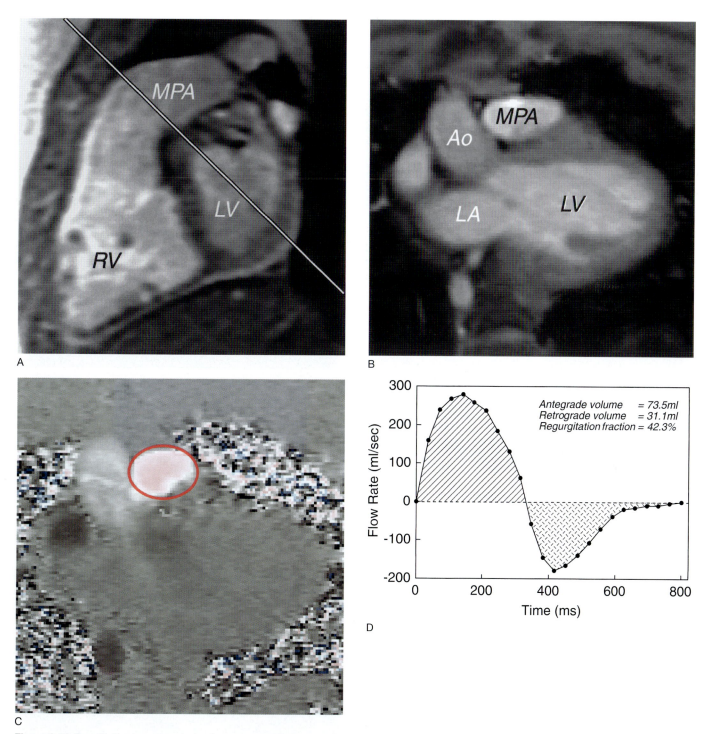

Figure 9.42 Quantitative assessment of pulmonary regurgitation by velocity-encoded cine MRI in a 26-year-old patient with repaired tetralogy of Fallot. (A) An imaging plane is placed across the main pulmonary artery (MPA) (multiphase gradient echo cine MR). (B) Magnitude image showing bright signal in the proximal main pulmonary artery (MPA). (C) The corresponding phase image contains the velocity and directional data. Using a computer workstation, a region of interest (red oval) is placed around the main pulmonary artery. (D) The systolic flow-time integral (area under the curve) above the baseline yields the antegrade flow volume and the diastolic flow-time integral below the baseline corresponds to the regurgitant flow volume. Regurgitation fraction is calculated as the ratio of retrograde (regurgitant volume) to antegrade volume.

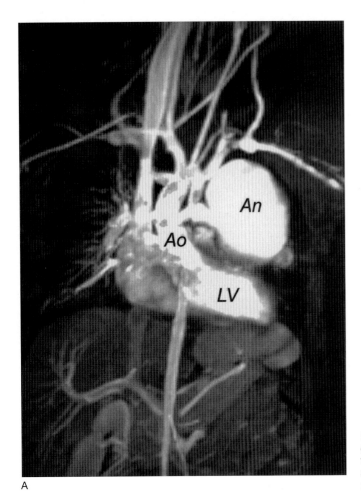

A

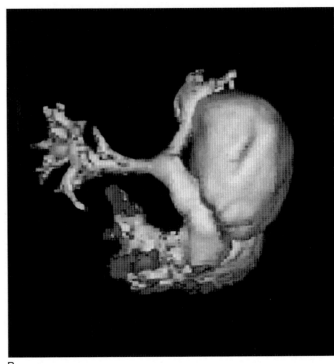

B

Figure 9.43 (A) Subvolume maximal intensity projection (MIP) image of gadolinium-enhanced three-dimensional MRA in an infant with repaired tetralogy of Fallot showing a large aneurysm of the main pulmonary artery (An). (B) Three-dimensional surface rendering demonstrating the relationship between the aneurysm and the branch pulmonary arteries.

dedicated workstations using a variety of image display techniques, including rapid construction of intuitive three-dimensional models.

MYOCARDIAL ISCHAEMIA AND VIABILITY

Although traditionally the diagnosis of myocardial ischaemia has not been a focus of imaging in congenital heart disease, it clearly has relevance in patients who have congenital and acquired coronary abnormalities (e.g. anomalous origin of the left coronary artery, pulmonary atresia with intact ventricular septum and Kawasaki disease) (Figure 9.44). Moreover, myocardial ischaemia is an important diagnostic challenge in postoperative and in adult CHD. Several MRI techniques for imaging the coronary arteries with sufficient resolution to detect stenotic lesions are under evaluation with some encouraging initial results. However, the optimal approach and clinical utility will probably remain in evolution for the next few years.

MRI techniques are also available for assessment of regional left ventricular myocardial perfusion. After a rapid intravenous gadolinium contrast injection, ultrafast, multislice imaging with an

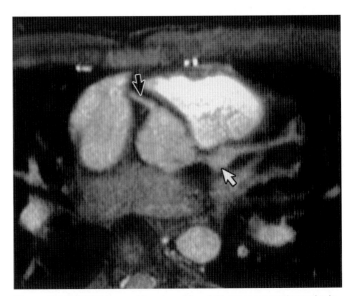

Figure 9.44 ECG-triggered free-breathing MR coronary angiography in a patient with Kawasaki disease. Note the aneurysm in the proximal left coronary artery (white arrow) and the somewhat ectatic proximal right coronary artery (black arrow).

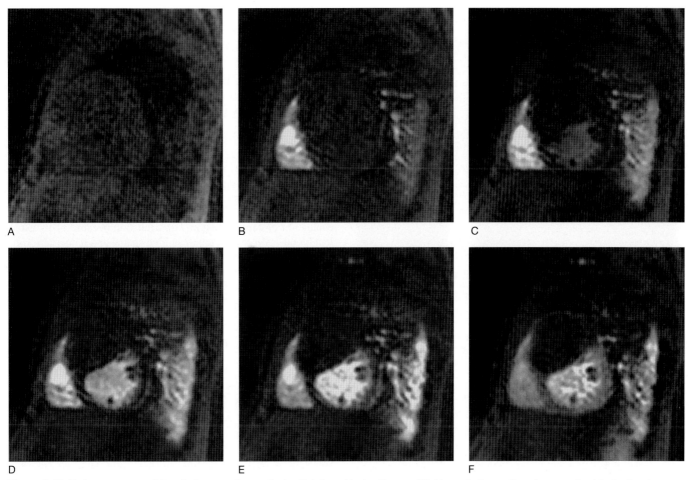

Figure 9.45 First-pass myocardial perfusion scan in a patient with left ventricular fibroma. (A) At onset of scan there is no contrast in the heart. (B) Arrival of contrast in the right ventricle. (C) Arrival of contrast in the pulmonary veins and early enhancement of left ventricular cavity. (D) Arrival of contrast in the left ventricular cavity (notice the unenhanced left ventricular myocardium). (E) Arrival of contrast in the left ventricular myocardium (notice the hypoperfused tumour in the anterolateral aspect of the septum). (F) Late myocardial enhancement with hypoperfused tumour.

echo-planar pulse sequence is performed during a 20–30 second breath-hold to image the first-pass of contrast through the myocardium (Figure 9.45). Stress perfusion imaging, which has improved sensitivity and specificity for detection of coronary artery stenosis over rest perfusion alone, can be achieved either by administering a coronary vasodilator (e.g. adenosine or dipyridamole) or at peak heart rate induced by dobutamine or other vasoactive drugs. The advantages of MRI perfusion over nuclear techniques include superior spatial resolution without the use of ionizing radiation. Alternatively, cine MRI can be used to detect focal wall motion abnormalities with pharmacological stress-induced ischaemia. Initial studies have demonstrated that for dobutamine stress studies, MRI is superior to transthoracic echocardiography, primarily as a result of its superior image quality.

Finally, there are a variety of MRI techniques that have been used to assess myocardial viability. In particular, there is growing evidence showing that hyperenhanced myocardial regions observed after the administration of gadolinium contrast agents are indicative of irreversible myocardial injury (Figure 9.46). Studies in animal models and in human subjects assessing the utility of this technique in the diagnosis and management of myocardial ischaemia are encouraging, and large-scale clinical trials are underway.

APPROACH TO MRI EVALUATION OF CONGENITAL HEART DISEASE

GENERAL CONSIDERATIONS

The indications for cardiac MRI in patients with congenital and acquired paediatric heart disease are rapidly expanding. In general, the clinical reasons for a cardiac MRI examination may fall into one or more of the following three categories: (1) when transthoracic echocardiography is incapable of providing the required diagnostic information; (2) as an alternative to diagnostic cardiac catheterization with its associated discomfort, ionizing radiation exposure, contrast agent load, risks of morbidity and mortality, and high cost; and (3) for MRI's unique capabilities such as tissue imaging, myocardial tagging and vessel-specific flow quantification.

Detailed pre-examination planning is crucial given the wide array of imaging sequences available and the often complex nature of the clinical, anatomical and functional issues in patients with CHD. The importance of a careful review of the patient's medical

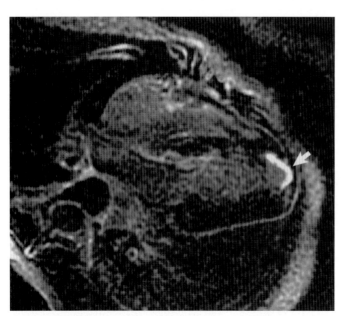

Figure 9.46 Assessment of myocardial viability in an infant who underwent resection of myocardial tumour. Non-viable myocardium produced bright signal (arrow) on an ECG-triggered, post-gadolinium, delayed enhancement, inversion recovery T1-weighted gradient echo sequence. Notice the dark signal from the viable left ventricular myocardium.

history, including details of all cardiovascular surgical procedures, interventional catheterizations, findings of previous diagnostic tests and current clinical status, cannot be overemphasized. As is the case with echocardiography and cardiac catheterization, cardiovascular MRI examination of CHD is an interactive diagnostic procedure that requires on-line review and interpretation of the data by the supervising physician. The unpredictable nature of the anatomy and haemodynamics often require adjustment of the examination protocol, modification of imaging planes, adding, deleting or changing sequences, and adjustment of imaging parameters. Reliance on standardized protocols and post-hoc reading alone in these patients might result in incomplete or even erroneous interpretation.

Sedation is often required in young patients who cannot cooperate with a cardiac MRI examination. Most patients younger than 5–6 years require sedation, some patients between 6 and 10 years of age are capable of cooperation, while most children older than 10 years can undergo a cardiac MRI study without sedation provided their mental development is age-appropriate and they are not claustrophobic. Screening for sedation need is part of the scheduling process for cardiac MRI and consultation with the referring cardiologist and parents is advised. Both conscious sedation and general anaesthesia have been successfully used in cardiac MRI. In our experience, the advantages of general anaesthesia include a better safety profile (secured airways and close monitoring by a paediatric anaesthetist), ability to suspend respiration leading to improved image quality and a shorter examination time, and control over duration of sedation. The disadvantages of this approach include a higher cost and availability of skilled anaesthesia personnel.

ASSESSMENT OF CARDIOVASCULAR ANATOMY

GRADIENT ECHO CINE MRI

Evaluation of cardiovascular anatomy and function in CHD are often inseparable. In general, an ECG-gated gradient echo cine MRI sequence is prescribed across the anatomy of interest to yield a stack of contiguous cross-sectional slices that can be displayed on a computer workstation in a multilocation, multiphase (cine loop) format. Imaging may be performed in an axial or coronal plane, following by oblique planes as necessary. ECG-gated steady-state free precession cine MRI is the sequence of choice for evaluation of cardiac anatomy and function because of its excellent blood-myocardium contrast, high spatial and temporal resolutions, and short acquisition time. Steady-state free precession, however, is relatively insensitive to flow disturbances secondary to stenotic or regurgitant jets and is highly sensitive to magnetic field inhomogeneities. Alternatively, a segmented k-space fast (turbo) gradient echo sequence can be prescribed when further delineation of abnormal flow jets is desirable or when implantable devices produce severe imaging artifacts.

CONTRAST-ENHANCED THREE-DIMENSIONAL MRA

Gadolinium (Gd)-enhanced 3D MRA is ideally suited for imaging of extracardiac vascular anatomy. Examples of common clinical applications include imaging of the aorta and its branches, pulmonary arteries, pulmonary veins, systemic veins, aorto-pulmonary and venous-venous collaterals, systemic-to-pulmonary artery shunts, conduits and vascular grafts. Although this technique is mostly used for imaging of extracardiac anatomy, we have found it useful in the evaluation of intra-atrial systemic and pulmonary baffles (e.g. Mustard or Senning operations and after Fontan procedures), as well as for imaging of the outflow tracts (e.g. repaired tetralogy of Fallot (TOF) and the arterial switch operation) (Figure 9.47). In addition, MRA clearly delineates the spatial relationships between vascular structures, the tracheobronchial tree, chest wall, spine, and other landmarks that may be useful for planning interventional catheterization or surgical procedures.

SPIN ECHO

Spin echo sequences, most commonly breath-hold fast (turbo) spin echo with double inversion recovery, are seldom used as the primary imaging technique for assessment of cardiac anatomy. Standard or fast spin echo are used primarily for tissue imaging. Examples include: myocardial and mediastinal tissue imaging (e.g. cardiac tumours); vessel wall imaging (e.g. aortic dissection); assessment of the myocardium for fatty infiltration or other pathological changes (e.g. arrhythmogenic right ventricular cardiomyopathy); and imaging of the pericardium (e.g. constrictive pericardium) (Figure 9.48). Another clinical application of spin echo imaging is to minimize image artifacts secondary to implanted devices (Figure 9.49).

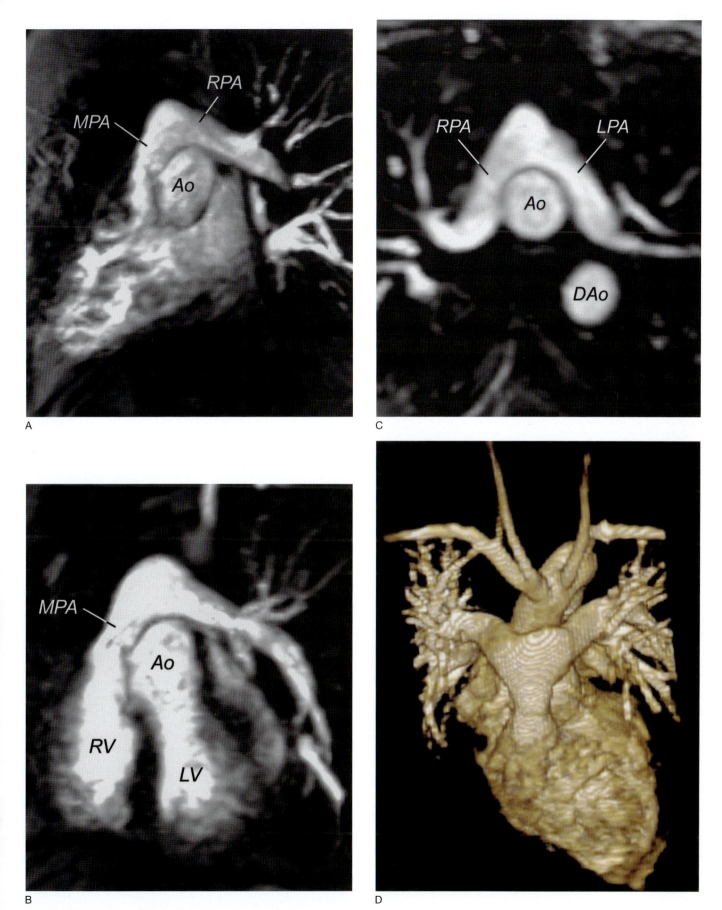

Figure 9.47 Gadolinium-enhanced 3D MRA in a patient with D-loop transposition of the great arteries, status post-arterial switch operation. (A) Sub-volume MIP image in an oblique sagittal plane showing the main (MPA) and right (RPA) pulmonary arteries. (B) Leftward angulation of the imaging plane shows the left pulmonary artery. (C) Axial plane MIP image demonstrates the left (LPA) and right (RPA) pulmonary arteries wrapped around the ascending aorta (Ao) (Lecompte manoeuvre). (D) Three-dimensional volume reconstruction provides enhanced perception of the relationships between the great vessels.

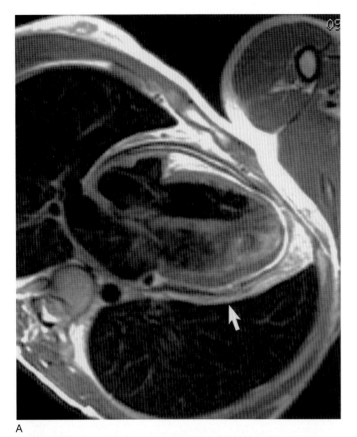

A

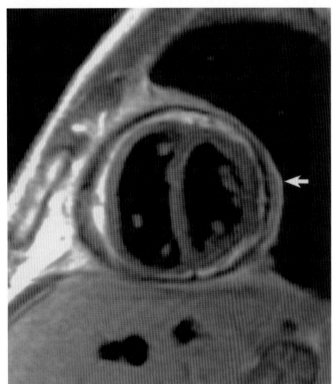

B

Figure 9.48 ECG-triggered breath-hold proton density-weighted fast spin echo with double inversion recovery images showing a markedly thickened pericardium (arrows) in a 13-year-old girl with constrictive pericarditis. (A) Four-chamber plane; (B) short-axis plane.

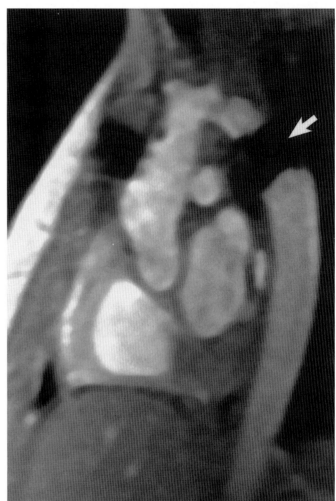

A

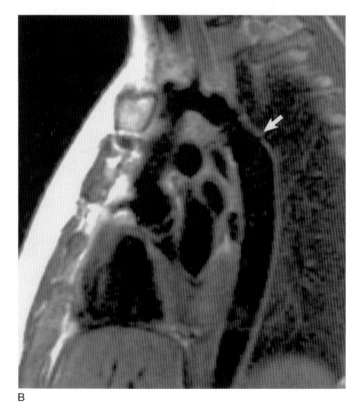

B

Figure 9.49 Image artifact (arrow) due to an endovascular stent placed in the aortic isthmus for treatment of recurrent coarctation of the aorta. (A) Gradient echo image. (B) Fast spin echo with double inversion recovery showing a markedly reduced image artifact (arrow).

VENTRICULAR FUNCTION

The principal MRI sequence used for evaluation of ventricular function is gradient echo cine MRI. An ECG or VCG-triggered segmented *k*-space fast (also termed 'turbo') gradient recall echo sequence has been used extensively during the 1990s and its accuracy and reproducibility in measuring left and right ventricular volumes, mass and ejection fraction have been extensively validated. A newer gradient echo imaging sequence, steady-state free precession, has been shown to provide a sharper contrast between the blood pool and the myocardium and to reduce motion-induced blurring during systole. Most modern cine MRI techniques utilize retrospective gating techniques that allow reconstruction of 20–30 images throughout the cardiac cycle.

Quantitative evaluation of ventricular function is achieved by obtaining a series of contiguous cine MRI slabs that cover the ventricles in short-axis (Figure 9.50). By tracing the blood-endocardium boundary, the slab's volume is calculated as the product of its cross-sectional area and thickness (which is prescribed by the operator). Ventricular volume is then determined by summation of the volumes of all slabs. The process can be repeated for each frame in the cardiac cycle to obtain a continuous time-volume loop or may be performed only on a diastolic and a systolic frame to calculate diastolic and systolic volumes. From this data one can calculate left and right ventricular ejection fractions and stroke volumes. Since the patient's heart rate at the time of image acquisition is known, one can calculate left and right ventricular output. Ventricular mass is calculated by tracing the epicardial borders, subtracting the endocardial volumes, and multiplying the resultant muscle volume by the specific gravity of the myocardium (1.05 g/mm^3). Most manufacturers of MRI scanners and some third party companies offer software packages that automatically perform the above calculations. Development of

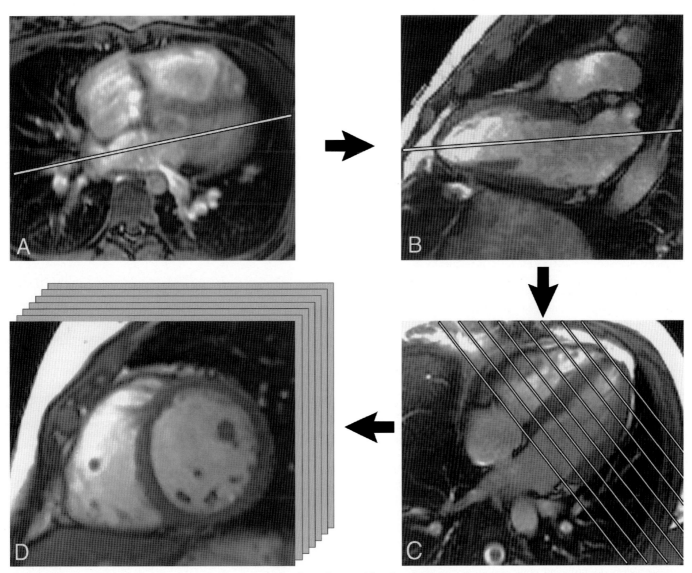

Figure 9.50 Cine MRI technique for assessment of ventricular dimensions and function. (A) Using a localizing image in the axial plane; an imaging plane is placed parallel to the left ventricular septal surface. (B) Two-chamber plane; (C) four-chamber plane; (D) short-axis plane. To obtain complete coverage of the ventricles, 12 contiguous imaging slabs are placed from the plane of the atrioventricular (AV) valves through the cardiac apex.

algorithms for automatic border detection has facilitated the application of these techniques, but further refinements are required to improve its accuracy. Because of its accurate spatial and temporal registration of data, MRI measurements of chamber dimensions have become the accepted reference standard to which other methods are compared.

Gradient echo cine MRI is also used to evaluate regional wall motion abnormalities and segmental wall thickening. Dobutamine stress MRI has been reported to be a useful test in adults with coronary artery disease. More recently, the use of an MRI-compatible supine cycle ergometer has been reported to allow assessment of ventricular function and valve regurgitation response to exercise.

Another approach to MRI evaluation of ventricular function and myocardial mechanics is based on myocardial tagging. Using a preparatory radiofrequency gradient echo pulse sequence such as spatial modulation of magnetization (SPAMM), the spin of the protons in selected parts of the image volume are flipped in such a way as to render them incapable of producing a signal. This results in stripes of signal void (dark stripes) across the image (Figure 9.41). Similarly, two sets of orthogonal stripes (tags) can be placed, producing a grid across the image. The grid or stripes are placed at the onset of the R wave of the ECG and is followed by a gradient echo cine MRI sequence. As the myocardium moves during the cardiac cycle, the tags follow it and their rotation, translation and deformation can be tracked allowing for calculation of myocardial strain and strain rate. This can be done during systole or diastole and in two or three dimensions. A recently described technique for the analysis of myocardial tagging data, harmonic phase imaging (HARP), greatly shortens the analysis time because it does not require manual tracing of the tags.

FLOW ANALYSIS

Velocity-encoded cine MRI (VEC MRI) is frequently used in functional MR evaluation of congenital heart disease for quantitative assessment of blood flow. Site-specific quantification of flow rate, flow velocity, stroke volume and minute flow can, in principle, be measured across any blood vessel within the central cardiovascular system. An imaging plane is prescribed perpendicular to the vessel of interest and two sets of multiphase images are reconstructed following a VEC MRI acquisition: a set of 'magnitude images' that provide anatomical information and a set of 'phase images' in which the velocity information is encoded (Figure 9.42). For each acquisition, the operator prescribes the field of view, matrix size and slice thickness, which, in turn, determine spatial resolution. *In vitro* studies have shown that the number of pixels included within the cross-sectional area of the vessel is crucial for accurate measurements of flow rate by VEC MRI. The accuracy of flow rate quantification decreases once the number of pixels per vessel cross-section is less than 16. Other variables such as the angle between the prescribed imaging plane and flow direction, velocity encoding range, flip angle and slice thickness must also be considered. Other known caveats of quantitative assessment of blood flow by VEC MRI include flow aliasing and dephasing secondary to turbulent flow. Aliasing can be avoided by prescribing a velocity encoding range higher than the maximal velocity within the target vessel. Avoiding dephasing secondary to

turbulent blood flow can be achieved by shortening the echo time, prescribing a thinner slice thickness or repositioning the imaging slice proximal or distal to the turbulent jet.

Clinically, VEC MRI is used to quantify cardiac output, pulmonary-to-systemic flow ratio, valvar regurgitation, differential lung perfusion, AV valve inflow and a variety of other clinical scenarios (Figure 9.51). Pharmacological stress can be used to provide additional information on functional reserve. For example, using either dipyridamole of adenosine for vasodilatation of the coronary vascular bed, coronary flow reserve can be assessed. Three-dimensional flow vector mapping is a useful adjunct to cine flow imaging because it provides dynamic 3D flow maps that can detect abnormal flow patterns regardless of the presence of turbulent flow jets (Figure 9.52).

MRI-GUIDED CARDIOVASCULAR INTERVENTIONS

The advent of real-time MRI now allows MRI-guided cardiovascular interventional procedures. Potential advantages of this approach include reducing or eliminating exposure to biologically harmful x-ray radiation, improved three-dimensional imaging capabilities of blood flow, vessel wall and the surrounding soft tissue, improved accuracy of delivering and positioning therapeutic devices (e.g. balloon, stent, gene-carrying vehicle, etc.), and the ability to instantly evaluate the effect of the intervention. Although the potential of MRI-guided cardiovascular interventions is promising, further research and development are required to improve spatial and temporal resolutions, adapt the MR hardware to facilitate cardiac interventional procedures, adapt the user interface for intuitive and responsive in-room scanning, and develop a wide range of MRI-compatible guidewires, catheters, stents, coils, occluding devices, needles, blades and other devices currently available to interventional cardiologists in the catheterization laboratory.

FURTHER READING

Bax JJ, Lamb H, Dibbets P et al. Comparison of gated single-photon emission computed tomography with magnetic resonance imaging for evaluation of left ventricular function in ischemic cardiomyopathy. American Journal of Cardiology 2000; 86:1299–1305.

Be'eri E, Maier SE, Landzberg MJ et al. In vivo evaluation of Fontan pathway flow dynamics by multidimensional phase-velocity magnetic resonance imaging. Circulation 1998; 98:2873–2882.

Bellenger NG, Burgess MI, Ray SG et al. Comparison of left ventricular ejection fraction and volumes in heart failure by echocardiography, radionuclide ventriculography and cardiovascular magnetic resonance; are they interchangeable? European Heart Journal 2000; 21:1387–1396.

Bellenger NG, Marcus NJ, Davies C et al. Left ventricular function and mass after orthotopic heart transplantation: a comparison of cardiovascular magnetic resonance with echocardiography. Journal of Heart and Lung Transplantation 2000; 19:444–452.

Carr JC, Simonetti O, Bundy J et al. Cine MR angiography of the heart with segmented true fast imaging with steady-state precession. Radiology 2001; 219:828–834.

Evans AJ, Iwai F, Grist TA et al. Magnetic resonance imaging of blood flow with a phase subtraction technique. In vitro and in vivo validation. Investigational Radiology 1993; 28:109–115.

Fogel MA. Assessment of cardiac function by magnetic resonance imaging. Pediatric Cardiology 2000; 21:59–69.

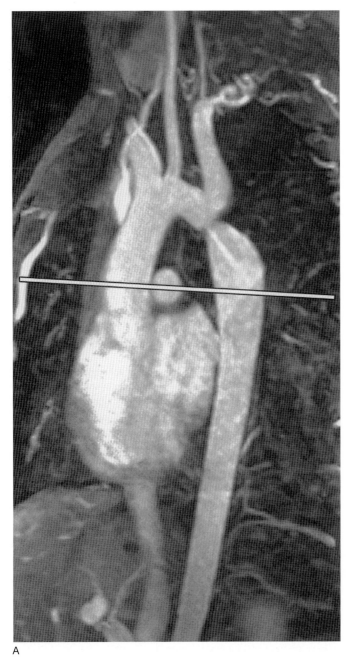

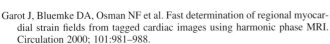

A

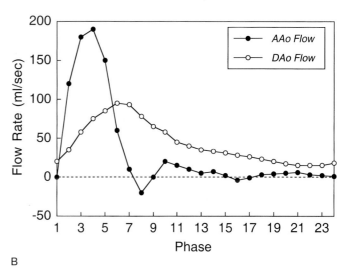

B

Figure 9.51 Velocity-encoded cine MRI (VEC MRI) evaluation of aortic coarctation. (A) An imaging plane is prescribed perpendicular to the ascending and descending aorta. (B) Flow-time curves obtain across the ascending and descending aorta in a patient with severe coarctation. The flow curve in the descending aorta is characterized by delayed onset peak flow, decreased acceleration rate and prolonged deceleration.

Garot J, Bluemke DA, Osman NF et al. Fast determination of regional myocardial strain fields from tagged cardiac images using harmonic phase MRI. Circulation 2000; 101:981–988.

Geva T. Future directions of congenital heart disease imaging. Pediatric Cardiology 2002; 23:117–121.

Greil G, Geva T, Maier SE et al. Effect of acquisition parameters on the accuracy of velocity encoded cine magnetic resonance imaging blood flow measurements. Journal of Magnetic Resonance Imaging 2002; 15: 47–54.

Greil GF, Powell AJ, Gildein HP et al. Gadolinium-enhanced three-dimensional magnetic resonance angiography of pulmonary and systemic venous anomalies. Journal of American Colloid Cardiology 2002; 39:335–341.

Greil GF, Stuber M, Botnar RM et al. Coronary magnetic resonance angiography in adolescents and young adults with kawasaki disease. Circulation 2002; 105:908–911.

Haber I, Metaxas DN, Axel L et al. Three-dimensional motion reconstruction and analysis of the right ventricle using tagged MRI. Medical Image Analysis 2000; 4:335–355.

Kim RJ, Wu E, Rafael A et al. The use of contrast-enhanced magnetic resonance imaging to identify reversible myocardial dysfunction. New England Journal of Medicine 2000; 343:1445–1453.

Klein C, Nekolla SG, Bengel FM et al. Assessment of myocardial viability with contrast-enhanced magnetic resonance imaging: comparison with positron emission tomography. Circulation 2002; 105:162–167.

Kuhl HP, Bucker A, Franke A et al. Transesophageal 3-dimensional echocardiography: in vivo determination of left ventricular mass in comparison with magnetic resonance imaging. Journal of the American Society of Echocardiography 2000; 13:205–215.

Laddis T, Manning WJ, Danias PG et al. Cardiac MRI for assessment of myocardial perfusion: current status and future perspectives. Journal of Nuclear Cardiology 2001; 8:207–214.

Lamb HJ, Singleton RR, van der Geest RJ et al. MR imaging of regional cardiac function: low-pass filtering of wall thickness curves. Magnetic Resonance Medicine 1995; 34:498–502.

Manning WJ, Stuber M, Danias PG et al. Coronary magnetic resonance imaging: Current status. Current Problems in Cardiology 2002; 27:275–333.

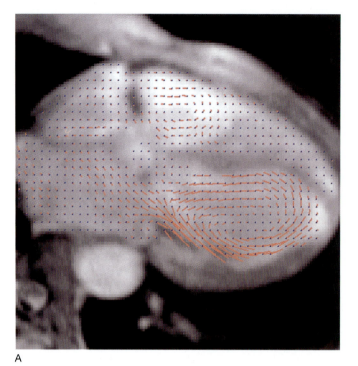 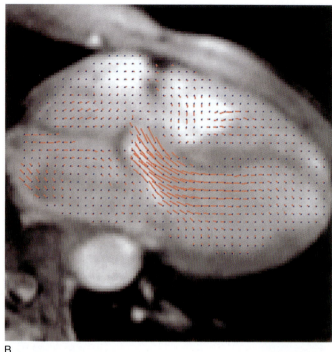

A

B

Figure 9.52 Three-dimensional flow vector map showing intracardiac diastolic (A) and systolic (B) flow pattern. The orientation of the vector corresponds to the instantaneous in-plane direction of blood flow whereas the vector's length is proportional to instantaneous velocity.

Masui T, Katayama M, Kobayashi S et al. Gadolinium-enhanced MR angiography in the evaluation of congenital cardiovascular disease pre- and postoperative states in infants and children. Journal of Magnetic Resonance Imaging 2000; 12:1034–1042.

Nagel E, Lehmkuhl HB, Bocksch W et al. Noninvasive diagnosis of ischemia-induced wall motion abnormalities with the use of high-dose dobutamine stress MRI: comparison with dobutamine stress echocardiography. Circulation 1999; 99:763–770.

Nayak KS, Pauly JM, Kerr AB et al. Real-time color flow MRI. Magnetic Resonance Medicine 2000; 43:251–258.

Ohno Y, Kawamitsu H, Higashino T et al. Time-resolved contrast-enhanced pulmonary MR angiography using sensitivity encoding (SENSE). Journal of Magnetic Resonance Imaging 2003; 17:330–336.

Panting JR, Gatehouse PD, Yang GZ et al. Abnormal subendocardial perfusion in cardiac syndrome X detected by cardiovascular magnetic resonance imaging. New England Journal of Medicine 2002; 346:1948–1953.

Pelc NJ, Herfkens RJ, Shimakawa A et al. Phase contrast cine magnetic resonance imaging. Magnetic Resonance Quarterly 1991; 7:229–254.

Plein S, Bloomer TN, Ridgway JP et al. Steady-state free precession magnetic resonance imaging of the heart: comparison with segmented k-space gradient-echo imaging. Journal of Magnetic Resonance Imaging 2001; 14:230–236.

Powell AJ, Geva T. Blood flow measurement by magnetic resonance imaging in congenital heart disease. Pediatric Cardiology 2000; 21:47–58.

Powell AJ, Maier SE, Chung T et al. Phase-velocity cine magnetic resonance imaging measurement of pulsatile blood flow in children and young adults: in vitro and in vivo validation. Pediatric Cardiology 2000; 21:104–110.

Rajagopalan S, Prince M. Magnetic resonance angiographic techniques for the diagnosis of arterial disease. Cardiology Clinics 2002; 20:501–512, v.

Reichek N. MRI myocardial tagging. Journal of Magnetic Resonance Imaging 1999; 10:609–616.

Roest AA, Helbing WA, Kunz P et al. Exercise MR imaging in the assessment of pulmonary regurgitation and biventricular function in patients after tetralogy of fallot repair. Radiology 2002; 223:204–211.

Schwitter J, DeMarco T, Kneifel S et al. Magnetic resonance-based assessment of global coronary flow and flow reserve and its relation to left ventricular functional parameters: a comparison with positron emission tomography. Circulation 2000; 101:2696–2702.

Setser RM, Fischer SE, Lorenz CH et al. Quantification of left ventricular function with magnetic resonance images acquired in real time. Journal of Magnetic Resonance Imaging 2000; 12:430–438.

Weiger M, Pruessmann KP, Boesiger P et al. Cardiac real-time imaging using SENSE. SENSitivity Encoding scheme. Magnetic Resonance Medicine 2000; 43:177–184.

THE NEONATE WITH A CONGENITAL HEART DISEASE

Denise Kitchiner, Cinzia Crawley

The frequency of antenatal diagnosis of congenital heart disease has increased but the majority of infants still present after birth with one of the following:

- cyanosis, with or without respiratory distress
- heart failure, with or without cyanosis
- cardiovascular collapse
- an associated lesion or syndrome
- an abnormal clinical sign detected on routine examination.

During fetal life the pulmonary vascular resistance is high and the pulmonary arterial and aortic pressures are equal. In the normal fetal circulation, blood shunts from right to left atrium across the oval foramen and from pulmonary artery to descending aorta through the arterial duct. At birth, there is a fall in pulmonary vascular resistance leading to a marked increase in pulmonary blood flow. The age of presentation in neonates with congenital heart disease depends on how the abnormal heart responds to the high pulmonary vascular resistance at birth, and the gradual fall of this resistance over the subsequent weeks. Closure of the arterial duct in the first week or two of life determines the presentation in infants with duct-dependent lesions. It is helpful to consider the timing of presentation (Table 9.3) together with the clinical, electrocardiographic and radiographic findings (Table 9.4).

PRESENTATION WITH CYANOSIS WITHOUT RESPIRATORY DISTRESS

This is usually due to transposition of the great arteries or pulmonary atresia. The latter occurs with a ventricular septal defect (a variant of tetralogy of Fallot) or with an intact ventricular septum. Less common causes include tricuspid atresia and other complex lesions with decreased pulmonary blood flow.

TRANSPOSITION OF THE GREAT ARTERIES

This is the commonest cyanotic lesion presenting in the neonatal period. The aorta arises from the right ventricle and pulmonary artery from the left ventricle. Deoxygenated blood returning to the right atrium passes via the right ventricle back into the aorta (Figures 9.53 and 9.54). Oxygenated blood returning from the pul-

Table 9.3 Timing and mode of presentation of congenital heart disease in the neonate

	EARLY 0–24 h High pulmonary vascular resistance, arterial duct open	INTERMEDIATE 4 h to 2 weeks Duct closing – 'duct dependent' lesions present	LATE After 2 weeks Duct closed Pulmonary vascular resistance continues to fall; lesions with a left-to-right shunt present
Cyanosis without congestive failure or respiratory distress	TGA with very restrictive oval foramen	*Duct dependent for pulmonary blood flow*, e.g. Pulmonary atresia with or without VSD Critical pulmonary stenosis (with right-to-left interatrial flow) Tricuspid atresia with small VSD ^Complex lesions with severe pulmonary stenosis *Duct dependent for mixing* TGA	Tetralogy of Fallot with severe pulmonary stenosis§ ^Complex lesions with pulmonary stenosis
Cyanosis with congestive failure or respiratory distress	Obstructed total anomalous pulmonary venous connection (usually infradiaphragmatic) Severe Ebstein's anomaly	Partially obstructed total anomalous pulmonary venous connection Pulmonary arteriovenous fistulas (rare)	*Mixed circulations with unobstructed pulmonary blood flow*, e.g. Unobstructed TAPVC (cardiac or supracardiac) Common arterial trunk Tricuspid atresia with a large VSD Some complex lesions with high pulmonary blood flow*
Collapse/shock		*Left heart obstruction*, e.g. Aortic coarctation or interruption Hypoplastic left heart syndrome Aortic stenosis	
Congestive cardiac failure (without cyanosis)		Left heart obstruction with a left-to-right shunt, e.g. Aortic coarctation ± VSD *Systemic arteriovenous fistulas*, e.g. cerebral	*Left-to-right shunts*, e.g. Large VSD or PDA Complete AV septal defect Aortopulmonary window Complex lesions **

Adapted from Forfar and Arneil's. Textbook of paediatrics, 6th edn. © Elsevier Ltd 2003.
NB. It is important to use this table as a guideline only – each condition can present unusually late or early! Tachyarrhythmias – usually SVT – can present with heart failure or collapse at any of these age groups, as can myocardial failure due to heart muscle disease such as hypertrophic cardiomyopathy or myocardial ischaemia secondary to perinatal distress. Cardiovascular collapse in the first few hours is usually related to such myocardial dysfunction; sepsis and metabolic disease should be considered.
PDA, patent arterial duct; TAPVC, total anomalous pulmonary venous connection; TGA, transposition of the great arteries (those with a small oval foramen and those without a ventricular septal defect present earlier); VSD, ventricular septal defect.
§ In tetralogy of Fallot, only the most severe present as a cyanotic neonate. The less severe forms present with cyanotic spells or a loud murmur on routine check.
^ Examples of complex lesions with low pulmonary blood flow include:
   1. any single ventricle with severe pulmonary or subpulmonary stenosis; and
   2. double outlet right ventricle with severe pulmonary stenosis.
* Examples of complex lesions with high pulmonary blood flow and cyanosis include:
   1. double outlet right ventricle with transposed great arteries; and
   2. pulmonary atresia with large aortopulmonary collateral arteries or large arterial duct.
** Examples of complex lesions with high pulmonary blood flow without cyanosis include:
   1. single ventricle without pulmonary stenosis; and
   2. double outlet right ventricle with normally related great arteries and without pulmonary stenosis.

Table 9.4 Flow chart for the differential diagnosis of central cyanosis (assessment of whether pulmonary blood flow is increased or diminished combined with the electrocardiographic findings helps to narrow the diagnostic possibilities)

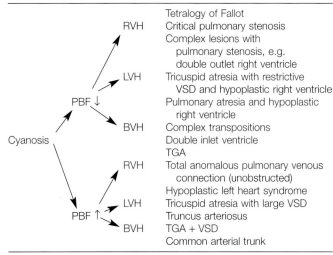

	RVH	Tetralogy of Fallot
		Critical pulmonary stenosis
		Complex lesions with pulmonary stenosis, e.g. double outlet right ventricle
PBF ↓	LVH	Tricuspid atresia with restrictive VSD and hypoplastic right ventricle
		Pulmonary atresia and hypoplastic right ventricle
	BVH	Complex transpositions
		Double inlet ventricle
		TGA
	RVH	Total anomalous pulmonary venous connection (unobstructed)
		Hypoplastic left heart syndrome
PBF ↑	LVH	Tricuspid atresia with large VSD
		Truncus arteriosus
	BVH	TGA + VSD
		Common arterial trunk

Cyanosis

Adapted from Forfar and Arneil's. Textbook of paediatrics, 6th edn. © Elsevier Ltd 2003.
PBF, pulmonary blood flow; RVH, right ventricular hypertrophy; LVH, left ventricular hypertrophy; BVH, biventricular hypertrophy; TGA, transposition of great arteries; VSD, ventricular septal defect.

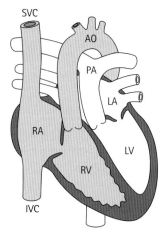

Figure 9.53 Transposition of the great arteries (atrioventricular concordance, arterioventricular discordance). Shading indicates desaturated/unoxygenated blood. SVC, superior vena cava; IVC, inferior vena cava; AO, aorta; LA, left atrium; PA, pulmonary artery; RA, right atrium; RV, right ventricle; LV, left ventricle. (Reproduced with permission from Forfar and Arneil's. Textbook of paediatrics, 6th edn. © Elsevier Ltd 2003.)

monary veins to the left atrium and left ventricle is directed back into the pulmonary arteries. Survival depends on mixing at atrial level via a patent oval foramen, and at arterial level via the patent arterial duct. Simple transposition indicates that there are no significant additional cardiac lesions. Complex transposition describes those infants with associated lesions such as a ventricular septal defect, pulmonary stenosis or aortic coarctation.

Cyanosis is detected in the first few days of life, becoming more obvious as the arterial duct closes (Table 9.3). If the atrial communication is small, the infant deteriorates rapidly and will die if the duct is not re-opened with intravenous prostaglandin, or the foramen enlarged by atrial septostomy. Chest radiography shows increased pulmonary vascularity (Figure 9.55), unlike other cyanotic conditions that present early with reduced pulmonary blood flow (Tables 9.3 and 9.4). This is because there are both left-to-right and right-to-left shunting at atrial and ductal levels, combined with hypoxia causing myocardial dysfunction. The upper mediastinum is narrow because the aorta lies anterior and slightly to the right of the pulmonary artery. The 'egg on side' appearance of the heart is not usually seen in the neonatal period because of the thymic shadow. Echocardiography shows the pulmonary artery arising from the left ventricle and the aorta from the right ventricle (Figure 9.56) with a characteristic parallel relationship of the great vessels. Additional lesions must be identified.

BALLOON ATRIAL SEPTOSTOMY

This is usually performed to enlarge the oval foramen and promote mixing at this level. A balloon septostomy catheter is passed from the right atrium across the oval foramen to the left atrium. The

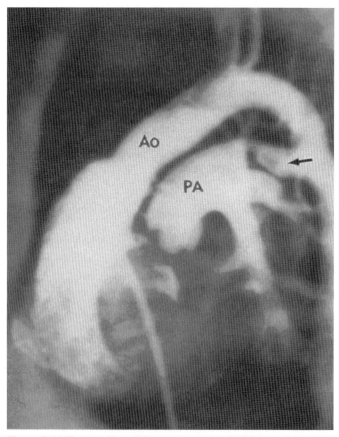

Figure 9.54 Transposition of the great vessels with intact ventricular septum. Right ventriculogram, lateral projection, shows the aorta (Ao) arising from the right ventricle. The aorta lies anteriorly and ascends parallel to the main pulmonary artery (PA). The pulmonary artery is filling via a patent arterial duct (arrow).

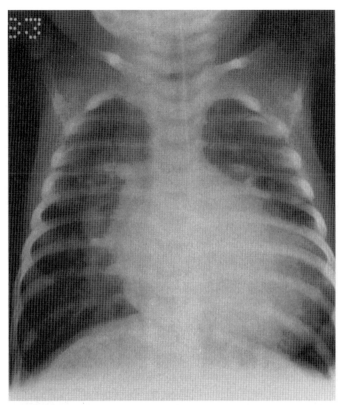

Figure 9.55 Transposition of the great arteries. Neonate with cyanosis. The lungs are plethoric. The heart is enlarged. The pulmonary trunk is not visible.

balloon is inflated and pulled back, tearing the interatrial septum (Figure 9.33).

ARTERIAL SWITCH OPERATION

This is performed early in the neonatal period using cardiopulmonary bypass (Figure 9.57). The arterial trunks are transected, the main pulmonary artery pulled forward, and the ascending aorta moved posteriorly such that the branch pulmonary arteries straddle the ascending aorta. The coronary arteries are removed and resutured into the new ascending aorta. The commonest complication is narrowing of the branch pulmonary arteries as they stretch over the aorta (Figure 9.47).

PULMONARY ATRESIA WITH VENTRICULAR SEPTAL DEFECT

This represents the severe end of the spectrum of tetralogy of Fallot. Most children with this condition have stenosis rather than atresia of the right ventricular outflow tract. They present outside the neonatal period and are therefore described later. Pulmonary atresia denotes complete obstruction between the right ventricle and pulmonary arteries, which are supplied by the arterial duct. Alternatively, collateral arteries from the aorta, major aortopulmonary collateral arteries (MAPCAs), supply sections of the lungs and connect with the true pulmonary arteries (Figure 9.58). The

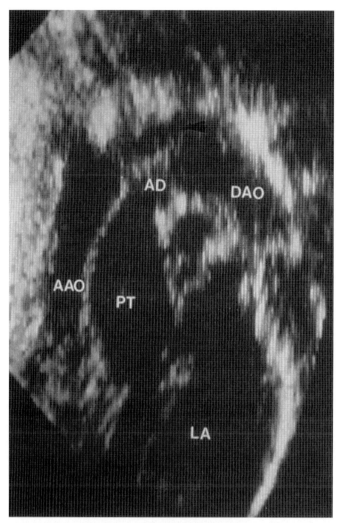

Figure 9.56 Transposition of the great arteries. Parasternal long axis two-dimensional echocardiogram shows ascending aorta (AAO) anteriorly and parallel to main pulmonary artery (PT). The arterial duct (AD) is patent. DAO, descending aorta; LA, left atrium. (Courtesy of Dr A.N. Redington.)

right and left pulmonary arteries may or may not be confluent, and are usually small. The aorta overrides a large ventricular septal defect (Figures 9.59 and 9.60).

When the infant is dependent on the arterial duct, cyanosis develops as it closes in the first days of life (Table 9.3). Major aortopulmonary collateral arteries provide a more stable source of pulmonary blood flow and cyanosis may be mild. A few infants have excessive pulmonary blood flow from these collateral vessels and present in heart failure with minimal cyanosis. Almost 50% of children have 22q11 chromosome deletion. Chest radiography shows pulmonary oligaemia (Table 9.4). Right ventricular hypertrophy may produce a 'boot-shaped' appearance to the heart and 25–30% of infants have a right aortic arch (Figure 9.101). Echocardiography shows the subaortic ventricular septal defect and identifies the central pulmonary arteries. Cardiac catheterization and angiography is needed, prior to definitive surgery, to accurately demonstrate the pulmonary arterial anatomy and aortopulmonary collateral arteries.

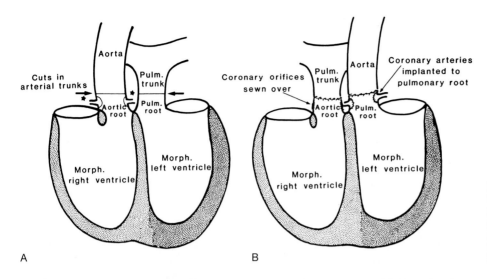

A   B

Figure 9.57 Diagrammatic representations of the arterial switch (A) before and (B) after the procedure. Morph., morphological; Pulm., pulmonary. (Reproduced with permission from Andersen RH et al. Paediatric cardiology; 2nd edn. Edinburgh: Churchill Livingstone; 2000:1308)

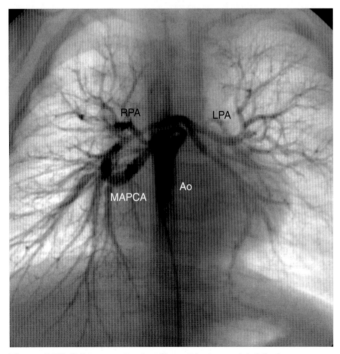

Figure 9.58 Pulmonary atresia with ventricular septal defect. Angiogram in the descending aorta (Ao) showing a major aortopulmonary collateral artery (MAPCA) supplying sections of the lungs and connecting with the true left (LPA) and right (RPA) pulmonary arteries.

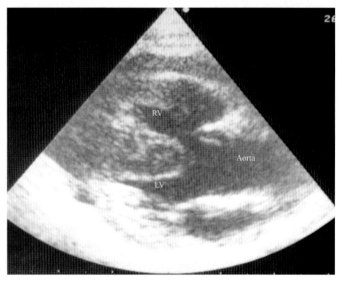

Figure 9.59 Echocardiogram of a child with tetralogy of Fallot showing a large ventricular septal defect (VSD) between left (LV) and right (RV) ventricles, with aortic override (Aorta).

lar septal defect and placing a conduit from right ventricle to pulmonary artery, is usually performed later.

INFANTS WITH DUCT-DEPENDENT PULMONARY CIRCULATION

A shunt is performed usually from the right innominate or subclavian artery to the right pulmonary artery (Figure 9.61), the modified Blalock–Taussig shunt.

INFANTS WITH MAJOR AORTOPULMONARY COLLATERAL ARTERIES

The aim is to connect important MAPCAs to the central pulmonary arteries. Definitive surgery, which consists of closing the ventricu-

PULMONARY ATRESIA WITH INTACT VENTRICULAR SEPTUM/CRITICAL PULMONARY VALVE STENOSIS

In this condition, the pulmonary valve is imperforate or has a tiny orifice and the ventricular septum is intact. The right ventricle and tricuspid valve are abnormal and may be severely hypoplastic. Pulmonary blood flow depends on the arterial duct. Cyanosis is caused by right-to-left shunting at atrial level, through a stretched oval foramen. In some infants, the small, hypertensive right ventricle has fistulous connections with the coronary arteries.

Neonates present with cyanosis and rapid clinical deterioration when the arterial duct closes (Table 9.3). Severe tricuspid

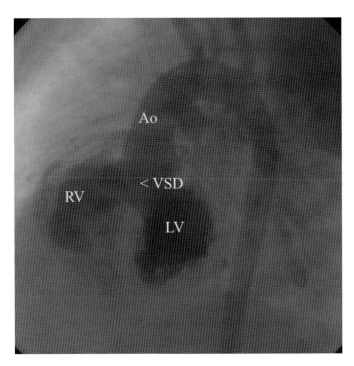

Figure 9.60 Angiogram of a child with tetralogy of Fallot, the aorta overriding the large ventricular septal defect (VSD) between the left (LV) and right (RV) ventricles.

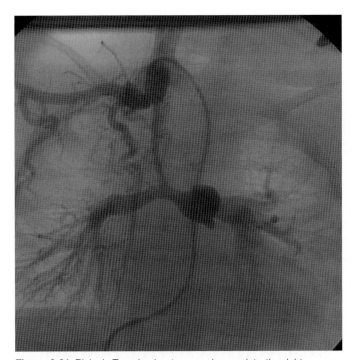

Figure 9.61 Blalock–Taussig shunt: an angiogram into the right subclavian artery (RSA) at the site of the shunt showing contrast filling the shunt and the pulmonary arteries. The pulmonary valve is atretic. PA, pulmonary artery; RPA, right pulmonary artery. (Reproduced with permission from Forfar and Arneil's. Textbook of paediatrics, 6th edn. © Elsevier Ltd 2003.)

regurgitation may be present. Chest radiography shows pulmonary oligaemia, with cardiomegaly due to right atrial enlargement if tricuspid regurgitation is severe (Table 9.4). Echocardiography shows right ventricular hypertrophy with a varying degree of hypoplasia. Abnormalities of the tricuspid valve can be seen, and pulmonary arteries fill through the arterial duct. Infants with critical stenosis have some flow through the pulmonary valve. If coronary fistulas are demonstrated with continuous colour Doppler signals within the right ventricular wall, or suspected because of enlarged coronary origins, cardiac catheterization will delineate them more clearly. Right ventricular angiography will define the right ventricular cavity and the stenosed or atretic valve.

Initial intervention consists of a systemic-to-pulmonary shunt (Figure 9.61), transcatheter perforation and balloon dilation of the stenosed or atretic valve (Figure 9.37) or surgical valvotomy. The ultimate clinical course depends on the size of the right ventricle. Infants with critical pulmonary valve stenosis and some with atresia will have a right ventricle of adequate size and, with relief of the obstruction, it will eventually function well. If the right ventricle is hypoplastic, the heart has functionally only a left ventricle. Palliation for all children with a single ventricle circulation is outlined later.

TRICUSPID ATRESIA

This spectrum of conditions has in common an absent right atrioventricular connection (Figure 9.62). Survival requires a large oval foramen, allowing systemic and pulmonary venous return to mix in the left atrium. There are many anatomical and haemodynamic variations, depending on the size of the ventricular septal defect and right ventricle, and the ventriculoarterial connections (Figure 9.63). If the ventricular septal defect is small, there will be reduced pulmonary blood flow (discussed below). If the

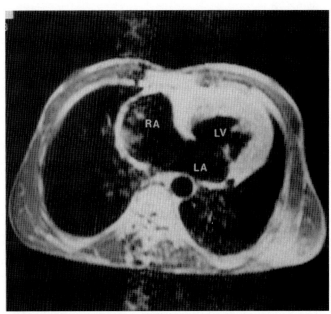

Figure 9.62 Tricuspid atresia. MRI scan shows absent right atrioventricular connection. The right atrium (RA) connects with the left atrium (LA) via an atrial septal defect (ASD). LV, left ventricle.

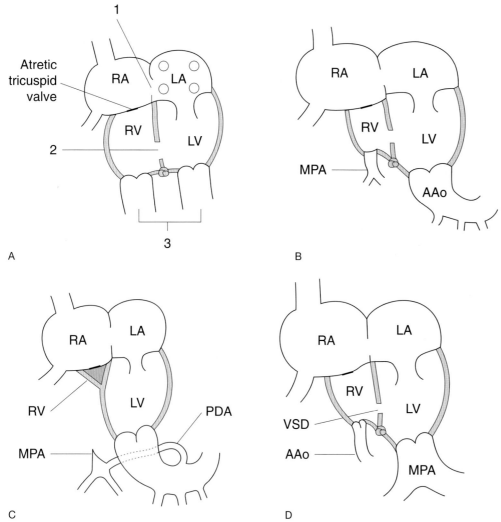

Figure 9.63 Tricuspid atresia: anatomical variations and physiological implications. (A) The basic structural elements are identified with an atretic tricuspid valve and the three key anatomical-pathophysiological factors: (1) status of the atrial septal defect (ASD), (2) size of the ventricular septal defect (VSD) and (3) great artery connections (normal or transposed). (B) A common form of tricuspid atresia with a large ASD, small-to-moderate VSD resulting in a small right ventricle (RV) and, with normally related great arteries, a small (stenotic) main pulmonary artery (MPA). This patient is likely to have inadequate pulmonary blood flow and need a neonatal shunt. (C) When there is no VSD and normally related great arteries, the RV is absent and MPA is atretic; pulmonary blood flow is dependent on ductal patency. Such patients always need a systemic-to-pulmonary shunt. (D) A small VSD and transposition results in hypoplasia of the RV and aorta; effectively, this is hypoplastic left heart syndrome. (Reproduced with permission from Skinner J, Alverson D, Hunter S (eds). Echocardiography for the neonatologist. Edinburgh: Churchill Livingstone; 2000:186.)

ventricular septal defect is large, excessive pulmonary blood flow will result in cyanosis and heart failure. When the pulmonary artery arises from the left ventricle and the aorta from the hypoplastic right ventricle, this constitutes a form of hypoplastic 'left' heart syndrome.

TRICUSPID ATRESIA WITH REDUCED PULMONARY BLOOD FLOW

In this condition, flow is to the pulmonary arteries either through a restrictive ventricular septal defect from the left to the right ventricle and pulmonary artery or through an arterial duct if the pulmonary valve is atretic (Figure 9.63). Neonates present with cyanosis in the first few days of life (Table 9.3). The lung fields are oligaemic on chest radiography (Table 9.4). Echocardiography demonstrates the absent tricuspid valve and other relevant anatomy.

The neonate usually requires a systemic-to-pulmonary shunt to provide a reliable source of pulmonary blood flow. The absent tricuspid valve means that the heart has functionally only a left ventricle. The child will have a single ventricle circulation and palliation is outlined under this condition.

PRESENTATION WITH CYANOSIS AND RESPIRATORY DISTRESS

The combination of cyanosis with respiratory distress at birth usually indicates a lung problem such as meconium aspiration syndrome, neonatal pneumonia, or surfactant deficiency in the pre-term infant. Chest radiography may indicate pneumonia or aspiration with areas of focal atelectasis, hyperexpanded or under-developed lungs, a pneumothorax or diaphragmatic hernia. Two uncommon congenital heart lesions that present in this way are Ebstein's anomaly and obstructed total anomalous pulmonary venous connection.

EBSTEIN'S ANOMALY

The tricuspid valve is displaced down the interventricular septum, towards the apex of the right ventricle, resulting in 'atrialization' of this chamber (Figure 9.64). This degree of displacement and the severity of valve dysplasia dictate the clinical spectrum. Antenatally, a dilated right heart may occupy much of the thorax resulting in pulmonary hypoplasia. There is usually an associated atrial septal defect. A ventricular septal defect and pulmonary stenosis also occur.

The most severe form results in marked tricuspid regurgitation and a poorly functioning thin-walled right ventricle. This reduces forward flow across the pulmonary valve and causes right-to-left shunting at atrial level. At birth, the infant is markedly cyanosed due to reduced pulmonary blood flow (Table 9.3), complicated by severe respiratory distress due to pulmonary hypoplasia. Chest radiography shows a markedly enlarged heart with oligaemic lung fields (Figure 9.65). Echocardiography defines the severity of the lesion and associated defects (Figure 9.66). Mild forms are asymptomatic, presenting with cyanosis, a murmur or supraventricular tachycardia due to Wolf–Parkinson–White syndrome.

At the severe end of the clinical spectrum, early mortality is high and long-term outlook poor. Infants with a small right ventricle require management similar to others with a single ventricle circulation. Children with a milder form of the condition have a better outlook but some require surgery to the tricuspid valve in later life.

TOTAL ANOMALOUS PULMONARY VENOUS CONNECTION

The pulmonary veins join to form a confluence behind the left atrium and drain into the right atrium to mix with the deoxygenated

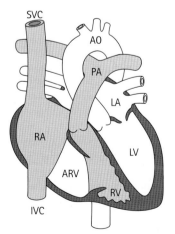

Figure 9.64 Ebstein's anomaly. The shaded area represents the atrialized portion of the right ventricle (ARV) resulting from the displacement of the septal and posterior leaflets. (Reproduced with permission from Forfar and Arneil's. Textbook of paediatrics, 6th edn. © Elsevier Ltd 2003.)

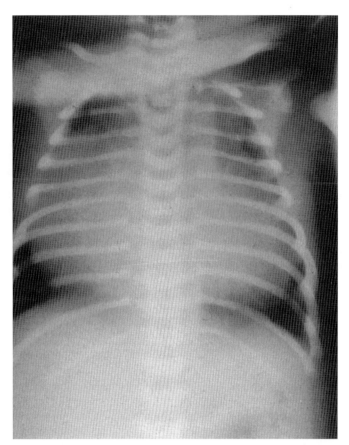

Figure 9.65 Ebstein's anomaly. The chest radiograph shows gross cardiomegaly and pulmonary oligaemia.

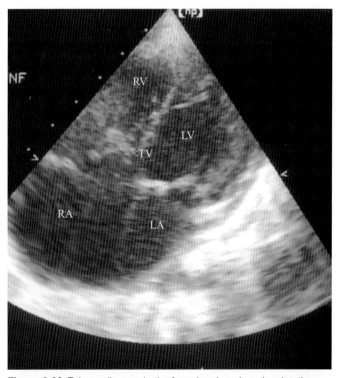

Figure 9.66 Echocardiogram in the four-chamber view showing the tricuspid valve (TV) inserted lower down the interventricular septum in the right ventricle (RV) producing tricuspid regurgitation and right atrial (RA) enlargement.

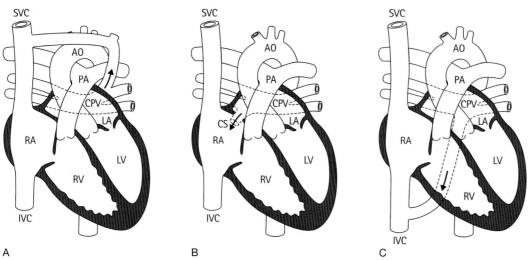

Figure 9.67 Total anomalous pulmonary venous connection. The three common varieties are shown: (A) supracardiac with the four pulmonary veins draining into a common pulmonary venous channel (CPV) and then via a vertical (ascending) vein to the innominate vein and the right heart; (B) cardiac with the pulmonary veins draining directly to the coronary sinus (CS) as shown or directly to the right atrium (not shown); (C) infracardiac draining into the inferior vena cava or portal vein. (Reproduced with permission from Forfar and Arneil's. Textbook of paediatrics, 6th edn. © Elsevier Ltd 2003.)

blood returning from the body. The route from the pulmonary venous confluence can be of three types (Figure 9.67). The clinical picture and timing of presentation depends on whether an obstruction prevents free drainage of the pulmonary venous blood into the right heart (Table 9.3). Infants with obstruction present shortly after birth with respiratory distress, cyanosis and cardiac failure. Those without obstruction, present at 2–8 weeks of age with mild cyanosis and progressive cardiac failure.

OBSTRUCTED TOTAL ANOMALOUS PULMONARY VENOUS CONNECTION

The infracardiac type is almost always severely obstructed (Figure 9.68). The infant becomes unwell shortly after birth as the pulmonary venous obstruction results in severe pulmonary venous hypertension, cyanosis, cardiac failure and respiratory distress. Chest radiography shows pulmonary venous hypertension, and the heart is not greatly enlarged. The streaky appearance due to the prominent pulmonary veins can easily be mistaken for lung disease such as meconium aspiration syndrome. Differentiation from persistent pulmonary hypertension of the newborn can be difficult on echocardiography since the left atrium and ventricle are under-filled in both conditions, and compressed by the enlarged right ventricle. There is right-to-left flow across the atrial septum. Diagnosis depends on recognizing the pulmonary venous chamber behind the left atrium draining into a vessel, which passes inferiorly below the diaphragm.

Ventilatory and circulatory support may be necessary followed by urgent surgery. The pulmonary venous chamber is opened into the back of the left atrium, and the abnormal connecting vein ligated. There is a risk of pulmonary vein stenosis, which is extremely difficult to manage successfully.

PRESENTATION WITH CYANOSIS AND CARDIAC FAILURE

This rare presentation may be caused by unobstructed total anomalous pulmonary venous connection, tricuspid atresia with a large ventricular septal defect, or common arterial trunk.

UNOBSTRUCTED TOTAL ANOMALOUS PULMONARY VENOUS CONNECTION

The majority of supracardiac and infracardiac types (Figure 9.67) are unobstructed. All systemic and pulmonary venous return mixes in the right atrium resulting in mild cyanosis that may be difficult to detect clinically. As pulmonary vascular resistance falls, the infant presents with congestive cardiac failure due to excessive pulmonary blood flow (Table 9.3). Chest radiography shows cardiomegaly with pulmonary plethora (Figure 9.69). The supracardiac type frequently has a broad mediastinum due to the ascending vein – the 'snowman' appearance (Figure 9.70). Management includes treatment for cardiac failure and early surgical correction.

TRICUSPID ATRESIA WITH EXCESSIVE PULMONARY BLOOD FLOW

In this condition, there is absence of the right atrioventricular connection, the great vessels are normally related and there is a large ventricular septal defect. Systemic venous return passes across the atrial septum to mix with pulmonary venous blood in the left atrium. All venous return then passes into the left ventricle (Figure 9.63). As the ventricular septal defect is non-restrictive, blood passes into the right ventricle and pulmonary arteries. As

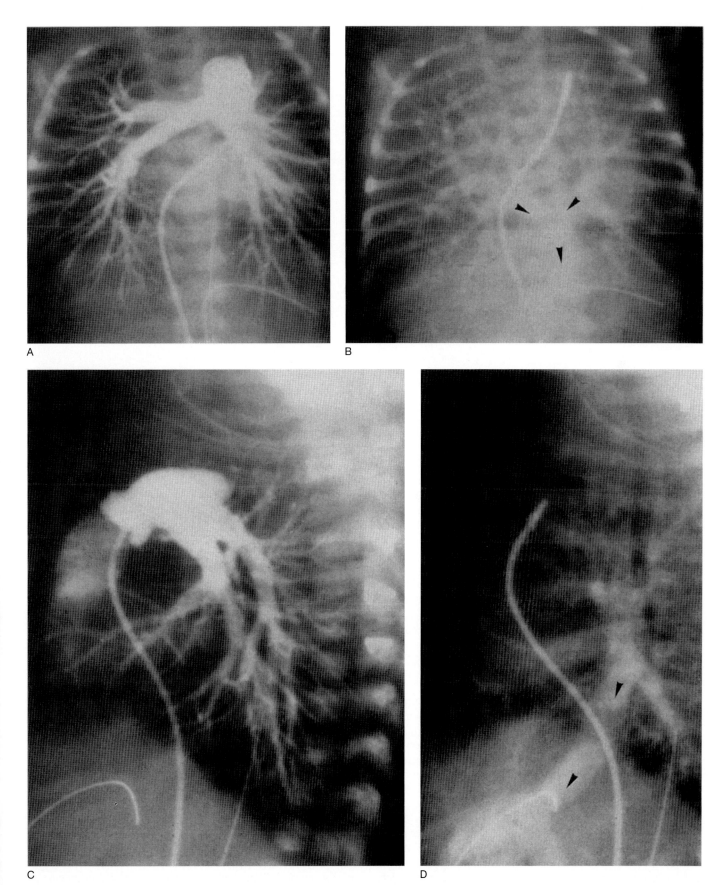

A

B

C

D

Figure 9.68 Infracardiac total anomalous pulmonary venous connection. (A,C) Arterial phase of pulmonary angiogram is normal. (B,D) Venous phase shows all the pulmonary veins draining into a retrocardiac venous confluence, and then into a common vein, which traverses the diaphragm to reach the portal vein. Arrowheads show the direction of flow.

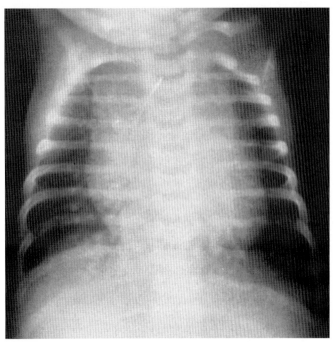

Figure 9.69 Supracardiac total anomalous pulmonary venous connection. The lungs are plethoric. The superior mediastinum is widened by dilated systemic veins.

pulmonary vascular resistance falls over the first few weeks of life, pulmonary blood flow increases. Infants present with mild cyanosis and congestive cardiac failure after 2 weeks of age (Table 9.3). Chest radiography shows plethoric lung fields (Table 9.4). Echocardiography shows the anatomical features necessary to make the diagnosis.

Initially, a pulmonary artery band is needed to limit pulmonary blood flow. As the tricuspid valve is atretic, the right ventricle can never function as a normal ventricle and the management is that of a child with a single ventricle circulation.

COMMON ARTERIAL TRUNK (TRUNCUS ARTERIOSUS)

The common arterial trunk fails to divide embryologically into aortic and pulmonary components. The truncal valve, which overrides a large ventricular septal defect, is commonly abnormal and may have more than three leaflets. Type 1 has a common origin of the pulmonary arteries from the arterial trunk (Figure 9.71), in type 2 they arise separately from the back of the trunk, and in type 3 they arise separately from the lateral walls of the trunk. Aortic coarctation or interruption is occasionally present.

Congestive cardiac failure occurs after 2 weeks of age due to the excessive pulmonary blood flow as pulmonary vascular resistance falls and there is mild cyanosis. Approximately 40% of children have chromosome 22q11 deletion. Chest radiography shows cardiomegaly and plethora, and 30% have a right aortic arch. Echocardiography shows the ventricular septal defect with overriding truncal valve similar to that in tetralogy of Fallot but the pulmonary arteries can be seen arising from the arterial trunk (Figure 9.72). Doppler echocardiography is used to assess truncal

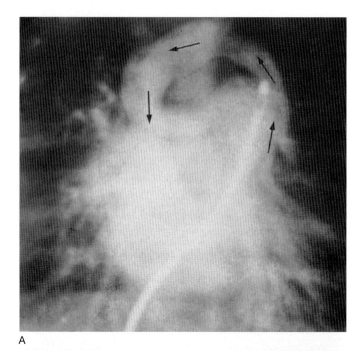

A

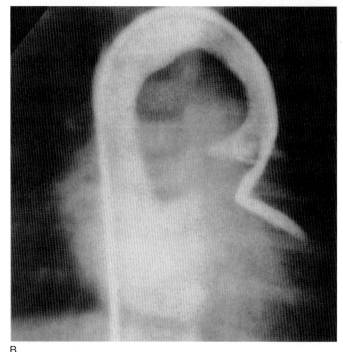

B

Figure 9.70 Supracardiac total anomalous pulmonary venous connection. (A) The venous phase of a pulmonary arteriogram shows that all the pulmonary veins converge to a vertical vein on the left, which drains into the right atrium via the brachiocephalic vein and superior vena cava. The arrows indicate the direction of flow. (B) Retrograde injection into the vertical vein.

valve regurgitation and stenosis. Cardiac catheterization is unnecessary unless late presentation suggests irreversible pulmonary hypertension.

Cardiac failure is treated medically and early surgery is necessary because the large left-to-right shunt rapidly produces pulmonary hypertension. The ventricular septal defect is closed and

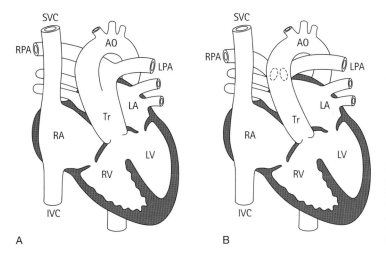

Figure 9.71 Common arterial trunk: (A) in type 1 the pulmonary arteries arise from the truncus (Tr) with a common origin; (B) in type 2 the pulmonary arteries arise separately from the back. In type 3 (not shown) the pulmonary arteries are more widely reported at origins and arise posteriorly/laterally from the trunk. (Reproduced with permission from Forfar and Arneil's. Textbook of paediatrics, 6th edn. © Elsevier Ltd 2003.)

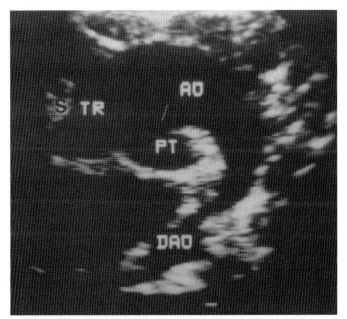

Figure 9.72 Common arterial trunk, type 1. Two-dimensional echocardiogram shows a persistent common arterial trunk (TR) overriding the ventricular septum (S) and dividing into ascending aorta (AO) and pulmonary trunk (PT). DAO, descending aorta.

a valved conduit is placed from the right ventricle to the pulmonary artery branches, which are detached from the trunk. Prognosis is poor if the truncal valve is stenotic or markedly regurgitant. The right ventricle to pulmonary artery conduit will need to be replaced as the child grows.

PRESENTATION WITH CARDIOVASCULAR COLLAPSE

The most common cardiac causes are the left heart obstructive lesions. Other conditions include cardiomyopathy, supraventricular tachycardia, myocardial ischaemia following perinatal distress or anomalous origin of the left coronary artery, and pericardial effusion with tamponade. Other causes of collapse in the neonate include sepsis, respiratory and metabolic disease. Clinically and on chest radiography, cardiomegaly is usually present with cardiac causes, and is rare in other conditions.

LEFT HEART OBSTRUCTIVE LESIONS

These are most commonly due to severe aortic coarctation, aortic arch interruption, hypoplastic left heart or critical aortic stenosis. Mitral valve or pulmonary vein stenosis is rare in isolation. All the left heart obstructions share common clinical features related to duct closure, resulting in a fall in flow in the aorta with decreased perfusion of vital organs. Presentation is usually within 48 h of birth and deterioration is extremely rapid with poor peripheral perfusion resulting in delayed capillary refill time, poor pulses and low blood pressure. The infant is usually tachypnoeic, the liver is enlarged and urine output poor. Chest radiography shows cardiomegaly with a combination of pulmonary plethora and oedema. The echocardiographic findings are described under the individual lesions. Intravenous prostaglandin reopens the arterial duct but the rapid deterioration means that these infants often require intensive support. The specific management of individual conditions is discussed below.

AORTIC COARCTATION

Narrowing of the aorta occurs between the left subclavian artery and the origin of the arterial duct. This is usually due to a shelf-like obstruction but it can be tubular (Figure 9.73) and is sometimes associated with hypoplasia of the transverse aorta (Figure 9.74). Most infants with coarctation have other lesions, commonly a bicuspid aortic valve, ventricular septal defect or mitral valve anomaly. Infants present in the first 2 weeks with rapid onset of cardiac failure progressing to cardiovascular collapse. In milder forms, the presentation is more insidious, with failure to thrive and cardiac failure. The femoral pulses are absent. The right arm blood pressure is higher than that recorded in the legs. Turner's syndrome should be considered in girls with coarctation. Echocardiography

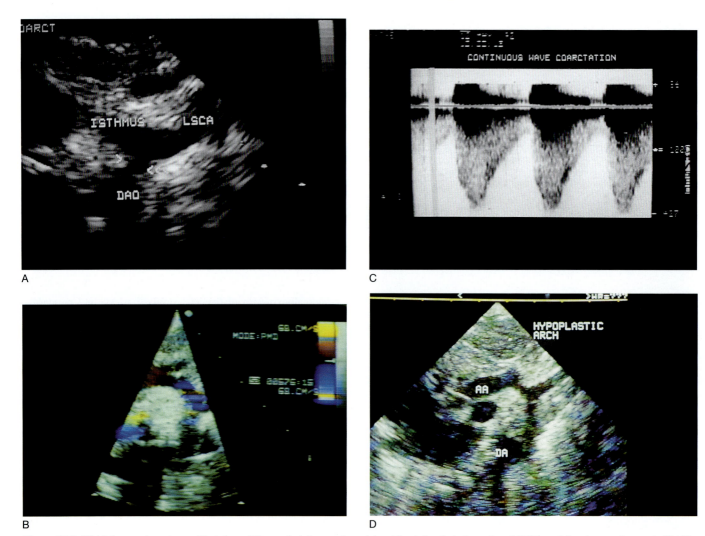

Figure 9.73 (A) High parasternal magnified view of the aortic isthmus, the origin of the left subclavian artery (LSCA) and the descending aorta (DAO). The narrowed area of the coarctation is arrowed. (B) Suprasternal view of an infant with coarctation. The arch is a reasonable size and the area of coarctation was identified by turbulence on the colour flow map. (C) Continuous wave Doppler from the descending aorta via the suprasternal approach. The classical continuous flow seen in coarctation is present. The peak velocity is high and the diastolic velocity never returns to the baseline. (D) Hypoplastic aortic arch in a child who also had coarctation of the aorta. Following surgery, there is still narrowing of the isthmus. AA, ascending aorta; DA, descending aorta. (Reproduced with permission from Skinner J, Alverson D, Hunter S (eds). Echocardiography for the neonatologist. Edinburgh: Churchill Livingstone; 2000:216.)

defines the area of narrowing with turbulent flow seen on colour Doppler. The Doppler flow pattern through the coarctation has a characteristic 'saw-tooth' appearance with flow continuing into diastole – the diastolic tail (Figure 9.73C). The right ventricle and pulmonary artery are enlarged and left ventricular dysfunction may be present. Associated lesions will also be seen.

Surgery is performed when the infant has been stabilized and the acidosis corrected. Repair is usually through a lateral thoracotomy, and consists of excision of the coarctation with end-to-end anastomosis of the aorta. Cardiopulmonary bypass is not necessary unless there is hypoplasia of the transverse aortic arch.

HYPOPLASTIC LEFT HEART

The left ventricle is small with hypoplasia or atresia of the mitral and aortic valves, and ascending aorta. Systemic circulation depends on flow through the arterial duct, which is supplied by the right ventricle and pulmonary artery. The infant presents with profound collapse (Table 9.3) when the duct closes. Echocardiography reveals a small left ventricle with stenotic or atretic mitral and aortic valves, and a hypoplastic aortic arch. The right atrium and ventricle are enlarged, as is the pulmonary artery. There is retrograde flow from the arterial duct around the aortic arch to the ascending aorta.

An increasing number of infants have an antenatal diagnosis of this condition and are started on prostaglandin infusion soon after birth. The high-risk, palliative Norwood operation (Figure 9.75) is performed in the first days of life if the infant is well enough. The aorta is enlarged using part of the pulmonary artery and the distal pulmonary artery is detached and supplied by an aortopulmonary shunt. Subsequent surgery is similar to that for other children with a single ventricle circulation. Survival through infancy can now be expected in over 50%.

CRITICAL AORTIC STENOSIS

The aortic valve is thickened, dysplastic and markedly stenotic. Presentation is similar to infants with a hypoplastic left heart. Echocardiography distinguishes it from the other similar conditions. There is an adequate-sized left ventricle, which is either hypertrophied or dilated with reduced function. The aortic valve is thickened with restricted opening and turbulence is seen on colour Doppler. The Doppler velocity across the valve may be increased, or reduced because of poor ventricular function. Once the infant has been stabilized, transcatheter balloon aortic valvuloplasty (Figure 9.76) or open surgical valvotomy is performed. The results are similar from the two procedures but recurrence of the stenosis occurs, which requires further intervention later in life.

INTERRUPTION OF THE AORTIC ARCH

Interruption of the aortic arch describes a complete occlusion, which may occur beyond the left subclavian (type A), between the left common carotid (type B) and the left subclavian arteries or between the carotid arteries (type C). Other cardiac lesions such as a ventricular septal defect and subaortic stenosis are often present. The infant presents with cardiovascular collapse in the first few days of life when the arterial duct closes. Over 50% of infants with type B interruption have chromosome 22q11 deletion. Interruption of the aortic arch is visible on echocardiography and cardiac catheterization is seldom necessary for diagnosis. Repair of the aortic arch is performed on cardiopulmonary bypass, usually with closure of the associated ventricular septal defect.

PRESENTATION WITH CARDIAC FAILURE WITHOUT CYANOSIS

A number of conditions present in early infancy with cardiac failure. These children usually present outside the neonatal period and are discussed later. These conditions include ventricular septal defect, atrioventricular septal defect, aortopulmonary window and persistent arterial duct. Occasionally, infants with cardiomyopathy present in the neonatal period and failure can also be caused by supraventricular tachycardia.

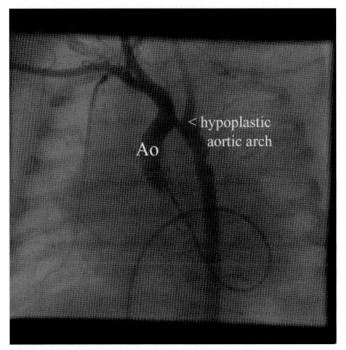

Figure 9.74 Aortic (Ao) angiogram showing hypoplasia of the transverse aortic arch (arrow).

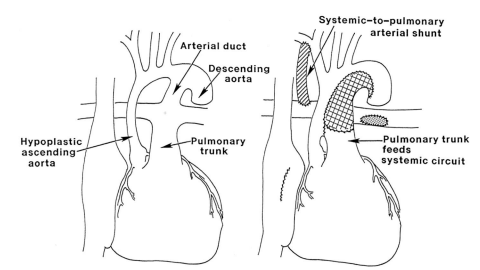

Figure 9.75 These diagrams show the arrangement of the circulations before and after the classical Norwood procedure, which is the first stage of palliative surgery. (Reproduced with permission from Andersen RH et al. Paediatric cardiology; 2nd edn. Edinburgh: Churchill Livingstone; 2000:1205)

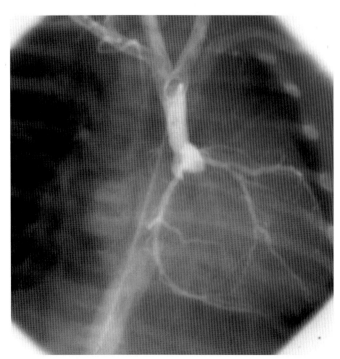

Figure 9.76 Critical aortic stenosis. The opacified coronary arteries indicate the enlargement of the heart. There is a small jet of negative contrast through the narrowed aortic valve.

PRESENTATION WITH AN ASSOCIATED LESION OR SYNDROME

The commoner syndromes likely to be associated with congenital heart disease are shown in Table 9.2. Congenital heart disease should always be considered in infants with a syndrome or dysmorphology.

PRESENTATION WITH AN ASYMPTOMATIC MURMUR

Congenital heart lesions that cause a systolic murmur audible from birth are aortic and pulmonary stenosis and tetralogy of Fallot. A small ventricular septal defect is the most common cause of an asymptomatic murmur audible as the right ventricular and pulmonary artery pressures fall after birth. Tricuspid or mitral regurgitation cause a pansystolic murmur, most commonly in myocardial ischaemia following perinatal distress, but can represent an isolated valve lesion, or be part of a more complex condition such as an atrioventricular septal defect. All these conditions are more common outside the neonatal period and will be discussed in the following section.

MISCELLANEOUS COMPLEX LESIONS

CONGENITALLY CORRECTED TRANSPOSITION OF THE GREAT ARTERIES

This rare lesion is characterized by discordance of both the atrioventricular and the ventriculoarterial connection (Figure 9.77). Systemic venous return passes from the right atrium through the mitral valve into a morphological left ventricle from which the pulmonary artery arises. Pulmonary venous return passes from the left atrium, through the tricuspid valve, into the morphological right ventricle and thence into the aorta. The aorta is usually located anterior and to the left of the pulmonary artery. Ventricular septal defect and pulmonary stenosis are the most frequently associated lesions and dextrocardia is also common. Associated cardiac lesions usually dictate the clinical presentation and course. If a large ventricular septal defect is present heart failure develops early. Those patients with a ventricular septal defect and pulmonary stenosis present with cyanosis and clinically resemble tetralogy of Fallot. In the absence of associated defects, the condition may not be recognized for many years but left-sided atrioventricular valve (tricuspid) regurgitation may develop progressively. Radiologically, the condition may be suspected by the presence of a straight upper left heart border produced by the left-sided anterior aorta. Echocardiography will determine the abnormal atrioventricular and ventriculoarterial connections and define any associated abnormality.

The management is usually that of the associated lesion. Severely cyanosed infants require a systemic-to-pulmonary shunt. For those with heart failure secondary to a large ventricular septal defect, pulmonary artery banding may be indicated. Closure of the ventricular septal defect is associated with a high incidence of complete heart block (30%) and significant mortality. Because of gradual deterioration of the systemic right ventricle and progressive tricuspid regurgitation, surgery, to restore the left ventricle to pump to the systemic circulation, has been performed. This can be achieved by means of the double switch operation (Figure 9.77).

DOUBLE INLET (SINGLE) VENTRICLE

Both atria are connected with a dominant ventricle, usually the left ventricle, and the other ventricle is rudimentary (Figure 9.78). The main ventricle usually has the morphology of a left ventricle with two inlet valves and the right ventricle is a small outflow chamber. The ventriculoarterial connection can vary but most commonly the aorta arises from the rudimentary chamber, and the pulmonary artery from the main ventricular chamber. The outlet chamber communicates with the main ventricular chamber via a ventricular septal defect. The severity of any associated pulmonary stenosis determines the presentation and the management is the same as for other children with a single ventricle circulation.

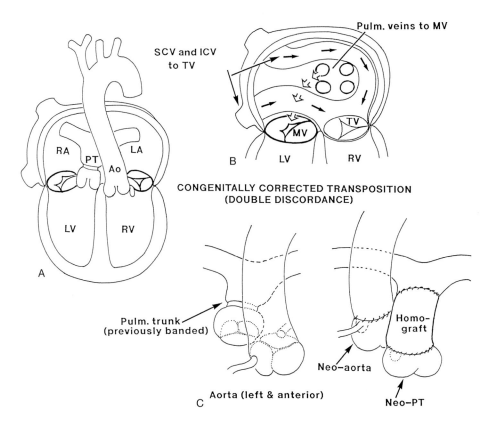

CONGENITALLY CORRECTED TRANSPOSITION
(DOUBLE DISCORDANCE)

Figure 9.77 The steps involved in the so-called double switch procedure involve, first, banding of the pulmonary trunk (PT) unless associated lesions have already 'prepared' the left ventricle (A). An atrial redirection procedure (B) is then combined with an arterial switch (C). This then produces both physiological and anatomical correction. Ao, aorta; LA, left atrium; LV, left ventricle; MV, mitral valve; pulm., pulmonary; RA, right atrium; RV, right ventricle; SVC and ICV, superior and inferior caval veins; TV, tricuspid valve. (Reproduced with permission from Andersen RH et al. (eds). Paediatric cardiology, 2nd edn. Edinburgh: Churchill Livingstone; 2000:1342)

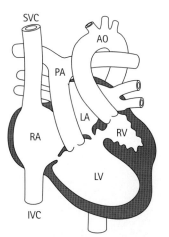

Figure 9.78 Double inlet ventricle or single ventricle. In the most common variety as here both atrioventricular valves connect to a morphologically normal left ventricle (LV) and the right ventricle is represented by a small rudimentary outflow chamber from which the aorta arises. There is usually arterioventricular discordance. (Reproduced with permission from Forfar and Arneil's. Textbook of paediatrics, 6th edn. © Elsevier Ltd 2003.)

DOUBLE OUTLET RIGHT VENTRICLE

The aorta and pulmonary artery both arise from the right ventricle. There are two common types. In one variation, there is a large ventricular septal defect, with no pulmonary stenosis. This is commonly associated with a posterior pulmonary artery and an anterior aorta. The ventricular septal defect is related to the large pulmonary valve and has obvious similarities to transposition with

a large ventricular septal defect (known as the Taussig–Bing malformation). In the other variation, there is a large ventricular septal defect with pulmonary stenosis and the features mimic the tetralogy of Fallot. Depending upon the associated lesions, the clinical features mimic other lesions such as transposition, ventricular septal defect, or tetralogy of Fallot. Echocardiography defines the anatomy and excludes other conditions.

Infants with high pulmonary blood flow require pulmonary artery banding whereas those with severe cyanosis, because of restrictive pulmonary blood flow, may require a Blalock–Taussig shunt. Definitive repair depends upon the site of the ventricular septal defect. Occasionally, only an intracardiac patch may be required but in other children, arterial switch and closure of a ventricular septal defect, or major reconstruction with the use of a conduit, may be necessary.

THE SINGLE VENTRICLE CIRCULATION

A number of conditions have in common one ventricle providing the majority of the cardiac output to the body and lungs. Palliation is directed towards allowing the functional ventricle to supply the systemic circulation. Blood returning from the superior and inferior caval veins is directed into the pulmonary arteries, driven by the central venous pressure and the negative forces generated by inspiration and ventricular diastole.

The cardiac lesion may give rise to:

- Inadequate pulmonary blood flow (tricuspid atresia or double inlet left ventricle with pulmonary stenosis, pulmonary atresia with intact ventricular septum and hypoplastic right ventricle, severe Ebstein's anomaly);

- Inadequate systemic blood flow (hypoplastic left heart, tricuspid atresia with transposition); and
- Unrestricted pulmonary blood flow (double outlet right ventricle with hypoplastic left ventricle).

At birth, the arterial duct compensates for inadequate pulmonary or systemic circulation and symptoms develop when the duct closes. Infants with inadequate pulmonary blood flow present with cyanosis. Those with inadequate systemic blood flow present with cardiovascular collapse. Those with unrestricted pulmonary blood flow present with signs of heart failure as the pulmonary vascular resistance falls. Treatment involves at least three staged procedures.

Optimizing systemic and pulmonary blood flow. Effective early palliation is critical. From infancy the blood flow into the lungs must be adequate but at low pressure. Neonates with inadequate pulmonary blood flow require a systemic to pulmonary (modified Blalock–Taussig) shunt (Figure 9.61). Those with inadequate systemic blood flow require a Norwood or other similar operation (Figure 9.75). Those with excessive pulmonary blood flow require a pulmonary artery band around the main pulmonary artery to reduce pulmonary blood flow (Figure 9.79). A few infants have a cardiac lesion that results in optimal systemic and pulmonary blood flow in that they have pulmonary stenosis and unobstructed systemic blood flow.

The definitive palliative procedure for all children with a single ventricle is the Fontan operation. This is usually carried out in two further stages.

Superior (bidirectional) cavo-pulmonary anastomosis relieves the systemic ventricle of chronic volume and pressure loads that occur regardless of the type of neonatal palliation. It usually decreases the cyanosis and reduces the risks at subsequent surgery. It is performed at 6–12 months of age. The superior caval vein is anastomosed to the proximal right pulmonary artery (Figure 9.80). If a left superior vena cava is present, this is anastomosed to the left pulmonary artery at the same procedure. If a Blalock–Taussig shunt is present, it is ligated. Residual lesions that increase the risk of subsequent surgery, such as pulmonary artery narrowing or re-coarctation, are corrected. The superior cavo-pulmonary anastomosis is well tolerated, even when combined with other procedures. During early childhood, the relative size of the lower body increases, and the ratio of blood returning from the inferior and superior caval veins alters. This results in increasing cyanosis, which may also occur due to venous collaterals that develop between the upper and lower body.

Completion of modified Fontan operation is usually performed at 2–5 years of age. The inferior vena cava is anastomosed to the pulmonary arteries, either by a baffle that is created inside the lateral wall of the right atrium or by an extracardiac conduit (Figure 9.81). Creation of a small hole or fenestration between this tunnel or conduit and the left-sided (systemic) circulation produces a small right-to-left shunt. This lowers the central venous pressure, preventing severe venous congestion in the postoperative period but producing systemic desaturation. The fenestration can be closed at a later time.

Prognosis depends on the underlying condition, the success of the various interventions and the long-term function of the systemic ventricle. The postoperative period may be protracted with high central venous pressure, ascites, pleural effusions and poor cardiac output. The quality of life in survivors is satisfactory but

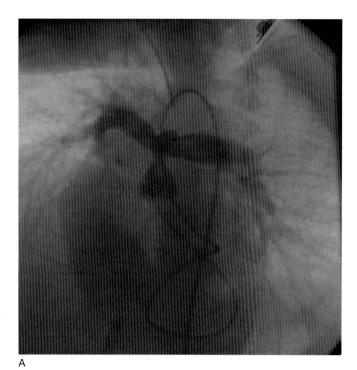

A

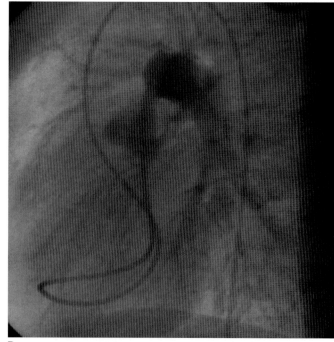

B

Figure 9.79 Pulmonary artery band: an angiogram into the main pulmonary artery (A) shows the constriction from the pulmonary artery band distal to the pulmonary valve, before the bifurcation into right and left pulmonary arteries. (B) A lateral projection of the same angiogram. LPA, left pulmonary artery; MPA, main pulmonary artery; RPA, right pulmonary artery. (Reproduced with permission from Forfar and Arneil's. Textbook of paediatrics, 6th edn. © Elsevier Ltd 2003.)

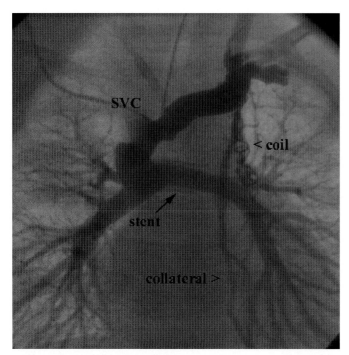

Figure 9.80 The superior cavo-pulmonary anastomosis. The angiogram in the superior caval vein shows the connection to the proximal right pulmonary artery. Contrast also fills the innominate vein on the left. Coils have been used to occlude some of the collateral veins from the innominate vein. An intravascular stent was expanded in the proximal left pulmonary artery at the time of surgery. LPA, left pulmonary artery; RPA, right pulmonary artery; SVC, superior caval vein. (Reproduced with permission from Forfar and Arneil's. Textbook of paediatrics, 6th edn. © Elsevier Ltd 2003.)

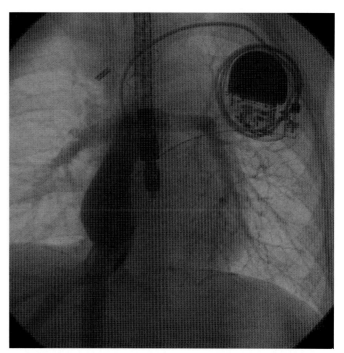

Figure 9.81 The Fontan operation. The angiogram shows the lateral tunnel connecting the inferior caval vein to the pulmonary arteries. The position of the connection between the superior caval vein and the pulmonary arteries is shown by the pacemaker lead, which passes from the subclavian vein, via the superior caval vein to the atrial wall. The transoesophageal probe is visible in the oesophagus. LPA, left pulmonary artery; RPA, right pulmonary artery; SVC, superior caval vein; TOE, transoesophageal echocardiographic probe. (Reproduced with permission from Forfar and Arneil's. Textbook of paediatrics, 6th edn. © Elsevier Ltd 2003.)

a number of late complications account for a continuing mortality. Reports of thromboembolism, both pulmonary and systemic (if a fenestration is present), have resulted in the use of long-term anticoagulation. Arrhythmias can produce significant haemodynamic deterioration. The only option for a child with a failing 'Fontan' circulation is heart transplant.

FURTHER READING

Anderson RH, Baker EJ, Macartney FJ et al. Pediatric cardiology, 2nd edn. Edinburgh: Churchill Livingstone; 2002.

Andrews R, Tulloh R, Sharland G et al. Outcome of staged reconstructive surgery for hypoplastic left heart syndrome following antenatal diagnosis. Heart 2001; 85:474–477.

Freedom RM, Hamilton R, Yoo SJ et al. The Fontan procedure: analysis of cohorts and late complications. Cardiology in the Young 2000; 10:307–325.

Goldmuntz E, Clark BJ, Mitchell LE et al. Frequency of 22q11 deletions in patients with conotruncal defects. Journal of the American College of Cardiology 1998; 32:492–498.

Mahle WT, Spray TL, Wernovsky G et al. Survival after reconstructive surgery for hypoplastic left heart syndrome: a 15-year experience from a single institution. Circulation 2000; 102 (Suppl 3):136–141.

Nollert G, Fischlein T, Bouterwek S et al. Long-term survival in patients with repair of tetralogy of Fallot: 36-year follow-up of 490 survivors of the first year after surgical repair. Journal of the American College of Cardiology 1997; 30:1374–1383.

Penny DJ, Shekerdemian LS. Management of the neonate with symptomatic congenital heart disease. Archives of Disease in Childhood 2001; 84:F141–145.

Prêtre R, Tamisier D, Bonhoeffer P et al. Results of the arterial switch operation in neonates with transposed great arteries. Lancet 2001; 357:1826–1830.

Ryan AK, Goodship JA, Wilson DI et al. Spectrum of clinical features associated with interstitial chromosome 22q11 deletions: a European collaborative study. Journal of Medical Genetics 1997; 34:798–804.

Skinner J, Alverson D, Hunter S. Echocardiography for the neonatologist. Edinburgh: Churchill Livingstone; 2000.

Tweddell JS, Litwin SB, Thomas JP, Mussatto K. Recent advances in the surgical management of the single ventricle patient. Pediatric Clinics of North America 1999; 46:465–480.

Tworetzky W, McElhinney DB, Reddy VM et al. Improved outcome after fetal diagnosis of hypoplastic left heart syndrome. Circulation 2001; 103:1269–1273.

INFANTS AND CHILDREN WITH CONGENITAL HEART DISEASE

ACYANOTIC ABNORMALITIES CAUSING OUTFLOW OBSTRUCTION

PULMONARY STENOSIS

Obstruction to flow occurring between the right ventricle and pulmonary circulation can occur at the subvalvar, valvar or supravalvar level or may occur in the peripheral pulmonary arteries. Pulmonary valve stenosis is the most common type. Noonan's syndrome is associated with pulmonary stenosis in which, unlike the more common form of valve stenosis, the valve is often thickened and dysplastic. In primary pulmonary valve stenosis, the pulmonary valve leaflets are thickened and fused resulting in impaired movement, with incomplete opening (Figure 9.82). Subvalvar stenosis occurs most often in association with a stenotic pulmonary valve due to hypertrophy of the right ventricle and infundibulum (Figure 9.83). Isolated subvalvar obstruction is rare. 'Supravalvar' stenosis with narrowing at the sinotubular junction can be isolated or occur in association with valvar stenosis. The latter is seen often in Noonan's syndrome. Peripheral pulmonary artery stenosis occurs as part of complex cardiac conditions, e.g. Fallot's tetralogy or with various syndromes including congenital rubella, Alagille's and Williams syndrome (Figure 9.84).

PATHOPHYSIOLOGY

The pressure in the right ventricle becomes elevated to an extent that is dependent on the severity of obstruction. The ventricle hypertrophies and the right atrial pressure may become elevated. In some patients, there may be an associated defect in the atrial septum with a resulting right-to-left shunt if right atrial pressure becomes elevated. This can lead to central cyanosis.

PRESENTATION

Most children are asymptomatic and are identified because of an incidental murmur found on routine examination for some other purpose. Cyanosis may be seen if there is an ASD and severe stenosis and in the neonate with critical pulmonary stenosis. Shortness of breath, chest pain and syncope are found less often and tend to indicate severe stenosis.

If a child has the clinical features of the above mentioned syndromes then obstruction at all levels should be carefully sought.

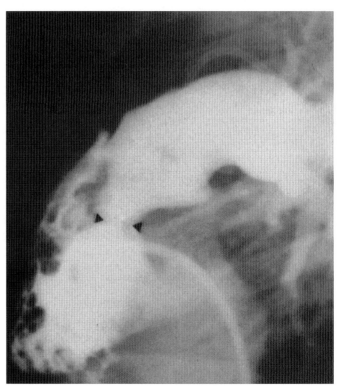

Figure 9.83 Subvalvar pulmonary stenosis. The lateral projection of the right ventriculogram shows discrete narrowing of the infundibulum (arrowheads). The right ventricle is hypertrophied.

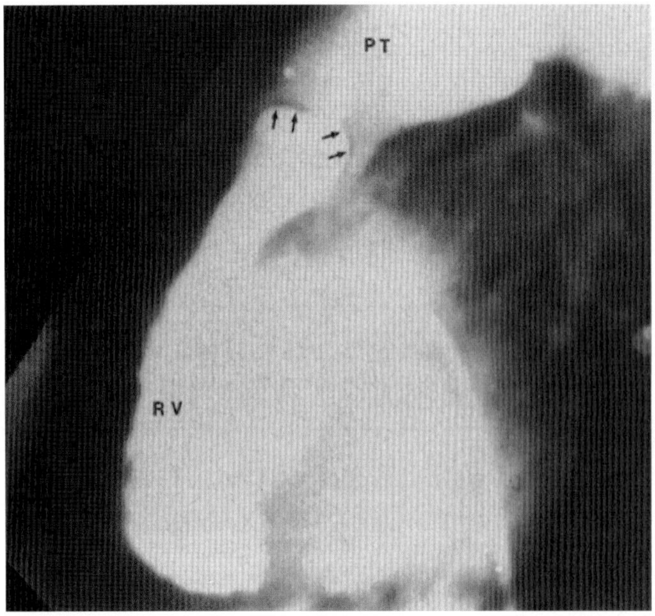

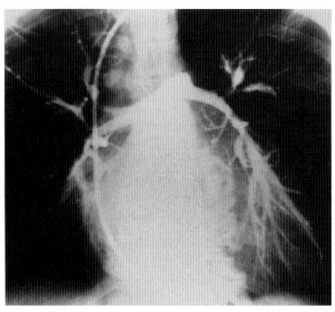

Figure 9.84 Peripheral pulmonary artery stenoses in an infant with Williams syndrome.

Figure 9.82 Pulmonary valve stenosis. Right ventriculogram, lateral projection in systole, shows thickened, doming pulmonary valve leaflets (arrows). The pulmonary trunk (PT) is dilated. RV, right ventricle.

INVESTIGATIONS

Chest radiograph

Most often the heart is normal in size with normal or subtly decreased pulmonary vascularity. The right ventricle may be enlarged. Classical enlargement of the main and left pulmonary artery is seen in valvar stenosis and is independent of the severity of the stenosis (Figure 9.85). When a right-to-left shunt is present pulmonary vascularity may be diminished. If congestive failure is present then the heart may be enlarged. The main pulmonary artery may appear enlarged in adolescents and young adults with a normal heart and is an important normal variant.

Echocardiography

Abnormalities of the pulmonary valve leaflets with thickening and altered motion can be seen. The pulmonary valve may demonstrate doming during systole. Poststenotic dilation of the main and branch pulmonary arteries are often easily seen. Right ventricular hypertrophy and qualitative analysis of the degree of stenosis from the Doppler flow can be assessed.

MANAGEMENT

In some cases, pulmonary stenosis will resolve spontaneously. However, management with percutaneous balloon valvuloplasty

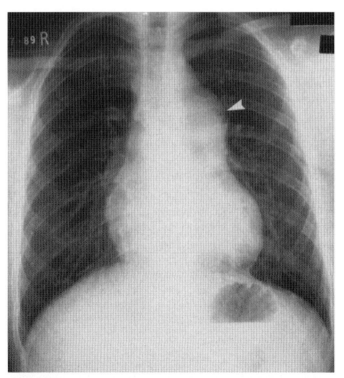

Figure 9.85 Pulmonary valve stenosis. The pulmonary trunk and left pulmonary artery (arrowhead) are dilated. The right pulmonary artery, peripheral pulmonary vessels and heart size are normal.

may be necessary. If the valves are dysplastic or other cardiac anomalies are present then surgical repair may be undertaken.

AORTIC STENOSIS

As with pulmonary stenosis, outflow obstruction may be at valvar most frequently, subvalvar and supravalvar level. More than one level of obstruction may occur. When aortic valve stenosis is isolated then the valve that is thickened is usually bicuspid. Poststenotic dilation of the ascending aorta may occur. A bicuspid aortic valve without stenosis occurs in 2% of the population. Subaortic stenosis is usually due to fibromuscular tissue below the aortic valve. Muscular subaortic obstruction occasionally occurs. Supravalvar stenosis is due to localized or diffuse thickening and narrowing of the ascending aorta. It is commonly associated with Williams syndrome or a positive family history (autosomal dominant inheritance) but 25% of cases are sporadic (Figure 9.86). Coronary artery abnormalities can occur.

CLINICAL FEATURES

Critical aortic stenosis is covered in the neonatal section.

Children may have an unobstructed bicuspid aortic valve. In those with obstruction presentation depends on the severity.

Most children are incidentally discovered to have aortic stenosis due to the finding of a murmur. Symptoms are not common but include syncope, chest pain and shortness of breath on exertion. Sudden death may occur with severe stenosis and may be due to arrhythmias.

INVESTIGATION

Chest radiography may be normal. Cardiomegaly when present is usually seen with heart failure. Poststenotic dilatation of the ascending aorta produces a prominent ascending aorta (Figure 9.87). It can be seen in mild stenosis due to a bicuspid valve and may be due to an associated abnormality of the wall of the ascending aorta. A rounded apex due to left ventricular hypertrophy may be evident and the left atrium may be enlarged. Calcification is not usually seen in children. Echocardiography shows the site of obstruction and whether left ventricular hypertrophy is present. The peak Doppler velocity beyond the valve provides a reliable indication of the severity of stenosis. Turbulence occurs on colour Doppler at the level of obstruction. Cardiac catheterization is not necessary for diagnosis but is undertaken as part of therapeutic balloon dilatation of the aortic valve.

MANAGEMENT

Stenosis at the aortic valve level progresses with time. Progression may be rapid in the early few years of life or during adolescence. Percutaneous balloon dilatation or surgical valvotomy may be undertaken. In the former restenosis and aortic regurgitation occur. Once severe aortic regurgitation develops, or if obstruction cannot be relieved, valve replacement is necessary. The Ross procedure is the operation of choice in children. The aortic valve is replaced

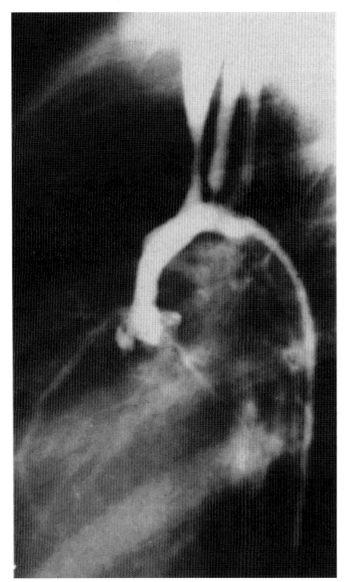

Figure 9.86 Supravalvar stenosis. Root aortogram showing a hypoplastic ascending aorta with strictures at the arterial origins. This infant had Williams syndrome.

by the patient's own pulmonary valve, and a homograft replaces the pulmonary valve. Subaortic stenosis is rarely relieved by balloon dilatation and requires surgery if the gradient reaches 40 mmHg. Localized supravalvar aortic stenosis responds well to surgery and re-operation is rarely necessary.

COARCTATION OF THE AORTA

Coarctation of the aorta is part of a spectrum of abnormalities ranging from a discrete narrowing at one end to an interrupted aortic arch at the other extreme where there is either complete discontinuity or an occluded cord between the ends of the aortic arch.

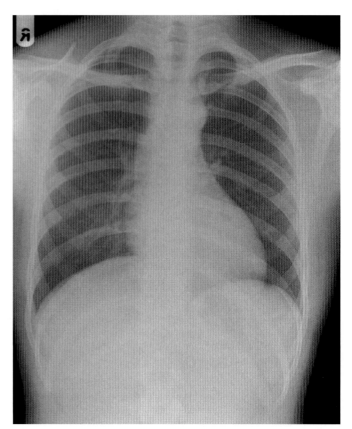

Figure 9.87 Prominent ascending aorta classically associated with a bicuspid aortic valve.

The 'infantile type' of coarctation is mainly tubular hypoplasia, in which there is a longer symmetrical segment of narrowing of the aortic arch in association with a more discrete distal narrowing, a patent ductus arteriosus plus or minus an intracardiac defect. Coarctation may form part of the hypoplastic left heart syndrome. The infantile type, interrupted aortic arch and hypoplastic left heart are considered in the neonatal section.

In the older child, discrete coarctations of the aorta are more commonly found. These are variably described as juxtaductal and postductal depending on the relationship of the narrowing to the insertion of the ductus or ligamentum arteriosum. They most commonly occur distal to the left subclavian artery and at or just beyond the ligamentum arteriosum, i.e. juxta- or post-ductal in location. Rarely, they are found proximal to the left subclavian artery. The isthmus is by definition that part of the aorta between the left subclavian artery and the site of insertion of the ductus or ligamentum arteriosus. Associated cardiovascular lesions more commonly found in the neonate due to early presentation include VSD, mitral valve abnormalities and bicuspid aortic valve. Discrete coarctation has been described in association with a right-sided and double aortic arch. Bicuspid aortic valves often become calcified, regurgitate and predispose to infective endocarditis.

The older child with a discrete coarctation is often asymptomatic and discovered due to the incidental finding of hypertension, which may be very severe, or a murmur. Coarctation is also associated with an increased incidence of Berry aneurysm.

INVESTIGATION

Chest radiograph

The heart is typically normal in size. In some cases, the ascending aorta is prominent just above the right hilum, particularly if there is an associated bicuspid aortic valve (Figure 9.87). A classically described notch often difficult to appreciate on the chest radiograph may be seen between the prestenotic dilation of the distal transverse arch and the poststenotic dilation of the descending thoracic aorta. This area of abnormality corresponds to the often described figure of 3 sign (Figure 9.88), the mid portion of the 3 representing the notch or site of narrowing. The reverse 3 sign is the corresponding finding on the barium swallow.

The presence and number of collaterals depends on the site and severity of narrowing and on the presence of associated abnormalities. They can be seen as early as infancy. Rib notching due to pressure erosion from the collateral vessels on the adjacent ribs is rarely seen before the age of 7–8 years. They are classically seen posteriorly from the 4th to 8th ribs (Figure 9.89). Dilated internal mammary arteries may cause retrosternal notching.

Echocardiography

This is accurate in the neonate and infant but due to a limited acoustic window may be difficult in the older child. Assessment of other intracardiac abnormalities can be obtained. The site and size of the coarctation can be assessed. Doppler studies may provide

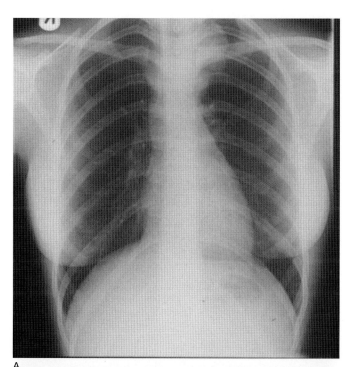

A

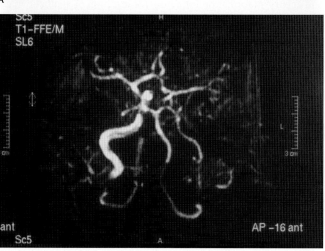

C

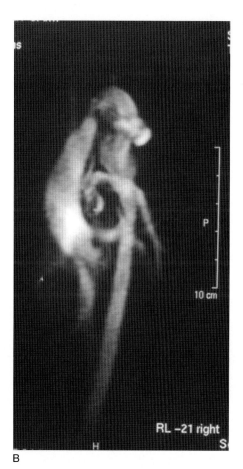

B

Figure 9.88 (A) Chest radiograph showing the typical dilatation of the distal arch of the aorta secondary to the narrowed coarcted area of the aorta. (B) Corresponding MR angiogram of a 14-year-old girl who presented with hypertension; lateral projection. (C) MR cerebral angiogram of the circle of Willis showing a right-sided Berry aneurysm.

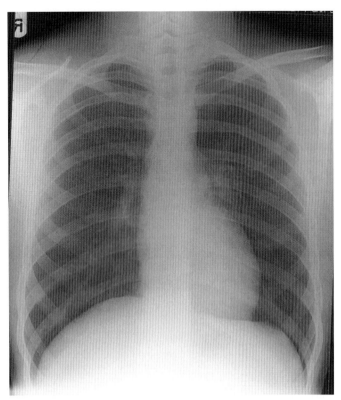

Figure 9.89 Chest radiograph demonstrates rib notching of the posterior aspect of the 4th and 5th ribs bilaterally. A stent is present in the descending aorta at the site of the coarctation.

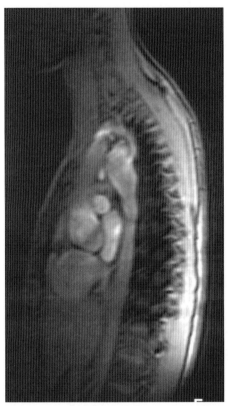

Figure 9.90 Sagittal oblique cine gradient echo of the thoracic aorta shows a typical coarctation in a juxtaductal position.

an assessment of the pressure gradient across the stenosis using the modified Bernoulli equation and derived from the maximal flow velocity. Continuous wave Doppler may demonstrate high flow across the coarctation as well as a classical diastolic tail when the stenosis is tight.

Magnetic resonance imaging

Qualitative and quantitative information can be obtained with MRI. The site and extent of stenosis, and relationship to the subclavian arteries and collateral vessels can all be demonstrated. Sagittal oblique T1 spin echo dark blood imaging and cine gradient echo white blood sequences are useful (Figure 9.90). Dynamic enhanced imaging gives an excellent three-dimensional view of the coarctation and collaterals. Velocity encoded phase contrast imaging gives information on the peak pressure gradient and measurements of left ventricular function can be obtained. In many cases, it can replace angiography.

Cardiac catheterization

Cardiac catheterization is now mainly used for treatment of the lesion by stenting or balloon angioplasty in children who on other imaging are deemed suitable.

MANAGEMENT

Management of the coarctation may be by balloon angioplasty, stenting or surgical repair depending on the severity and complexity of the lesion. Three different operations can be performed: a subclavian flap, resection and end-to-end anastomosis or insertion of a prosthetic patch aortoplasty. Postoperative complications include restenosis with the former two operations and aneurysm formation following the insertion of synthetic material. Balloon angioplasty is the preferred method following restenosis due to the higher postoperative mortality and morbidity with reoperations.

MITRAL STENOSIS

Congenital mitral valve stenosis is the most common type of mitral valve obstruction in the young population. It may occur with a central or asymmetrical orifice. Various components of the mitral valve may be abnormal including the leaflets, annulus, commissures, chordae tendinae and papillary muscles. In parachute mitral valve, which is relatively common the chordae tendinae insert onto a single rather than two papillary muscles resulting in obstruction. Congenital mitral stenosis is most often associated with coarctation of the aorta and aortic valve stenosis. Outcome tends to be influenced by associated abnormalities. The chest radiograph demonstrates left atrial enlargement and, in some cases, pulmonary venous hypertension. Echocardiography can assess the various components of the mitral valve, associated abnormalities, the presence of left atrial thrombus, coexisting mitral incompetence, as well as quantitative analysis derived from velocity measurements.

ACYANOTIC ABNORMALITIES CAUSING INCREASED VOLUME LOAD

VENTRICULAR SEPTAL DEFECT (VSD)

A ventricular septal defect is the most common congenital heart abnormality. The incidence of isolated ventricular septal defects is approximately 3.6–5.5 cases per 1000 live births. It may exist as a single abnormality or in association with other defects.

It is important to understand the anatomy of the right ventricle as the nomenclature and surgical approach is usually from the right ventricular side. The ventricular septum is divided into membranous and muscular parts. The membranous septum is the smallest of the three portions and lies closely related to the junction of the right and non-coronary cusp of the aortic valve. It is partially covered by the septal leaflet of the tricuspid valve, which may balloon through the defect partially closing it. The membranous septum is surrounded on all sides by muscular septum. It is well seen on the short axis parasternal view on echocardiography beneath the tricuspid valve and between the right and non-coronary cusps of the aortic valve. Most defects involving the membranous septum extend to involve the adjacent muscular septum and are therefore named perimembranous defects. They form the majority of ventricular septal defects.

The muscular septum is divided into three parts, which radiate from the membranous septum. The outlet part lies superiorly extending inferiorly from the papillary muscle of the conus to superiorly between the aortic and pulmonary valves. The trabecular portion extends from the membranous septum inferiorly to the apex forming the bulk of the muscular septum. It can be seen inferiorly on echocardiography in the parasternal long axis view, which also images the more superior infundibular or outlet septum. The third part of the muscular septum is the inlet septum extending from the membranous septum inferiorly between the tricuspid and mitral valves. Muscular defects are divided into inlet, outlet or trabecular depending on location. If multiple defects exist within the trabecular part of the membranous septum then it gives a Swiss cheese effect.

The size of the VSD is conventionally compared with the size of the aortic valve opening. Large defects, similar or larger than the aortic orifice, are non-restrictive in that they do not create resistance to flow. The systolic pressure in both ventricles is therefore similar. Small VSDs are typically restrictive, resulting in the pressure in the right ventricle being normal or slightly increased.

IMAGING FINDINGS

Chest radiograph

The chest radiographic findings depend on the size of the ventricular septal defect. When small, the chest radiograph may be normal. With larger defects cardiomegaly due to enlargement of the left atrium and left ventricle and in some cases right ventricle occurs. Pulmonary plethora due to the shunt is seen. The aorta is typically small. In untreated cases, pulmonary hypertension occurs. The chest radiograph reflects this. There is a decrease in the heart size as the shunt reverses to become right to left. Prominent central pulmonary arteries and peripheral pulmonary artery pruning develops. The patient then develops Eisenmenger syndrome, the reverse of normal flow across the defect. This is only seen in untreated cases.

Echocardiography

The size, number and position of the VSD can be determined. Colour Doppler imaging is useful in demonstrating small defects. With small defects the velocity is often greater than 4 m/s due to a normal right ventricular pressure. When the defects are large the left atrium and left ventricle are dilated and the velocity across the shunt decreases as right ventricular pressure increases.

Catheterization

This is rarely required except to evaluate associated lesions or on the child who presents late with pulmonary hypertension.

MANAGEMENT

Many of the smaller and particularly the muscular types of VSDs close spontaneously. Indications for surgery include failure to thrive, congestive heart failure and pulmonary hypertension. Other indications include endocarditis and aortic regurgitation though the latter is more common in adults with residual defects. Aortic prolapse tends to occur with the outlet muscular VSDs. When surgery is not indicated because of the presence of multiple muscular defects or chronic lung problems then a pulmonary artery band may be applied to limit pulmonary flow and the subsequent development of pulmonary hypertension.

ATRIAL SEPTAL DEFECT

ANATOMY

The atria are made up of four components, i.e. the venous part, vestibule, appendage and septal surface. The vestibule supports the AV valve. The septal surface of the right atrium is made up of the floor of the oval fossa and the surrounding muscle. The septum secundum is an infolding between the SVC and right pulmonary

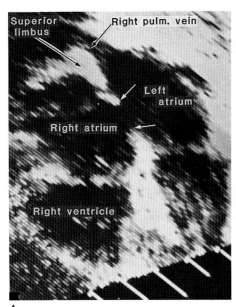

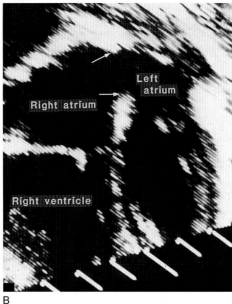

Figure 9.91 Cross-sectional echocardiograms of atrial septal defects (between arrows) in the subcostal view. (A) The typical location of a secundum defect and (B) the sinus venosus defect is superior to the intact rim of the oval fossa. (Reproduced with permission from Andersen RH et al. (eds). Paediatric cardiology, 2nd edn. Edinburgh: Churchill Livingstone; 2000:916).

veins. It forms the upper rim of the fossa. Only part of the septal surface of the atria truly separates the two atria. This is due to the infolding of the septum related to the SVC and IVC.

There are four types of atrial septal defects, classified according to their position within the septum. The most common type is the ostium secundum defect, situated in the region of the fossa ovalis (Figure 9.91). Ostium primum defects occur at the lower part of the septum and are partial AVSDs; they are discussed under that heading. Sinus venosus defects occur in the superior and posterior part of the atrial septum and are associated with partial anomalous venous drainage of the right upper pulmonary vein to the superior vena cava or right atrium.The defect lies outside the fossa ovalis and the SVC usually overrides the defect, which has the superior rim of the fossa ovalis as its inferior border (Figure 9.92). Sinus venosus defects involving the inferior vena cava are even less common. The coronary sinus travels in the atrioventricular groove. It normally drains into the right atrium adjacent to the inferior aspect of the atrioventricular groove. There may be partial absence of the roof of the coronary sinus as it passes close to the left atrium causing a direct communication. The mouth of the coronary sinus in the right atrium tends to be enlarged.

PHYSIOLOGY

The volume of left-to-right shunt depends on the size of the defect and the relative compliance of the ventricles. This determines the size of the right atrium, right ventricle, pulmonary artery and left atrium that receive the excessive blood flow. Pulmonary hypertension does not develop until adult life. A patent oval foramen is not usually haemodynamically significant but if the right atrial pressure is increased due to another cardiac abnormality, right-to-left shunting can occur with systemic desaturation. It may also be a cause of paradoxical systemic emboli.

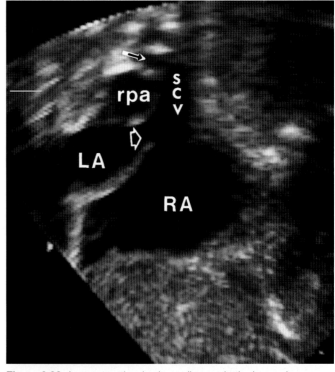

Figure 9.92 A cross-sectional echocardiogram in the long-axis subcostal view shows the pathognomonic feature of a superior sinus venosus defect (open arrow). There is overriding and bi-atrial connection of the SVC. Note the anomalous drainage of the right upper pulmonary vein (small arrow). LA, left atrium; RA, right atrium; RPA, right pulmonary artery. (Reproduced with permission from Andersen RH et al. (eds). Paediatric cardiology, 2nd edn. Edinburgh: Churchill Livingstone; 2000:916).

CLINICAL FEATURES

Presentation may be with an asymptomatic murmur or symptoms of tiredness, exertional dyspnoea or recurrent chest infections with large defects. Undiscovered defects may result in right heart failure or pulmonary hypertension.

INVESTIGATIONS

The chest radiograph may be normal when the shunt is small. Large atrial septal defects characteristically result in cardiomegaly with pulmonary plethora and an enlarged main pulmonary artery (Figure 9.93). The right atrium and ventricles are enlarged and the aorta is classically small and inconspicuous. With the development of pulmonary hypertension and Eisenmengers, the shunt will reverse to become right to left. The pulmonary vascularity may become normal and the main and branch pulmonary arteries are enlarged with peripheral pruning (Figure 9.94). This is seen in the older child.

Echocardiography confirms the size and type of defect together with a large right atrium, right ventricle and pulmonary artery. The four-chamber view will differentiate the various types of ASD. The velocity across the pulmonary valve is usually normal but may be increased due to flow. Cardiac catheterization is seldom necessary for diagnosis, except for sinus venosus defects when the pulmonary venous drainage is unclear. Similar anatomical information can be obtained with MRI.

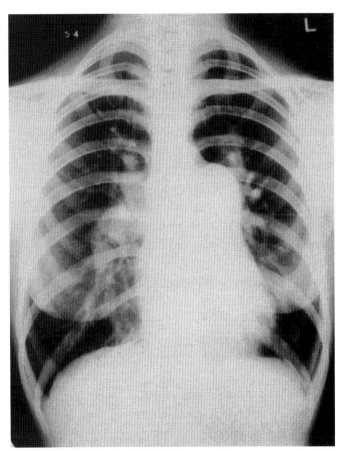

Figure 9.94 Pulmonary arterial hypertension. The central pulmonary arteries are very large. The peripheral arteries are pruned. This patient had Eisenmenger ASD.

Pulmonary artery pressures are normal or slightly elevated and the increase in oxygen content between systemic veins and pulmonary artery allows the left-to-right shunt ratio to be calculated. Angiography can identify the site of pulmonary venous drainage. Transoesophageal echocardiography also defines the defect and pulmonary veins.

MANAGEMENT AND PROGNOSIS

Many of the secundum defects and smaller defects will close spontaneously. Defects of more than 8 mm are unlikely to close. Percutaneous transcatheter closure of central defects with adequate supporting margins can be performed (Figure 9.95). Results are comparable to surgical closure. Surgical closure can be performed by either direct suture or patch.

FURTHER READING

Durongpisitkul K, Tang NL, Soongswang J, Laohaprasitiporn D, Nanal A. Predictors of successful transcatheter closure of atrial septal defect by cardiac magnetic resonance imaging. Pediatric Cardiology Dec 2003; 15 (Epub ahead of print).

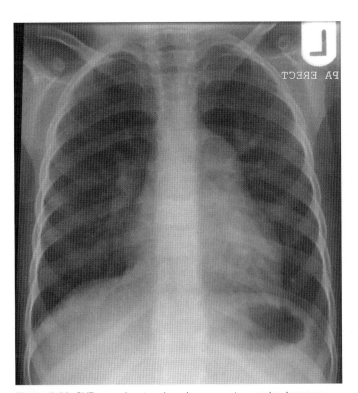

Figure 9.93 CXR, prominent main pulmonary artery and pulmonary plethora due to an atrial septal defect.

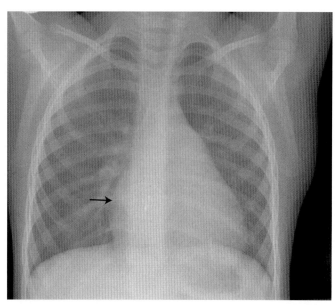

Figure 9.95 CXR, occlusion device in the interatrial septum across the ASD.

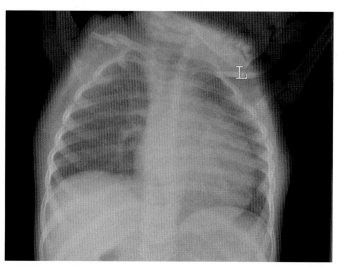

Figure 9.96 Chest radiograph shows an enlarged heart and pulmonary plethora due to a patent ductus arteriosus.

Durongpisitkul K, Soongswang J, Laohaprasitiporn D et al. Comparison of atrial septal defect closure using amplatzer septal occluder with surgery. Pediatric Cardiology 2002; 23:36–40.

Fischer G, Stieh J, Uebing A et al. Experience with transcatheter closure of secundum atrial septal defects using the Amplatzer septal occluder: a single center study in 236 consecutive patients. Heart 2003; 89:199–204.

PATENT ARTERIAL DUCT

ANATOMY

The ductus arteriosus is a normal structure usually connecting the pulmonary artery and descending aorta (Figure 9.96). When the aortic arch is right sided the arterial duct may also be right sided connecting the right pulmonary artery to the descending aorta. Rarely, there are bilateral ducts. A patent ductus arteriosus usually closes in the first few days of life by contraction of smooth muscle due to a combination of factors. This is delayed in premature infants, those born at high altitudes or who have other causes of relative hypoxia as with severe pulmonary disease. Associated congenital heart defects may be present.

Premature infants

Premature infants with and without associated lung disease have an increased incidence of patent ductus arteriosus. The incidence increases with very low birth weight. A frequent clinical presentation is deterioration several days postdelivery in a premature infant who is recovering from respiratory distress syndrome. A murmur may be intermittent. Other causes of lung disease need to be excluded. The chest radiograph in these infants may only show progressive cardiomegaly, pulmonary plethora or failure may not be evident. The echocardiogram enables an assessment of progressive enlargement of the left atrium, left ventricle and PDA. In those infants without lung disease a murmur may be heard from 24 h after birth. The infant may be asymptomatic or develop congestive heart failure if the shunt is large. The chest radiograph may be normal or demonstrate pulmonary plethora or oedema. Echocardiography usually demonstrates the shunt. Management may be with medical therapy until closure, transcatheter closure or surgical ligation.

Term infants and older children

A patent ductus arteriosus can be isolated, occur in association with congenital rubella infection or be familial. The presentation depends on the size of the duct. When small, it may be picked up as an asymptomatic murmur. The chest radiograph is often normal and the diagnosis is made by echocardiography. Larger ducts present as poor weight gain, irritability, recurrent chest infections and congestive failure. The chest radiograph will show cardiomegaly with enlargement of the left atrium, left ventricle and main pulmonary artery. Pulmonary plethora with superimposed pulmonary oedema may be evident. If left untreated those who survive may develop improvement in the clinical picture with reduction in heart size and pulmonary vascularity. This typically occurs around 18 months of age. These are sinister findings and indicate the development of irreversible pulmonary hypertension with reversal of the shunt. Endocarditis is a rare complication. Management includes catheter closure if the duct is not large, i.e. less than 5–6 mm or surgical closure (Figure 9.97). Late presentation with irreversible pulmonary hypertension is an absolute contraindication to duct closure.

ATRIOVENTRICULAR SEPTAL DEFECT

ANATOMY

Atrioventricular septal defects (AVSDs) represent a spectrum of conditions that have in common a deficiency of the atrioventricular septum and adjacent valves. It is particularly common in infants with Down's syndrome. All have a reduced ventricular septal length from apex to inlet, a goose neck deformity of the left ventricular outflow tract, which is best appreciated on angiography. It is due to the aortic valve not being wedged between the abnormal AV valve and abnormalities in the position of the conduction system. The AVSD has been classified for simplicity into complete and incomplete forms. A partial atrioventricular septal defect is often described as an ostium primum atrial septal defect associated with an abnormal AV valve containing two valve annuli. Often, the anterior leaflet of the left AV valve has a cleft. Less often, an interventricular communication is present. Classification becomes confusing and an intermediate AVSD is variably used to describe these slightly more complex partial defects. A complete atrioventricular septal defect consists of an AV valve with a common annulus and usually five leaflets. An atrial and/or ventricular septal component may be present (Figure 9.98). The lesion was previously called an endocardial cushion defect or common atrioventricular canal.

PARTIAL DEFECTS

Partial defects usually have two separate atrioventricular valves at the same level. Children with partial atrioventricular septal defects have haemodynamics similar to an atrial septal defect. There is virtually always a cleft in the anterior leaflet of the mitral valve, which may cause regurgitation. Symptoms occur early when there is significant mitral regurgitation. The regurgitant jet may pass directly from the left ventricle to the right atrium.

Occasionally, left ventricular outflow tract obstruction or a hypoplastic ventricle can complicate the clinical picture. Tetralogy of Fallot, double outlet right ventricle transposition of the great vessels and heterotaxia, especially with asplenia, may coexist. Down's syndrome is present in over 65% of children with a

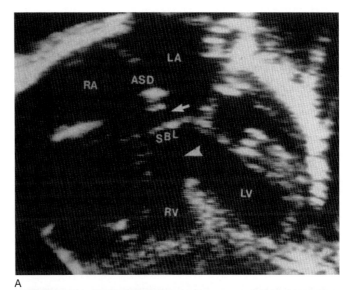

A

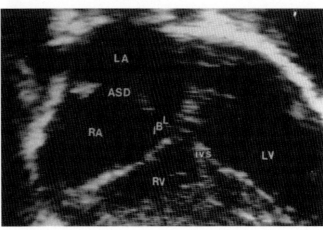

B

Figure 9.98 Echocardiogram of an infant with a complete AVSD. The patient also has a secundum ASD. Four-chamber two-dimensional views. (A) The interatrial component of the defect (arrow) lies above the superior bridging leaflet (SBL) of the common atrioventricular valve, and the interventricular component of the defect (arrowhead) lies below this leaflet. (B) The inferior bridging leaflet (IBL) of the common valve is attached to the crest of the interventricular septum (IVS). RA, right atrium; RV, right ventricle; LA, left atrium; LV, left ventricle.

Figure 9.97 Chest radiograph demonstrates an occlusion device in a patent ductus arteriosus.

complete atrioventricular septal defect and 25% of those with a partial defect.

COMPLETE DEFECTS

In the complete atrioventricular septal defect, there is a single (common) atrioventricular valve. They are physiologically similar to a ventricular septal defect.

The atrioventricular valves are always regurgitant. If this is severe, the haemodynamic effect adds to that of the septal defect.

INVESTIGATIONS

The chest radiograph usually demonstrates an enlarged heart with pulmonary plethora resulting from left-to-right shunting (Figure 9.99). Echocardiography identifies the anatomical type of atrioventricular septal defect and the size of the atrial and ventricular components. It allows evaluation of ventricular size and balance, atrioventricular valve regurgitation and other cardiac lesions. It also provides information on the degree of pulmonary hypertension. Cardiac catheterization may be required to assess pulmonary vascular resistance in older infants and children. Angiography defines the atrial and ventricular septal defects and atrioventricular valve regurgitation.

MANAGEMENT AND PROGNOSIS

Partial atrioventricular septal defects are closed surgically slightly later and preferably as soon as left AV regurgitation is demon-

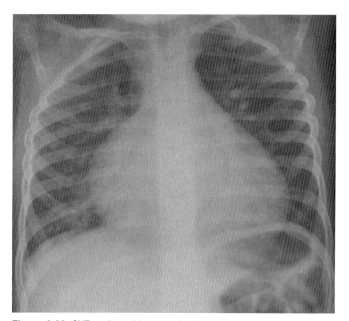

Figure 9.99 CXR, enlarged heart and pulmonary plethora due to an AVSD.

strated. Complete atrioventricular septal defects require surgery at 3–6 months of age or earlier if congestive failure complicates the clinical picture. Pulmonary artery banding may be performed to defer definitive surgery in infants with other lesions or when surgery carries a high risk. At the time of definitive surgery the left atrioventricular valve is repaired to reduce regurgitation and improve outcome. Re-operation is occasionally necessary for left atrioventricular valve regurgitation or stenosis, or left ventricular outflow tract obstruction. A few patients require a pacemaker for complete heart block after surgery, or develop late supraventricular tachyarrhythmias.

AORTOPULMONARY WINDOW

This rare congenital abnormality is a defect between the ascending aorta and pulmonary trunk above valve level. It most often occurs between the left lateral wall of the aorta and the right side of the pulmonary trunk. Presentation is usually with congestive failure in the neonatal period or infancy. The chest radiograph may demonstrate cardiomegaly and pulmonary plethora but can be normal when the communication is small. The diagnosis is usually made with echocardiography when other associated cardiac abnormalities can be identified. The presence of two separate valves allows differentiation from a common trunk. Magnetic resonance imaging will demonstrate the lesion. Early surgery is warranted in order to prevent irreversible damage to the pulmonary vascularity.

CORONARY ARTERY FISTULA

A fistula may occur between the branches of a coronary artery and an adjacent vessel or heart chamber. It is a rare abnormality and is often an isolated finding. The right coronary artery is the most commonly involved often with drainage into the right atrium or ventricle. A left-to-right shunt develops. It may be haemodynamically insignificant and asymptomatic. Heart failure is rare. Dyspnoea or chest pain may be due to 'stealing' of blood from the coronary circulation. Often it is discovered due to the finding of a murmur, which mimics a patent ductus but in an unusual location. The chest radiograph may be normal or demonstrate cardiomegaly or an unusual contour due to the presence of a large fistula. Echocardiography may demonstrate the fistula. Cardiac angiography may be required for a more detailed assessment and for therapeutic embolization.

RUPTURED ANEURYSM OF VALSALVA

Congenital aneurysm of the aortic sinus of Valsalva is a rare abnormality due to weakness of the wall. The right sinus is the most often involved and it may rupture into the right ventricle or atrium producing a left-to-right shunt. Symptoms of heart failure develop acutely. The findings on the chest radiograph are non-specific and include vascular congestion. Diagnosis is made by echocardiography and treatment is surgical.

MITRAL REGURGITATION

Mitral regurgitation may occur in association with a large number of congenital and acquired conditions, e.g. AVSD, VSD, PDA, coarctation of the aorta, rheumatic endocarditis, Marfan syndrome, Kawasaki disease and many other conditions. As an isolated congenital abnormality it is rare. It may be found with mitral valve prolapse, a cleft or prolapsed mitral valve.

Clinical presentation depends on associated lesions. Symptoms and signs of congestive failure occur earlier in infants and children than adults. The chest radiograph may demonstrate left atrial and left ventricular enlargement as well as signs of pulmonary venous congestion. Echocardiography will demonstrate the morphology of the regurgitant valve and enable an assessment of the severity of the regurgitation based on calculations of regurgitant jet width and area on colour Doppler. Indirect findings based on left atrial and left ventricular size are also useful. Cardiac catheterization is rarely necessary. Management is mainly medical but surgical in severe cases. Conservative surgical reconstruction or valvuloplasty is preferred over valve replacement in infants and children.

AORTIC REGURGITATION

Aortic regurgitation rarely occurs in isolation in children. It may occur with a congenitally stenotic bicuspid valve, a subaortic ventricular septal defect or following endocarditis or rheumatic fever. The chest radiograph will demonstrate cardiomegaly, enlargement of the left atrium and a prominent ascending aorta. It may, however, be normal. Echocardiography will demonstrate the abnormality and enable an assessment of severity from the left ventricular size at end diastole. In severe isolated aortic regurgitation, surgical repair is required. The Ross procedure involves replacing the aortic valve with a pulmonary homograft. This has the advantage of not requiring anticoagulation and being less susceptible to endocarditis than a prosthetic aortic valve replacement.

TRICUSPID REGURGITATION

Tricuspid regurgitation is usually associated with Ebstein's anomaly (Figure 9.100).

PULMONARY REGURGITATION

Trivial regurgitation detected on colour Doppler echocardiography is a normal finding. Isolated pulmonary regurgitation is rare. It may occur in Marfan syndrome, following repair of Fallot's tetralogy or as a result of pulmonary hypertension. Absence of the pulmonary valve in tetralogy of Fallot causes severe pulmonary regurgitation with markedly dilated pulmonary arteries.

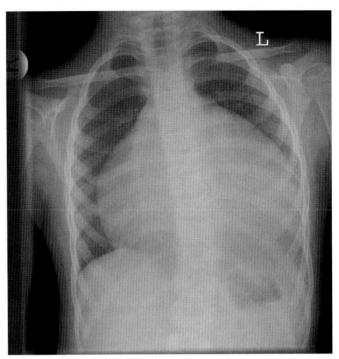

Figure 9.100 CXR, enlarged heart with pulmonary oligaemia in a child with Ebstein's anomaly.

CYANOTIC LESIONS

FALLOT'S TETRALOGY

Tetralogy of Fallot (TOF) is the commonest cause of cyanotic congenital heart disease presenting beyond the neonatal period, though in western society it is unusual not to diagnose this at birth. It is characterized by right ventricular outflow (RVOT) obstruction, an overriding aorta, ventricular septal defect and right ventricular hypertrophy.

RVOT obstruction characteristically occurs in a subpulmonic or infundibular position and it is generally agreed that this is due to deviation of the conal, outlet or infundibular septum in a cephalad and anterior direction. Subpulmonic narrowing may occur in association with obstruction at the valvar, supravalvar and peripheral pulmonary artery levels. The left pulmonary artery is more commonly involved than the right, seen as asymmetrical pulmonary vascularity on a preoperative chest radiograph.

In most cases of Fallot's tetralogy, the VSD is perimembranous, occurring below the right and non-coronary cusps of the aortic valve; it can be seen on a parasternal long-axis view or in more detail in the short-axis view just below the aortic valve. The VSD is classically non-restrictive, i.e. non-obstructive. An AVSD less commonly occurs and most often in association with trisomy 21. The overriding aorta is also related to the displacement of the infundibular septum. If the aorta lies 50% or less over the right ventricle then it is called overriding, whereas if it is >50% over the right ventricle then a double outlet right ventricle (DORV) is present. Another method of distinguishing DORV and Fallot's tetralogy is by identifying a subaortic and subpulmonic conus in the former. The parasternal long-axis view on echo or the equivalent MRI view demonstrate the overriding aorta well. Right ventricular hypertrophy occurs secondary to the subpulmonic obstruction.

ASSOCIATED FINDINGS

The aortic arch is right sided in 25% of cases. There may be an associated aberrant subclavian artery, important for the surgeon to know about when considering a Blalock shunt connecting the subclavian artery to the pulmonary artery, which is usually performed on the side opposite the arch. There is an association with a secundum ASD, AVSD especially in children with Down's syndrome, anomalous origin of the anterior descending artery from the right coronary artery and enlargement of the conus branch of the right coronary artery. Anomalies of the coronary arteries are particularly important for the surgeon to know about when considering right ventriculotomy. Absence of the pulmonary valve or of a branch pulmonary artery can occur.

PATHOPHYSIOLOGY

After birth blood flow to the lungs increases due to a reduction in pulmonary vascular resistance. In an infant or child with Fallot's tetralogy, blood flow to the lungs may be via a narrowed ventricular outflow tract only. In others with moderate to severe outflow obstruction, pulmonary flow may be dependent on a single or bilateral arterial ducts or major aortopulmonary collateral arteries (MAPCAs). Discussion in this section will be limited to cases with right ventricular outflow obstruction without MAPCAs or patent duct. In most cases, the VSD is large and consequently the pressure within the right and left ventricle are equal. If the resistance of the right ventricular outflow is less than systemic then a left-to-right shunt will occur and the child will not appear cyanosed (pink tetralogy). The more severe the right ventricular outflow obstruction with pulmonary resistance increasing to systemic resistance, then the greater the right-to-left shunt. If systemic resistance decreases, e.g. with administration of anaesthetic agents, then the pressure within both ventricles drops leading to a decrease in pulmonary blood flow. Pulmonary blood flow depends on the degree of resistance to pulmonary outflow as well as systemic vascular resistance. In most cases, the pulmonary artery pressure is normal or low.

INVESTIGATIONS

The heart is usually normal in size. There is a concavity in the pulmonary bay due to a small pulmonary trunk. The apex is often elevated due to right ventricular hypertrophy. In approximately 25% of cases of TOF the aortic arch is right sided. An upper right superior mediastinal opacity is then seen indenting the right side of the trachea. This finding together with concavity of the pulmonary bay and an elevated apex due to right ventricular hypertrophy describe the classical chest radiographic findings of a boot-shaped heart (Figure 9.101). Pulmonary vascularity is most often reduced but

may be asymmetrical due to unilateral peripheral pulmonary stenosis. There are, however, varying degrees of severity of the components of TOF (right ventricular hypertrophy, right ventricular outflow obstruction, overriding aorta and VSD). In less severe cases, the right ventricular outflow obstruction may be mild such that the interventricular shunt is balanced or left to right with normal or increased pulmonary vascularity. In pulmonary atresia and VSD, the most severe type of TOF, the main pulmonary artery is absent and systemic collateral vessels arise from the aorta and supply the lung. The pulmonary vascularity has a bizarre and slightly disorganized appearance on the chest radiograph (Figure 9.102).

Echocardiography will demonstrate all the features of tetralogy and enable assessment of associated anomalies (Figure 9.103). Doppler is useful to assess the size and direction of the VSD. Doppler velocity will determine the pressure gradient between the right ventricle and pulmonary artery. Cardiac catheterization and angiography may be performed to assess the pulmonary and coronary arteries.

MANAGEMENT

Interventional procedures include balloon dilatation of the right ventricular outflow tract which may be performed as a palliative procedure prior to definitive operation or following complete repair to dilate a residual narrowing. Coil embolization of systemic collaterals to the lung segments with a dual supply may be performed. A modified Blalock–Taussig shunt, between the subclavian artery and pulmonary artery, may be performed as a palliative procedure in those patients with small pulmonary arteries in order to allow further growth. Complications include chylothorax, diaphragmatic paralysis and a seroma related to the shunt. There

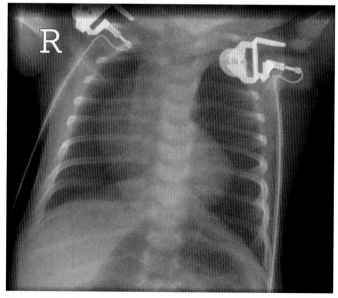

Figure 9.101 Classical boot-shaped heart in Fallot's tetralogy. Concavity in the pulmonary bay, right aortic arch and elevated apex due to right ventricular hypertrophy.

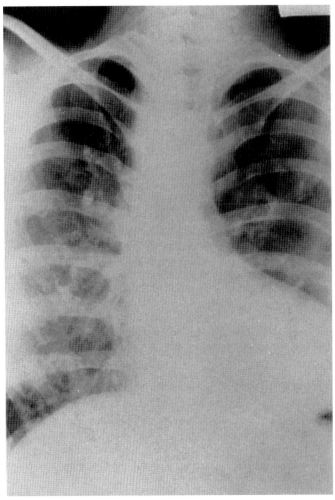

Figure 9.102 A patient with pulmonary atresia and systemic supply to the lungs. The main pulmonary arteries are not visible. Large disorganized vessels are seen at the hila. The aortic arch is right sided.

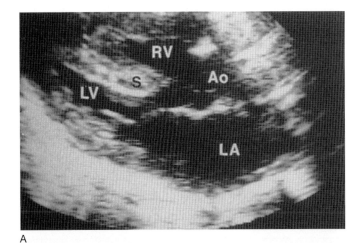

A

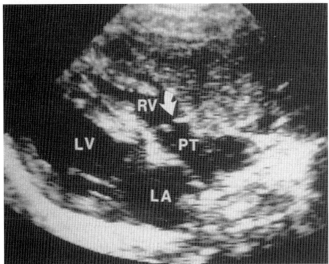

B

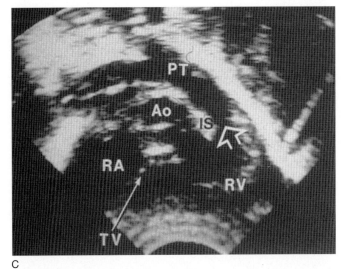

C

Figure 9.103 Tetralogy of Fallot: (A,B) long-axis views and (C) a short-axis view. The long-axis views show a hypertrophied RV, a large aortic root (Ao), which overrides the septum (s). A subaortic intraventricular septal defect and thickened pulmonary valve leaflets (arrow) are also visible. The short-axis view shows infundibular stenosis (open arrow) due to anterior displacement of the infundibular septum (IS).

is now the tendency to perform a primary repair in the first year of life. The ventricular septal defect is closed and the right ventricular outflow tract is enlarged by muscle resection, pulmonary valvotomy and occasionally by patch augmentation, which can be extended to include the branch pulmonary arteries.

PULMONARY ATRESIA AND VENTRICULAR SEPTAL DEFECT

Pulmonary atresia with ventricular septal defect is often described as the severe form of TOF. Pulmonary blood flow then depends on a persistent arterial duct or major systemic collaterals often arising from the aorta (MAPCAs). Surgical repair is determined by the presence of confluent branch pulmonary arteries; when present a pulmonary conduit may be used to attach the confluent pulmonary arteries to the right ventricle. On the other hand, if the branch pulmonary arteries do not join and are therefore non-confluent, then the MAPCAs can be joined to the right ventricle in the unifocalization procedure. MRI can demonstrate the branch pulmonary artery size, whether they are confluent and the presence and origin of MAPCAs without the need for radiation.

TETRALOGY OF FALLOT WITH ABSENT PULMONARY VALVE

This condition is characterized by severe pulmonary regurgitation and aneurysmal dilatation of the pulmonary arteries (Figure 9.104). The enlarged arteries may compress the adjacent bronchi. Surgery is aimed at reducing the size of the pulmonary arteries.

MISCELLANEOUS CONDITIONS

VASCULAR RINGS

The trachea and airways can be compressed by various vascular structures, significant and symptomatic ones present with stridor, respiratory distress or feeding difficulties. Often seen is an aberrant right subclavian artery arising below the ductus from the aorta and crossing behind the oesophagus. It is asymptomatic and may be found incidentally on barium studies or cross-sectional imaging (Figure 9.105).

There are five important anomalies: vascular rings, aberrant right subclavian artery, innominate arterial compression, aberrant left pulmonary artery and the less common absence of the pulmonary valve. The pattern of indentation of the trachea and oesophagus is useful in confirming the presence of vascular compression and gives guidance on the likely cause.

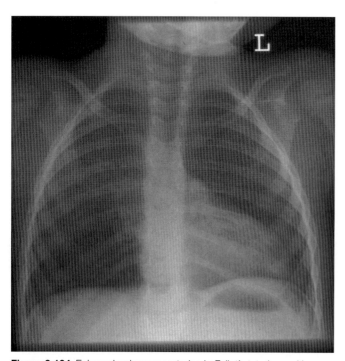

Figure 9.104 Enlarged pulmonary arteries in Fallot's tetralogy with absent pulmonary valve.

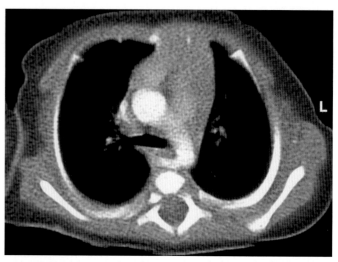

Figure 9.105 Contrast-enhanced CT shows an aberrant right subclavian artery coursing posterior to the oesophagus and trachea.

The two most common vascular rings include a double aortic arch and a right aortic arch with an aberrant left subclavian artery and a left ligamentum arteriosum.

DOUBLE AORTIC ARCH

Both right and left aortic arches are present; the right aortic arch is characteristically the larger of the two and gives off the right subclavian and common carotid arteries either as a common brachiocephalic artery or as two separate vessels. The left arch is usually smaller in size and may in fact be atretic beyond the origin of the great vessels, which include the left common carotid and left subclavian arteries.

The arches unite posteriorly to form the descending aorta which is usually left sided.

A chest radiograph may demonstrate right-sided indentation of the trachea by the right aortic arch. The barium swallow will also demonstrate a right-sided indentation on the AP view as well as a lower left indentation due to the smaller and more anterior left arch. Posterior indentation of the oesophagus on the lateral view will alert the radiologist to the presence of a vascular ring (Figure 9.106). Further imaging should be with MRI, which has the advantage of demonstrating the airways and fibrous atretic left arch as well as enabling multiplanar and three-dimensional imaging. Most double aortic arches are not associated with intracardiac abnormalities. Dynamically enhanced CT imaging will provide similar information as MRI.

It is important to inform the surgeon of the relative sizes of the aortic arches as the side of thoracotomy usually coincides with the smaller arch.

RIGHT AORTIC ARCH, ABERRANT LEFT SUBCLAVIAN ARTERY AND LIGAMENTUM OR DUCTUS

The trachea is encircled by the right aortic arch, posterior aberrant left subclavian artery and ligamentum or ductus passing from the

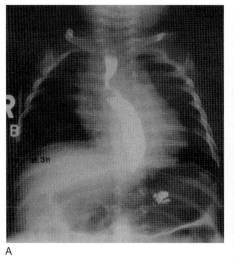
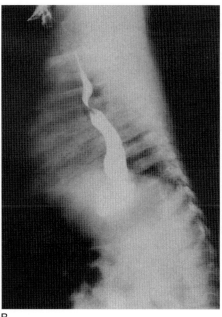
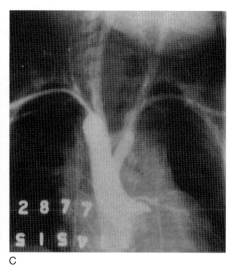

Figure 9.106 Double aortic arch. (A) Barium oesophogram showing compression of both sides of the oesophagus and (B) lateral view showing the posterior compression. (C) Corresponding aortogram showing a persistent double arch. The right is larger and more cephalad.

aberrant left subclavian to the more anterior left pulmonary artery. In order, the great vessels arising from the right aortic arch are, from anterior to posterior, the left common carotid artery, right brachiocephalic artery and lastly left subclavian artery, which passes posterior to the oesophagus. The aberrant subclavian artery may be associated with a diverticulum near its origin, often referred to as a Kommerell diverticulum.

In comparison, mirror image branching of the great vessels arising from a right aortic arch is often associated with congenital heart disease but does not usually cause a vascular ring. It describes the branching pattern in order from anterior to posterior, left brachiocephalic artery, right common carotid artery and lastly the right subclavian artery.

LESS COMMON VASCULAR RINGS

Other less common causes of a vascular ring include a left aortic arch and right descending aorta with a right ligamentum, a right aortic arch and left descending aorta with a left ligamentum and a right aortic arch with mirror image branching and a ductus diverticulum and ligament arising from the right descending thoracic aorta.

A mediastinal mass may be the first clue to the diagnosis. A cervical aortic arch is one that arises above the level of the clavicles. It may be right or left sided and associated with a normal branching pattern or occur with an aberrant subclavian artery and ductus diverticulum, the latter forming a vascular ring. The descending aorta may descend on the side opposite the arch. Magnetic resonance imaging or dynamic enhanced CT will demonstrate the position of the arch and descending aorta, define the branching pattern and assess the relationship to the trachea.

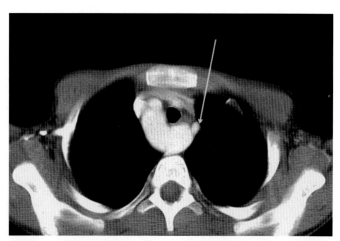

Figure 9.107 Axial contrast-enhanced image of the upper mediastinum shows a right aortic arch and aberrant left subclavian artery (white arrow) arising from a diverticulum.

ABERRANT LEFT SUBCLAVIAN ARTERY

Most cases of right aortic arch with an aberrant left subclavian artery are asymptomatic (Figure 9.107). If a patent ductus or ligamentum connects from the aberrant left subclavian artery to the left pulmonary artery then a vascular ring is formed.

ABERRANT RIGHT SUBCLAVIAN ARTERY

A left aortic arch with an aberrant right subclavian artery is a fairly common incidental finding occurring in approximately 0.5% of the population. Posterior indentation only of the oesophagus is demonstrated on barium swallow and is characteristically seen as an oblique shallow indentation crossing from a left inferior direction to a right superior position. It is the last vessel to arise from the aortic arch and passes directly behind the oesophagus. It may rarely cause dysphagia but does not cause stridor.

A Kommerell diverticulum was originally described in association with an aberrant right subclavian artery and left aortic arch, the right subclavian artery arising from the diverticulum and directly from the descending aorta.

PULMONARY SLING

A pulmonary sling occurs when the left pulmonary artery arises from the right pulmonary artery. It passes posteriorly between the trachea and oesophagus. The right main bronchus may be compressed as the left pulmonary artery passes over it and this may in turn lead to hyperinflation of the right lung (Figure 9.108). The relative overinflation of the right lung may also be due to a hypoplastic or small aberrant left pulmonary artery. Tracheal rings with stenosis of the distal trachea are common associations.

INNOMINATE ARTERY COMPRESSION

A controversial entity, it is thought to occur when there is anterior compression of the trachea by an innominate artery. Absence of the pulmonary valve is discussed above (see 'Fallot's tetralogy').

FURTHER READING

Berdon WE. Rings, slings, and other things: vascular compression of the infant trachea updated from the mid-century to the millennium – the legacy of Robert E. Gross, MD, and Edward B.D. Neuhauser, M.D. Radiology 2000; 216:624–634.

MARFAN SYNDROME

Marfan syndrome is a connective tissue disorder involving multiple systems including the skeletal, ocular, pulmonary, skin and central nervous system. The cardiovascular involvement, present in almost all patients, is an important cause of morbidity. Progressive enlargement of the aortic root and aortic dissection are

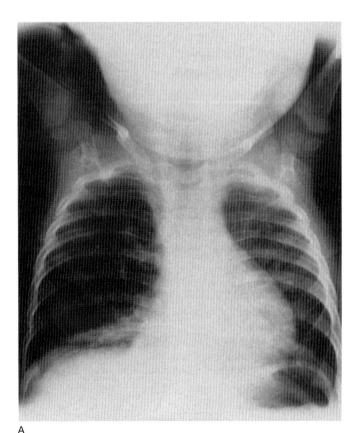
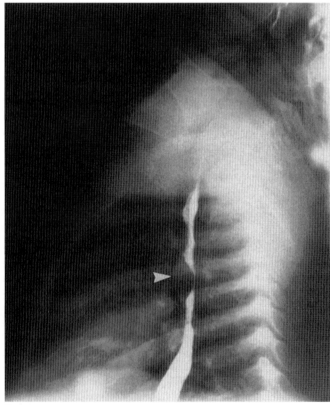

A

B

Figure 9.108 Anomalous origin of the left pulmonary artery. (A) There is hyperinflation of the right lung with collapse consolidation of the right middle lobe. (B) Barium oesophagram shows the anomalous left pulmonary artery as an oval density (arrowhead) compressing the oesophagus anteriorly, lying behind the trachea.

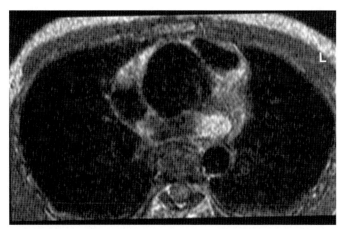

Figure 9.109 Axial ECG gated T1-weighted SE of the heart demonstrates an enlarged ascending aorta in a patient with Marfan syndrome.

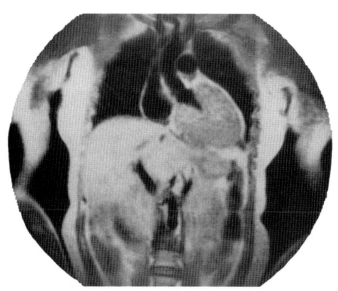

Figure 9.110 MRI of a patient with hypertrophic cardiomyopathy. Note the diffuse severe hypertrophy of the left ventricle with a small ventricular cavity.

the major complications that require monitoring. Transthoracic echocardiography and MRI are important modalities in assessing the aortic root size (Figure 9.109). Measurements are typically obtained at the valve annulus, aortic sinus and sinotubular junction.

Other complications include aortic regurgitation, mitral prolapse and regurgitation, and abdominal aortic aneurysm.

ACQUIRED DISEASES

INFECTIVE ENDOCARDITIS

Infective endocarditis is an important cause of morbidity and mortality. It is a well known complication of underlying congenital heart disease both pre- and postoperatively, particularly following the insertion of a prosthetic shunt. Premature neonates and any child with central venous lines are further groups at risk. Endocarditis is also described in children without an obvious underlying risk factor. High flow abnormalities, particularly ventricular septal defect, a patent ductus arteriosus and aortic stenosis predispose to endocarditis. The postoperative risk in the former two conditions is negligible following complete repair of solitary defects, however there is a significant residual risk of endocarditis postoperatively in patients with valvar aortic stenosis, particularly following insertion of a prosthetic valve. The risk of endocarditis is relatively low in isolated pulmonary stenosis, atrioventricular septal defect, atrial septal defect and pulmonary stenosis.

A high index of suspicion is important as the clinical presentation is often non-specific and variable. Positive blood cultures and the demonstration of vegetations on the cardiac structures or lines by echocardiography confirm the diagnosis. Magnetic resonance imaging, particularly gradient echo sequences, is emerging as a useful diagnostic tool in demonstrating vegetations. Complications include valve regurgitation, mycotic aneurysm formation, aortic root abscess and fistula, congestive heart failure, and systemic and pulmonary abscess formation.

HEART MUSCLE DISEASE

HYPERTROPHIC CARDIOMYOPATHY

Often familial, in hypertrophic cardiomyopathy there is idiopathic thickening of a non-dilated left ventricle.

The majority of patients do not have left outflow obstruction. The degree of ventricular myocardial thickening varies amongst patients and it may be asymmetrical. Anterior systolic motion of the mitral valve is highly specific for the condition though not a sensitive indicator. Myocardial ischaemia is common. Patients become symptomatic in early adulthood. Sudden mortality due to ventricular arrhythmia is highest is childhood. Most children are asymptomatic prior to the fatal event.

The chest radiograph may be normal or may demonstrate a bulky heart. Cardiomegaly is only usually seen late in the course of the disease. Echocardiography usually demonstrates myocardial thickening, particularly involving the septum, anterior systolic motion of the mitral valve and early closure of the aortic valve. MRI may also demonstrate the left ventricular muscle bulk (Figure 9.110).

MYOCARDITIS

Myocarditis is inflammation of the cardiac muscle, which causes disordered contractility and may lead to failure. Most identifiable causes are due to a viral infection; other causes include connective tissue disorders, drugs and Kawasaki disease. The chest radiograph demonstrates generalized cardiomegaly and pulmonary oedema. A dilated poorly functioning left ventricle is seen with echocardiography. The differential diagnosis includes other causes of congestive failure including hypoxia and hypoglycaemia in the neonatal period.

ARRHYTHMOGENIC RIGHT VENTRICULAR DYSPLASIA-CARDIOMYOPATHY

This is a primary muscle disorder that predominantly involves the right ventricle. It may be picked up incidentally as an abnormal ECG tracing or present as exercise-induced or spontaneous tachycardia. Often there is a positive family history. It is an important condition to recognize as it may result in ventricular arrhythmias or lead to sudden death in young patients. The muscle, particularly the free wall of the right ventricle, becomes replaced by fibrofatty tissue. Echocardiography may demonstrate enlargement of the right ventricle as well as dyskinesia of the ventricular wall. Angiography although invasive may also show localized areas of altered motion of the right ventricular wall. Magnetic resonance imaging is emerging as a useful non-invasive tool for diagnosis. ECG gated T1 spin echo and cine gradient echo sequences are useful in showing fatty replacement of the muscle as well as focal areas of hypokinesia, respectively. Aneurysms or dilatation of the right ventricle or right ventricular outflow tract may be evident. Fatty replacement, seen as high signal on the T1-weighted sequences, may not be present in every case.

CARDIAC TUMOURS

Primary cardiac tumours are rare in children. Clinical presentation is with symptoms of outflow obstruction or from emboli. They may be discovered antenatally. Rhabdomyomas are the commonest type. Other tumours include fibromas in all age groups, teratomas in neonates and infants and myxomas in older children. Congestive failure may be the presentation in newborns and simulate a hypoplastic left heart. Rhabdomyomas are often multiple and have an association with tuberous sclerosis. They most often involve the ventricles. Children with rhabdomyomas may be asymptomatic or have symptoms related to outflow obstruction of the right or left side of the heart. Arrhythmias may cause sudden death. On echo, they are homogeneous solid echogenic masses. They may spontaneously regress in time. Surgical excision is necessary if life-threatening arrhythmias or outflow obstruction causes severe haemodynamic disturbances.

Fibromas tend to be single and involve the interventricular septum or free wall of the left ventricle. Like rhabdomyomas they tend to be homogeneous and echogenic on echocardiography.

Teratomas are most often intrapericardial and involve the base of the heart. They are more often right sided and compress adjacent structures. They are often found between the ascending aorta and SVC. They are heterogeneous with cystic and calcified elements. They may be benign or malignant; malignant lesions may infiltrate the cardiac structures or great vessels. The main differential is a bronchogenic cyst. Bronchogenic cysts do not contain neural elements and are cystic without solid elements. Pericardial effusions are often associated with intrapericardial teratomas.

Myxomas are benign solitary tumours, which mainly occur in the atria particularly on the left (Figure 9.111). They may cause obstruction to pulmonary venous or atrioventricular flow or produce distal emboli.

The heart may be invaded by non-Hodgkin's lymphoma, neuroblastoma or leukaemia, as well as by other tumours.

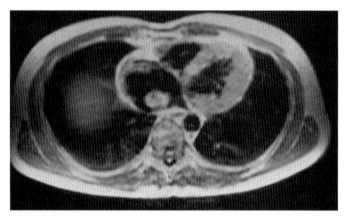

Figure 9.111 Left atrial myxoma. MRI scan demonstrates a pedunculated mass in the left atrium.

RHEUMATIC FEVER AND RHEUMATIC HEART DISEASE

The incidence of rheumatic fever in developed countries is again rising. It remains an important condition due to the subsequent development of rheumatic heart disease. Diagnosis can be difficult due to the non-specific presentation. Clinical signs include a fleeting arthritis, sore throat and a rash.

A pancarditis, which is usually clinically silent, occurs in approximately 50% of children and is more common in children under 3 years of age. The diagnosis of cardiac involvement is made by echocardiography with colour Doppler flow. Progressive mitral valve thickening and chordal shortening or a combination of aortic and mitral incompetence with cusp thickening are changes specific for acute rheumatic fever. Pericardial effusion or reduced ejection fraction are non-specific.

RHEUMATIC HEART DISEASE

The risk of rheumatic heart disease increases with increasing severity of initial cardiac involvement and younger age at the time of the initial attack. The mitral valve is most often involved followed by the aortic valve. Isolated aortic valve disease is rare.

Mitral regurgitation is the commonest lesion in children with rheumatic heart disease. In older children and adults, it may be associated with mitral stenosis. The appearances on the radiograph are cardiomegaly with an enlarged left atrium. As disease progresses interstitial pulmonary oedema develops. Echocardiography confirms enlargement of the left atrium and left ventricle and colour Doppler shows the presence of regurgitation and gives an estimate of its severity. The mitral valve leaflets are thickened and tethered. Fibrosis and calcification of the valve and reduced mobility of the leaflets is also seen. M-mode echocardiography demonstrates a reduced closure rate of the anterior mitral valve leaflet. The Doppler signal shows an increased velocity and reduced rate of pressure fall across the valve throughout diastole, a quantitative assessment of which can be obtained.

MANAGEMENT

Indications and timing of mitral and aortic valve surgery remain controversial. Because of the possibility of valve replacement, it is desirable to defer surgery if possible until the child is fully grown. However, deterioration in left ventricular function is an indication for surgery. Annuloplasty may be performed for mitral regurgitation, or surgical or balloon valvotomy for mitral stenosis. Valve replacement is required for severe aortic regurgitation.

FURTHER READING

Abernethy M, Bass N, Sharpe N et al. Doppler echocardiography and the early diagnosis of carditis in acute rheumatic fever. Australian and New Zealand Journal of Medicine 1994; 24:530–535.

Olivier C. Rheumatic fever – is it still a problem? Journal of Antimicrobial Chemotherapy 2000; 45:13–21.

Rocha P, Freitas S, Alvares S. Rheumatic fever – a review of cases. Revista Portuguesa de Cardiologia 2000; 19:921–928.

Saxena A. Diagnosis of rheumatic fever: current status of Jones Criteria and role of echocardiography. Indian Journal of Pediatrics 2000; 67(3 Suppl):S11–14.

Tani LY, Veasy LG, Minich LL, Shaddy RE. Rheumatic fever in children younger than 5 years: is the presentation different? Pediatrics 2003; 12:1065–1068.

Vasan RS, Shrivastava S, Vijayakumar M et al. Echocardiographic evaluation of patients with acute rheumatic fever and rheumatic carditis. Circulation 1996; 94:73–82.

PERICARDIAL DISEASE

NORMAL PERICARDIUM

The normal pericardium is a flask-shaped structure extending from the diaphragm to the proximal aspect of the great vessels to include the pulmonary bifurcation and exclude the aortic arch. Posteriorly, it includes the proximal portions of the pulmonary veins and inferiorly the inferior vena cava. It encases the proximal superior vena cava. It consists of superficial parietal and deep visceral layers separated by a small amount of fluid. Deep to the visceral layer is epicardial fat, which is best appreciated on MRI, particularly over the anterior aspect of the heart. In a few locations at sites of pericardial reflections the pericardial space and fluid may appear slightly prominent on CT and MRI. These include the transverse or superior sinus posterior to the ascending aorta, the preaortic recess anterior to the main pulmonary artery and a small recess posterior to the left pulmonary artery. A further small recess may be seen immediately above the right atrial appendage located anterior to the ascending aorta. These are normal findings.

PERICARDITIS AND PERICARDIAL EFFUSION

Pericarditis can be caused by infectious or non-infectious inflammatory conditions.

The clinical presentation includes fever, malaise and chest pain. The most common cause of pericarditis in older children and adolescents is viral, often associated with a myocarditis. Bacterial and tuberculous pericarditis are rare in developed countries. Pericarditis occurs as part of the pancarditis of rheumatic fever and Kawasaki disease. Pericarditis and pericardial effusions are found in children with chronic renal failure, collagen diseases, particularly systemic lupus erythematosus and juvenile rheumatoid arthritis, and after cardiac surgery. In children with leukaemia or other malignancies, pericardial effusion may occur early due to pericardial infiltration or later as a result of mediastinal irradiation. No cause is found in a third of cases. A haemorrhagic pericardial effusion may be caused by chest trauma. Moderate to large effusions are most common in neoplastic, viral, idiopathic, uraemic and collagen disorders and are rare with rheumatic pericarditis and Kawasaki disease. A small volume is relatively more significant in a younger child, and rapid accumulation is more likely to produce cardiac tamponade.

Pericardial infection may occur following surgery or result from purulent mediastinitis.

IMAGING

The chest radiograph may demonstrate globular enlargement of the cardiac silhouette with a large pericardial effusion (Figure 9.112). Pericardial calcification occurs with constrictive pericarditis but is very rare in children. Pericardial calcification is well demonstrated by CT. Echocardiography is the most sensitive technique to assess the presence and size of a pericardial effusion. The parietal pericardium is normally separated from the myocardium by an echo-free space of 2 mm; an increase above this indicates an effusion. Pericardial fluid may be echogenic in haemorrhagic or purulent collections. Collapse of the free wall of the right ventricle indicates increased intrapericardial pressure and may be an early sign of tamponade. The normal pericardium has a low signal line outlined by adjacent fat or myocardium on ECG gated spin echo MR imaging. Pericardial thickening and the amount and distribution of pericardial fluid can be assessed if echocardiography is unsatisfactory. Characterization of the nature of fluid by signal intensity is unreliable as movement artifact alters the signal.

PERICARDIOCENTESIS

Where bacterial infective pericarditis is suspected, blood cultures should be performed and pericardiocentesis is mandatory. The fluid should be examined for cells and organisms and cultured for bacteria, viruses, mycobacteria and fungi. When appropriate, serological evidence of a viral infection or autoimmune disease should be sought.

Pericardiocentesis is essential and urgent in children with overt tamponade and should be considered if echocardiography shows cardiac compression. Except in an emergency this is usually carried out in the cardiac catheterization theatre under ultrasound and fluoroscopic guidance with electrocardiographic monitoring. A sub-xiphoid approach is usually used. It is advisable to leave a drain in situ until the effusion has resolved. Constriction is rare in children and is usually due to tuberculous pericarditis, which may be calcified.

CONGENITAL ABSENCE OF THE PERICARDIUM

Complete or partial absence of the pericardium are rare defects often discovered incidently. Partial defects are of importance

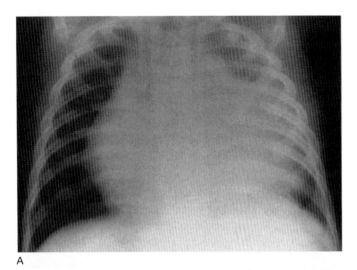

A

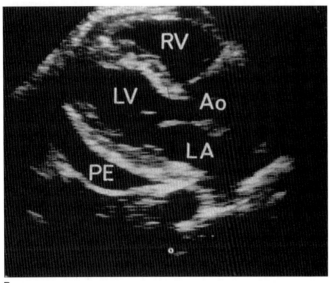

B

Figure 9.112 Pericardial effusion. (A) Chest x-ray showing the enlarged cardiac outline with the characteristic contours. (B) Long axis view of the echo shows an echo-free fluid collection (PE) behind the heart. RV, right ventricle; LV, left ventricle; Ao, aorta; LA, left atrium.

because of the association with herniation and torsion of adjacent structures, e.g. the atrial appendage, great vessels and coronary arteries.

Partial defects are most often left sided. Complete absence of the left pericardium may result in leftward shift of the heart. A partial defect on the left may manifest as a left upward bulge of the cardiac silhouette in the region of the main pulmonary artery on the chest radiograph, resulting from herniation of the left atrial appendage through the defect.

On MRI a left defect will be demonstrated by absence of the pericardium. Herniation of structures through the defect may be appreciated.

PERICARDIAL MASSES

The most common benign pericardial mass is a pericardial cyst, most often located in the cardiophrenic sulcus on the right. These

cysts have signal characteristics of fluid on MRI and may be seen to be surrounded by low signal pericardium. They do not tend to communicate with the pericardial cavity.

Malignant pericardial tumours are rare. Teratoma is the most frequent primary lesion and occurs in infancy in particular.

PNEUMOPERICARDIUM

Pneumopericardium may be iatrogenic, traumatic or occur following assisted ventilation of the premature infant. On the chest radiograph, it is seen as a variable thickness lucency and, in some instances, the pericardium may be outlined. Classically, it extends beneath the heart and above the diaphragm in the midline and does not extend above the great vessels, unlike a pneumomediastinum. Small collections of air are often not clinically relevant and resolve spontaneously. Large collections may need to be drained urgently because of the risk of cardiac tamponade.

PULMONARY OEDEMA

Pulmonary oedema in children may be cardiogenic or non-cardiogenic. Cardiogenic oedema may be acute or chronic. The underlying pathology is abnormal accumulation of fluid in the pulmonary interstitium, air spaces or both. Non-cardiogenic pulmonary oedema tends to be acute with a mixture of interstitial and alveolar oedema. The heart size is normal. Causes include meningococcal septicaemia, renal failure, head injury, drowning and acute upper airways obstruction.

Cardiogenic oedema is usually due to volume overload of the left ventricle or pulmonary venous obstruction. The presence of cardiomegaly depends on the underlying cause.

Radiographically, the earliest changes are loss of clarity of the pulmonary vessels due to the oedema and accumulation of fluid in the perivascular lymphatic spaces. Oedema of the bronchial walls occurs, which is often described as peribronchial cuffing. As oedema progresses, air space shadowing develops as fluffy hazy opacities. Fluid becomes visible in the pulmonary fissures and frank pleural effusions develop. Exceptionally, this may become loculated in the interlobar fissures and may be confused with a 'mass'. Its location and pleural-based characteristics should avoid confusion.

With chronic raised pulmonary venous pressure in older children, on an erect chest radiograph one may see upper lobe blood diversion.

FURTHER READING

Beghetti M, Gow RM, Haney I et al. Pediatric primary benign cardiac tumors: a 15 year review. American Heart Journal 1997; 134:1107–1114.
Mok GC, Menahem S. Large pericardial effusions of inflammatory origin in childhood. Cardiology in the Young 2003; 13:131–136.

KAWASAKI DISEASE

Kawasaki disease or mucocutaneous lymph node syndrome, first described in Japan, is a disease of unknown aetiology, suspected but not proven to be infectious in nature. It predominantly affects children less than 5 years of age. Presentation is with a sudden onset of fever, a subsequent skin rash, conjunctivitis, cervical lymphadenopathy, and swelling and redness of the hands and feet. The acute phase lasts around 10 days. It is characterized pathologically by a generalized vasculitis involving the gastrointestinal, genitourinary and neurological systems as well as causing arthralgia. Signs of acute endocarditis, myocarditis or pericarditis may be present. Coronary artery aneurysms may be evident as early as 10 days from the onset of the illness. They develop in 15–25% of affected children. Sudden death may occur due to cardiac arrhythmias, ruptured coronary aneurysm or myocardial infarction. The myocardial infarction may be silent. Coronary artery aneurysms tend to involve the proximal parts of the vessels as well as branching points.

Many of the aneurysms will regress with time. Thrombosis, stenosis and no change in size of the aneurysm may also occur. Initially, management is aimed at reducing the inflammation and includes aspirin and intravenous gamma globulin. Further management may include thrombolysis, interventional procedures of the coronary arteries or coronary bypass surgery.

IMAGING

The chest radiograph is often normal. Occasionally, the coronary artery aneurysms will calcify. Echocardiography may demonstrate mitral valve regurgitation, a pericardial effusion and dilation to aneurysmal formation of the proximal aspect of the coronary arteries. Radionuclide imaging may demonstrate areas of ischaemia or infarction.

It is generally recommended that myocardial radionuclide stress tests and echocardiography and, in some cases, angiography be performed to follow-up the course of coronary artery lesions. Coronary magnetic resonance angiography is emerging as a noninvasive tool in assessing coronary arteries and may replace coronary angiography.

TAKAYASU'S ARTERITIS

This is a chronic inflammatory condition of the aorta and major branches. It has a predilection for the aortic arch and great vessels, abdominal aorta, renal and pulmonary arteries. The clinical picture in the acute stages is non-specific with vague constitutional symptoms and an elevated sedimentation rate. A high index of suspicion is necessary for its diagnosis. In the healing phase occlusion, stenosis and aneurysms form in the involved vessels. It is mainly found in non-Caucasian females in the mid to late teens. MRI, CT and angiography may demonstrate mural thickening in the acute phase. In the chronic phase, the CXR may demonstrate cardiomegaly, dilation of the aortic arch and calcification of the aortic wall. Vessel stenoses, aneurysmal dilation and occlusion can be imaged by echocardiography, CT, MRI or angiography. Mortality is high amongst children.

MIDDLE AORTIC SYNDROME

The middle aortic syndrome, a rare condition, was first described in 1963 by Sen et al. At that time the term was used to descibe a narrowing below the isthmus in the thoracic aorta. It has variously been used to describe both sub- and supradiaphragmatic aortic nar-

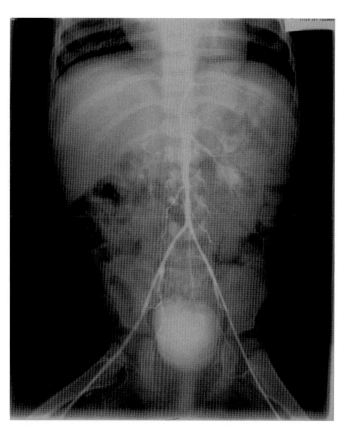

Figure 9.113 Narrowing of the abdominal aorta in middle aortic syndrome.

rowing. In the former, renal and visceral involvement and in the latter thoracic aortic narrowing near the diaphragm occur. The subdiaphragmatic lesions in children typically present with hypertension refractory to treatment. It may first present with congestive heart failure. The aetiology is obscure. It has been described in association with Williams syndrome, neurofibromatosis, Turner's syndrome and some believe it is a variant of Takayasu's arteritis. The involved vessels can be imaged using CT, MRI or angiography (Figure 9.113).

FURTHER READING

Applegate KE, Goske MJ, Pierce G et al. Situs revisited: imaging of the heterotaxy syndrome. Radiographics 1999; 19:837.

Araoz P, Eklund HE, Welch TJ et al. CT and MR imaging of primary cardiac malignancies. Radiographics 1999; 19:1421.

Babbit DB, Cassidy GE, Godard JE. Rib notching in aortic coarctation during infancy and childhood. Radiology 1974; 110:169.

Becker C, Soppa C, Fink U et al. Spiral CT angiography and 3D reconstruction in patients with aortic coarctation. European Radiology 1997; 7:1473.

Berdon WE, Baker DH. Vascular anomalies and the infant lung: rings, slings and other things. Seminars in Roentgenology 1972; 7:39.

Bisset GS III, Strife JL, McCloskey J. MR imaging of coronary artery aneurysms in a child with Kawasaki disease. American Journal of Roentgenology 1989; 152:805–807.

Bremerich J, Reddy GP, Higgins CB. MRI of supracristal ventricular septal defects. Journal of Computed Assisted Tomography 1999; 23:13.

Celiker A, Qureshi SA, Bilgic A. Transcatheter closure of patent arterial ducts using controlled-release coils. European Heart 1997; 18:359.

Chen SJ, Li YW, Wu MH et al. CT and MRI findings in a child with constrictive pericarditis. Pediatric Cardiology 1998; 19:295.

Cheng CF, Wang JK, Wu MH. Morphological characterization of ventricular septal defect with posterior deviation of the outlet septum. Cardiology 1998; 89:134.

Choe YH, Kim YM, Han BK et al. MR imaging in the morphologic diagnosis of congenital heart disease. Radiographics 1997; 17:403.

Driscoll DJ. Left-to-right shunt lesions. Pediatric Clinics of North America 1999; 46:355.

Elliott LP (ed). Cardiac imaging in infants, children, and adults. Philadelphia: J P Lippincott; 1991.

Ferencz C, Neill CA, Broughman JA et al. 1989 Congenital cardiovascular malformations associated with chromosome abnormalities: an epidemiologic study. Journal of Pediatrics 1989; 114:79.

Garver KA, Hernandez RJ, Vermilion RP et al. Images in cardiovascular medicine: Correlative imaging of aortopulmonary window: demonstration with echocardiography, angiography, and MRI. Circulation 1997; 96:1036.

Greenberg SB, Marks LA, Eshaghpour EE. Evaluation of magnetic resonance imaging in coarctation of the aorta: the importance of multiple imaging planes. Pediatric Cardiology 1997; 18:345.

Jaffe RB. Magnetic resonance imaging of vascular rings. Seminars in Ultrasound CT MR 1990; 11:206.

Jaffe RB. Radiographic manifestations of congenital anomalies of the aortic arch. Radiologic Clinics of North America 1991; 29:319.

Kitchiner D, Jackson M, Walsh K et al. Prognosis of supravalvar aortic stenosis in 81 patients in Liverpool (1960–1993). Heart 1886; 75:396.

Kovalchin JP, Forbes TJ, Nihill MR et al. Echocardiographic determinants of clinical course in infants with critical and severe pulmonary valve stenosis. Journal of American College of Cardiology 1997; 29:1095.

Kuhn JP, Slovis TL, Haller JO (eds). Caffey's pediatric diagnostic imaging, vol. 2, 10th edn. Philadelphia: Mosby Inc; 2003.

McAllister HA Jr, Hall RJ, Cooley DA. Tumors of the heart and pericardium. Current Problems in Cardiology 1999; 24:57.

Meisner H, Guenther T. Atrioventricular septal defect. Pediatric Cardiology 1998; 19:276.

Miller SW. Imaging pericardial disease. Radiologic Clinics of North America 1989; 27:1113.

Mirowitz SA, Gutierrez FR, Canter CE et al. Tetralogy of Fallot: MR findings. Radiology 1989; 171:207–212.

Newman B, Meza MP, Towbin RB et al. Left pulmonary artery sling: diagnosis and delineation of associated tracheobronchial anomalies with MR. Pediatric Radiology 1996; 26:661.

O'Rourke RA. Aortic valve stenosis: a common clinical entity. Current Problems in Cardiology 2000; 69:562.

Seminars in Nuclear Medicine 1999; 29 (whole Journal).

Senocak F, Oxme S, Bilgic A et al. Partial anomalous pulmonary venous return: evaluation of 51 cases. Japanese Heart Journal 1994; 35:43.

Tentolouris K, Kontozoglou T, Trikas A et al. Fixed subaortic stenosis revisited: congenital abnormalities in 72 new cases and review of the literature. Cardiology 1999; 92:4.

Van Son JA, Schneider P, Falk V. MR findings in Shone's complex of left heart obstructive lesions. Pediatric Radiology 1998; 28:841.

White CS, Laskey WK, Stafford JL et al. Coronary MRA: Use in assessing anomalies of coronary artery origin. Journal of Computed Assisted Tomography 1999; 23:203.

Winer-Muram HT, Tonkin ILD. The spectrum of heterotaxic syndromes. Radiologic Clinics of North America 1989; 27:1147.

SECTION | 10

THE GASTROINTESTINAL TRACT

Introduction

David A Stringer

Radiological investigation remains an essential source of information for the clinicians investigating infants and children with gastrointestinal tract disorders. As with any investigation, especially that utilizing ionizing radiation, the value of the information that can be obtained should be carefully considered in conjunction with the clinical findings.

Following a detailed clinical evaluation that includes a history and physical examination, it is common for gastrointestinal problems to require a plain film as the initial investigation of choice. Plain radiography is frequently useful as it delineates bowel gas and may aid rapid cost effective diagnosis in many children. It can also help to further evaluate the need for other investigations, such as contrast studies or ultrasound. Other more invasive studies are rarely necessary for evaluation of the gastrointestinal tract.

The aim of every radiological study should be to obtain the maximum amount of information with the minimum of harm to the infantile child. Hence, any plain film examination should use either fast rare earth screens or low-dose digital technology to reduce radiation dosage. Similarly, fluoroscopic studies should only be undertaken using low-dose techniques such as last image hold, cine loop technology, frame grab technology and pulsed fluoroscopy, all of which can considerably reduce fluoroscopic dose. Above all, a careful fluoroscopic technique can allow a very satisfying rapid evaluation of the paediatric gastrointestinal tract.

Because children tend to be smaller and have less fat than adults this makes ultrasound a superb choice of imaging technology in children and it is able to show many bowel abnormalities, especially when there is a mass lesion such as in hypertrophic pyloric stenosis.

Further techniques, including CT, are rarely indicated. When utilized low-dose CT techniques should be used (see Chapter 1.4). When CT is considered, the value of MRI should also be analyzed, as it does not involve radiation.

FURTHER READING

Dobranowski J, Stringer DA, Somers S, Stevenson GW. Procedures in gastrointestinal radiology. New York: Springer-Verlag; 1990.

Stringer DA and Babyn P. Paediatric gastrointestinal imaging and intervention, 2nd edn. Hamilton: B.C. Decker Inc.; 2000.

Various authors. Imaging of the paediatric gastrointestinal tract. In: Walker WA, Durie PR, Hamilton JR et al. (eds) Paediatric gastrointestinal disease, 3rd edn. Hamilton: B.C. Decker Inc.; 2000:1538–1682.

Techniques and Contrast Media used to Image the Gastrointestinal Tract

David A Stringer, Helen R Nadel

Plain films and contrast examinations remain the most important radiological investigation for the gastrointestinal tract, and other investigations have a value when there are specific indications. Each modality will be discussed in turn.

PLAIN FILM

Low-dose techniques should be used as discussed in the introduction. The aim of the examination should be to gain the maximum amount of information with the minimum amount of radiation and patient discomfort.

The technique in infants is somewhat different than that for older children. The images can be taken with the baby in the incubator. Decubitus rather than erect films may be useful; usually the left side down decubitus is the most useful. Bowel gas is very helpful in evaluating the bowel in children of all ages, especially in the neonate. The technique of inversion of the baby to evaluate length of anorectal malformation should no longer be performed, as the test is unreliable as well as being barbarous. A useful technique in children suspected of having rectosigmoid Hirschsprung's disease is the prone cross-table lateral film of the rectosigmoid region as this may demonstrate the zone of transition.

CONTRAST MEDIA AND FLUOROSCOPY

GENERAL CONSIDERATIONS

The infant or child should be kept warm and wrapped securely in a blanket or in a commercially designed cradle. Careful holding of the child is often necessary and care should be taken to keep the operator's hands out of the x-ray beam. Videotape recording, last image hold, frame grab and cine loop techniques are useful in reducing dose, along with pulsed fluoroscopy.

Endoscopic techniques have decreased the number of fluoroscopic studies performed in adults but fluoroscopy still plays a major role in the evaluation of the paediatric gastrointestinal tract. The most commonly performed studies are single contrast upper or lower gastrointestinal tract examinations and a variety of contrast media can be used.

CONTRAST MEDIA

The easiest, cheapest most commonly available contrast medium is air. The presence of gas within the bowel can be most useful in delineating abnormalities, particularly a proximal high atresia. Occasionally, it is worthwhile injecting air to delineate the bowel better and, if necessary, this can be instilled by nasogastric tube or per rectum. In addition, air is now the contrast of choice for intussusception reduction. This is considered further in Chapter ••.

There are a variety of other intraluminal contrast media that can be used in the gastrointestinal tract but most commonly a dilute barium sulphate solution is used.

In the evaluation of the upper gastrointestinal tract, single contrast techniques are generally used, as cancers and ulcers are much less common in children; gross morphological structure is more important. In neonates low osmolar water soluble contrast is mainly used and in the older child with taste buds who refuses barium, it can be used safely and with high-quality images. A dilute barium sulphate solution can generally be used unless there is concern of perforation or aspiration. For a single contrast barium meal and follow-through, barium sulphate is usually given in an approximately 85% w/v concentration. For those under 1 year of age, it can be mixed with a sterile dextrose solution, as it is often a replacement for a meal. If perforation or aspiration is suspected then a low osmolar water-soluble contrast can be used, but Gastrografin (meglumine diatrizoate) should never be used in the upper gastrointestinal tract because if aspiration occurs it can lead to rapid pulmonary oedema and death. The low non-ionic contrast media can be extremely useful, especially as the newer iso-osmolar contrast appear in the renal tract only if there is a perforation or a very abnormal bowel mucosa.

For single contrast enemas in infants a water-soluble low-osmolar contrast is usually preferred as the conditions being investigated are usually very different from those in older infants and children and so require a different technique. These media are much safer than barium suspension, as young infants are more susceptible to perforation. In particular, the very low birth weight premature infant requires very careful handling indeed. Enema evaluation in these critically ill infants is best performed using an iso-osmolar water-soluble contrast media.

Gastrografin is a hyperosmolar liquorice-flavoured medium that has been advocated for treatment of meconium ileus. Unfortunately, Gastrografin is very hyperosmolar, which rapidly draws fluid from the extracellular compartment into the lumen of the bowel. This can have catastrophic haemodynamic effects. In addition, Gastrografin contains a wetting compound called Tween 90 that has been shown to sometimes cause an acute fulminant colitis. Some experienced paediatric radiologists still use Gastrografin safely in a dilute form to good effect; however, in the authors' opinion this medium should not be used except by the most experienced, as there are such significant risks, and especially as a Cystic Fibrosis Foundation Consensus Conference of experts brought together to assess the treatment of meconium ileus found that there is no scientific evidence to suggest that Gastrografin has a better effect than a low-osmolar water-soluble contrast media.

UPPER GASTROINTESTINAL TRACT STUDIES

The standard upper gastrointestinal tract examinations are the barium swallow, barium meal or barium follow-through. The child is best examined following a fast according to Table 10.2.1. These examinations are well described in other texts and only some of the more unusual examinations will be discussed here.

VIDEO-PRONE OESOPHOGRAM

A video-prone oesophogram is the logical examination of choice if a H-type tracheo-oesophageal fistula is clinically suspected. Barium sulphate should be used, as a very dense medium is needed to evaluate these often tiny fistulae. Care should be taken that aspiration is avoided or at least kept to a minimum.

Table 10.2.1 Fasting of infants and children prior to upper GI tract studies

Age	Fasting time
Under 1 month	Usual time interval between feeds, i.e. time procedure for when next feed is due
1 month to 1 year	4 h
1 year to 8 years	6 h
Over 8 years	8 h

SMALL BOWEL ENEMA (ENTEROCLYSIS) VERSUS BARIUM FOLLOW-THROUGH

Enteroclysis can demonstrate small bowel beautifully. However, it is an unpleasant procedure requiring intubation of the jejunum and has an increased radiation dose compared to a conventional small bowel follow-through. With other newer techniques available for the more complex case, enteroclysis is no longer indicated in children.

A small bowel follow-through is a useful screening evaluation for some small bowel disorders. It is best performed with 85% w/v barium with films taken prone every 20–30 min depending on rate of passage of barium. The majority of examinations take approximately 90 min but can take much longer. The terminal ileum is best evaluated by the radiologist under fluoroscopy. Sometimes the peroral pneumocolon, with rectal insufflation of gas can be very helpful in delineating the terminal ileum. It is a quick, well-tolerated procedure in older children.

LOWER GASTROINTESTINAL TRACT STUDIES

CONTRAST ENEMA

The majority of studies are unprepared single contrast studies using low-density barium or water-soluble contrast media. In defunctional bowel, water-soluble contrast should be used unless the density of barium is required such as in defecatory proctograms. If used it should be washed out by enemas.

The formal double contrast enema uses a high-density barium with air insufflation following 2 days of bowel preparation and so is reserved for those suspected of having inflammatory bowel disease or polyps where endoscopy is not indicated; however, this situation is very rare.

COMPLICATIONS OF FLUOROSCOPIC EXAMINATIONS

ASPIRATION

If aspiration is suspected clinically then the initial study can be performed using an iso-osmolar non-ionic contrast media, while carefully monitoring the child with suction available. If no aspiration occurs then barium can be substituted. Gastrografin should never be used in the upper gastrointestinal tract because if aspiration occurs it can lead to rapid pulmonary oedema and death.

BARIUM IMPACTION

Barium impaction can occur with Hirschsprung's disease or if there is considerable faecal loading in the large bowel. Care should be taken not to overfill the bowel with barium and the patient, parents and nursing staff should be informed that following any barium procedure they should ensure a good evacuation, using laxatives if necessary. Of course, if water-soluble contrast media is used no impaction can occur.

PERFORATION AND BARIUM PERITONITIS

When assessing infants and children for contrast study, care should be taken in evaluating the possible risk of perforation. It is only the unwary who would perform a contrast examination in any infant or child who has clinical evidence of peritonism. If the radiologist is concerned over possible potential for perforation this should be discussed in detail with the referring clinician to make a mutual decision on whether an examination is still indicated despite this perceived risk.

Perforation with either a low osmolar water-soluble contrast media or air is preferable to a barium perforation, where the risk of peritonitis is much higher. If perforation does occur then it should be promptly recognized and the clinician informed, with rapid referral to a paediatric surgeon.

In patients with suspected intussusception, a paediatric surgeon should have examined the child and be aware of the case prior to any attempted intussusception reduction, because if perforation occurs treatment can then be expedited. In intussusception reduction, air is preferable to barium and in experienced hands gives the best and safest results. If a perforation occurs with air a wide bore needle should be at hand to perforate the anterior abdominal wall to relieve any gaseous pressure effects on the cardiovascular system. Perforations during air enema have been shown to be small, more easily repaired and with no clinical sequelae. Hence, quite aggressive intussusception reduction techniques can be used, if agreed by the paediatric surgeon.

ULTRASOUND

Ultrasound is often thought to be less useful in the gut than in the solid organs. It has a significant value, however, in assessing peristalsis, the presence of free fluid, bowel wall thickness and the nerutence glands. However, ultrasound is useful in evaluating the presence of appendicitis, intussusception or mass lesion. When these conditions are clinically suspected, the technique of graded compression sonography is an excellent method of examining all quadrants of the abdomen, especially in infants. Also a mass lesion, such as a mesenteric, duplication or ovarian cyst, or abscesses can be readily detected.

Hypertrophic pyloric stenosis of infancy can be reliably diagnosed using ultrasound. It is best to fill the stomach with a clear fluid, such as sterile 10% dextrose water, so that one can assess the peristalsis of the stomach and the passage of fluid through the pylorus.

Ultrasound of bowel is useful in assessing bowel thickness, hernia sac contents and some inflammatory diseases such as typhlitis and other necrotizing enteropathies. Doppler sonography is also helpful in looking for bowel inflammation as indicated by an increase in vascularity of the bowel wall.

NUCLEAR MEDICINE

Scintigraphic studies for the investigation of gastrointestinal disorders are performed mainly with a variety of technetium 99m (Tc 99m) based radiopharmaceuticals. Depending on the examination, the radiopharmaceuticals are introduced intravenously or are ingested. Images are performed using standard gamma camera technology and the addition of single photon emission tomography (SPECT) can sometimes be helpful. These examinations are well tolerated by the patients and rarely require sedation. Distraction techniques can be helpful in the longer studies to help immobilize the child. The radiation burden for many of the tests is similar to other standard imaging diagnostic procedures. Preparation for most of the studies is similar. Fasting is appropriate for age and the guidelines in Table 10.2 1 for UGI contrast examinations can be applied to GI scintigraphic studies.

For gastric emptying and gastro-oesophageal reflux studies, oral technetium 99m sulphur colloid is used, as the sulphur colloid is not absorbed from the gastrointestinal tract. Also, if it is aspirated into the lungs, it remains as a localized area that is readily detectable and is eventually cleared by action of the cilia. Technetium 99m sulphur colloid is given orally mixed in the patient's food. The patient is imaged under the camera in the supine position. Once the feeding is complete, the patient is imaged continuously in the supine position for 1 h. It is best to digitize the images so that contrast may be enhanced to show minimal degrees of reflux or small foci of aspiration.

To assess for aspiration, images of the thorax to visualize the lungs are taken at approximately 1 h and 4 h after the dynamic reflux images.

The salivagram examination is a relatively simple way to assess for direct aspiration of saliva. In this examination, a small amount of radiocolloid similar to that used for reflux scan is placed on the tongue and allowed to mix with oral secretions. Anterior images of the thorax with the patient supine are collected in the computer at 30-s intervals to 1 h or terminated earlier if aspiration with visualization of the tracheobronchial tree is obtained.

Scintigraphic evaluation of gastric emptying time is the 'gold standard' for quantitatively assessing abnormal gastric motility. Scintigraphic techniques utilize radiolabelled standard meals of mainly solid or mixed meals.

There is a wide variation in normal values and the results are influenced by, among other factors, meal sugar and protein content, time of day, medications, age and gender of the patient. Normal values in infants and children vary with age and size and each laboratory must ensure that they develop meaningful ranges for these values generally in the range of T1/2 of 45–90 min +/− 30 min. Results can be expressed as a T1/2 or per cent residual at 60 or 90 min or both. In infants and children it has been recommended that per cent residual at 60 min be used as emptying value with 50% emptied by 90 min.

A child with painless rectal bleeding can be evaluated with technetium 99m pertechnetate Meckel scintigraphy. Ectopic gastric mucosa in duplication cysts, enteric cysts and Barrett oesophagus can also give a positive test. The pertechnetate is taken up primarily in the superficial mucous-secreting cells. For an optimal study, the patient should not have ingested a laxative or aspirin for 5 days prior to the scan. A barium study should not be performed for at least 48 h prior to the scan as retained barium can interfere with visualization of the gastric mucosa. Pharmaceuticals such as pentagastrin, glucagon and cimetidine or ranitidine given as premedication prior to the test can augment the sensitivity of the study. Pentagastrin increases the gastric excretion of radionuclide. Glucagon decreases intestinal peristalsis thereby preventing spillage of gastric contents into the bowel and so can be useful in conjunction with pentagastrin use. Cimetidine or ranitidine are H2 receptor antagonists, which decrease gastric output by approximately 50% in the resting state and also decrease the volume of secreted gastric juice and pepsin. The clinical effect is to inhibit the secretion of pertechnetate into the gastric lumen.

A flow study is performed at the time of the injection and is useful for detecting vascular lesions, such as haemangiomas, as the cause of bleeding. It is important that the patient empty the bladder both prior to and at 30 min during the study, as there is renal excretion of pertechnetate into the bladder that can obscure a small Meckel diverticulum lying behind the bladder. Uptake in the diverticulum usually parallels the course of uptake in the stomach. Diverticula are mobile and although most often located in the right lower quadrant, can move about the abdomen during the examination. Transit of contents of the diverticulum, dilution of radiopharmaceutical by bowel content, insufficient gastric mucosa, impaired vascular supply and poor positioning can be potential causes for uncommon false-negative studies. Sometimes a repeat study in a few weeks after a negative study may identify a site of ectopic gastric mucosa. This may be due to necrosis of the mucosa at the time of the acute bleed,which then heals and will again take up the pertechnetate. Careful positioning ensuring the entire bladder is included on the images and the use of additional positional and postvoid images will minimize false-negative studies. SPECT can also sometimes be helpful. Imaging the thorax in young infants and children is also included to look for other sites of potential ectopic gastric mucosa, such as a bronchopulmonary foregut duplication. Bowel ulceration and inflammation and renal activity may also be a cause of false-positive results. Because pertechnetate is taken up by the thyroid gland, choroid plexus and salivary glands, potassium perchlorate at 10 mg/kg is administered after the study is completed to competitively inhibit the uptake, and thereby reduce radiation to the thyroid.

If the bleeding is acute, technetium 99m-labelled red blood cells (Tc-99mRBC) are used for a bleeding study. Detection rates are excellent when the patient is bleeding with a minimum rate of 0.1 ml/min to 0.5 ml/min to visualize the bleeding lesion. Imaging must be performed at the time the patient is actively bleeding. Tc-99mRBC studies allow intermittent surveillance of the abdomen over a 24-h period. Colonic activity will be noted at 24 h in the presence of an upper GI bleeding site, with no significant colonic activity if there has not been bleeding in the previous 24 h. Dynamic cine viewing of the continuously acquired imaging is essential to assess for small areas of activity that show rapid

intestinal transit. Barium and contrast can interfere with visualization on scintigraphic examination, therefore a Meckel scan or Tc-99mRBC study should be performed before barium GI examination or angiography, and a Meckel scan should be done before a Tc-99mRBC study.

Tc-SC can be used to detect an acute bleeding site. It will circulate in the vascular compartment with a half-life of 2.5–3.5 min and will extravasate at actively bleeding sites before it is cleared by the reticuloendothelial system. Because of this rapid background clearance, a 99m-Tc-SC scan will detect even smaller bleeding volumes between 0.05 and 0.1 ml/min. However, the bleeding site must be visualized early in the study due to the rapid liver uptake of radionuclide from the blood.

Radiolabelled autologous white blood cells can be used to determine whether there is active inflammation in the colon with good sensitivity, specificity and diagnostic accuracy. Radioactive labelled white blood cells (WBCs) will leave the circulation at sites of infection and migrate into the infected tissues as part of the normal host response. While both 111-indium-WBC and Tc-99m HMPAO can be used for inflammation imaging, the latter has more favourable imaging parameters for standard gamma cameras and better dosimetry. When assessing patients with Crohn's disease for the presence of extraintestinal complications such as sepsis, abscess or fistulae, labelled white blood cell studies are best used as complementary tools to ultrasound and computed tomography (CT) scanning. Abscesses will be visualized as intensely abnormal focal accumulations of white blood cells on late images at 24 h.

More recently there have been reports of the use of positron emission tomography (PET) for evaluation of inflammatory bowel disease. This may be an adjunctive technique in those centres that have the availability of clinical PET imaging. This technique will identify areas of bowel inflammation with good sensitivity and is technically easier than labelled white blood cell studies.

Helicobacter pylori infection has been causally implicated in many GI disorders. The wide interest in this bacterium has spawned many investigations of its relationship, if any, with other gastrointestinal diseases such as inflammatory bowel disease. The diagnosis of *Helicobacter pylori* infection can be achieved using invasive methods that require the use of endoscopy to provide tissue samples for rapid urease tests, culture and histological examination. Non-invasive testing can be achieved by blood sampling for antibody tests and urea breath testing using carbon-14 (C-14) or carbon-13 (C-13).

The non-invasive testing using breath tests are painless and can be performed in children who are old enough to follow simple instructions for ingestion and blowing through a straw. Both C-13 and C-14 urea breath tests for the diagnosis of *H. pylori* infection can be utilized. Both tests take advantage of the fact that *H. pylori* produces urease, which is needed to break down labelled urea. Gastric urease activity can then be measured and used as an indicator of the presence of infection. Both tests rely on the measurement of labelled carbon dioxide exhaled by the patient after consuming a standard dose of labelled urea. When C-14 urea is used it is excreted in the breath as labelled carbon dioxide or in the urine.

Neuroendocrine tumours or APUDomas can involve the intestinal tract and pancreas and are divided into two groups, the carcinoids and endocrine pancreatic tumours, which are described by their hormone production and include VIPomas, gastrinomas, insulinomas, somatostatinomas and non-functioning islet cell tumours. The best radiopharmaceutical for imaging these tumours depends on the metabolic characteristics of the tumour and recent advances now allow for use of mainly radiolabelled MIBG, vasointestinal peptide and indium-111 pentetreotide. Unexpected lesions can be localized that were not seen on CT and magnetic resonance imaging (MRI) and can indicate whether treatment with somatostatin analogues or other specific radiotherapy should be carried out.

COMPUTED TOMOGRAPHY

Low-dose CT techniques should always be used in children with the exact dose and technique dependent on the diagnostic information required; every examination should be tailored to the specific child and clinical problem. CT is an invasive procedure that usually requires sedation, oral contrast and intravenous contrast. In children, fast scanning techniques are highly recommended to reduce motion artifacts.

MAGNETIC RESONANCE IMAGING

The main disadvantages of using MRI are the image degradation by respiratory, peristaltic or cardiac motion, difficulty of monitoring sick infants and children, the need for sedation in many children, and the length and cost of examination. MRI of the gut in children is still being evaluated and may become more important in the future.

ANGIOGRAPHY AND INTERVENTIONAL TECHNIQUES

Angiography and interventional techniques are generally not required for gastrointestinal disease but may be useful in specific complex cases.

FURTHER READING

Dobranowski J, Stringer DA, Somers S, Stevenson GW. Procedures in gastrointestinal radiology. New York: Springer-Verlag; 1990.

Schiepers C, Becker W (eds). Diagnostic nuclear medicine. Berlin: Springer-Verlag; 2000.

Skehan SJ, Issenman R, Mernagh J, Nahmias C, Jacobson K. 18F-fluorodeoxyglucose positron tomography in diagnosis of paediatric inflammatory bowel disease. Lancet 1999; 354:836–837.

Stringer DA and Babyn P. Paediatric gastrointestinal imaging and intervention, 2nd edn. Hamilton: B.C. Decker Inc.; 2000.

Various authors. Imaging of the paediatric gastrointestinal tract. In: Walker WA, Durie PR, Hamilton JR et al. (eds) Paediatric gastrointestinal disease, 3rd edn. Hamilton: B.C. Decker Inc.; 2000:1538–1682.

Interventional Techniques

Peter G Chait, Devon Jacobson

Paediatric Interventional Radiology (PIR) has become an integral part of the care of patients in most major paediatric hospitals. The role of the PIR physician has increased, encompassing clinical care, interacting with referral services and becoming the responsible physicians for the interventional services provided.

The extent of PIR procedures has increased as a direct result of the improvement of imaging technology, including ultrasound, fluoroscopy, computed tomography (CT) and the emergence of interventional magnetic resonance imaging (MRI). There has also been a rapid advancement in technology with the development of numerous new catheters, wires, balloons and other devices.

The provision of a PIR service requires dedication and commitment. The Toronto Hospital for Sick Children's Image Guided Therapy Department currently has four rooms, four PIR staff carrying out non-neurological interventional procedures, two fellows and a full complement of nurses, technologists and administrative staff.

In order to maintain such a service and to cope with the large volume of patients, several services have been developed to maintain the large patient groups, in particular, enterostomy access where a paediatrician, PIR staff, nurse clinicians, discharge planners, dieticians and occupational therapists work together to cover the complete needs of this group of patients. Services provided include preprocedure investigation, admission, postprocedure care and follow-up long-term care. We have also developed this system in our Vascular Access Service (Hospital for Sick Children, Toronto) and, to a lesser extent, in caecostomy patients where we have a dedicated caecostomy nurse. One of the other significant improvements that has taken place over the last few years is that a paediatrician has become part of our interventional team, who takes part in the pre- and postprocedure rounds with the interventional radiologists. The paediatrician is involved with the care of patients and admissions and discharges. Clinics are also run with the paediatricians, PIR staff and other relevant physicians.

FURTHER READING

Chait P. Future directions in interventional pediatric radiology. Pediatric Clinics of North America 1997; 44:763–782.
Diament MJ, Boechat MI, Kangarloo H. Interventional radiology in infants and children: clinical and technical aspects. Radiology 1985; 154:359–361.
Goldberg MA, Mueller PR, Saini S et al. Importance of daily rounds by the radiologist after interventional procedures of the abdomen and chest. Radiology 1991; 180:767–770.
Hoffer FA, Fellows KE, Wyly JB, Lock JE. Therapeutic catheter procedures in pediatrics. Pediatric Clinics of North America 1985; 32:1461–1476.
Hubbard AM, Fellows KE. Pediatric interventional radiology: current practice and innovations. Cardiovascular and Interventional Radiology 1993; 16:267–274.
Katzen BT, Kaplan JO, Dake MD. Developing an interventional radiology practice in a community hospital: the interventional radiologist as an equal partner in patient care. Radiology 1989; 170:955–958.
Ring EJ, Kerlan RK Jr. Inpatient management: a new role for interventional radiologists. Radiology 1985; 154:543.
Towbin RB, Ball WS Jr. Pediatric interventional radiology. Radiologic Clinics of North America 1988; 26:419–440.
vanSonnenberg E, Wittich GR, Edwards DK et al. Percutaneous diagnostic and therapeutic interventional radiologic procedures in children: experience in 100 patients. Radiology 1987; 162:601–605.
White RI Jr, Rizer DM, Shuman KR et al. Streamlining operation of an admitting service for interventional radiology. Radiology 1988; 168:127–130.

CONSENT

Informed consent is obtained from the patient and parent, prior to all procedures. Consent for anaesthesia is obtained independently. The procedures are explained and the potential risks and complications outlined and discussed with the parents and patient.

FURTHER READING

Bartholome WG. A new understanding of consent in pediatric practice: consent, parental permission, and child assent. Pediatric Annals 1989; 18:262–265.
Leikin SL. Minors' assent or dissent to medical treatment. Journal of Pediatrics 1983; 102:169–176.

PROCEDURE PLANNING

PREPROCEDURE CARE

The referring physician must relate the reason for the referral, patient's pertinent history, physical findings and diagnostic work-up. Further imaging should be ordered if necessary. Immediately prior to the procedure, the patient's chart and imaging should be reviewed. A specific history of drug or environmental allergies is essential. Previous sedation and anaesthetic records should also be reviewed. Laboratory studies usually ordered are coagulation profile, platelet count and haemoglobin. Additional tests are obtained as needed for specific procedures. In conjunction with the referring physician and anaesthetist, decisions are made as to whether preprocedure transfusions with platelets, fresh frozen plasma or packed cells should be given. Patients undergoing sedation or having general anaesthetic must not take solids 8 h before and clear fluids 2 h before the procedure.

Table 10.3.1 Guidelines for preprocedure correction of bleeding abnormalities (reproduced from Chait P et al. Pediatric gastrointestinal imaging and intervention. Hamilton: Decker; 2000:100–105)

Defect	Parameter	Treatment
Qualitative platelet dysfunction	Bleeding time (normal <8–9 min)	Desmopressin (DDAVP), 0.3 g/kg over 30 min, or transfuse 1 unit platelets/5–10 kg (for an increase of 40 000–70 000), or cryoprecipitate, 1 unit/10 kg
cause: congenital or acquired qualitative or quantitative platelet dysfunction		
	Platelet count	Transfuse 1 unit platelets/5–10 kg (for an increase of 40 000–70 000)
Extrinsic pathway Identify with increased PT and increased INR, usually seen with warfarin administration, nutritional (vitamin K deficiency) and DIC	PT, INR	Hold warfarin (replace with heparin) Vitamin K1: 2 mg (infants), 5–10 mg (children), im or sq Fresh frozen plasma: 10–15 ml/kg
Intrinsic pathway Identify with increased PTT, often as a result of heparin or inoxaparin (low molecular weight heparin) treatment	PTT	Hold heparin Fresh frozen plasma: 10–15 ml/kg

INR, international normalized ratio; PT, prothrombin time; PTT, partial thromboplastin time; im, intramuscular; sq, subcutaneous.

In most paediatric gastrointestinal interventional procedures, preprocedure prophylactic antibiotics are given; for example, in upper GI procedures, a first generation cephalosporin (kefazolin 40 mg/kg) is used as a single dose preprocedure. Patients requiring intervention in the colon or in those requiring biliary manipulation are given a combination of gentamycin 2.5 mg/kg, ampicillin 50 mg/kg or metronidazole 10 mg/kg as a single preprocedure dose, and the same doses are continued three times a day, depending on the procedure and how complicated it is. In children who require cardiac prophylaxis, a combination of ampicillin 50 mg/kg and gentamycin 2.5 mg/kg is administered 30 min before starting the procedure. They then receive a repeat dose of intravenous ampicillin 25 mg/kg 6 h following the procedure. Patients who are allergic to penicillin and cephalosporin receive vancomycin 20 mg/kg over an hour and gentamycin 2.5 mg/kg. Guidelines for preprocedure correction of bleeding abnormalities are given in Table 10.3.1.

FURTHER READING

Cantani A. Latex allergy in children. Journal of Investigational Allergology and Clinical Immunology 1999; 9:14–20.

Moneret-Vautrin DA, Beaudouin E, Widmer S et al. Prospective study of risk factors in natural rubber latex hypersensitivity. Journal of Allergy and Clinical Immunology 1993; 92:668–677.

Pandit UA, Pandit SK. Fasting before and after ambulatory surgery. Journal of Perianesthesiology and Nursing 1997; 12:181–187.

Phillips S, Daborn AK, Hatch DJ. Preoperative fasting for paediatric anaesthesia. British Journal of Anaesthesia 1994; 73:529–536.

Schreiner MS, Triebwasser A, Keon TP. Ingestion of liquids compared with preoperative fasting in pediatric outpatients. Anesthesiology 1990; 72:593–597.

Soreide E, Holst–Larson H, Veel T, Steen PA. The effects of chewing gum on gastric content prior to induction of general anesthesia. Anesthesia and Analgesia 1995; 80:985–989.

Splinter WM, Schaefer JD. Unlimited clear fluid ingestion two hours before surgery in children does not affect volume or pH of stomach contents. Anaesthesia in Intensive Care 1990; 18:522–526.

PERIPROCEDURAL CARE

Procedure planning including the position of the patient and the use of a tilting table are part of the initial set-up. Decubitus position would be used for patients undergoing transrectal abscess drainage; for biopsy of a retroperitoneal mass a decubitus or prone position might be used. The position of the monitors, ultrasound machine, iv poles, anaesthetist's support staff and nurses, and technologists must also be considered. Patient temperature is important and maintaining the correct temperature in neonates is usually obtained by elevating the room temperature using conventional airwarmers, warming blankets, saline bags, radiant lights or by covering the patient with plastic wrap. The pooling of wet antiseptic solutions during preparation of the patient should also be reduced to minimize cooling and skin irritation. Ultrasound gel and barium can be warmed prior to procedures.

PROTECTION FROM RADIATION

The dangers of radiation exposure when working in an interventional suite are significantly decreased with modern pulsed fluoroscopy and careful colimation. A lead apron and thyroid shield should be worn during any fluoroscopic procedure. Prescription and non-prescription lead goggles are available for eye protection. Whenever possible, images should be saved rather than exposures taken to reduce radiation. The use of thin compliant lead gloves can reduce the dose to the hands by 50%.

SEDATION, ANALGESIA AND ANAESTHESIA

The approach to the type of sedation or anaesthesia depends largely on the procedure to be performed, the complexity of the case and local policy. Most procedures are performed under sedation when feasible. In Canada where nurse anaesthetists do not exist, spe-

Table 10.3.2 Commonly used medications for sedation in interventional radiology at the Hospital for Sick Children, Toronto (repoduced with permission from Temple M, Chait P, Connolly B. Pediatric anesthesia: principles and practice. Toronto: McGraw-Hill; 2002:1389)

Drug	Dosage	Maximum	Onset	Duration	Reversal Agent
Pentobarbital	4–6 mg/kg iv Given slowly and titrated to desired effect	200 mg	1–5 min	1–4 h	None available
Chloral hydrate	80–100 mg/kg po Dose may be repeated 40 mg/kg/dose in 1 h Neonate dose: 50 mg/kg Lethargic or very ill Neonate dose: 25 mg/kg	2 g/dose	30–60 min	2–8 h	None available
Midazolam po Midazolam iv	0.3–0.5 mg/kg po 0.05 mg/kg iv For supplement to Nembutal	20 mg 0.15 mg/kg	10–30 min 1–1.5 min	1–2 h 15–80 min	Flumazenil Dosage: 0.01 mg/kg May repeat in 1–3 min as required May repeat in 1–3 min intervals as required
Diazemuls/diazepam Lorazepam	0.1 mg/kg iv titrated to effect 0.05 mg/kg SL	20 mg iv 4 mg SL	1.5–3 min 30–60 min	2–6 h 3–4 h	Maximum dose/injection: 1 mg/dose Maximum total dose: 2 mg or 0.05 mg/kg (whichever is less) Onset: 30–60 s Duration: dependent on dose administered Requires 3 h recovery
Meperidine hydrochloride	0.5–1.5 mg/kg/dose iv Given slowly and titrated to desired effect	2 mg/kg/dose or 100 mg dose (whichever is less)	1–5 min	2–4 h	Naloxone hydrocholride Dose: 0.001–0.01 mg/kg iv Beginning with 0.001 mg/kg increments
Morphine sulphate	0.05–0.1 mg/kg iv over 2–3 min	May be repeated q 15 min	1–5 min	1–3 h	Maximum dose: 0.01 mg/kg/dose or 1 mg/dose. Titration is key Onset: iv 1–2 min Duration: 45 min Requires 3 h recovery

Abbreviations: po, orally; iv, intravenous; sl, sublingual.

cially trained interventional nurses can sedate healthy patients under the direction of the interventional radiologist.

The most common contraindication to nurse-administered sedation includes uncorrected, complex congenital cardiac abnormalities, tachycardia, oxygen saturation less than 95% in room air, pulmonary insufficiency (i.e. pneumonia, pleural effusion) and an absent gag reflex.

For some children, their cardiovascular reserve is so compromised that any degree of sedation or anaesthesia is risky; these procedures are performed without sedation but with local anaesthetic alone and 'anaesthesia stand-by'. By this we mean that an anaesthetist is present during the case to ensure a safe airway and cardiovascular system and adequate analgesia while the radiologist concentrates on the procedure at hand. Choice of anaesthetic is determined by the procedure performed, the comfort level of the operator and the nature of the child.

Due to a higher volume workload and acuity of patients, a full anaesthetic list is run daily in the interventional suite at the Hospital for Sick Children, Toronto The choice of anaesthesia is determined by the anaesthetist who must take into account the interventional requirements for the procedure and overall safety of the patient.

Good communication at the beginning of the day prior to the commencement of the cases is useful in planning the radiological and anaesthetic requirements. In several instances, local anaesthetic alone may be considered the safest option for the children undergoing minimally invasive procedures. In general, most paediatric procedures that are very painful or require the patient to be

completely mobilized will require deep sedation or general anaesthesia. In both cases, the procedure should be performed under the supervision of an anaesthetist. General anaesthesia may also be indicated for lengthy procedures and for procedures where the area of interest is close to vital structures. However, some neonates or patients with oropharyngeal abnormality may be poor candidates for tracheal interventions. In these cases, local anaesthesia or light sedation may be required.

Sedated patients are monitored continuously for blood pressure, ECG and pulse oximetry. Visual monitoring by physicians, nurses and technologists is by far the most important way of ensuring safety and avoiding complications. Regardless of the level of sedation chosen, full resuscitation and anaesthetic equipment with suction should be readily available. A wide variety of medications are available for anaesthesia and sedation. Radiologists tend to use a limited selection of drugs for sedation and analgesia (see Table 10.3.2).

Infants weighing less than 5 kg may be given an oral dose of chloral hydrate 80 mg/kg followed by intravenous morphine. In young children weighing 5–20 kg, intravenous pentobarbital 3 mg/kg iv followed by intravenous meperidine 1 mg/kg may be given and repeated once if necessary. In older children or adolescents, sedation would include intravenous diazemul 0.1 mg/kg followed by intravenous meperidine (1 mg/kg) and repeated as necessary. Sedation for anxious patients undergoing short, relatively painless procedures is usually achieved with oral midazolam. The use of local anaesthetics, even in sedated and anaesthetized patients, improves postprocedure recovery and decreases pain experienced at the operative site. Local anaesthetic should be administered through a 27-gauge needle with minimal discomfort. The patient acceptance is improved if the site is prepared with topical Emla® cream or Ametop® gel. Emla® patches may also be used in neonates but not where there is an open skin wound or mucosa. To decrease the pain of subcutaneous injection, the pH of lidocaine can be raised with a 1 to 9 mixture of injectable sodium biocarb. The maximum dosage of 1% lidocaine is 0.5 ml/kg. For longer durations of analgesia, 0.25% bupivacaine (maximum dose 1 ml/kg) is used instead of lidocaine. Local anaesthetic with epinephrine 1 in 100 000 can be used to cause vasoconstriction. This results in prolonged anaesthetic effect and decreases bleeding. Epinephrine should not be used in areas where there is an end artery such as a digit, the nose and the penis.

FURTHER READING

Lowrie L, Weiss AH, Lacombe C. The pediatric sedation unit: a mechanism for pediatric sedation. Pediatrics 1998; 102:E30.

Ronchera CL, Marti-Bonmati L, Poyatos C et al. Administration of oral chloral hydrate to paediatric patients undergoing magnetic resonance imaging. Pharmaceutisch Weekblad Scientific Edition 1992; 14:349–352.

Russell SC, Doyle E. A risk-benefit assessment of topical percutaneous local anaesthetics in children. Drug Safety 1997; 16:279–287.

Sectish TC. Use of sedation and local anesthesia to prepare children for procedures. American Family Physician 1997; 55:909–916.

Sievers TD, Yee JD, Foley ME et al. Midazolam for conscious sedation during pediatric oncology procedures: safety and recovery parameters. Pediatrics 1991; 88:1172–1179.

Strain JD, Harvey LA, Foley LC, Campbell JB. Intravenously administered pentobarbital sodium for sedation in pediatric CT. Radiology 1986; 161:105–108.

Strain JD, Harvey LA, Foley LC, Campbell JB. IV Nembutal: safe sedation for children undergoing CT. American Journal of Roentgenology 1988; 151:975–979.

Temple M, Chait P, Connolly B. Interventional radiology: radiology considerations. In: Bissonnette B et al., eds. Pediatric anesthesia: principles and practice. Toronto: McGraw-Hill; 2002:1389.

POSTPROCEDURE MANAGEMENT

Immediately upon completion of the procedure, the time, date and type of medication used are recorded and the patient monitoring records are signed by the PIR physician. A brief written note is placed in the chart and its outcome, any complications and recommendations are noted. Postprocedure orders are also recorded. The parents are then seen and the procedure is explained and the results conveyed. At The Hospital for Sick Children, Toronto, if patients are awake enough, they are sent straight back to the ward or to the recovery room, or to the postanaesthesia care unit (PACU) if they require further monitoring.

Patients are followed-up on the ward until they are stable or until the tube is removed. Patients with long-term catheter placements are seen until such a time as the catheter is working satisfactorily and, subsequently, only when necessary and for tube maintenance.

Table 10.3.3 Comparative evaluation of image guidance systems (reproduced from Chait P et al. Pediatric gastrointestinal imaging and intervention. Hamilton: Decker; 2000:100–105)

	Advantages	Disadvantages
Fluoroscopy	Availability Rapid localization Needle tip easily visualized Real time	Poor tissue differentiation Ionizing radiation Not portable No quantitative depth measurement
Ultrasonography	Rapid localization Rapid multiplanar imaging No ionizing radiation Portable	Needle difficult to visualize Limited anatomical information Obscured by gas or bone More technically demanding
Computed tomography	Needle tip easily seen Fine anatomical detail No interference from overlying viscus or gas CT fluoroscopy allows real-time imaging	Expensive Ionizing radiation Not portable Longer procedure time

TECHNIQUE

CHOICE OF IMAGING

The majority of paediatric interventional procedures are performed using a combination of ultrasound (US) and/or fluoroscopy. The advent of CT fluoroscopy has rendered procedures under CT guidance faster, less cumbersome and with 'real-time visualization' but with a significantly higher radiation dose. A comparative evaluation of image guidance systems is given in Table 10.3.3.

ULTRASONOGRAPHY

Ultrasound guidance is ideal for paediatric patients due to the limited amount of subcutaneous and intraperitoneal fat. Furthermore, ultrasound uses no ionizing radiation and is a 'real-time' modality. The technology has advanced and the quality of the images obtained with high frequency linear and curvilinear probes has improved dramatically, allowing most of our percutaneous biopsies and accesses to be performed under ultrasound alone. Ultrasound is, however, not ideal in lesions that are deep or difficult to visualize, or where there is intervening gas or bony structures.

FLUOROSCOPY

Fluoroscopy is generally used for guidance where there is a difference in density between structures. For example, gas interfaced between distended gastric lumen can be easily seen and punctured percutaneously under fluoroscopic guidance. Dilatation, stenting and vascular procedures are also performed primarily under fluoroscopic guidance. In many cases, the initial puncture is performed under ultrasound guidance, followed by fluoroscopic guidance for final catheter, stent or other device placement.

COMPUTED TOMOGRAPHY

The use of CT is limited and is used primarily where lesions are close to vital structures or where other imaging modalities, such as ultrasound or fluoroscopy, are not capable of achieving the desired results. CT fluoroscopy has increased the accuracy but one must always be aware of the significant dose of radiation that the patient and the operator are exposed to.

MAGNETIC RESONANCE IMAGING

Interventional MRI is in its infancy and is not available in most centres for paediatric interventional procedures.

FURTHER READING

Silverman SG, Tuncali K, Adams DF et al. CT fluoroscopy-guided abdominal interventions: techniques, results, and radiation exposure. Radiology 1999; 212:673–681.

The Oesophagus

Veronica Donoghue, Eilish L Twomey

TRACHEOESOPHAGEAL FISTULA AND OESOPHAGEAL ATRESIA

The incidence of oesophageal atresia is 2.4 per 10 000 births. The incidence in Caucasians is nearly double that of non-white populations. The risk of a second affected infant is 0.5–2% but it increases to 20% if more than one sibling is affected. The risk of oesophageal atresia occurring in the offspring of an affected adult is 3–4%. Oesophageal atresia is usually sporadic. The aetiology of oesophageal atresia and a tracheoesophageal fistula (TOF) is uncertain. The trachea and oesophagus are formed from the primitive foregut, a common channel in early uterine life. Division into trachea and oesophagus occurs by ingrowth of paired lateral ridges. Fistula formation may be due to failure of fusion of these lateral ridges. Atresia may occur as a result of differential growth rates of the epithelial lining of the oesophagus and its mesenchymal wall, causing stretching and interruption of the epithelium. These anomalies occur in the first 5 weeks of embryogenesis.

Tracheoesophageal fistula and oesophageal atresia are classified as follows (see Figure 10.4.1):

(A) Oesophageal atresia without fistula (7.8%).
(B) Oesophageal atresia with proximal fistula (0.8%).
(C) Oesophageal atresia with distal fistula (85.8%).
(D) Oesophageal atresia with fistula to both pouches (1.4%).
(E) H-type fistula without atresia (4.2%).

Presentation is usually in the first few hours of life with excessive oral secretions, choking and sometimes cyanosis. Typically, symptoms become more pronounced during the first feed. The abdomen may be distended due to air passing through the distal fistula into the stomach, possibly leading to respiratory distress. In the rare cases of atresia without a fistula or atresia with a proximal fistula, the abdomen will be scaphoid and gasless. The H-type fistula often presents later in childhood with recurrent respiratory infections, although it can present in the neonate.

Oesophageal atresia may be diagnosed by antenatal ultrasound (US). This is suspected on the basis of maternal polyhydramnios, little or absent stomach fluid and the proximal oesophageal pouch seen as a central anechoic area in the fetal neck or upper chest. The presence and size of a tracheoesophageal fistula will determine the amount of stomach and gastrointestinal fluid seen. Associated anomalies in other systems may also be identified. Atresias may be multiple and involve the oesophagus, duodenum and anus.

In the majority of patients, the site of the atresia is between the proximal and middle thirds of the oesophagus with a gap of varying length between the atretic pouches. The proximal oesophagus forms a blind pouch, which is distended with air indicating the diagnosis on plain radiographs. Confirmation can be accomplished by passing a radiopaque feeding tube, a reprobal tube, through the nose to the level of the atresia. This curls when it approaches the blind end of the proximal pouch (Figure 10.4.2). Chest films should include the upper abdomen to assess the presence of air in the stomach, which indicates the presence of a distal fistula. If a lateral film is obtained, there is usually considerable anterior displacement of the upper trachea but this view is not routinely indicated. When there is a proximal fistula, it is located in the anterior wall of the oesophagus and in such cases the proximal pouch is not distended. Rarely, when there is atresia with a proximal fistula, there may be communication with the distal pouch via a further distal fistula. If a fine nasogastric tube is used to identify the upper pouch, it may pass through the fistulas into the lower oesophagus and give the appearance of continuity of the oesophagus. To avoid this pitfall, a reprobal tube is normally used.

In oesophageal atresia with a distal fistula, the length of the gap between the oesophageal segments is usually short and primary repair is possible. When there is atresia with no distal fistula, there is usually a long gap (in the order of five vertebral bodies) between the proximal and distal oesophageal segments. During the first months of life, growth of the oesophageal segments tends to lessen the gap, making a delayed primary repair feasible. A gastrostomy is established for feeding in the meantime. The H-type fistula can be at any level, although the majority occur between C7 and T2 vertebral bodies.

Routine contrast examinations are not required in the neonate with oesophageal atresia and tracheoesophageal fistulas. Occasionally, a small volume of non-ionic contrast medium may be injected into the proximal oesophageal pouch to demonstrate a proximal fistula. This should be suspected in the presence of a short or narrow proximal pouch due to decompression by the fistula, and can usually be adequately identified at surgery without preoperative imaging. Contrast injection should be undertaken carefully to avoid aspiration or respiratory distress secondary to pouch distension. The absence of air in the gastrointestinal tract usually implies that there is no distal fistula. Occasionally, however, a narrow or occluded distal fistula is discovered at surgery that did not allow passage of air to the stomach.

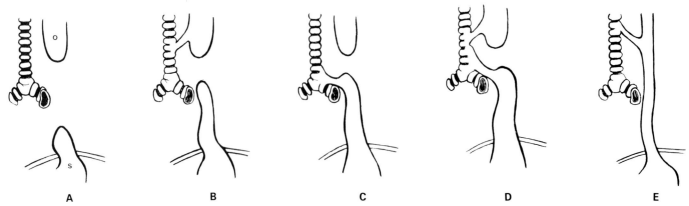

Figure 10.4.1 Oesophageal atresia and tracheoesophageal fistula. (A) Atresia without fistula, (B) atresia with proximal fistula, (C) atresia with distal fistula, (D) atresia with fistula to both pouches and (E) H-type fistula without atresia.

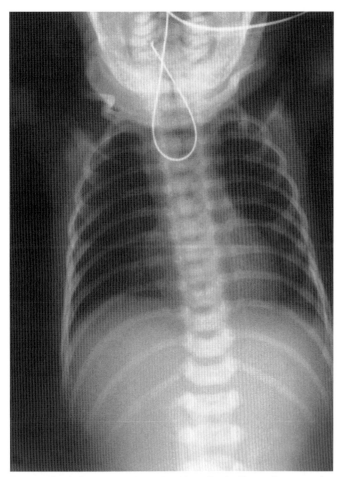

Figure 10.4.2 Oesophageal atresia without fistula. The radiopaque tube curls as it approaches the blind end of the proximal pouch. No air is present in the stomach, indicating there is no fistula.

Radiological examination of infants with a possible H-type fistula should be performed under fluoroscopic control in a prone position. The infant is placed prone on a pad on the step of an erect fluoroscopic table and firmly held if horizontal fluoroscopy is otherwise impossible. A feeding tube with end holes is introduced through the nose. The examination is begun with the tip of the tube in the distal oesophagus. Non-ionic contrast medium is injected through the tube, with enough pressure to distend the oesophagus as the tube is slowly withdrawn. The examination is recorded on video to allow for review of the fluoroscopy and spot films obtained, if possible. If contrast appears in the trachea or lungs, it is very important to be certain if the contrast went through a fistula or was aspirated. If the examiner is uncertain, the examination must be repeated after the trachea is cleared of contrast. The H-type fistula characteristically runs an upwardly oblique course; this is more accurately described as an N-type fistula (Figure 10.4.3). H-type fistulas are commonly demonstrated by contrast studies; however, bronchoscopy or oesophagoscopy are more sensitive methods and may be indicated to confirm the diagnosis. This is particularly so in an older child where a prone tube oesophagram is inappropriate or when contrast studies are normal in the setting of suggestive symptoms.

Computed tomography (CT), either direct sagittal acquisition or axial acquisition with multiplanar reconstructions, is occasionally used in preoperative evaluation of these neonates. It is not routinely indicated but may demonstrate the precise location of a fistula and the length of the gap between the oesophageal segments. In neonates with long-gap atresia, accurate assessment of the length of gap is important to allow sufficient time for adequate growth of the oesophageal segments and consequently optimal timing of primary surgical repair. Alternative techniques to assess the length of the gap include the introduction of a stiff feeding tube or bougie into the proximal pouch with delineation of the distal pouch by bougie, flexible endoscope or contrast media refluxed from a gas-distended stomach (Figure 10.4.4).

A right-sided aortic arch occurs in approximately 5% of patients with oesophageal atresia and influences the choice of side for thoracotomy. The usual thoracotomy approach for repair of atresia is via the right side. If a right-sided arch is present and identified, a left thoracotomy is usually preferred.

If primary anastomosis is impossible, oesophageal replacement with a gastric interposition, gastric tube or, more rarely, colon transplant is performed. The gastric tube is made from the greater curvature of the stomach and is usually placed in the anterior mediastinum. In colonic replacement, a portion of the colon is interposed between the proximal oesophagus and stomach.

Most surgeons advocate an extrapleural approach for oesophageal atresia – tracheoesophageal fistula repair to avoid

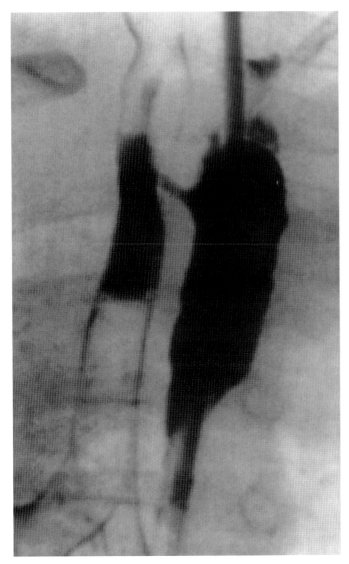

Figure 10.4.3 H-type tracheoesophageal fistula. The fistula runs an upwardly oblique course.

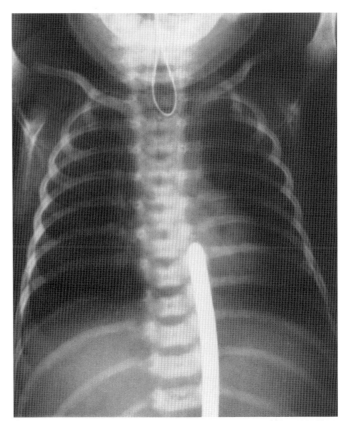

A

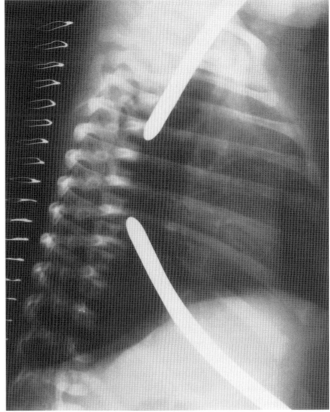

B

Figure 10.4.4 Oesophageal atresia. (A) A feeding tube has been introduced from above and a metal bougie from below (via a gastrostomy) to determine the length of the atretic segment. (B) The same infant some weeks later showing a shorter gap. A radiopaque marker is included in the image to correct for radiographic magnification.

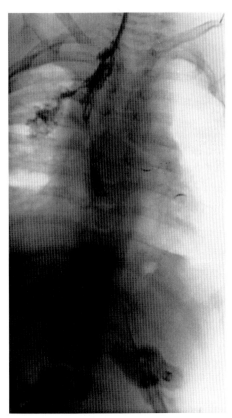

Figure 10.4.5 Postoperative leak. Water-soluble contrast media is seen to leak at the level of the anastomosis and collect in the extrapleural space of the right hemithorax.

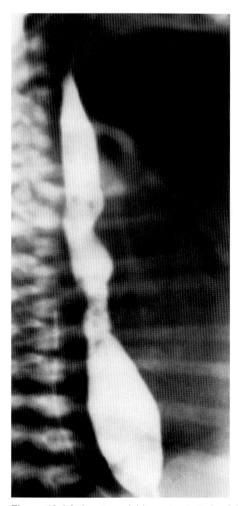

Figure 10.4.6 A water-soluble contrast study of the oesophagus after surgical repair shows a satisfactory anastomosis.

opening the pleural cavity and consequently empyema formation in the event of an anastomotic breakdown. A mediastinal drain is usually placed for the immediate postoperative period. The incidence of anastomotic leaks is approximately 15%. Most leaks are clinically insignificant and up to 95% close spontaneously. A low osmolar contrast swallow examination is commonly performed 5–7 days postoperatively, to exclude anastomotic leaks (Figures 10.4.5 and 10.4.6). Extrapleural fluid collections due to a significant leak look similar to pleural effusions on chest radiographs. They are associated with an increased risk of stricture formation and occasionally recurrent tracheoesophageal fistula.

POSTREPIR COMPLICATIONS

Clinically significant stricture formation at the anastomotic site is a common postoperative complication. It is related to surgical technique, ischaemia at the oesophageal ends, anastomotic leak and gastroesophageal reflux. Traditionally, dilatation has been performed with bougies at oesophagoscopy under general anaesthesia. An alternative is dilatation with inflatable balloon catheters (Figure 10.4.7). Food bolus impaction may occur when the child is older.

Rarely, a tracheoesophageal fistula may recur in the early postoperative period, usually in the setting of an anastomotic leak. Occasionally it may not be recognized for months or even years. The symptoms are similar to those seen with an H-type fistula and

careful contrast examination or bronchoscopy is required to detect the recurrent fistula (Figure 10.4.8).

Oesophageal dysmotility after repair of oesophageal atresia is common and is probably due to both congenital oesophageal motor dysfunction and acquired abnormality as a result of surgical manipulation or vagal disruption. The commonest manifestation of this is gastroesophageal reflux. Many of these children undergo antireflux procedures to avoid further morbidity associated with acid reflux.

Tracheomalacia is a further problem in these infants and is thought by some to be due to chronic intrauterine compression of the trachea by a distended upper oesophageal pouch. Fluoroscopy allows dynamic evaluation of the degree of tracheal collapse during respiration and, if there is doubt, bronchoscopy with or without bronchography will confirm.

Owing to oesophageal dysmotility, with or without proximal dilatation above the anastomosis, there is poor clearance of oesophageal content in the supine position and at night overspill with aspiration pneumonia may occur. This poor clearance will not be appreciated unless the examination is done in the supine position.

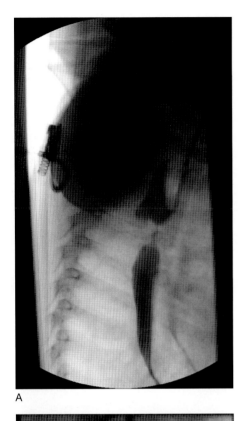

A

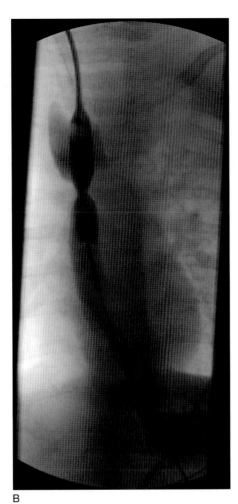

B

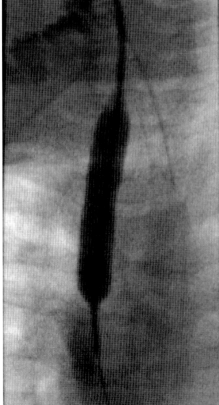

C

Figure 10.4.7 Oesophageal stricture postatresia repair. (A) A contrast oesophagogram outlines a tight stricture at the anastomotic site. (B) An inflated balloon crosses the stricture with a characteristic waist seen during the dilatation procedure. (C) Later in the dilatation procedure the waist is no longer seen. (Images courtesy of Dr Bairbre Connolly, The Hospital for Sick Children, Toronto.)

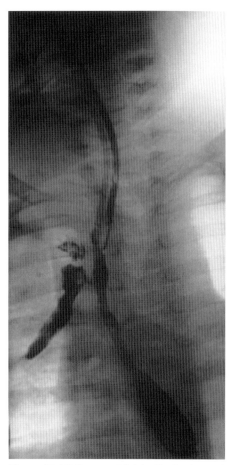

Figure 10.4.8 Recurrent fistula. Contrast examination of the oesophagus shows filling of the trachea and right bronchus through a recurrent tracheoesophageal fistula at the anastomotic site.

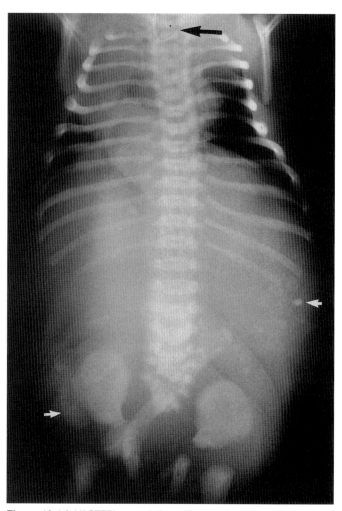

Figure 10.4.9 VACTERL association with oesophageal atresia (black arrow). This infant demonstrates dextrocardia, and lower lumbar and sacral vertebral anomalies. The infant also had an ectopic anus. There is calcification of meconium in the peritoneal cavity, the result of intrauterine perforation (white arrows). There is a left pneumothorax.

VACTERL ASSOCIATION

Between 50% and 70% of infants with oesophageal atresia have associated anomalies, most commonly congenital heart disease. The acronym VACTERL refers to a spectrum of associated congenital malformations that include vertebral abnormalities, anal atresia, cardiac defects, tracheoesophageal fistula, (o)esophageal atresia, renal anomalies and radial limb abnormalities (Figure 10.4.9). This is also known as the VATER syndrome. The work-up of these children should include echocardiography and renal US. Table 10.4.1 lists the common and uncommon associated congenital anomalies seen with oesophageal atresia and tracheoesophageal fistulas. In the last half century, the overall survival rate of infants with oesophageal atresia has improved from less than 40% to between 84% and 95%. Presently, mortality is usually associated with low birth weight (<1500 g), severe cardiac or other congenital anomalies or ventilator dependency.

FURTHER READING

Donnelly LA, Frush DP, Bisset GS. The appearance and significance of extrapleural fluid after EA repair. American Journal of Roentgenology 1999; 172:231–233.

Engum SA, Grosfeld JL, West KW et al. Analysis of morbidity and mortality in 227 cases of esophageal atresia and/or tracheoesophageal fistula over two decades. Archives of Surgery 1995; 130:502.

Farrant P. The antenatal diagnosis of oesophageal atresia by ultrasound. British Journal of Radiology 1980; 53:1202.

Harris J, Kallen B, Robert E. Descriptive epidemiology of alimentary tract atresia. Teratology 1995; 52:15.

Iuchtman M, Brereton R, Spitz L et al. Morbidity and mortality in 46 patients with the VACTERL association. Isreali Journal of Medical Science 1992; 28:281.

Pletcher BA, Friedes JS, Breg WR et al. Familial occurrence of esophageal atresia with and without tracheoesophageal fistula: report of two unusual kindreds. American Journal of Medical Genetics 1991; 39:380.

Puri P, Ninan GK, Blake NS et al. Delayed primary anastomosis for esophageal atresia: 18 months' to 11 years' follow-up. Journal of Pediatric Surgery 1992; 27:1127.

Spitz L. Esophageal atresia: past, present and future. Journal of Pediatric Surgery 1996; 31:19.

Tovar JA, Diez Pardo JA, Murcia J et al. Ambulatory 24-hour manometric and pH metric evidence of permanent impairment of clearance capacity in patients with esophageal atresia. Journal of Pediatric Surgery 1995; 30:1224.

Table 10.4.1 VACTER associations

	Common	Uncommon
Cardiovascular	Patent ductus arteriosus	Right aortic arch
	Ventricular septal defect	Atrial septal defect
		Fallot's tetralogy
		Dextrocardia
		Double aortic arch
		Total anomalous pulmonary venous drainage
		Coarctation of the aorta
		Transposition of the great vessels
Skeletal	Vertebral	Sternal
	Rib	Congenital dislocation of the hip
	Radial	Club feed
		Polydacthy
Pulmonary		Lobar hypoplasia
		Lobar agenesis
		Unilateral pulmonary hypoplasia
		Unilateral pulmonary agenesis
		Pulmonary sequestration
		Tracheal agenesis
		Tracheal stenosis
		Oesophageal lung
Gastrointestinal	Anorectal atresia	Duodenal stenosis
	Duodenal atresia	Malrotation of bowel
		Hypertrophic pyloric stenosis
		Oesophageal duplication cyst
		Congenital oesophageal stenosis
		Anal stenosis
Genitourinary	Unilateral renal genesis	Horseshoe kidney
	Renal dysplasia	
Miscellaneous	Down's syndrome	Pierre Robin syndrome
		Goldenhar anomaly

LARYNGOTRACHEO-ESOPHAGEAL CLEFT

This is a rare anomaly with a cleft of variable size through the larynx, cricoid cartilage and the trachea. The most severe form is a common tube for the trachea and oesophagus (oesophagotrachea) (Figure 10.4.10). Presentation is early with choking on feeding, excessive mucous, aspiration and respiratory distress. Anomalies such as oesophageal atresia and tracheoesophageal fistula may be associated. The diagnosis is made by laryngoscopy. A barium swallow may first identify an unsuspected lesion. The diagnosis of cleft larynx should be considered if contrast medium easily fills the upper trachea on a swallow. A small cleft may be difficult to identify by contrast studies and the definitive method of diagnosis is endoscopy.

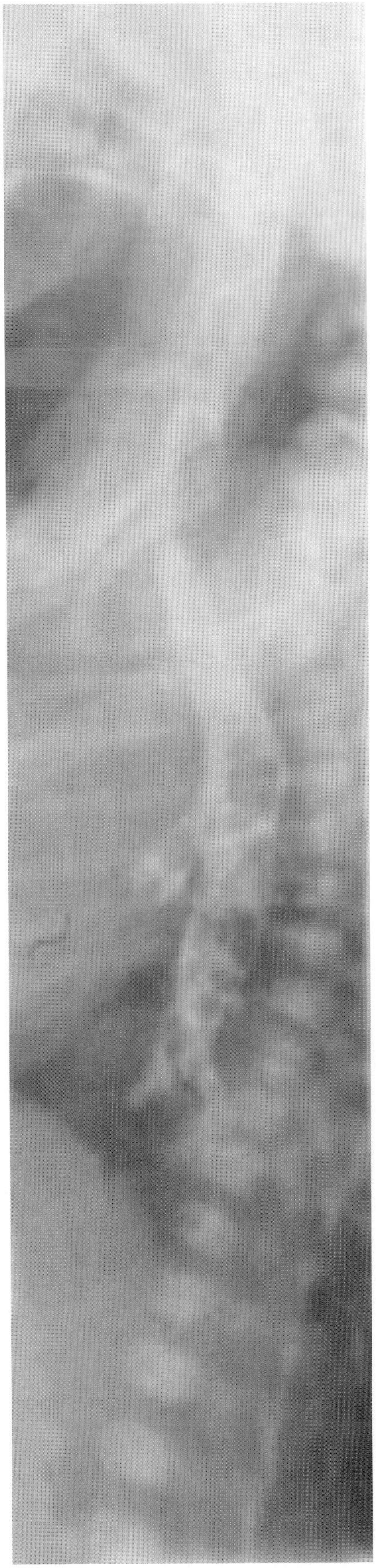

Figure 10.4.10 An infant with a laryngotracheal oesophageal cleft. Note filling of both trachea and oesophagus on water-soluble contrast swallow.

FURTHER READING

Burroughs N, Leap LL. Laryngotracheoesophagal cleft: report of a case successfully treated and review of the literature. Pediatrics 1974; 53:516–522.
Morgan CL, Grossman H, Leonidas J. Roentgenographic findings in a spectrum of uncommon tracheoesophageal anomalies. Clinical Radiology 1979; 30:353–358.

PHARYNGEAL PERFORATION

Passage of a nasogastric tube may inadvertently result in retropharyngeal perforation by the tube, which then passes into the mediastinum (Figure 10.4.11). The tube passage is halted and this may simulate a tracheoesophageal fistula with an upper pouch on x-ray. The injection of water-soluble non-ionic contrast will show the typical appearance of mediastinal contrast.

GASTROESOPHAGEAL REFLUX

The neonatal lower oesophageal sphincter is shorter and functionally more immature than that of the older child or adult. During early neonatal life gastroesophageal reflux may be considered physiological. The lower oesophageal sphincter rapidly matures in the first 6–7 weeks of life, regardless of the gestational age of the neonate. Predisposing factors to continued and severe gastroesophageal reflux include a short intra-abdominal oesophagus, hiatus hernia (Figure 10.4.12), oesophageal atresia, bronchopulmonary dysplasia and coexisting neurological disorders.

The role of imaging in these infants is to rule out conditions that may cause similar symptoms such as gastric outlet obstruction or malrotation. Barium or non-ionic water-soluble studies are the initial investigation in most centres. Severe reflux is usually

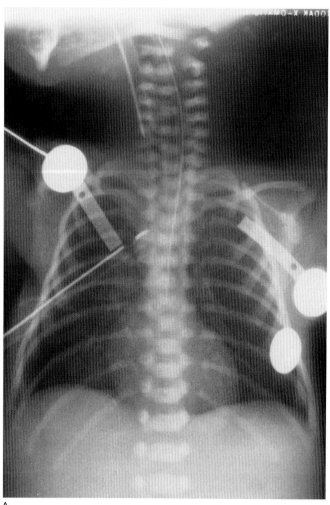

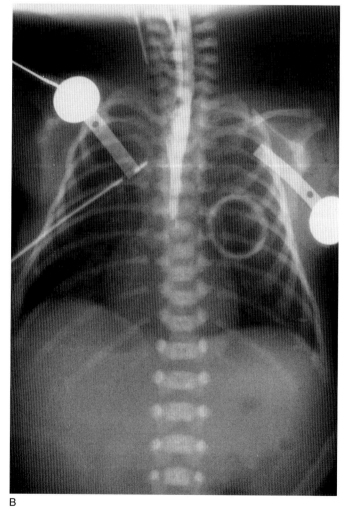

A

B

Figure 10.4.11 Oesophageal perforation. (A) Without contrast. (B) Contrast swallow. Iatrogenic retropharyngeal perforation with nasogastric tube in the mediastinum. The tube is too low to be in an atretic oesophagus. The contrast swallow shows typical appearances of mediastinal contrast. Right pneumothorax drain *in situ*.

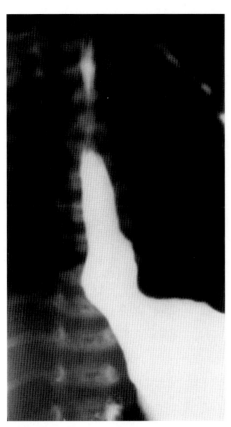

Figure 10.4.12 Gastroesophageal reflux. There is oesophageal irregularity suggesting oesophagitis and a small hiatus hernia.

demonstrated but small degrees of reflux may not. The level of the reflux should be recorded.

Severe gastroesophageal reflux may not be demonstrated by barium studies due to the short screening time and the non-physiological nature of the study conditions. In particular, there is low sensitivity for demonstrating oesophagitis. A radionuclide 'milk scan' is more sensitive for the detection of reflux, probably related to the extended observation of the examination. Similarly, colour Doppler sonography is a sensitive indicator of gastroesophageal reflux but lacks criteria for determination of reflux severity. Twenty-four-hour pH monitoring is considered the gold standard for diagnosis of pathological gastroesophageal reflux.

Treatment consists of adopting a semi-seated position 24 h a day and thickening of feeds. Other measures include frequent feeds of small volume to decrease gastric distension.

Complications of severe gastroesophageal reflux include failure to thrive, stricture formation in the oesophagus and aspiration pneumonia.

FURTHER READING

Boix-Ochoa J, Canals J. Maturation of the lower esophagus. Journal of Pediatric Surgery 1976; 11:749.

Jang HS, Lee JS, Lim GY. Correlation of color Doppler sonographic findings with pH measurement in gastroesophageal reflux in children. Journal of Clinical Ultrasound 2001; 29:212–217.

Orenstein SR. Gastroesophageal reflux. Pediatric Review 1992; 13:174.

Sondheimer JM. Continuous monitoring of distal esophageal pH: a diagnostic test for gastroesophageal reflux in infants. Journal of Pediatrics 1980; 96:804.

ENTERIC DUPLICATIONS AND CYSTS

The histology of the mucosal lining of the cyst determines the nature of a foregut duplication cyst. These are subdivided into bronchogenic cysts, enteric cysts and neurenteric cysts. The oesophagus is the second most common site of gastrointestinal duplications after ileal duplication. Enteric cysts are lined by oesophageal or gastric mucosa and have a smooth muscle wall. These cysts occur in the posterior mediastinum or neck and frequently cause pressure effects on the adjacent oesophagus or airway (Figure 10.4.13). Enteric cysts are often integrated within the oesophageal wall and may rarely communicate with the lumen. Rarely, the cyst extends into the abdomen and may communicate with the lumen of the stomach, small bowel or pancreatic duct. Acidic secretions from gastric mucosal lining may cause ulceration and haemorrhage with an acute presentation due to expansion and mass effect, or anaemia.

Neurenteric cysts have a gastrointestinal mucosal lining and are associated with vertebral anomalies. There may be a connection with the spinal canal such as a fibrous track or fistula to the dura. These cysts carry the risk of spinal cord compression or meningitis, although they may be asymptomatic at presentation. The vertebral anomalies are commonly butterfly vertebrae, hemivertebra or anterior spina bifida and are located superior to the neurenteric cyst. The anomalies may cause scoliosis or kyphoscoliosis.

The cysts are usually detectable on plain radiography of the chest with or without associated vertebral anomalies. A contrast swallow may depict the lesion's proximity to the oesophagus but is rarely diagnostic. CT or MRI is helpful for surgical planning. The cyst is non-enhancing with a homogeneous near-water attenuation on CT. It has low signal on T1-weighted and high signal on T2-weighted images on MRI. Spinal MRI or, rarely, CT contrast myelography is indicated in the presence of vertebral anomalies to delineate the anatomy.

Bronchogenic cysts are described here as these too are part of the spectrum of bronchopulmonary foregut malformations. Bronchogenic cysts may present in the neonatal period if they cause airway compression, or may be discovered later in life. They become symptomatic if they enlarge or become infected and compress the airways. They may also be discovered incidentally on radiographs (Figure 10.4.14). Bronchogenic cysts are most frequently located in the subcarinal region but can occur anywhere along the trachea. When they occur in the vicinity of a bronchus they may cause lobar collapse or obstructive emphysema. The cysts are fluid filled and are smooth-walled masses both on x-ray and cross-sectional imaging.

FURTHER READING

Ildstad ST, Tollerud DJ, Weiss RG et al. Duplications of the alimentary tract. Clinical characteristics, preferred treatment and associated malformations. Annals of Surgery 1988; 208:184–189.

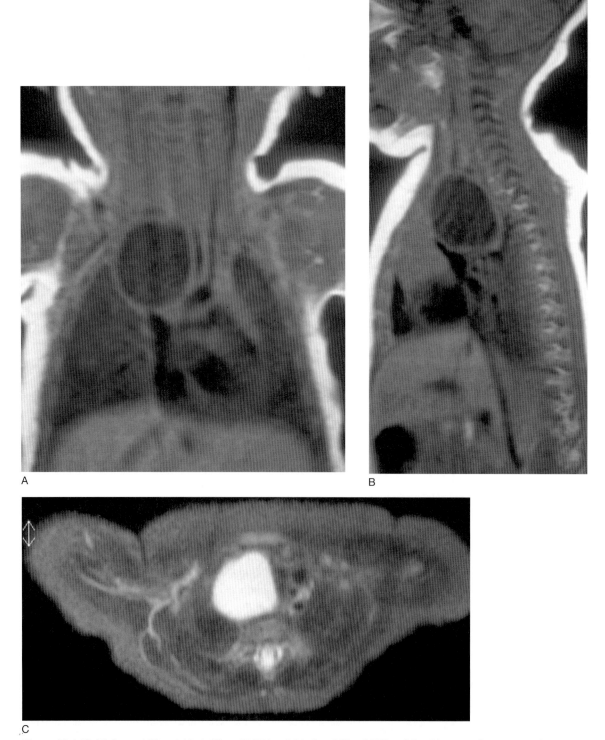

A

B

C

Figure 10.4.13 (A) Coronal T1-weighted, (B) sagittal T1-weighted and (C) axial T2-weighted images of a neonate who presented with stridor. The MR images demonstrate typical appearance of a proximal oesophageal duplication cyst displacing the trachea and causing the airway obstruction.

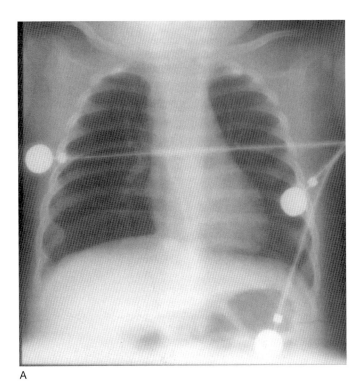

A

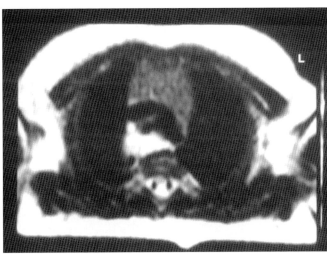

B

Figure 10.4.14 (A) Radiograph and (B) MRI of a 2-week-old infant with stridor. On the x-ray there is subtle widening of the mediastinal shadow and slight overinflation of the lungs. The T2-weighted MRI shows the high signal within the bronchogenic cyst.

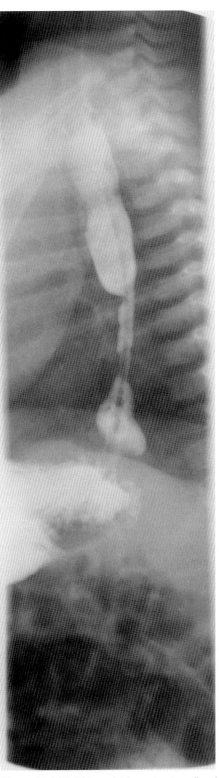

Figure 10.4.15 Water-soluble contrast swallow in a 3-week-old infant with marked feeding difficulties. There is narrowing of the lower one-third of the oesophagus with a normal hiatus. There was no reflux on the study. This segmental narrowing is typical of a congenital oesophageal stenosis at this age.

Superina RA, Ein SH, Humphreys RP. Cystic duplications of the esophagus and neurenteric cysts. Journal of Pediatric Surgery 1984; 19:527–530.

Weiss LM, Fagelman D, Warhit JM. CT demonstration of an esophageal duplication cyst. Journal of Computer Assisted Tomography 1983; 7:716–718.

CONGENITAL OESOPHAGEAL STENOSIS

Congenital oesophageal stenosis is a rare condition that must be differentiated from acquired stenosis due to gastroesophageal reflux or, in older children, ingestion of caustic agents. It may occur in the setting of oesophageal atresia and tracheoesophageal fistula or other congenital anomalies. There are three described patterns: a membranous web or diaphragm, fibromuscular hypertrophy (Figure 10.4.15) and stenosis secondary to tracheobronchial remnants within the oesophageal wall. The commonest location is the mid or lower oesophagus. Symptoms of dysphagia and vomiting usually occur or become pronounced when solid food is introduced to the diet. At the time of diagnosis the oesophageal narrowing may be erroneously attributed to undiagnosed gastro-esophageal reflux or achalasia, and oesophageal manometry or pH monitoring may be required to establish the correct diagnosis. The treatment options include oesophageal dilatation by bougienage or balloon dilatation, or surgical resection. Oesophageal webs and stenosis due to tracheobronchial remnants are treated by surgical excision and reanastomosis.

FURTHER READING

Neilson IR, Croitoru DP, Guttman FM et al. Distal congenital esophageal stenosis associated with esophageal atresia. Journal of Pediatric Surgery 1991; 26:478.

Yeung CK, Spitz L, Brereton RJ et al. Congenital esophageal stenosis due to tracheo-bronchial remnants: a rare but important association with esophageal atresia. Journal of Pediatric Surgery 1992; 27:852.

The Stomach

Veronica Donoghue, Eilish L Twomey

INTERPRETATION OF THE NEONATAL ABDOMINAL RADIOGRAPH

In the normal term neonate, air is present in the stomach within a few seconds of the first breath, in the proximal small bowel within minutes, the distal small bowel by 3h, the caecum by 4–6h and the rectum by 24h. The passage of air is delayed in many situations. These include traumatic delivery, septicaemia, hypoglycaemia and hypoxia. All these conditions may cause ileus and thus also delayed passage of meconium. Bowel obstruction will present early in high lesions but commonly is not evident until 24h with more distal lesions. Absence of bowel gas is often seen in infants who are mechanically ventilated, have drug-induced neuromuscular paralysis or who are on nasogastric suction.

The initial radiological examination in an infant presenting with obstructive bowel symptoms is an anteroposterior (AP) supine abdominal radiograph. This should cover the abdomen from diaphragm to pubis and include the hernial orifices. A decubitus film will identify fluid levels and a pneumoperitoneum if necessary. When scrutinizing the radiograph one should attempt to identify the presence of gas throughout the bowel, remembering that the patterns of jejunum and ileum and colon are not established in neonates. The presence of rectal gas indicates patency of the gastrointestinal tract unless there has been a rectal examination or a rectal washout. Absence of rectal gas, an indicator of possible Hirschsprung's disease, is a common normal finding in premature babies. The sigmoid colon in an infant is intra-abdominal and not pelvic and may lie in the right iliac fossa and cause confusion of interpretation. The umbilical cord or an umbilical hernia may cause central opacities.

MICROGASTRIA

Congenital microgastria is a very rare anomaly in which the fetal rotation of the stomach fails and the greater and lesser curves are not distinguishable. The stomach is small, tubular and midline in position (Figure 10.5.1). Gastroesophageal reflux is common and the oesophagus is often dilated. Presentation is with feeding difficulties and non-bilious vomiting. It may be seen in association with other anomalies such as asplenia, Hirschsprung's disease and intestinal atresias.

FURTHER READING

Gorman B, Shaw DG. Congenital microgastria. British Journal of Radiology 1984; 57:260–262.
Hockberger O, Swoboda W. Congenital microgastria. A follow-up observation over six years. Pediatric Radiology 1974; 2:207–208.
Kessler H, Smulewicz JJ. Microgastria associated with agenesis of the spleen. Radiology 1973; 107:393–396.
Shackelford GD, McAlister W, Brodeur AE et al. Congenital microgastria. American Journal of Roentgenology 1973; 188:72–76.

GASTRIC ATRESIA

Almost all gastric atresias occur at the pylorus or antrum. They are thought to be due to localized vascular occlusion in fetal life and not to failure of recanalization of the intestinal tract. The condition may occasionally be familial and is inherited in an autosomal recessive manner. There are three types:

1. complete atresia, with no connection between the atretic ends;
2. complete atresia, with a fibrous band connecting the atretic ends; and
3. gastric membrane or diaphragm.

Gastric membranes may lead to incomplete intestinal obstruction, due to perforations of variable size in the membrane. In this instance, gas is seen in the distal intestine. All other types of atresia lead to a gas-filled distended stomach on abdominal radiographs.

Functional gastric dilatation is seen occasionally and may be accompanied by a paucity of distal gas in the intestine. These appearances may be caused by sepsis, neurological impairment or generalized disorders of gastrointestinal motility and should not be

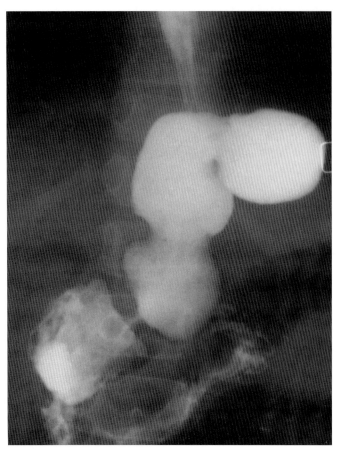

Figure 10.5.1 Congenital microgastria. The barium meal shows a small tubular stomach.

confused with true gastric atresia. Gastric atresia may be associated with multiple other gastrointestinal atresias, particularly of the colon, and a contrast enema should be a routine part of preoperative investigation.

Rarely, gastric atresia may be a complication of epidermolysis bullosa but seldom in neonates. The 'atresia' is due to scar formation.

FURTHER READING

Cremin BJ. Congenital pyloric antral membranes in infancy. Radiology 1969; 92:509–512.
Jinkins JR, Ball TI, Clements JL Jr et al. Antral mucosal diaphragms in infants and children. Pediatric Radiology 1980; 9:69–72.
Melham RE, Salem G, Mishalany H et al. Pyloro-duodenal atresia – a report of three families with similarly affected children. Pediatric Radiology 1975; 3:1–5.

GASTRIC RUPTURE

Spontaneous rupture of the stomach is a well-described but rare occurrence in neonates and carries a high mortality rate (Figure 10.5.2A). The aetiology is unclear but appears to occur in associ-

ation with indomethacin use, gastric ischaemia, peptic ulceration or gastric distension secondary to distal obstruction or mechanical ventilation. Presentation is usually in the first week of life, in a previously well neonate. Abdominal radiographs show a gross pneumoperitoneum with the ligamentum falciparum outlined by air. The free air in the peritoneum is sometimes referred to as the 'football sign'. It may result from any intestinal perforation in infants. Absence of the gastric air–fluid level is often noted on decubitus views. A further rare cause of gastric perforation is volvulus of the stomach with gastric outlet obstruction (Figure 10.5.2B). Caecal perforation may also occur spontaneously in neonates. As for gastric perforation, the diagnosis is made at surgery.

FURTHER READING

Lloyd JR. The aetiology of gastrointestinal perforations in the newborn. Journal of Pediatric Surgery 1969; 4:77–84.
Pochaczevsky R, Bryk D. New roentgenographic signs of neonatal gastric perforation. Radiology 1972; 102:147–148.
Rosser SB, Clark CH, Elechi EN. Spontaneous neonatal gastric perforation. Journal of Pediatric Surgery 1982; 17:390–394.

GASTRIC DUPLICATION CYSTS

Gastric duplication cysts are an uncommon cause of vomiting in the neonate. They most commonly occur in the antropyloric region of the stomach. Ultrasound (US) shows an inner echogenic mucosa with a hypoechoic muscular wall, which is diagnostic. The gastric mucosal lining of the cyst may ulcerate and haemorrhage and echogenic debris may be seen within the cyst on sonography.

FURTHER READING

Gupta AK, Berry M, Mitra DK. Gastric duplication cyst in children: report of two cases. Pediatric Radiology 24:346–347.
Moccia WA, Astacio JE, Kaude JV. Ultrasonographic demonstration of gastric duplication in infancy. Pediatric Radiology 1981; 11:52–54.

PYLOROSPASM

In this condition, peristalsis is present in the stomach but the distal antrum and pylorus fail to relax to allow emptying of the stomach. Vomiting may be projectile in nature and associated with poor feeding. Ultrasound of the pylorus shows normal dimensions. It is important to differentiate this condition from hypertrophic pyloric stenosis as the treatment of pylorospasm is expectant. At US the gastric antrum is identified, the pylorus fails to open but the pyloric canal dimensions and wall thickness are normal. Similar findings are identified on contrast studies. There may be extensive to and fro peristalsis in the stomach.

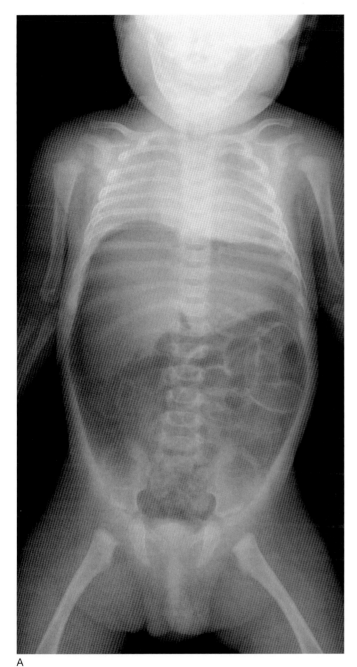

A

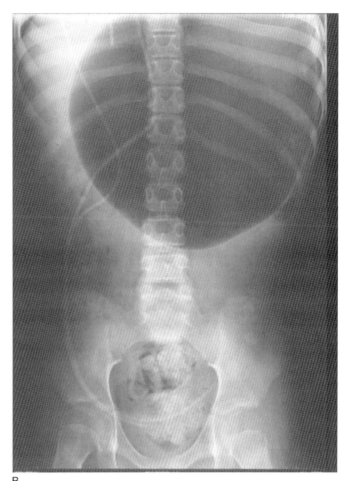

B

Figure 10.5.2 (A) Infant who sustained a massive pneumoperitoneum due to spontaneous gastric rupture. Note huge amount of free air and the ligamentum falciparum outlined by air. (B) An older child showing typical appearances of gastric volvulus.

FOCAL FOVEOLAR HYPERPLASIA

This is a rare condition in which there is hypertrophy of the foveolar cells in the gastric antrum and it causes gastric outlet obstructive symptoms. It has been described in association with prostaglandins used for treating congenital heart disease. It resolves spontaneously. The diagnosis is usually made with US where the hypertrophic mucosa is seen. This is discussed further in Chapter 10.12.

The Duodenum

Veronica Donoghue, Eilish L Twomey

The differentiation of small from large bowel on plain radiographs in the neonate can be impossible due to the absence of distinguishing features such as haustral folds, which do not develop until about 6 weeks. The sigmoid colon in a neonate can be an inferior relation of the liver and can lie predominantly in the right side of the abdomen (Figure 10.6.1). This is due to absence of the normal pelvic cavity in the neonate. Although the rectum can be identified, particularly on a lateral view, the presence of gas within the rectum may be the result of digital rectal examination and should not be taken to indicate continuity of the gut. In the presence of clinical signs of high intestinal obstruction such as bilious vomiting and plain abdominal radiographs, which are not characteristic of complete duodenal obstruction, contrast medium studies are indicated to provide information about the location and type of obstruction, of which malrotation and duodenal stenosis are the most likely causes. A corroborative sign of high obstruction is the to-and-fro movement of contrast medium in the duodenum with duodenogastric reflux. The causes of duodenal obstruction in the newborn are listed in Table 10.6.1.

DUODENAL ATRESIA, STENOSIS AND WEBS

Duodenal atresia results from a failure of gut recanalization and not from an intrauterine vascular accident, which appears to be the aetiology of jejunal and ileal atresia. Atresia occurs more commonly than duodenal webs, although they appear to have the same aetiology. Webs may be complete or incomplete. Duodenal stenosis is rare. Eighty per cent of these duodenal lesions occur just distal to the ampulla of Vater.

Associated anomalies are found in half of all patients with duodenal atresia. Down's syndrome is present in 30% of patients. Other associated conditions include congenital heart disease, malrotation, anorectal anomalies or other gastrointestinal atresias. When duodenal atresia and oesophageal atresia without fistula occur together the abdomen appears gasless on radiographs. Ultrasound (US) shows a grossly dilated fluid-filled stomach and proximal duodenum.

Antenatal diagnosis is often possible due to identification of the dilated stomach and duodenum in the upper abdomen. Polyhydramnios is seen in 40% of infants. Clinical presentation is usually with bilious vomiting in the first hours of life. The presentation may be delayed if the obstruction is incomplete, as is the case with duodenal stenosis or incomplete duodenal webs. The vomiting is non-bilious in the 20% of neonates with atresia just proximal to the ampulla of Vater.

In duodenal atresia, the abdominal radiograph is diagnostic showing gaseous distension of the stomach and proximal duodenum without distal gas, the so-called 'double-bubble' appearance (Figures 10.6.2 and 10.6.3). No further radiological investigation is required. If the child has vomited just before the radiograph is taken the 'double bubble' may be lost but a wait of 30 min will restore it. Distal gas in the intestine is seen with duodenal stenosis, incomplete duodenal web or rarely in the presence of a complete atresia where a Y-shaped bile duct inserts both proximal and distal to the atresia.

If partial obstruction is seen on abdominal radiographs an upper gastrointestinal study is appropriate to differentiate duodenal stenosis (Figure 10.6.4) or web from other causes of high neonatal intestinal obstruction such as malrotation with volvulus or obstructing Ladd's bands. The duodenal web is often difficult to demonstrate; the characteristic intraluminal diverticulum or 'windsock' appearance often does not develop until later in life (Figure 10.6.5). Some surgeons request a contrast enema preoperatively to rule out additional intestinal atresias. The colon should have a normal calibre in duodenal atresia and therefore demonstration of a microcolon indicates a distal atresia.

FURTHER READING

Crowe JE, Sumner TE. Combined esophageal and duodenal atresia without tracheoesophageal fistula: characteristic radiographic changes. American Journal of Roentgenology 1978; 130:167–168.

Fonkalsrud EW, de Lorimar AA, Hays DM. Congenital atresia and stenosis of the duodenum. A review compiled from the members of the Surgical Section of the American Academy of Pediatrics. Pediatrics 1969; 43:79–83.

Kassner EG, Sutton AL, De Groot TJ. Bile duct anomalies associated with duodenal atresia: paradoxical presence of small bowel gas. American Journal of Roentgenology 1972; 116:577–583.

Table 10.6.1 Causes of duodenal obstruction in the newborn

Intrinsic	*Extrinsic*
Duodenal atresia	Ladd's bands
Duodenal stenosis	Midgut volvulus with malrotation
Duodenal web or diaphragm	Annular pancreas
	Duplication
	Haematoma
	Preduodenal portal vein

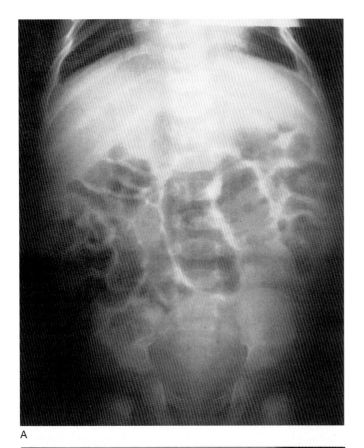

A

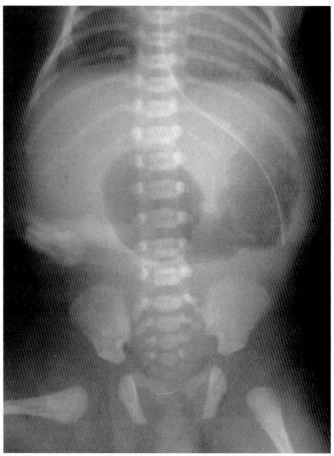

Figure 10.6.2 Duodenal atresia. Supine radiograph shows the characteristic 'double bubble' sign.

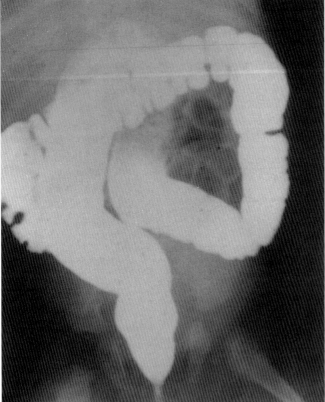

B

Figure 10.6.1 (A) Supine abdominal radiograph shows gas-filled loops of bowel in the mid and right abdomen. (B) Redundant colon is seen at barium enema with the sigmoid colon lying to the right side.

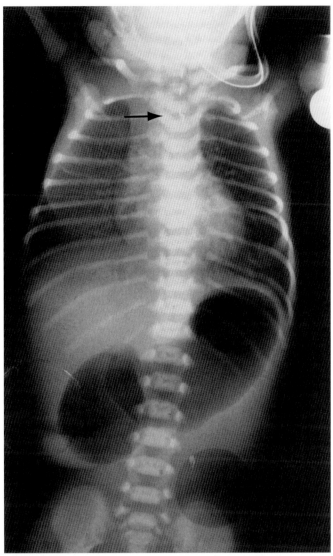

Figure 10.6.3 Duodenal atresia. A 'double bubble' is seen in the upper abdomen. Note the oesophageal atresia with an associated tracheoesophageal fistula. There is an artifact from an incubator hole in the lower left abdomen.

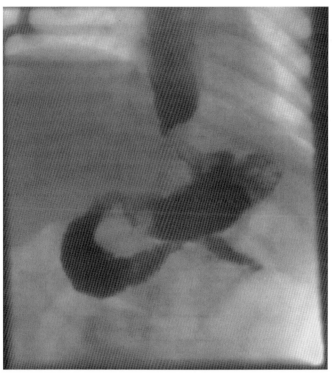

Figure 10.6.4 Three-week-old infant with duodenal stenosis. Contrast study shows a mildly dilated duodenum typical of the early findings in duodenal stenosis. If left untreated the proximal duodenum can massively dilate and, in older children, presents as failure to thrive, vomiting and halitosis secondary to the undigested food.

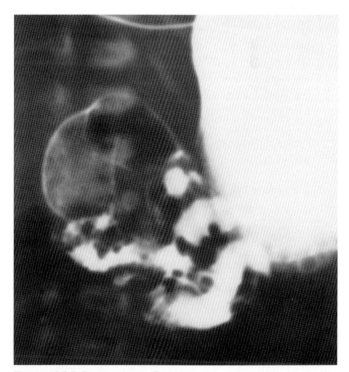

Figure 10.6.5 Duodenal web. There is an incomplete obstruction at the level of the ampulla of vater and dilatation of the proximal duodenum. An incomplete diaphragm was found at surgery.

ANNULAR PANCREAS

Annular pancreas is often incidentally discovered at surgery in the neonate with duodenal atresia or stenosis. Annular pancreas often coexists with these conditions, although the primary cause of duodenal obstruction is thought to be the atresia or stenosis. The degree of duodenal obstruction may be partial or complete. Annular pancreas results from failure of the ventral part of pancreas to rotate completely around the duodenum and fuse with the dorsal portion. Ultrasound or computed tomography (CT) may demonstrate a ring of pancreatic tissue surrounding the second part of duodenum and contiguous with the pancreas. The diagnosis is usually made in the neonatal period. If the pancreatic ring is incomplete there may be little or no associated symptoms and presentation may be delayed into adulthood.

FURTHER READING

Inamoto K, Ishikawa Y, Itoh N. CT demonstration of annular pancreas: case report. Gastrointestinal Radiology 1983; 8:143–144.
Merrill JR, Raffensperger JG. Pediatric annular pancreas: twenty years experience. Journal of Pediatric Surgery 1976; 11:921–925.
Orr LA, Powell RW, Melhem RE. Sonographic demonstration of annular pancreas in the newborn. Journal of Ultrasound Medicine 1992; 11:373–375.

PREDUODENAL PORTAL VEIN

This rare abnormality results from the portal vein lying anterior to the duodenum causing indentation and compression. The gut is drained in uterine life by the right and left vitelline veins, which are connected by three venous channels. The middle channel normally persists as the portal vein and follows a course posterior to the duodenum. A preduodenal portal vein occurs as a result of abnormal persistence of the inferior channel.

Over 85% of infants with a preduodenal portal vein have associated malformations such as malrotation with bands, situs inversus, intrinsic duodenal obstruction, biliary atresia and annular pancreas. The radiological findings depend on the degree of obstruction. The diagnosis may be suspected due to an indentation on the duodenum between the first and second parts. Doppler ultrasound or contrast-enhanced CT may demonstrate the portal vein in this anomalous position. Frequently, the diagnosis is made at surgery for an associated anomaly. It is important that the anomalous vein is recognized and not transected, especially as it may lie contained in a peritoneal band.

FURTHER READING

Fernandes ET, Burton EM, Hixson SD et al. Preduodenal portal vein: surgery and radiographic appearance. Journal of Pediatric Surgery 1990; 25: 1270–1272.
Georgacopulo P, Vigi V. Duodenal obstruction due to a preduodenal portal vein in a newborn. Journal of Pediatric Surgery 1980; 15:339–340.
Johnson GF. Congenital preduodenal portal vein. American Journal of Roentgenology 1971; 112:93–99.

The Small Bowel

Veronica Donoghue, Eilish L Twomey

The small bowel of the neonate is quite different in appearance from that of the older child. It is difficult to identify the valvulae conniventes and also to distinguish jejunum from ileum. Peristalsis is usually quite marked and the transit time to large bowel is often shorter than in the older child or adult.

JEJUNOILEAL ATRESIA AND STENOSIS

Small bowel atresia is more common than duodenal or colonic atresia and usually occurs as an isolated anomaly of the gastrointestinal tract. There are four types of small bowel atresia:

type 1 – membranous or web-like atresia;
type 2 – atresia with a fibrous cord connecting the atretic bowel ends;
type 3 – total atresia with an associated V-shaped defect in the mesentery;
type 4 – multiple atresias.

Small bowel stenosis, which appears to be a form fruste of atresia, is much less common than complete atresia. The atresia is caused by intrauterine ischaemic injury, in contrast to duodenal atresia, which appears to be a failure of recanalization. An unusual variant of type 3 atresia is termed apple peel (Christmas tree) atresia. In this form, there is proximal jejunal atresia with a large mesenteric defect and shortening of the small bowel distal to the atresia. This shortened bowel is spiralled around its blood supply from collaterals of the ileocolic artery, giving the characteristic apple peel appearance. The aetiology is most likely due to intrauterine occlusion of the distal superior mesenteric artery. The shortened small bowel leads to significant nutritional problems. A form of multiple intestinal atresias from the stomach to the rectum is recognized with an autosomal recessive pattern of inheritance. Plain film radiography may demonstrate calcification of intraluminal contents in the intervening segments of bowel.

The diagnosis of small bowel atresia may be suggested on antenatal ultrasound (US) with the presence of polyhydramnios and dilated fluid-filled loops of bowel. These findings are non-specific and the diagnosis is usually not confirmed until after birth. The neonate most often presents with bilious vomiting, abdominal distension and failure to pass meconium, although the latter will depend on the site and intrauterine timing of the atresia. Meco-

nium may be passed if the atresia is located in the jejunum and occurred late in intrauterine life.

The number and location of gas-filled loops of bowel may indicate the site of the atresia. A few loops in the left upper quadrant suggest a high intestinal obstruction such as the jejunum or proximal ileum (Figure 10.7.1 and Figure 10.7.2). If the atresia is in the proximal jejunum only one or two loops of small bowel will be seen – the so-called 'triple bubble' sign.

A low intestinal atresia in the distal ileum will usually result in many dilated loops of bowel throughout the abdomen (Figure 10.7.3). Multiple air–fluid levels are usually seen in decubitus

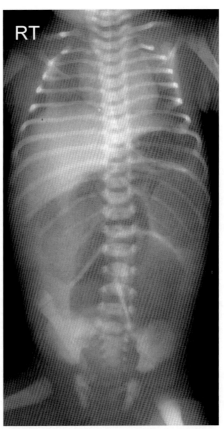

Figure 10.7.1 Infant with mid jejunal atresia showing massively dilated loops of jejunum but only about four 'bubbles', which indicates a high obstruction.

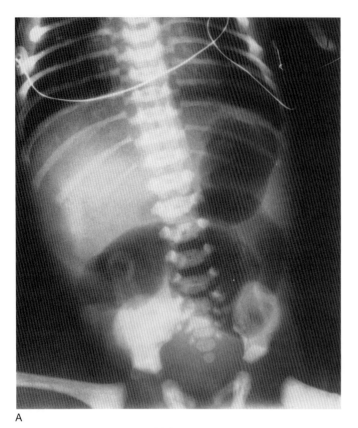

A

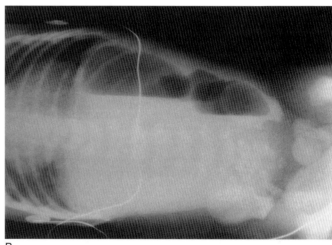

B

Figure 10.7.2 Jejunal atresia. (A) Supine radiograph shows approximately three dilated gas-filled loops indicating a high gastrointestinal obstruction. (B) Air–fluid levels on a decubitus radiograph confirm bowel obstruction.

films, which may suggest the diagnosis as these occur less often in meconium ileus. In some instances, gas mixed with meconium can produce a 'soap bubble' appearance, although this is more commonly seen with meconium ileus. The loop just proximal to the atresia is often grossly distended (Figure 10.7.3C) and occasionally may be filled with fluid giving the impression of a mass on plain radiography (Figure 10.7.4).

In utero perforation at the time of the ischaemic insult resulting in meconium peritonitis may cause speckled peritoneal calcification. Intramural calcification may be seen and probably indicates intrauterine bowel necrosis. Rarely, extensive intraluminal calcification may occur (Figure 10.7.5).

Additional imaging is not usually required in the presence of a high intestinal obstruction. A contrast enema is required for further evaluation of low bowel obstruction to distinguish between a large or small bowel obstruction. The most common causes of neonatal distal small bowel obstruction are ileal atresia and meconium ileus. Water-soluble low osmolar contrast media is introduced via a soft rectal catheter. In distal ileal atresia, an unused colon (microcolon) is seen with a very small calibre but the rectum is distensible, distinguishing it from the microcolon occasionally found in long segment Hirschsprung's disease. Care must be taken not to precipitate colonic perforation by forceful injection of contrast media.

The calibre of the colon depends on the amount of succus entericus reaching it *in utero*. In distal small bowel obstruction, this will be negligible resulting in a microcolon. In the presence of jejunal atresia, the colon will be more normal in size. Hence, a microcolon in the presence of high bowel obstruction indicates a second, more distal atresia. The ileocaecal valve is rarely competent in the neonate and in normal infants contrast medium, once it enters the small bowel, will flow freely. In distal ileal atresia, contrast stops at the atresia and does not enter the proximal dilated bowel, as is seen with meconium ileus (Figure 10.7.3E). An 'apple peel' atresia (Figure 10.7.6) may be suspected if the contrast-filled distal ileum adopts a spiral pattern. This diagnosis is very likely if there is also evidence of high intestinal obstruction and a microcolon. Abdominal US may have a role in distinguishing meconium ileus from ileal atresia. In the latter condition, the dilated bowel contains fluid and gas whereas echogenic bowel contents are prominent in meconium ileus.

Surgical treatment involves resection of the atretic or stenotic portion of intestine with reanastomosis. The proximal dilated bowel may remain dilated for some time postoperatively with altered motility. Consequently, delayed passage of contrast media may be evident in the presence of a widely patent anastomosis.

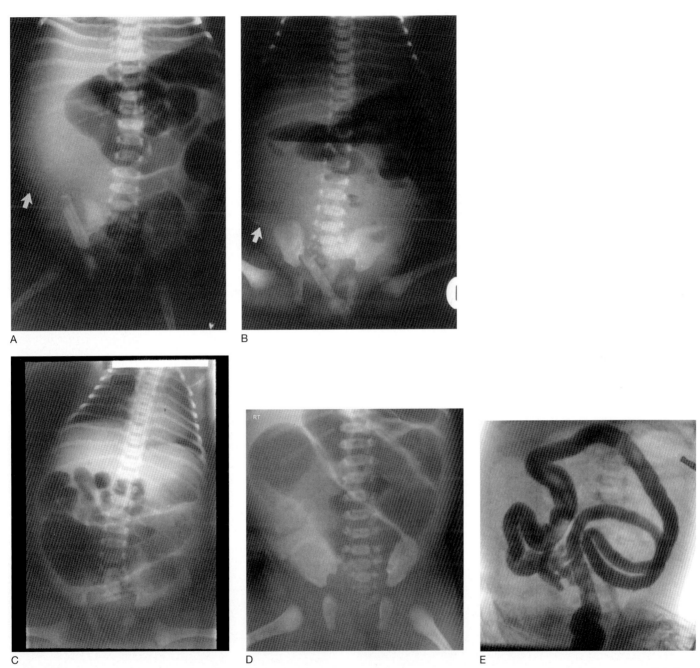

Figure 10.7.3 Three different infants with ileal atresia showing different radiographic appearances. Infant 1: a supine radiograph shows many dilated loops of bowel (A) and an erect radiograph demonstrates multiple gas–fluid levels in keeping with ileal atresia (B). Note calcification of meconium (arrow) within the peritoneal cavity due to antenatal bowel perforation, most likely the result of a vascular insult. Infant 2: note the long dilated loop of bowel proximal to the atresia with meconium but with relatively collapsed bowel more proximally (C). Infant 3: in this infant there are only a few dilated loops, which would suggest a higher atresia (D,E) but the contrast enema (E) shows the typical microcolon appearance of an ileal atresia. Note the distended rectum, which distinguishes it from Hirschsprung's disease. Note also the blind-ending atretic ileum.

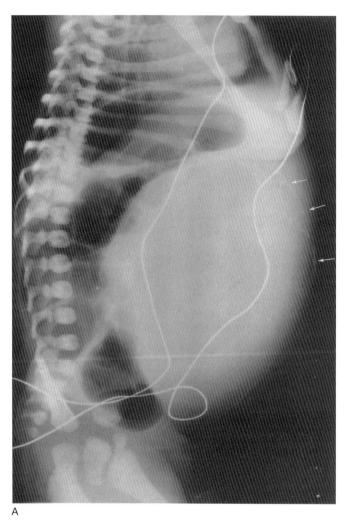

A

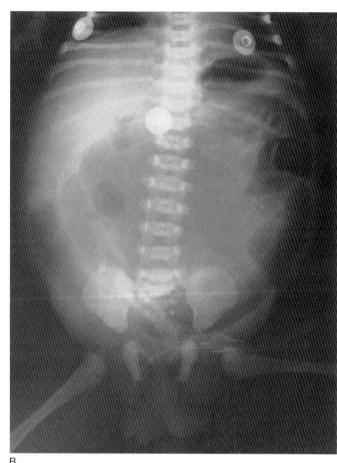

B

Figure 10.7.4 Ileal atresia with pseudocyst formation. (A) The pseudocyst consists of grossly dilated loops of small bowel which are fluid filled but will also contain meconium. These are displacing the more proximally distended bowel around it. Note the peritoneal calcification due to meconium peritonitis (small white arrows). (B) Same child some hours later showing air within the pseudocyst indicating perforation.

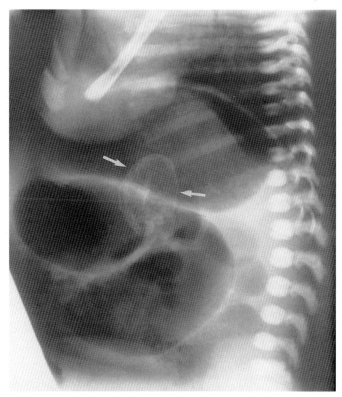

Figure 10.7.5 Ileal atresia with intraluminal calcification of meconium within the small intestine.

FURTHER READING

Aharon M, Kleinhaus U, Lichtig C. Neonatal intramural intestinal calcifications associated with bowel atresia. American Journal of Roentgenology 1978; 130:999–1000.

Berdon WE, Baker DH, Santulli TV et al. Microcolon in newborn infants with intestinal obstruction. Its correlation with the level and time of onset of obstruction. Radiology 1968; 90:878–885.

Daneman A, Martin DJ. A syndrome of multiple intestinal atresias with intraluminal calcification. A report of a case and a review of the literature. Pediatric Radiology 1979; 8:227–231.

de Lorimer AA, Fonkalsrud EW, Hays DM. Congenital atresia and stenosis of the jejunum and ileum. Surgery 1969; 65:819–827.

Leonidas JC, Amoury RA, Ashcraft KW et al. Duodenojejunal atresia with 'apple peel' small bowel. A distinct form of intestinal atresia. Radiology 1976; 118:661–665.

Neal MR, Siebert JJ, Vanderzalm T et al. Neonatal ultrasonography to distinguish between meconium ileus and ileal atresia. Journal of Ultrasound Medicine 1997; 16:263–266.

Schiavetti E, Massotti G, Torricelli M et al. 'Apple peel' syndrome. A radiological study. Pediatric Radiology 1984; 14:380–383.

MECONIUM ILEUS

Meconium ileus is distal intestinal obstruction seen in neonates due to impaction of thick, tenacious meconium in the distal ileum. It almost always occurs in children with cystic fibrosis but it has also been documented in children with abnormal intestinal motility or pancreatic insufficiency due to aplasia or ductal stenosis. Ten to twenty per cent of patients with cystic fibrosis present with meconium ileus and there may be a family history of the recessive condition.

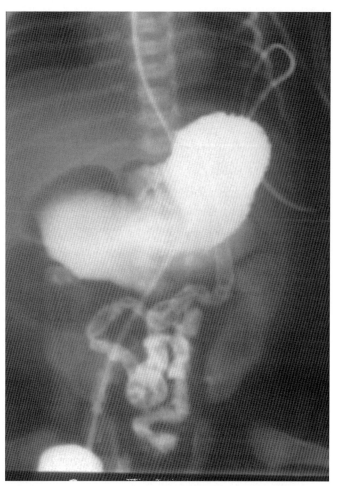

Figure 10.7.6 Contrast studies of an infant with 'apple peel' atresia. Contrast had originally been introduced into the stomach, which showed a proximal jejunal atresia. The contrast enema shows the typical appearances of a narrow, unfixed bowel lying centrally, as seen in 'apple peel' atresia.

Presentation is usually within the first 24 h of life with a clinical picture of bilious vomiting, abdominal distension and failure to pass meconium. The abdominal radiograph shows dilated gas-filled loops of bowel consistent with low intestinal obstruction. A mottled gaseous or 'soap-bubble' appearance may be seen in the right lower quadrant due to a mixture of air and meconium (Figure 10.7.7). This sign is not specific, however, and may be seen in any cause of distal intestinal obstruction. A paucity of air–fluid levels due to the viscosity of the meconium is reported to be suggestive of meconium ileus but similarly this is not a sensitive or specific sign.

Meconium ileus may become complicated by volvulus, intestinal atresia and perforation with meconium peritonitis or pseudocyst formation. Evidence of complicated meconium ileus may be seen on plain radiographs as pneumoperitoneum or ascites. If bowel perforation has occurred, diffuse speckled peritoneal calcifications indicate previous intrauterine perforation with meconium peritonitis (Figure 10.7.8). This may be seen over the liver, under the diaphragm or in the scrotum. A localized perforation forms a meconium pseudocyst, which may have peripheral curvilinear calcifications seen on plain radiographs (Figure 10.7.9). The term pseudocyst also refers to a necrotic and adherent mass of twisted

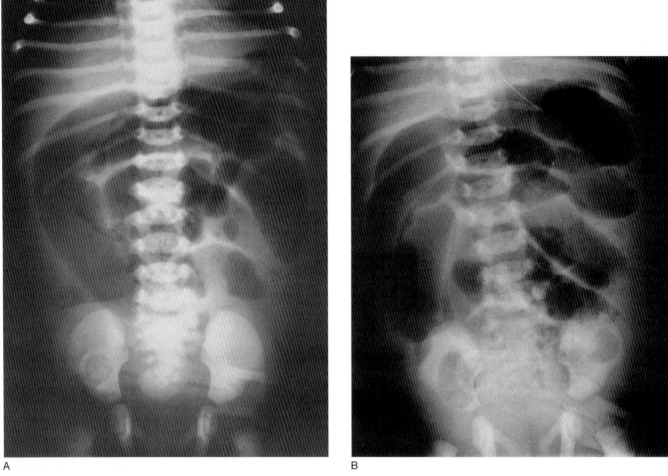

A   B

Figure 10.7.7 Meconium ileus. (A) A supine radiograph shows numerous dilated air-filled loops of bowel. (B) An erect radiograph shows the paucity of air–fluid levels suggestive of meconium ileus. Note the 'soap bubble' appearance on the left side of the abdomen.

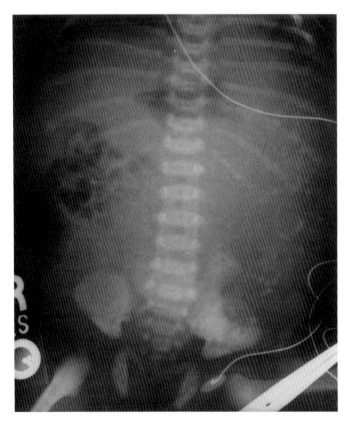

Figure 10.7.8 Meconium peritonitis. An abdominal radiograph demonstrates speckled calcifications throughout the peritoneum consistent with intrauterine bowel perforation with meconium peritonitis.

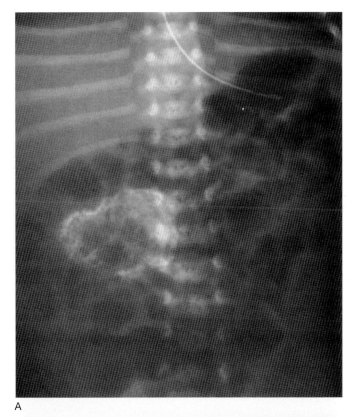

A

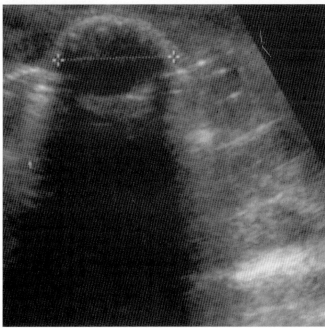

C

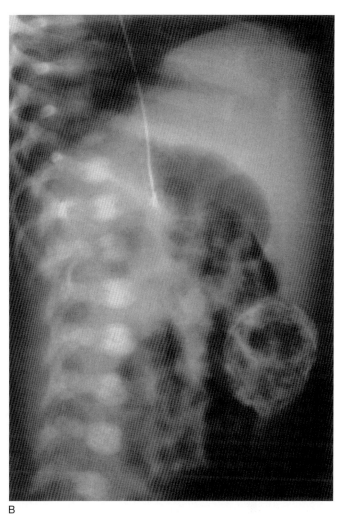

B

Figure 10.7.9 Meconium pseudocyst. (A,B) Supine and lateral abdominal radiographs show a well delineated calcified mass in the right flank. There is no pneumoperitoneum. (C) Ultrasound demonstrates the pseudocyst with peripheral calcification.

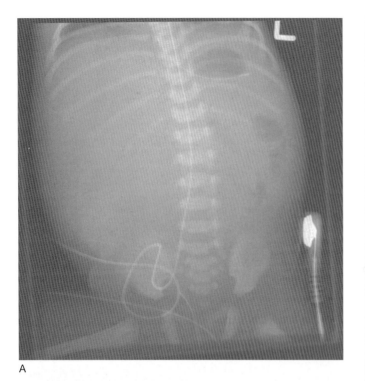

A

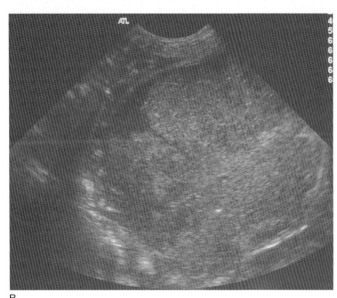

B

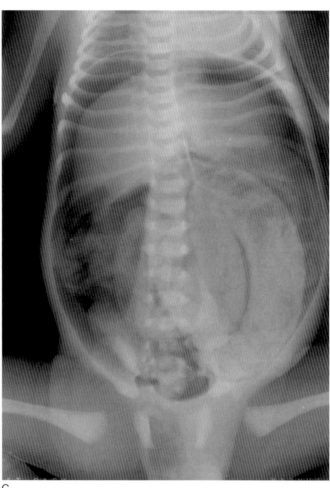

C

Figure 10.7.10 (A) Radiograph, (B) ultrasound and (C) delayed radiograph showing the appearances of a meconium-filled pseudocyst in an infant with cystic fibrosis. (A) Note the large central abdominal mass-like lesion displacing a couple of air-filled loops around it, mainly on the left. (B) Ultrasound shows typical appearances of meconium but note also no separate bowel loops can be identified, indicating that this already had perforated, and the meconium lay within the 'meconium cyst'. (C) Image shows massive pneumoperitoneum following perforation of a meconium cyst.

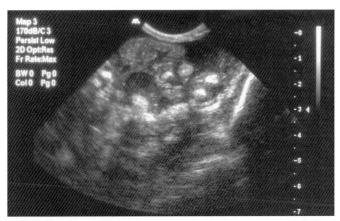

Figure 10.7.11 Image of abdomen in a neonate with cystic fibrosis showing echobright meconium.

bowel and its viscous contents, which may be seen as a mass on radiographs. It may initially be gasless and appear solid but air may slowly enter the 'mass' and cause a loculated pneumoperitoneum (Figure 10.7.10). Volvulus is caused by the weight of the meconium-packed bowel.

Ultrasound, either antenatally or in the neonate, can detect abnormal bowel dilatation and echogenic bowel contents in infants with meconium ileus (Figure 10.7.11). Complications such as meconium peritonitis or pseudocyst may be identified as echogenic material lying outside bowel loops, with or without associated calcification.

Definitive diagnosis is made by a low osmolar water-soluble contrast enema. A microcolon is seen. Reflux of contrast into the distal ileum shows multiple filling defects of inspissated meconium. Further filling of the small bowel outlines the dilated and meconium-filled ileum (Figure 10.7.12). This feature distinguishes the condition from distal ileal atresia.

Once the diagnosis is established a therapeutic enema should be undertaken to help the passage of sticky meconium and so relieve the obstruction. In the past, this was undertaken by means of a dilute gastrograffin (diatrizoate meglumine) enema. The choice of contrast media is controversial but gastrograffin continues to be used by many radiologists. An expert group convened by the Cystic Fibrosis Foundation Consensus Conference found no scientific evidence that gastrograffin was superior to other water-soluble low osmolar contrast media in the treatment of meconium ileus. Gastrograffin is hyperosmolar and causes considerable fluid shift into the bowel lumen, even when used in a dilute form. This may cause hypotension or circulatory collapse in newborn infants and extreme care must be taken with fluid and electrolyte balance. Additionally, Tween 90, an agent found in some diatrizoate meglumine preparations, is associated with acute fulminant colitis. In view of such considerations, many radiologists currently favour the use of low osmolar agents in these infants.

The aim is to introduce the contrast medium into the dilated small bowel proximal to the obstructing inspissated meconium but care must be taken to avoid over distension of the microcolon. Several attempts may be made (1–2 enemas in 24 h) as long as there is progressive clinical improvement in the neonate in terms of degree of abdominal distension and passage of meconium. The infant's fluid and electrolyte balance must be carefully attended to before, during and after each procedure. The reported success rate for relieving meconium ileus is 50–60%, with a perforation rate of

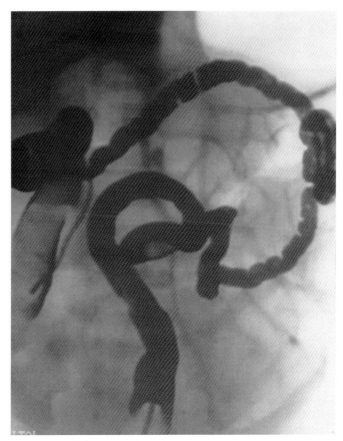

Figure 10.7.12 Meconium ileus. Contrast enema outlines a functional microcolon. The terminal ileum is dilated and filled with meconium. Note the small pellets of meconium frequently found in the microcolon.

3–10%. These figures must be viewed with caution as they often include infants who have functional bowel obstruction due to failure to pass the initial meconium – the so-called meconium plug syndrome. Enema successfully treats almost all this latter group. If signs of obstruction are not relieved or perforation/peritonitis develop further attempts at therapeutic enema should be abandoned. In such unsuccessful cases, surgery often reveals complicated meconium ileus.

Though liver and gallbladder disease may be found in children with cystic fibrosis, they are not a feature in the neonatal period.

FURTHER READING

Auburn RP, Feldman SA, Gadacz TR et al. Meconium ileus secondary to partial aplasia of the pancreas: report of a case. Surgery 1969; 65:689–693.

Caniano DA, Beaver BL. Meconium ileus: a fifteen year experience with forty-two neonates. Surgery 1987; 102:699.

Fakhoury K, Durie PR, Levison H et al. Meconium ileus in the absence of cystic fibrosis. Archives of Disease in Childhood 1992; 67:1204–1206.

Hurwitt ES, Arnheim EE. Meconium ileus associated with stenosis of the pancreatic ducts. A clinical, pathologic, and embryological study. American Journal of Disease in Childhood 1972; 64:443.

Kao SCS, Franken EA Jr. Nonoperative treatment of simple meconium ileus: a survey of the Society for Pediatric Radiology. Pediatric Radiology 1995; 25:97–100.

Leonidas JC, Berdon WE, Baker DH et al. Meconium ileus and its complications: a reappraisal of plain film roentgen diagnostic criteria. American Journal of Roentgenology 1970; 108:598–609.

Willi U, Reddish JM, Teele RL. Cystic fibrosis: its characteristic appearance on abdominal sonography. American Journal of Roentgenology 1980; 134:1005–1010.

ANOMALIES OF INTESTINAL ROTATION AND FIXATION

The term malrotation encompasses a wide variety of anomalies of intestinal rotation and mesenteric fixation – non-rotation, malrotation and reverse rotation. Additionally, malrotation occurs as an integral part of diaphragmatic hernia, gastroschisis and omphalocele.

Knowledge of the embryology of normal intestinal development is essential for an understanding of the types of malrotation encountered. In early intrauterine life, the gut is a single U-shaped loop, arranged with the omphalomesenteric artery (this will become the superior mesenteric artery) as its central axis (Figure 10.7.13). The duodenojejunal or prearterial loop is located above and anterior to the artery. The ileocolic or postarterial loop is located below and behind the artery. Before 6 weeks' gestation, the duodenum initially rotates 90° anticlockwise to lie to the right of the artery. The ileocolic loop also rotates 90° in the same direction to lie to the left of the artery. During the 6th week of gestation, the liver is growing rapidly and fills the greater part of the abdominal cavity. Accommodation for the bowel is sought elsewhere and the developing gut moves into the umbilical cord. During the 6th week the duodenum rotates another 90° anticlockwise to lie posterior to the artery, while the rest of the midgut is in the umbilical cord. By the 10th to 12th weeks of gestation, the intestine slides back into the peritoneal cavity and the final 90° anticlockwise rotation of the duodenum and 180° anticlockwise rotation of the caecum and colon occurs. Thus, the 270° rotation results in the third part of the duodenum located posterior to the superior mesenteric artery and the duodenojejunal flexure to the left of the artery. The colon is the last portion of the gastrointestinal tract to rotate completely. The transverse colon comes to lie anterior to the superior mesenteric artery and the caecum descends into the right lower quadrant. The process is completed by fixation of the bowel by the mesentery. Normally, the small bowel mesentery is broad based, with its attachment extending from the duodenojejunal flexure (ligament of trietz) to the ileocaecal valve. This wide base prevents the small intestine from twisting around the superior mesenteric artery.

The normal location of the duodenojejunal flexure is to the left of the spine and at the level of the duodenal bulb. Any deviation from this location must be considered abnormal, with the exception of some specific pitfalls outlined below. Non-rotation results in both the duodenojejunal flexure and duodenum being located entirely to the right of the spine. In partial rotation of the duodenum, the duodenojejunal flexure approximates the midline.

The caecum is normally located in the right lower quadrant. In non-rotation of the colon, it is found in the left lower quadrant or in the midline. In partial rotation, it is located in either the right or left upper quadrants. Rotation of the duodenum and caecum occur as distinct and separate processes at different stages of development and as such malrotation may occasionally involve only one of them, the other being normally located. Malrotation may involve just the duodenum or caecum; however, in most cases, both are abnormal in location.

Reverse rotation is a rare anomaly in which the duodenum and colon rotate clockwise about the superior mesenteric artery. This results in the duodenum being anterior to the superior mesenteric artery and the transverse colon posterior. The mesenteric vessels may cause mid-colonic obstruction and abnormal fixation renders midgut volvulus a possibility.

Malrotation of the gut does not in itself cause symptoms or complications, however the frequently associated malfixation and narrowed mesenteric base may result in clockwise volvulus about the superior mesenteric artery causing bowel obstruction and vascular compromise (Figure 10.7.14). This is a true emergency as bowel necrosis may supervene with loss of the entire jejunum and ileum. Some types of malrotation are associated with higher incidences of volvulus. In a symptomatic infant, the identification of malro-

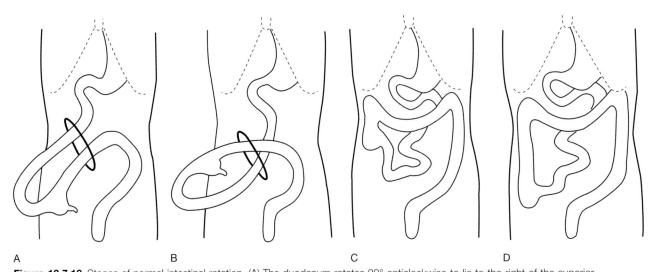

A	B	C	D

Figure 10.7.13 Stages of normal intestinal rotation. (A) The duodenum rotates 90° anticlockwise to lie to the right of the superior mesenteric artery. The distal large bowel also rotates 90° anticlockwise. (B) The duodenum rotates another 90° anticlockwise. The duodenojejunal flexure lies in the midline posterior to the artery. (C) The duodenum has rotated its last 90° anticlockwise and the duodenojejunal flexure now lies to the left of the midline. The caecum continues its rotation. (D) Normally rotated and fixed bowel.

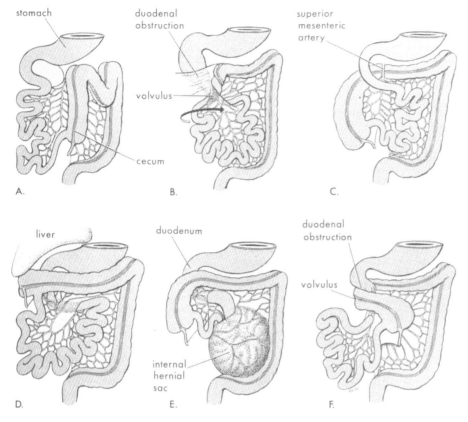

stomach

duodenal
obstruction

superior
mesenteric
artery

volvulus

cecum

A.

B.

C.

liver

duodenum

duodenal
obstruction

volvulus

internal
hernial
sac

D.

E.

F.

Figure 10.7.14 Midgut volvulus. Schematic drawing of forms of pathological midgut rotation. (A) Non-rotation, (B) rotation and volvulus, (C) reverse rotation, (D) normal rotation but high caecum, (E) mesenteric hernia and (F) midgut volvulus. Types (B) and (F) are the most frequent presentations in the neonatal period because of the duodenal obstruction. The others may remain asymptomatic or present at any age with volvulus, secondary to the short mesentery and malfixation. (Reproduced with permission from The Developing Human, 3rd edn. W. B. Saunders.)

tated bowel should be treated as a surgical emergency. Direct radiological evidence of volvulus may not be evident as volvulus may be partial or intermittent. Other causes of bowel obstruction and vomiting in a child with malrotation include condensations of peritoneum that cross the duodenum (Ladd's bands) or, rarely, internal hernias. In approximately 10% of children with malrotation, an intrinsic duodenal obstruction is found such as a web or atresia.

Two-thirds of children with malrotation will present in the first week of life. Presentation is usually with bilious vomiting and at surgery volvulus is usually present. This clinical pattern in a neonate is highly suspicious for malrotation and volvulus. Symptoms in the older child may be subtle, often non-specific abdominal pain, and this combined with a lower index of suspicion means diagnosis may be delayed with catastrophic results.

Plain radiographs may be diagnostic and may obviate the need for further imaging prior to surgery. The presence of partial duodenal obstruction (dilatation of the stomach and proximal duodenum with gas in distal non-distended loops) in a neonate with bilious vomiting suggests the diagnosis of malrotation with volvulus. This appearance may occur in duodenal atresia with an incomplete diaphragm, however it is a much less common occurrence. Occasionally, duodenal obstruction is complete and appearances mimic the 'double bubble' seen in complete duodenal atresia. Gastric dilatation may be prominent due to its greater distensibility and appearances may erroneously suggest gastric outlet obstruction (Figure 10.7.15). The bowel gas pattern may be normal on occasion and prompt evaluation by means of an upper gastrointestinal examination is essential. It may also show the typical

appearances of the small bowel on the right and colon on the left (Figure 10.7.16).

The abdominal radiograph may also show a pattern of ileus or small bowel obstruction, which when malrotation is present is usually due to volvulus and closed-loop obstruction. A gasless abdomen with fluid-filled bowel loops may also indicate volvulus (Figure 10.7.17). These signs are non-specific but are also indicators of bowel necrosis.

The location of the duodenojejunal flexure is of critical importance in the upper gastrointestinal examination. It is vital to obtain a true anterior–posterior view of the upper abdomen with the first pass of contrast medium through the proximal small bowel. The antrum of the stomach should not be overfilled, to avoid obscuring the flexure. An abnormally located duodenojejunal junction is the most accurate indicator of malrotation. It should be located to the left of the left vertebral pedicle at L2 and at or almost at the level of the duodenal bulb. The duodenojejunal junction is mobile in children and may be pushed inferiomedially by an overdistended stomach, chronic bowel dilatation, enlarged spleen or in the presence of a nasojejunal tube. Attempts to correct these pitfalls should be made to allow for a true assessment of the duodenojejunal flexure position. The position of the duodenojejunal flexure is to the right of the spine in non-rotation and near the midline in partial rotation of the duodenum (Figure 10.7.18). In both types, the flexure is located below the level of the duodenal bulb. If duodenal obstruction is complete, contrast may not pass far enough to identify the duodenojejunal flexure but this is irrelevant as surgery is then indicated.

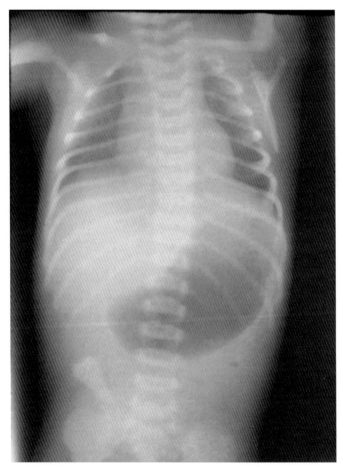

Figure 10.7.15 Midgut malrotation with volvulus. A supine radiograph demonstrates a gasless abdomen other than a gas-filled and distended stomach. Note the absence of duodenal gas, which contrasts with its usual finding in intrinsic duodenal obstruction.

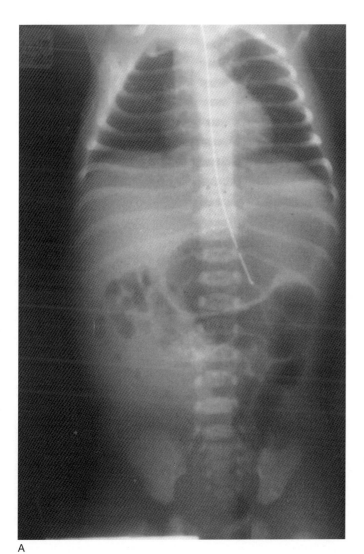

A

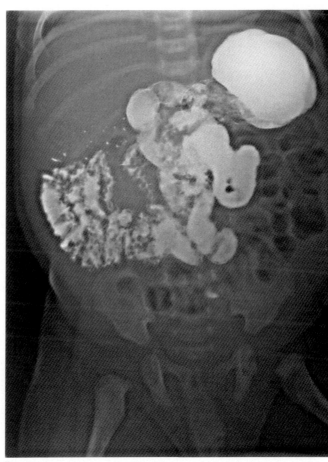

B

Figure 10.7.16 Images of two infants with malrotation showing (A) the small bowel gas on the right, with the colonic gas centrally and to the left and (B) a contrast study showing the small bowel on the right but note the dilatation of the duodenum and proximal jejunum due to the associated volvulus.

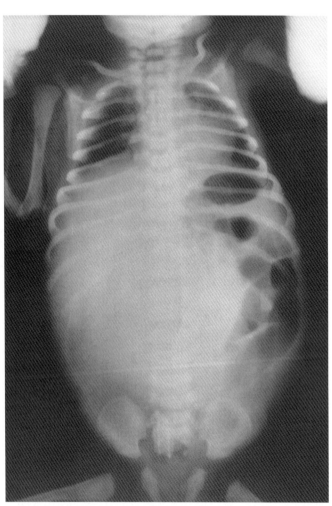

Figure 10.7.17 Malrotation with volvulus. A supine abdominal film demonstrates gas-filled loops of bowel that are displaced to the left of the abdomen by a mass, which represents the midgut volvulus. There is pneumoperitoneum localized to the right lower quadrant. The perforation has occurred in ischaemic bowel secondary to volvulus.

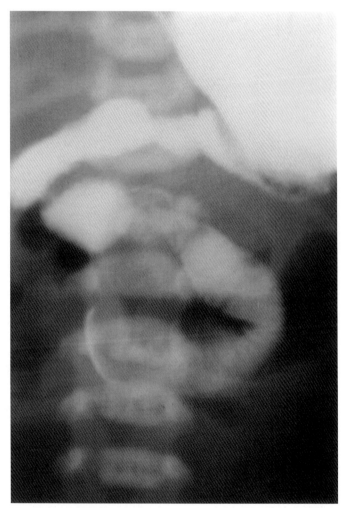

Figure 10.7.18 Partial rotation of the duodenum. Upper gastrointestinal contrast examination demonstrates the duodenojejunal flexure overlying the left vertebral pedicle and below the level of the pylorus.

The normal duodenum is a retroperitoneal structure and on lateral views it lies behind the level of the stomach, with the fourth part of duodenum superimposed on the second part of duodenum. A malrotated duodenum is seen to course anteriorly, losing this important superimposed relationship. Because of partial obstruction there may be to-and-fro peristalsis in the duodenum. Thus, a lateral view of the contrast-filled duodenum is an important additional view in the upper gastrointestinal study. An abnormal position of the duodenojejunal flexure may be the only indication of malrotation, as in 16% of cases the caecum occupies its normal position in the right lower quadrant.

In spite of the obstruction being in the duodenum, the duodenum may not be very dilated. A further pattern is one of air in the stomach only. The abdomen x-ray may be normal in malrotation and, if clinically suspected, upper gastrointestinal tract contrast studies are mandatory.

In malrotation, the jejunum commonly occupies the right side of the abdomen, however this is not an indication of malrotation of itself as the jejunum in a normal child is relatively mobile and may be seen to the right of the spine. If the diagnosis is uncertain after the upper gastrointestinal study a contrast enema may be undertaken to determine the caecal location. In the past, a contrast enema was the first investigation performed to evaluate for malrotation. This practice has been replaced by upper gastrointestinal examination due to its greater sensitivity and specificity for malrotation. It should be remembered that the caecum may be mobile in neonates and may be seen in the right upper quadrant in the absence of malrotation. This normal variant should be distinguished from partial rotation of the caecum where the caecum occupies a more midline position with a transverse orientation. Occasionally, the upper gastrointestinal study is normal and the only indication of malrotation is an abnormally located caecum. Although this combination is rare, it underlines the importance of performing both an upper and lower contrast study if the diagnosis is uncertain or if there is strong clinical suspicion of malrotation despite a normal result from one study.

In malrotation with volvulus, the duodenum may be partially or completely obstructed with little or no contrast medium passing this region. A beaked tapering of the obstructed duodenum may be evident with complete obstruction. More commonly, the volvulus is intermittent with incomplete bowel obstruction and contrast medium fills the proximal small bowel. The characteristic 'corkscrew' appearance of the duodenum and jejunum is seen due to their clockwise twisting around the mesenteric artery (Figure 10.7.16B and Figure 10.7.19). Occasionally a 'Z-shaped' duodenum and proximal jejunum is seen, which is also suspicious for obstructing Ladd's bands or volvulus.

Ultrasound of the superior mesenteric artery and vein may reveal reversal of their normal orientation in patients with malrotation. The superior mesenteric artery is normally located to the left of the vein. When the superior mesenteric vein is to the left of the artery, malrotation may be present (Figure 10.7.20). The vessels should be assessed as distally as possible from the superior mesenteric vein–splenic vein confluence and in a direct anterior–posterior orientation to avoid errors. This sign is not sensitive, however, as a third of patients with malrotation demonstrate normal artery–vein orientation. Conversely, abnormal orientation does not definitely indicate malrotation and an upper gastrointestinal study is required to evaluate the midgut rotation. Occasionally, the superior mesenteric vein and its mesentery are seen

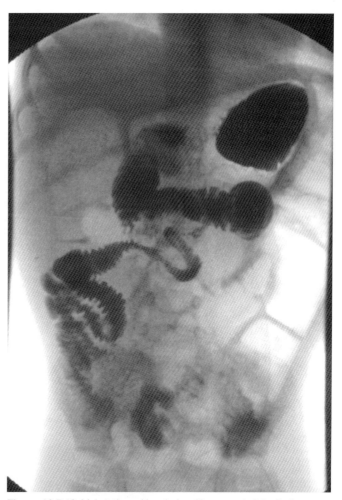

Figure 10.7.19 Malrotation with volvulus. Upper gastrointestinal contrast examination reveals cork-screwing of the proximal small bowel as it twists around the superior mesenteric artery. Note also dilated duodenum.

to rotate clockwise about the artery on colour Doppler US (Figure 10.7.21). This is termed the 'whirlpool' sign and in a symptomatic infant indicates malrotation with volvulus. Less frequently, only the pulsatile superior mesenteric artery is seen due to compression of the vein in the presence of volvulus.

Malrotation in the neonate is a surgical emergency because of the high incidence of associated volvulus. At surgery, the volvulus is reduced, peritoneal bands are divided and a Ladd's procedure is performed to elongate the mesenteric base. This involves placing the intestine in a non-rotated position – the small bowel to the right of the spine and the colon to the left.

FURTHER READING

Beasley SW, de Campo JF. Pitfalls in the radiological diagnosis of malrotation. Australasian Radiology 1987; 31:376–383.

Berdon WE, Baker DH, Bull S et al. Mid gut malrotation and volvulus: which films are most helpful? Radiology 1970; 96:375–383.

Long FR, Kramer SS, Markowitz RI et al. Radiographic patterns of intestinal malrotation in children. Radiographics 1996; 16:547–556.

Pracos JP, Sann L, Genin G et al. Ultrasound diagnosis of midgut volvulus: the whirlpool sign. Pediatric Radiology 1992; 22:18–20.

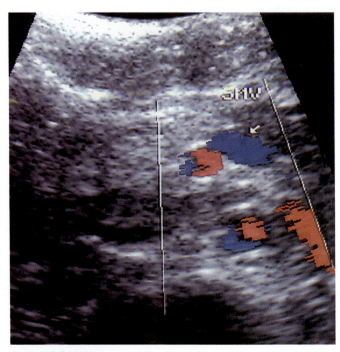

Figure 10.7.20 Abnormal relationship of the superior mesenteric artery and vein. The superior mesenteric vein (arrow) should normally lie on the right of the artery.

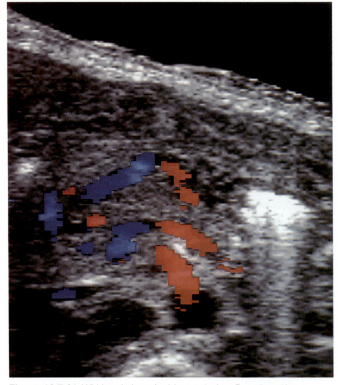

Figure 10.7.21 Whirlpool sign of midgut volvulus. Doppler colour ultrasound demonstrates the superior mesenteric vein (and the midgut it drains) swirling clockwise about the centrally placed superior mesenteric artery, indicating midgut volvulus.

Richardson WR, Martin LW. Pitfalls in the surgical management of the incomplete duodenal diaphragm. Journal of Pediatric Surgery 1969; 4:303–312.

Slovis TL, Klein MD, Watts FB Jr. Incomplete rotation of the intestine with a normal cecal position. Surgery 1980; 87:325–330.

Snyder QH, Chaffin L. Embryology and pathology of the intestinal tract: presentation of 40 cases of malrotation. Annals of Surgery 1954; 140:368–380.

Taylor GA, Teele RL. Chronic intestinal obstruction mimicking malrotation in children. Pediatric Radiology 1985; 15:392–394.

Zerin JM, DiPietro MA. Superior mesenteric vascular anatomy at US in patients with surgically proved malrotation of the midgut. Radiology 1992; 183:693–694.

OMPHALOCELE

In omphalocele (exomphalos), there is herniation of abdominal viscera into the base of the umbilical cord. The herniated viscera are contained within a sac of peritoneum and amnion (Figures 10.7.22 and 10.7.23). Occasionally, the liver may herniate into the omphalocele, accompanied by variable lengths of intestine. Malposition of the abdominal viscera and malrotation of the bowel is an integral part of the condition. Routine preoperative radiographs are not usually required but the contents can be determined by ultrasonography if necessary. Of more importance in these infants is the detection of associated anomalies, which occur in two-thirds of children. These most commonly include cardiac anomalies, chromosomal anomalies (trisomy 13 and 18) and Beckwith–Wiedeman syndrome. The mortality rate for children with omphalocele is nearly three times that of gastroschisis and is due to associated anomalies rather than the abdominal wall abnormality. The diagnosis is often made *in utero,* and in countries in which abortion is practised, if found to be associated with chromosomal abnormalities or if very large, is considered an indication for abortion.

GASTROSCHISIS

In gastroschisis, bowel herniates through a paraumbilical defect usually located to the right of the umbilicus. It too may be diagnosed *in utero*. It is easily distinguished from an omphalocele as the umbilicus is normal and the herniated bowel does not possess a peritoneal/amnion covering. A fibrous peel is seen coating the loops of herniated bowel. More than half of all neonates with gastroschisis are premature. Gastroschisis occurs twice as commonly as omphalocele in live births; however, when all births are considered omphalocele has a greater incidence due to associated anomalies. Gastrointestinal abnormalities associated with gastroschisis include malrotation, shortened gut, small bowel atresia, dysmotility, gastroesophageal reflux and increased risk of necrotizing enterocolitis. While these anomalies cause significant morbidity, the prognosis for survival is favourable.

Both omphalocele and gastroschisis, if large, may cause respiratory embarrassment when the contents are replaced within the peritoneum and the abdominal wall closed. Other postoperative complications include ileus, adhesion obstruction or short bowel complications if resection of compromised bowel has occurred.

FURTHER READING

Blane CE, Wesley JR, DiPietro MA et al. Gastrointestinal complications of gastroschisis. American Journal of Roentgenology 1985; 144:589–591.

Mayer T, Black R, Matlak ME et al. Gastroschisis and omphalocele. Annals of Surgery 1980; 192:783–787.

Ramsden WH, Arthur RJ, Martinez D. Gastroschisis: a radiological and clinical review. Pediatric Radiology 1997; 27:166–169.

Tibboel D, Raine P, McNee M et al. Developmental aspects of gastroschisis. Journal of Pediatric Surgery 1986; 21:865–869.

NEONATAL INTUSSUSCEPTION

Neonatal intussusception is rare and is more likely to be due to a pathological lead point such as Meckel's diverticulum, mucosal polyp or tumour mass. Clinical signs are usually non-specific and include vomiting, abdominal distension and bloodstained stools. Plain radiographs may show small bowel obstruction (Figure 10.7.24). If the intussusception is longstanding or occurred *in utero*, ascites or pneumoperitoneum may be seen. The diagnosis is confirmed by abdominal US and air enema reduction should be cautiously attempted bearing in mind that obstruction may have been prolonged or a lead point may be present. The reduction rates are lower than in older infants.

FURTHER READING

Cipel L, Fonkalsrud EW, Gyepes MT. Ileo-ileal intussusception in the newborn. Report of a radiologically diagnosed case. Radiology 1977; 6:39–42.

Newman J, Schuh S. Intussusception in babies under 4 months of age. Canadian Medical Association Journal 1987; 136:266–272.

Patriquin HB, Afshani E, Effman E et al. Neonatal intussusception: report of 12 cases. Radiology 1977; 125:463–466.

SEGMENTAL DILATATION OF SMALL BOWEL

Congenital segmental dilatation of the small bowel is a rare condition in which the calibre of the bowel is increased locally, without obstruction or thickening of the muscle wall. The passage of intestinal contents through the dilated segment is not delayed unless there is a coexistent problem. A variety of persistent but non-specific symptoms are reported with the condition.

Plain radiographs of the abdomen show an isolated dilated loop of bowel with an air–fluid level (Figure 10.7.25). The characteristic finding on barium studies of the small bowel is a localized dilatation of the small bowel lumen. In the absence of complications, the transit time of contrast medium is not delayed. The condition may be associated with an omphalocele, Meckel's diverticulum or malrotation. Surgical excision is curative.

FURTHER READING

Bell MJ, Ternberg JL, Bower RJ. Ileal dysgenesis in infants and children. Journal of Pediatric Surgery 1982; 17:395–399.

Brown A, Carty H. Segmental dilatation of the ileum. British Journal of Radiology 1984; 57:371–374.

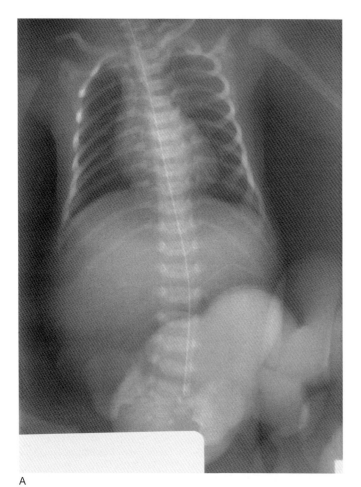

A

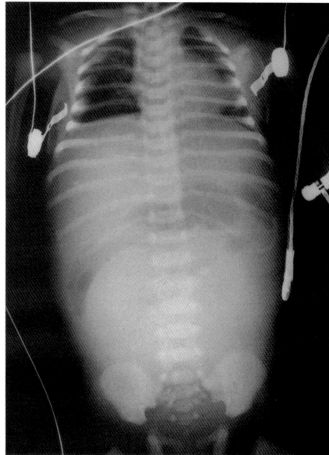

B

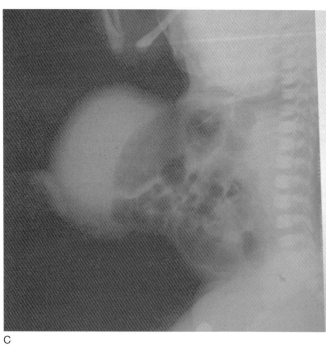

C

Figure 10.7.22 (A) A large omphalocele. (B) Postrepair radiograph. Note the elevation of the diaphragms and the paucity of bowel gas. The repositioning of the contents of the omphalocele leads to these features. (C) Another infant showing a moderately sized omphalocele.

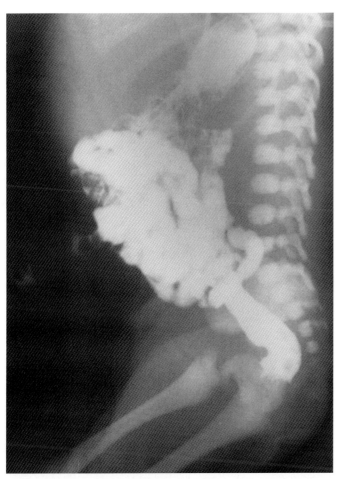

Figure 10.7.23 A small omphalocele. A small bowel barium study demonstrates the limited extent of bowel herniation into the omphalocele.

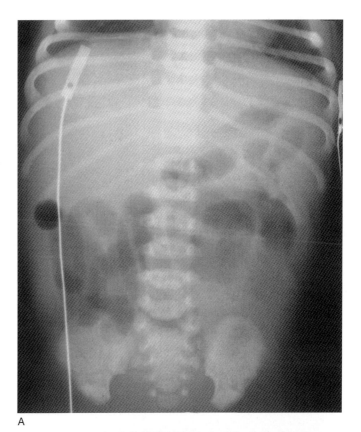

A

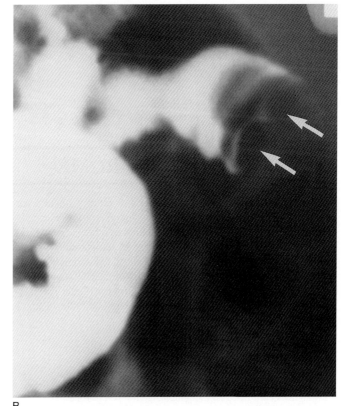

B

Figure 10.7.24 (A) Neonate with intussusception. Presentation was with abdominal distension and bleeding per rectum. (B) Contrast enema examination outlines an intussusception (arrows) which was successfully reduced hydrostatically.

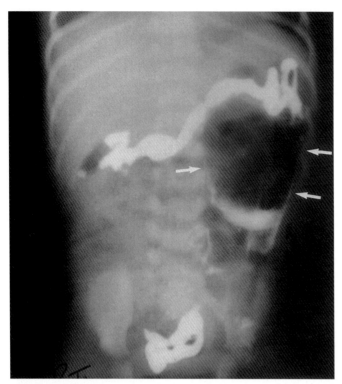

Figure 10.7.25 Segmental dilatation of small bowel. Contrast examination shows barium in a localized segment of markedly dilated bowel, with a gas–barium level.

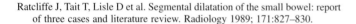

Ratcliffe J, Tait T, Lisle D et al. Segmental dilatation of the small bowel: report of three cases and literature review. Radiology 1989; 171:827–830.

SHORT BOWEL SYNDROME

The small intestine may be shortened as a result of surgical resection for conditions such as volvulus, congenital atresias (especially the 'apple peel' type of small bowel atresia) or other surgical interventions. Shortened small bowel is seen in association with gastroschisis. Congenital short bowel as an isolated anomaly is rare. Contrast studies show generalized dilatation of the small bowel loops with prominence of the mucosal folds (Figure 10.7.26). Motor activity of the bowel may be disordered and transit time is usually rapid.

FURTHER READING

Sansaricq C, Chen WJ, Manka M et al. Familial congenital short small bowel with associated defects. A long term survival. Clinical Pediatrics 1984; 23:453–455.

Tiu CM, Chou YH, Pan HB et al. Congenital short bowel. Pediatric Radiology 1984; 14:343–345.

Touloukian RJ, Smith GJ. Normal intestinal length in preterm infants. Journal of Pediatric Surgery 1983; 18:720–723.

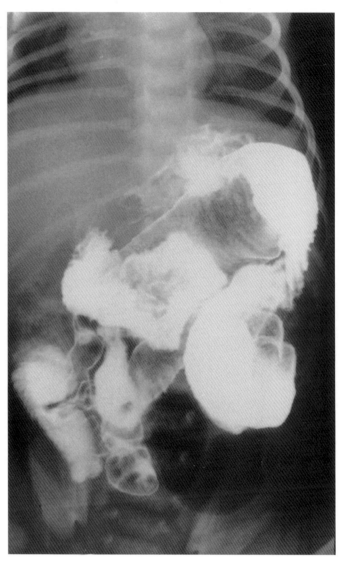

Figure 10.7.26 Short bowel syndrome. Water-soluble upper gastrointestinal examination outlines a short small bowel with dilatation of some of the loops.

DUPLICATION CYSTS

Duplication cysts may occur anywhere throughout the gastrointestinal tract but are most commonly found in the distal ileum, followed by the oesophagus and duodenum. They are spherical or tubular structures with a wall of smooth muscle that is usually continuous with the muscle of the adjacent bowel. They are lined with intestinal epithelium, which may be the same type as the adjacent bowel or may have ectopic tissue such as gastric mucosa or pancreatic tissue. The cysts typically do not communicate with the bowel lumen but this is occasionally seen in the tubular type of duplication cyst. The diagnosis may be made antenatally.

Symptoms associated with duplication cysts include abdominal pain, a palpable mass or abdominal distension with bowel obstruc-

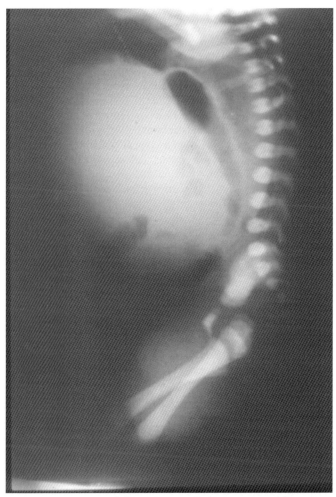

Figure 10.7.27 Lateral radiograph of abdomen in an infant with a very large duplication cyst displacing bowel around it.

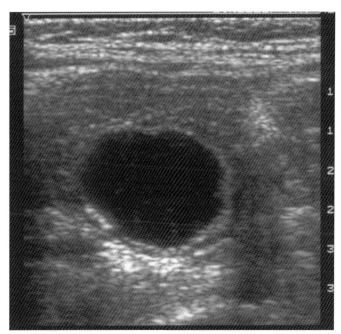

Figure 10.7.28 Ultrasound of right upper quadrant with a small duplication cyst showing the typical 'gut signature' of the double wall.

tion. Rarely, intussusception may occur with the duplication cyst acting as a lead point.

A soft tissue mass may be seen on abdominal radiographs, with or without signs of proximal bowel obstruction. It may also displace loops of intestine around it (Figure 10.7.27). Ultrasound usually establishes the diagnosis, showing a well-defined unilocular cystic mass with a characteristic gut signature. The 'gut signature' (Figure 10.7.28) refers to an inner echogenic layer (mucosa) and an outer hypoechoic layer (smooth muscle wall) and is virtually pathognomonic of duplication cysts. Occasionally, debris is seen within the cyst due to haemorrhage or secretions from the mucosal lining. Careful evaluation with high-resolution ultrasound may occasionally reveal peristalsis within the wall of the cyst. In the presence of a gastric mucosal lining, technetium 99m sodium pertechnetate will be taken up and this study may be of value when the diagnosis is uncertain. Barium studies may show displaced or obstructed loops of bowel but seldom produce filling of the cyst lumen. MRI studies show the cyst as high signal on T2-weighted images with the wall of low signal. The differential diagnosis includes mesenteric cyst and, in girls, ovarian cysts. Mesenteric cysts are lymphangiomas. They are frequently septated and do not have the gut signature. Neonatal ovarian cysts similarly do not have gut signature.

FURTHER READING

Barr LL, Hayden CK Jr, Stansberry SK et al. Enteric duplication cysts in children: are their ultrasonographic wall characteristics diagnostic? Pediatric Radiology 1990; 20:26–28.

Gilchrist AM, Sloan JM, Logan CJH et al. Gastrointestinal bleeding due to multiple ileal duplications diagnosed by scintigraphy and barium studies. Clinical Radiology 1990; 41:134–136.

Macpherson RI. Gastrointestinal tract duplications: clinical, pathologic, etiologic and radiologic considerations. Radiographics 1993; 13:1063–1080.

Spottswood SE. Peristalsis in duplication cyst: a new diagnostic sonographic finding. Pediatric Radiology 1994; 24:344–345.

Teele RL, Henschke CI, Tapper D. The radiographic and ultrasonographic evaluation of enteric duplication cysts. Pediatric Radiology 1980; 10:9–14.

MILK ALLERGY

This condition usually results from intolerance of cows' milk. Clinically, the infant presents with diarrhoea and vomiting. Contrast studies demonstrate flocculation of the barium, dilated small bowel loops and increased transit time. The appearances resemble those observed in coeliac disease.

FURTHER READING

Liu HY, Whitehouse WM, Giday Z. Proximal small bowel transit pattern in patients with malabsorption induced by bovine milk protein ingestion. Radiology 1975; 115:415–420.

Walker-Smith J. Cow's milk protein intolerance: transient food intolerance of infancy. Archives of Disease in Childhood 1975; 50:347–350.

HERNIA

Hernias that may present in the neonatal period include both internal and external hernias. These are described elsewhere in the book but are mentioned here for completeness. External hernias are in the umbilical and inguinal locations. Internal hernias include congenital diaphragmatic hernias (CDH) of both Morgagni and Bochdalek varieties and more rarely hiatal hernias of both the sliding and paraoesophageal types. CDH usually presents clinically in the neonatal period but occasionally small ones may be discovered incidentally on radiographs. Similar remarks apply to hiatal lesions but these are more often found incidentally.

Umbilical hernias are due to a portion of intestine protruding through the umbilicus. They may occur due to severe abdominal distension and will regress with resolution of this. They also occur spontaneously and will regress by about 6 months. They are a recognized association of Beckwith–Wiedemann syndrome. On x-ray they appear as a central abdominal soft tissue opacity.

Inguinal hernias often present in the first month of life. They result from persistent patency of the processus vaginalis. This is patent in about 80% of infants at birth but in less than 20% by age two. The persistent processus may contain herniated bowel, which may even extend into the scrotum. Indirect inguinal hernias are the commonest cause of bowel obstruction in infants beyond the immediate birth period. These hernias may contain a testis or an ovary. There is a 95% male and 80% right-sided dominance. When the hernia contains bowel gas they are easily identified on abdominal radiographs but when incarcerated or fluid-filled they are more difficult to identify. The scrotum loses the normal symmetrical V shape formed by the inguinoscrotal folds. Ultrasound of the inguinal canal will when necessary confirm the diagnosis by identifying the bowel and testis or ovary if present.

The Colon

Veronica Donoghue, Eilish L Twomey

In the newborn, the haustral pattern of the colon is less prominent than that seen in the older child or adult, or absent entirely. In addition, the sigmoid colon is often more redundant (see Figure 10.6.1) and often lies entirely to the right. The caecum may be higher and more medial than usual. A further finding is rectal herniation through a patent processus vaginalis into the inguinal canal, referred to as the 'rectal ear'.

NECROTIZING ENTEROCOLITIS

Necrotizing enterocolitis is primarily a disease of premature neonates. It occurs commonly in the first week of life. Neonates of younger gestational age may have a more delayed onset. The precise aetiology is uncertain although mucosal damage, bacterial invasion and inflammatory response are the most likely mechanisms of bowel wall injury and necrosis.

The clinical findings include blood or bile-stained aspirates, blood per rectum, diarrhoea, abdominal distension, hypotension, shock and apnoea. Laboratory investigations reveal thrombocytopenia, neutropenia and metabolic acidosis. Treatment is commenced as soon as necrotizing enterocolitis is suspected. Enteral feeding is stopped with decompression of the bowel by nasogastric suction. Broad-spectrum intravenous antibiotics are commenced. Anteroposterior (AP) and cross-table lateral radiographs of the abdomen are obtained. A left side down decubitus view, an alternative to the cross-table lateral film, is less sensitive in the detection of intraperitoneal air than the cross-table lateral and involves unnecessary repositioning of the ill neonate.

The role of radiology is to confirm the diagnosis and to monitor the course of the disease. Serial radiographs, the timing being determined clinically, are important to help determine the appropriate time to stop treatment or for timely surgical intervention in the event of deterioration. The earliest and most common radiographic sign of necrotizing enterocolitis is gaseous bowel distension. In neonates, pneumatosis intestinalis is diagnostic of necrotizing enterocolitis (Figure 10.8.1). It may be cystic (submucosal) or linear (intramuscular or subserosal) in appearance, depending on the intramural location of the gas. Cystic pneumatosis can be difficult to differentiate from air mixed with meconium. However, a bubbly stool pattern is rare in the first weeks of life (Figure 10.8.2). Pneumatosis tends to be an early rather than late finding and may be fleetingly seen. It can occur anywhere from the oesophagus to rectum but is commonly seen involving the ileum and right colon. The correlation between the presence and extent of pneumatosis and the severity of necrotizing enterocolitis is poor.

Associated radiographic signs include separation of bowel loops due to wall thickening and loss of symmetry of bowel gas distribution within the abdomen or a persistently isolated dilated bowel loop. Findings associated with a poor outcome include ascites and portal venous gas. Radiographic signs of ascites include a gasless abdomen or relatively few centrally located gas-containing loops and separation of bowel loops. Ultrasound (US) is often utilized to detect intraperitoneal fluid and to localize it with accuracy for paracentesis. Ultrasound is particularly sensitive in the detection of gas in the portal vein or within smaller portal branches in the liver parenchyma. It should be remembered that gas passing through an umbilical venous catheter might give rise to portal venous gas in the absence of necrotizing enterocolitis (Figure 10.8.3). Gas in the bowel wall and abscess formation are also detected by US.

The presence of a pneumoperitoneum is an absolute indication for surgery and indicates full thickness bowel wall necrosis with perforation. When there is a large quantity of free air, it may be identified on supine radiographs as a central lucency with air outlining the falciform ligament in the right upper quadrant (football sign) (Figure 10.8.4). Air delineating both sides of the bowel wall (lumenal and peritoneal aspects of the wall) is referred to as Rigler's sign (Figue 10.8.5). The cross-table lateral view is best to demonstrate small amounts of free intraperitoneal air, which is seen as triangular lucencies between loops of bowel deep to the anterior abdominal wall (Figure 10.8.6). A loculated pneumoperitoneum may also be seen and air may collect in the subhepatic space. Only 63% of patients with surgically proven perforation, however, demonstrate a radiographically detectable pneumoperitoneum.

In equivocal cases, low osmolar contrast studies have been advocated in the diagnosis of necrotizing enterocolitis. Contrast is administered via a nasogastric tube and serial portable radiographs obtained. Necrotizing enterocolitis is suspected on the basis of mucosal irregularity and ulceration with wide separation of the contrast-opacified bowel loops due to mural thickening.

Non-ionic low osmolar contrast medium is not absorbed by normal gastrointestinal mucosa but does occur in the presence of

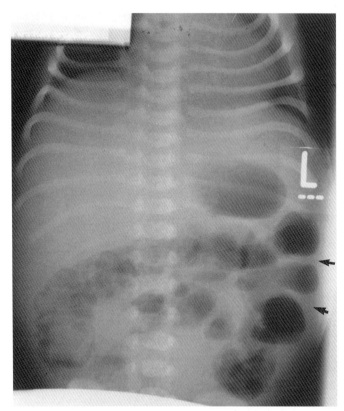

Figure 10.8.1 Necrotizing enterocolitis. Erect radiograph of the abdomen shows separation of bowel loops (arrows) and intramural gas.

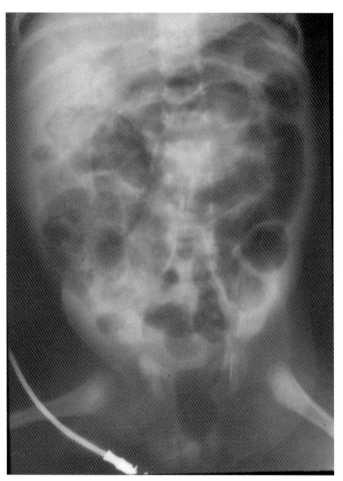

Figure 10.8.3 Portal venous gas is present in the liver. Note also intramural gas.

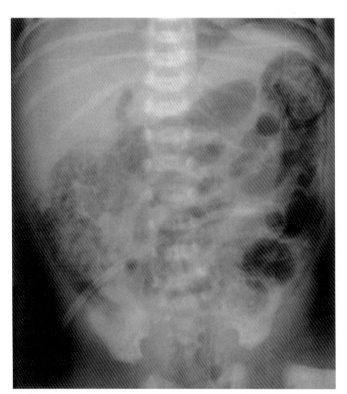

Figure 10.8.2 Necrotizing enterocolitis. Note the diffuse pneumatosis intestinalis and portal venous gas.

bowel necrosis or perforation. Contrast media is subsequently excreted via the kidneys. The absorbed contrast medium may be detected by laboratory assessment of serum or urine but also by computed tomography (CT) analysis of urine for increased attenuation coefficient. This method may help in the identification of those infants with bowel necrosis and impending perforation.

In 1978, Bell introduced a now widely practised system of grading necrotizing enterocolitis: stage 1 refers to suspected or early disease, stage 2 refers to definite necrotizing enterocolitis and stage 3 refers to advanced disease with bowel necrosis.

While pneumoperitoneum is an absolute indication for surgery with resection of non-vital bowel, other recognized indications are clinical deterioration despite aggressive medical management, fixed dilated loops on radiographs, abdominal mass, erythematous abdominal wall, portal venous gas and ascites. Occasionally, if a neonate is too unwell or small to undergo surgery despite the presence of ascites or an intra-abdominal abscess, percutaneous drainage may be performed with delayed resection of necrotic bowel.

The incidence of strictures after necrotizing enterocolitis is increasing as the mortality rate from the disease decreases. The commonest site is the colon, particularly the left colon and splenic flexure (Figure 10.8.7). The strictures are commonly single but

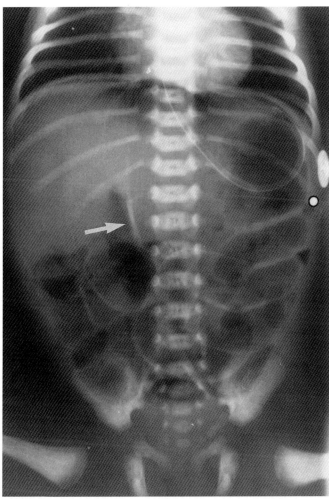

Figure 10.8.4 Necrotizing enterocolitis with bowel perforation. A supine radiograph shows the falciform ligament outlined by air (white arrow).

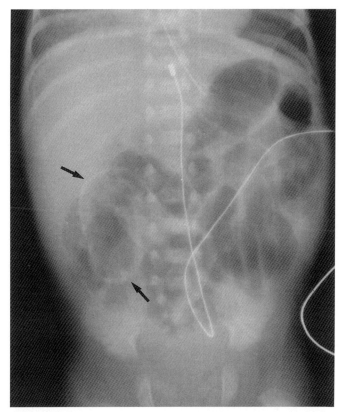

Figure 10.8.5 An infant with necrotizing enterocolitis showing a typical Rigler's sign with gas outlining the bowel wall (arrows).

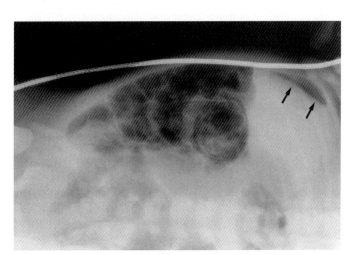

Figure 10.8.6 Necrotizing enterocolitis. A lateral decubitus radiograph shows bowel wall thickening and intramural air. There is a small collection of air over the liver (arrows) indicating pneumoperitoneum.

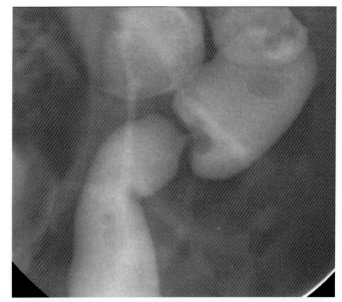

Figure 10.8.7 Colonic stricture. Barium enema shows a persistent focal narrowing in the sigmoid colon postnecrotizing enterocolitis.

multiple strictures can occur (Figure 10.8.8). Strictures may resolve spontaneously, particularly if they occur relatively soon after the acute episode of necrotizing enterocolitis. Clinically, they are suspected in an infant with constipation, recurrent intermittent obstruction, acute obstruction or low-grade rectal bleeding. A contrast enema should be performed to assess the cause of these symptoms. As some strictures are very short, great care needs to be taken during fluoroscopy to show the continuity of the bowel lumen without overlapping loops obscuring pathology. At times, an upper intestinal study with follow-through films may be more revealing than an enema. A contrast study of the distal bowel to ensure a normal calibre is routine in infants that have undergone a defunctioning enterostomy before closure of the stoma. Balloon dilatation of colonic strictures is considered inappropriate following necrotizing enterocolitis.

Other complications of necrotizing enterocolitis include enterocyst formation (a stagnant loop of bowel located between two strictures), lymphoid hyperplasia, internal fistulas, adhesions and malabsorption. A short bowel syndrome may occur if there is extensive surgical resection.

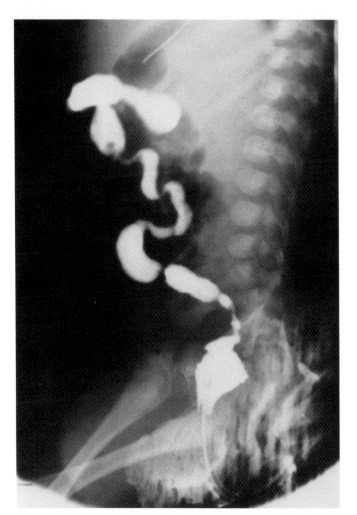

Figure 10.8.8 Multiple strictures. Necrotizing enterocolitis resulting in multiple colonic strictures in this infant.

FURTHER READING

Daneman A, Woodward S, deSilva M. The radiology of neonatal necrotizing enterocolitis: a review of 47 cases and the literature. Pediatric Radiology 1978; 7:70.

Donoghue V, Kelman CG. Transient portal venous gas in necrotizing enterocolitis. British Journal of Radiology 1982; 55:681–683.

Ein SH, Marshall DG, Girvan D. Peritoneal drainage under local anesthesia for perforations from necrotizing enterocolitis. Journal of Pediatric Surgery 1977; 12:963–967.

Frey EE, Smith W, Franken EA Jr et al. Analysis of bowel perforation in necrotizing enterocolitis. Pediatric Radiology 1987; 17:380–382.

Janik JS, Ein SH, Mancer K. Intestinal stricture after necrotizing enterocolitis. Journal of Pediatric Surgery 1981; 16:438.

Kosloske AM. Indications for operation in necrotizing enterocolitis revisited. Journal of Pediatric Surgery 1994; 29:663.

Patton W, Willmann JK, Lutz AM et al. Worsening enterocolitis in neonates: diagnosis by CT examination of urine after enteral administration of iohexol. Pediatric Radiology 1999; 29:95–99.

HIRSCHSPRUNG'S DISEASE

In this condition, there is an absence of ganglia in the submucosal and intramuscular plexuses of the colon. The aganglionosis always involves the anus including the internal anal sphincter and extends proximally for a variable distance.

In normal intrauterine development, neuroenteric cells migrate from the neural crest to the upper end of the gastrointestinal tract by 5 weeks and then proceed in a caudal direction. These cells reach the rectum by 12 weeks and commence the intramural migration from Auerbach's (myenteric) plexus to the submucosal plexus. Hirschsprung's disease is caused by abnormal neural crest cell migration resulting in arrested distal migration of these cells.

The disease has a strong male predominance with a male-to-female ratio of 4 : 1. The transition zone to normal ganglionic colon is located in the rectosigmoid region in 73–81% of cases; a longer segment of colon is involved in 10–24% and the total colon is aganglionic in 3–9% of cases. The male-to-female ratio approaches 1:1 in long segment disease. Furthermore, the familial incidence is increased in index cases with long segment involvement. Down's syndrome occurs in approximately 5–16% of patients with Hirschsprung's disease. This group have a poorer prognosis for bowel continence postsurgery and there is an increased incidence of enterocolitis. Coexistent atresia of the small or large bowel is another important association, although it is rare.

One hundred per cent of full-term and 99% of premature neonates pass meconium in the first 48 h of life. Failure to do so is highly suggestive of Hirschsprung's disease. Other clinical signs include abdominal distension and poor feeding with bilious vomiting. Hirschsprung's disease complicated by life-threatening enterocolitis presents with explosive diarrhoea, abdominal distension and fever and may progress to perforation with peritonitis. Hirschsprung's disease is usually diagnosed in Western society in the neonatal period. Delayed diagnosis still occurs with a history of constipation since birth, failure to thrive or acute enterocolitis.

Abdominal radiographs reveal distal bowel obstruction with a paucity of rectal air (Figure 10.8.9). These radiographic findings are non-specific; Table 10.8.1 outlines the differential diagnosis of low bowel obstruction in the neonate. Pneumoperitoneum occurs in approximately 4% of infants with Hirschsprung's disease due to

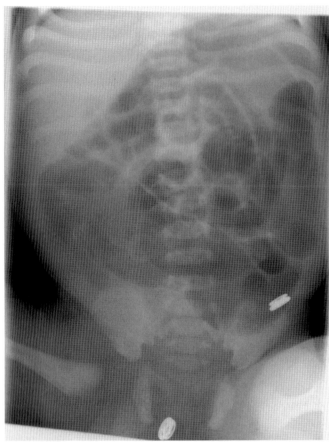

Figure 10.8.9 Hirschsprung's disease. A supine radiograph shows dilated loops of bowel with relatively little rectal gas.

Table 10.8.1 Differential diagnosis of neonatal distal bowel obstruction

Mechanical	Functional
Imperforate anus	Hirschsprung's disease
Colonic or ileal atresia	Neuronal intestinal dysplasia
Meconium ileus	Meconium plug syndrome
Ileal stenosis	Small left colon syndrome
Neonatal intussusception	Megacystis-microcolon intestinal hypoperistalsis syndrome
	Hypothyroidism
	Prematurity
	Sepsis and Electrolyte imbalance

colonic perforation. This complication usually occurs in patients with long segment or total colonic disease.

Rectal examination should not be performed prior to the enema examination as this may mask a low-lying zone of transition from aganglionic to normal colon. No bowel preparation is needed. The catheter should be inserted just inside the anal margin without inflating the balloon. Low osmolar water-soluble contrast medium is preferable as the risk of barium peritonitis is avoided in the event of colonic perforation. The bowel is filled slowly with the infant in a lateral position. The diagnosis is made if there is an inverted cone-like transition zone between the narrow aganglionic distal bowel and proximally dilated normal colon (Figure 10.8.10).

A characteristic transition zone may not always be precisely demarcated. In such cases, the aganglionic portion of distal bowel

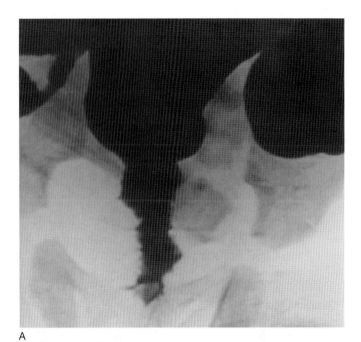

A

B

Figure 10.8.10 Hirschsprung's disease. (A) Frontal and (B) lateral views of the rectosigmoid colon at enema examination reveal a funnel-shaped transition zone at the rectosigmoid junction. Note the abnormal saw-toothed mucosal pattern in the rectum due to disordered muscular contractions.

may be identified by an irregular saw-toothed mucosal pattern attributed to disordered contractions in the aganglionic colon. The aganglionic bowel may be of normal calibre and appear narrowed only by comparison with the more dilated proximal bowel (Figure 10.8.11). The rectosigmoid index can be used to detect Hirschsprung's disease confined to the rectum – this compares the ratio of the rectal diameter to the sigmoid diameter and is considered abnormal if the sigmoid colon is more dilated than the rectum (index <1).

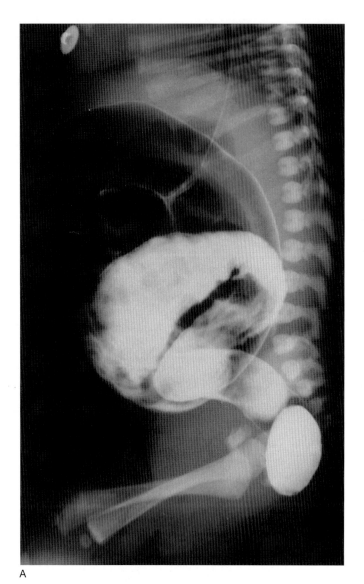

A

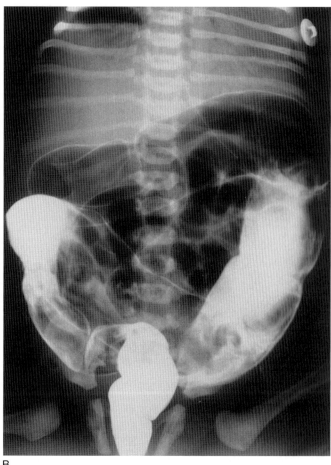

B

Figure 10.8.11 Hirschsprung's disease. Lateral (A) and supine (B) films taken during contrast enema examination. The proximal sigmoid and descending colon are very dilated in comparison to the distal sigmoid colon and rectum. The sigmoid colon is filled with meconium. The transition zone is at proximal sigmoid colon level.

A 24-h delayed film may help in equivocal cases, although opinion is divided about this aspect of the examination. Signs observed in Hirschsprung's disease include delayed retention of contrast media, contrast media mixed with stool or a more obvious transition zone than that seen on immediate films. In the first weeks of life, a contrast enema may fail to show a transition zone and in these neonates, the associated signs or delayed radiographs may be helpful. Histological confirmation of the transition zone is essential at surgery, as the proximal extent of the colonic aganglionosis may not correlate exactly with the transition zone identified radiologically.

If the neonate demonstrates clinical signs of enterocolitis, an enema examination may not be undertaken due to the risk of perforation. Enterocolitis is a potentially fatal complication and may occur before or after the surgical treatment of Hirschsprung's disease. Occasionally, an enema will show signs of unsuspected enterocolitis such as colonic dilatation, thickening

of the haustral folds, mucosal oedema and ulceration. The presence of the intestinal cut-off sign on plain radiographs (described as gaseous intestinal distension with abrupt cut-off at the level of the pelvic brim) is a more specific indicator of Hirschsprung's enterocolitis.

Confirmation of Hirschsprung's disease is achieved by means of a suction biopsy. This is an accurate test with a very low incidence of complications and may be performed without anaesthetic. The sample should be taken 2 cm above the dentate line, as below this the normal anus has relative hypoganglionosis. Contrast enema examinations may be safely performed 24 h after a suction biopsy, although ideally the enema should precede a biopsy.

A further test that may help in equivocal cases is anorectal manometry. This relies on anal sphincter reflex relaxation in response to distension of the rectum and is absent in patients with Hirschsprung's disease. A caveat is that this reflex may not be fully developed in the first weeks of life. A normal result, however, will

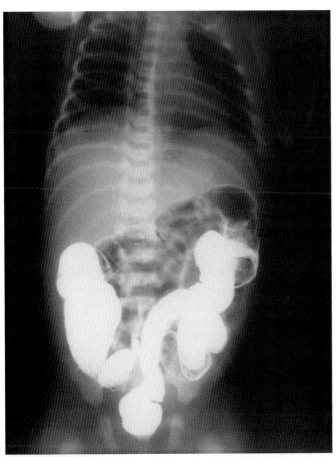

Figure 10.8.12 Hirschsprung's disease. Contrast enema in a neonate with total aganglionosis demonstrates normal colonic calibre without a transition zone.

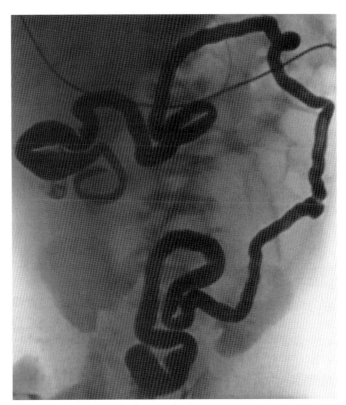

Figure 10.8.13 Hirschsprung's disease. Total colonic Hirschsprung's disease is seen in this neonate as a complete microcolon with no transition zone.

help exclude Hirschsprung's disease. The reported accuracy and reliability of this test varies with the age of the infant and the experience of the operator.

The enema may be non-diagnostic in patients with total colonic aganglionosis or ultrashort disease. In total colonic aganglionosis the diagnosis is often delayed and the incidence of complications before and after surgical treatment is increased. The contrast enema usually shows a normal colonic calibre but a microcolon may be seen (Figures 10.8.12 and 10.8.13). While the characteristic transition zone is absent, a question mark colon may be identified due to colonic shortening with rounding of the hepatic and splenic flexures. The colonic wall may appear irregular with abnormal contractions seen throughout. Additionally, there may be impaction of meconium throughout the colon giving a double contrast effect to the contrast enema. In rare cases, the aganglionic region extends to the small bowel to a variable extent. Total intestinal aganglionosis is extremely rare and invariably fatal.

In ultrashort disease, the enema may fail to show a transition zone and suction biopsy above 3 cm may show some ganglion cells. The diagnosis is usually made by anal manometry and the surgical treatment is anorectal myectomy.

Surgical treatment of Hirschsprung's disease may be undertaken in a one-step procedure with resection of the aganglionic segment and confirmation of ganglia in the proximal bowel. There are three commonly performed techniques for reanastomosis: direct reanastomosis with the rectal stump (Swenson procedure); pull-through of the normal colon with an enlongated cuff of aganglionic rectum (Soave procedure); or fashioning of a mixed ganglionic/aganlionic pouch from the rectum and normal colon (Duhamel procedure). In low birth weight neonates or those with complicating medical conditions, treatment is usually by diverting colostomy with delayed resection of the aganglionic segment.

Complications following surgical treatment include incontinence and constipation above anastomotic strictures.

FURTHER READING

Clark DA. Times of first void and first stool in 500 newborns. Pediatrics 1977; 60:457.

Elhalaby EA, Coran AG, Blane CE et al. Enterocolitis associated with Hirschsprung's disease: a clinical-radiological characterization based on 168 patients. Journal of Pediatric Surgery 1995; 30:76–83.

Holschneider AM et al. The development of anorectal continence and its significance in the diagnosis of Hirschsprung's disease. Journal of Pediatric Surgery 1976; 11:151.

Ikeda K et al. Long segment aganglionosis (Hirschsprung's disease) in brothers. Shujutsu 1968; 22:806.

Ito Y, Donahoe P, Hendren W. Maturation of the rectoanal response in premature and perinatal infants. Journal of Pediatric Surgery 1977; 12:477.

Newman B, Nussbaum A, Kirkpatrick JA Jr. Bowel perforation in Hirschsprung's disease. American Journal of Roentgenology 1987; 148: 1195–1197.

Quinn FM, Surana R, Puri P. The influence of trisomy 21 on outcome in children with Hirschsprung's disease. Journal of Pediatric Surgery 1994; 29:781.

Swenson O, Sherman JO, Fisher JH. Diagnosis of congenital megacolon: an analysis of 501 patients. Journal of Pediatric Surgery 1973; 8:587.

Vane D, Grosfeld J. Hirschsprung's disease, experience with the Duhamel operation in 195 cases. Pediatric Surgery International 1986; 1:95.

INTESTINAL NEURONAL DYSPLASIA

Patients with intestinal neuronal dysplasia are often clinically indistinguishable from those with Hirschsprung's disease but rectal biopsy shows hyperplasia of ganglion cells in the submucosal and myenteric plexuses rather than aganglionosis. The imaging findings are not well described but often mimic Hirschsprung's disease (Figure 10.8.14). Older children present with a history of constipation, rectal bleeding and pseudo-obstruction and the enema shows a megacolon. Peristaltic activity is present but uncoordinated and when observed by US is often vigorous. The diagnosis is established by histopathology of biopsy specimens. The condition may be localized or widespread, with extension to involve the small bowel. Occasionally, intestinal neuronal dysplasia may accompany Hirschsprung's disease. Treatment initially is conservative, with laxatives and enemas as needed. The natural history is one of periods of improvement and relapse but slow improvement in symptoms occurs with maturity. Surgery is occasionally needed for intractable cases.

FURTHER READING

Puri P, Wester T. Intestinal neuronal dysplasia. Seminars in Pediatric Surgery 1998; 7:181–186.

Scharli AF, Meier-Ruge W. Localized and disseminated forms of neuronal intestinal dysplasia mimicking Hirschsprung's disease. Journal of Pediatric Surgery 1981; 16:164–170.

Schofield DE, Yunis EJ. Intestinal neuronal dysplasia. Journal of Pediatric Gastroenterology and Nutrition 1991; 12:182–189.

NEONATAL FUNCTIONAL COLONIC OBSTRUCTION

Meconium plug syndrome and small left colon syndrome are related entities in the spectrum of neonatal functional colonic obstruction. They present within 1–2 days of life with abdominal

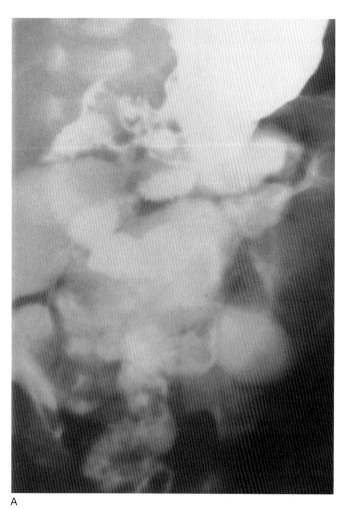

A

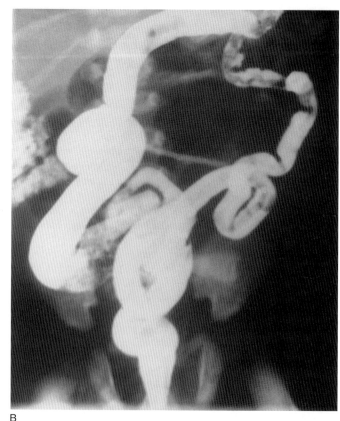

B

Figure 10.8.14 (A) Upper and (B) lower gastrointestinal contrast study in an infant with intestinal neuronal dysplasia. Note the dilatation of the mid small bowel with more proximal relatively normal calibre bowel, the narrow calibre colon. Proven case of intestinal dysplasia.

distension, failure to pass meconium and, occasionally, vomiting, which may be bilious. They are due to transient colonic inertia, with failure of normal peristalsis in a normally innervated colon. Plain radiographic findings are non-specific showing distal bowel obstruction with no gas seen in the distal colon or rectum. The exact aetiology is unknown, however there are described associations with maternal diabetes, prematurity, sepsis, traumatic delivery and the administration of magnesium sulphate or psychotropic drugs in the antenatal period. The two conditions will be considered separately for clarity.

MECONIUM PLUG SYNDROME

This is the most frequent cause of delayed passage of meconium in infants. In this condition, contrast enema examination is both diagnostic and therapeutic. Low osmolar contrast medium should be used, with careful attention to hydration of the neonate.

The colon is usually of normal calibre. The meconium plug occupies the rectosigmoid region but may extend throughout the colon (Figure 10.8.15). The meconium can be seen as one continuous plug or may occur as discrete meconium lumps. Stimulation of the rectum by the enema or, occasionally, digital rectal examination precipitates passage of the plug and subsequently a normal evacuation pattern is established.

Differentiation should be made between meconium plug syndrome and meconium ileus. The latter term is reserved for bowel obstruction secondary to inspissated meconium in the distal small bowel and proximal colon, most often seen in patients with cystic fibrosis.

SMALL LEFT COLON SYNDROME

This is really a variant of functional colonic obstruction. In this condition, contrast enema examination demonstrates a microcolon limited to the descending and rectosigmoid colon with transition to normal colonic calibre in the region of the splenic flexure. Typically, there is improvement in clinical and radiological findings in a matter of hours or, occasionally, days. The condition sometimes mimics Hirschsprung's disease due to the transition zone to normal calibre colon in the region of the splenic flexure (Figure 10.8.16). Characteristically, once a normal bowel pattern is established in patients with neonatal functional colonic obstruction it remains normal. Patients with Hirschsprung's disease will have ongoing difficulties. If there is any suspicion of Hirschsprung's disease further evaluation by means of suction biopsy or anal manometry should be performed.

FURTHER READING

Amodio J, Berdon W, Abramson S et al. Microcolon of prematurity: a form of functional obstruction. American Journal of Roentgenology 1986; 146:239–244.

Berdon WE, Slovis TL, Campbell JB et al. Neonatal small left colon syndrome; its relationship to aganglionosis and meconium plug syndrome. Radiology 1977; 125:457–462.

Le Quesne GE, Reilly BJ. Functional immaturity of the large bowel in the newborn infant. Radiologic Clinics of North America 1975; 13:331–342.

Pockaczesky R, Leonidas JC. The meconium plug syndrome; roentgen evaluation and differentiation from Hirschsprung's disease and other pathologic states. American Journal of Roentgenology 1974; 120:342–352.

INSPISSATED MILK CURD SYNDROME

Intestinal obstruction secondary to milk curd is a condition resulting from feeding concentrated, incorrectly reconstituted powdered milk to infants. It differs from other causes of neonatal intestinal obstruction in that there is normal passage of meconium before the obstruction develops.

Plain abdominal radiographs show distended loops of colon and distal small bowel, in which the milk curds may be outlined by air. Most infants can be managed conservatively. Introduction of water-soluble low osmolar contrast medium per rectum into the region of the inspissated curds will help their evacuation, as will adequate rehydration. On rare occasions, the intraluminal masses of milk curds are associated with local mucosal necrosis and perforation needing surgical treatment (Figure 10.8.17).

FURTHER READING

Cook RCM, Rickham PP. Neonatal intestinal obstruction due to milk curds. Journal of Pediatric Surgery 1969; 4:599–605.

Cremin BJ, Smythe PM, Cywes S. The radiological appearance of the 'inspissated milk syndrome'. A cause of intestinal obstruction in infants. British Journal of Radiology 1970; 43:856–858.

Konvolinka CW, Frederick J. Milk curd syndrome in neonates. Journal of Pediatric Surgery 1989; 24:497–498.

MEGACYSTIS–MICROCOLON– HYPOPERISTALSIS SYNDROME

Megacystis–microcolon–hypoperistalsis syndrome is a rare cause of functional intestinal obstruction in the newborn. The condition predominantly occurs in females but males can be affected also, though this is very rare. The exact aetiology is unknown and the condition is almost always fatal.

There is abdominal distension caused by a massively distended non-obstructed bladder. This is usually evident on plain abdominal radiographs. No mechanical bladder neck or urethral obstruction is present and vesicoureteric reflux does not occur. There is commonly dilatation of the ureters and pelvicalyceal system.

The bowel is markedly shortened to approximately one-third of normal length and is often malrotated. The proximal small bowel is dilated with absent or ineffective peristalsis throughout the bowel. Contrast enema shows a microcolon. The condition is generally refractory to therapy.

FURTHER READING

Berdon WE, Baker DH, Blanc WA et al. Megacystis-microcolon-hypoperistalsis syndrome; a rare cause of intestinal obstruction in the newborn. American Journal of Roentgenology 1976; 126:957–964.

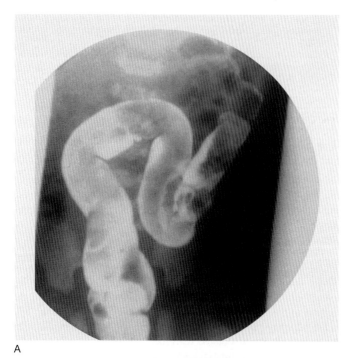

A

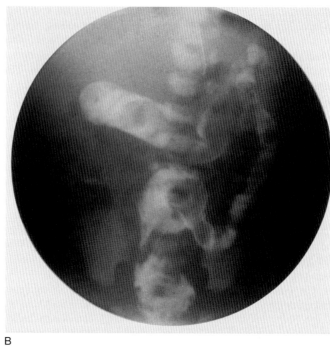

B

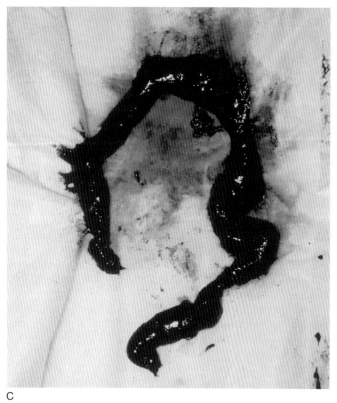

C

Figure 10.8.15 Meconium plug syndrome. (A) The obstructing meconium plug is seen impacted in the rectosigmoid and descending colon. (B) Contrast media outlines the colon after evacuation of the plug during the enema examination. (C) Typical appearance of an evacuated plug.

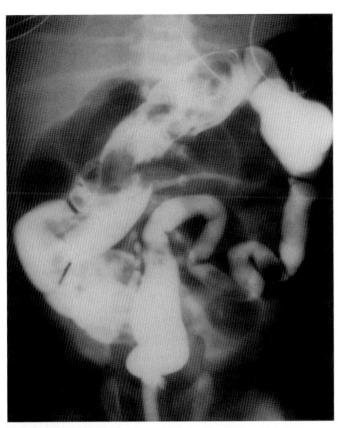

Figure 10.8.16 Small left colon syndrome. The colon returns to a normal calibre in the region of the splenic flexure.

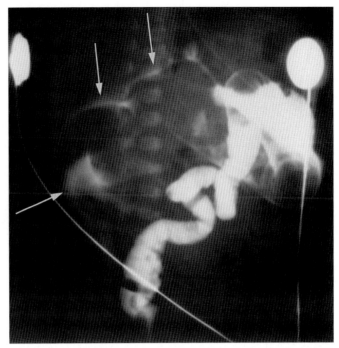

Figure 10.8.17 Inspissated milk curd syndrome. Water-soluble contrast enema examination demonstrates a 'milk mass' in the distal transverse colon causing obstruction at this level. There is associated perforation with spill of contrast into the peritoneal cavity (arrows).

Krook OM. Megacystis-microcolon-hypoperistalsis syndrome in a male infant. Radiology 1980; 136:649–650.

Patel R, Carty H. Megacystis-microcolon-hypoperistalsis syndrome: a rare cause of intestinal obstruction in the newborn. British Journal of Radiology 1980; 53:249–252.

Young LW, Yunis EJ, Girdany BR et al. Megacystis-microcolon-intestinal hypoperistalsis syndrome: additional clinical, radiologic, surgical and histopathologic aspects. American Journal of Roentgenology 1981; 137:749–755.

ANORECTAL ANOMALIES

The incidence of anorectal anomalies is 1 in 5000 live births. There is a slight male predominance with approximately 60% of cases occurring in boys. There have been several systems of classification of these anomalies, however none has gained consistent international recognition. A practical concept is division of the lesions into high, intermediate or low in terms of the relationship of the distal rectal pouch to the pelvic floor (puborectalis muscle). High and intermediate lesions are treated with diverting colostomy with a delayed definitive repair, while low lesions are repaired by anoplasty. Correct classification of the anomaly is essential to avoid an erroneous deep perineal exploration in a high lesion and a colostomy in a low anomaly.

A more descriptive but simple classification system was developed by an international symposium of paediatric surgeons in Melbourne in 1970 and introduced into the literature by Gans.

Anorectal anomalies are subdivided into four categories. Ectopic anus is the most common abnormality and occurs when the terminal bowel opens at an abnormal location such as the perineum, scrotum, vulva, vestibule, urethra, vagina or cloaca (Figures 10.8.18 and 10.8.19). This anomaly results from failure of the hindgut to descend properly to join the anus, instead emptying ectopically through a fistula. Fistulas of this nature from the distal rectal pouch are more correctly termed an ectopic anus. The anal dimple and external anal sphincter are usually present to some degree. In imperforate anus, the terminal bowel ends blindly and no fistula exsists. There are two types – anal atresia and anorectal atresia – depending on the length of the atretic portion. The third category is rectal atresia. In this condition, the anus is present and open, however a variable segment of the rectum above it is atretic and no fistula exsists. Anal or rectal stenoses are the final entity in this classification and refer to incomplete atresia.

The survival and quality of life of children with anorectal anomalies often depends more on associated abnormalities of other systems. These are found in approximately half of the children, the incidence being greater in children with high anorectal anomalies. Associated anomalies may manifest as part of the VACTERL pattern (vertebral, anal, cardiac, tracheoesophageal, renal and limb anomalies). Lumbosacral vertebral abnormalities are common in children with anorectal malformation, reported in 10% and 25% of children with low and high lesions, respectively (Figure 10.8.20). Sacral agenesis, hemivertebrae and fusion anomalies are seen. In recent times, evaluation of these children by MRI and US has revealed an incidence of occult dysraphism and cord abnormalities in up to 50%. Abnormalities encountered included thickened filum, fibrolipoma, tethered cord and

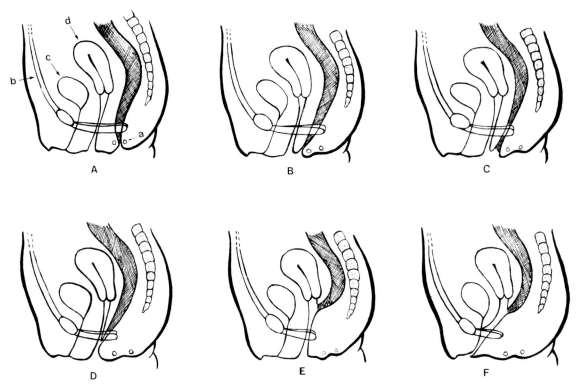

Figure 10.8.18 Ectopic anus in female infant: (A) normal female infant, (B) anoperineal fistula, (C) rectovestibular fistula, (D) low rectovaginal fistula, (E) high rectovaginal fistula and (F) rectocloacal fistula. a, external anal sphincter; b, puborectalis sling; c, bladder; d, uterus.

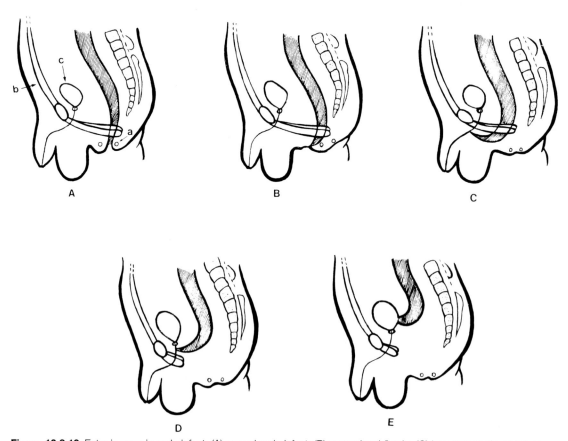

Figure 10.8.19 Ectopic anus in male infant: (A) normal male infant, (B) anoperineal fistula, (C) low rectouretheral fistula, (D) high rectouretheral fistula and (E) rectovesical fistula. a, external anal sphincter; b, puborectalis sling; c, bladder.

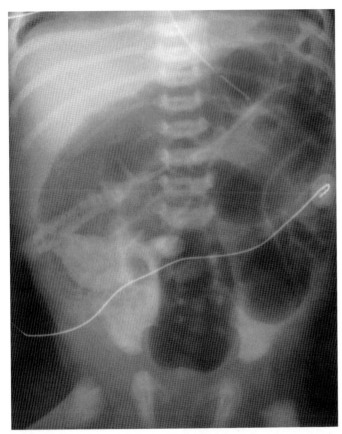

Figure 10.8.20 Anorectal atresia. This plain radiograph demonstrates several sacral vertebral anomalies in the presence of a high anorectal atresia.

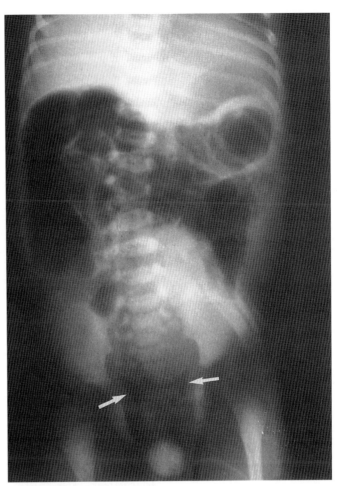

Figure 10.8.21 Ectopic anus in a male infant. Note air in the bladder (white arrows) indicating a rectovesical fistula.

syringohydromyelia. These conditions may contribute to poor bowel and bladder continence in the postoperative period. The Currarino triad is a rare collection of associated anomalies and includes an anorectal malformation, lumbosacral abnormalities and a presacral mass, which may be a teratoma, anterior meningocele or enteric cyst.

Cardiovascular abnormalities, most commonly tetralogy of Fallot and ventricular septal defect, are seen in 12–22% of infants with anorectal anomalies. The principal gastrointestinal abnormalities encountered are oesophageal atresia, with or without tracheoesophageal fistula, duodenal atresia and Hirschsprung's disease. Urological anomalies are common in this population, seen in 20% of children with low lesions and 60% of those with high lesions. The commonest anomalies include vesicoureteric reflux, renal agenesis and renal dysplasia. One-third of female children with anorectal anomalies will have genital abnormalities such as bicornuate uterus, uterine didelphus or vaginal septum. Cryptorchidism is seen in approximately one-fifth of males with anorectal anomalies.

Anorectal malformations are usually diagnosed early in the neonatal period due to failure to pass meconium or, more commonly, due to an absent or abnormal anal dimple. Initial assessment is primarily concerned with differentiation of a high (or intermediate) lesion from a low lesion in order to plan early surgery. It may be possible to do so by careful clinical examination. The rectal pouch terminates in a high position in two-thirds of boys and in a low position in two-thirds of girls with anorectal anomalies. Radiology alone is unreliable in differentiating high

from low anomalies but it plays an important role in conjunction with clinical evaluation.

Abdominal radiographs will show distal bowel obstruction. In males, gas may be seen in the bladder and rarely in the vagina in female infants, confirming an associated fistula (Figures 10.8.21 and 10.8.22). It is important to allow enough time for gas to reach the rectum, i.e. at least 12 h after birth. A prone cross-table lateral view taken with a pillow beneath the neonate to elevate the buttocks may be helpful (Figure 10.8.23). This examination is controversial due to well-documented inaccuracies; however, in individual cases it can be informative and it allows for assessment of the lumbosacral spine. Gas in the rectum outlines the distal extent of the hindgut and bony landmarks indicate the puborectalis, in order to classify the anomaly as high or low. The puborectalis muscle was thought to coincide with a line drawn from the mid symphysis pubis to the sacrococcygeal junction. This pubococcygeal line is now believed to be too high and the 'M' line running horizontal to it, dividing the lower third and upper two-thirds of the ischium, is suggested as being more accurate (Figure 10.8.24). Impaction of meconium in the distal rectal pouch can make a low anomaly appear high and conversely straining, crying or excessive distension of a high rectal pouch may be seen as a low lesion.

Ultrasound of the perineum can measure the rectal pouch–perineal distance to help classify the anomaly. It is suggested that

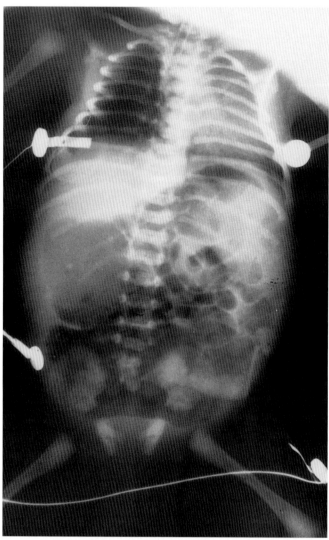

Figure 10.8.22 Anorectal atresia. There is calcified meconium in the colon in the right upper quadrant. The child had a large rectourethral fistula and the calcification is due to the mixture of urine and meconium.

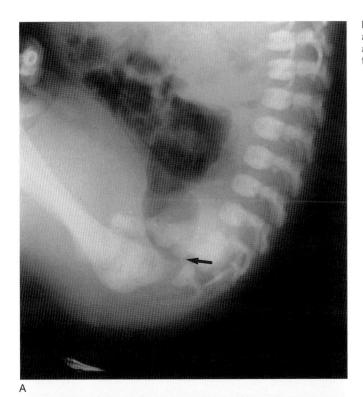

A

Figure 10.8.23 (A) Ectopic anus. Lateral radiograph demonstrates an air-filled distal rectal pouch ending blindly above the ischium, indicating a high lesion (arrow). (B) Low lesion. Note air in the distal pouch almost touches the barium on the anus.

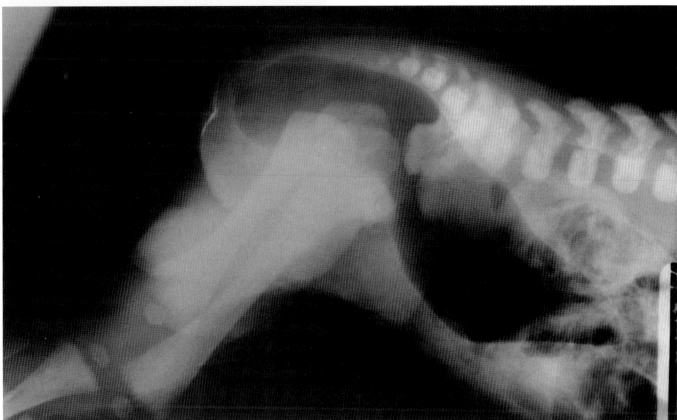

B

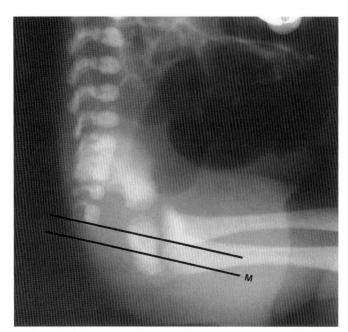

Figure 10.8.24 M line drawn through the junction of the upper two-thirds and lower one-third of the ischium. This corresponds to the level of the puborectalis muscle and determines a high or a low lesion. Note in this child the high lesion, also fusion of the lower sacral segments.

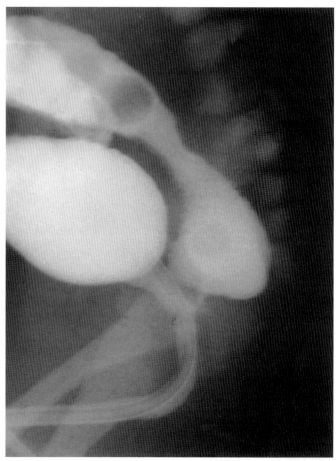

Figure 10.8.25 Rectouretheral fistula in an infant with ectopic anus. The rectal pouch fills with contrast media instilled via the uretheral catheter. There is a large fistula from the prostatic urethra to the rectal pouch.

a distance of less than 10 mm indicates a low lesion and can be safely treated by anoplasty, while a distance greater than 10–15 mm should be diverted with a colostomy. The reliability of US has not been determined; however, it is likely to be subject to the same inaccuracies as plain radiography.

Direct puncture of the anus and injection of contrast media into the rectal pouch is occasionally useful but is not routinely favoured.

Initial assessment of the neonates should include detection of associated fistulas, additional anomalies and the degree of development of the sphincter muscle complex. This is usually undertaken after diverting colostomy. Micturating cystography will delineate many fistulas in males and also detects associated vesicoureteric reflux, which may be a further cause of long-term morbidity (Figure 10.8.25). A vaginogram may be required in females to demonstrate possible fistulas. Fistulas can also be depicted by distal loopogram studies in children with a defunctioning colostomy. This is the preferred type of examination in many centres. It allows for localization of the distal rectal pouch. Ultrasound of the abdomen should be performed early for evaluation of the renal tract.

Evaluation of the spine may be performed by plain radiography and US. However, increasingly, these children undergo early MRI studies to simultaneously assess the rectal pouch position in relation to the puborectalis and to detect associated vertebral, spinal cord or genitourinary anomalies. MRI allows for direct visualization of the muscles of the pelvic floor in contrast to other modalities. The sphincter muscle complex (puborectalis and external anal sphincter) is usually well developed in children with low anomalies. Those with intermediate or high anomalies have variable development of one or both elements of the sphincter muscle complex with important sequelae in terms of postoperative bowel continence. In patients with sacral agenesis, the muscle complex may be in an anomalous location and preoperative awareness of this is valuable. T1-weighted images in three orthogonal planes are the standard sequences obtained. Meconium appears uniformly hyperdense on these images with excellent contrast to the rectal wall and surrounding musculature of the pelvic floor. MRI has low sensitivity for the detection of fistulas, however T2-weighted sequences and dynamic contrast-enhanced sequences or the use of bowel contrast (Vaseline or corn oil instilled into the distal colostomy loop) may improve detection.

Definitive repair of high or intermediate anomalies is usually undertaken in the first year of life. Posterior sagittal anorectoplasty is performed from a perineal approach with utilization of both the external anal sphincter and puborectalis for continence. In most patients, it is possible to mobilize the distal bowel adequately from below for the pull-through procedure, however a combined abdominoperineal approach may be required. Prior to surgery, a distal colonogram is performed by catheterization of the defunctioned colon. A moderately sized (11F) balloon catheter is inserted into the proximal colostomy, the balloon inflated and a hand injection of contrast performed. The aim is to achieve sufficient distension to fill a recto urethra, vesical or vaginal fistula (Figure 10.8.26).

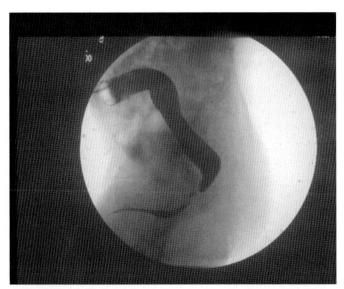

Figure 10.8.26 Distal colonogram prior to pull-through to repair an anorectal atresia. Note the large fistula to the urethra with some reflux into the bladder.

FURTHER READING

Cortes D, Thorup JM, Nielsen OH et al. Cryptorchidism in boys with imperforate anus. Journal of Pediatric Surgery 1995; 30:631.

Currarino G, Coln D, Votteler T. Triad of anorectal, sacral and presacral anomalies. American Journal of Roentgenology 1981; 137:395–398.

Donaldson JS, Black CT, Reynolds M et al. Ultrasound of the distal pouch in infants with imperforate anus. Journal of Pediatric Surgery 1989; 24:465–468.

Gans SL. Classification of anorectal anomalies: a critical analysis. Journal of Pediatric Surgery 1970; 5:511–513.

Hall R, Fleming S, Gysler M et al. The genital tract in female children with imperforate anus. American Journal of Obstetrics and Gynecology 1985; 151:169.

McHugh K, Dudley NE, Tam P. Pre-operative MRI of anorectal anomalies in the newborn period. Pediatric Radiology 1995; 25:S33–S36.

McLorie GA, Sheldon CA, Fleisher M et al. The genitourinary system in patients with imperforate anus. Journal of Pediatric Surgery 1987; 22:1100–1104.

Partridge JP, Gough MH. Congenital abnormalities of the anus and rectum. British Journal of Surgery 1961; 49:37.

Rivosecchi M, Lucchetti MC, Zaccara A et al. Spinal dysraphism detected by magnetic resonance imaging in patients with anorectal anomalies: incidence and clinical significance. Journal of Pediatric Surgery 1995; 30:488.

Sato Y, Pringle KC, Bergman RA et al. Congenital anorectal anomalies: MR imaging. Radiology 1988; 168:157–162.

COLONIC ATRESIA

Three types of colonic atresia are recognized:

type 1 – membranous occlusion;
type 2 – atresia connected by a thin atretic band; and
type 3 – complete atresia with no connecting band.

In types 2 and 3, there is an associated mesenteric defect, similar to that seen in small intestinal atresia. Type 3 is the most common atresia encountered. Colonic stenosis represents an incomplete form of atresia and occurs less frequently. The aetiology is most likely an intrauterine vascular insult to a normally formed colon. The condition presents in the first 1–2 days of life with progressive abdominal distension, vomiting and failure to pass meconium due to complete colonic obstruction. Radiographically, the colon proximal to the atresia is often massively dilated. Occasionally, the proximally dilated colon ruptures with a resultant pneumoperitoneum. A contrast enema reveals a distal microcolon (Figure 10.8.27). The blind-ending distal colon may curl on itself to form a hook sign. In the presence of a type 1 atresia, the blind-ending distal colon when filled with contrast material may bulge into the proximal dilated colon to give a windsock or club-shaped appearance.

FURTHER READING

Bley WR, Franken EA Jr. Roentgenology of colon atresia. Pediatric Radiology 1973; 1:105–108.

Selke AC Jr, Jona JZ. The hook sign in type 3 congenital colonic atresia. American Journal of Roentgenology 1978; 131:350–351.

Winters WD, Weinberger E, Hatch EI. Atresia of the colon in neonates: radiographic findings. American Journal of Roentgenology 1992; 159:1273–1276.

COLONIC DUPLICATION

This is rare and is usually tubular affecting a variable length of colon. It may be in communication with the normal lumen at both ends, or blind at one end. At enema, contrast fills both lumina (Figure 10.8.28).

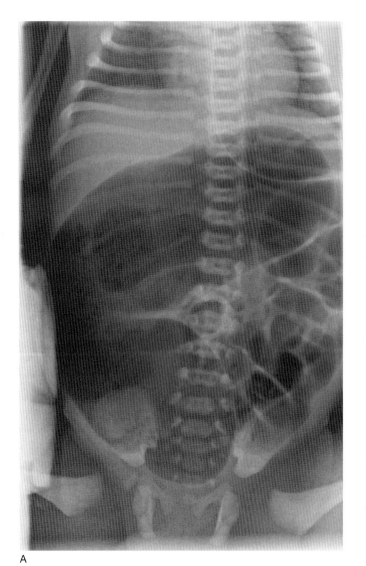

A

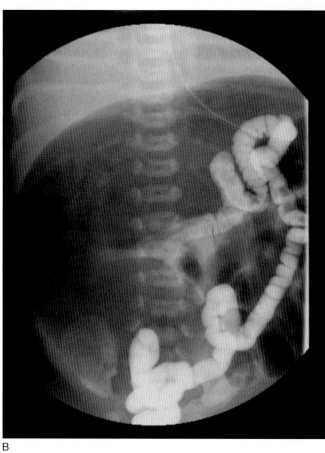

B

Figure 10.8.27 Colonic atresia. (A) Abdominal radiograph showing a massively dilated colon proximal to the atresia and (B) the corresponding contrast enema. The contrast enema outlines a microcolon ending abruptly at the site of atresia.

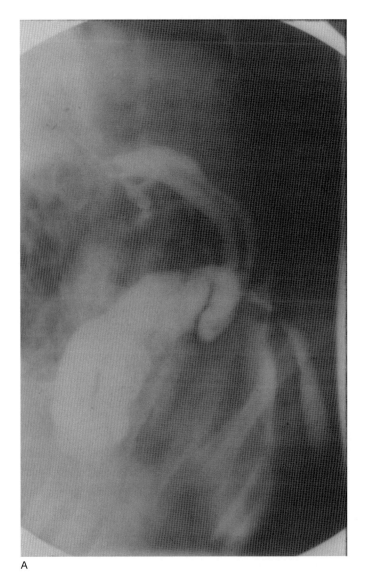

A

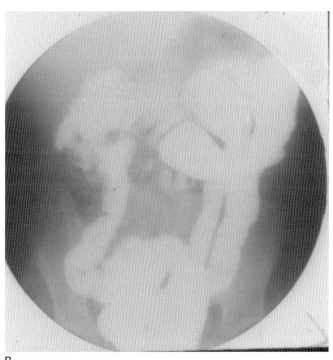

B

Figure 10.8.28 (A,B) Two images of an infant with tubular duplication of the colon. Note filling of two lumina in the sigmoid and descending colon.

The Salivary Glands and Tongue

Sambasiva R Kottamasu, David A Stringer

DISORDERS OF SALIVARY GLANDS IN CHILDREN

There are three pairs of main salivary glands: the parotid, the submandibular and the sublingual. In addition, numerous minor salivary glands are present beneath the mucous membrane of the upper digestive tract. The secretions of the parotid glands are totally serous; the submandibular gland secretions are partly serous and partly mucous; and the secretions of the sublingual gland are almost completely mucous. Disorders of salivary glands are less common in children. Inflammatory lesions are the most common but calculi, neoplasms and miscellaneous conditions also occur.

It is appropriate to use ultrasonography (US) as the initial imaging study for evaluation of salivary gland lesions in children. In most cases, US permits differentiation of intraglandular and extraglandular lesions and may suggest the correct diagnosis. Vascular lesions can be well demonstrated by colour Doppler imaging. If the mass has deep extension or bony involvement, further imaging with CT or MRI is necessary.

IMAGING

The salivary glands in children may manifest a variety of lesions and are often evaluated with plain radiography, sialography, ultrasonography (US), scintigraphy, contrast enhanced computed tomography (CT) and magnetic resonance imaging (MRI). Radiographs are useful for evaluation of salivary calculi, calcification within a mass/neoplasm and bony involvement. Sialography is reserved for evaluation of recurrent pain or swelling in a salivary gland and detecting calculi. It is performed with water-soluble contrast. Films, which may include tomographs, are taken during filling and washout following stimulation of salivary secretions with lemon juice. Successful sialography requires patient cooperation. The orifice of the parotid duct lies above the second upper molar in the mucous membrane of the cheek. The submandibular orifices are in the mucosa of the floor of the mouth on either side of the frenulum. Scintigraphy is helpful for functional evaluation of the salivary glands and for differentiation of various benign and malignant neoplasms. US assesses the size of the salivary gland and vascularity, distinguishes diffuse from focal disease and cystic from solid lesions, and guides fine-needle

aspiration. However, further evaluation with CT or MRI may be needed to better define the nature and deep extent of the disease and bony involvement. CT is helpful for evaluation of most paediatric parotid diseases including acute inflammation, abscess, calculi and most solid masses. A mass associated with facial nerve symptoms should be evaluated with MRI. More recently, MR sialography shows promise as an investigative tool to evaluate the duct system.

FURTHER READING

Garcia CJ, Flores PA, Arce JD, Chuaqui B, Schwartz DS. Ultrasonography in the study of salivary gland lesions in children. Pediatric Radiology 1998; 28:418–425.
Lowe LH, Stokes LS, Johnson JE et al. Swelling at the angle of the mandible: imaging of the paediatric parotid gland and periparotid region. Radiographics 2001; 21:121–127.

CONGENITAL DISORDERS

Salivary gland agenesis is an extremely uncommon congenital anomaly. It is usually unilateral but bilateral cases have been described as a rare cause of profound xerostomia.

FURTHER READING

Ferreira AP, Gomez RS, Castro WH et al. Congenital absence of lacrimal puncta and salivary glands: report of a Brazilian family and review. American Journal of Medical Genetics 2000; 94:32–34.
Goldenberg D, Flax-Goldenberg R, Joachims HZ, Peled N. Misplaced parotid glands: bilateral agenesis of parotid glands associated with bilateral accessory parotid tissue. Journal of Laryngology and Otology 2000; 114:883–885.

RANULA

Ranula is a mucocele originating from the sublingual salivary gland. There are two main forms of ranula: simple and plunging. The simple ranula presents as an intraoral slow-growing nontender mass, usually on one side of the mouth, and is more frequent than the plunging ranula. The plunging ranula represents a mucus escape reaction occurring from disruption of the sublingual salivary gland. The precise aetiology of their predisposition is unknown, although local trauma or inherent mylohyoid dehiscence may play important roles. A ranula is transonic on ultrasound and has well-defined margins. CT shows a low attenuation mass.

On MRI, ranulas were all well-defined, homogeneous masses giving low signal on T1-weighted and markedly high signal on T2-weighted images (Figure 10.9.1). While simple ranulas are all confined to the sublingual space, plunging ranulas are centred on the submandibular space and thus present as a neck mass. They extend into the sublingual space anteriorly, producing a so-called tail sign, and/or into the parapharyngeal space. Although they sometimes fill a considerable part of the parapharyngeal space, displacement of surrounding muscles or vessels is usually slight.

FURTHER READING

Ugboko VI, Hassan O, Prasad S, Amole AO. Congenital ranula. A report of two cases. Journal for Oto-rhino-laryngology and its Related Specialities 2002; 64:294–296.

Kurabayashi T, Ida M, Yasumoto M et al. MRI of ranulas. Neuroradiology 2000; 42:917– 922.

TRAUMA AND FOREIGN BODIES

Trauma involving the parotid gland is rare and is usually caused by penetrating injuries or fractures of the facial skeleton; rupture of the parotid gland rarely occurs. Introduction of a foreign body into the parotid gland, either from the oral cavity or through the skin, is extremely uncommon.

FURTHER READING

Smith OD, McFerran DJ, Antoun N. Blunt trauma to the parotid gland. Emergency Medicine Journal 2001; 18:402–403.

SIALOLITHIASIS

Sialolithiasis is an uncommon disorder in childhood; initially asymptomatic and symptoms may appear gradually. These can vary from moderate discomfort to severe pain with large glandular swelling accompanied by trismus. The correct interpretation of symptoms and a proper investigation for localization of salivary stones are important for effective treatment. Investigation starts with radiographs, which should include a floor of mouth view for suspected submandibular disease (Figure 10.9.2). Ultrasound, using high-resolution probes, is a sensitive technique for demonstrating sialectasis. This appears as multiple sonolucent lesions within the gland. Acoustic shadowing occurs with stones. A water-soluble sialogram shows calculi as filling defects (Figure 10.9.3). Care must be taken to ensure that air bubbles are not introduced into the duct as these may simulate stones.

MR sialography performed using a heavily T2-weighted, two-dimensional, fast spin-echo technique and a surface coil with contiguous 3-mm axial images and fat suppression have a sensitivity of 69% in revealing calculus disease and may replace contrast sialography. However, the sensitivity increases to 100% when MR sialograms are correlated with plain radiographs. MR sialography

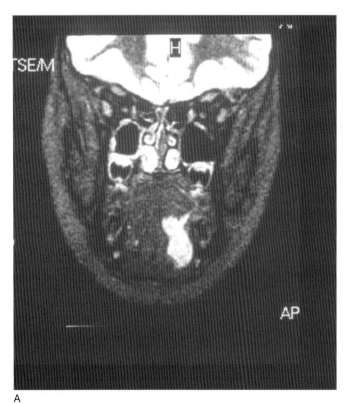

A

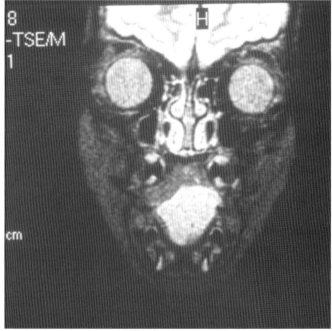

B

Figure 10.9.1 (A,B) Two children with ranulas. (A) Typical appearance of a plunging ranula; (B) ranula confined to the floor of the mouth.

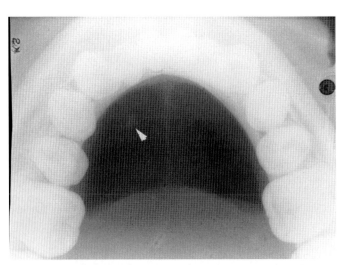

Figure 10.9.2 Calculus: Intraoral view showing stone in orifice of left submandibular gland (arrow).

accurately reveals stricture, sialectasis and neoplasm. Overall, MR sialography plus radiographs is reported to have a sensitivity, specificity and diagnostic accuracy of 100%, 88% and 96%, respectively, in revealing salivary duct abnormalities.

In patients with sialolithiasis on conventional T1-weighted, fast spin-echo fat-suppressed T2-weighted and short inversion time-inversion recovery sequences, MRI findings include evidence of acute ductal obstruction during a symptomatic phase or chronic obstruction associated with fatty replacement of the parenchyma in symptom-free periods.

FURTHER READING

Becker M, Marchal F, Becker CD et al. Sialolithiasis and salivary ductal steno-sis: diagnostic accuracy of MR sialography with a three-dimensional extended-phase conjugate-symmetry rapid spin-echo sequence. Radiology 2000; 217:347–358.

Varghese JC, Thornton F, Lucey BC et al. A prospective comparative study of MR sialography and conventional sialography of salivary duct disease. American Journal of Roentgenology 1999; 173:1497–1503.

INFLAMMATORY AND INFECTIOUS CONDITIONS

Acute sialadenitis is relatively frequent in children but does not require imaging routinely. It may be caused by organisms such as *Streptococcus viridans*, staphylococcus and pneumococcus. It may be associated with lymphadenopathy.

CHRONIC RECURRENT PAROTITIS

Chronic recurrent parotitis (CRP) is a rare inflammatory disease of unknown aetiology characterized by recurrent episodes of uni-lateral or bilateral parotid swelling, pain and inflammation associ-ated with fever and malaise over a period of years. Sialography depicts ductal strictures or ectasia and excludes sialolithiasis

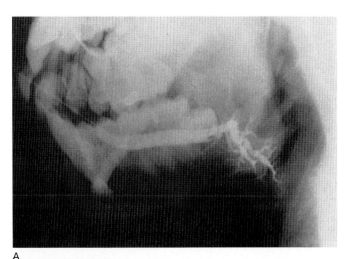

A

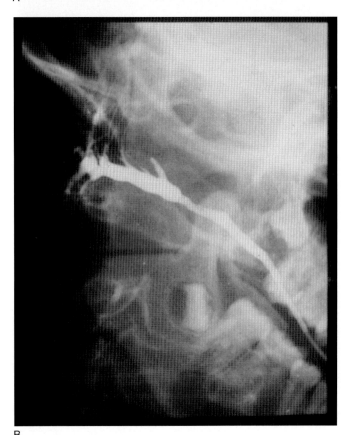

B

Figure 10.9.3 (A) Calculus; there is gross dilatation of the main submandibular and branch ducts proximal to the obstructing stone. (B) Parotid sialogram showing a mid-duct stricture with a small defect due to a calculus and proximal dilatation.

(Figure 10.9.4). Histologically, sialectasis and stricturing occur in the distal ducts, whereas inflammation is noted in the gland and duct epithelium. Inflammation usually resolves spontaneously during adolescence. MRI of the parotid glands shows diffuse contrast enhancement during acute inflammation and cysts are encountered in children who have suffered multiple episodes of inflammation. Characteristic sialectasis of the distal ducts may be

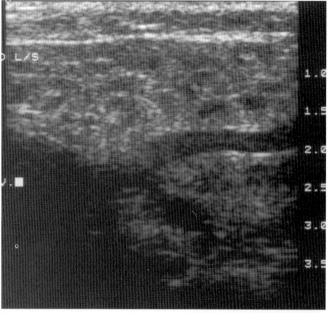

A

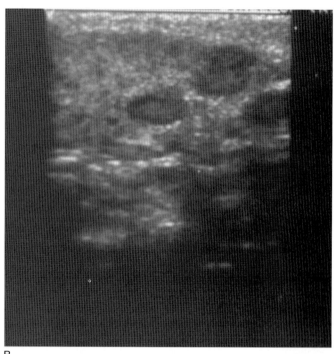

B

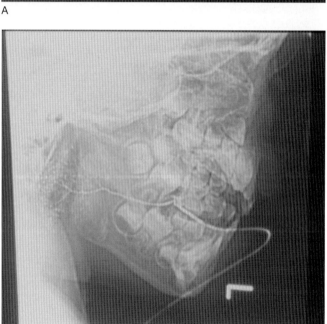

C

Figure 10.9.4 (A) Ultrasound of the parotid glands showing sialectasis. The small hypoechoic regions represent the sialectasis. (B) The left gland has, in addition, enlargement of lymphoid tissue within the gland, due to infection. (C) Parotid sialogram demonstrates dilated acini due to sialectasis.

demonstrated by imaging during the acute phase of the disease. Abscesses rarely occur.

FURTHER READING

Huisman TA, Holzmann D, Nadal D. MRI of chronic recurrent parotitis in childhood. Journal of Computed Assisted Tomography 2001; 25:269–273.

Menauer F, Jager L, Leunig A, Grevers G. Role of diagnostic imaging in chronic recurrent parotitis in childhood. Laryngorhinootologie 1999; 78:497–499.

SALIVARY GLAND ABNORMALITIES IN HIV-POSITIVE PATIENTS

HIV-positive children may present with bilateral gland enlargement. Sonography most frequently shows hypoechoic foci, hyperechoic striae and the enlargement of intraparotid and adjacent lymph nodes. Lymphoepithelial cysts and parenchymal lymphoproliferation in the parotid glands have been reported.

FURTHER READING

Goddart D, Francois A, Ninane J et al. Parotid gland abnormality found in children seropositive for the human immunodeficiency virus (HIV). Pediatric Radiology 1990; 20:355–357.

SJÖGREN'S SYNDROME

Sjögren's syndrome (SS) is a progressive autoimmune disorder mainly affecting the exocrine glands, particularly the salivary and lacrimal glands. Its precise aetiology is unknown, although several contributing factors have been identified. One theory is that the condition results from complications related to infection with the Epstein–Barr virus. A genetic marker specific for Sjögren's syndrome, HLA-DR4, has been identified. Sjögren's syndrome is uncommon in children and occurs most often in association with autoimmune diseases (secondary Sjögren's syndrome) and may present with recurrent parotitis, keratoconjunctivitis sicca or pronounced and early tooth decay associated with xerostomia. The diagnosis of primary Sjögren's syndrome largely depends on the results of biopsy of the lower lip or the presence of anti-SS antibodies.

Sialectasis of parotid terminal ducts is common. Sialogram findings vary from a slightly narrowed ductal system to multiple peripheral ductal ectasia and completely destroyed parenchyma.

Scintigraphy is abnormal in about one-third and severely abnormal in approximately half of those cases. For the diagnosis of Sjögren syndrome, salivary gland scintigraphy showed higher sensitivity than MR sialography. On the other hand, MR sialography showed higher specificity and positive predictive value than salivary gland scintigraphy. Overall, diagnostic accuracy is 83% for MR sialography and 72% for salivary gland scintigraphy.

FURTHER READING

Aguilera S, Lobo G, Ladron de Guevara D, Zerboni A. Salivary gland scintigraphy in Sjögren syndrome and its relation with the result of lip biopsy. Comparative study with a control population. Review of Medicine in Children 2000; 128:877–886.
Stiller M, Golder W, Doring E, Kliem K. Diagnostic value of sialography with both the conventional and digital subtraction techniques in children with primary and secondary Sjögren's syndrome. Oral Surgery, Oral Medicine, Oral Pathology, Oral Radiology and Endodontics 1999; 88:620–627.
Tonami H, Higashi K, Matoba M et al. A comparative study between MR sialography and salivary gland scintigraphy in the diagnosis of Sjögren syndrome. Journal of Computed Assisted Tomography 2001; 25:262–268.

NEOPLASMS

Tumours of the salivary glands are uncommon in children and are most commonly benign. They present clinically as mass lesions. The most frequent benign tumours are haemangiomas (Figures 10.9.5 and 10.9.6) or pleomorphic adenomas. Haemangiomas often contain calcified phleboliths. Other less common benign neoplasms include lymphangioma, transonic on ultrasound, Warthin's

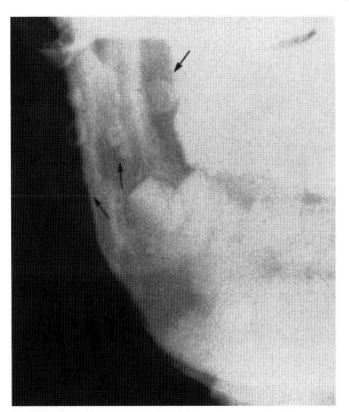

Figure 10.9.5 Haemangioma of the right parotid gland. Multiple calcified phleboliths are present.

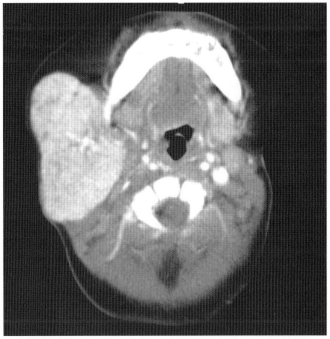

Figure 10.9.6 Parotid haemangioma. On arterial phase CT, there is marked enhancement of a markedly enlarged right parotid gland. (Courtesy of Dr Doug Jamieson.)

Table 10.9.1 Salivary gland neoplasms in children

Benign
Haemangioma
Lymphangioma
Pleomorphic adenoma
Neurofibroma
Warthin's tumour
Haemangioendothelioma
Intraductal papilloma

Malignant
Epidermoid carcinoma
Lymphoma
Leukaemia
Rhabdomyosarcoma
Sialoblastoma

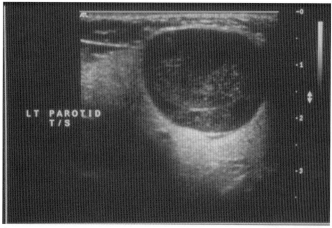

A

tumour, neurofibroma and intraductal papilloma (Table 10.9.1). Malignant tumours include rhabdomyosarcoma and mucoepidermoid carcinoma. Benign or malignant tumours may arise from other structures within the gland, e.g. neural tumours (Figure 10.9.7). Lymphoma and leukaemia can also affect the salivary glands. Sialoblastoma is an extremely rare salivary tumour diagnosed at birth or shortly thereafter with significant variability in histological appearance and clinical course. Investigation of all lesions is by US, CT and/or MRI with final histological confirmation. Cross-sectional imaging is required to identify the margins of the lesion, its extent, the relationship to the facial nerve and any associated lymphadenopathy.

FURTHER READING

Bentz BG, Hughes CA, Ludemann JP, Maddalozzo J. Masses of the salivary gland region in children. Archives of Otolaryngology and Head and Neck Surgery 2000; 126:1435–1439.

Choi DS, Na DG, Byun HS et al. Salivary gland tumours: evaluation with two-phase helical CT. Radiology 2000; 214:231–236.

Goto TK, Yoshiura K, Nakayama E et al. The combined use of US and MR imaging for the diagnosis of masses in the parotid region. Acta Radiologica 2001; 42:88–95.

Siddiqi SH, Solomon MP, Haller JO. Sialoblastoma and hepatoblastoma in a neonate. Pediatric Radiology 2000; 30:349–351.

FUNCTIONAL ABNORMALITIES OF SALIVARY GLANDS

Decreased salivation occurs with Down's syndrome, graft versus host disease, total body irradiation for bone marrow transplantation and thalassaemia. Drooling beyond the age of 4 years is pathological. Imaging is not required.

FURTHER READING

Bagesund M, Richter S, Agren B, Ringden O, Dahllof G. Scintigraphic study of the major salivary glands in paediatric bone marrow transplant recipients. Bone Marrow Transplant 2000; 26:775–779.

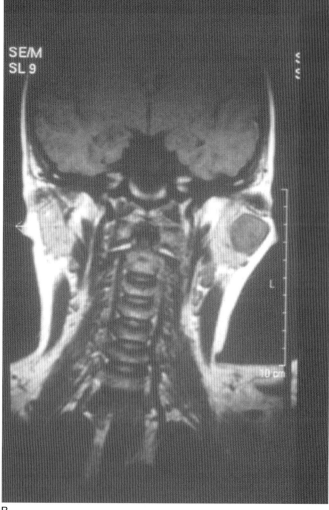

B

Figure 10.9.7 (A) Ultrasound and (B) MR images showing a well-defined left parotid mass. Histology showed this to be a schwannoma.

VASCULAR MALFORMATIONS

These may occur anywhere in the body. Haemangioma of the parotid gland is described above. Vascular malformations of the floor of the mouth, tongue, face and facial bones are classified and managed as described in Chapter 8. Vascular malformations of the mouth are very unpleasant as they may present with recurrent bleeding from repetitive minor trauma.

DISORDERS OF THE TONGUE IN CHILDREN

IMAGING

Most abnormalities of the tongue, such as infectious and inflammatory disorders, are apparent from direct inspection. Fluoroscopy can be useful in the investigation of sleep apnoea in children (see chapter 10.10). It may show glossoptosis, in which the tongue moves posteriorly during sleep and abuts the posterior pharynx and is a cause of airway obstruction and oxygen desaturation. Other abnormalities may be shown during these studies, such as macroglossia, or micrognathism or retrognathism (as in Pierre Robin syndrome or Rubinstein–Taybi syndrome).

Ultrasonography and technetium pertechnetate scintigraphy are useful if a mass lesion such as sublingual thyroid is suspected but for more complex lesions such as haemangiomas and lymphangiomas MRI is required.

INFECTIOUS AND INFLAMMATORY DISORDERS

Infectious and inflammatory disorders are often readily diagnosed clinically. Occasionally, unusual infections can occur, such as systemic cysticercosis, a serious disease in endemic areas, and may present with multiple nodules on the tongue.

BENIGN MASSES AND CONGENITAL LESIONS

A variety of congenital abnormalities and mass lesions are described. The tongue may be double, associated with cleft palate. There are also a variety of congenital benign masses, including haemangioma, vascular malformation (Figure 10.9.8), lymphatic malformation, dermoid cyst, hamartoma, choristoma (foregut duplication cyst), and lingual cyst, lingual thyroid or lingual tonsil. Lingual cyst may contain respiratory or gastric epithelium. Thyroglossal duct cyst (TGDC) is one of the more common causes of a paediatric neck mass and is rarely lingual. Lymphangiomas are very common vascular lesions, which may be macrocystic, microcystic or of mixed types. Lymphangiomas are most frequent in the

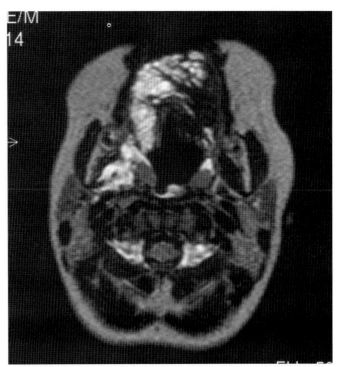

Figure 10.9.8 Vascular malformation, which involved the left side of the tongue extending into the floor of the mouth.

head and neck. Lymphangiomas in the tongue cause macroglossia. Aggressive fibromatosis and infantile myofibromatosis of the tongue is rare.

Primary, acquired benign lingual neoplasms are less common and include mucous cyst, polyp, squamous papilloma, teratoma, neurothecoma and benign epithelial cyst.

Cystic masses are well demonstrated by US. More complex lesions require CT and MRI. Haemangiomas and lymphangiomas typically demonstrate signal that is isointense to muscle on T1-weighted and increased signal on T2-weighted images making it impossible to distinguish between them. Scintigraphy with 99m-technetium pertechnetate is useful in delineating a lingual thyroid, a rare developmental disorder due to failure of descent of the gland early in the course of embryogenesis. Scintigraphy demonstrates absence of thyroid gland in normal location and evidence of an ectopic thyroid in posterior aspect of the tongue; US or MRI may reveal a soft tissue mass at the base of the tongue.

Aggressive fibromatosis on MRI shows a well-defined mass, mildly hypointense on T1-weighted and minimally hyperintense on T2-weighted images.

MALIGNANT NEOPLASMS

These uncommon lesions in children include lymphoma of Waldeyer's ring (invariably non-Hodgkin's lymphomas), squamous cell carcinoma, adenoid cystic carcinoma and a variety of sarcomas.

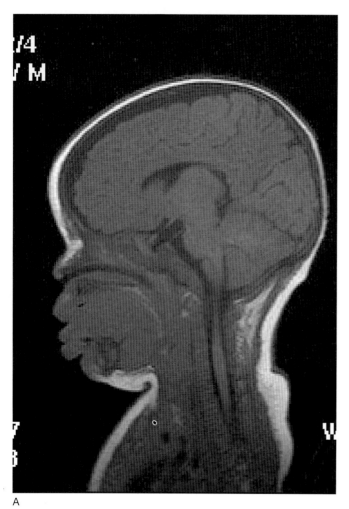

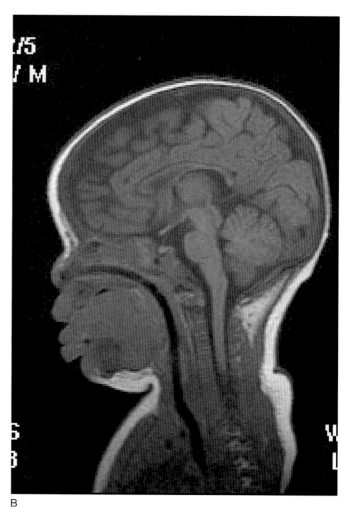

A   B

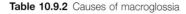

Figure 10.9.9 (A,B) Sagittal MRI scans showing enlarged tongue.

Table 10.9.2 Causes of macroglossia

Beckwith–Wiedemann syndrome
Double tongue
Down's syndrome
Glycogen storage disease
Haemangioma
Hypothyroidism
Lymphangioma
Mucopolysaccharidosis

MACROGLOSSIA

Macroglossia is enlargement of the tongue (Figure 10.9.9). This may cause drooling at the mouth or obstruction to the airways. It may occur secondary to mass lesions as previously discussed. Haemorrhage into a lymphangioma or sudden enlargement of a proliferative haemangioma may be life threatening.

There are also a variety of syndromes associated with macroglossia (Table 10.9.2).

The classic manifestations in Beckwith–Wiedemann syndrome (BWS) include visceromegaly, macroglossia, tumour predisposition and other congenital abnormalities.

FURTHER READING

Britto JA, Ragoowansi RH, Sommerlad BC. Double tongue, intraoral anomalies, and cleft palate – case reports and a discussion of developmental pathology. Cleft Palate Craniofacial Journal 2000; 37:410–415.

Donnelly LF, Jones BV, Strife JL. Imaging of paediatric tongue abnormalities. American Journal of Roentgenology 2000; 175:489–493.

Johnson JC, Coleman LL. Magnetic resonance imaging of a lingual thyroid gland. Pediatric Radiology 1989; 19:461–462.

Murayama S, Manzo RP, Kirkpatrick DV, Robinson AE. Squamous cell carcinoma of the tongue associated with Fanconi's anemia: MR characteristics. Pediatric Radiology 1990; 20:347.

Saul SH, Kapadia SB. Primary lymphoma of Waldeyer's ring. Clinicopathologic study of 68 cases. Cancer 1985; 56:157–166.

The Pharynx

*Sambasiva R Kottamasu,
David A Stringer*

INTRODUCTION

Imaging of the pharynx includes conventional radiographs, fluoroscopy with or without oral contrast, radionuclide imaging, ultrasound, computed tomography and magnetic resonance imaging. Plain radiographs of the airway are often used as the initial diagnostic technique in children with airway obstruction. The advantages of computed tomography (CT) and magnetic resonance imaging (MRI) are their multiplanar capability and ability to diagnose submucosal disease and localized as well as regional complications. CT is advantageous due to its fast imaging protocol and wide availability but MRI is superior due to its excellent soft tissue contrast.

NORMAL ANATOMY

The pharynx is a musculomembranous tube and may be subdivided from above downward into three parts: the nasopharynx, oropharynx and hypopharynx. The nasopharynx lies behind the nose and above the soft palate. The oropharynx extends from the soft palate to the level of the hyoid bone. It opens anteriorly into the mouth, while in its lateral wall, between the two pillars, is the palatine tonsil. The hypopharynx extends from the level of the hyoid bone to the level of the cricoid cartilage, where it is continuous with the oesophagus. The muscles of the pharynx include superior, middle and inferior constrictors, which insert posteriorly into a median raphe. The inferior fibres of the inferior constrictor comprise the cricopharyngeus. The adenoid is midline lymphoid tissue in the nasopharynx that is not visible in the newborn but is recognizable in infants over 6 months of age, becomes prominent in early childhood and disappears in early adulthood.

IMAGING OF CHILDREN WITH SWALLOWING DIFFICULTIES

VIDEOFLUOROSCOPIC STUDY OF SWALLOWING

Children with neurological disorders and dysphagia are at high risk for silent aspiration. The videofluoroscopic modified barium swallow (VMBS) delineates the oral, pharyngeal and upper oesophageal phases of the swallow and evaluates for aspiration. VMBS can provide valuable information regarding the most appropriate food textures and rates of oral feeding for children with feeding difficulties and may prevent chronic aspiration and malnutrition. A change in the position of the patient's head may eliminate aspiration during a modified barium swallow study.

Abnormalities seen include impairment of the oral phase: poor or absent lip seal, slow bolus formation and slow transit, and oral residue after swallowing, pooling of liquid barium in the hypopharynx prior to swallowing, delay of cricopharyngeal relaxation, aspiration of liquids (often silent), aspiration of purées and pooling of purées in the pharynx after swallowing (Figure 10.10.1).

RADIONUCLIDE SALIVAGRAM

A radionuclide salivagram is an effective study for demonstrating aspiration of oral secretions. Following sublingual administration of 300 microcuries of technetium 99m sulphur colloid in a drop of saline, serial images are obtained for 60 min and evaluated for tracer activity in the major airways and lung parenchyma.

Recurrent aspiration causing pneumonias can be demonstrated as aspirated tracer activity in trachea, bronchi or lung parenchyma.

FURTHER READING

Bar-Sever Z, Connolly LP, Treves ST. The radionuclide salivagram in children with pulmonary disease and a high risk of aspiration. Pediatric Radiology 1995; 25:S18–S183.
Darrow DH, Harley CM. Evaluation of swallowing disorders in children. Otolaryngology Clinics of North America 1998; 31:405–418.
Wright RE, Wright FR, Carson CA. Videofluoroscopic assessment in children with severe cerebral palsy presenting with dysphagia. Pediatric Radiology 1996; 26:720–722.

IMAGING OF CHILDREN WITH OBSTRUCTIVE SLEEP APNOEA

Dynamic sleep fluoroscopy, ultrasound and cephalometric radiography, nasopharyngeal endoscopy and 3D CT, and ultrafast MR imaging have all been used to evaluate sleep apnoea. Nasopharyngeal endoscopy was more reliable in identifying all the obstructive nasopharyngeal processes compared to conventional cephalometric studies. 3D CT and MRI are reserved for investigation of craniofacial malformations. Ultrafast MRI can assess function.

Glossoptosis (posterior displacement of the tongue abutting the posterior pharynx) is a frequent cause of airway obstruction in paediatric patients referred for fluoroscopic sleep studies (see Chapter ••).

FURTHER READING

Donnelly LF, Strife JL, Myer CM 3rd. Glossoptosis (posterior displacement of the tongue) during sleep: a frequent cause of sleep apnea in paediatric patients referred for dynamic sleep fluoroscopy. American Journal of Roentgenology 2000; 175:1557–1560.
Donnelly LF, Casper KA, Chen B. Correlation on cine MR imaging of size of adenoid and palatine tonsils with degree of upper airway motion in asymptomatic sedated children. American Journal of Roentgenology 2002; 179:503–508.
Fernbach SK, Brouillette RT, Riggs TW, Hunt CE. Radiologic evaluation of adenoids and tonsils in children with obstructive sleep apnea: plain films and fluoroscopy. Pediatric Radiology 1983; 13:258–265.
Suto Y, Matsuo T, Kato T et al. Evaluation of the pharyngeal airway in patients with sleep apnea: value of ultrafast MR imaging. American Journal of Roentgenology 1993; 160:311–314.

IMAGING OF CHILDREN WITH SPEECH DISORDERS

Evaluation of the velopharynx is useful in a variety of speech disorders. Videofluoroscopy, nasendoscopy and MRI have all been used with different effectiveness. Videofluoroscopy can be performed in a variety of planes; lateral, frontal, basal and Towne's projections to assess incompetence during connected speech. Barium is usually given to coat the pharynx. MRI has the advantage of no radiation and multiplanar capability, but is expensive and time consuming and requires a lot of cooperation.

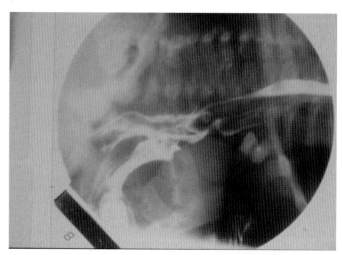

Figure 10.10.1 Nasal escape and aspiration. Infant with feeding difficulties showing nasal escape of barium and aspiration on videofluoroscopic swallow.

Table 10.10.1 Pharyngeal neoplasms in children

Benign
Juvenile nasopharyngeal angiofibroma
Haemangioma
Lymphangioma
Teratoma

Malignant
Nasopharyngeal carcinoma
Rhabdomyosarcoma
Primary lymphoma of Waldeyer's ring
Malignant mesenchymoma

FURTHER READING

Stringer DA, Witzel MA. Velopharyngeal insufficiency on multiview videofluoroscopy: a comparison of projections. American Journal of Roentgenology 1986; 146:15–19.

CONGENITAL DISORDERS

A basal encephalocele must be considered in the differential diagnosis of airway obstruction in the newborn and is associated with bony deformities of the skull base. CT and MRI show a heterogeneous mass involving the pharynx and parapharyngeal space (Figure 10.10.2).

Branchial cleft anomalies are the most common congenital anomaly and present either as a cyst, fistula or sinus (Figure 10.10.3). If the branchial cleft remains patent without a communication to the pharyngeal pouch and to the skin, a cyst develops; if there is communication a fistula develops (Figure 10.10.3); and if the branchial cleft does not communicate with the pharyngeal pouch, but extends to the skin, a sinus forms (Figure 10.10.4).

Second branchial cleft and pharyngeal pouch anomalies are the most common. Fistulae and sinuses may present with mucoid drainage during infancy or childhood. A sinus or fistula can be injected with water-soluble contrast via a fine catheter such as a

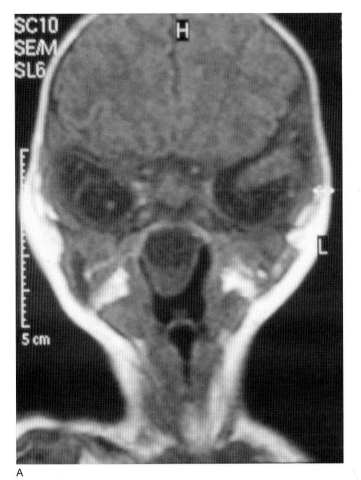

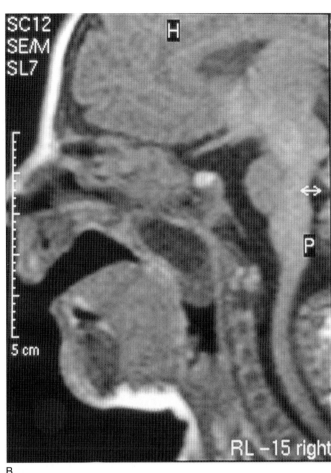

Figure 10.10.2 (A) Coronal and (B) sagittal T1-weighted images of infant who presented with obstructed feeding. The pharyngeal mass shows the typical appearance of a transphenoidal encephalocele.

sialogram catheter (Figure 10.10.5) and the study may be combined with a CT examination. A fistula typically extends from the tonsillar region to the anterior border of the sternomastoid in the lower neck. It extends between internal and external carotid arteries (Figure 10.10.3). Cysts are usually superficial in the neck, are lined with stratified squamous epithelium and can be demonstrated well on ultrasound (US) or CT evaluation of the neck (Figure 10.10.6). A cyst is typically anechoic on US, but may be echogenic if it contains desquamated epithelial cells or is infected.

Third and fourth branchial remnants are rare and often present diagnostic and therapeutic challenges. They may result in cysts and abscesses that are in close contact or involving the thyroid gland and are usually left sided and may communicate with the tip of the pyriform sinus. CT, MRI and pharyngoscopy all play a role in evaluation of these complex anomalies.

FURTHER READING

Kottamasu SR, Stringer DA. The oesophagus (congenital and developmental anomalies of the pharynx and oesophagus). In: Stringer DA, Babyn P, eds. Paediatric gastrointestinal imaging and intervention. 2nd edn. Hamilton: B.C. Decker Inc.; 2000:171–174.

Liberman M, Kay S, Emil S et al. Ten years of experience with third and fourth branchial remnants. Journal of Pediatric Surgery 2002; 37:685–690.

TRAUMA AND FOREIGN BODIES

Foreign body ingestion is common, especially in the young child, but even the older child or adult may swallow a piece of bone, especially fish bone. A plain film is the initial investigation, along with clinical examination. If this does not solve the problem, a contrast swallow or occasionally CT or MRI will demonstrate the object (Figure 10.10.7). It should be remembered that fish bones may be very radiolucent, and plastic and aluminium (e.g. fizzy drink can tops) can have the same radiodensity as soft tissues.

Penetrating injury to the oral cavity and pharynx, although rare, may cause serious morbidity and mortality in the paediatric population, because they may involve the mediastinum or neurovascular structures and may require surgery (Figure 10.10.7). Pharyngeal perforation is a rare though recognized occurrence in

A
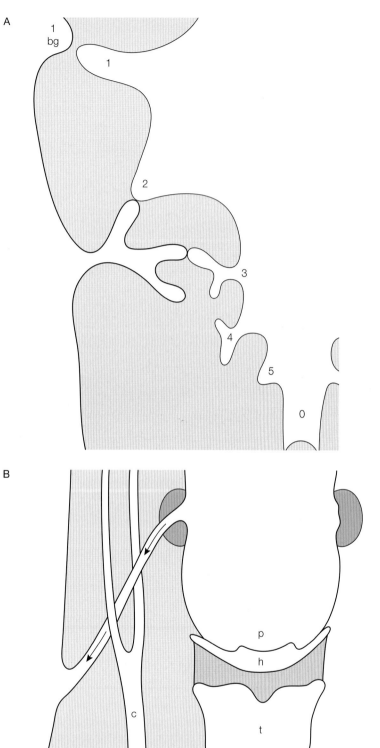

B

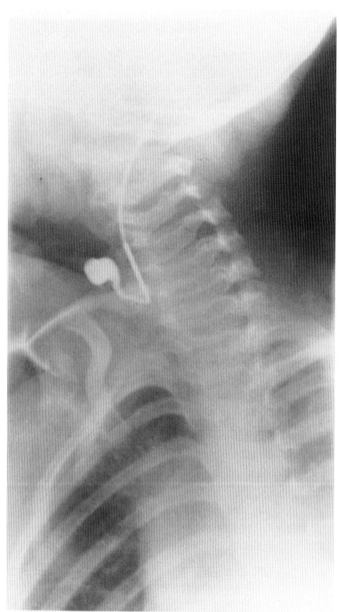

Figure 10.10.4 Branchial sinus. Sinogram of a branchial sinus. Contrast injected via a sialographic cannula fills a fluid sac. The child presented with chronic discharge from the sinus.

Figure 10.10.3 (A) A schematic drawing of development of branchial arches and grooves. This becomes the external acoustic meatus by term. The other grooves, which lie opposite the second, third and fourth arches form the cervical sinus that is obliterated by term as the neck develops. bg, branchial grooves; o, oesophagus. (B) Schematic drawing of the position of a branchial sinus fistula. p, pharynx; h, hyoid bone; t, thyroid cartilage; c, common carotid artery.

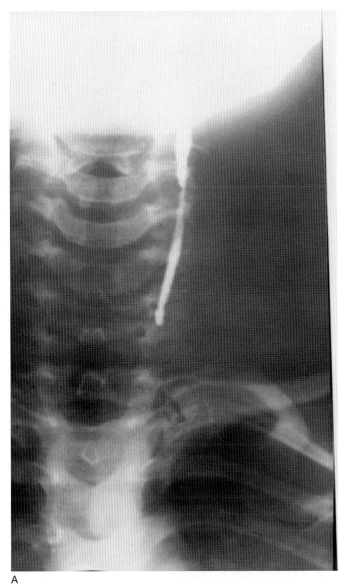

A

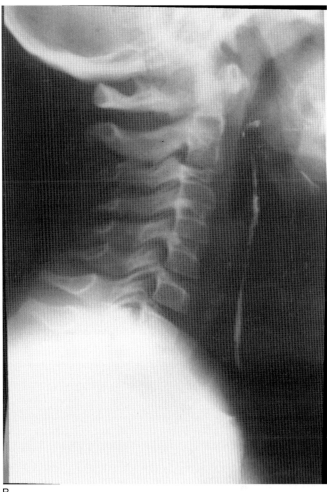

B

Figure 10.10.5 Second branchial cleft fistula. Anteroposterior (AP) (A) and lateral (B) view of a sinogram showing the position of the fistula, anterior to the sternocleidomastoid muscle.

child abuse. It occurs by insertion of a finger or sharp object into the mouth.

Iatrogenic perforation of the pharynx following endotracheal intubation and feeding tube manipulation is increasingly recognized, particularly in newborn preterm infants (Figure 10.10.8). The perforation often occurs in the pharynx and a feeding tube may extend through the mediastinum and on into the abdomen.

FURTHER READING

Alford BR, Chenault DI, Danziger J. Detection of foreign bodies with computerized tomography. Archives of Otolaryngology 1979; 105:203–204.

Schoem SR, Choi SS, Zalzal GH, Grundfast KM. Management of oropharyngeal trauma in children. Archives of Otolaryngology and Head and Neck Surgery 1997; 123:1267–1270.

INFLAMMATORY AND INFECTIOUS DISEASES

The commonest inflammatory and infectious diseases are pharyngitis, tonsillitis and cervical lymphadenitis but these usually do not require radiological investigation. However, the complications, such as retropharyngeal abscess, or unusual conditions, such as Crohn's disease, tularaemia and graft versus host disease often require radiological investigation.

Retropharyngeal space infection, now a relatively rare entity since the introduction of modern antibiotics, has traditionally been described to occur in children less than 4 years of age with suppurative disorders of the ear, nose and throat. The child with retropharyngeal cellulites and/or abscess appears ill and presents

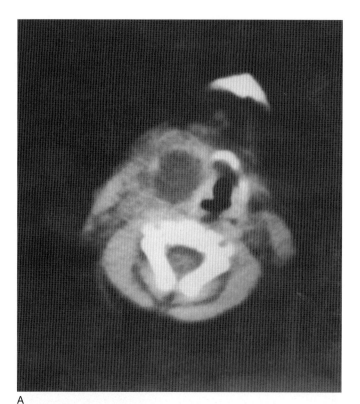

A

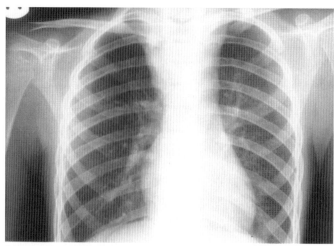

A

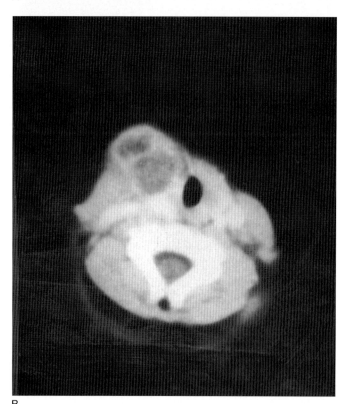

B

Figure 10.10.6 Branchial cyst. (A) Without contrast, (B) with contrast. Child aged 6 months with recent onset of left neck mass. The mass was transonic on ultrasound and thought to be a cystic hygroma. CT performed to show its extent and relationship to the great vessels. The mass has contrast enhancement of the borders due to infection. There is some compression of the trachea. The cyst lies anterior to the carotid artery and anterior to the sternocleidomastoid muscle.

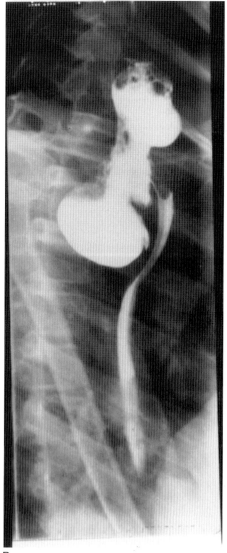

B

Figure 10.10.7 Foreign body perforation. (A) A widened mediastinum secondary to a mediastinal abscess from traumatic perforation of the pharynx. Three-month-old history of increasing dysphagia. (B) Contrast swallow (same child). A large pseudodiverticulum of the pharynx extends into the proximal thorax and displaces the oesophagus anteriorly. At surgery a plastic toy coin was found in the pseudodiverticulum/abscess cavity. The child required a colonic interposition.

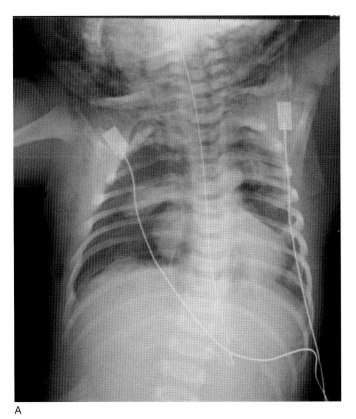

A

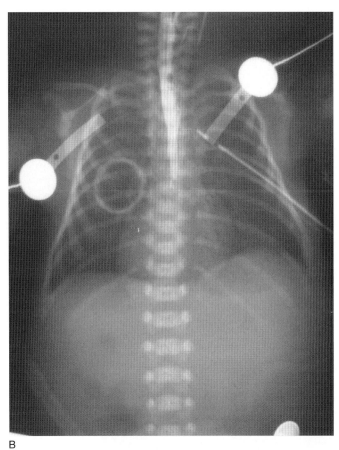

B

Figure 10.10.8 (A) Radiograph and (B) contrast study. Traumatic perforation of the pharynx by nasogastric tube. Note pneumomediastinum on x-ray and hold up of contrast in the mediastinum. This contrast was not in the oesophagus but was extraluminal and in the mediastinum.

with swallowing difficulty and drooling. Neck soft tissue radiographs are useful to exclude a foreign body or airway obstruction (Figure 10.10.9). On lateral radiographs, a soft tissue mass must be distinguished from apparent soft tissue mass due to tracheal buckling related to the expiratory phase of respiration and/or flexion of the neck. CT and MRI are useful in complicated cases (Figure 10.10.10).

FURTHER READING

Gianoli GJ, Espinola TE, Guarisco JL, Miller RH. Retropharyngeal space infection: changing trends. Otolaryngology and Head and Neck Surgery 1991; 105:92–100.

Vogl TJ, Mack MG, Balzer J, Diebold T. Inflammatory diseases of the pharynx. The imaging findings and diagnostic strategy. Radiologe 2000; 40:619–624.

DIVERTICULA

Traction and pulsion (Zenker's) diverticula in the pharynx are uncommon in children but are occasionally seen in older children.

They consist of a posterolateral outpouching through Killian's dehiscence, a site of potential weakness at the junction of the middle third and inferior third of the inferior constrictor, the inferior third also being known as the cricopharyngeus. Acquired diverticula may be secondary to trauma, particularly in neonates, caused by iatrogenic perforation during endotracheal intubation or passage of a nasogastric tube.

NEOPLASMS

The commonest neck mass in childhood is lymphadenopathy. The diagnosis is usually clinically obvious and ultrasound can be useful to demonstrate lymph node abscess formation. True pharyngeal neoplasms are rare in childhood. Ultrasound can be useful initially if there is a neck mass but CT and/or MRI (especially contrast-enhanced fat suppression MRI) are the investigations of choice.

Nasopharyngeal benign tumours are mesenchymal and include juvenile nasopharyngeal angiofibroma, haemangioma, lymphangioma and the rare teratoma.

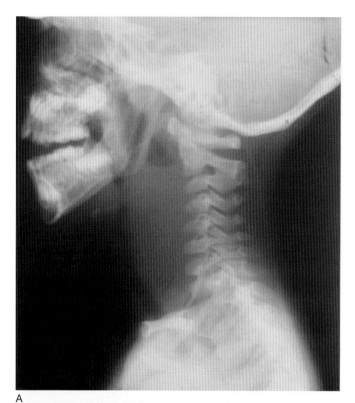

A

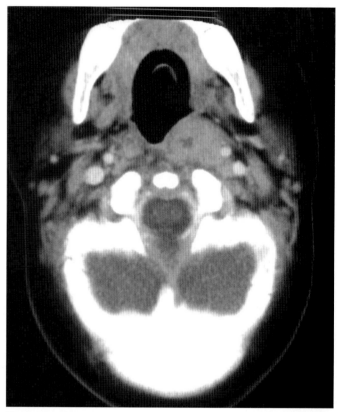

Figure 10.10.10 Contrast enhanced CT shows an enhancing mass in the retropharynx on the left with a poorly enhancing irregular centre. This was a *Staphylococcus aureus* retropharyngeal abscess with a pus centre. (Courtesy of Dr Doug Jamieson.)

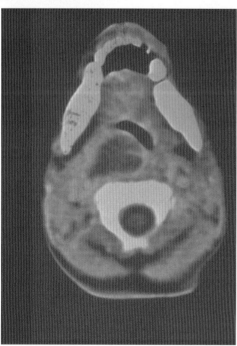

B

Figure 10.10.9 (A) Four-year-old boy with a retropharyngeal abscess. There is swelling with an air fluid level in the retropharyngeal soft tissues at the level of C2. (B) CT scan of a different child showing large retropharyngeal abscess.

Nasopharyngeal angiofibroma is a benign neoplasm, mainly of adolescent males, characterized by epistaxis and local aggressive growth (10.10.11). In advanced cases, the tumour may extend intracranially. The diagnosis by CT is based upon the site of origin

of the lesion in the pterygopalatine fossa and the posterior nasal cavity, erosion of the upper medial pterygoid plate, and intense enhancement after contrast. The characteristic features on MRI are due to the high vascularity of the tumour causing signal voids and strong postcontrast enhancement. MRI shows the preoperative soft tissue extent of angiofibroma optimally but its more important application is to show any residual or recurrent tumour postoperatively and to monitor the effects of radiotherapy.

Haemangioma and lymphangioma may present as an enlarging mass in the pharynx. Macrocystic and microcystic lymphangiomas occur; the former being commonly referred to as cystic hygroma. Larger lesions can be very extensive and extend to involve the floor of the mouth and tongue. Lymphangiomas frequently contain haemangiomatous elements and so their appearance on Doppler ultrasound, CT and MRI can be similar to that of haemangiomas with marked vascularity on Doppler ultrasound and vivid CT and MRI enhancement after intravenous contrast. The larger lymphangiomas demonstrate decreased signal relative to muscle on T1-weighted images. They are hyperintense on T2-weighted images and may show enhancement of walls and septations after gadolinium.

FURTHER READING

Lloyd G, Howard D, Lund VJ, Savy L. Imaging for juvenile angiofibroma. Journal of Laryngology and Otology 2000; 114:727–730.

Ussmuller J, Hartwein J. Intramuscular hemangioma of the posterior wall of the pharynx. Diagnosis and differential diagnosis. Laryngorhinootologie 1992; 71:568–571.

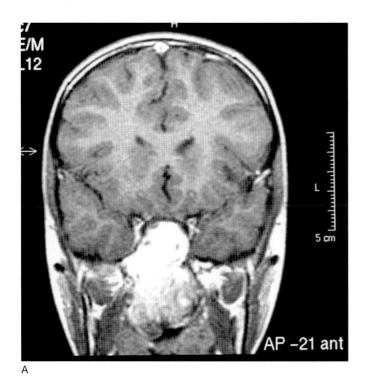

A

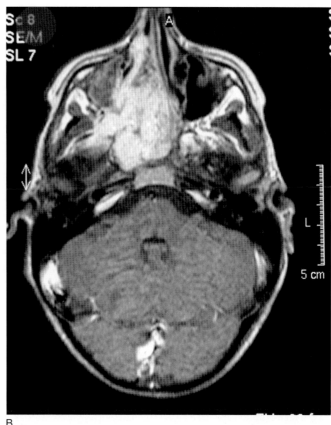

B

Figure 10.10.11 T2-weighted sequences. (A) Coronal and (B) axial showing large hyperintense pharyngeal mass typical of a nasopharyngeal angiofibroma.

MALIGNANT NEOPLASMS

Malignant neoplasms of the pharynx are rare in children; the least uncommon are rhabdomyosarcoma, nasopharyngeal carcinoma and lymphoma.

Rhabdomyosarcoma is the most common nasopharyngeal malignancy in childhood in Caucasians. The median age of presentation of rhabdomyosarcoma is 5–6 years and thus significantly younger than the age of presentation of a nasopharyngeal carcinoma. Lymph node metastases may occur with rhabdomyosarcoma but are usually unilateral and smaller by comparison with the typical conglomerate masses associated with nasopharyngeal carcinoma. Nasopharyngeal carcinoma is the most common epithelial carcinoma in children. It is more common in Chinese but is uncommon in Caucasians. Both rhabdomyosarcomas and nasopharyngeal carcinomas cause local bony erosion. CT and MRI are both required for staging and complete evaluation. Follow-up imaging should be according to the tumour protocols. The prognosis for nasopharyngeal carcinoma is better than rhabdomyosarcoma.

Pharyngeal lymphoma usually affects Waldeyer's ring, with involvement of tonsil and nasopharynx, and is usually non-Hodgkin's lymphoma. These tumours are frequently associated with disseminated lymphoma, extranodal disease, particularly involving the gastrointestinal tract, and have a variable prognosis.

Ultrasound can be useful initially if there is a neck mass but CT (Figure 10.10.12) and/or MRI (especially contrast-enhanced fat suppression MRI) are the investigations of choice for the initial assessment. Care should be taken to evaluate any tumour extension locally into adjacent spaces, bones and skull. Gallium is useful for follow-up and assessing the presence of other disease.

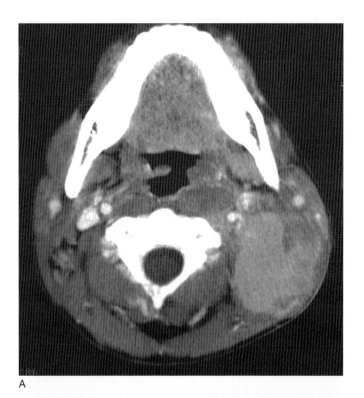

A

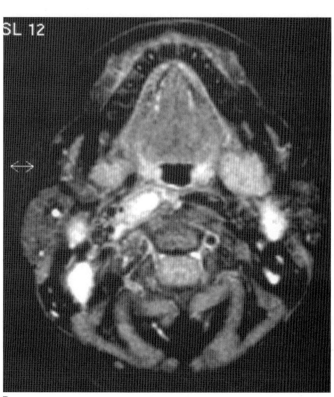

B

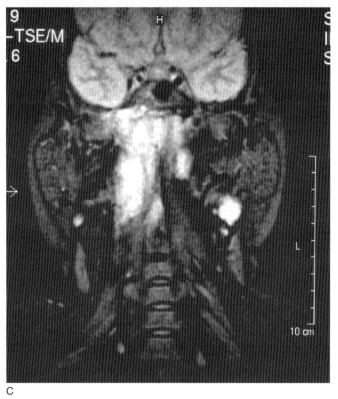

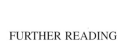

C

Figure 10.10.12 (A) Contrast enhanced CT shows a poorly enhancing mass in the left nasopharynx with adjacent enhancing lymph nodes. (Courtesy of Dr Doug Jamieson.) (B) Axial and (C) coronal T2-weighted MRI scans demonstrating high signal in the retropharynx on the right, which on biopsy proved to be nasopharyngeal carcinoma.

FURTHER READING

Barakos JA, Dillon WP, Chew WM. Orbit, skull base, and pharynx: contrast-enhanced fat suppression MR imaging. Radiology 1991; 179:191–198.

Cheung YK, Sham JS, Chan FL, Leong LL, Choy D. Computed tomography of paranasopharyngeal spaces: normal variations and criteria for tumour extension. Clinical Radiology 1992; 45:109–113.

Saul SH, Kapadia SB. Primary lymphoma of Waldeyer's ring. Clinicopathologic study of 68 cases. Cancer 1985; 56:157–166.

The Oesophagus

Theresa E Geley, Ingmar Gaßner

INTRODUCTION

The oesophagus is a muscular tube composed of outer longitudinal and inner circular muscle fibres and lined by stratified squamous epithelium. The upper oesophageal sphincter (UOS) and lower oesophageal sphincter (LOS) control the function of its upper and lower end, respectively. The cricopharyngeus muscle composes the UOS, which is the horizontal portion of the inferior pharyngeal constrictor (Figure 10.11.1). The LOS is not a distinct muscular entity but is defined as a high-pressure zone in the oesophagogastric region. At rest, the oesophageal body is normally collapsed with both sphincters closed to prevent retrograde flow of oesophageal and gastric content. With swallowing, the UOS relaxes followed by relaxation of the LOS shortly thereafter and the primary peristaltic contraction propagates down the oesophagus traversing its length to push the bolus distally from the mouth.

The oesophagus in infants and children is similar to the adult oesophagus but there are a few important radiological differences. The normal extrinsic imprints of aorta, left main stem bronchus and the posterior border of left atrium are usually less prominent in infants than in adults; not only extrinsic structures such as the heart but also expiration may cause displacement of the entire distal oesophageal segment. Pharyngoesophageal contractions (i.e. the radiological equivalent of the pharyngoesophageal sphincter or cricopharyngens) in children are transient findings and not responsible for dysphagia (Fig. 10.11.1).

Air is frequently present in the oesophagus on chest radiographs, especially in neonates. Persistent or unusually marked filling and dilatation of the oesophagus is abnormal and may indicate tracheoesophageal fistula or gastroesophageal reflux. Dyspnoeic infants often have considerable air in the oesophagus related to the negative intrapleural pressure in respiratory distress.

The oesophageal calibre is very variable. The entire oesophagus is often filled on rapid swallowing of liquids and all or parts of the oesophagus may transitorily dilate to an extent that would be seen as abnormal in an adult. Rapid repeated swallows in infants and children will inhibit a propagating primary peristaltic wave and may be mistaken for peristaltic disruption. In such oesophagrams, secondary peristalsis, initiated by local oesophageal stimulation or distension, may be noted beginning near the diaphragm and cause both provisional and retrograde flow of contrast.

FURTHER READING

Giedion A, Nolte K. The non obstructive pharyngo-esophageal cross roll. Annals of Radiology 1973; 16:129–135.

INFLAMMATION

INFECTIVE OESOPHAGITIS

Infectious diseases involving the oesophagus are less frequent in infants and children than peptic oesophagitis associated with gastroesophageal reflux. Infectious agents such as tuberculosis, histoplasmosis, meningococcosis or syphilis have been reported as causes of oesophagitis in children but their occurrence is rare.

The most common causes of infectious oesophagitis that are likely to be encountered clinically are *Candida albicans* followed by herpes simplex and cytomegalovirus. Clinically, significant oesophagitis usually occurs when underlying malignancy, debilitating illness, diabetes, or treatment with radiation, steroids or other cytotoxic agents impairs the host's immune system. Association of candida with local oesophageal stasis due to achalasia or strictures or impaired oesophageal peristalsis has been recognized as well as the development of candida and herpes oesophagitis in otherwise healthy individuals. Cytomegalovirus has been found almost exclusively in patients suffering from acquired immune deficiency syndrome (AIDS) and shows similar radiological and clinical features to herpes infection. Concomitant candida and herpes oesophagitis has been documented, which may be the cause of persistent oesophagitis despite adequate therapy and most likely results from superinfection of herpetic ulcers.

Patients with oesophagitis typically present with acute odynophagia, characterized by severe substernal chest pain during swallowing or dysphagia and less commonly upper gastrointestinal bleeding. The presence of oropharyngeal candidiasis or herpetic lesions should suggest the possibility of oesophageal involvement. Usually this can be cured with appropriate therapy but rarely complicating strictures develop and balloon dilatation may be needed. The use of anti-inflammatory agents is reported to avoid this complication of stricture formation.

A double contrast oesophagogram may demonstrate the wall of the oesophagus to be thick and the mucosa to be irregular with

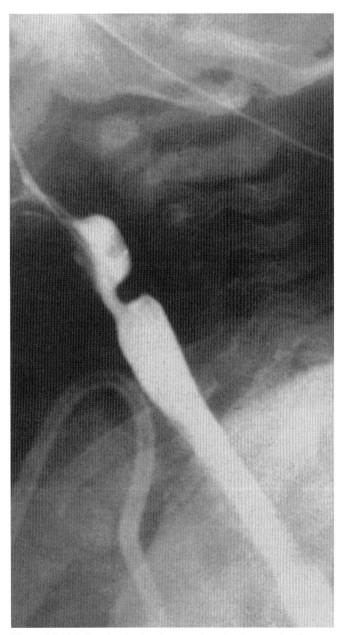

Figure 10.11.1 Prominent cricopharyngeal contraction causing the posterior indentation of the oesophagus ('pharyngoesophageal cross roll').

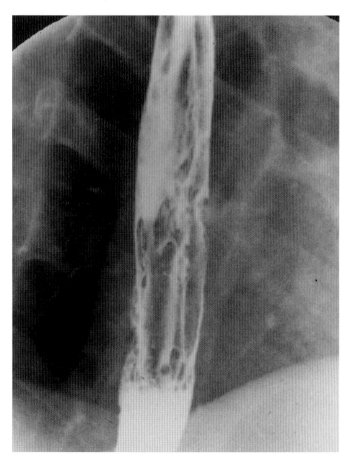

Figure 10.11.2 Early and later monilial oesophagitis. As the infection develops, the raised nodules representing monilial plaques become more defined.

discrete mucosal plaques or nodules. This appearance is initially likely to be due to oedema but later in the course of infection plaques of fungi will produce similar appearances. All these findings may be seen with candidiasis as well as herpes (Figure 10.11.2 and 10.11.3). Discrete ulcers on otherwise normal mucosa are very suggestive of herpes oesophagitis. Many children with oesophagitis unfortunately will not tolerate double-contrast studies as it requires cooperation. Children under 5 years of age frequently have serious difficulties in swallowing the effervescent agents, especially when given with barium. Other imaging techniques such as endoscopy during which biopsies are performed should be considered even though these require general anaesthetic.

On single-contrast studies a common but non-specific finding of oesophagitis is dysmotility. Extreme spasm can lead to so-called pseudodiverticula. Other changes consist of extensive mucosal oedema with either linear or cobblestone appearance or diffuse ulceration. The adhesion of barium to the oesophageal mucosa for several hours points towards a diagnosis of oesophagitis.

The characteristic endoscopic appearance of candida oesophagitis consists of patchy white plaques covering a frail, erythematous mucosa. In more advanced disease, ulceration and necrosis may be seen. Early herpes oesophagitis has a characteristic appearance of blisters or vesicles that subsequently rupture to form discrete, punched-out ulcers on the mucosa. With advanced herpes oesophagitis the ulcers may become covered by fibrinous exudate or pseudomembranes and may be indistinguishable from candidiasis. Endoscopic mucosal biopsies and brushing are usually necessary to determine the aetiology and direct appropriate therapy. A differential diagnosis should include reflux oesophagitis, intramural diverticulosis, non-infective oesophagitis and technical artifact such as undissolved effervescent agent air bubbles and debris. Rarely, the radiological appearance mimics varices but the clinical history should clarify the situation.

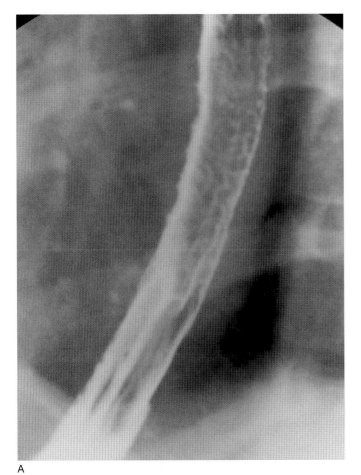

A

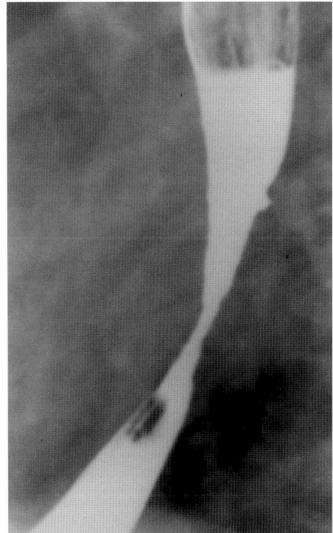

B

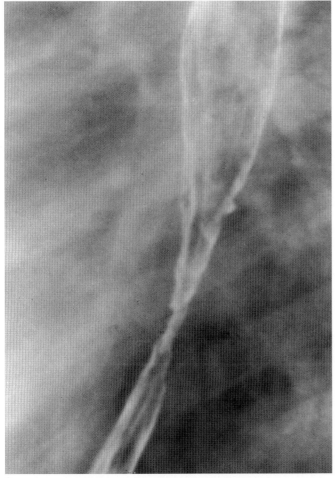

C

Figure 10.11.3 *Candida albicans* and herpes virus oesophagitis.
(A) Double-contrast oesophagogram shows the mucosa to be irregular,
ulcerated and nodular due to combined fungal and viral infections in an
immunosuppressed child with leukaemia. Stricture rapidly developed as
seen on subsequent single-contrast (B) and double-contrast
(C) examinations. From Stringer DA, Babyn PS. Paediatric
Gastrointestinal Imaging and Intervention 2e. Hamilton: BC Decker Inc.
© 2000.

FURTHER READING

Chowhan NM. Injurious effects of radiation on the esophagus. American Journal of Gastroenterology 1990; 85:115–120.
Gefter WB, Laufer I, Edell S et al. Candidiasis in the obstructed esophagus. Radiology 1981; 138:25–28.
Isaac DW, Parham DM, Patrick CC. The role of esophagoscopy in diagnosis and management of esophagitis in children with cancer. Medical and Pediatric Oncology 1997; 28:299–303.
Levine MS, Macones AJ Jr, Laufer I. Candida esophagitis: accuracy of radiographic diagnosis. Radiology 1985; 154:581–587.

NON-INFECTIVE OESOPHAGITIS

EPIDERMOLYSIS BULLOSA

Epidermolysis bullosa is a rare hereditary skin disease in which minimal trauma causes separation of the epidermis and dermis with subsequent bullae formation. Two main forms of the disease, the dystrophic and the simplex forms, have been described.

The dystrophic form includes several variants, with either autosomal dominant or autosomal recessive traits. The dominant varieties are characterized by the formation of bullae on friction sites in later infancy or early childhood, which heal with scarring. These scars tend to become keloidal or hyperplastic. Mucous membranes are not affected and hair and teeth develop normally. In the potentially lethal, autosomal recessive variants, large bullae or raw denuded areas are present at birth and the resulting scars are distinct and mutilating. Mucous membranes are severely involved and hair, nails and teeth are commonly abnormal.

Epidermolysis bullosa simplex also includes several variants with the majority being inherited by autosomal dominant transmission. Blisters may be present at birth but often become more apparent on sites of friction when the child becomes mobile. They quickly rupture and heal with no subsequent scarring. The mucous membranes may occasionally be involved but do not show gross changes. The disease usually subsides at puberty.

Depending on the genetic type, blisters in oesophageal involvement may either heal without permanent damage or ulcerate and progress to strictures or, rarely, to webs. On barium studies, the upper half of the oesophagus often shows a smooth short stricture, possibly because of oesophageal compression by the aortic arch, which exacerbates the traumatic effect of swallowed food at this level. These strictures may be present even when the skin is relatively clear and may remain unchanged in size for many years despite variations in dysphagic symptoms. The radiological appearance is similar to other causes of oesophagitis and the following may be seen: diffuse inflammatory changes, motility disorders, small blisters or bullae seen as constant nodular-filling defects, oesophageal ulcers, scars, pseudodiverticula, transverse and circumferential webs, shortening of the oesophagus with development of traction hiatal hernia and gastroesophageal reflux, perforation, and complete obstruction of the oesophageal lumen (Figure 10.11.4).

FURTHER READING

Agha FP, Francis IR, Ellis CN. Esophageal involvement in epidermolysis bullosa dystrophica: clinical and roentgenographic manifestations. Gastrointestinal Radiology 1983; 8:111–117.
Ergun GA, Lin AN, Dannenberg AJ et al. Gastrointestinal manifestations of epidermolysis bullosa. A study of 101 patients. Medicine (Baltimore) 1992; 71:121–127.
Kabakian HA, Dahmash NS. Pharyngoesophageal manifestations of epidermolysis bullosa. Clinical Radiology 1978; 29:91–94.

PEMPHIGUS

Pemphigus is characterized by the development of autoantibodies against epidermal structures leading to superficial erosions and blisters on both epidermis and mucosa. It is rare in children but should be kept in mind whenever severe oral ulcers not due to candida or herpes persist. Barium studies may reveal oedema, spasm or superficial ulceration in the early stages of oesophageal involvement, while subsequent scarring may present itself by the development of webs or strictures.

FURTHER READING

Agha FP, Raji MR. Esophageal involvement in pemphigoid: clinical and roentgen manifestations. Gastrointestinal Radiology 1982; 7:109–112.
Al-Kutoubi MA, Eliot C. Oesophageal involvement in benign mucous membrane pemphigoid. Clinical Radiology 1984; 35:131–135.
Schissel DJ, David-Bajar K. Esophagitis dissecans superficialis associated with pemphigus vulgaris. Cutis 1999; 63:157–160.

EOSINOPHILIC OESOPHAGITIS

Eosinophilic gastroenteritis is an uncommon condition of unknown aetiology characterized by peripheral eosinophilia and eosinophilic infiltration of the gastrointestinal tract. The vast majority of cases show mucosal involvement of the gastric antrum and small intestine. Rarely, associated eosinophilic oesophagitis has been described. Recently, an isolated form of eosinophilic oesophagitis has been reported that occurs in adults and children.

At presentation, symptoms are similar to those of gastroesophageal reflux and encompass vomiting, pain and dysphagia. Dysphagia, due to upper oesophageal narrowing, may be intermittent or progressive. Allergy, particularly food allergy, is an associated finding in most patients and acute episodes of dysphagia are often precipitated by specific food allergens.

Findings on barium examination vary from normal to irregular mucosa and one or more segmental strictures in the upper thoracic oesophagus near the aortic arch (Figure 10.11.5). Nodularity or ulceration may be found within the narrowed segment. Rarely, polypoid lesions may be found analogous to those found in the stomach or duodenum.

Endoscopy may reveal a subtle granularity with furrows or rings. Differentiation from gastroesophageal reflux disease is approached by analyzing peripheral eosinophil density and response to therapeutic trials.

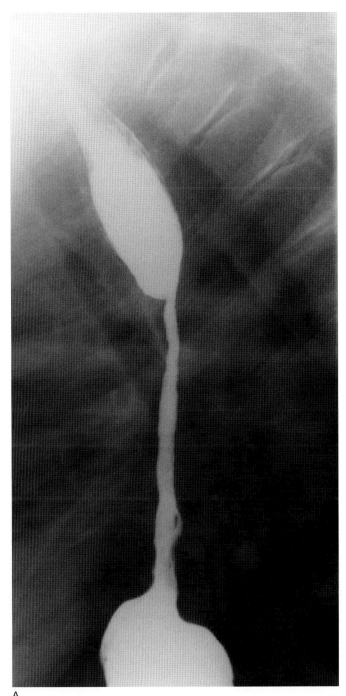

A

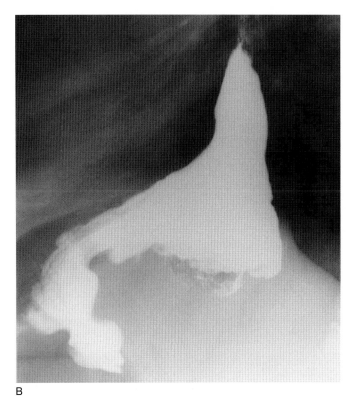

B

Figure 10.11.4 Epidermolysis bullosa dystrophica. (A) Long stricture beginning in the upper thoracic oesophagus. (B) Tractional hiatal hernia due to concomitant shortening of the oesophagus.

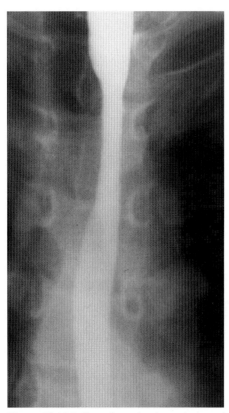

Figure 10.11.5 Oesophageal stricture from eosinophilic gastroenteritis. A long stricture with a tapered upper end is present in the mid-oesophagus.

FURTHER READING

Feczko PJ, Halpert RD, Zonca M. Radiographic abnormalities in eosinophilic esophagitis. Gastrointestinal Radiology 1985; 10:321–324.
Orenstein SR, Shalaby TM, Di Lorenzo C et al. The spectrum of pediatric eosinophilic esophagitis beyond infancy: a clinical series of 30 children. American Journal of Gastroenterology 2000; 95:1422–1430.

PEPTIC OESOPHAGITIS

Peptic oesophagitis, the result of gastroesophageal reflux, is in its early stage best assessed by endoscopy. Endoscopy will document irregularity of the mucosa and fine ulcerations. By the time radiological signs, such as very irregular ragged mucosal appearance and thickening of the oesophageal wall and strictures are present, the disease is fairly advanced. As can be expected, most of the changes occur in the distal third or half of the oesophagus. Unless associated with a large hiatus hernia and encountered in the neonatal period or early infancy the overall problem of advanced oesophagitis and stricture formation is not very common.

FURTHER READING

Robertson D, Aldersley M, Shepherd H et al. Patterns of acid reflux in complicated oesophagitis. Gut 1987; 28:1484–1488.
Rode H, Millar AJ, Brown RA et al. Reflux strictures of the esophagus in children. Journal of Pediatric Surgery 1992; 27:462–465.

CROHN'S DISEASE

Crohn's disease rarely affects the oesophagus in children. The radiological appearance is similar to that in adults with patchy mucosal ulceration and stricture formation. Although Crohn's disease affects primarily the small bowel and colon, the earliest morphological lesions of Crohn's disease, aphthous ulcers, may be detected in the oesophagus by means of double-contrast oesophagography. These aphthous ulcers appear radiologically as punctate, slit-like or ring-like collections of barium surrounded by radiolucent halos of oedematous mucosa. Aphthous ulcers may occur as isolated lesions in the oesophagus or may be associated with other, more advanced changes of Crohn's disease such as localized or diffuse oesophagitis or areas of deep ulceration.

With more advanced disease, severe oesophagitis, manifested by thickened folds and pseudomembranes, transverse or longitudinal intramural tracks similar to those found with granulomatous colitis, and oesophageal perforation may be seen. Progressive scarring may eventually lead to the development of strictures. Gastrointestinal radiographic studies are reported to frequently fail in the detection of upper gastrointestinal lesions and endoscopy should, therefore, be considered in all children and adolescents with Crohn's disease. Superficial ulceration seen during endoscopy and the histological finding of focal inflammation are representative for upper gastrointestinal Crohn's disease in paediatric patients. It is important to take biopsies from normal-appearing mucosa since histological changes might otherwise be missed.

FURTHER READING

Decker GA, Loftus EV Jr, Pasha TM et al. Crohn's disease of the esophagus: clinical features and outcomes. Inflammatory Bowel Disease 2001; 7:113–119.
Lenaerts C, Roy CC, Vaillancourt M et al. High incidence of upper gastrointestinal tract involvement in children with Crohn disease. Pediatrics 1989; 83:777–781.
Schmidt-Sommerfeld E, Kirschner BS, Stephens JK. Endoscopic and histologic findings in the upper gastrointestinal tract of children with Crohn's disease. Journal of Pediatric Gastroenterology and Nutrition 1990; 11:448–454.

BEHÇETS DISEASE

This multisystem disorder is of unknown aetiology and is characterized by recurrent oral and genital ulcers, ocular inflammation, arthritis, thrombophlebitis, neurological abnormalities, skin lesions, fever and colitis. The condition is rare in children. Pathologically, there is vasculitis of small and medium-sized arteries with cellular infiltrations leading to necrosis and obliteration of the vessel lumen. Involvement of the oesophagus has occasionally been reported as severe oesophagitis, which can progress to stricture formation. Discrete superficial ulcers in the mid and distal oesophagus may be seen on double-contrast oesophagography but have to be differentiated from herpes oesophagitis since Behçet's disease is often treated with immunosuppressive agents. Involvement of the ileum and colon closely resembles Crohn's disease.

FURTHER READING

Lebwohl O, Forde KA, Berdon WE et al. Ulcerative esophagitis and colitis in a pediatric patient with Behçet's syndrome. Response to steroid therapy. American Journal of Gastroenterology 1977; 68:550–555.

INTRAMURAL OESOPHAGEAL PSEUDODIVERTICULOSIS

This disease is extremely rare in children and primarily involves the upper oesophagus. The aetiology is not fully understood. A high percentage of patients have associated strictures suggesting a pressure-related transport of intraluminal material into the adnexal glands leading to metaplasia and gland dilatation. Others have postulated that ductal dilatation results from plugging and obstruction of the ducts or, alternatively, from extrinsic compression of the ducts due to chronic oesophagitis or corrosive injury. In addition, infection may be involved in the development since candida is frequently present.

The oesophagogram demonstrates multiple, flask-shaped outpouchings in longitudinal rows parallel to the long axis of the oesophagus. These pseudodiverticula extend 2–3mm from the oesophagus lumen. In half of cases, bridging may occur between adjacent pseudodiverticula, which produce discrete intramural tracks. These tracks might be mistaken for large flat ulcers in the oesophagus. Massive ductal dilatation or sealed-off perforation of the ducts may result in irregular extraluminal collection of barium. Such a ductal perforation may lead to the development of a perioesophageal inflammation or abscess, which is described as oesophageal peridiverticulitis. Ninety per cent of patients have associated strictures, most frequently in the upper third of the oesophagus. In such cases, the pseudodiverticula extend above and below the level of the stricture. Oesophageal pseudodiverticulosis as a localized phenomenon in the distal oesophagus is often associated with gastroesophageal reflux and hiatus hernia. The disorder may occasionally be recognized on computed tomography (CT) by thickening of the oesophageal wall with intramural gas collection and irregularity of the lumen.

FURTHER READING

Boyd RM, Bogoch A, Greig JH et al. Esophageal intramural pseudodiverticulosis. Radiology 1974; 113:267–270.

Bruhlmann WF, Zollikofer CL, Maranta E et al. Intramural pseudodiverticulosis of the esophagus: report of seven cases and literature review. Gastrointestinal Radiology 1981; 6:199–208.

Canon CL, Levine MS, Cherukuri R et al. Intramural tracking: a feature of esophageal intramural pseudodiverticulosis. American Journal of Roentgenology 2000; 175:371–374.

Lupovitch A, Tippins R. Esophageal intramural pseudodiverticulosis: a disease of adnexal glands. Radiology 1974; 113:271–272.

Markle BM, Hanson K. Esophageal pseudodiverticulosis: two new cases in children. Pediatric Radiology 1992; 22:194–195.

MOTILITY DISORDERS

Oesophageal motility disorders are usually classified as primary or secondary types. In primary motility disorders, the oesophagus is the primary or only organ involved. Secondary oesophageal motility disorders result from a variety of systemic diseases or from physical or chemical injury.

PRIMARY OESOPHAGEAL MOTILITY DISORDERS

ACHALASIA

Achalasia, the best known of the primary oesophageal motility disorders, is characterized by the failure of normal relaxation of the lower oesophageal sphincter (LOS) associated with uncoordinated contractions of the thoracic oesophagus. It is a condition that primarily affects adolescents and adults and familial cases have been reported. Children under the age of 4 years comprise less than 5% of patients. Previous congenital oesophageal stenosis may occur with tracheoesophageal fistula and may be associated to cartilaginous rings or remnants. Such rings and remnants here should be kept in mind in cases of early presenting achalasia (Figures 10.11.6 and 10.11.7).

The aetiology of achalasia is unknown but in some cases a decrease in ganglion cell number in the distal oesophagus has been noted. Thus, achalasia appears to be a neurogenic disorder. The heightened response of oesophageal muscles to cholinergic stimulation supports evidence of denervation hypersensitivity.

Symptoms, which are insidiously progressive, include difficulty in swallowing, chronic regurgitation of undigested food, aspiration pneumonia and failure to thrive. Secondary stasis oesophagitis is common and may be associated with ulceration. Achalasia may also be a precursor of oesophageal carcinoma.

Achalasia is characterized manometrically by the absence of primary peristalsis, elevated or normal resting LOS pressures, and incomplete or absent LOS relaxation.

In the early stages, x-ray findings are scant. The dilatation of the oesophagus is only mild and, therefore, not seen on plain chest radiographs. In more advanced cases, oesophageal dilatation may become massive and an air–fluid level is frequently seen in the upright chest x-ray. The stomach gas bubble is frequently absent. The food- or fluid-filled oesophagus might suggest a mediastinal mass. Barium studies show absence of primary peristalsis and a widened, food-filled oesophagus with sigmoid appearance. Typically, the lower end of the oesophagus has a smooth, tapered, beak-like deformity, which reflects the persistently narrowed gastroesophageal junction. The absence of propulsive peristaltic waves or bizarre contractions of the oesophagus above the beak helps to distinguish achalasia from peptic oesophagitis. Persistent aspiration may result in pneumonia and bronchiectasis. In advanced cases, oesophagitis may be noticed.

At endoscopy, the oesophagus will be dilated with generally reduced or absent peristalsis. A secondary form of achalasia associated with carcinoma of the gastroesophageal junction has been reported. Biopsy specimens may, therefore, be obtained during endoscopy to distinguish between primary achalasia and secondary forms due to carcinoma.

Recently, ultrasound has become more frequently used in the study of patients with achalasia, because it can demonstrate the characteristic dilatation of the distal oesophagus in association with a normal wall thickness (Figure 10.11.8). Marked thickening

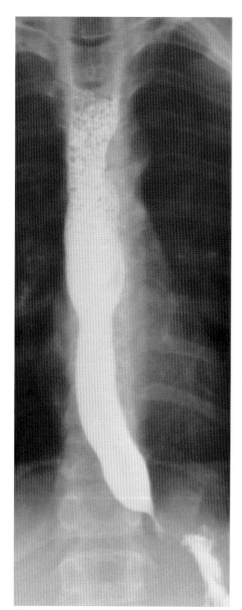

A

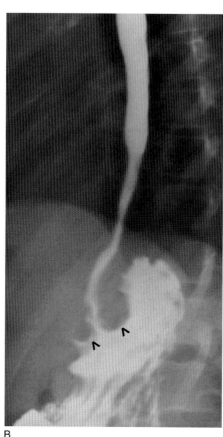

B

Figure 10.11.6 Achalasia. There is a moderately dilated oesophagus with retained secretions and smooth, tapered beak-like appearance at the level of the oesophageal hiatus. Repetitive non-peristaltic contractions were seen at fluoroscopy. (B) After Heller myotomy and fundoplication the gastric wrap produces narrowing of the distal oesophagus and a fundal mass with a smooth contour (v).

of the distal oesophageal wall is found in leiomyomatosis or malignant tumours.

Treatment consists of balloon dilatation of the distal sphincter, which may result in a significant improvement in symptoms for many years. Endoscopic ultrasonographically guided botulin toxin injections into the lower oesophageal sphincter may be beneficial but are not superior to balloon dilatation. Because there is always a risk of oesophageal perforation, mucosal tears or relapse after balloon dilatation, some specialists prefer primary surgical treatment using the method of laparoscopic Heller myotomy (see Figure 10.11.16).

FURTHER READING

Aichbichler BW, Eherer AJ, Petritsch W et al. Gastric adenocarcinoma mimicking achalasia in a 15-year-old patient: a case report and review of the literature. Journal of Pediatric Gastroenterology and Nutrition 2001; 32:103–106.

Bergami GL, Fruhwirth R, Di Mario M et al. Contribution of ultrasonography in the diagnosis of achalasia. Journal of Pediatric Gastroenterology and Nutrition 1992; 14:92–96.

Blam ME, Delfyett W, Levine MS et al. Achalasia: a disease of varied and subtle symptoms that do not correlate with radiographic findings. American Journal of Gastroenterology 2002; 97:1916–1923.

Hurwitz M, Bahar RJ, Ament ME et al. Evaluation of the use of botulinum toxin in children with achalasia. Journal of Pediatric Gastroenterology and Nutrition 2000; 30:509–514.

Ip KS, Cameron DJ, Catto-Smith AG et al. Botulinum toxin for achalasia in children. Journal of Gastroenterology and Hepatology 2000; 15:1100–1104.

Mehra M, Bahar RJ, Ament ME et al. Laparoscopic and thoracoscopic esophagomyotomy for children with achalasia. Journal of Pediatric Gastroenterology and Nutrition 2001; 33:466–471.

Muehldorfer SM, Schneider TH, Hochberger J et al. Esophageal achalasia: intrasphincteric injection of botulinum toxin A versus balloon dilation. Endoscopy 1999; 31:517–521.

Pineiro-Carrero VM, Sullivan CA, Rogers PL. Etiology and treatment of achalasia in the pediatric age group. Gastrointestinal Endoscopy Clinics of North America 2001; 11:387–408, viii.

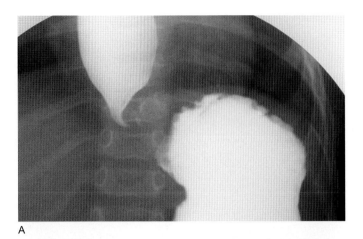

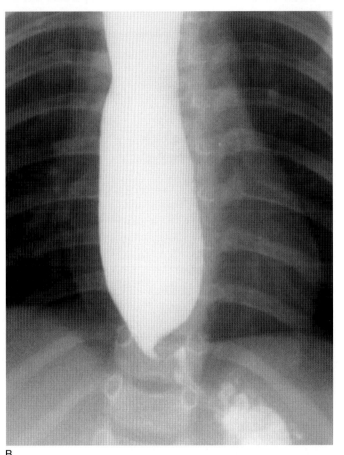

Figure 10.11.7 Seven-month-old female with congenital oesophageal stenosis (tracheobronchial remnants) in the distal oesophagus. (A) The dilated oesophagus with distal beak-like deformity mimics that of achalasia. (B) The kink at the level of cardia and the young age point towards a congenital anomaly.

SECONDARY OESOPHAGEAL MOTILITY DISORDERS

COLLAGEN VASCULAR DISEASE

The collagen vascular diseases are a group of acquired multisystem disorders of unknown origin with a pathoimmunological basis and inflammatory changes in connective tissue. The most frequently encountered collagen diseases involving the oesophagus in children are scleroderma and dermatomyositis.

SCLERODERMA

Generalized scleroderma is a systemic disease characterized by fibrosis and degenerative changes in the skin, synovium and parenchyma of multiple organs. In about one-third of affected children the oesophagus, in particular the lower third, will be involved resulting in pain and dysphagia. Loss of normal motility and coordination are early signs of oesophageal involvement but are not unique to this disease. In more advanced stages, complete atony and dilatation of the oesophagus may develop and sacculation may be seen. Reflux oesophagitis, strictures and Barrett's oesophagus are complications due to the malfunctioning of the gastroesophageal junction. Gastrointestinal involvement in children with scleroderma is more frequent than clinical symptoms may suggest. Modalities for assessing oesophageal dysfunction are oesophageal manometry, cine-oesophagography and oesophageal transit scintigraphy. These three diagnostic modalities are approximately equal in their ability to demonstrate the severity of oesophageal involvement. High-resolution ultrasound is also reported to be useful in evaluation of cervical oesophageal motility.

FURTHER READING

Klein HA, Wald A, Graham TO et al. Comparative studies of esophageal function in systemic sclerosis. Gastroenterology 1992; 102:1551–1556.

Takebayashi S, Matsui K, Ozawa Y et al. Cervical esophageal motility: evaluation with US in progressive systemic sclerosis. Radiology 1991; 179:389–393.

Weber P, Ganser G, Frosch M et al. Twenty-four hour intraesophageal pH monitoring in children and adolescents with scleroderma and mixed connective tissue disease. Journal of Rheumatology 2000; 27:2692–2695.

DERMATOMYOSITIS

Dermatomyositis is characterized by degeneration of muscle fibres with a chronic inflammatory reaction and a distinct skin rash. Muscle weakness is variable and commonly affects the proximal muscle groups of all four limbs. Involvement of the pharynx and upper oesophagus leads to poor clearing of contrast from the pharynx, diminished peristalsis in the upper oesophagus and nasal regurgitation at barium examination. Recently, Laskin et al. described a case of dermatomyositis associated with a dilated, atonic oesophagus, delayed gastric emptying and intestinal mucosal thickening. Dermatomyositis in childhood tends to 'burn out' but may leave severe restriction of limb movement due to

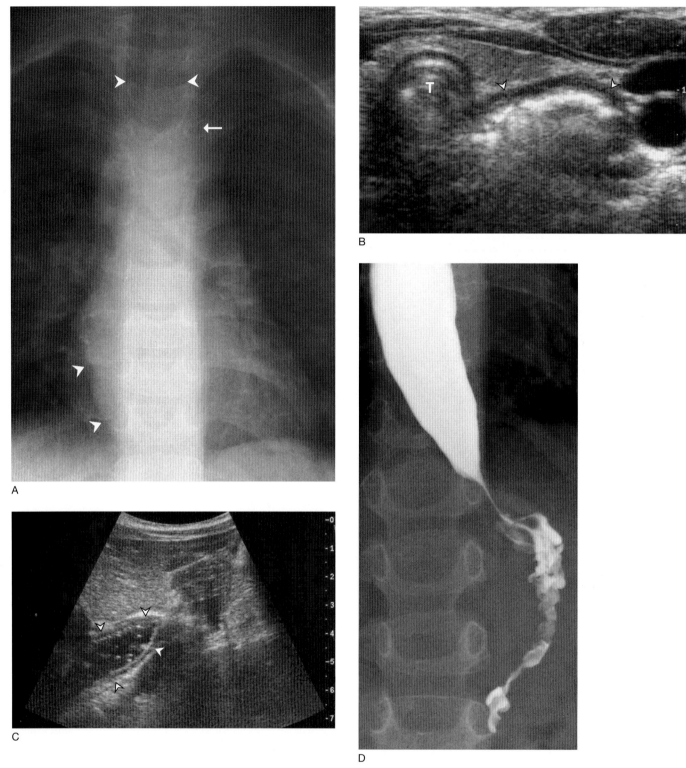

Figure 10.11.8 Five-year-old boy with triple A (achalasia–ACTH insensitivity–alacrima) syndrome. (A) Chest x-ray: parenchymal changes due to recurrent aspiration. The oesophagus (arrowheads) is dilated with a gas–fluid level (arrow). The stomach gas bubble is absent. (B,C) Ultrasonography: transverse scan at cervical level (B) and longitudinal scan at the level of the gastroesophageal junction (C) show a thick-walled, markedly dilated oesophagus (arrowheads); trachea (T). (D) Oesophagram: dilated, aperistaltic oesophagus with tapered, beak-like lower end. The stomach is contracted without gas bubble.

calcification in and around muscles. Complications such as ulcerations or spontaneous perforation of the oesophagus are reported.

FURTHER READING

Horowitz M, McNeil JD, Maddern GJ et al. Abnormalities of gastric and esophageal emptying in polymyositis and dermatomyositis. Gastroenterology 1986; 90:434–439.
Laskin BL, Choyke P, Keenan GF et al. Novel gastrointestinal tract manifestations in juvenile dermatomyositis. Journal of Pediatrics 1999; 135:371–374.
Pachman LM. An update on juvenile dermatomyositis. Current Opinion in Rheumatology 1995; 7:437–441.
Thompson JW. Spontaneous perforation of the esophagus as a manifestation of dermatomyositis. Annals of Otology, Rhinology and Laryngology 1984; 93:464–467.

CHAGAS' DISEASE

The only form of achalasia with known aetiology is Chagas' disease caused by American trypanosomiasis, a zoonosis transmitted by bloodsucking insects. It is a major health problem of South America but is extremely uncommon outside endemic areas. In Chagas' disease, the organism *Trypanosoma cruzi* causes inflammation of the mucosa and submucosa and destroys the nerve cells of the myenteric plexus. Manometrical and radiological features are identical to those in primary achalasia.

FURTHER READING

Dantas RO, Aprile LR, Aben-Athar CG et al. Esophageal striated muscle contractions in patients with Chagas' disease and idiopathic achalasia. Brazilian Journal of Medical and Biological Research 2002; 35:677–683.

FAMILIAL DISORDERS

STEINERT'S MYOTONIC DYSTROPHY

Steinert's myotonic dystrophy is an autosomal dominant hereditary condition, which usually appears with clinical symptoms of muscle weakness and atrophy in adult life. In the child, psychomotor retardation may occur and the pharyngo-oesophageal motility may be severely deranged in both amplitude and coordination. As in other inherited myopathies, barium studies demonstrate distension and hypotonicity of the oesophagus and impaired propulsive peristalsis. Transit studies may quantify oesophageal involvement.

FURTHER READING

Ham HR, Piepsz A, Georges B et al. Evaluation of esophageal transit in children and in infants by means of Krypton-81m. Pediatric Radiology 1985; 15:161–164.
Lecointe-Besancon I, Leroy F, Devroede G et al. A comparative study of esophageal and anorectal motility in myotonic dystrophy. Digestive Disease Science 1999; 44:1090–1099.
Modolell I, Mearin F, Baudet JS et al. Pharyngo-esophageal motility disturbances in patients with myotonic dystrophy. Scandinavian Journal of Gastroenterology 1999; 34:878–882.
Turpin JC, Morice J. Myotonic dystrophy severity (Steinert's disease) [author's translation]. La Semaine de Hopitaux 1980; 56:335–340.

GRANULOMATOUS DISEASE

Granulomatous disease is an inherited condition of abnormal phagocyte function that results in a chronic and persistent, indolent inflammatory reaction within tissues exposed to viable microbes. In this condition, thickening and narrowing of the antrum is more common but similar changes may be seen in the oesophagus. Radiographic, endoscopic and motility studies may reveal a markedly atonic oesophagus with varying function of the lower oesophageal sphincter. Oesophageal stricture has also been reported. Pharmacological therapy and oesophageal dilatations are usually unsuccessful in establishing adequate oesophageal function. Corticosteroid therapy is justified in preventing life-threatening obstruction.

FURTHER READING

Chin TW, Stiehm ER, Falloon J et al. Corticosteroids in treatment of obstructive lesions of chronic granulomatous disease. Journal of Pediatrics 1987; 111:349–352.
Renner WR, Johnson JF, Lichtenstein JE et al. Esophageal inflammation and stricture: complication of chronic granulomatous disease of childhood. Radiology 1991; 178:189–191.

FAMILIAL DYSAUTONOMIA

Familial dysautonomia (Riley–Day syndrome) is an autosomal recessive disorder pathologically characterized by a specific disturbance of the nervous system and aberrations in autonomic nervous system function. The disease is expressed in infancy by poor sucking and swallowing, excessive sweating, defective lacrimation, insensitivity to pain, autonomic crisis with attacks of cyclic vomiting, generalized seizures and impaired intellectual function. Aspiration pneumonia may occur due to impaired swallowing or secondary to the dysfunction of the distal oesophagus. Distension of the small bowel or colon is also described.

FURTHER READING

Axelrod FB, Nachtigal R, Dancis J. Familial dysautonomia: diagnosis, pathogenesis and management. Advances in Pediatrics 1974; 21:75–96.
Grunebaum M. Radiological manifestations in familial dysautonomia. American Journal of Diseases of Childhood 1974; 128:176–178.

THE TRIPLE A SYNDROME

The triple A syndrome (Allgrove's syndrome) is an autosomal recessive multisystem disorder in which ACTH insensitivity is associated with achalasia and alacrima. Various neurological symptoms such as hyper-reflexia, muscle weakness, dysarthria and ataxia together with impaired intelligence and abnormal autonomic function, particularly postural hypotension, may be associated (Figure 10.11.8).

FURTHER READING

Clark AJ, Metherell L, Swords FM et al. The molecular pathogenesis of ACTH insensitivity syndromes. Annales D Endocrinologie (Paris) 2001; 62:207–211.

Grant DB, Barnes ND, Dumic M et al. Neurological and adrenal dysfunction in the adrenal insufficiency/alacrima/achalasia (3A) syndrome. Archives of Disease in Childhood 1993; 68:779–782.

Moore PS, Couch RM, Perry YS et al. Allgrove syndrome: an autosomal recessive syndrome of ACTH insensitivity, achalasia and alacrima. Clinical Endocrinology (Oxford) 1991; 34:107–114.

IDIOPATHIC INTESTINAL PSEUDO-OBSTRUCTION

Functional disorders of the gastrointestinal tract may manifest with signs and symptoms suggesting mechanical obstruction. Although the name of the syndrome suggests primary involvement of the small and large bowel, the oesophagus, stomach and bladder can be involved as well. With oesophageal involvement, the patient's major complaint will be dysphagia and absence of normal peristalsis with intermittent irregular contractions will be documented at barium studies.

FURTHER READING

Anuras S, Mitros FA, Soper RT et al. Chronic intestinal pseudoobstruction in young children. Gastroenterology 1986; 91:62–70.

Schuffler MD, Pope CE 2nd. Esophageal motor dysfunction in idiopathic intestinal pseudoobstruction. Gastroenterology 1976; 70:677–682.

Schuffler MD, Rohrmann CA Jr, Templeton FE. The radiologic manifestations of idiopathic intestinal pseudoobstruction. American Journal of Roentgenology 1976; 127:729–736.

TRAUMA TO THE OESOPHAGUS

CORROSIVE OESOPHAGITIS

This injury most commonly follows ingestion of household cleaning products such as alkalis, acids, bleaches and detergents but burns related to microwave overheated baby food may also be seen. The degree of injury depends on the nature, concentration and volume of the corrosive agent as well as the duration of tissue contact. Alkalis produce a severe, deep liquefaction necrosis that affects all layers of the oesophagus. Since alkalis have no taste, a child may ingest a significant amount. Acid agents produce a coagulative necrosis and a thick eschar that usually limits the depth of the injury to the mucosa and superficial muscular layers; owing to their bitter taste, the total ingested volume is usually smaller.

Both alkalis and acids can cause severe gastritis. Mouth lesions are commonly present but it has to be stressed that their absence does not exclude oesophageal lesions. Any swelling of the epiglottis or oedema of the airway should be viewed with alarm and measures to ensure airway patency should be implemented. Corrosive oesophagitis is characterized pathologically by three phases of injury: an acute necrotic phase, an ulcerative granulation phase and a final phase of cicatrization and stricture formation. The main and potentially lethal complications of caustic ingestion are mediastinitis and oesophageal perforation. The time of greatest risk of spontaneous perforation of a caustic injured oesophagus is 7–26 days after ingestion. The risk of stricture formation is related

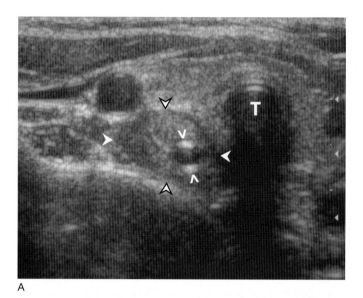

A

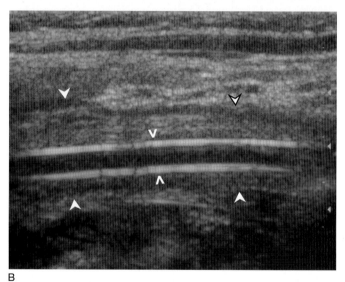

B

Figure 10.11.9 Lye ingestion. Ultrasonography 24 h after ingestion. (A) Transverse and (B) longitudinal scan at cervical level: the mucosa is markedly asymmetrically swollen and fits the nasogastric tube tightly (v). Oesophagus (arrowheads); trachea (T).

directly to the severity of the injury and occurs in up to 30% of cases. The incidence of reflux also increases regardless of an associated hiatus hernia. Rarely, tracheoesophageal and oesophagoaortic fistulas may develop.

Endoscopy has generally been advocated as the best means of assessing the extent and severity of oesophageal injury and it is recommended that it is performed in all patients within 48 h. The risk of oesophageal perforation, however, demands a very cautious approach and it should be kept in mind that radiological studies may also provide valuable information during both the acute and chronic stages of the disease. Ultrasonography (US) can reveal an increased wall thickness of the pharynx, the oesophagus and the cardia (Figure 10.11.9). Chest and abdominal radiographs to identify air leaks should be obtained routinely on children who have

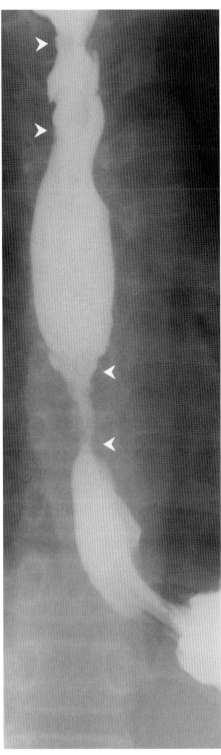

Figure 10.11.10 Advanced strictures due to lye ingestion. There are two long segmental strictures (arrowheads) in the upper and lower oesophagus. The presence of long segment narrowing in the cervical or thoracic oesophagus is characteristic of prior caustic injury.

ingested caustic agents. With milder injuries the x-rays are normal. In more severe cases, plain chest films taken in the acute phase will show a dilated gas-filled, atonic oesophagus or, if oesophageal perforation has occurred, mediastinal widening, pneumomediastinum and/or pleural effusions.

Oesophagography using a non-ionizing water-soluble contrast medium should be performed to exclude the presence of a leak. In the acute phase, the contrast appearances vary from being normal to almost complete obstruction to the passage of contrast by mucosal oedema. Single contrast oesophagography may underestimate the damage. It may show a rigid, narrow oesophagus with a variable degree of ulceration, a dilated atonic or an irritable oesophagus with tertiary waves. Swallowing incoordination may cause aspiration. In less severely affected children, it may be possible to perform a double-contrast study. Double-contrast studies may show shallow ulcers or even transverse folds related to contractions of the muscularis mucosae, which may eventually develop into sites of stenosis. When stenosis occurs, it usually involves a long segment and appears as a smooth, tapered narrowing (Fig. 10.11.12). The stricture must be assessed on a supine swallow as the length may be overestimated in the erect position. However, some strictures have an irregular contour or eccentric areas of sacculation because of asymmetrical scarring (see Figure 10.11.10). The development of short segment strictures and webs are less frequent. It has to be kept in mind that sporadic cases of carcinoma can arise in corrosive strictures years after the initial injury.

FURTHER READING

Appelqvist P, Salmo M. Lye corrosion carcinoma of the esophagus: a review of 63 cases. Cancer 1980; 45:2655–2658.

Martel W. Radiologic features of esophagogastritis secondary to extremely caustic agents. Radiology 1972; 103:31–36.

Muhlendahl KE, Oberdisse U, Krienke EG. Local injuries by accidental ingestion of corrosive substances by children. Archives of Toxicology 1978; 39:299–314.

Muhletaler CA, Gerlock AJ Jr, de Soto L et al. Acid corrosive esophagitis: radiographic findings. American Journal of Roentgenology 1980; 134:1137–1140.

Reeder JD, Kramer SS, Dudgeon DL. Transverse esophageal folds: association with corrosive injury. Radiology 1985; 155:303–304.

Wilsey MJ Jr, Scheimann AO, Gilger MA. The role of upper gastrointestinal endoscopy in the diagnosis and treatment of caustic ingestion, esophageal strictures, and achalasia in children. Gastrointestinal Endoscopy Clinics of North America 2001; 11:767–787, vii–viii.

OESOPHAGEAL FOREIGN BODY

The strong natural desire to learn provokes children to put all sorts of objects into their mouth to investigate their texture. Coins are generally the most commonly swallowed objects by children less than 5 years. Most swallowed objects pass through the intestinal tract without complications. Foreign bodies that become lodged in the oesophagus usually do so at one of three levels of physiological narrowing. Most frequently, foreign bodies impact at the level of the cricopharyngeal muscle and the thoracic inlet (on chest x-rays grave foreign bodies will be seen at the level of the clavicles). Alternatively, the foreign body may get stuck at the level of the carina and aortic arch or most distantly just proximal to the gas-

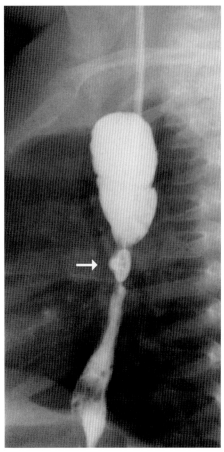

Figure 10.11.11 Oesophageal stricture following oesophageal atresia repair secondary to the anastomotic repair and to reflux oesophagitis. A press button (arrow) is lodged at the site of stenosis.

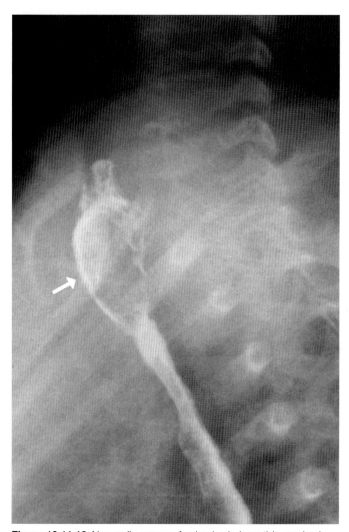

Figure 10.11.12 Non-radio-opaque foreign body (carrot) in proximal oesophagus. Contrast material outlines the non-opaque piece of carrot (arrow).

troesophageal sphincter (foreign body will be two to four vertebral bodies above the gastric bubble). Lodging of material at any other site should suggest an underlying oesophageal anomaly such as congenital or acquired strictures, webs or extrinsic masses (Figure 10.11.11).

The patient's history with an attack of coughing, drooling and choking commonly guides diagnosis. Foreign bodies in the oesophagus usually cause pain, dysphagia and sometimes dyspnoea due to compression of the larynx. Some cases, however, may be unsuspected especially those located high in the oesophagus or the hypopharynx, and present after an initial symptom-free interval with signs of oesophageal obstruction due to oedema and inflammation, chronic respiratory distress, recurrent pneumonia or failure to thrive. Complications include stenosis, ulceration and perforation.

Radio-opaque foreign bodies are easily diagnosed on plain films. A combination of abdomen, chest and lateral neck radiographs is taken. A barium swallow is needed for radiolucent or low-radiodensity material such as some food, fish bones, plastic, non-leaded glass or aluminium can tops (Figure 10.11.12). Coins and other flat objects in the oesophagus usually lie in the coronal plane while those in the trachea lie in the sagittal plain with the flat surfaces facing sideways (Figure 10.11.13). Foreign bodies

usually pass spontaneously but the child may still have a feeling of something 'sticking'. Before surgical or balloon removal is attempted, an x-ray should be done to ensure that the object has not passed into the stomach. Since a foreign body impacted in the oesophagus is unlikely to pass spontaneously, smooth, small and otherwise non-injurious objects may be removed retrograde with the aid of Foley catheters. Because the balloon does not firmly grab the object it may slip away during the procedure and once the object is pulled to the oropharynx the patient is at risk of tracheobronchial aspiration. The use of a wire retrieval basket advanced through a placed soft tube with an open tip may overcome these difficulties. An orogastric tube with a magnet can be used for the removal of magnetic objects (Figure 10.11.14). Immediate endoscopic removal is recommended for sharp-edged foreign bodies to avoid perforation and is the method of choice for all objects in many centres.

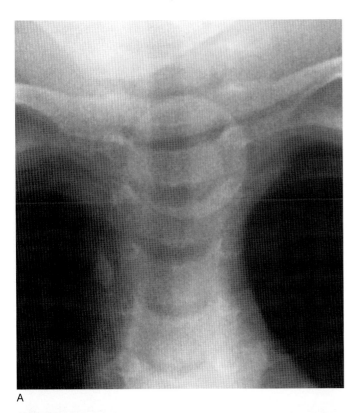

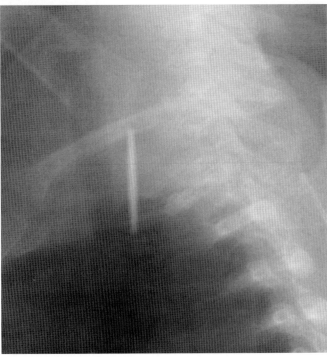

Figure 10.11.13 (A,B) Aluminium coin in the proximal oesophagus. The coin lies, as other flat objects, typically in the coronal plane.

FURTHER READING

Brown EG, Hughes JP, Koenig HM. Removal of foreign bodies lodged in esophagus by a Foley catheter without endoscopy: success with two cases. Clinical Pediatrics 1972; 11:468–471.
McGahren ED. Esophageal foreign bodies. Pediatric Review 1999; 20:129–133.
Neilson IR. Ingestion of coins and batteries. Pediatric Review 1995; 16:35–36.

OESOPHAGEAL RUPTURE AND PERFORATION

Oesophageal rupture can be a complication of extensive corrosive oesophagitis, ingestion of pointed foreign bodies, iatrogenic intervention, external (blunt or penetrating) trauma or increased intraluminal pressure facilitated by cricopharyngeal spasm. Blunt external trauma such as blast injuries compresses the oesophageal wall leading to an increase in the intraluminal oesophageal pressure beyond tolerance. Iatrogenic interventions that may cause oesophageal perforation are positive pressure ventilation in neonates, intraluminal tube insertion, balloon dilatation or endoscopic manoeuvres (Figure 10.11.15). Perforation of the posterior pharyngeal wall at the pharyngoesophageal junction has been described in the newborn after delivery. The resulting intense spasm of the cricopharyngeus muscle leads to not only clinical but also radiographic behaviour similar to oesophageal atresia (Figure 10.11.16).

Radiological differentiation from the blind pouch of oesophageal atresia is best achieved with contrast studies, which show a greater distance between the pouch and the trachea and a more irregular outline of the traumatic track. Contrast cannot be aspirated from the mediastinal track.

Oesophageal perforation may be manifest on plain chest films as mediastinal widening, cervical emphysema, pneumomediastinum and/or hydropneumothorax depending on the site of perforation. When oesophageal perforation is suspected in patients who have normal or equivocal plain films, a limited water-soluble contrast study should be performed to document the presence of perforation. CT may be helpful for further characterization of the extent and nature of the perforation. In cases of perforation of the cervical oesophagus, endoscopy is as effective as water-soluble contrast studies.

FURTHER READING

Eklöf O, Lohr G, Okmian L. Submucosal perforation of the esophagus in the neonate. Acta Radiologica Diagnostica 1969;8:187–192.
Heller RM, Kirchner SG, O'Neill JA. Perforation of the pharynx in the newborn: a near look-alike for esophageal atresia. American Journal of Roentgenology 1977; 129:335–337.
White RK, Morris DM. Diagnosis and management of esophageal perforations. American Surgery 1992; 58:112–119.

IATROGENIC OESOPHAGITIS

Iatrogenic oesophagitis may result from radiation or medication and shows features such as abnormal motility, mucosal oedema, stricture formation, ulceration and pseudodiverticulum or fistula formation.

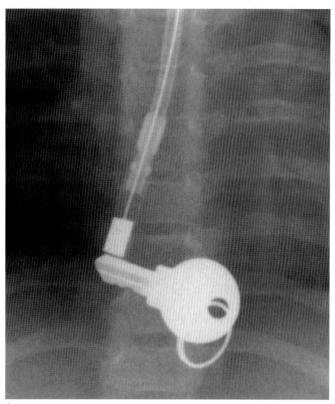

A

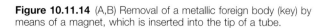

Figure 10.11.14 (A,B) Removal of a metallic foreign body (key) by means of a magnet, which is inserted into the tip of a tube.

B

FURTHER READING

Lepke RA, Libshitz HI. Radiation-induced injury of the esophagus. Radiology 1983; 148:375–378.

RADIATION OESOPHAGITIS

Oesophageal damage is the major limiting factor for high-dose, external beam radiation to the chest. An acute and a chronic stage of radiation oesophagitis are described. Most patients have clinical evidence of oesophagitis shortly after the onset of radiotherapy. Acute radiation oesophagitis is usually self-limited without permanent sequelae. During that period, radiological or endoscopic examinations are rarely necessary. Chronic radiation injury to the oesophagus may cause dysphagia several months after completion of radiotherapy. Dysphagia may result from abnormal oesophageal motility or, less commonly, from the development of strictures. Usually, abnormal motility can be recognized less than 4 months and strictures more than 4 months after radiotherapy. Both the acute and the chronic effects of radiation on the oesophagus may be affected by adjuvant chemotherapy, which increases the likelihood and accelerates the development of radiation-induced injuries.

A clinically distinct type of oesophagitis has been recognized with low doses of mediastinal radiation in patients who simultaneously or sequentially receive either adriamycin or actinomycin D. These patients suffer from recurrent episodes of oesophagitis during each course of chemotherapy. The radiographic findings are non-specific, ranging from subtle alterations in motility to severe ulceration with irreversible stricture formation.

Acute radiation oesophagitis may manifest itself by superficial ulcers or a granular appearance of the mucosa. In chronic radiation injury, stricture formation, ulcers and, in severe cases, tracheoesophageal and oesophagobronchial fistulas caused by radiation necrosis can be demonstrated.

FURTHER READING

Boal DK, Newburger PE, Teele RL. Esophagitis induced by combined radiation and adriamycin. American Journal of Roentgenology 1979; 132:567–570.
Chowhan NM. Injurious effects of radiation on the esophagus. American Journal of Gastroenterology 1990; 85:115–120.

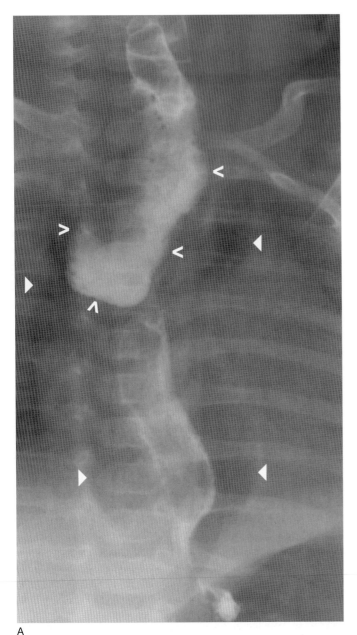
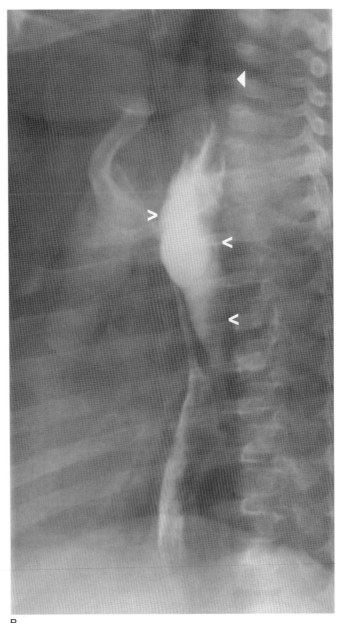

A   B

Figure 10.11.15 (A,B) Iatrogenic pharyngoesophageal perforation (oesophagoscopy) after scald. Swallowed contrast material enters the retroesophageal space with formation of a cavity extending into the mediastinum (v). There is also a pneumomediastinum (arrowheads).

Lepke RA, Libshitz HI. Radiation-induced injury of the esophagus. Radiology 1983; 148:375–378.

DRUG-INDUCED OESOPHAGITIS

Many medications have been implicated in oesophagitis and include doxycylin and quinidine. In older children, tetracycline, which is frequently used to treat acne, can produce local, self-limiting oesophagitis. Drug-induced oesophagitis is caused by a local chemical injury of the mucosa and usually occurs in the mid-oesophagus, presumably as a result of delayed passage of the medication at this level due to extrinsic compression of the oesophagus by the aortic arch. Symptoms of drug-induced oesophagitis develop rapidly within several hours or days after taking the medication. The timely relationship between ingestion of the offending medication and the onset of oesophagitis helps to discriminate drug-induced oesophagitis from herpes oesophagitis, which may present with identical radiological features. Drug-induced oesophagitis is generally benign and will improve after cessation of medication. However, many antibiotics and other medications may rarely cause a severe generalized disease called toxic epidermal necrolysis, which has a high mortality rate and may cause strictures as a consequence of oesophagitis.

On endoscopy, the oesophageal mucosa shows evidence of friability and redness as well as erosion, ulcers and, rarely,

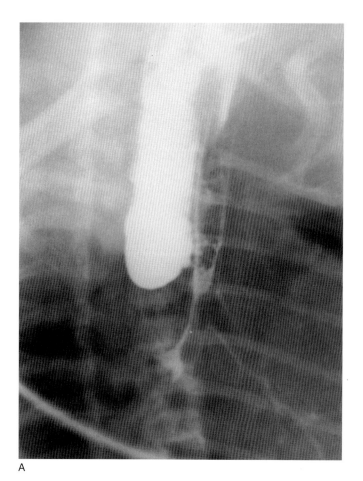

A

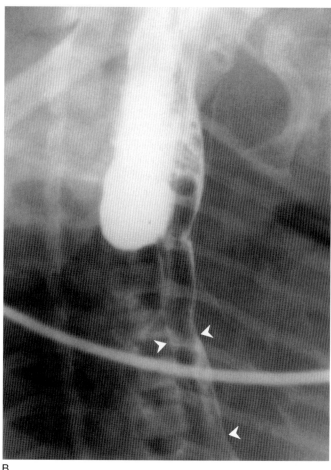

B

Figure 10.11.16 One-day-old female newborn with pharyngoesophageal perforation caused by the obstetrician's finger during breech delivery. (A) The contrast medium in the retroesophageal space fills a large sinus that mimics a proximal pouch of oesophageal atresia. (B) Shortly thereafter the true oesophageal lumen is also outlined with contrast material (arrowheads).

strictures. Single-contrast barium studies may demonstrate deep ulcers and strictures but are rarely able to detect superficial areas of ulceration. With double-contrast barium examinations, however, shallow ulcers and other mucosal changes can be detected in older children.

FURTHER READING

Bott S, Prakash C, McCallum RW. Medication-induced esophageal injury: survey of the literature. American Journal of Gastroenterology 1987; 82:758–763.

Carter FM, Mitchell CK. Toxic epidermal necrolysis – an unusual cause of colonic perforation. Report of a case. Diseases of the Colon and Rectum 1993; 36:773–777.

Eng J, Sabanathan S. Drug-induced esophagitis. American Journal of Gastroenterology 1991; 86:1127–1133.

Jaspersen D. Drug-induced oesophageal disorders: pathogenesis, incidence, prevention and management. Drug Safety 2000; 22:237–249.

GRAFT-VERSUS-HOST DISEASE

In graft-versus-host disease (GVHD), donor T-cells react against host major histocompatibility complex antigens predominately in the skin, gastrointestinal tract and liver. An acute (developing 7–14 days post-bone marrow transplant) and a chronic (developing more than 100 days post-bone marrow transplant) form are recognized. Oesophageal involvement may occur in severe forms of acute GVHD in association with a toxic, epidermal necrolysis-like erythroderma. In chronic GVHD, the immunological process causes desquamation and sloughing of the oesophagus. Subsequent scarring may lead to the development of webs, ring-like narrowing, abnormalities of oesophageal motility and smoothly tapering strictures. Symptoms include dysphagia, odynophagia, substernal chest pain and weight loss.

In chronic GVHD, barium studies may demonstrate an oesophagus with an irregular, serrated contour due to mucosal desquamation and sloughing. With the development of scarring, webs or strictures are usually seen in the cervical oesophagus. Other patients may develop ring-like or smoothly tapering strictures in the mid and upper oesophagus. The characteristic desquamation is best documented by endoscopy.

FURTHER READING

McDonald GB, Sullivan KM, Schuffler MD et al. Esophageal abnormalities in chronic graft-versus-host disease in humans. Gastroenterology 1981; 80:914–921.

BOERHAAVE'S SYNDROME

Spontaneous oesophageal rupture or so-called Boerhaave's syndrome appears most commonly in middle-aged males and is caused by increased luminal pressure during retching or vomiting with a closed glottis. Clinical signs are excruciating chest pain, mediastinitis and sometimes rupture into the left pleural space. It is rare in children and when it does occur it is more likely to happen in the neonatal period. Increased intraluminal pressure leading to neonatal oesophageal perforation may be encountered *in utero* during delivery and will then present within the first day of life. Symptoms include respiratory distress due to tension hydropneumothorax, choking spells and difficulty in feeding. Haematemesis may occur.

The radiographic appearances are different in neonates from those in children and adults. In neonates, mediastinal gas is less common and, due to the more right-sided position of the neonatal oesophagus, a right-sided pneumothorax or hydropneumothorax is seen.

FURTHER READING

Inculet R, Clark C, Girvan D. Boerhaave's syndrome and children: a rare and unexpected combination. Journal of Pediatric Surgery 1996; 31:1300–1301.

MALLORY–WEISS SYNDROME

Upper gastrointestinal haemorrhage resulting from a laceration in the mucosa of the gastroesophageal junction is occasionally reported in children. Mucosal tears, best seen endoscopically, may be accompanied by gastritis, duodenitis with or without *Helicobacter pylori* infection, *Helicobacter pylori*-positive duodenal ulcer, gastroesophageal reflux disease and bronchial asthma. A history of violent retching or vomiting followed by haematemesis usually suggests the diagnosis. Barium studies may reveal linear fissures in the distal oesophagus. Endoscopic electrocoagulation of actively bleeding Mallory–Weiss tears if required is the treatment of choice.

FURTHER READING

Bak-Romaniszyn L, Malecka-Panas E, Czkwianianc E et al. Mallory–Weiss syndrome in children. Diseases of the Esophagus 1999; 12:65–67.
Papp JP. Electrocoagulation of actively bleeding Mallory–Weiss tears. Gastrointestinal Endoscopy 1980; 26:128–130.

OESOPHAGEAL NEOPLASM

Both benign and malignant primary tumours of the oesophagus are extremely uncommon in children and include leiomyomas, oesophageal papillomas, squamous cell carcinomas and adenocarcinomas.

BENIGN NEOPLASM

OESOPHAGEAL LEIOMYOMATOSIS

Oesophageal leiomyomatosis is a rare, benign neoplastic disorder in which proliferation of smooth muscle leads to marked circumferential wall thickening of a sizable portion of the oesophagus. This condition is found predominantly in children and young adults. Oesophageal leiomyomatosis can occur as an isolated finding or may be associated with hereditary nephritis (Alport's syndrome), with hypertrophic osteoarthropathy or with leiomyomas elsewhere in the body. Presenting symptoms such as dysphagia, dyspnoea and retrosternal pain usually overlap with more common oesophageal disorders. Barium studies may reveal narrowing of the distal oesophagus covered by smooth mucosa with varying degrees of proximal dilatation. Circumferential oesophageal wall thickening is seen on CT and ultrasound (Figure 10.11.17).

Oesophageal leiomyomatosis should be differentiated from another closely related condition known as idiopathic muscular hypertrophy of the oesophagus. This disease is characterized by non-neoplastic expansion of smooth muscle in the wall of the oesophagus, normal motility, normal oesophagoscopy and no or only minor problems in swallowing. Barium studies can reveal a corkscrew appearance with innumerable non-peristaltic contractions or an achalasia-like appearance.

FURTHER READING

Cochat P, Guibaud P, Garcia Torres R et al. Diffuse leiomyomatosis in Alport syndrome. Journal of Pediatrics 1988; 113:339–343.
Demian SD, Vargas-Cortes F. Idiopathic muscular hypertrophy of the esophagus. Postmortem incidental finding in six cases and review of the literature. Chest 1978; 73:28–32.
Guest AR, Strouse PJ, Hiew CC et al. Progressive esophageal leiomyomatosis with respiratory compromise. Pediatric Radiology 2000; 30:247–250.
Kirk VG, McFadden S, Pinto A et al. Leiomyoma of the esophagus associated with bronchial obstruction owing to inflammatory pseudotumor in a child. Journal of Pediatric Surgery 2000; 35:771–774.
Kreczy A, Gassner J, Mikuz G. Idiopathic hypertrophy of the oesophagus in children. A case report and review of the literature. Virchows Archives A Pathological Anatomy Histopathology 1990; 417:81–84.
Lee H, Morgan K, Abramowsky C et al. Leiomyoma at the site of esophageal atresia repair. Journal of Pediatric Surgery 2001; 36:1832–1833.
Rabushka LS, Fishman EK, Kuhlman JE et al. Diffuse esophageal leiomyomatosis in a patient with Alport syndrome: CT demonstration. Radiology 1991; 179:176–178.
Thorner P, Heidet L, Moreno Merlo F et al. Diffuse leiomyomatosis of the esophagus: disorder of cell–matrix interaction? Pediatric Developmental Pathology 1998; 1:543–549.

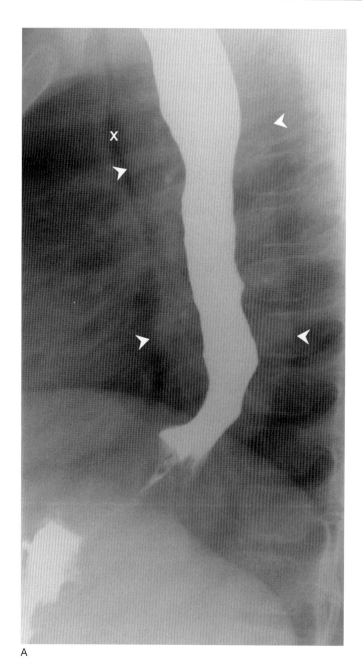

A

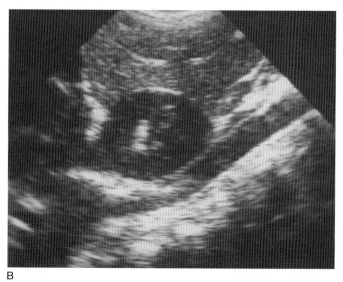

B

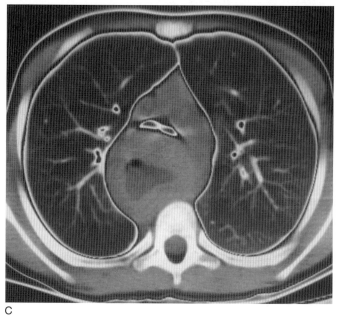

C

Figure 10.11.17 Oesophageal leiomyomatosis. Six-year-old girl with dysphagia, recurrent respiratory infections and attacks of dyspnoea with cyanosis. Oesophagectomy was unavoidable. (A) Oesophagography reveals a dilated, extremely thick-walled oesophagus (arrowheads) with narrowing near the gastroesophageal junction. The trachea (x) is compressed. (B) Longitudinal ultrasound scan at the level of the gastroesophageal junction shows massive thickening of the oesophageal wall. (C) CT scan shows the thick-walled oesophagus compressing the carina.

OESOPHAGEAL PAPILLOMAS

Oesophageal papillomas usually occur as solitary lesions, ranging from 0.5 to 1.5 cm in size. Rarely, multiple oesophageal papillomas have been reported in children in association with recurrent respiratory involvement known as oesophageal papillomatosis. Because of the small size of the lesions double-contrast is preferable to single-contrast studies and may show multiple filling defects (Figure 10.11.18). Endoscopy is the method of choice for detection of oesophageal papillomas and is recommended in patients with significant laryngeal lesions or postcricoid involvement.

FURTHER READING

Batra PS, Hebert RL 2nd, Haines GK 3rd et al. Recurrent respiratory papillomatosis with esophageal involvement. International Journal of Pediatric Otorhinolaryngology 2001; 58:233–238.

Odze R, Antonioli D, Shocket D et al. Esophageal squamous papillomas. A clinicopathologic study of 38 lesions and analysis for human papillo-

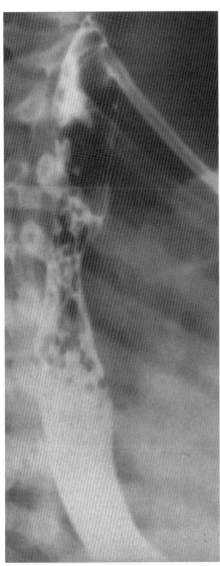

Figure 10.11.18 Oesophageal papillomatosis. The multiple defects are due to tiny polyps. This child had involvement of the pharynx and upper airways as well.

mavirus by the polymerase chain reaction. American Journal of Surgical Pathology 1993; 17:803–812.

MALIGNANT TUMOURS

Carcinomas of the oesophagus are extremely rare in children. Squamous cell carcinomas following primary achalasia and an unusual case of a squamous cell carcinoma arising from an oesophageal duplication cyst have been reported. Barrett's oesophagus predisposes to the development of adenocarcinoma, which represents 0.05% of all malignant paediatric gastrointestinal tumours.

FURTHER READING

Sasaki H, Sasano H, Ohi R et al. Adenocarcinoma at the esophageal gastric junction arising in an 11-year-old girl. Pathology International 1999; 49:1109–1113.
Singh S, Lal P, Sikora SS et al. Squamous cell carcinoma arising from a congenital duplication cyst of the esophagus in a young adult. Diseases Esophagus 2001; 14:258–261.
Zotter H, Schwinger W, Kerbl R et al. Management of a 16-year-old boy with adenocarcinoma at the esophageal gastric junction. Medical and Pediatric Oncology 2001; 37:557.

DIFFERENTIAL DIAGNOSIS

EXTRINSIC COMPRESSION

Extrinsic compression may mimic a benign oesophageal neoplasm. Vascular rings such as double aortic arch, pulmonary artery sling or right aortic arch with aberrant left pulmonary artery, lymphadenopathy, thyromegaly, aortic aneurysms and left atrial enlargement are among the reported causes of extrinsic oesophageal compression (Figures 10.11.19, 10.11.20, 10.11.21, 10.11.22).

FURTHER READING

Cappell MS. Endoscopic, radiographic, and manometric findings associated with cardiovascular dysphagia. Digestive Disease Science 1995; 40:166–176.
Gilliland MD, Scott LD, Walker WE. Esophageal obstruction caused by mediastinal histoplasmosis: beneficial results of operation. Surgery 1984; 95:59–62.

OESOPHAGEAL VARICES

Oesophageal varices are usually secondary to portal hypertension. Portal vein obstructions due to thrombosis secondary to sepsis and/or dehydration and hepatic cirrhosis are the most frequent cause of portal hypertension. A rare congenital form also exists. Variceal bleeding may be the presenting symptom in children with congenital hepatic fibrosis associated with polycystic renal disease. A case of cytomegalovirus hepatitis leading to non-cirrhotic sinusoidal fibrosis and the association of oesophageal varices with congenital asplenia and total anomalous pulmonary venous return have been reported.

Although endoscopy is the primary investigation for identifying oesophageal varices, they may be seen incidentally on imaging performed for other reasons. If oesophageal varices cause sufficient irregularity of the oesophagus, paraspinous widening may be seen on chest radiographs but this is rare. Doppler imaging with colour flow mapping allows demonstration of the haemodynamics of the varices and the treatment response. On barium studies the varices appear as serpinginous filling defects in the barium column. Varices alternately distend and collapse with peristalsis, respiration and varying degrees of oesophageal distension (Figure 10.11.23 and Figure 10.11.24). This changeable nature on fluoroscopy allows differentiation from lymphoma deposits or inflammatory conditions that may be manifested by thickened tortuous, longitudinal folds.

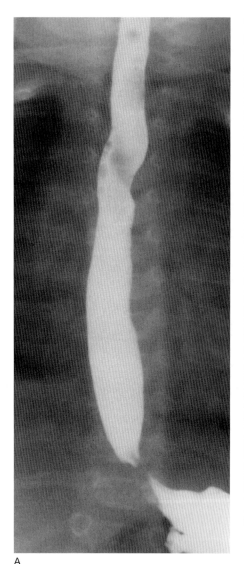

A

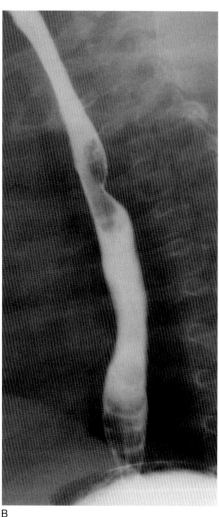

B

Fig 10.11.19 Left aortic arch with aberrant right subclavian artery. Characteristic oblique oesophageal indentation on frontal (A) and slightly triangular small indentation on lateral (B) view.

Variceal bleeding is not only the commonest presentation of portal hypertension but also the most common cause of severe gastrointestinal bleeding in childhood. Early treatment such as sclerotherapy is needed to reduce mortality and morbidity in these patients.

FURTHER READING

Chen HY, Chen SJ, Li YW et al. Esophageal varices in congenital heart disease with total anomalous pulmonary venous connection. International Journal of Card Imaging 2000; 16:405–409.

Ghishan FK, Greene HL, Halter S et al. Noncirrhotic portal hypertension in congenital cytomegalovirus infection. Hepatology 1984; 4:684–686.

Harinck E, Fernandes J, Vervat D. Congenital esophageal varices in identical twins without portal hypertension. Journal of Pediatric Surgery 1971; 6:488.

McKiernan PJ. Treatment of variceal bleeding. Gastrointestinal Endoscopy Clinics of North America 2001; 11:789–812, viii.

Zargar SA, Javid G, Khan BA et al. Endoscopic ligation compared with sclerotherapy for bleeding esophageal varices in children with extrahepatic portal venous obstruction. Hepatology 2002; 36:666–672.

DUPLICATION CYSTS

Most oesophageal cysts are congenital duplication cysts caused by abnormal embryological development in which islands of cells are sequestered from the primitive foregut. Oesophageal duplications cannot always be differentiated clinically or radiographically from bronchogenic cysts. Duplication cysts are posterior, while most bronchogenic cysts are in the middle mediastinum. They may be located anywhere along the length of the oesophagus and may extend transdiaphragmatically. Both may cause airway narrowing and respiratory symptoms or may be an incidental finding on routine chest radiographs or antenatal ultrasound. The size of these cysts is very variable. Association of oesophageal duplication cysts with pulmonary cystic malformations, oesophageal atresia and vertebral defects has been described. They usually appear on oesophagograms as submucosal masses that are indistinguishable from solid mesenchymal tumours. Ultrasound, CT and magnetic resonance imaging (MRI) are helpful as they demonstrate that duplication cysts and bronchogenic cysts are fluid-filled structures

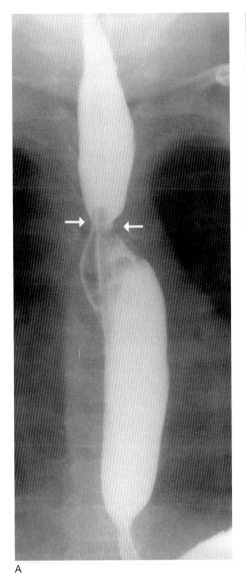

A

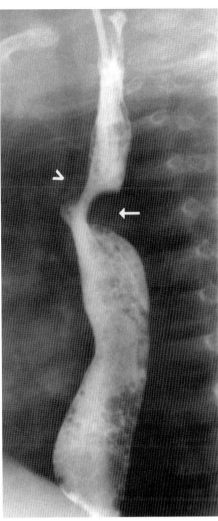

B

Figure 10.11.20 Double aortic arch.
(A) Frontal oesophagram: both sides of the oesophagus are intended by the two arches (arrows). (B) Lateral oesophagram: large posterior indentation by the retroesophageal component of the double aortic arch (arrow). The anterior wall of the trachea (v) is intended at the level of the aortic arch.   *Continued*

(Figure 10.11.25 and Figure 10.11.26). A complication of duplication cysts is sudden increase in size due to haemorrhage as duplication cysts may contain gastric mucosal cells.

The development of neurenteric cysts is not completely understood but seems to be due to an imperfect separation of the notochord. The resulting malformation is a cystic structure usually found in the posterior mediastinum, which is connected to the spinal canal either through a fibrous tract or a fistula. Resulting vertebral anomalies such as butterfly vertebrae with anterior spina bifida or hemivertebrae are always above the cyst (Figure 10.11.27).

FURTHER READING

Beardmore H, Wiglesworth F. Vertebral anomalies and alimentary duplications: clinical and embryological aspects. Pediatric Clinics of North America 1958; 5:457–474.

Kitano Y, Iwanaka T, Tsuchida Y et al. Esophageal duplication cyst associated with pulmonary cystic malformations. Journal of Pediatric Surgery 1995; 30:1724–1727.

McCullagh M, Bhuller AS, Pierro A et al. Antenatal identification of a cervical oesophageal duplication. Pediatric Surgery International 2000; 16:204–205.

Snyder ME, Luck SR, Hernandez R et al. Diagnostic dilemmas of mediastinal cysts. Journal of Pediatric Surgery 1985; 20:810–815.

Stringer MD, Spitz L, Abel R et al. Management of alimentary tract duplication in children. British Journal of Surgery 1995; 82:74–78.

Rafal RB, Markisz JA. Magnetic resonance imaging of an esophageal duplication cyst. American Journal of Gastroenterology 1991; 86:1809–1811.

TRACTION AND PULSION DIVERTICULA

True oesophageal diverticula consist of only mucosa without a muscular layer. These diverticula are due to herniations through congenitally potentially weak areas of the muscular wall of the oesophagus. The most common locations include the pharyngoesophageal junction (Zenker's diverticulum), the mid-oesophagus and the distal oesophagus just above the oesophageal hiatus (epiphrenic diverticulum). Zenker's diverticula are occasionally

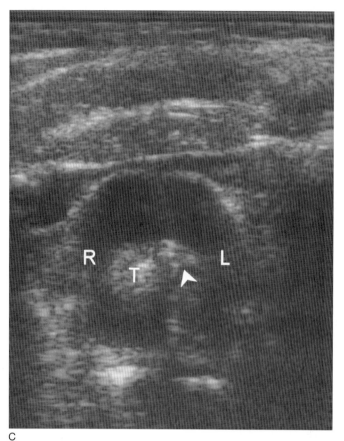

C

Figure 10.11.20, cont'd (C) Axial ultrasound at the level of aortic arches shows the vascular ring. Right (R), left (L) aortic arch; oesophagus (arrowhead); trachea (T).

seen in older children and may cause difficulty in swallowing, with possible aspiration during sleep.

The radiological appearance of diverticula is similar to that seen in adults with a posterolateral outpouching of mucosa/submucosa through the Killian's dehiscence. The diverticulum may compress the upper oesophagus or grow to occlude the lumen. Diverticula at the mid-oesophagus are thought to be pulsion diverticula or traction diverticula caused by scarring of carinal lymph nodes in tuberculosis or histoplasmosis. An epiphrenic diverticulum is very rare and an underlying condition such as Ehlers–Danlos syndrome should be considered.

A pseudodiverticulum may occur from unrecognized oesophageal perforation and be associated with mediastinitis.

FURTHER READING

Kaye MD. Oesophageal motor dysfunction in patients with diverticula of the mid-thoracic oesophagus. Thorax 1974; 29:666–672.

Toyohara T, Kaneko T, Araki H et al. Giant epiphrenic diverticulum in a boy with Ehlers–Danlos syndrome. Pediatric Radiology 1989; 19:437.

GASTROESOPHAGEAL REFLUX

GASTROESOPHAGEAL REFLUX AND GASTROESOPHAGEAL REFLUX DISEASE

Gastroesophageal reflux (GOR), defined as the passage of gastric contents into the oesophagus, is a common, self-limited process in infants that usually resolves by 6–12 months of age. The main mechanisms of GOR are transient lower oesophageal sphincter (LOS) relaxation and periods of low/absent LOS pressure. Vomiting, spitting up or regurgitation are the most common clinical signs. There is no need to perform any radiological evaluation in the otherwise healthy infants of 1 month to 1 year of age. Effective, conservative management involves thickened feedings, prone positioning and parental reassurance.

Gastroesophageal reflux disease (GORD), defined as symptoms or complications of GOR, is a less common, more serious pathological process that usually warrants medical management and diagnostic evaluation. Clinical manifestations of GORD in children include vomiting, poor weight gain, dysphagia, abdominal or retrosternal pain, oesophagitis and respiratory disorders. GORD is usually found in association with hiatus hernia and other disorders affecting oesophageal motility and is a common complication following successful repair of oesophageal atresia and tracheoesophageal fistula.

The diagnosis of GORD is made based upon the child's history and a variety of diagnostic procedures, which include the standard upper gastrointestinal barium study, pH-probing, scintigraphy, micromanometric methods, non-invasive breath tests and endoscopy. The selection of procedures is usually individualized and based on the clinical situation and availability. Since all of these tests have advantages and disadvantages, more than one is performed in each patient, but it is almost universally agreed that pH monitoring is the most sensitive study for detecting acidic reflux and determining the duration of its presence. However, some authors state that most reflux episodes that occur in infants are non-acidic and are therefore undetectable by standard pH-probe monitoring. A combination of pH monitoring with intraoesophageal impedance measurement is recommended to allow a more precise detection of bolus movement within the oesophagus.

The first step when dealing with infants who present with signs of GORD is the evaluation of the anatomy of the oesophagus, the stomach and stomach outlet, and the exclusion of a hiatus hernia, gastric outlet obstruction and malrotation. Determination of gastric outlet abnormalities such as antral webs, pyloric stenosis, pylorospasm or gastric ulcer disease is best achieved with ultrasound in infants and barium studies in older children. In infants with malrotation and complete or incomplete duodenal obstruction, contrast studies are required for definite diagnosis. The gastroesophageal junction itself can easily be visualized with ultrasound in both infants and older children. In the longitudinal plane, gross reflux, which is sonolucent or echogenic fluid, depending on the gastric content and the wide cardia, are clearly visible (Figure 10.11.28).

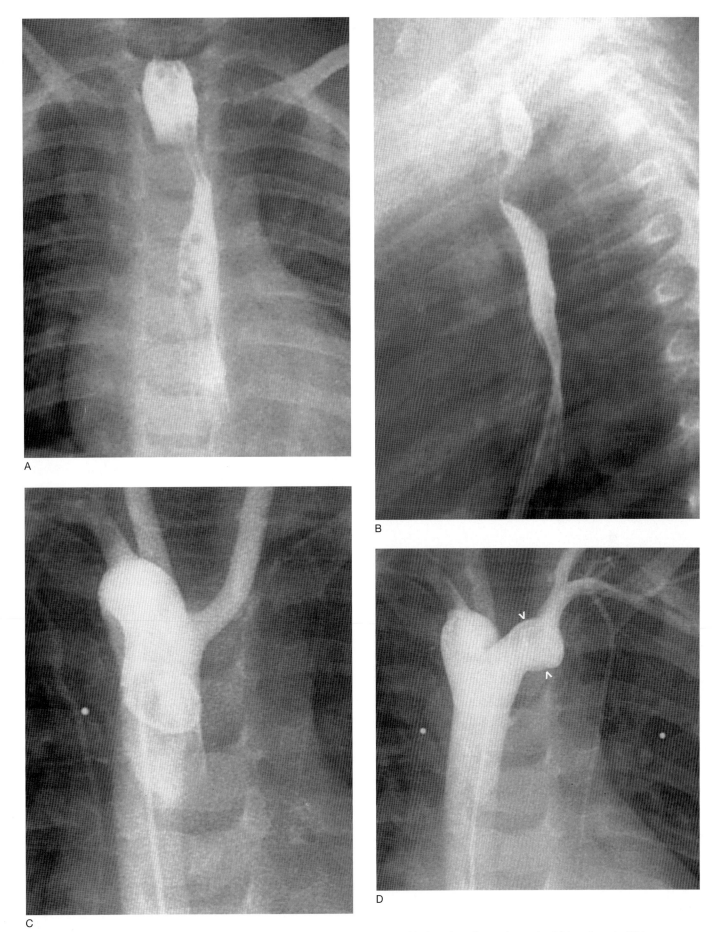

Figure 10.11.21 Right aortic arch with aberrant left subclavian artery. (A) Right lateral indentation of oesophagus by right aortic arch. (B) Large posterior indentation of oesophagus from aortic (Kommerrell) diverticulum. Aortogram demonstrates (C) right aortic arch and right descending aorta as well as (D) a large aortic (Kommerrell) diverticulum (v) at the junction of the right aortic arch and right descending aorta.

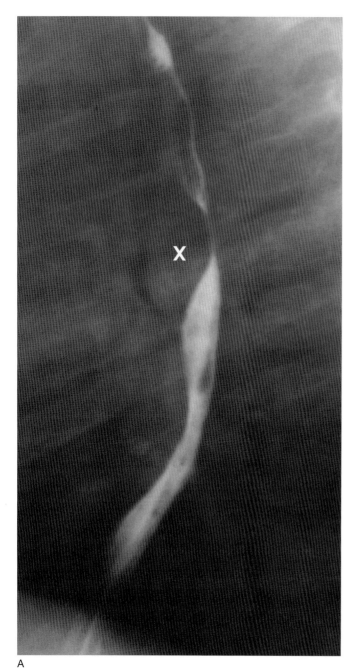

A

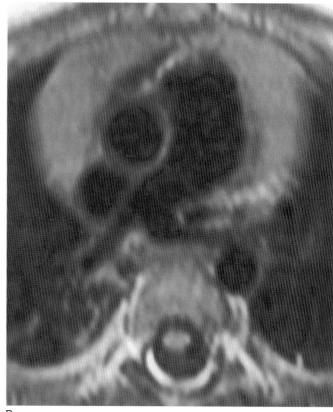

B

Figure 10.11.22 Aberrant left pulmonary artery (pulmonary artery sling). (A) Oesophagram: the aberrant left pulmonary artery (x) is seen as an oval mass between the trachea and oesophagus. Note characteristic anterior indentation of the oesophagus. (B) MRI findings. Axial T1-weighted image. The left pulmonary artery arises from the right pulmonary artery and crosses to the left lung posterior to the trachea and in front of the oesophagus.

The patient is examined in the recumbent position but partially rotated towards the examiner. A shortening of the subdiaphragmatic part of the oesophagus, an obtuse His' angle, and the demonstration of a slow, trickling reflux of the gastric content are described for GORD. No criteria for evaluating the severity of GOR on ultrasound or characteristic sonographic features of reflux oesophagitis are yet established.

An upper GI series demonstrates the upper gastrointestinal tract from the oral cavity to the jejunum. On barium studies severe oesophagitis is seen as ulceration, which may be superficial, deep or sometimes confluent. Oesophageal strictures occur but less frequently than might be expected. The full extent of these strictures is only seen with contrast studies. Strictures may improve with treatment of the reflux. In children with severe reflux, the gastroesophageal junction is often seen to be wide and lax (Figure 10.11.29). However, the upper GI series is not reliable in detecting gastroesophageal reflux itself since gastroesophageal reflux results from multiple transient relaxations of the LOS that occur at random and as intermittent episodes and might therefore be missed during the brief period of observation. The sensitivity of fluoroscopic detection of gastroesophageal reflux may be increased with provocation manoeuvres such as coughing, the Valsalva manoeuvre, rolling from the supine to the right lateral position and the water-siphon test.

Gastroesophageal scintigraphy is an alternative technique that appears to be far more accurate than conventional barium studies.

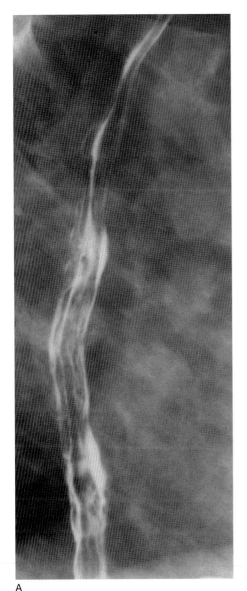

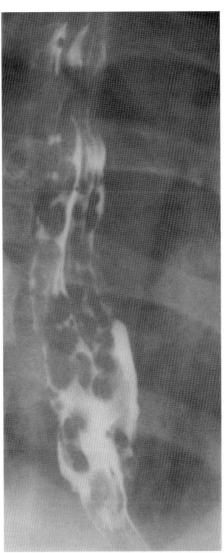

Figure 10.11.23 Oesophageal varices. Changeable nature of varices at fluoroscopy: the varices are collapsed in (A) and distended to numerous serpiginous vermiform filling defects in (B).

A

B

It additionally may demonstrate reflux-associated aspiration, a possible cause of recurrent chest infections. For gastroesophageal scintigraphy, the radiopharmaceutical is mixed with the usual meal formula or juice and administered to the patient after fasting for a minimum of 6 h. Images of the upper abdomen and chest are obtained in the supine and left lateral decubitus positions during a recording period of 60–90 min. At 3–4 h, a 5-min image of the chest is obtained to document radioactive material in the lungs.

The ^{13}C-acetate breath test, which already has been validated in adults, is a non-invasive and non-radioactive alternative method and its results closely correlate with those of scintigraphy in a paediatric population.

CONDITIONS ASSOCIATED WITH GASTROESOPHAGEAL REFLUX

Gastroesophageal reflux can be an isolated problem but it occurs with increased frequency in children with neuromuscular disorders, repair of oesophageal atresia and tracheoesophageal fistula, cystic fibrosis and collagen–vascular diseases. An increased incidence of peptic oesophagitis and strictures is found in these children (Figure 10.11.30 and Figure 10.11.31). Most children with isolated GOR outgrow the process but those with underlying abnormalities are less likely to do so. Some of these children require surgical augmentation of the LOS with gastric wrap around the lower oesophagus, called fundoplication.

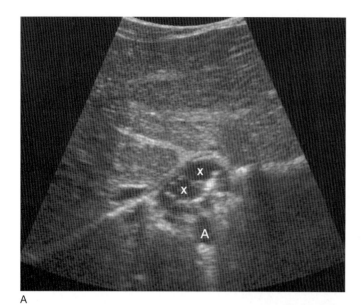

A

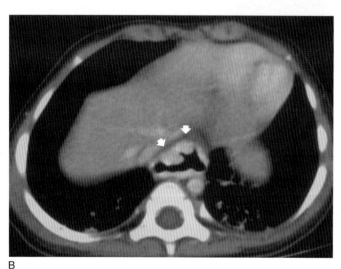

B

Figure 10.11.24 Oesophageal varices. (A) Ultrasound findings: transverse scan at the level of cardia. The varices (x) protrude into the oesophageal lumen. Aorta (A). (B) CT findings: during infusion of intravenous contrast there was medium dense enhancement of the large varices in the wall of the oesophagus (arrows).

FURTHER READING

Delbende B, Perri F, Couturier O et al. 13C-octanoic acid breath test for gastric emptying measurement. European Journal of Gastroenterology and Hepatology 2000; 12:85–91.

Dutta HK, Grover VP, Dwivedi SN et al. Manometric evaluation of postoperative patients of esophageal atresia and tracheo-esophageal fistula. European Journal Pediatric Surgery 2001; 11:371–376.

Fotter R, Hollwarth M, Uray E. Correlation between manometric and roentgenologic findings of diseases of the esophagus in infants and children. Progress in Pediatric Surgery 1985; 18:14–21.

Gomes H, Menanteau B. Gastro-esophageal reflux: comparative study between sonography and pH monitoring. Pediatric Radiology 1991; 21:168–174.

Jang HS, Lee JS, Lim GY et al. Correlation of color Doppler sonographic findings with pH measurements in gastroesophageal reflux in children. Journal of Clinical Ultrasound 2001; 29:212–217.

Madi-Szabo L, Kocsis G. Examination of gastroesophageal reflux by transabdominal ultrasound: can a slow, trickling form of reflux be responsible for reflux esophagitis? Canadian Journal of Gastroenterology 2000; 14:588–592.

Norrashidah AW, Henry RL. Fundoplication in children with gastroesophageal reflux disease. Journal of Paediatrics and Child Health 2002; 38:156–159.

Orenstein SR. An overview of reflux-associated disorders in infants: apnea, laryngospasm, and aspiration. American Journal of Medicine 2001; 111 (Suppl 8A):60S–63S.

Pearl RH, Robie DK, Ein SH et al. Complications of gastroesophageal antireflux surgery in neurologically impaired versus neurologically normal children. Journal of Pediatric Surgery 1990; 25:1169–1173.

Salvia G, De Vizia B, Manguso F et al. Effect of intragastric volume and osmolality on mechanisms of gastroesophageal reflux in children with gastroesophageal reflux disease. American Journal of Gastroenterology 2001; 96:1725–1732.

Simanovsky N, Buonomo C, Nurko S. The infant with chronic vomiting: the value of the upper GI series. Pediatric Radiology 2002; 32:549–550.

Wenzl TG, Moroder C, Trachterna M et al. Esophageal pH monitoring and impedance measurement: a comparison of two diagnostic tests for gastroesophageal reflux. Journal of Pediatric Gastroenterology Nutrition 2002; 34:519–523.

ANAEMIA

Haemorrhage is the major manifestation of reflux oesophagitis and may be reflected in the presence of occult blood in the stool, haematemesis and, rarely, melaena. Iron-deficiency anaemia may develop in severe cases. Complaints of substernal pain are rare but dysphagia may cause irritability and anorexia in advanced cases.

FURTHER READING

Bohmer CJ, Niezen-de Boer MC, Klinkenberg-Knol EC et al. Gastroesophageal reflux disease in intellectually disabled individuals: leads for diagnosis and the effect of omeprazole therapy. American Journal of Gastroenterology 1997; 92:1475–1479.

Buchta RM, Bickerton R. A case of profound iron deficiency anemia owing to corrosive esophagitis in a 20-year-old developmentally delayed male. Journal of Adolescent Health 1994; 15:592–594.

Vinton NE. Gastrointestinal bleeding in infancy and childhood. Gastroenterology Clinics of North America 1994; 23:93–122.

RECURRENT RESPIRATORY SYMPTOMS

The coincidence of recurrent respiratory symptoms and GOR is a well-known phenomenon in children. GOR is also thought to play a causative role in subglottic stenosis, recurrent croup, apnoea, chronic cough bronchospasm and asthma. It is an important inflammatory cofactor in chronic sinusitis/otitis/bronchitis, in laryngomalacia and possibly in true vocal cord nodules and recurrent choanal stenosis. Recurrent pulmonary aspiration can lead to permanent lung damage with bronchiectasis and rarely pulmonary fibrosis. Twenty-four-hour oesophageal pH studies to evaluate GOR are recommended in patients presenting with chronic respiratory symptoms. With this method, however, only acid and alkaline GOR can be detected. Gastroesophageal reflux with an oesophageal pH within the physiological range may, despite being clinically relevant, be unrecognized by pH-metry. Demonstration of aspirated gastrointestinal content by gastroesophageal scintigraphy is the best evidence that the pulmonary problems are due to reflux. Despite frequent observation of respiratory symptoms,

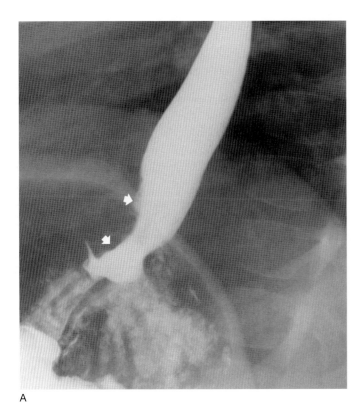

A

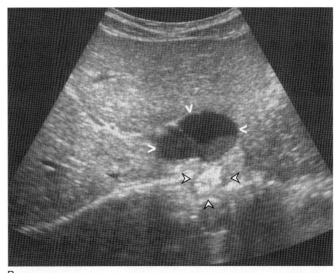

B

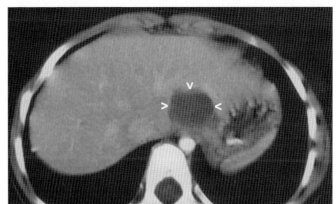

C

Figure 10.11.25 Oesophageal duplication cyst at the level of cardia. (A) Oesophagram shows evidence of an extrinsic intending mass (arrows). (B) Axial ultrasound scan at the level of cardia shows the cyst with fluid and debris (v) adjacent to the oesophageal wall (arrowheads). (C) Contrast-enhanced CT scan: fluid-filled cyst (v) at the gastroesophageal junction.

demonstration of aspirated radionuclide in the lungs is less frequently found. The absence of demonstrable aspiration may indicate that the respiratory symptoms depend on an involuntary mechanism of vagal type but does not exclude aspiration.

FURTHER READING

Bibi H, Khvolis E, Shoseyov D et al. The prevalence of gastroesophageal reflux in children with tracheomalacia and laryngomalacia. Chest 2001; 119:409–413.

Latini G, Del Vecchio A, De Mitri B et al. Scintigraphic evaluation of gastroesophageal reflux in newborns. La Pediatria Medica e Chirugica 1999; 21:115–117.

Sheikh S, Stephen T, Howell L et al. Gastroesophageal reflux in infants with wheezing. Pediatric Pulmonology 1999; 28:181–186.

Suskind DL, Zeringue GP 3rd, Kluka EA et al. Gastroesophageal reflux and pediatric otolaryngologic disease: the role of antireflux surgery. Archives of Otolaryngology: Head and Neck Surgery 2001; 127:511–514.

Wenzl TG, Silny J, Schenke S et al. Gastroesophageal reflux and respiratory phenomena in infants: status of the intraluminal impedance technique. Journal of Pediatric Gastroenterology and Nutrition 1999; 28:423–428.

APNOEA ATTACK, LARYNGOSPASM, NEAR-MISS COT DEATH AND SUDDEN INFANT DEATH SYNDROME

Reflux-induced apnoea affects nearly 1% of infants and involves laryngospasm as well as aspiration of milk. Both occurrences are suggested to be involved in acute life-threatening events (near-miss sudden infant death syndrome and sudden infant death syndrome). From epidemiological data, the role of gastroesophageal reflux in the aetiology of these life-threatening events is still unclear.

FURTHER READING

Gomes H, Lallemand P. Infant apnea and gastroesophageal reflux. Pediatric Radiology 1992; 22:8–11.

Orenstein SR. An overview of reflux-associated disorders in infants: apnea, laryngospasm, and aspiration. American Journal of Medicine 2001;111 (Suppl 8A):60S–63S.

Page M, Jeffery H. The role of gastroesophageal reflux in the aetiology of SIDS. Early Human Development 2000; 59:127–149.

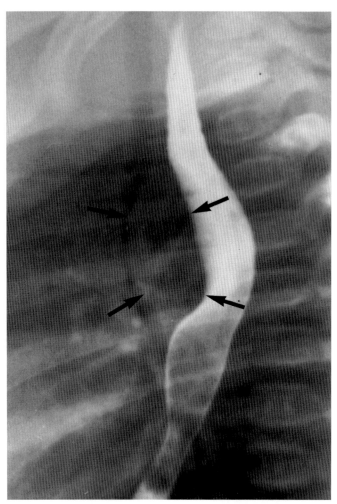

Figure 10.11.26 Bronchogenic cyst. Rarely, a bronchogenic cyst appears as a mass (arrows) between the oesophagus and the trachea, mimicking an aberrant left main pulmonary artery. From Strunger DS, Babyn PS. Paediatric Gastrointestinal Imaging and Intervention 2e. Hamilton: BC Decker Inc. © 2000.

Vandenplas Y, Hauser B. Gastroesophageal reflux, sleep pattern, apparent life threatening event and sudden infant death. The point of view of a gastroenterologist. European Journal of Pediatrics 2000; 159:726–729.

COWS' MILK SENSITIVE REFLUX OESOPHAGITIS

Cows' milk sensitive reflux oesophagitis is an emerging clinical entity in children, normally indistinguishable from primary GOR apart from the response to dietary antigen exclusion. Preliminary studies provide evidence to suggest a pathogenesis in which specific recruitment of T-cells and eosinophils may contribute to oesophageal dysmotility.

FURTHER READING

Butt AM, Murch SH, Ng CL et al. Upregulated eotaxin expression and T cell infiltration in the basal and papillary epithelium in cows' milk associated reflux oesophagitis. Archives of Disease in Childhood 2002; 87:124–130.

SANDIFER'S SYNDROME

Opisthotonus and maintenance of other abnormal head posturing in association with gastroesophageal reflux is known as Sandifer's syndrome. The manoeuvres are not due to neurological impairment but may be a mechanism to protect the airway or reduce acid reflux-associated pain. Symptoms cease with successful treatment.

HERBST TRIAD

Children with this diagnosis have digital clubbing and hypoproteinaemia associated with their GOR. After GOR is corrected, the other abnormalities disappear.

FURTHER READING

Herbst JJ, Johnson DG, Oliveros MA. Gastroesophageal reflux with protein-losing enteropathy and finger clubbing. American Journal of Disease in Childhood 1976; 130:1256–8.
Sacher P, Stauffer UG. The Herbst triad: report of two cases. Journal of Pediatric Surgery 1990; 25:1238–1239.

THE INFLAMMATORY POLYP-FOLD COMPLEX

The inflammatory polyp-fold complex is an uncommon endoscopic or radiological finding in children associated with reflux oesophagitis. In this complex, an inflammatory polyp at the gastroesophageal junction is present, often in continuity with a prominent gastric fold. Histologically, there is an inflammatory infiltrate in otherwise normal gastric and oesophageal mucosa.

FURTHER READING

Bishop PR, Nowicki MJ, Subramony C et al. The inflammatory polyp-fold complex in children. Journal of Clinical Gastroenterology 2002; 34:229–232.

TRANSVERSE FOLDS IN THE OESOPHAGUS – THE FELINE OESOPHAGUS

Fine transverse folds of the oesophagus are well described as a transient motor phenomenon seen in older children and adults with or without gastroesophageal reflux. They appear to be due to contraction of the muscularis mucosa and are thought to have little, if any, significance (Figure 10.11.32). Thin transverse folds or striations above the level of the aortic arch, producing a spiculated or serrated appearance in profile, are considered a normal variant in the adult oesophagus on double-contrast radiographs.

FURTHER READING

Cho KC, Gold BM, Printz DA. Multiple transverse folds in the gastric antrum. Radiology 1987; 164:339–341.
Levine MS, Low V, Laufer I et al. Focal spiculation of the upper thoracic esophagus: normal variant at double-contrast esophagography. Radiology 1992; 183:807–809.

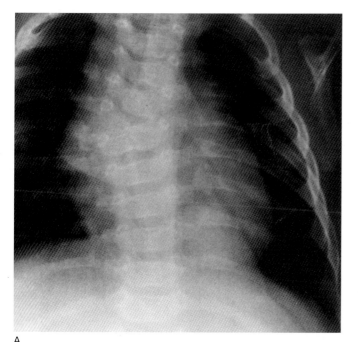

A

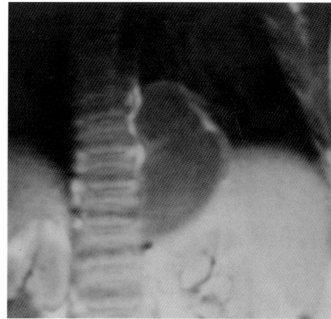

B

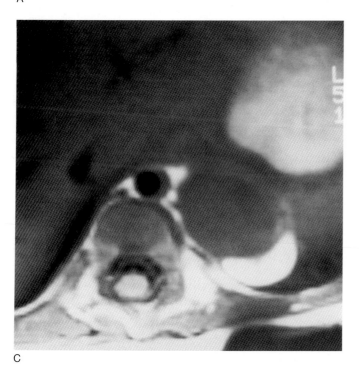

C

Figure 10.11.27 Neurenteric cyst. A large posterior mediastinal mass and associated mid-thoracic vertebral anomaly can be seen on the frontal chest radiograph (A). Coronal (B) and axial (C) MRI clearly shows the position of the mass adjacent to the thoracic vertebrae. From Stringer DA, Babyn PS. Paediatric Gastrointestinal Imaging and Intervention 2e. Hamilton: BC Decker Inc. © 2000.

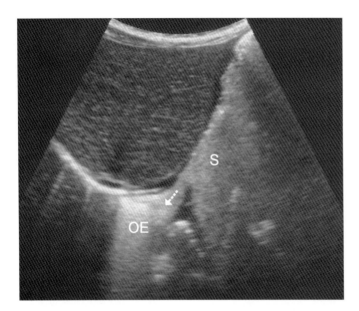

Figure 10.11.28 Gastroesophageal reflux. Ultrasonography: gastroesophageal reflux is seen as retrograde passage (arrow) of highly echogenic material towards the oesophagus (OE). S, stomach.

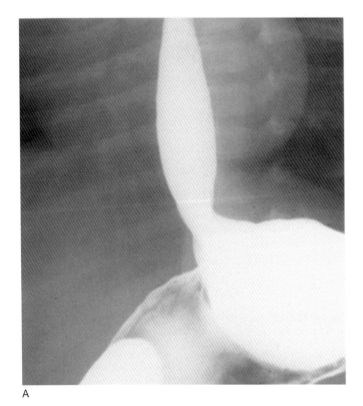

Figure 10.11.29 Gastroesophageal reflux. (A) A large volume of contrast material refluxes into the oesophagus. (B,C) The gastroesophageal junction is intermittently patulous (B).

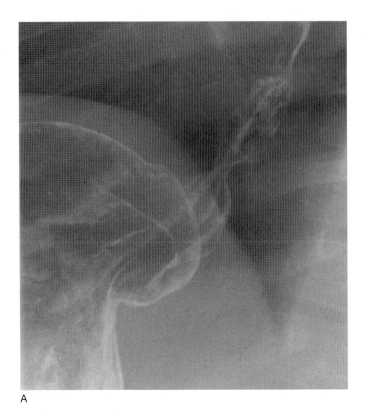

A

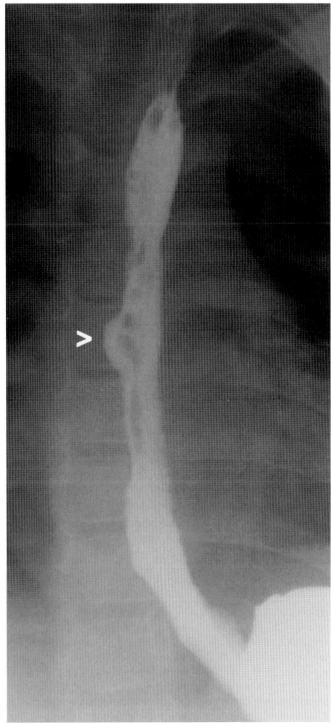

B

Figure 10.11.30 Sliding hiatal hernia with gastroesophageal reflux and deep ulcer from reflux oesophagitis. (A) Gastric rugae are seen in the hernia. (B) Severe oesophagitis with deep ulceration (v).

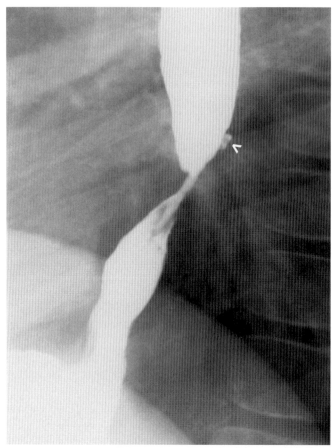

Figure 10.11.31 Peptic oesophageal stricture with ulcerations (v) at the proximal border due to longstanding gastroesophageal reflux since the newborn period. (Barrett's oesophagus could produce identical findings.)

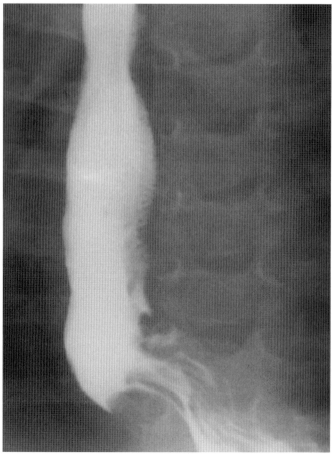

Figure 10.11.32 'Feline' oesophagus, gastroesophageal reflux disease. Multiple fine transverse folds are seen due to contractions of the longitudinally oriented muscularis mucosae. (Courtesy of Professor Ernst Richter, Hamburg, Germany.)

BARRETT'S OESOPHAGUS

Barrett's oesophagus is an acquired metaplastic condition in which there is replacement of the normal oesophageal mucosa with a gastric mucosa above the lower oesophageal sphincter. It is rare in childhood but carries the risk of malignant transformation into an adenocarcinoma. Patients who suffer from postoperative gastroesophageal reflux after correction of oesophageal atresia seem to be at risk for developing this metaplastic condition since it is predominantly acquired as a protective mechanism against longstanding gastroesophageal reflux and subsequent reflux oesophagitis. However, a non-acid peptic cause for the development of Barrett's oesophagus has also recently been described.

On double-contrast barium oesophagograms, the classic radiological feature consists of a high oesophageal stricture or ulcer often associated with a sliding hiatal hernia or gastroesophageal reflux. The unusual location of these strictures and ulcers can be attributed to the fact that they occur in the proximal zone of columnar metaplasia near the squamocolumnar junction. A reticular mucosal pattern associated with a stricture has also been described

as a relatively specific sign. The strictures may appear as ring-like constrictions or, less commonly, as smooth, non-distensible, tapered narrowing of the mid-to-distal oesophagus. In addition, focal mural deformity associated with fixed transverse folds and limited distensibility of the oesophagus may be found. Since both the specificity and sensitivity of radiographic findings in Barrett's oesophagus are limited, endoscopy and biopsy are required to diagnose this condition. At endoscopy, Barrett's oesophagus may be recognized by the presence of velvety, pinkish red islands or tongues of columnar mucosa extending above the gastroesophageal junction.

FURTHER READING

Heine RG, Cameron DJ, Chow CW et al. Esophagitis in distressed infants: poor diagnostic agreement between esophageal pH monitoring and histopathologic findings. Journal of Pediatrics 2002; 140:14–19.

Krug E, Bergmeijer JH, Dees J et al. Gastroesophageal reflux and Barrett's esophagus in adults born with esophageal atresia. American Journal of Gastroenterology 1999; 94:2825–2828.

The Stomach

Kamaldine Oudjhane

THE NORMAL STOMACH

The stomach is the widest segment of the digestive tract and lies below the left hemidiaphragm. The barium meal study is the classical imaging modality, followed by sonography, which can assess the stomach as early as the 14th week of gestation. The stomach is more transverse in position and of conoidal form in the infant. It gradually gains the longitudinal hook-shaped type in the older child. The stomach acts as a double organ, the fundus and the body are a reservoir, the antrum is more active in mixing food. A shallow peristalsis starts from the body towards the pylorus. Poor gastric mucosal coating on barium studies in children is related to an excess of gastric mucus. The gastric rugae or mucosal folds are not commonly seen in the neonate. They are more pronounced in the fundus and along the greater curvature. A lateral or right anterior oblique positioning of the patient helps in visualizing the pylorus and antrum on barium studies, since these areas are more posterior than in the adults. A 'waterfall' or 'cascade' type of stomach is not uncommon with the barium outlining the fundus as a pocket posterior to the body, which is more to the right and at an inferior level (Figure 10.12.1). This is not to be taken as gastric volvulus.

The gastroesophageal junction includes a sphincter around the gastroesophageal vestibule held by a phrenicoesophageal membrane. The non-distensible portion of the distal oesophagus should lie below the diaphragm and can be assessed by ultrasonography (US) (Figure 10.12.2). The muscle tone at the gastroesophageal junction does not mature until 8 weeks after birth. Some reflux is common in all infants, normal or physiological. Sonography outlines a gastric mucosa thickness of 3 mm or less (Figure 10.12.3). Higher resolution US can demonstrate at least four layers: an echogenic mucosa, a hypoechoic muscularis mucosa, an echogenic submucosa and a hypoechoic circular muscularis. Normal pylorus has a muscle thickness of 2 mm or less, with peristalsis through the channel. A variable amount of air is swallowed, especially with crying. In the supine position, air is seen in the antrum. There are challenges for the quantitative assessment of the gastric emptying rate with scintigraphy use of technetium (Tc) sulphur colloid mixed with food. The stomach empties more rapidly with liquids than with digestible or indigestible solids. Emptying is more prolonged with large meals and is at a slower rate with cows' milk versus human milk.

FURTHER READING

Gomes H, Lallemand A, Lallemand P. Ultrasonography of the gastroesophageal junction. Pediatric Radiology 1993; 23:94–99.
Heyman S. Gastric emptying in children. Journal of Nuclear Medicine 1998; 39:865–869.
Stringer DA, Daneman A, Brunelle F et al. Sonography of normal and abnormal stomach (excluding hypertrophic pyloric stenosis) in children. Journal of Ultrasound Medicine 1986; 5:183–188.

CONGENITAL ANOMALIES

GASTRIC MALPOSITION

The stomach is usually in the left upper quadrant in a situs solitus along with expected left cardiac apex and left-sided aorta and spleen. In polysplenia syndrome, gastric location may be on the left or right side of the abdomen or is indeterminate. A common abnormality is the intrathoracic stomach, with left diaphragmatic hernia; placement of a nasogastric tube with or without opacification helps confirm it. The stomach may project to the right of the dorsal spine, associated with hernia of the diaphragm hiatus. Such a situation favours volvulus of the stomach.

HIATAL HERNIA

There are two types of herniation of the stomach through the diaphragm hiatus. A paraoesophageal or rolling hiatal hernia, which is often large, is frequently asymptomatic. A chest radiograph may show a large air-containing mass usually over the right cardiophrenic angle (Figure 10.12.4). The sliding type of hiatal hernia is more common (Figure 10.12.5) but is less frequently seen in childhood than in adults. Incompetence of the lower oesophageal sphincter is usually associated with the condition. Barium meals demonstrate the type of hernia and potential complications such as gastroesophageal reflux and peptic oesophageal stricture (Figure 10.12.6). The oesophagus appears kinked. The stomach may be almost completely intrathoracic with rotation of its body along its longitudinal axis with a pylorus directed inferiorly. This organoaxial gastric volvulus results in pyloric obstruction. Symptomatic gastroesophageal reflux is a

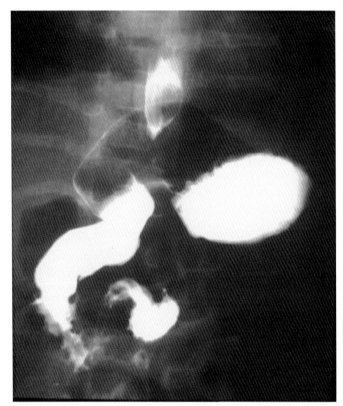

Figure 10.12.1 'Waterfall stomach'. Contrast fills first the fundus then cascades into the body and antrum.

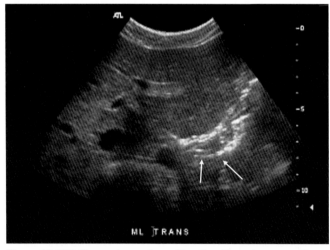

Figure 10.12.2 The gastroesophageal junction. Normal sonographic appearance (arrows), transverse view. The central echogenic mucosal outline is surrounded by hypoechoic muscularis.

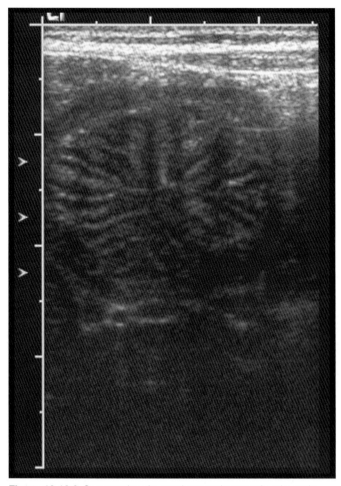

Figure 10.12.3 Sonography of normal stomach: smooth echogenic mucosal folds in an empty stomach.

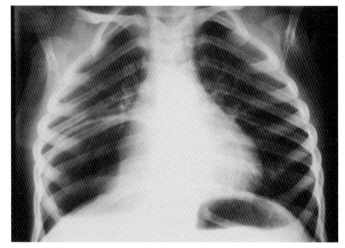

Figure 10.12.4 Hiatal hernia. A chest radiograph shows a round lucency projecting right to the dorsal spine, above the diaphragm.

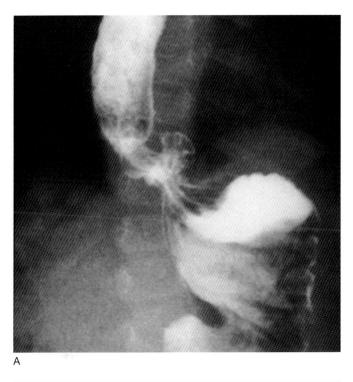

A

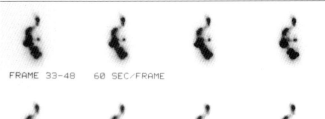

FRAME 33-48   60 SEC/FRAME

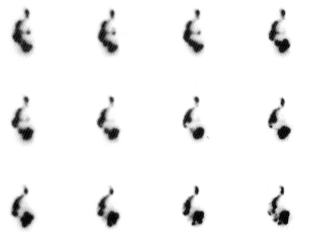

B

Figure 10.12.5 Hiatal hernia in an 11-month-old infant with omphalocele. (A) Barium meal demonstrates a sliding hiatal hernia. (B) Radionuclide scan depicts a severe oesophageal reflux in this baby who is failing to thrive.

good indication for surgical repair of the hernia. A fundoplication procedure such as the Nissen method acts as an antireflux measure. The plain postoperative radiograph can show a pseudotumour projecting into the fundus due to the wrapping of the fundus around the distal oesophagus with closure of the His angle. A barium meal outlines a narrow channel at the gastroesophageal junction sur-

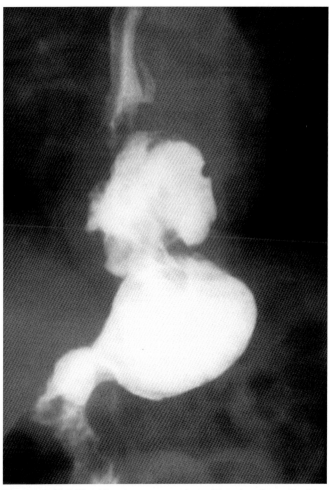

Figure 10.12.6 Hiatal hernia, paraoesophageal type in a 6-month-old infant. The contrast study outlines an incarcerated hernia above the diaphragm level, with spontaneous gastroesophageal reflux.

rounded by a mass effect. Postoperative complications may occur with dysphagia and failure of normal belching ability and inability to vomit. This is due to too tight wrap around. On the other hand, a paraoesophageal hernia may follow a Nissen repair (Figure 10.12.7).

GASTRIC VOLVULUS

Normal gastric fixation is obtained with the gastrohepatic, gastrophrenic, gastrosplenic and gastrocolic ligaments. The retroperitoneal position of the duodenum permits fixation of the stomach inferiorly. A diaphragmatic or ligamentous anomaly favours gastric volvulus. Asplenia is another associated condition. There are two types of gastric volvulus. The organoaxial variety is defined by rotation of the stomach along the longitudinal axis of its body. Symptoms are related to gastric outlet obstruction. Hyperaeration of the GI tract after enterocolitis seems to be a triggering factor. Radiography shows gas distension of the intestinal tract. A barium meal study outlines the characteristic uppermost position of the great curvature with the antropyloric axis pointing inferiorly. Prone

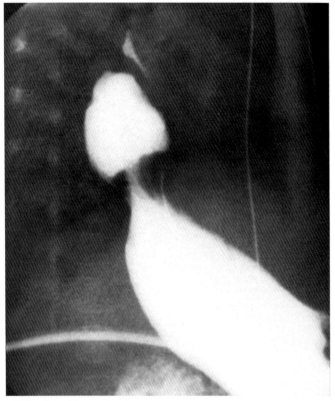

Figure 10.12.7 Hiatal hernia, postoperative appearance of a failed Nissen fundoplication with paraoesophageal hernia in a 3-month-old infant.

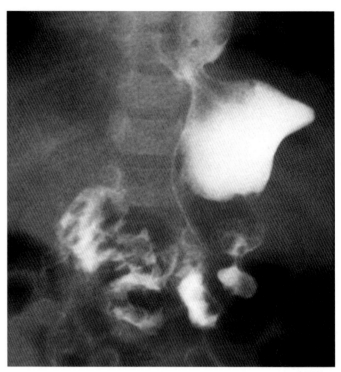

Figure 10.12.8 Microgastria in a 10-month-old infant with severe GE reflux. 10 cm³ of barium outline a small vertically oriented stomach with easy reflux in dilated oesophagus. The pylorus is positioned downward.

positioning seems to alleviate the abnormal shape of the stomach. Prominent vomiting is usually related to associated conditions such as hiatal hernia or pyloric stenosis.

Mesenteroaxial volvulus may occur at any age; it has acute onset, with feeding intolerance, retching without vomiting and epigastric pain. Severe distension with air–fluid levels and a beaked displaced antrum are the classical radiographic signs. Placement of a nasogastric tube may be precluded because of obstruction at the gastroesophageal junction. Mesenteroaxial volvulus is considered a surgical emergency and if left undiagnosed, the torsion results in strangulation, necrosis and gastric perforation.

MICROGASTRIA

Microgastria is a very rare congenital anomaly. It may be isolated or be part of the VACTERL sequence, or be seen with asplenia or mid-gut malrotation. The stomach is small, more vertical than normal with a pylorus pointing downward. There is frequent gastroesophageal reflux and a dilated oesophagus (Figure 10.12.8.). A small or absent fetal stomach after the 18th week of gestation is associated with a guarded prognosis. An absent stomach is seen in fetuses with oesophageal atresia or neurological conditions. A karyotype is appropriate when multiple morphological abnormalities are encountered.

GASTRIC ATRESIA/ANTROPYLORIC MEMBRANE

Gastric atresia is thought to result from failure of recanalization of the GI tract. A congenital familial form of gastric diaphragm has been described with an autosomal recessive inheritance pattern. An incomplete form may mimic pyloric stenosis and includes a diaphragm or membrane at the pylorus or antrum. A complete obstruction is evident with the absence of air distal to the stomach on the radiographs. Pyloric atresia has been reported in patients with epidermolysis bullosa and can occur in association with agenesis of the gallbladder and atresias at other segments of the intestine. Antenatal diagnosis of atresia is possible with evidence of isolated fetal gastric distension and polyhydramnios. On barium meal study, the antral diaphragm can be defined if a diagnostic pitfall of mucous strands is avoided (Figure 10.12.9). Sonography may outline it through a true sagittal approach of the stomach.

GASTRIC DUPLICATION

Gastric duplications constitute 7% of the enteric duplications (Figure 10.12.10). Three types are described:

- a non-communicating cystic form, usually arising from the greater curvature, presenting as a mass, often mistaken as a pancreatic pseudocyst;

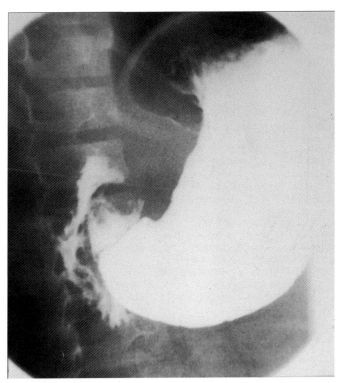

Figure 10.12.9 Antral web. 15-month-old infant with intermittent vomiting. The contrast study outlines the diaphragm in the antrum.

- a communicating tubular form is much rarer, parallel to the greater curvature;
- a very rare variety is a pedunculated cyst hanging from the stomach wall.

A cystic duplication may become communicating after peptic ulceration. The most frequent presentation is within the first 3 months of life with vomiting, an epigastric mass and haematemesis. At US, the definition of the typical bowel layers of the wall of the cyst is diagnostic. At CT, a cystic mass may have a liquid or mucoid content. Scintigraphy is useful. Correlative imaging is necessary in cases with associated anomalies of pancreatitis or ectopic spleen. True complete gastric duplication, carcinoma in a duplication cyst or multiple gastric cystic duplications are rarely encountered. Gastric diverticula correspond to communicating duplications. A pseudodiverticulum is thought to be related to herniation through a parietal gastric deficiency such as in patients with Ehlers–Danlos syndrome.

PANCREAS HETEROTOPIA

Aberrant pancreatic tissue in the gastric antrum is a cause of partial gastric outlet obstruction. Presenting symptoms include cyclic postprandial pain and vomiting. An upper GI study may delineate a smooth filling defect rising from the greater curvature with possible prolapse into the duodenum. Central umbilication may be seen in the mass.

FURTHER READING

Allison JW, Johnson JF, Barr LL et al. Induction of gastroduodenal prolapse by antral heterotopic pancreas. Pediatric Radiology 1995; 25:50–51.

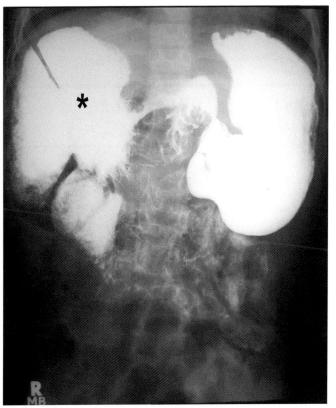

Figure 10.12.10 Gastric duplication in a 6-year-old boy. Postoperative barium meal study demonstrating normal situs of the stomach and opacification of another viscus in the right upper abdominal quadrant (*), after cyst-enterostomy. Preoperative diagnosis was confirmed by a positive nuclear Meckel scan in the right upper abdomen and gastric mucosal lining of the duplication on histology.

Al-Salem AH. Intrathoracic gastric volvulus in infancy. Pediatric Radiology 2000; 30:842–845.

Andiran F, Tanyel FC, Balkanci F et al. Acute abdomen due to gastric volvulus: diagnostic value of a single plain radiograph. Pediatric Radiology 1995; 25:S240.

Berrocal T, Torres J, Gutierrez J et al. Congenital anomalies of the upper gastrointestinal tract. Radiographics 1999; 19:855–872.

Dittrich JR, Spottswood SE, Jolles PR. Gastric duplication cyst. Scintigraphy and correlative imaging. Clinical Nuclear Medicine 1997; 22:93–96.

Dolan DR, Smith LT, Sybert VP. Prenatal detection of epidermolysis bullosa letalis with pyloric atresia in a fetus by abnormal ultrasound and elevated alpha fetoprotein. American Journal of Medical Genetics 1993; 47:395–400.

Heller RE, Fernbach SK. Two apparent suprarenal masses. Two cases in children: heterotaxy syndrome with spleen lying in suprarenal space and gastric duplication cyst lying in suprarenal space. Pediatric Radiology 2000; 30:400–403.

Koumanidou C, Montemarano H, Vakaki M et al. Perforation of multiple gastric duplication cysts: diagnosis by sonography. European Radiology 1999; 9:1675–1677.

Lund DP, Compton C. A 3 week-old girl with pyloric stenosis and an unexpected operative finding. Massachusetts General Hospital Case Records. Case 26-1999. New England Journal of Medicine 1999; 341:679–684.

Materne R, Clapuyt P, Saintmartin C et al. Gastric cystic duplication communicating with a bifid pancreas: a rare cause of recurrent pancreatitis. Journal of Pediatric Gastroenterology and Nutrition 1998; 27:102–105.

McKenna KM, Goldstein RB, Stringer MD. Small or absent fetal stomach: prognostic significance. Radiology 1995; 197:729–733.

McPherson RI. Gastrointestinal tract duplications: clinical, pathologic, etiologic and radiologic considerations. Radiographics 1993; 13:1063–1080.

Okoye BO, Patrikh DH, Buick RG et al. Pyloric atresia: five new cases, a new association, and a review of the literature with guidelines. Journal of Pediatric Surgery 2000; 35:1242–1245.

Pelizzo G, Lembo MA, Franchella A et al. Gastric volvulus associated with congenital diaphragmatic hernia, wandering spleen and intrathoracic left kidney: CT findings. Abdominal Imaging 2001; 26:306–308.

Segal SR, Sherman NH, Rosenberg HK et al. Ultrasonographic features of gastrointestinal duplications. Journal of Ultrasound Medicine 1004; 13:863–870.

GASTROESOPHAGEAL REFLUX

Gastroesophageal reflux is the retrograde passage of gastric contents into the oesophagus. It is different from regurgitation of food from the stomach to the mouth or vomiting. It may be considered normal when it is transient and/or of small volume. Major reflux is associated with clinical features such as heartburn, dysphagia, failure to thrive and iron deficiency anaemia. More confusing respiratory symptoms may be present, including asthma, apnoeas, acute life-threatening episodes or stridor. Many imaging modalities have been used in the work-up of gastroesophageal reflux. A standard upper GI study provides functional information on swallowing and gastric emptying and may show obstruction down to the duodenojejunal junction. Oesophageal pH monitoring is the 'gold standard' method in demonstrating acid reflux. Scintigraphy with milk scan demonstrates several episodes of reflux (Figure 10.12.5B) and possible lung aspiration. Gastroesophageal reflux is more frequent in children with cerebral palsy. In Sandifer's syndrome, there is an involuntary torsion spasm of the head and neck with abnormal posturing, in relation to massive gastroesophageal reflux.

FURTHER READING

Hanaa A, Alkhawari HA, Sinan TS et al. Diagnosis of gastrooesophageal reflux in children: comparison between oesophageal pH and barium examinations. Pediatric Radiology 2002; 32:765–770.

Hirsch W, Kedar R, Preib U. Color Doppler in the diagnosis of the gastroesophageal reflux in children: comparison with pH measurements and B mode ultrasound. Pediatric Radiology 1996; 26:232–235.

Miller JH. Upper gastrointestinal tract evaluation with radionuclides in infants. Radiology 1991; 178: 326–327.

Rudolph C, Mazur L, Lipjack G et al. Guidelines for evaluation and treatment of gastrooesophageal reflux in infants and children. Recommendations of the North American Society for Pediatric Gastroenterology and Nutrition. Journal of Pediatric Gastroenterology and Nutrition 2001; 32:S1–S29.

GASTRIC OUTLET OBSTRUCTION (Table 10.12.1)

There are many causes of delayed gastric emptying, including infections (bacterial toxins), myopathy, neuronal dysfunctions (vagotomy or central disorder), medications (anticholinergic) and metabolic disorders (hypocalcaemia, hypothyroidism). An anatomical obstruction must be searched for, such as hypertrophic pyloric stenosis, duodenal stenosis or malrotation.

FURTHER READING

Babyn P, Peled N, Manson D et al. Radiologic features of gastric outlet obstruction in infants after long term prostaglandin administration. Pediatric Radiology 1995; 25:41–43.

Callahan MJ, McCauley RG, Patel H et al. The development of hypertrophic pyloric stenosis in a patient with prostaglandin-induced foveolar hyperplasia. Pediatric Radiology 1999; 29:748–751.

Cohen HL, Zinn HL, Haller JO et al. Ultrasonography of pylorospasm: findings may simulate hypertropic pyloric stenosis. Journal of Ultrasound Medicine 1998; 17:705–711.

Hanquinet S, Damry N, Dassonville M et al. Gastric outlet obstructions: unusual ultrasonographic findings in the pyloric and antral regions. Pediatric Radiology 1995; 25:S163–S166.

Kobayashi N, Aida N, Nishimura G et al. Acute gastric outlet obstruction following the administration of prostaglandin: an additional case. Pediatric Radiology 1997; 27:57–59.

PYLORIC STENOSIS

The incidence of this frequent condition is 1 in 300 live births. It is more prevalent in males than in females, with a ratio of 5:1 and is more frequent in white than in black or oriental children. Instances of familial cases have been observed. Pyloric stenosis has been reported after erythromycin ingestion, in stressed babies with brain tumours or hydrocephalus, and in eosinophilic gastroenteritis or after prostaglandin-induced foveolar hyperplasia. It is seen following placement of transpyloric feeding tubes and its frequency is increased in children with tracheoesophageal fistula. Pyloric stenosis is defined by hypertrophy of the circular muscular fibres of the pylorus. Its aetiology is unknown but possible causes include gastric hypersecretion with resulting duodenal irritation and pylorospasm. Hyperplasia of the antral mucosa is a constant associated feature.

Immunohistochemical studies have shown there to be a decrease or absence of the glial cells with poor intrinsic innervation of the muscle layers of the pylorus. Clinically, postprandial projectile and alimentary vomiting begins around the third week of life. The appetite is, however, maintained. Weight loss, dehydration and hypochloremic alkalosis will develop as the vomiting persists. Constipation is usual but jaundice is rarely seen. Haematemesis is related to prepyloric gastric ulceration or oesophagitis. Diagnosis can certainly be made on purely clinical grounds, with the palpation of an 'olive' mass in the subhepatic region in an infant with the appropriate history. Antral peristaltic waves can be observed. The mass is reported in up to 80% of cases, however, the past decades have seen an increasing reliance on diagnostic tests, first with barium meal studies and now with sonography.

A simple plain radiograph in upright position delineates an air–fluid level in the stomach. Paucity of intestinal gas is related to dehydration. Gastric pneumatosis, of benign prognosis, is secondary to increased stomach pressure. An upper GI study is a very reliable diagnostic method, demonstrating dynamic and morphological signs of hypertrophic pyloric stenosis. Gastric distension can be so severe that a nasogastric tube placement is necessary for decompression. There is a delay in gastric emptying and opacifi-

Table 10.12.1 Gamut: the gastric outlet obstruction

1. Hypertrophic pyloric stenosis
2. Tumour
3. Chemical gastritis
4. Gastric volvulus
5. Antral diaphragm/atresia
6. Chronic granulomatous disease
7. Foveolar antral hyperplasia
8. Malposition of gastrostomy tube

cation of the pyloric channel. The pylorus is elongated and narrow (string sign) and this is constantly seen throughout the examination. The pylorus turns upward to the patient's left. A double track sign refers to the squeezing of the channel lumen by hypertrophic muscle (Figure 10.12.11). There is indentation on the antrum (shoulder sign) (Figure 10.12.12) and on the duodenal bulb (mushroom or umbrella sign) (Figure 10.12.13). The antrum is beaked if barium does not pass into the canal. An air contrast view of the pylorus, with the patient in oblique position or after manual compression, will outline the mass effect on the antrum as an 'olive on end' image. In less than 10% of cases, the diagnosis is more difficult with unusual appearances of the antropyloric area: funnel shape of the channel, asymmetrical impression on the cephalic aspect of the pylorus or spiculated narrowing of the canal. The barium study may also show hiatal hernia, a prepyloric membrane or gastroesophageal reflux.

Sonography is the imaging modality of choice in an infant with clinical presumption of pyloric stenosis with the sensitivity and specificity of this method approaching 100%. A high-frequency linear array transducer (5 MHz or greater) is used. The gallbladder, which is adjacent to the pylorus, is a good landmark. Classical signs of hypertrophic pyloric stenosis parallel the radiographic findings (Figure 10.12.14). The hypoechoic pyloric muscle is at least 3 mm thick and the elongated pyloric canal is at least 12 mm thick, muscle thickness being the most specific and sensitive sign for pyloric stenosis. The hypertrophic muscle may look non-uniform on transverse scanning of the pylorus. This is related to the sonographic artifact of anisotropic effect, because of the

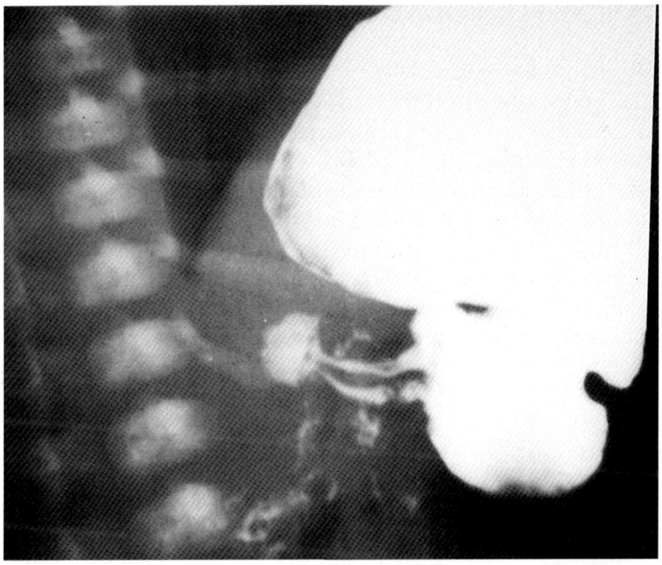

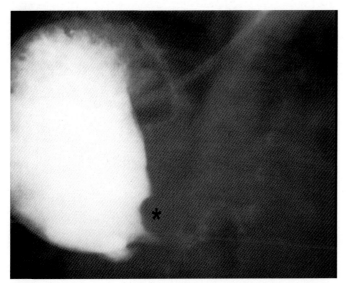

Figure 10.12.11 Pyloric stenosis: double track sign on an upper GI study.

Figure 10.12.12 Pyloric stenosis: barium meal showing the shoulder sign (*) due to indentation of the hypertrophic pyloric muscle on the antrum.

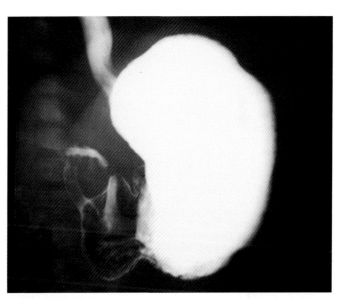

Figure 10.12.13 Pyloric stenosis: indentation of hypertrophic muscle on the duodenal bulb (umbrella or mushroom sign) seen on an upper GI study.

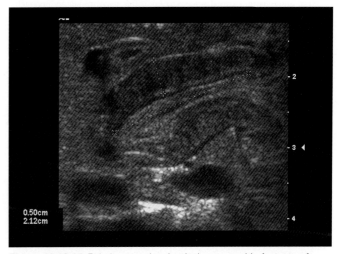

Figure 10.12.14 Pyloric stenosis: classical sonographic features of elongated and thickened hypoechoic pyloric muscle.

orientation of the muscle fibres. The pylorus may take a curved shape and it indents on the antrum. Redundant pyloric mucosa may protrude into the antrum (mucosal nipple sign). Antral peristalsis stops at the pylorus and gastric contents fail to pass into the duodenum.

US measurements support the visual impression of the echographic diagnosis; however, two possible pitfalls need to be recognized. First, pseudothickening of the muscle is related to tangential scanning through a contracted antrum. Second, gastric overdistension makes the examination difficult. This is solved by stomach decompression, feeding the patient with sugar water and scanning through the liver window. A challenge may occur in the case of a younger or premature neonate. Intermediate size of the muscle thickness (<3 mm) may represent early hypertrophy. Correction of the biochemical emergencies is a first priority then repeat US or even upper GI study can be performed after 24 h if necessary. In the postoperative patient, the muscle thickness gradually regresses to normal by 8 weeks following a successful pyloromyotomy.

FURTHER READING

Breaux CW, Hodd JS, Georgeson KE. The significance of alkalosis and hypochloremia in hypertrophic pyloric stenosis. Journal of Pediatric Surgery 1989; 24:1250–1252.

Godbole P, Sprigg A, Dickson JAS et al. Ultrasound compared with clinical examination in infantile hypertrophic pyloric stenosis. Archives of Disease in Childhood 1996; 75:335–337.

Haider S, Spicer R, Grier D. Ultrasound diagnosis in infantile hypertrophic pyloric stenosis. Determinants of pyloric length and the effect of prematurity. Clinical Radiology 2002; 57:136–139.

Hernanz-Schulman M, Sells LL, Ambrosino MM et al. Hypertrophic pyloric stenosis in the infant without a palpable olive: accuracy of sonographic diagnosis. Radiology 1994; 193:771–776.

Hernanz-Schulman M, Dinuaer P, Ambrosino MM et al. The antral nipple sign of pyloric mucosal prolapse: endoscopic correlation of a new sonographic observation in patients with pyloric stenosis. Journal of Ultrasound Medicine 1995; 14:283–290.

Hernanz-Schulman M, Neblett III WW, Polk DB et al. Hypertrophic pyloric mucosa in patients with hypertrophic pyloric stenosis. Pediatric Radiology 1998; 28:901.

Ito S, Tamura K, Nagae J et al. Ultrasonographic diagnostic criteria using scoring for hypertrophic pyloric stenosis. Journal of Pediatric Surgery 2000; 35:1714–1718.

Levine D, Edwards DK. The olive on end: a useful variant of the "shoulder" sign in the barium xray diagnosis of idiopathic hypertrophic pyloric stenosis. Pediatric Radiology 1992; 22:275–276.

Lijima T, Okamatsu T, Matsumura M et al. Hypertrophic pyloric stenosis associated with hiatal hernia. Journal of Pediatric Surgery 1996; 31:272–279.

Milla PJ. Motor disorders including pyloric stenosis. In: Walker WA, Durie PR, Hamilton JR, Walker-Smith JA, Watkins JB (eds). Pediatric gastrointestinal disease. Pathophysiology, diagnosis, management, 3rd edn. Hamilton: BC Decker Inc.; 2000:415–423.

Neilson D, Hollman AS. The ultrasonic diagnosis of infantile hypertrophic pyloric stenosis: technique and accuracy. Clinical Radiology 1994; 49:246–247.

Ozsvath RR, Poustchi-Amin M, Leonidas JC et al. Pyloric volume: an important factor in the surgeon's ability to palpate the pyloric "olive" in hypertrophic pyloric stenosis. Pediatric Radiology 1997; 27:175–177.

Poon TSC, Zhang A, Cartmill T et al. Changing patterns of diagnosis and treatment of infantile hypertrophic pyloric stenosis: a clinical audit of 303 patients. Journal of Pediatric Surgery 1996; 31:1611–1615.

Spevak MR, Ahmadjian JM, Kleinman PK et al. Sonography of hypertrophic pyloric stenosis: frequency and cause of non-uniform echogenicity of the thickened pyloric muscle. American Journal of Roentgenology 1992; 158:129–132.

OTHER CAUSES

ANTROPYLORIC DYSKINESIA

Pylorospasm or antropyloric dyskinesia is a functional disorder often seen in milk allergy or some forms of gastritis. The normal antrum peristalsis is of a systolic type with change in volume with stable length. In the case of pylorospasm, there is a persisting contraction. With barium studies, there is no indirect signs of pyloric stenosis. The gastric folds are thickened and there is delay in gastric emptying. On US, the pyloric muscle is less than 3 mm thick and the antral mucosa is thickened. Infants with pylorospasm respond to medical therapy (metoclopramide).

FOCAL FOVEOLAR MUCOSAL HYPERPLASIA

Focal foveolar mucosal hyperplasia develops following prostaglandin E1 and E2 (PGE1 and PGE2) therapy in infants with congenital heart disease to ensure patency of the ductus arteriosus. Persistent asymptomatic gastric distension can be seen within 48 h of initiation of treatment. Gastric outlet obstruction develops in association with long-term prostaglandin prescription (Figure 10.12.15). The antrum is narrow with a polypoid mucosal outline on an upper GI study. On US, the mucosal hyperplasia with thickening of mucosal folds correlates with histological findings of impacted interfoveolar mucin products and dilated mucosal glands (Figure 10.12.16). The obstruction disappears after therapy is

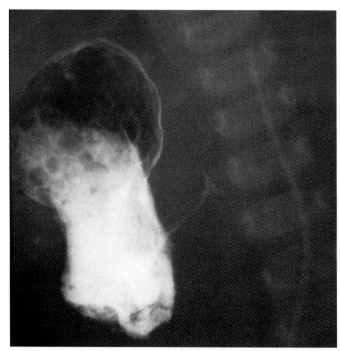

Figure 10.12.15 Foveolar mucosal hyperplasia. Upper GI study in a 10-week-old infant with gastric outlet obstruction and narrow elongated pylorus, with a history of necrotizing enterocolitis and prostaglandin therapy.

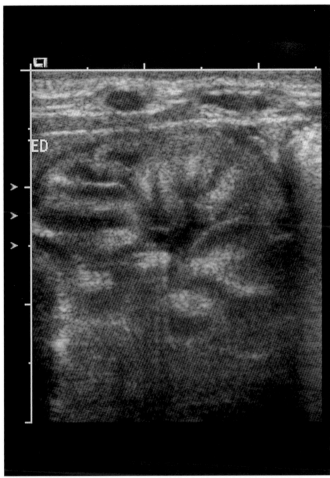

Figure 10.12.16 Prostaglandin-induced mucosal hyperplasia. Long-term prostaglandin therapy for hypoplastic left-heart syndrome. Vomiting. US depicts thickened mucosal folds, as distinct from Figure 10.12.3, which shows a normal stomach.

discontinued. True pyloric stenosis has been reported in the case of prostaglandin-induced foveolar hyperplasia.

Other rare causes of gastric outlet obstruction include gastro-duodenal intussusception from rare tumours, chronic granulomatous disease and extrinsic compression of the pylorus.

GASTRITIS

PEPTIC GASTRIC ULCER

Gastric ulcers are rare and are less common than duodenal ulcers. Stress ulcers may occur in response to burns, trauma or sepsis. *Helicobacter pylori*, a motile spiral organism, has been implicated in gastritis and peptic ulceration. The majority of infected persons remain asymptomatic. The mode of transmission is most likely person-to-person, probably from oropharyngeal secretions. The diagnosis is by culture, silver stain and the urease test. Abdominal pain is usual followed by possible haematemesis, vomiting and anaemia. Neonates and infants have a high perforation rate.

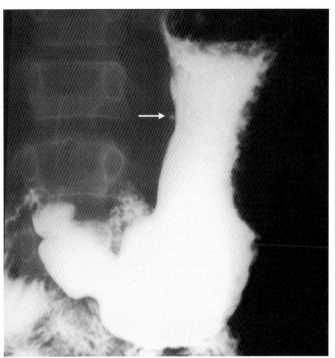

Figure 10.12.17 Peptic ulcer disease in an adolescent. The ulcer (arrow) is located at the upper zone of the lesser curvature.

Endoscopy remains the diagnostic 'gold standard'. A double-contrast barium study is, however, a very good screening method. A single-contrast study may show an ulcer as an outpouching in the lesser curvature (Figure 10.12.17). A large ulcer may be associated with folds radiating from a central niche. Multiple ulcers cause scarring and a thick gastric wall is evident on US. Sonography is useful in the follow-up of known lesions. Delay in gastric emptying in infants is related to the thickened deformed antropyloric region. Zollinger–Ellison syndrome is suspected in a patient with ulcer pain and watery diarrhoea. It includes severe peptic ulceration, gastric hypersecretion and pancreatic islet cell tumour. Gross hypertrophy of the gastric rugal folds is seen on barium meal examination. Small bowel follow-through studies may show a non-specific malabsorptive pattern with small bowel ulcerations.

FURTHER READING

Cello JP. Helicobacter pylori and peptic ulcer disease. American Journal of Roentgenology 1995; 164:283–286.
Chelimsky G, Czinn S. Peptic ulcer disease in children. Pediatrics in Review 2001; 22:349–354.
Ernst PB, Gold BD. Helicobacter pylori in childhood: new insights into the immunopathogenesis of gastric disease and implications for managing infection in children. Journal of Pediatric Gastroenterology and Nutrition 1999; 28:462–743.
O'Hara SM. Acute gastrointestinal bleeding. Radiology Clinics of North America 1997; 35:879–895.

GASTRITIS/CLASSIFICATION

Inflammation of the stomach wall has multiple aetiologies. The primary form includes eosinophilic gastritis; the varioliform includes gastritis and Crohn's disease. Secondary gastritis is related to medications (steroids, aspirin, non-steroidal anti-inflammatory drugs (NSAIDs)), local infections and stressed patients with sepsis and burns. Endoscopy is the definite modality for diagnosis with a possibility of tissue biopsy. Radiological diagnosis is best made with the double-contrast technique. Radiological classification of gastritis includes the erosive, corrosive, emphysematous and miscellaneous forms.

EROSIVE GASTRITIS

The erosive form of gastritis is seen in adolescents who take aspirin. On double-contrast meal study, there is a varioliform pattern of erosions with small punctate or slit-like collections of barium surrounded by a radiolucent halo of mucosal oedema. These lesions are mostly in the antrum, with a size of 3–11 mm. On US, thickening of the gastric wall is shown. This finding, however, is non-specific and is also present in gastric malignancy and portal hypertension gastropathy.

CORROSIVE GASTRITIS

The corrosive form of gastritis is secondary to ingestion of acid but also occurs in up to 20% of patients following alkali ingestion. Endoscopy allows assessment of extent of the lesions but may fail because of oedema at the gastroesophageal junction. Barium studies and US may delineate the sequelae of inflammation with fibrosis and aperistaltic narrowing in the antrum. Sonography with fluid distension of the stomach may demonstrate submucosal thickening from fibrosis. Acute iron ingestion causes diffuse thickening of the gastric wall with a non-specific ileus.

EMPHYSEMATOUS GASTRITIS

Emphysematous gastritis is associated with gas in the stomach wall. It occurs rarely in infants, usually following gastroenteritis. Other causes include pneumatosis intestinalis or are secondary to bowel obstruction, gastric volvulus or after endoscopy. Plain radio-graphs or CT demonstrate the gas tracking within the wall.

MISCELLANEOUS GASTRITIS

CROHN'S DISEASE

Crohn's disease of the stomach is rare but when present it usually produces mucosal irregularity and antral narrowing. Subtle umbilicated aphthae may be the earliest signs on a double-contrast study. Gastric involvement in Crohn's disease is very rare but may be associated with a poor prognosis.

EOSINOPHILIC GASTROENTERITIS

This causes a nodular pattern of the mucosal outline of the antrum. Toxoplasmosis and candidiasis infection may affect the stomach in immunodepressed children. Toxoplasmosis may manifest with antrum narrowing. Other causes of stomach involvement in AIDS patients include lymphoma as well as cryptosporidiosis and cytomegalovirus infection.

MÉNÉTRIER DISEASE

This disease is rare in childhood. It is a giant hypertrophic gastritis with prominent gastric folds, excess of mucous secretions, protein-losing enteropathy and clinical peripheral oedema. Symptoms include nausea, vomiting and loose bowel movements. There are two forms of the disease: acute and chronic. The acute form, which is self-limiting, is usually seen in childhood. An association with cytomegalovirus and *Helicobacter pylori* has been reported. The incidence of gastric carcinoma may be higher in Ménétrier disease. The radiological diagnosis is made by demonstration of hypertrophic tortuous gastric folds in the fundus and body of the stomach.

HENOCH–SCHÖNLEIN PURPURA

This condition may cause antral wall thickening and gastric outlet obstruction (Figure 10.12.18).

CHRONIC GRANULOMATOUS DISEASE

This disease is an inherited defect in neutrophil function. Recurrent infections with granuloma and abscess formation may affect many organs (liver, lungs, lymph nodes). Gastric involvement manifests as antrum narrowing. A stiff and narrow antropyloric area is observed on sonography.

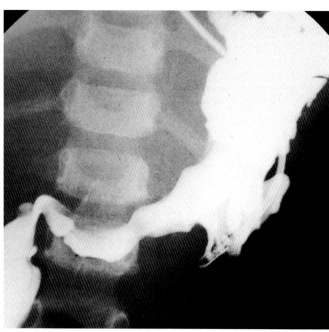

Figure 10.12.18 Henoch–Schönlein purpura in a 4-year-old boy with abdominal pain, vomiting, haematemesis and purpura in the buttocks and feet. The upper GI shows irregular narrowing of a thick antrum.

FURTHER READING

Aviram G, Kessler A, Reif S. Corrosive gastritis: sonographic findings in the acute phase and follow-up. Pediatric Radiology 1997; 27:805–806.

Manson DE, Stringer DA, Durie PR et al. The radiologic and endoscopic investigation and etiologic classification of gastritis in children. Journal of the Canadian Association of Radiology 1990; 41:201–206.

Sferra TJ, Pawel BR, Qualman SJ et al. Menetrier disease of childhood: role of cytomegalovirus and transforming growth factor alpha. Journal of Pediatrics 1996; 128:213–219.

Smith FJ, Taves DH. Gastroduodenal involvement in chronic granulomatous disease of childhood. Journal of the Canadian Association of Radiology 1992; 43:215–217.

Takaya J, Kawamura Y, Kino M et al. Menetrier's disease evaluated serially by abdominal ultrasonography. Pediatric Radiology 1997; 27:178–180.

GASTRIC NEOPLASMS

All forms of gastric neoplasms are rare. They are less frequent than extrinsic indentation of the stomach by mass lesions such as pancreatic pseudocyst, splenic or choledochal cyst, GI duplication cyst, splenomegaly, haematoma due to trauma or a bleeding diathesis, retroperitoneal tumour or lymphangioma. Symptoms are those of a feeding intolerance. Clinical suspicion of a mass is best approached first by sonography.

BENIGN TUMOURS

BENIGN LYMPHOID HYPERPLASIA

This is a rare entity. It is usually associated with immunoglobulin abnormalities. At US there is a thickened antrum and a barium meal study delineates gastric nodules.

INTRAMURAL GASTRIC HAEMATOMA

This is a rare manifestation of haemophilia that might present as a mass.

PANCREATIC REST

Pancreatic rest is located within the gastric mucosa; it may mimic a gastric neoplasm.

POLYPS

Gastric polyps have been reported in children with different conditions such as Coffin–Siris syndrome or Cowden's disease. Gastric polyps can be part of polyposis syndromes such as Gardner's syndrome, Peutz–Jeghers syndrome or familial polyposis. In the latter, many gastric polyps are regenerative. Adenomatous polyps are seen in Gardner's syndrome. Double-contrast studies demonstrate small polyps but endoscopy is necessary. Gastric inflammatory pseudotumours or plasma cell granulomas simulate malignancy and present with fever, pain and anaemia.

Other rare tumours are often mesenchymal; they are seen in adolescents and include lipoma, neurofibroma, haemangioma or carcinoid.

GASTRIC TERATOMA

Gastric teratoma usually presents in infancy with a strong male predominance. A palpable mass is responsible for abdomen distension, respiratory distress and haematemesis. Preoperative diagnosis is difficult since renal or hepatic tumours and adrenal haemorrhage mimic the teratoma of the stomach. US and CT show a well-defined mass with cystic and solid components with areas of fat and calcification (Figure 10.12.19).

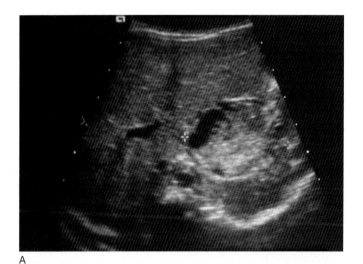

A

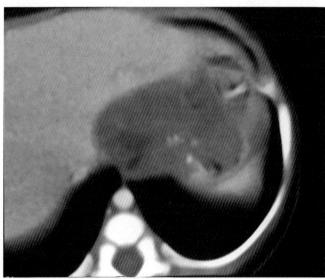

B

Figure 10.12.19 Gastric teratoma in a neonate with vomiting for 2 weeks. (A) US shows a complex mass at the wall of the lesser gastric curvature. (B) CT: focal fat and calcifications identified.

MALIGNANT TUMOURS

GASTRIC CARCINOMA

Gastric carcinoma is rare in childhood. *Helicobacter pylori* has been implicated in its pathogenesis. Carcinoma is associated with familial polyposis coli and has an increased incidence in children who recover from therapy for other malignancies.

LYMPHOMA

Gastric lymphoma may be present in children (Figure 10.12.20); it is usually the B-cell type. *Helicobacter pylori* may play a role in the development of the non-Hodgkin variety.

LEIOMYOSARCOMA

Coexistence of gastric and oesophageal leiomyosarcoma, pulmonary chondroma and functional extra-adrenal paraganglioma constitute the Carney's triad (Figure 10.12.21). Children with ataxia-telangiectasia have an increased incidence of lymphoma of the GI tract. Barium studies of gastric malignancies demonstrate nodular mass lesions, mucosal irregularity and ulceration and thickening of the gastric wall. Cross-sectional imaging modalities delineate the size and extent of the mass.

FURTHER READING

Al-Hilaly N, Kwiatkowski D, Gould S et al. Gastric leiomyosarcoma presenting as severe iron-deficiency anaemia. Journal of Pediatric Gastroenterology and Nutrition 1999; 29:354–357.

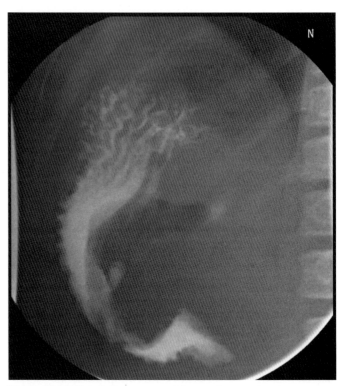

Figure 10.12.21 Leiomyosarcoma at the greater curvature in a teenager with Carney's triad. The upper GI study shows a large mass with ulcer.

Dunlap JP, James CA, Maxson RT et al. Gastric teratoma with intramural extension. Pediatric Radiology 1995; 25:383–384.
Gupta AK, Berry M, Mitra DK. Ossified gastric leiomyoma in a child: a case report. Pediatric Radiology 1995; 25:48–49.
Harned RK. The hamartomatous polyposis syndromes: clinical and radiological features. American Journal of Roentgenology 1995; 164:565–571.
Hoppin AG. Esophageal and gastric neoplasms. In: Walker WA, Durie PR, Hamilton JR, Walker-Smith JA, Watkins JB (eds). Pediatric gastrointestinal disease. Pathophysiology, diagnosis, management, 3rd edn. Hamilton: BC Decker Inc.; 2000:405–414.
Levine MS, Elmas N, Furth EF et al. Helicobacter pylori and gastric MALT lymphoma. American Journal of Roentgenology 1996; 166:86–88.

MISCELLANEOUS GASTRIC PATHOLOGY

BEZOARS

Bezoars are formed from ingested materials, which collect in the stomach and small bowel. There are three main types of bezoars: lactobezoars, trichobezoars and miscellaneous bezoars. Lactobezoars are due to undigested milk curds, mostly occurring in infancy, because of incorrectly reconstituted powdered milk (Figure 10.12.22). Abdominal distension is common. Medical treatment ensures a favourable course. Phytobezoars are formed from fibres, for example, from persimmon, coconut fibres or celery. Fibre accumulation may occur in patients who have had partial gastrectomy or gastrojejunostomy. Myotonia dystrophica

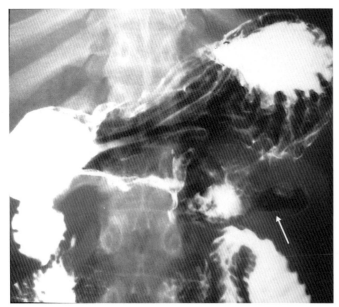

Figure 10.12.20 Gastric lymphoma in a 17-year-old boy with non-Burkitt lymphoma with ulcerated infiltrative mass along the greater curvature (arrow).

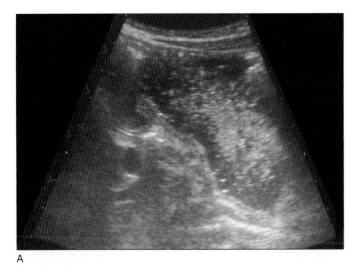
A
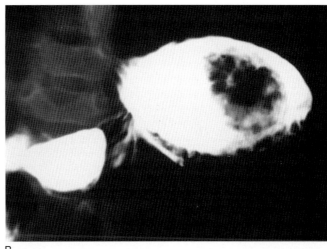
B

Figure 10.12.22 Lactobezoar in a 6-month-old infant. (A) US: echogenic contents in the stomach. (B) Barium study outlining the formed milk curds.

may induce a food bezoar because of decreased gastric peristalsis. Trichobezoars, mainly affecting females, are far commoner in childhood than in adults. They usually occur in emotionally disturbed children. Anorexia, loss of weight, vomiting, foul breath, alopecia and abdominal mass are the main physical findings. Miscellaneous bezoars are of a more solid character, including shellac, tar and dirt. Complications of bezoars include ulceration, perforation, abscess, haematemesis and intestinal obstruction. Rapunzel syndrome refers to the manifestation of long tail trichobezoars presenting as an obstruction from a mass in the stomach and small bowel. On plain radiographs, a mottled gastric shadow mimics food. The bezoar is a heterogeneously echogenic mass. A trichobezoar may get barium coating in its crevices. Treatment of gastric trichobezoar is usually surgical despite attempts at endoscopic removal.

FOREIGN BODY INGESTION

The majority of cases of ingestion of foreign bodies occur in children between 6 months and 5 years of age, coins being the most common. In older children, ingestion is usually accidental or associated with psychiatric disorders. Sharp objects include needles, pins, batteries and toy parts (Figure 10.12.23). Caustic substance or acid ingestion will result in a corrosive effect. Usually an intragastric foreign body is passed within 4–7 days. Disc batteries are differentiated from coins because of their double density profile and a step-off lateral outline on radiographs. Mercury poisoning is a theoretical concern. Zinc-based coins, when retained in the stomach, may develop radiolucent corrosions and constitute an indication for endoscopic removal. Abdominal radiographs may be helpful in identifying radiopaque iron tablets (Figure 10.12.24) but are not mandatory for the management of an overdose. Complications are rare and are mainly antral strictures. Sharp objects may perforate the bowel and lead paint ingestion can cause lead poisoning. In practice, a radiographic foreign body survey assesses a wide area from mouth to rectum.

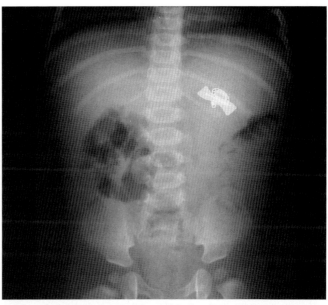

Figure 10.12.23 Foreign body ingestion. Swallowed metallic hair clip in the stomach.

GASTRIC DILATATION/ PNEUMATOSIS/RUPTURE

Gastric pneumatosis may be isolated but is usually associated with gastric outlet obstruction (Figure 10.12.25). Necrotizing enterocolitis is a common cause and may be accompanied by its other stigma, portal venous gas. Acute gastric dilatation may be accompanied by pneumatosis. It may represent ileus in response to various insults (Figure 10.12.26), abdominal trauma, diabetic ketoacidosis or a postoperative state after scoliosis surgery. Use of

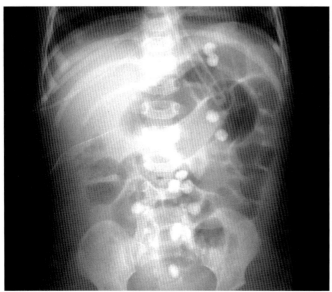

Figure 10.12.24 Iron pills ingestion: multiple radiopaque pills identified throughout the GI tract on this radiograph.

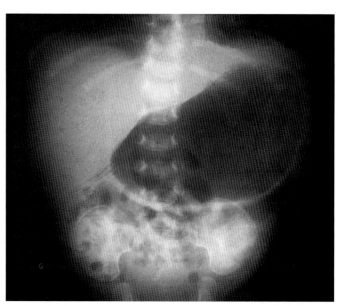

Figure 10.12.26 Acute gastric dilatation in an infant post-bone marrow transplant for severe combined immunodeficiency: early sign of gastric involvement of graft versus host disease.

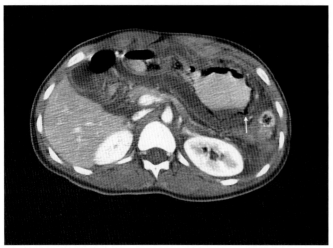

Figure 10.12.25 Gastric pneumatosis in an 11-year-old boy with cerebral palsy. Acute deterioration of respiratory distress and pneumoperitoneum. Thick oedematous gastric wall and mural pneumatosis (arrow) seen on CT. Patient with gastric outlet obstruction and superior mesenteric artery syndrome.

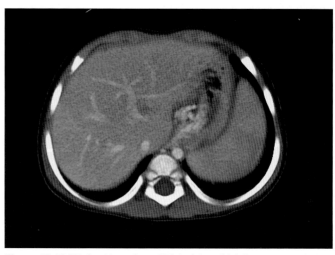

Figure 10.12.27 Gastric varices: CT depicts a thick lesser curvature and associated varices at the gastroesophageal junction area.

mydriatics in a newborn can result in severe acute distension. Initiation of prostaglandin therapy results in gastric dilatation within 48 h. Children with H-type tracheoesophageal fistula may present with severe gastric distension due to resuscitation. A more chronic condition is seen in neglected children and in pathological aerophagia or air swallowing. Gastric perforation is rare in blunt trauma. Spontaneous rupture of the stomach in neonates may occur in situations of stress with selective ischaemia, in peptic ulcer or with duodenal obstruction. Iatrogenic gastric perforation has been described with ventriculoperitoneal shunt tube or nasogastric tubes.

GASTRIC INFARCTION/VARICES

Gastric infarction should be included in the differential diagnosis of a dilated aperistaltic stomach. Predisposing factors include mesenteroaxial gastric volvulus and, in the neonate, the conjunction of broad antibiotic therapy and asphyxia state. Gastric varices are located in the submucosa of the fundus and upper part of the gastric body. They are associated with oesophageal varices in patients with portal hypertension (Figure 10.12.27). On plain radiograph or barium studies, they may manifest as polypoid projections in the fundus. Portal hypertensive gastropathy is an endoscopic entity with ectasia of mucosal and submucosal capillaries and venules. Only the most severe cases of gastropathy tend to bleed.

POSTOPERATIVE PROBLEMS

Percutaneous gastrostomy is replacing traditional methods of long-term enteral alimentation of sick and malnourished children. Potential complications include malposition or migration of the catheter or a leak. This is assessed by fluoroscopy with injection of iso-osmolar water-soluble contrast medium. Gastrojejunostomy tubes have a risk of jejunal intussusception. Children with neurological impairment may suffer gastric and intestinal dysmotility following gastrostomy. This presents as pain and retching. It is often only related to feeding. Contrast studies should initially be done with water-soluble contrast but then followed by 'a feeding study' in which the food is mixed with contrast and the child fed normally in an attempt to mirror the clinical situation in which symptoms occur. Poor gastric and intestinal peristalsis with delayed emptying are often seen.

FURTHER READING

Chen HR, Beierle EA. Gastrointestinal foreign bodies. Pediatric Annals 2000; 30:736–742.

Christoph CL, Poole CA, Kochan PS. Operative gastric perforation: a rare complication of ventriculoperitoneal shunt. Pediatric Radiology 1995; 25:S173–S174.

Donnelly LF, Paterson A. Feeding intolerance secondary to marked hepatosplenomegaly compressing the stomach in children. Pediatric Radiology 2000; 30:653.

Everson GW, Oudjhane K, Young LW et al. Effectiveness of abdominal radiographs in visualizing chewable iron supplements following overdose. American Journal of Emergency Medicine 1989; 7:459–463.

Hyams JS, Treem WR. Portal hypertensive gastropathy in children. Journal of Pediatric Gastroenterology and Nutrition 1993; 17:13–18.

Kawano S, Tanaka H, Daimon Y et al. Gastric pneumatosis associated with duodenal stenosis and malrotation. Pediatric Radiology 2001; 31:656–658.

Koplewitz BZ, Daneman A, Fields S et al. Case 29: Gastric trichobezoar and subphrenic abscess. Radiology 2000; 217:739–742.

Kriss VM, Desai NS. Relation of gastric distention to prostaglandin therapy in neonates. Radiology 1997; 203:219–221.

Lee JM, Jung SE, Lee KY. Small bowel obstruction caused by phytobezoar: MR imaging findings American Journal of Roentgenology 2002; 179:538–539.

Maves MD, Lloyd TV, Carithers JS. Radiographic identification of ingested disc batteries. Pediatric Radiology 1986; 16:154–156.

McLaughlin RF, So CB, Gray RR. Fluoroscopically guided percutaneous gastrostomy: current status. Journal of the Canadian Association of Radiology 1996; 47:10–15.

O'Hara S, Donnelly LF, Chuang E et al. Gastric retention of zinc-based pennies: radiographic appearance and hazards. Radiology 1999; 213:113–117.

Ripolles T, Garcie-Agonoyu J, Nartinez MJ et al. Gastrointestinal bezoars: sonographic and CT characteristics. American Journal of Roentgenology 2001; 177:65–69.

Sarici SU, Yurdakök M, Ünal S. Acute gastric dilatation complicating the use of mydriatics in a preterm newborn. Pediatric Radiology 2001; 31:581–583.

Saverymuttu AH, Corbishley CM, Maxwell JD et al. Thickened stomach – an ultrasound sign of portal hypertension. Clinical Radiology 1990; 41:17–18.

Sinzig M, Umschaden HW, Haselbach H et al. Gastric trichobezoar with gastric ulcer: MR findings. Pediatric Radiology 1998; 28:296.

West WM, Duncan ND. CT appearances of the Rapunzel Syndrome: an unusual form of bezoar and gastrointestinal obstruction. Pediatric Radiology 1998; 28:315–316.

Wollman B, D'Agostino HB, Walus-Wiele JR et al. Radiologic, endoscopic and surgical gastrostomy: an institutional evaluation and meta analysis of the literature. Radiology 1995; 197:699–704.

The Duodenum

Peter J Strouse

EMBRYOGENESIS

The duodenum originates from the caudal portion of foregut and cranial portion of midgut, demarcated by the origin of the bile duct. Early in development, at 5–6 weeks gestation, the lumen is obliterated by epithelium. Later in embryogenesis, by 8 weeks gestation, the lumen is recanalized. During rotation of the midgut, the doudenum assumes its C-loop course. Except for the first portion, the duodenum becomes fixed in the retroperitoneum.

NORMAL ANATOMY AND RADIOGRAPHIC APPEARANCE

The first portion of the duodenum, the duodenal bulb, is intraperitoneal. The remainder of the duodenum is retroperitoneal. The second portion of the duodenum descends to the right of the pancreatic head. The third portion extends back to the left, across the midline. The fourth portion then extends cephalad to meet the jejunum. The duodenojejunal junction, the ligament of Trietz, is normally to the left of the spine and at approximately the level of the pylorus. On a lateral view, the second through fourth portions of the duodenum project posteriorly near the spine, due to their retroperitoneal location. Together, the four portions of the duodenum form a C-loop, encircling the pancreatic head. The ampulla of Vater may be occasionally identified on barium studies along the medial margin of the second portion of the duodenum. Normal impressions on the duodenum may be seen due to the common bile duct, the gallbladder, and the superior mesenteric artery and spine. Proximally, the duodenal mucosa is smooth (Figure 10.13.1). The folds are more pronounced distally. Transit of barium through the duodenum is usually rapid. Substantial delay in passage of barium through the duodenum should raise concern for underlying pathology. Under normal circumstances, little gas is seen in the duodenum on radiographs.

CONGENITAL AND DEVELOPMENTAL

LATE PRESENTATION OF CONGENITAL DUODENAL OBSTRUCTION

Most congenital lesions causing duodenal obstruction present in the newborn or neonatal period. A detailed discussion is found in the chapter on the neonatal duodenum. Occasionally, when the obstruction is not complete, the patient may not present until a later age. Congenital abnormalities that may cause partial duodenal obstruction include duodenal stenosis, duodenal web and windsock diverticulum, annular pancreas and preduodenal portal vein. Frequently, these abnormalities coexist in the same patient (Figure 10.13.2). Some children with malrotation may also have chronic partial duodenal obstruction due to bands or a partial volvulus.

DUODENAL STENOSIS

Duodenal stenosis, like duodenal atresia, is probably the result of failure of recanalization of the duodenal lumen. Duodenal stenosis is less common than duodenal atresia. Most patients present in the neonatal period. The clinical severity and onset of symptoms in a patient with duodenal stenosis is dependent on the degree of obstruction. Children may remain relatively asymptomatic until they begin to eat solid food. Symptoms include vomiting, abdominal pain, failure to thrive and halitosis. Halitosis is due to retained undigested food. There is an association with trisomy 21. Radiographs of a patient with a delayed diagnosis of duodenal stenosis may show gaseous distension of the duodenum; the bowel gas pattern is otherwise normal. Occasionally, retained foreign bodies may be seen (Figure 10.13.3). The diagnosis is confirmed by an upper GI examination, showing dilatation of the duodenum proximal to the point of obstruction with an abrupt calibre change. The point of obstruction is usually in the second or third portion of the duodenum. Food debris or retained foreign bodies may be seen as filling defects within the dilated duodenum.

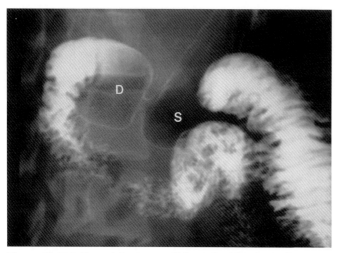

Figure 10.13.1 Normal duodenum. Oblique view shows a well distended normal duodenal bulb and proximal duodenum. The duodenal fold pattern is normal. S, stomach.

DUODENAL WEB OR DUODENAL DIAPHRAGM

Duodenal web or duodenal diaphragm produces a focal stenosis of the duodenum. The aetiology is also likely to be a failure of recanalization of the duodenal lumen. Usually the web is located near the ampulla of Vater. With time, pressure from duodenal contents and peristalsis may stretch the web distally producing a windsock-shaped obstructing membrane (intraluminal duodenal diverticulum) anchored proximally at its edges and containing a small aperture for passage of duodenal contents. The clinical severity and onset of symptoms in a patient with duodenal web or windsock diverticulum is dependent on the degree of obstruction. Most patients present in the neonatal period; however, patients with lesser obstruction may present later in childhood, even in adolescence. Symptoms include recurrent abdominal pain, nausea and vomiting, halitosis and failure to thrive. Plain films are usually normal but may show gaseous distension of the proximal duodenum. Proximal duodenal dilatation may also be seen on upper GI examination. In such cases, the duodenal web may be obvious. If the proximal duodenum is less dilated, the duodenal web may be subtle (Figure 10.13.4). The web may be seen as a thin, curvilinear filling defect, which may not be visible in all projections (Figure 10.13.5).

ANNULAR PANCREAS AND PREDUODENAL PORTAL VEIN

Annular pancreas and preduodenal portal vein are not infrequently associated with duodenal stenosis, duodenal web or malrotation. In fact, annular pancreas may be a secondary manifestation of maldevelopment of the duodenum. Annular pancreas is due to anomalous pancreatic tissue encircling the second portion of the duodenum. The abnormality is probably due to failure of normal dorsal migration of the ventral anlage of the embryonic pancreas to meet the dorsal anlage. With severe obstruction, or other associated lesions, children present as a neonate. Patients with less

severe obstruction may not present until later in life, even into adulthood. As with delayed presentation of forms of congenital duodenal obstruction, presenting symptoms are usually pain and vomiting. Radiographs are normal. On upper GI studies, a persistent waist is seen partially obstructing the second portion of the duodenum (Figure 10.13.6).

Preduodenal portal vein is rarely diagnosed preoperatively and rarely is the sole cause of duodenal obstruction. It is thus important for the surgeon to be cogniscent of the association of this anomaly with the other congenital lesions causing duodenal obstruction. Preduodenal portal vein is due to persistence of the inferior (ventral) anastomotic channel connecting the paired vitelline veins rather than the middle (dorsal) anastomotic channel. Radiographic findings depend on the associated anomaly. In the rare isolated preduodenal portal vein, an obstruction of variable degree is seen at the distal duodenal bulb or second portion of the duodenum.

FURTHER READING

Elliott GB, Kliman MR, Elliott KA. Pancreatic annulus: a sign or a cause of duodenal obstruction? Canadian Journal of Surgery 1968; 11:357–364.
Jadvar H, Mindelzun RE. Annular pancreas in adults: imaging features in seven patients. Abdominal Imaging 1999; 24:174–177.
Karoll MP, Ghahremani GG, Port RB et al. Diagnosis and management of intraluminal duodenal diverticulum. Digestive Disease Science 1983; 28:411–416.
Ladd AP, Madura JA. Congenital duodenal anomalies in the adult. Archives of Surgery 2001; 136:576–584.
McCarten KM, Teele RL. Preduodenal portal vein: venography, ultrasonography, and review of the literature. Annals of Radiology 1978; 21:155–160.
Rowe MI, Buckner D, Clatworthy HW Jr. Wind sock web of the duodenum. American Journal of Surgery 1968; 116:444–449.
Smith GV, Teele RL. Delayed diagnosis of duodenal obstruction in Down syndrome. American Journal of Roentgenology 1980; 134:937–940.
Sprinkle JD Jr, Hingsberger EA. Retained foreign body: association with elevated lead levels, pica, and duodenal anomaly. Pediatric Radiology 1995; 25:528–529.

LATE PRESENTATION OF MALROTATION

Most patients who develop symptoms related to malrotation will do so in the first month of life; however, some patients present with chronic symptoms later in life and, rarely, previously asymptomatic patients may present with acute symptoms due to volvulus. Chronic symptoms related to malrotation include abdominal pain, nausea and vomiting, failure to thrive and symptoms related to malabsorption. Regardless of age, it is important to demonstrate the normal duodenal course on an upper GI study and exclude malrotation as an aetiology for symptoms. A more detailed discussion of malrotation is found in the chapters on the neonatal duodenum and small bowel.

Radiographs are most commonly normal; bowel malposition may be suggested by noting a small bowel gas pattern exclusively in the right abdomen and colon to the left. Such cases may represent non-rotation in which the incidence volvulus and chronic symptoms is less than other forms of malrotation. Bands may produce duodenal or, rarely, colonic dilatation. In rare cases of volvulus beyond the neonatal period, findings include mass effect,

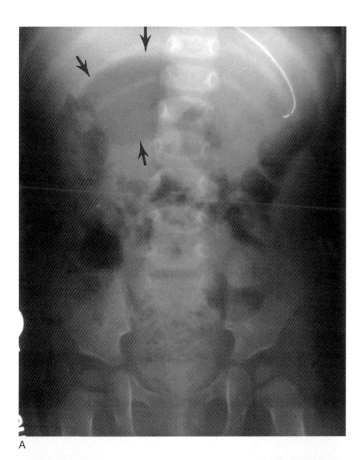

A

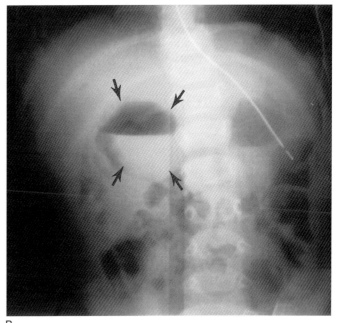

B

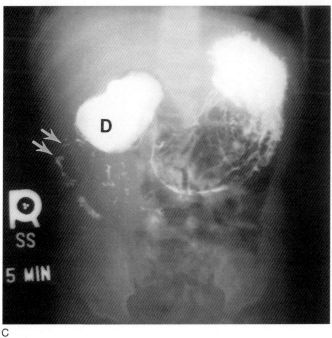

C

Figure 10.13.2 Delayed presentation of duodenal stenosis. The patient was 8 months old with a 3-week history of vomiting. Supine (A) and upright (B) abdominal films show distension of the proximal duodenum (arrows) with gas and fluid. (C) Upper GI study shows marked obstruction in the second portion of the duodenum (D). What little barium that does get past the stenosis shows malposition of proximal small bowel in the right upper abdomen (arrows). Duodenal stenosis and malrotation were surgically confined.

separation of loops due to bowel wall thickening and pneumatosis intestinalis due to ischaemia. As in neonates, upper GI is the preferred mode of diagnosis. The degree of abnormality on upper GI may be less pronounced in older patients than in patients presenting in the neonatal period. The normal distal duodenum should extend to the left of the spine and reach the level of the pylorus. Malrotated duodenum takes an anomalous course. Radiographic findings of volvulus include a beaked obstruction and a narrowed 'corkscrew' course of distal duodenum and proximal jejunum (Figure 10.13.7).

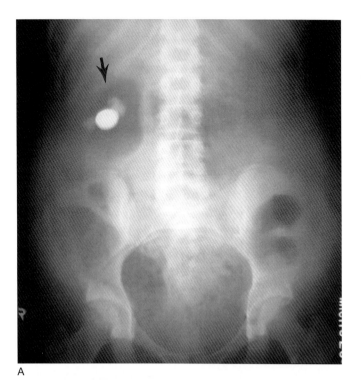

A

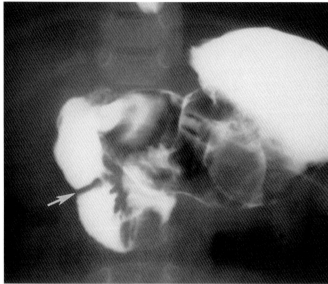

Figure 10.13.4 Duodenal web. 4-month-old male with trisomy 21 and persistent vomiting. A focal narrowing of the descending duodenum (arrow) was present throughout the examination.

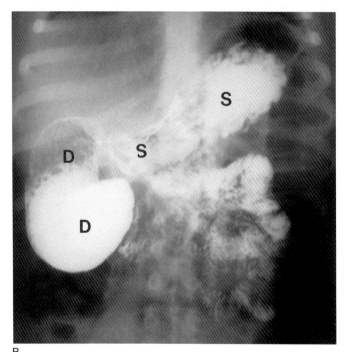

B

Figure 10.13.3 Late presentation of duodenal stenosis. Recurrent vomiting was noted in this 15-year-old with trisomy 21. (A) Retained foreign bodies are seen in dilated duodenum (arrow) on radiography. (B) Upper GI shows marked calibre change from dilated proximal duodenum (D) to normal calibre distal duodenum and jejunum. No malrotation was noted. S, stomach.

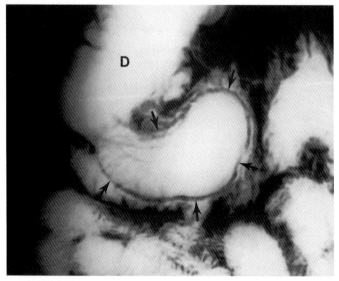

Figure 10.13.5 Intraluminal duodenal diverticulum. A windsock-shaped membrane (arrows) extends into the third portion of the duodenum. The proximal duodenum (D) is dilated. The patient was 20 years old with longstanding symptoms of epigastric pain, nausea and vomiting. Symptoms resolved after surgery. (Courtesy of V. Tsaloff, Petoskey, MI, USA.)

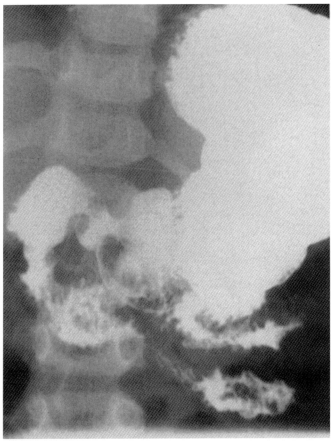

Figure 10.13.6 Annular pancreas. 6-year-old boy with symptoms of vomiting attacks since birth. There is narrowing of the second part of the duodenum. There was no associated malrotation.

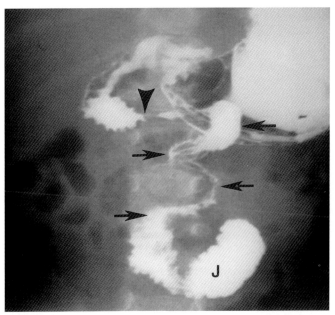

Figure 10.13.7 Malrotation with volvulus. Narrowing of the distal duodenum (arrowhead) is noted with a 'corkscrew' course (arrows) of proximal jejunum, extending inferiorly. J, proximal jejunum in the lower mid-abdomen.

FURTHER READING

Berdon WE. The diagnosis of malrotation and volvulus in the older child and adult: a trap for radiologists. Pediatric Radiology 1995; 25:101–103.

Dilley AV, Pereira J, Shi EC et al. The radiologist says malrotation: does the surgeon operate? Pediatric Surgery International 2000; 16:45–49.

Friedland GW, Mason R, Poole GJ. Ladd's bands in older children, adolescents, and adults. Radiology 1970; 95:363–368

Jackson A, Bisset R, Dickson AP. Malrotation and midgut volvulus presenting as malabsorption. Clinical Radiology 1989; 40:536–537.

Maxson RT, Franklin PA, Wagner CW. Malrotation in the older child: surgical management, treatment, and outcome. American Surgeon 1995; 61:135–138.

Pochaczevsky R, Ratner H, Leonidas JC et al. Unusual forms of volvulus after the neonatal period. American Journal of Roentgenology, Radium Therapy and Nuclear Medicine 1972; 114:390–393.

Powell DM, Othersen HB, Smith CD. Malrotation of the intestines in children: the effect of age on presentation and therapy. Journal of Pediatric Surgery 1989; 24:777–780.

Seashore JH, Touloukian RJ. Midgut volvulus. An ever-present threat. Archives of Pediatric and Adolescent Medicine 1994; 148:43–46.

Shimanuki Y, Aihara T, Takano H et al. Clockwise whirlpool sign at color doppler US: an objective and definite sign of midgut volvulus. Radiology 1996; 199:261–264.

Spigland N, Brandt ML, Yazbeck S. Malrotation presenting beyond the neonatal period. Journal of Pediatric Surgery 1990; 25:1139–1142.

Zissin R, Rathaus V, Oscadchy A et al. Intestinal malrotation as an incidental finding on CT in adults. Abdominal Imaging 1999; 24:550–555.

SITUS INVERSUS AND SITUS AMBIGUOUS

The incidence of malrotation is increased in patients with situs inversus, albeit very slightly and probably not of sufficient degree to warrant further investigation in patients who are asymptomatic. To exclude malrotation in a patient with situs inversus, the

As ultrasound and computed tomography (CT) are used extensively to image older children presenting with abdominal pain it is imperative to know the findings of malrotation on these modalities. Malposition of the superior mesenteric vein to the left of the superior mesenteric artery, rather than the normal rightward position, is a sign of malrotation but is neither sensitive nor specific (Figure 10.13.8). Nevertheless, identification of this finding warrants further investigation for malrotation. On careful inspection, the duodenal course can usually be identified on CT. Failure to identify the distal duodenum crossing the midline inferior to the superior mesenteric artery is another indication of malrotation. Frank malposition of small bowel or colon may be evident (Figure 10.13.8). Occasionally, volvulus may be evident on ultrasound or CT. Volvulus produces a mass in the central abdomen with a whorled appearance due to bowel and blood vessels wound around the mesenteric axis (Fig. 10.13.9).

It is important to remember that not all forms of malrotation produce symptoms. The anatomical abnormality reflects the stage in embryological development at which arrest occurs. The degree of fixation and breadth of the mesenteric pedicle determine the likelihood of volvulus occurring. Particularly in older children and adults, malrotation may be an incidental finding or potentially may be unrelated to patient symptoms (Figure 10.13.10).

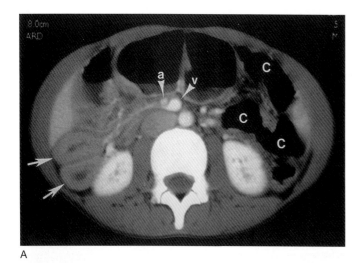

A

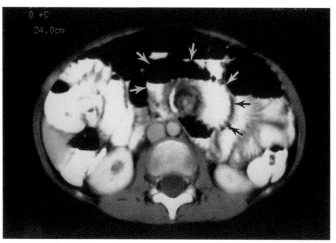

Figure 10.13.9 Malrotation with volvulus. 7-year-old with 2-year history of chronic, recurrent abdominal pain. CT shows a whorled appearance of bowel and blood vessels around the superior mesenteric artery in the mid-abdomen (arrows), consistent with volvulus.

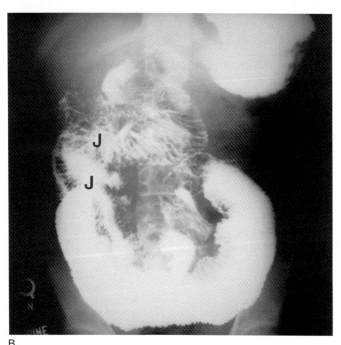

B

Figure 10.13.8 Malrotation. (A) CT was performed for abdominal pain. In retrospect, a history of symptoms of malabsorption was also obtained. Thick-walled small bowel loops (arrows) are seen on the right and colon (C) on the left. The duodenum was not seen to cross the midline. Superior mesenteric vein (v) is left of superior mesenteric artery (a). (B) Upper GI with small bowel follow-through confirms malrotation. Proximal jejunal (J) folds are diffusely thickened in the right upper quadrant.

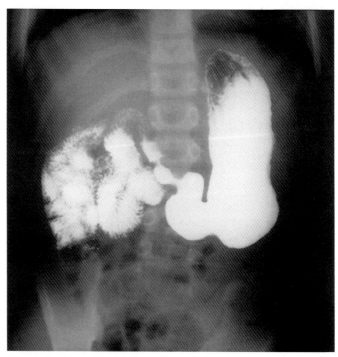

Figure 10.13.10 Malrotation. 12-year-old with chronic, recurrent abdominal pain. Malrotation was suspected when the appendix was not normally located at appendectomy. The appendix was normal. The upper GI shows duodenum and proximal jejunum in the right upper quadrant (non-rotation). No obstruction or volvulus is evident. Although a Ladd's procedure was performed, the patient's pain persisted and was probably unrelated to malrotation.

anatomy is shown to be in mirror image to that seen in a normal patient with normally placed organs (situs solitus) (Figure 10.13.11). Malrotation is nearly universal in patients with situs ambiguous. Situs ambiguous represents a spectrum of disease, including asplenia (bilateral right-sidedness) and polysplenia (bilateral left-sidedness) syndromes. Unfortunately, these children, particularly those with asplenia, are often afflicted with severe congenital heart disease. Sonography is usually performed to confirm asplenia or polysplenia. An upper GI study is recommended, when

patient condition permits, to confirm malrotation. The patient's overall condition relative to their congenital heart disease often determines whether and when surgery is pursued. Unfortunately, these infants may occasionally develop volvulus and present acutely.

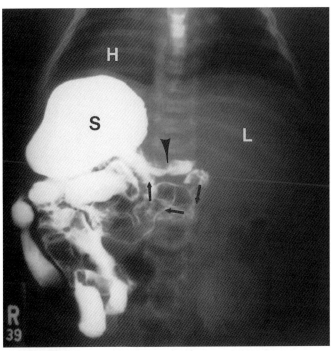

Figure 10.13.11 Situs inversus. Heart apex (H) and stomach (S) are on the right. Liver (L) is on the left. The duodenal course (arrows) is mirror image to normal. Proximal small bowel is in the right upper quadrant. Arrowhead, pylorus. (Courtesy of K. A. Garver, Ann Arbor, MI, USA.)

FURTHER READING

Applegate KE, Goske MJ, Pierce G et al. Situs revisited: imaging of the heterotaxy syndrome. Radiographics 1999; 19:837–852.

Cheikhelard A, De Lagausie P, Garel C et al. Situs inversus and bowel malrotation: contribution of prenatal diagnosis and laparoscopy. Journal of Pediatric Surgery 2000; 35:1217–1219.

Nakada K, Kawaguchi F, Wakisaka M et al. Digestive tract disorders associated with asplenia/polysplenia syndrome. Journal of Pediatric Surgery 1997; 32:91–94.

DUODENAL DUPLICATION

A detailed discussion of bowel duplication is found in Chapter 10.14. Approximately 5% of duplications are found at the duodenum. Duodenal duplications are usually cystic or spherical and located at the first or second portion of the duodenum. Rarely, the duplication may extend cephalad into the thorax. Duodenal duplications frequently cause widening of the C-loop. Occasionally, a more tubular duplication may parallel a length of duodenum. Many duodenal duplications are identified prenatally by obstetrical sonography. Some duplications present in the neonatal period and most within the first year of life. If a mass is suspected, sonography is the preferred modality. Most, but not all, duodenal duplication cysts will show a layered appearance, consisting of the internal hyperechoic mucosa with a more peripheral hypoechoic muscular layer (Figure 10.13.12). By identifying this characteristic 'gut signature' and excluding connection to the biliary tree, sonography is able to distinguish a duodenal duplication from a choledochal cyst, the chief differential diagnosis for a cystic mass located within the

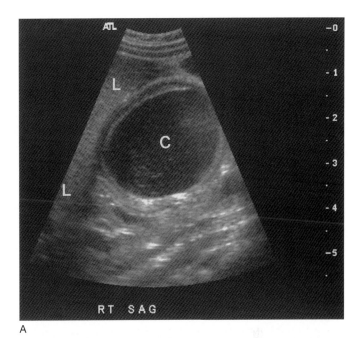

A

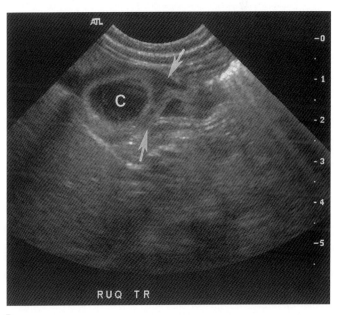

B

Figure 10.13.12 Duplication cyst. (A) The cyst (C) has an inner, hyperechoic layer (mucosa) and an outer, hypoechoic layer (muscle). Debris is present in the cyst. L, liver. (B) Note continuity of the muscular wall of the duplication cyst (C) with adjacent bowel wall (arrows).

C-loop of the duodenum. Findings on CT are less specific. A well-defined fluid attenuation mass is seen. An upper GI will demonstrate mass effect and distortion or widening of the duodenal C-loop by the duplication (Figure 10.13.13). Because the duplication is intimately related to the underlying duodenum, simple excision is not usually possible. Often, a segment of duodenum is removed and a duodenoduodenostomy or gastroduodenostomy is performed.

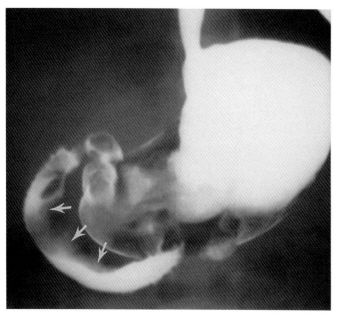

Figure 10.13.13 Duplication cyst. Mass effect widens the duodenal C-loop with slight effacement and dilatation (arrows).

FURTHER READING

Guibaud L, Fouque P, Genin G et al. CT and ultrasound of gastric and duodenal duplications. Journal of Computer Assisted Tomography 1996; 20:382–385.

Macpherson RI. Gastrointestinal tract duplications: clinical, pathologic, etiologic, and radiologic considerations. Radiographics 1993; 13:1063–1080.

Teele RL, Henschke CI, Tapper D. The radiographic and ultrasonographic evaluation of enteric duplication cysts. Pediatric Radiology 1980; 10:9–14.

DUODENAL DIVERTICULUM

Although duodenal diverticula are seen in up to 5% of upper GI examinations in adults, the diverticula are quite rare in children, indicating that they are acquired rather than congenital lesions. When seen in children, duodenal diverticula are usually an incidental finding.

INFECTION AND INFLAMMATION

DUODENITIS AND DUODENAL ULCER

Peptic ulcer disease is uncommon in children. With widespread use of endoscopy, radiographic diagnosis of a duodenal ulcer has become distinctly uncommon, particularly in children. If peptic ulcer disease is suspected, endoscopy is the preferred method of diagnosis. Nevertheless, duodenitis and duodenal ulcers will occasionally be diagnosed on upper GI examinations in children. If

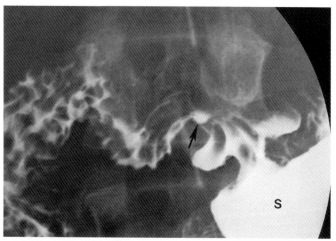

Figure 10.13.14 Duodenal ulcer. Deformity of duodenal bulb with small ulcer (arrow) and fold thickening in the postbulbar duodenum. S, stomach. (Courtesy of L. Paul Sonda, Ann Arbor, MI, USA.)

inflammatory disease or ulcer is a strong diagnostic possibility, performing the upper GI examination with a double-contrast technique will substantially increase diagnostic accuracy. Success of the technique is highly dependent on patient cooperation and patience, and persistence of the examining radiologist.

The aetiology of duodenal ulcers is multifactorial. In recent years, *Helicobacter pylori* has been identified as a causal organism. Treatment of ulcer disease thus often includes antibiotic coverage. Stress probably plays a role in ulcer development. Familial tendencies to peptic ulcer disease exist. Children with severe illness and those on steroid therapy are at increased risk of developing an ulcer. Increased secretion of acid by the stomach or inadequate buffering in the duodenum increases risk. Patients with inadequate pancreatic function, including patients with cystic fibrosis, may be at some increased risk for duodenal ulcer, although this is controversial.

The cardinal symptom of duodenal ulcer is pain; however, in children, particularly if younger, symptoms may be ill defined. Young children often present with feeding difficulty, vomiting or gastrointestinal haemorrhage. Older children are more likely to have the classic symptom of epigastric pain relieved by food. Many affected children have co-morbidities or other illnesses. Gastric ulcers are more common than duodenal ulcers in the young child. In older children and adolescents, duodenal ulcers outnumber gastric ulcers.

Careful evaluation of the duodenal bulb is necessary to delineate an ulcer. An ulcer produces a persistent barium collection (Figures 10.13.14 and 10.13.15). Double-contrast views of the duodenal bulb or profiled single-contrast views will show the ulcer. The duodenum should be assessed in multiple projections. The ulcer crater extends beyond the normal lumen. The collection persists on palpation; however, palpation may be limited in many patients due to the overlying rib cage or guarding by a less than cooperative patient. Duodenal ulcers in children are usually small. Adjacent fold thickening may be noted and the folds may radiate to the ulcer. With chronic ulcer disease the duodenal bulb is deformed, often taking a 'cloverleaf' appearance due to scarring.

Perforation of a duodenal ulcer in a child is very rare. Pneumoperitoneum or pneumoretroperitoneum may be seen. Clinically

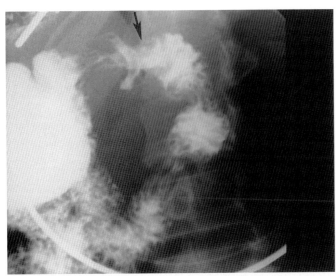

Figure 10.13.15 Duodenal ulcer. A small ulcer crater (arrow) is seen in poorly distended duodenal bulb. The patient had *Helicobacter pylori* infection.

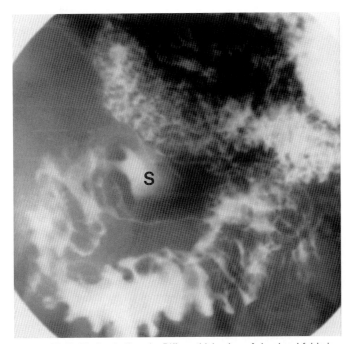

Figure 10.13.16 Cystic fibrosis. Diffuse thickening of duodenal folds is noted. S, stomach.

significant haemorrhage from a duodenal ulcer in a child is also quite rare, but unfortunately often compounds the clinical course of a child with other illnesses. If necessary, angiography with interventional techniques can be utilized to treat haemorrhage from an ulcer.

Duodenitis may precede the development of ulcers. Persistent thickened folds are seen on an upper GI examination. Evidence of inflammation in the form of duodenitis probably warrants endoscopic evaluation for an ulcer, even if an ulcer is not seen on the upper GI study. Peptic ulcer disease, however, is not the only cause of thickening of duodenal folds. Other inflammatory conditions including Crohn's disease, eosinophilic enteritis (idiopathic and non-idiopathic), infection and graft-versus-host disease may produce thickened duodenal folds. In children with cystic fibrosis, duodenal fold thickening is often present, although the pathogenesis of this finding is unknown (Figure 10.13.16). Duodenal fold thickening may also be seen with hypoproteinaemia and protein-losing enteropathy or with intramural haemorrhage.

FURTHER READING

Cox K, Ament ME. Upper gastrointestinal bleeding in children and adolescents. Pediatrics 1979; 63:408–413.

Drumm B, Rhoads JM, Stringer DA et al. Peptic ulcer disease in children: aetiology, clinical findings, and clinical course. Pediatrics 1988; 82:410–414.

Gold BD. Helicobacter pylori infection in children. Current Problems in Pediatrics 2001; 31:247–266.

Long FR, Kramer SS, Markowitz RI et al. Duodenitis in children: correlation of radiologic findings with endoscopic and pathologic findings. Radiology 1998; 206:103–108.

Nord KS, Rossi TM, Lebenthal E. Peptic ulcer in children: the predominance of gastric ulcers. American Journal of Gastroenterology 1981; 75:153–157.

Stringer MD, Veysi VT, Puntis JW et al. Gastroduodenal ulcers in the Helicobacter pylori era. Acta Paediatrica 2000; 89:1181–1185.

CROHN'S DISEASE

Duodenal Crohn's disease is most commonly diagnosed by endoscopy. Thus, although involvement of the proximal portion of small bowel is more prevalent in children with Crohn's disease than adults, radiographic demonstration of duodenal involvement is uncommon. In most cases, non-specific fold thickening is seen. Ulceration may be noted. Findings mimic peptic ulcer disease (Figure 10.13.17). Frequently, there is also fold thickening in the proximal jejunum. In most cases, the terminal ileum is also involved; however, in 10–15% of cases duodenal disease is seen without involvement of the terminal ileum.

FURTHER READING

Cameron DJ. Upper and lower gastrointestinal endoscopy in children and adolescents with Crohn's disease: a prospective study. Journal of Gastroenterology and Hepatology 1991; 6:355–358.

Griffiths AM, Alemayehu E, Sherman P. Clinical features of gastroduodenal Crohn's disease in adolescents. Journal of Pediatric Gastroenterology and Nutrition 1989; 8:166–171.

Grill BB, Lange R, Markowitz R et al. Delayed gastric emptying in children with Crohn's disease. Journal of Clinical Gastroenterology 1985; 7:216–226.

Lenaerts C, Roy CC, Vaillancourt M et al. High incidence of upper gastrointestinal tract involvement in children with Crohn disease. Pediatrics 1989; 83:777–781.

NEOPLASMS

Both primary and secondary neoplasms of the duodenum in children are exceedingly rare. Rarely, the duodenum may be involved in a child with lymphoma, specifically Burkitt's subtype (Figure

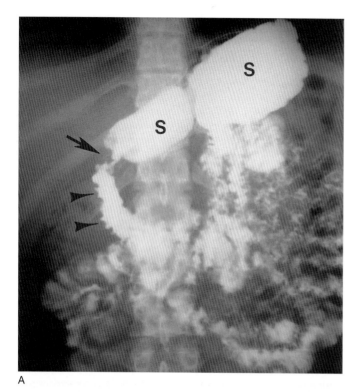

A

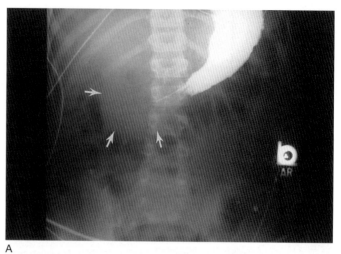

A

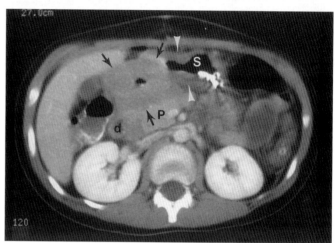

B

Figure 10.13.18 Lymphoma. (A) Upper GI shows complete gastric outlet obstruction. Note mass effect (arrows). (B) CT shows soft tissue mass (arrows) encasing the duodenum and pylorus. The distal gastric wall is thick (arrowheads). d, distal duodenum; P, pancreas; S, stomach.

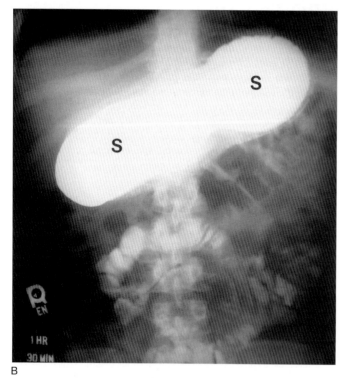

B

Figure 10.13.17 Duodenal Crohn's disease. (A) At initial presentation, irregular narrowing is seen at the antro-pyloric junction and proximal duodenum (arrows). Duodenal folds are thickened (arrowheads). Diffuse nodular fold thickening is seen in the jejunum in the left upper quadrant. (B) Nine months later, a 90-min film from small bowel follow-through shows near complete gastric outlet obstruction. S, stomach.

10.13.18). Rarely, the duodenum may be involved in a haemangioma or lymphangioma of the retroperitoneum. Intramural haemangiomas are rare (Figure 10.13.19). Extrinsic mass effect on the duodenum from neoplasms in the retroperitoneum or involving adjacent organs is more common than intrinsic involvement of the duodenum. Duodenal polyps may be seen with Peutz–Jeghers syndrome (see Figure 10.14.40) or rarely with familial adenomatous polyposis. Nodular filling defects produced by duodenal varices due to portal hypertension may mimic polyps (Figure 10.13.20).

FURTHER READING

Balikian JP, Nassar NT, Shamma'a MH et al. Primary lymphomas of the small intestine including the duodenum. American Journal of Roentgenology, Radiation Therapy and Nuclear Medicine 1969; 107:131–141.

Golding RL, Perri G. The radiology of gastrointestinal Burkitt's lymphoma in children. Clinical Radiology 1977; 28:465–468.

Lakhkar B, Abubacker S. Duodeno-jejunal hemangiomatosis. Indian Journal of Pediatrics 2000; 67:931–933.

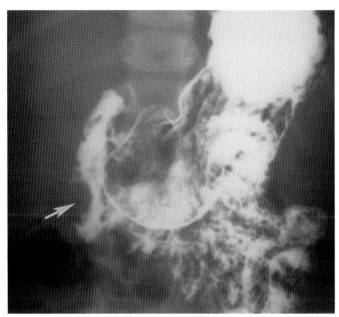

Figure 10.13.19 Intramural haemangioma. A focal filling defect (arrow) is seen in the second portion of the duodenum.

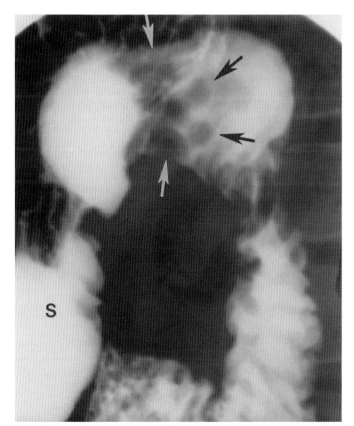

Figure 10.13.20 Duodenal varices. 12-year-old who developed portal hypertension after hepatic trisegmentectomy for hepatoblastoma. Nodular filling defects are seen in the postbulbar duodenum (arrows). S, stomach.

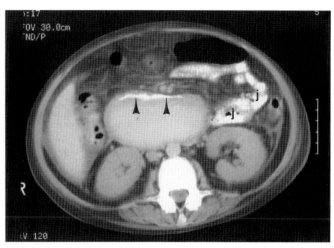

Figure 10.13.21 Duodenal haematoma. The patient had leukaemia. A large intramural mass compresses the duodenal lumen (arrowheads) anteriorly. Some contrast reaches the proximal jejunum (j).

Marshall DG, Kim F. Leiomyosarcoma of the duodenum. Journal of Pediatric Surgery 1987; 22:1007–1008.

Riggle KP, Boeckman CR. Duodenal leiomyoma: a case report of hematemesis in a teenager. Journal of Pediatric Surgery 1988; 23:850–851.

HAEMORRHAGE

DUODENAL HAEMATOMA (NON-TRAUMATIC)

Haemorrhage into the wall of the duodenum is most commonly seen as a consequence of traumatic injury. Traumatic injuries are discussed in greater detail in Chapter 10.16. Other disorders that may predispose a patient to intramural haemorrhage include Henoch–Schönlein purpura, haemophilia, anticoagulant therapy and children with suppressed platelet counts due to leukaemia, chemotherapy and idiopathic thrombocytopaenic purpura (ITP). The degree of pain varies and in the sick child may be masked by other complaints. Large haematomas may cause obstruction of the duodenal lumen and resultant vomiting. On ultrasound, larger haematomas may be seen as a mass of varying echotexture. Fresh haematoma tends to be hyperechoic whereas older haematoma tends to be hypoechoic. CT will show a mass impinging upon the duodenum (Figure 10.13.21). Fresh haematoma tends to be higher in attenuation whereas older haematoma tends to be lower in attenuation, near that of fluid. If an upper GI study is performed, mass effect, fold thickening and obstruction may be seen.

FURTHER READING

Hernanz-Schulman M, Genieser NB, Ambrosino M. Sonographic diagnosis of intramural duodenal hematoma. Journal of Ultrasound Medicine 1989; 8:273–276

Kagimoto S. Duodenal findings on ultrasound in children with Schönlein–Henoch purpura and gastrointestinal symptoms. Journal of Pediatric Gastroenterology and Nutrition 1993; 16:178–182.

Kawasaki M, Suekane H, Imagawa E et al. Duodenal obstruction due to Henoch–Schönlein purpura. American Journal of Roentgenology 1997; 168:969–970.

OBSTRUCTION

Most causes of duodenal obstruction have been discussed above: delayed presentation of congenital obstructive lesions including duodenal stenosis, delayed presentation of malrotation with volvulus or obstructing bands, rare neoplasms of the duodenum and duodenal haematoma.

SUPERIOR MESENTERIC ARTERY SYNDROME/CAST SYNDROME

Superior mesenteric artery syndrome is caused by apparent compression of the third portion of the duodenum between the superior mesenteric artery anteriorly and the spine posteriorly. This form of obstruction can be seen in children who are malnourished and in children who have lost weight, including children with a severe illness and adolescents with anorexia nervosa. Altered anatomy may contribute to the obstruction. Realignment of the spine due to surgical fusion or application of a body cast ('cast' syndrome) may precipitate the obstruction. It is probably the spine rather than the superior mesenteric artery that causes the obstruction. Children present with vomiting.

On an upper GI examination, the obstruction is seen as a vertically oriented impression on the third portion of the duodenum as it crosses the spine (Figure 10.13.22). The duodenum is mild to moderately dilated leading up to the point of obstruction. The obstruction is often partially relieved by placing the left side of the patient down.

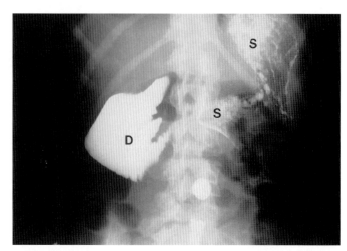

Figure 10.13.22 Superior mesenteric artery syndrome. 30-min film shows no barium beyond third portion at duodenum (D). The patient had a history of substantial recent weight loss due to illness. S, stomach.

Surgical management is rarely required. Placement of an enteric feeding tube beyond the point of obstruction and, if necessary, parenteral nutrition allows for adequate nutrition to promote weight gain and recovery.

FURTHER READING

Elbadaway MH. Chronic superior mesenteric artery syndrome in anorexia nervosa. British Journal of Psychiatry 1992; 160:552–554.

Ooi GC, Chan KL, Ko KF et al. Computed tomography of the superior mesenteric artery syndrome. Clinical Imaging 1997; 21:210–212.

Vaisman N, Stringer DA, Pencharz P. Functional duodenal obstruction (superior mesenteric artery or cast syndrome) in cerebral palsy. Journal of Parenteral and Enteral Nutrition 1989; 13:326–328.

Wilkinson R, Huang CT. Superior mesenteric artery syndrome in traumatic paraplegia: a case report and literature review. Archives of Physical Medicine and Rehabilitation 2000; 81:991–994.

The Small Bowel, Mesentery and Peritoneum

Peter J Strouse

SMALL BOWEL

EMBRYOGENESIS

The small bowel is a midgut derivative. The midgut also contributes the distal portion of duodenum, the caecum, the appendix and the proximal portion of colon. The embryonic midgut communicates with the yolk sac via the vitelline (omphalomesenteric) duct, which is later obliterated. Early on in development, the midgut is suspended by a short mesentery. Subsequently, the midgut and mesentery elongate. There is a normal herniation of midgut into umbilical cord at 6 weeks' gestation. At 10 weeks' gestation the midgut returns to the abdomen, undergoing a 270 degree counterclockwise rotation and achieving fixation with a broad mesenteric attachment from left upper quadrant to right lower quadrant. Additional discussion of small bowel development is found in the chapters on neonatal duodenum and small bowel.

TECHNIQUE AND INDICATIONS

Methods for evaluating the small bowel are presented in the chapter on techniques. Small bowel follow-through is the primary method for dedicated evaluation of the small bowel. Indications include small bowel obstruction, inflammatory bowel disease, chronic or recurrent abdominal pain and unexplained gastrointestinal blood loss. Today, studies are only rarely performed for malabsorption. Enteroclysis provides a more detailed evaluation of small bowel; however, it is more invasive and less well tolerated in children. Enteroclysis may be beneficial in problematic cases. Peroral pneumocolon can be used in conjunction with small bowel follow-through to enhance evaluation of the terminal ileum. Ultrasound and computed tomography (CT) can be used to evaluate many disorders of the small bowel, as illustrated in this chapter.

NORMAL ANATOMY AND RADIOGRAPHIC APPEARANCE

The jejunum extends from the ligament of Trietz in the left upper quadrant to the midabdomen where there is an imperceptible transition to ileum. The ileum continues from this point, joining the caecum at the ileocaecal valve in the right lower quadrant. Although the course of the small bowel can vary considerably, the jejunum is predominantly in the left upper quadrant and the ileum in the lower abdomen, occasionally coursing deep into the pelvis. Mucosal folds are more numerous in the jejunum and produce a feathery appearance. The ileal folds are less pronounced (Figures 10.14.1 and 10.14.2). The fold pattern develops with age. In infants, the jejunal and ileal fold patterns are more homogeneous. Lymphoid hyperplasia is commonly seen in the terminal ileum, producing a nodular appearance (Figure 10.14.3). This can be differentiated from inflammatory disease because the nodules are regular, the bowel is peristaltic and pliable, and no extrinsic mass effect is produced.

On abdominal radiographs of children, the amount of gas seen within small bowel will vary considerably. In infants, small bowel and colon are poorly distinguished by their fold pattern, although anatomical location helps in differentiation. In older children, small bowel and colonic fold patterns are more developed and identification of valvulae conniventes may aid in distinguishing small bowel from colon (Figure 10.14.4).

ABDOMINAL PAIN

The small bowel is but one of innumerable sources for abdominal pain in a child. Nevertheless, and guilty or not, the small bowel is commonly blamed for this symptom. Acute abdominal pain is a very common presenting symptom in children. Approximately 25% of children will seek medical attention for an episode of acute abdominal pain by the time they are 15 years of age. Approximately 5% of unscheduled paediatric office and emergency room visits will be for acute abdominal pain unrelated to trauma. Only a small fraction of children presenting with acute abdominal pain will have an organic aetiology. Clinical findings suggesting an underlying disease process include pain that is not per umbilical or localizes away from the umbilicus, fever, blood in the stool, a palpable mass or laboratory abnormalities including leukocytosis or an abnormal urinalysis.

The pathophysiology of abdominal pain is complex. Stretching, tension or rapid distention of an organ, such as small bowel, causes pain. Processes with slow onset are less painful. Inflammatory and ischaemic conditions cause pain through chemical mediators. Stress contributes to pain by altering intestinal tonus and other

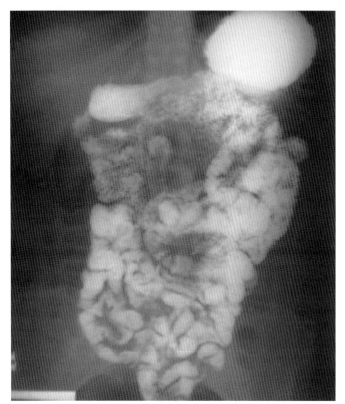

Figure 10.14.1 Normal small bowel follow-through. Folds are more prominent in the jejunum (upper left) than the ileum (lower right). Barium has not reached the caecum.

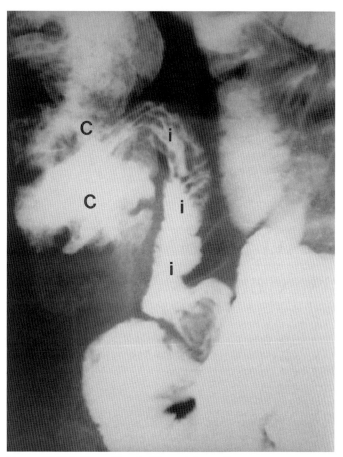

Figure 10.14.2 Normal terminal ileum. i, ileum; C, caecum.

effects. Visceral pain is mediated by sympathetic nerves and is poorly localized, often perceived as midline or periumbilical. Frequently, there are accompanying autonomic-mediated symptoms, including nausea, vomiting and pallor. If severe, visceral pain may be referred to a dermatome. Parietal pain, originating from the peritoneum, the diaphragm and abdominal wall, is well localized and dermatomal in distribution. The location of visceral pain, although poorly localized, is a guide to the organ of origin. Epigastric pain originates from foregut derivatives including stomach, duodenum, liver, biliary tree, spleen and pancreas. Periumbilical pain originates from midgut derivatives including small bowel, appendix and caecum. Infraumbilical and pelvic pain originates from hindgut derivatives including colon and rectum, as well as from pelvic organs and the kidneys.

The differential diagnosis for abdominal pain is myriad and varies considerably dependent on the age of the child. A differential diagnosis for abdominal pain is provided in Chapter 10.15. It is not infrequent for extra-abdominal conditions or systemic diseases to cause abdominal pain (Figure 10.14.5). The imaging of a child presenting with acute abdominal pain may include radiography, ultrasound and/or CT. Other imaging methods are infrequently utilized, unless symptoms suggest a specific diagnosis. Radiographs are particularly useful if gastrointestinal pathology is suspected. Ultrasound is helpful in many children and is preferred as no ionizing radiation is imparted. Both ultrasound and CT are best utilized when guided by clinical findings and suspicions. The importance of a good physical examination and history in guiding imaging cannot be overstated.

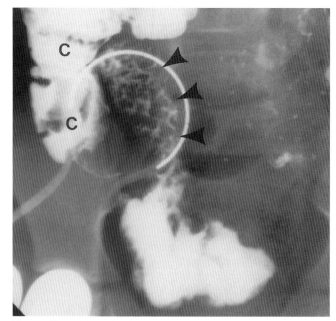

Figure 10.14.3 Lymphoid hyperplasia of the terminal ileum. Nodular filling defects are seen (arrowheads). The terminal ileum was peristaltic and pliable to palpation. A compression paddle is being applied. C, caecum.

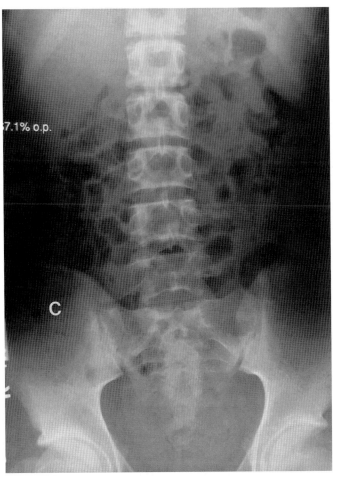

Figure 10.14.4 Normal small bowel gas pattern. Gas is seen within non-dilated small bowel loops. Normal valvulae conniventes are seen at several locations. There is a paucity of colonic gas in this patient. C, caecum, filled with faeces.

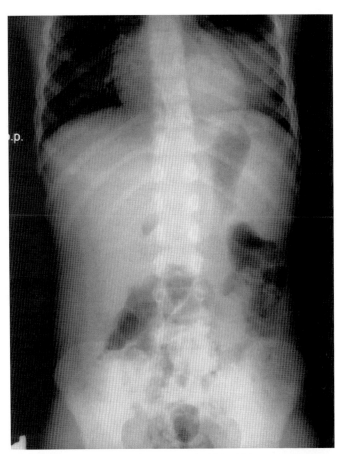

Figure 10.14.5 Left lower lobe pneumonia. This child presented with abdominal pain.

Chronic, recurrent abdominal pain is also a common presenting symptom in children. As many as 10% of children may suffer from chronic, recurrent abdominal pain. As with acute abdominal pain, the overwhelming majority of children with chronic, recurrent abdominal pain do not have an identifiable underlying organic aetiology. Perhaps the most common organic disease process presenting in this manner is Crohn's disease. Rarely, a child with malrotation may present later in childhood with a complaint of chronic, recurrent abdominal pain (see Figures 10.13.8 and 10.13.9). Clinical findings suggesting an underlying disease process include pain localized away from midline, weight loss, failure to thrive, growth failure, blood in stools, abnormal laboratory examinations and genitourinary tract symptoms.

FURTHER READING

Apley J. The child with abdominal pains, 2nd edn. Oxford: Blackwell Scientific; 1975.

Buchert GS. Abdominal pain in children: an emergency practitioner's guide. Emergency Medicine Clinics of North America 1989; 7:497–516.

Jones PF. The acute abdomen in infancy and childhood. Practioner 1979; 222:473–478.

Kao SCS, Franken EA. The child with abdominal pain. In: Hilton SvW, Edwards DK, eds. Practical pediatric radiology, 2nd edn. Philadelphia: W.B. Saunders; 1994:159–186.

Reynolds SL, Jaffe DM. Diagnosing abdominal pain in a pediatric emergency department. Pediatric Emergency Care 1992; 8:126–128.

Scholer SJ, Pituch K, Orr DP, Dittus RS. Clinical outcomes of children with acute abdominal pain. Pediatrics 1996; 98:680–685.

Siegel MJ, Carel C, Surratt S. Ultrasonography of acute abdominal pain in children. Journal of the American Medical Association 1991; 266:1987–1989.

van der Meer SB, Forget PP, Arends JW et al. Diagnostic value of ultrasound with recurrent abdominal pain. Pediatric Radiology 1990; 20:501–503.

CONGENITAL AND DEVELOPMENTAL

LATE PRESENTATION OF JEJUNAL OR ILEAL STENOSIS

Congenital jejunal and ileal stenoses are much less common than atresia. The majority of children will present in the neonatal period. Occasionally, and usually with less severe obstruction, a child may present later in infancy of early childhood. Symptoms include abdominal distension and vomiting. Imaging studies may show dilated bowel proximal to the obstruction; however, the point of obstruction may be difficult to demonstrate.

OMPHALOMESENTERIC DUCT ANOMALIES

The omphalomesenteric duct is normally obliterated by the fifth to sixth week of intrauterine life. Portions of the duct can persist in the infant. If the entire duct persists, the result is an omphalomesenteric fistula (persistent omphalomesenteric duct) (Fig. 10.14.6). The infant with a fistula will present with faecal material passing per the umbilicus. Contrast can be injected into the fistula to confirm the diagnosis and demonstrate the anatomy. Persistence of the umbilical end of the duct produces an umbilical sinus (omphalomesenteric sinus). Persistence of the small bowel end of the duct produces a diverticulum known as Meckel's diverticulum. Persistent patency within the mid-portion of the duct with occlusion at the umbilicus and at the small bowel produces an omphalomesenteric cyst. Finally, even with complete obliteration of the lumen, the remnant band (omphalomesenteric band) passing from small bowel to umbilicus may cause obstruction or act as a nidus for an obstruction due to distal small bowl volvulus. Occasionally, an omphalomesenteric polyp may form at the umbilicus due to remnant intestinal mucosa. The polyp, in itself, is not of clinical significance; however, it can be the harbinger of other underlying anomalies related to the omphalomesenteric duct.

MECKEL'S DIVERTICULUM

Meckel's diverticula are present in 1–3 % of persons. Only a fraction of those with Meckel's diverticula will develop symptoms related to it. Meckel's diverticula are located on the antimesenteric side of the distal ileum, usually within 60 cm of the ileocaecal valve. Most diverticula contain intestinal mucosa. Diverticula containing ectopic gastric mucosa are prone to producing symptoms. Asymptomatic Meckel's diverticula are rarely demonstrated radiographically (Fig. 10.14.7). A characteristic triangular fold pattern may be seen at the base of the diverticulum if it is seen on a small bowel follow-through or enteroclysis. Meckel's diverticula can present clinically with gastrointestinal bleeding, inflammation or obstruction.

Gastrointestinal bleeding is the most common clinical manifestation of a Meckel's diverticulum. Pain if present is usually a less prominent symptom. Perforation of a Meckel's diverticulum may present with abdominal wall swelling. When there is ectopic gastric mucosa within a Meckel's diverticulum, inflammation or ulceration is produced within the diverticula or within adjacent ileum. The resultant gastrointestinal bleeding is usually painless and intermittent; however, patients may present with sudden, massive bleeding. Gastrointestinal bleeding may also present as chronic anaemia. In the setting of acute bleeding, a nuclear medicine gastrointestinal bleeding scan with tagged red blood cells may be used to localize the source. Abdominal angiography is uncommonly performed, but may be used in patients with massive bleeding to both identify the source of bleeding and potentially treat it by embolization.

In the setting of recurrent bleeding or chronic anaemia, with suspicion for a Meckel's diverticulum, a nuclear medicine scan can be performed specifically to identify the ectopic gastric mucosa within the Meckel's diverticulum. The scan is performed with technetium 99m pertechnetate. Premedication with cimetidine or ranitidine decreases secretion by gastric epithelium, but not tracer uptake, thereby enhancing visualization. Uptake within a Meckel's

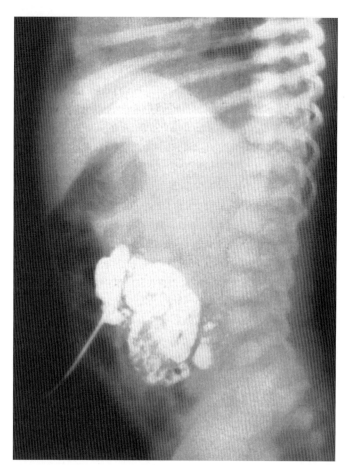

Figure 10.14.6 Omphalomesenteric fistula. Sinogram through a discharging umbilicus shows a fistula extending to the ileum.

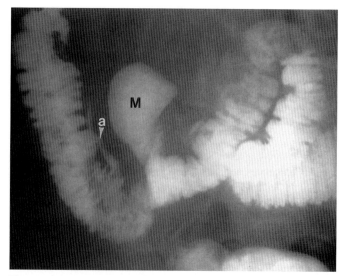

Figure 10.14.7 Meckel's diverticulum. Small bowel follow-through with filling of a large Meckel's diverticulum (M). a, appendix.

diverticulum is focal, parallels uptake in gastric mucosa of the stomach and is usually located in the right lower quadrant of the abdomen (Figure 10.14.8). Activity within the bladder may occasionally obscure a low-lying Meckel's diverticulum. False-negative scans occur when there is little or no gastric mucosa within the Meckel's diverticulum or when the mucosa has been severely damaged by inflammation or ischaemia. False-positive scans can be seen due to gastric mucosa within a duplication cyst, or occasionally with other pathologies that spuriously lead to tracer uptake.

Meckel's diverticulitis produces symptoms mimicking appendicitis, although pain tends to be closer to the midline than in classic appendicitis. Preoperative distinction from appendicitis is difficult, although demonstration of a normal caecum and appendix should suggest the diagnosis (Figures 10.14.9 and 10.14.10). Inflammation due to peptic acid from ectopic mucosa can lead to diverticulitis. As with the appendix, enteroliths may form within a Meckel's diverticulum, contributing to luminal obstruction and subsequent inflammation.

Meckel's diverticula may act as the lead point for an intussusception originating in the ileum, and potentially progressing into the colon (ileo–ileo–colic). Occasionally, the diverticulum may be identified by sonography as a fluid-filled structure within the intussusception. Meckel's diverticula can also produce small bowel obstruction due to inflammation, small bowel volvulus around an associated omphalomesenteric band, incarceration in a hernia or herniation of other bowel through the mesentery of the diverticulum. In each of these cases, it is unusual to diagnose the Meckel's diverticulum prospectively. Most obstructions related to Meckel's diverticula present in children less than 2 years of age.

Giant Meckel's diverticulum, or ileal dysgenesis, is not due to a persistence of a portion of the omphalomesenteric duct but rather, it is due to persistence of a portion of the adjacent embryonic gut. The result is a variably sized, segmental area of dilatation on the antimesenteric side of ileum. Symptoms vary but may represent the manifestation of bacterial overgrowth within the dilated segment. The diagnosis is rare. Findings are manifest on a small bowel study as a wide-necked saccular outpouching from the

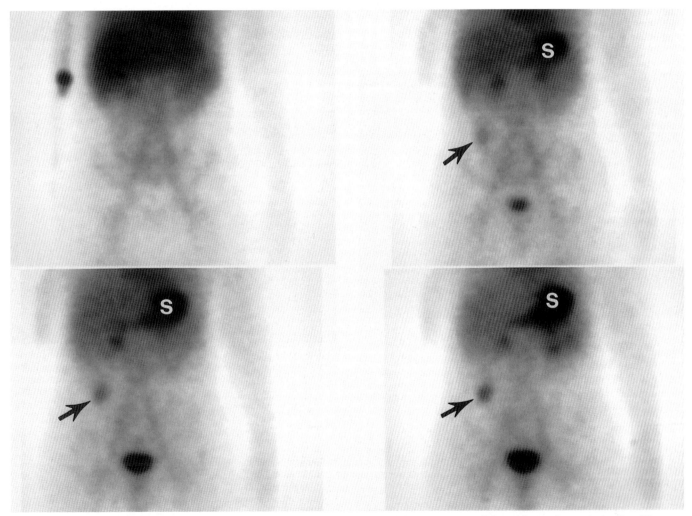

Figure 10.14.8 Meckel's diverticulum. The patient presented with painless bright red blood per rectum. Selected frames from a technetium 99m sodium pertechnetate scan shows focal uptake in the right lower quadrant (arrows) paralleling stomach activity (S), consistent with a Meckel's diverticulum containing gastric mucosa.

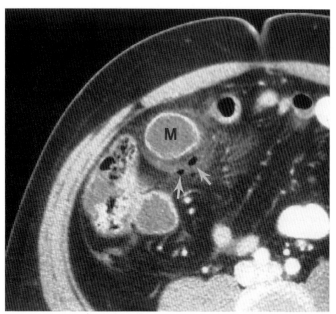

Figure 10.14.9 Perforated Meckel's diverticulitis. A blind ending, tubular, fluid-filled structure (M) was seen connecting to ileum. Inflammatory oedema is seen in adjacent fat. Note extraluminal gas from perforation (arrows). A normal appendix was identified on other images. (Courtesy of L. Paul Sonda, Ann Arbor, MI, USA.)

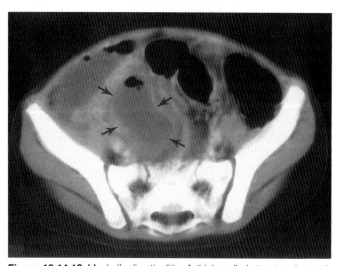

Figure 10.14.10 Meckel's diverticulitis. A thick-walled structure (arrows) with an air–fluid level did not connect with adjacent bowel. A torsed, inflamed Meckel's diverticulum was found at surgery.

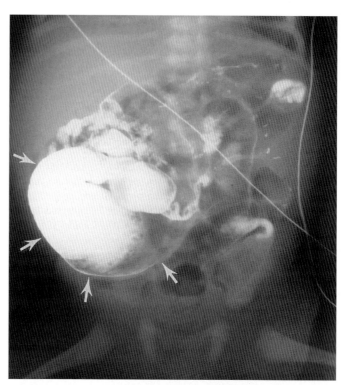

Figure 10.14.11 Ileal dysgenesis. A focal area of distended ileum (arrows) was non-obstructive. At surgery, a Meckel's diverticulum was also noted.

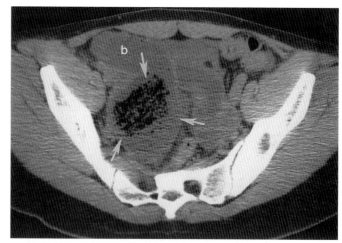

Figure 10.14.12 Giant Meckel's diverticulum. 22-year-old with episodic abdominal pain. CT without contrast shows a dilated bowel loop (arrows) containing mottled lucency centrally. This loop is in continuity with dilated small bowel (b). At surgery, a 7-cm saccular expansion of small bowel was found, located 45 cm proximal to the ileocaecal valve. A phytobezoar filled the lumen. (Courtesy of L. Paul Sonda, Ann Arbor, MI, USA.)

normal small bowel lumen or a segmental area of dilatation (Figures 10.14.11 and 10.14.12).

FURTHER READING

Brown A, Carty H. Segmental dilation of the ileum. British Journal of Radiology 1984; 57:371–374.

Dalinka MK, Wunder JF. Meckel's diverticulum and its complications, with emphasis on roentgenologic demonstration. Radiology 1973; 106:295–298.

Daneman A, Myers M, Shuckett B et al. Sonographic appearances of inverted Meckel diverticulum with intussusception. Pediatric Radiology 1997; 27:295–298.

DiSantis DJ, Siegel, Katz ME. Simplified approach to umbilical remnant abnormalities. Radiographics 1991; 11:59–66.

Fink AM, Alexopoulou E, Carty H. Bleeding Meckel's diverticulum in infancy: unusual scintigraphic and ultrasound appearances. Pediatric Radiology 1995; 25:155–156.

Gaisie G, Curnes JT, Scatliff JH et al. Neonatal intestinal obstruction from omphalomesenteric duct remnants. American Journal of Roentgenology 1985; 144:109–112.

Kutin ND, Allen JE, Jewett TC. The umbilical polyp. Journal of Pediatric Surgery 1979; 14:741–744.

Miller DL, Becker MH, Eng K. Giant Meckel's diverticulum. Radiology 1981; 140:93–94.

Moore TC. Omphalomesenteric duct malformations. Seminars in Pediatric Surgery 1996; 5:116–123.

Okazaki M, Higashihara H, Yamasaki S et al. Arterial embolization to control life-threatening hemorrhage from a Meckel's diverticulum. American Journal of Roentgenology 1990; 154:1257–1258.

Orenstein SR, Magill HL, Whitington. Ileal dysgenesis presenting with anemia and growth failure. Pediatric Radiology 1984; 14:59–61.

Pantongrag-Brown L, Levine MS, Buetow PC et al. Meckel's enteroliths: clinical, radiologic, and pathologic findings. American Journal of Roentgenology 1996; 167:1447–1450.

Plinio R, Gourtsoyiannis N, Bezzi M et al. Meckel's diverticulum: imaging diagnosis. American Journal of Roentgenology 1996; 166:567–573.

Rossi P, Gourtsoyiannis N, Bezzi N et al. Meckel's diverticulum: imaging diagnosis. American Journal of Roentgenology 1996; 166:567–573.

Sfankianakis GN, Conway JJ. Detection of ectopic gastric mucosa in Meckel's diverticulum and in other aberrations by scintigraphy: pathophysiology and 10-year clinical experience. Journal of Nuclear Medicine 1981; 22:647–654.

Vane DW, West KW, Grosfeld JL. Vitelline duct anomalies: experience with 217 childhood cases. Archives of Surgery 1987; 156:56–64.

DIVERTICULA

Apart from Meckel's diverticula, congenital diverticula of the small bowel are extremely rare. Such diverticula may, in fact, represent duplications in communication with the bowel lumen. Congenital diverticula are true diverticula, containing all layers of bowel wall. Small bowel diverticula can rarely be associated with syndromes, including Noonan syndrome, cutis laxa, Marfan's syndrome and Ehlers–Danlos syndrome. Acquired small bowel diverticula are very rarely seen in children. Acquired diverticula are usually false diverticula, herniating throughout the muscle layer adjacent to blood vessels. Pseudodiverticula can occasionally be seen related to inflammatory bowel disease and/or strictures.

FURTHER READING

Cumming WA, Simpson JS. Intestinal diverticulosis in Noonan's syndrome. British Journal of Radiology 1977; 50:64–65.

Fich A, Polliack G, Libson E. Gastrointestinal diverticulosis in association with Marfan syndrome. Journal of Medical Imaging 1989; 3:11–13.

Goltz RW, Hult AM. Generalized elastosis (cutis laxa) and Ehlers–Danlos syndrome (cutix hyperelastica): a comparative clinical and laboratory study. Southern Medical Journal 1965; 58:848–854.

DUPLICATION

Duplications (enteric cysts) contain gastrointestinal mucosa and smooth muscle. The mucosa does not necessarily correspond to the adjacent portion of the intestine. A single duplication may contain more than one type of mucosa. Approximately 15% of duplications contain gastric mucosa. Duplications are most commonly cystic and spherical. Tubular duplications, which communicate with the bowel lumen, are rare. Duplications may occur anywhere throughout the gastrointestinal tract; they are most common in the distal ileum. Approximately one-third of duplications are found at the distal ileum. Most patients have only a single duplication; however, there may be multiple duplications present. Duplications are uniformly found on the mesenteric side of the bowel.

The aetiology of gastrointestinal duplications is uncertain. Many theories have been proposed but none satisfactorily explains all duplications. Duplications increase in size due to the accumulation of secretions. When they reach a critical size, duplications usually present due to mass effect, which causes partial obstruction of the adjacent bowel lumen. Patients present with pain and sometimes vomiting. Occasionally, duplications can act as the lead point for an intussusception or as the focal point for a small bowel volvulus. In duplications containing gastric mucosa, patients may present with pain due to inflammation or, rarely, with gastrointestinal bleeding. Occasionally, duplications present as an asymptomatic, palpable mass. Most duplications present in the first year of life. Some present in the neonatal period. Some are identified on prenatal sonography.

Radiographs are usually normal unless the duplication is large enough to cause mass effect or intestinal obstruction. Ultrasound is the preferred mode of investigation. On sonography, uncomplicated duplications will be identified as a well-defined spherical or elliptical cystic mass. Debris may be seen within the fluid centre. Peristaltic contractions may occasionally be seen in the cyst wall. Characteristically, the wall of the cyst, being of gastrointestinal origin, has a double-layered appearance ('gut signature'), with an internal hyperechoic layer, the mucosa, and an external hypoechoic layer, representing smooth muscle (Figure 10.14.13). This double-layered appearance is not always present, particularly when inflammatory changes are present. Other structures of gastrointestinal origin, namely Meckel's diverticulum, may also bear this gut signature. Barium studies may show displacement of bowel or mass effect related to the duplication; however, some duplications are poorly delineated. Rarely, a tubular duplication is opacified by barium.

Duplications containing gastric mucosa will show activity on technetium 99m pertechnetate studies and thus must be considered within the differential diagnosis for focal uptake along with

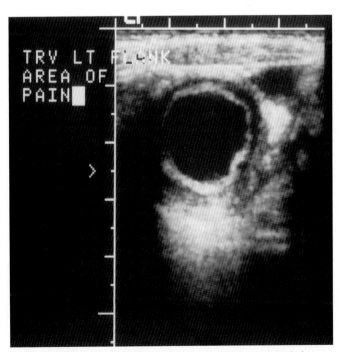

Figure 10.14.13 Duplication cyst. The cyst wall has a hyperechoic inner layer (mucosa) and a hypoechoic outer layer (muscle).

Meckel's diverticulum. Findings of a duplication on CT are less specific than with sonography as the characteristic layered appearance of the wall of the duplication is not delineated by CT. Nevertheless, if a cystic mass is identified adjacent to bowel, a duplication must be considered. On magnetic resonance imaging (MRI), duplication cysts have high signal on T2-weighted images and have smooth walls.

Treatment of a duplication cyst usually requires resection of the adjacent bowel as the walls of the duplication and the native bowel are intimately associated, sharing a muscular wall and blood supply. A mesenteric cyst is the main differential diagnosis for duplication cysts. The distinction is important as most surgeons will remove duplication cysts because of the complication of severe bleeding from contained gastric mucosa but mesenteric cysts, if symptomatic, may be left in situ.

FURTHER READING

Berrocal T, Lamas M, Gutierrez J. Congenital anomalies of the small intestine, colon, and rectum. Radiographics 1999; 19:1219–1236.

Macpherson RI. Gastrointestinal tract duplications: clinical, pathologic, etiologic, and radiologic considerations. Radiographics 1993; 13:1063–1080.

Peksoy I, Caner B, Kale G et al. Tc-99m pertechnetate scintigraphy for the detection of ileal duplication. Clinical Nuclear Medicine 1998; 23:233–234.

Spotswood SE. Peristalsis in duplication cyst: a new diagnostic sonographic finding. Pediatric Radiology 1994; 24:344–345.

Stern LE, Warner BW. Gastrointestinal duplications. Seminars in Pediatric Surgery 2000; 9:135–140.

Teele RL, Henschke CI, Tapper D. The radiographic and ultrasonographic evaluation of enteric duplication cysts. Pediatric Radiology 1980; 10:9–14.

OTHER CYSTS

Enteric non-duplication cysts are rare lesions, which have an enteric mucosal lining but no muscular lining. Imaging findings are non-specific; however, they will not have the characteristic double-layered appearance of a duplication cyst as they lack the hypoechoic muscular layer. Mesothelial cysts are also rare and also have the non-specific appearance of unilocular fluid-filled mass. They have a mesothelial lining.

FURTHER READING

Bento L, Martinez MA, Conde J et al. Mesothelial cysts of the peritoneum in children. Cirugia Pediatrica 1989; 2:140–142.

Ros PR, Olmsted WW, Moser RR Jr et al. Mesenteric and omental cysts: histologic classification with imaging correlation. Radiology 1987; 164:327–332.

CONGENITAL SHORT GUT SYNDROME

Congenital short gut syndrome is rare, particularly in the absence of associated congenital intestinal atresia. It may be associated with malrotation, perhaps representing an early volvulus with infarction and reconstitution of the lumen. Radiographs may show dilated bowel loops with air–fluid levels (Fig. 10.14.14). The diagnosis is suggested by rapid transit of barium through a diminished length of bowel. The existing bowel is dilated, partially fluid filled, and there is poor distinction between small bowel and colon.

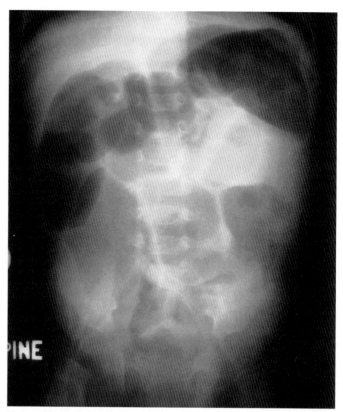

Figure 10.14.14 Congenital short gut syndrome. Bowel is diffusely dilated. Small bowel study showed short intestinal length with poor distinction of small bowel and colon. At surgery, it appeared that there was an auto-anastomosis of mid-jejunum to mid-colon, perhaps due to *in utero* volvulus.

FURTHER READING

Tiu CM, Chou YH, Pan HB et al. Congenital short bowel. Pediatric Radiology 1984; 14:343–345.

ACQUIRED ANATOMICAL ABNORMALITIES

ACQUIRED SHORT GUT SYNDROME

Short gut syndrome is usually the manifestation of small bowel resection for congenital atresia(s), gastroschisis, necrotizing enterocolitis, volvulus and occasionally other disorders. Severity of clinical manifestations is determined not only by the length of small bowel that remains but also its anatomy. Absence of the ileocaecal valve portends a worse prognosis. Symptoms are manifest as failure to thrive, with malabsorption and diarrhoea. Segmental areas of dilatation predispose to enteritis from bacterial overgrowth. Management of fluid and electrolytes is a constant challenge. The children are predisposed to gallstones, particularly with absence of the distal ileum, and renal stones, due to excessive resorption of oxalate. Hepatic disease is common due to reliance on supplemental parenteral nutrition.

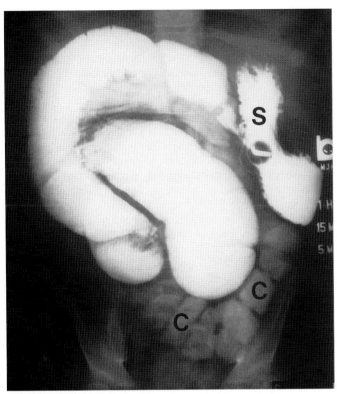

Figure 10.14.15 Acquired short gut syndrome. The patient, a 10-year-old boy, was born with gastroschisis and had a substantial length of small bowel resected. The entirety of the patient's remaining small bowel is opacified with barium. The small bowel is dilated, in part due to a partial obstruction at the enterocolonic anastomosis. The patient had clinical evidence of bacterial overgrowth. Faint barium reaches non-dilated colon (C). S, stomach, with gastrostomy.

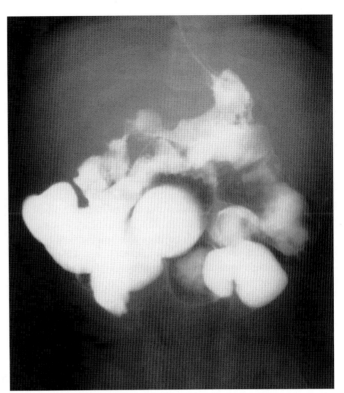

Figure 10.14.16 Acquired short gut syndrome. The patient is a 5-month-old status-post bowel resection for necrotizing enterocolitis. Dilated small bowel loops vary in calibre. The overall length of small bowel is diminished.

Barium studies will show the short anatomical length of small bowel (Figure 10.14.15). In general, the remaining small bowel is increased in calibre and mucosal folds increased in prominence. These findings, in part, may represent a compensatory mechanism to increase surface area for nutritional absorption. The calibre of the remaining small bowel may vary considerably and disordered transit may fragment the barium column (Figure 10.14.16).

FURTHER READING

Barksdale EM, Stanford A. The surgical management of short bowel syndrome. Current Gastroenterology Report 2002; 4:229–237.

Kalifa G, Devred P, Ricour C et al. Radiological aspects of the small bowel after extensive resection in children. Pediatric Radiology 1979; 8:70–75.

Parigi GB, Braheri R, Minniti S et al. How short must a bowel be to be a "short bowel"? Transplant Proceedings 1994; 26:1450.

Sigalet DL. Short bowel syndrome in infants and children: an overview. Seminars in Pediatric Surgery 2001; 10:49–55.

OTHER SMALL BOWEL SURGERIES

In addition to straightforward resections and end-to-end anastomoses, a number of surgical procedures may affect the paediatric small bowel. Roux-en-Y procedures are uncommon but are occasionally performed as part of the Kasai procedure for biliary atresia, liver transplantation and unusual situations where pylorus or duodenum is excluded. Gastric dissociation is a recently introduced procedure for intractable gastroesophageal reflux where the stomach is disconnected from the oesophagus and a roux-en-Y loop of jejunum is connected to the oesophagus, usually end-to-side. A gastrostomy is used for feeding. The operation may be complicated by leak at the oesophagojejunal anastomosis, obstruction of the jejunal loop or persistent jejunoesophageal reflux. In children with short gut syndrome, the Bianchi procedure or similar operation may be performed for bowel lengthening. Small bowel transplants are occasionally performed for children with short gut syndrome or other diffuse small bowel abnormality (i.e. intestinal neuronal dysplasia). Small bowel transplants are often performed in conjunction with transplantation of other organs, including liver and pancreas. Limited success of small bowel transplantation has prevented more widespread use. In addition to mechanical complications, these children are at risk for other complications associated with transplantation and immunosuppression, including infection and malignancy.

FURTHER READING

Bach DB, Levin MF, Vellet AD et al. CT findings in patients with small-bowel transplants. American Journal of Roentgenology 1992; 159:311–315.

Bianchi A. Experience with longitudinal intestinal lengthening and tailoring. European Journal of Pediatric Surgery 1999; 9:256–259.

Campbell WL, Abu-Elmagd K, Federle MP et al. Contrast examination of the small bowel in patients with small-bowel transplants: findings in 16 patients. American Journal of Roentgenology 1993; 161:969–974.

Park BK. Intestinal transplantation in pediatric patients. Progress in Transplantation 2002; 12:97–113.

Putnam P, Reyes J, Kocoshis S et al. Gastrointestinal posttransplant lymphoproliferative disease in children after small intestinal transplantation. Transplant Proceedings 1996; 28:2777.

ISCHAEMIA AND HAEMORRHAGE

MESENTERIC VASCULAR INSUFFICIENCY

Mesenteric vascular insufficiency is most common in the neonatal period as a consequence of necrotizing enterocolitis or as a complication of umbilical vascular catheterization. Children with hypoperfusion of gut related to congenital heart disease may develop ischaemic gut, which behaves in a similar way clinically to the necrotizing enterocolitis seen in neonates. This has been called mesenteric ischaemia of childhood (MIC). Mesenteric ischaemia may occur due to mechanical abnormalities including malrotation with volvulus, intussusception, obstruction and trauma. Embolic mesenteric occlusion may occur in children with congenital heart disease, polycythaemia, clotting disorders or with catheterization. Mesenteric ischaemia may rarely be seen in children with collagen vascular disorders, arteritis, nephrotic syndrome and meningococcaemia. Although atherosclerotic mesenteric occlusive disease does not present in childhood, children with idiopathic middle aortic syndrome or syndromic vascular disease (i.e. neurofibromatosis) may have mesenteric insufficiency due to aortic or branch vessel narrowing or occlusion.

Acute mesenteric insufficiency presents with pain, distension and vomiting. Blood may be noted in stools. Presentation may be catastrophic. Chronic mesenteric insufficiency is more cryptic in presentation. Chronic abdominal pain is commonly noted. The child may have malabsorption. Abdominal radiographs are often unrevealing. With advanced bowel ischaemia or infarction, bowel wall thickening of intramural gas may be noted. These findings are well delineated by CT. Ischaemic bowel wall may show dense enhancement with contrast. Catheter angiography or magnetic resonance angiography may be used to image the abdominal aorta and mesenteric vasculature.

FURTHER READING

Alpern MB, Glazer GM, Francis IR. Ischemic or infarcted bowel: CT findings. Radiology 1988; 166:149–152.

Hebra A, Brown MF, Hirschl RB et al. Mesenteric ischemia in hypoplastic left heart syndrome. Journal of Pediatric Surgery 1993; 28:606–611.

Meacham PW, Dean RH. Chronic mesenteric ischemia in childhood and adolescence. Journal of Vascular Surgery 1985; 2:878–885.

Zochondne D. Von Recklinghausen's vasculopathy. American Journal of the Medical Sciences 1984; 287:64–65.

PNEUMATOSIS INTESTINALIS

Pneumatosis intestinalis (intramural gas) may be curvilinear or multicystic in appearance. Dependent on aetiology, findings may involve the colon, small bowel or both. The colon is more frequently affected. In children, pneumatosis intestinalis is most commonly the consequence of necrotizing enterocolitis; this is covered in the neonatal gastrointestinal section of this text. In older children, various causes of mesenteric ischaemia, discussed previously, may result in pneumatosis intestinalis. Obstruction may lead to pneumatosis intestinalis, presumably due to increased intraluminal pressure and local mucosal disruption. Pneumatosis intestinalis may rarely be seen with severe gastroenteritis, heralding a poorer prognosis (see Figure 14.14.21). Children with cystic fibrosis will rarely develop asymptomatic pneumatosis intestinalis. Patients on steroids for collagen vascular disease or transplants occasionally also develop asymptomatic pneumatosis intestinalis for unclear reasons. Pneumatosis intestinalis is also occasionally seen in children with short gut syndrome and/or a history of gastroschisis repair; the reason for this is unclear. Idiopathic pneumatosis intestinalis is extremely rare in children.

The radiographic finding of pneumatosis intestinalis is nonspecific. Other radiological findings and clinical findings may help to determine the aetiology and clinical significance. On radiographs, curvilinear or circular lucency is seen paralleling the bowel wall (Figure 10.14.17). Cystic pneumatosis intestinalis appears bubbly or mottled and may be difficult to differentiate from faeces. Occasionally, CT may be used to confirm pneumatosis intestinalis. Portal venous gas is usually an ominous sign. Positional films are necessary to look for evidence of pneumoperitoneum, which may indicate perforation and a need for surgery.

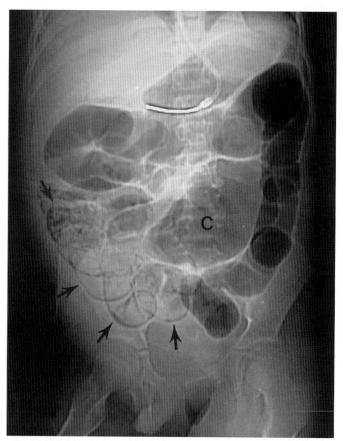

Figure 10.14.17 Pneumatosis intestinalis. CT scout image in a boy with chronic graft-versus-host disease on high-dose steroids. Diffuse intramural gas is seen in distal ileum. C, malpositioned caecum (no volvulus present).

FURTHER READING

Fenton LZ, Buonomo C. Benign pneumatosis in children. Pediatric Radiology 2000; 30:786–793.
Reynolds HL Jr, Gauderer MWL, Hrabovsky EE et al. Pneumatosis cytoides intestinalis in children beyond the first year of life: manifestations and management. Journal of Pediatric Surgery 1991; 26:1376–1380.
West KW, Rescoria FJ, Grosfeld JL et al. Pneumatosis intestinalis in children beyond the neonatal period. Journal of Pediatric Surgery 1989; 24:818–822.

INTRAMURAL HAEMORRHAGE

The most common cause of small bowel intramural haematoma is trauma. This is discussed in the chapter on gastrointestinal tract trauma. Minor trauma, often unnoticed, may cause bowel wall haematoma in patients with haemophilia, in patients with thrombocytopaenia due to malignancy and/or chemotherapy and in patients on anticoagulant therapy.

HENOCH–SCHÖNLEIN PURPURA

Henoch–Schönlein purpura (HSP), also known as anaphylactoid purpura, is a vasculitic disease of uncertain aetiology. Occasionally, a preceding infectious illness is noted. HSP most commonly occurs in children under 10 years old. HSP is characterized by a purpuric rash, arthritis, abdominal pain and, occasionally, transient renal insufficiency. Blood may be noted in stools. Abdominal symptoms not infrequently precede the purpuric rash rendering the diagnosis difficult. Imaging may show bowel wall thickening due to oedema and intramural haemorrhage. A 'stack of coins' appearance from intramural haemorrhage and inflammatory oedema is frequently seen on small bowel studies (Figure 10.14.18). Luminal narrowing may be significant. The abnormality may be diffuse,

segmental or localized. Proximal and mid-small bowel is commonly affected. Focal areas of intramural haemorrhage may act as a lead point for small bowel intussusception, occasionally progressing into the colon (ileo–ileo–colic). These intussusceptions may be difficult to reduce. Sonography can be used to demonstrate small bowel haematoma (Figure 10.14.19) or intussusception.

HSP, in general, is a self-limited process with a very good clinical outcome. Rarely, a severe complication may occur involving the gastrointestinal tract, the urinary tract or the brain. Patients are treated with steroids.

FURTHER READING

Connolly B, O'Halpin D. Sonographic evaluation of the abdomen in Henoch–Schölein purpura. Clinical Radiology 1994; 49:320–323.
Glasier CM, Siegel MJ, McAlister WH et al. Henoch–Schönlein syndrome in children: gastrointestinal manifestations. American Journal of Roentgenology 1981; 136:1081–1085.
Hu SC, Feeney MS, McNicholas M et al. Ultrasonography to diagnose and exclude intussusception in Henoch–Schönlein purpura. Archives of Disease in Childhood 1991; 66:1065–1067.
Siskind BN, Burrell MI, Pun H et al. CT demonstration of gastrointestinal involvement in Henoch–Schönlein syndrome. Gastrointestinal Radiology 1985; 10:352–354.

HAEMOLYTIC URAEMIC SYNDROME

Haemolytic uraemic syndrome (HUS), a necrotizing vasculitis, produces renal failure (uraemia), haemolytic anaemia and thrombocytopaenia. The disease is probably postinfectious in aetiology. There is a recognized association with an *Escherichia coli* 0157:H7 gastroenteritis and therefore outbreaks occur. A gastroenteritis-like prodrome is often seen with gastrointestinal symptoms including pain, vomiting and diarrhoea, which may be bloody. Later, patients

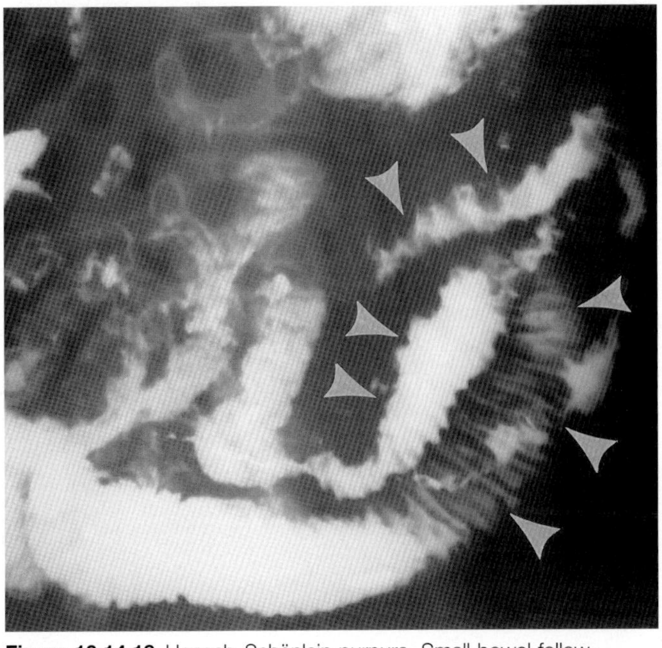

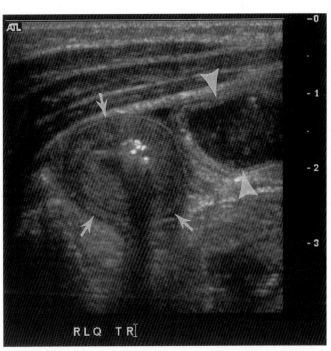

Figure 10.14.18 Henoch–Schönlein purpura. Small bowel follow-through shows fold thickening and separation of loops (arrowheads).

Figure 10.14.19 Henoch–Schönlein purpura. Ultrasound shows a thick-walled loop of ileum (arrows). Adjacent bowel is normal (arrowheads).

have fatigue, weakness, listlessness and decreased urine output. The disease affects both small and large bowel, although colonic disease often predominates. Bowel wall oedema or intramural haemorrhage may produce segmental fold thickening. The affected segment may act as the lead point of an intussusception. In severe cases, an adynamic ileus or obstruction may be seen. After the acute phase, strictures may occasionally form.

FURTHER READING

Kirks DR. The radiology of enteritis due to hemolytic-uremic syndrome. Pediatric Radiology 1982; 12:179–183.

INFECTION AND INFLAMMATION

GASTROENTERITIS

Infectious gastroenteritis is a common cause of illness and hospital admission in children throughout the world. In developed countries, gastroenteritis is usually viral and usually self-limited or easily treated. In underdeveloped countries, other pathogens are more common, medical care is poor and many children still die of gastroenteritis. Malabsorption may be a complication of severe gastroenteritis; however, it is usually transient.

In northern climates, viral gastroenteritis is seasonal, with a higher incidence of disease in the colder months. Rotavirus is the most commonly identified pathogen, although other viruses can cause similar illness. Children present with diarrhoea and vomiting. Except for the rare infant or child who develops problems due to late recognition and treatment of dehydration, most children with viral gastroenteritis do well. Cytomegalovirus may cause gastroenteritis in immunodeficient patients. A variety of agents can cause bacterial gastroenteritis including *Campylobacter*, *E. coli*, *Staphylococcus aureus*, *Salmonella typhi*, *Shigella*, *Vibrio cholera*, and *Yersinia enterocolitica*. Cholera is principally seen in Asia. Yersina is commonly seen in North America and is often acquired through the consumption of contaminated food or water. *Escherichia coli* gastroenteritis is often seen in outbreaks related to contaminated food or water.

Plain films will show diffuse gaseous distension of small and large bowel, with air–fluid levels on positional views – the pattern of an ileus (Figure 10.14.20). The amount of air versus fluid present varies considerably. Intramural gas may rarely be seen in severe infections, particularly if complicated by dehydration or sepsis (Figure 10.14.21). Similar abnormality is seen on CT. The findings are non-specific; however, imaging does often serve to exclude other processes such as appendicitis. The radiographic findings for *Yersinia enterocolitica* warrant special mention. *Yersinia enterocolitica* produces wall thickening and mucosal irregularity in the terminal ileum, which may be easily confused with Crohn's disease (Figure 10.14.22). There may be associated mesenteric lymph node enlargement. The diagnosis is made by identification of the organism in stools. Occasionally, other pathogens may also cause focal abnormality in the terminal ileum.

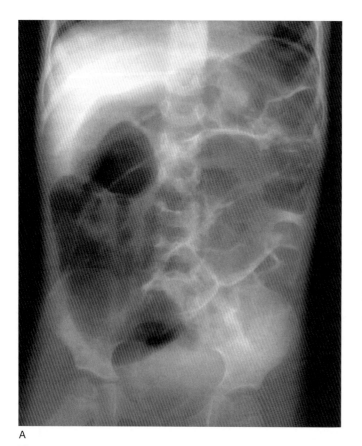

A

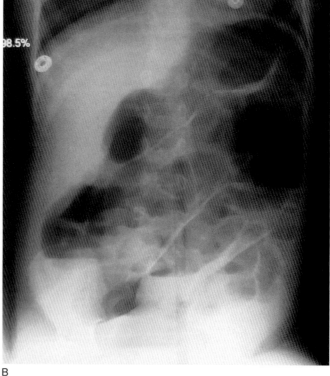

B

Figure 10.14.20 Viral gastroenteritis. (A) Radiographs show diffuse gaseous distension of bowel, predominantly colon. (B) The upright view shows multiple air–fluid levels.

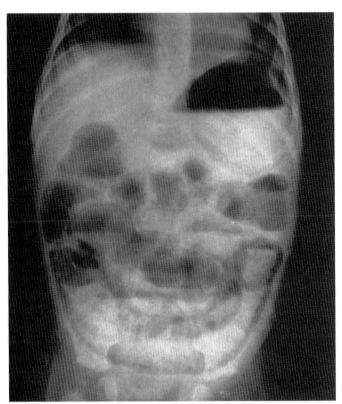

Figure 10.14.21 Gastroenteritis. There is diffuse pneumatosis of both stomach and the entire small bowel. The disease was fatal in this child from the Middle East.

FURTHER READING

Abdel-Haq NM, Asmar BI, Abuhammour WM et al. Yersinia enterocolitica infection in children. Pediatric Infectious Diseases Journal 2000; 19:954–958.

Balthazar EJ, Charles HW, Megibow AJ. Salmonella- and Shigella-induced ileitis: CT findings in four patients. Journal of Computer Assisted Tomography 1996; 20:375–378.

Hoogkamp-Korstanje JA, Stolk-Engelaar VM. Yersinia enterocolitica infection in children. Pediatric Infectious Diseases Journal 1995; 14:771–775.

Jelloul L, Fremond B, Dyon JF et al. Mesenteric adenitis caused by Yersinia pseudotuberculosis presenting as an abdominal mass. European Journal of Pediatric Surgery 1997; 7:180–183.

Lieberman JM. Rotavirus and other viral causes of gastroenteritis. Pediatric Annals 1994; 23:529–532, 534–535.

Matsumoto T, Iida M, Sakai T et al. Yersinia terminal iteitis: sonographic findings in eight patients. American Journal of Roentgenology 1991; 156:965–967.

Rodriguez-Baez N, O'Brien R, Qiu SQ et al. Astrovirus, adenovirus, and rotavirus in hospitalized children: prevalence and association with gastroenteritis. Journal of Pediatric Gastroenterology and Nutrition 2002; 35:64–68.

TUBERCULOUS ENTERITIS

Tuberculous enteritis may be due to a primary infection of small bowel, secondary to swallowed byproducts from a pulmonary infection or due to haematogenous spread. The disease is more common in underdeveloped countries but is occasionally seen in all parts of the world. One-third of the world's population is infected with tuberculosis. Children with immunodeficiency or malnutrition are predisposed. Most children with intestinal

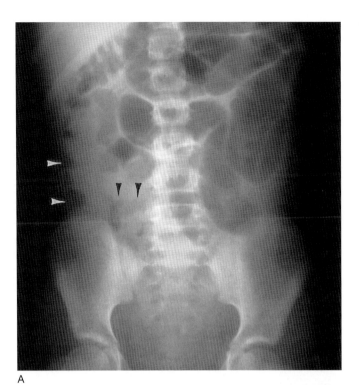

Figure 10.14.22 *Yersinia enterocolitica*. (A) Radiograph shows partial small bowel obstruction. A paucity of gas in the right lower quadrant and irregular gas within ascending colon and distal ileum (arrowheads) suggests abnormality. (B) CT shows thickening of the caecal wall (C) and wall of terminal ileum (arrowheads). (Courtesy of K. A. Garver, Ann Arbor, MI, USA.)

tuberculosis are substantially ill, both due to their underlying illness and to tuberculosis itself. Signs and symptoms include emaciation, abdominal distension, abdominal pain, vomiting and diarrhoea. Symptoms may be seen due to other areas of involvement, particularly the lungs. Lung disease is not invariably present. Diagnosis may be made by microbiological methods; however, these results may be delayed or low in yield. Skin testing is also performed; however, it is important to remember that in severely ill, immunodeficient or malnourished children, skin tests may be false negative.

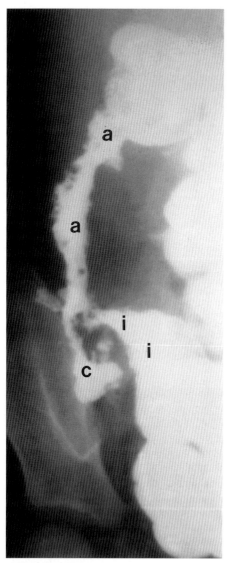

Figure 10.14.23 Ileocaecal tuberculosis. Narrowing and mucosal irregularity is seen in the terminal ileum (i), caecum (c) and ascending colon (a). (Courtesy of D. H. Jamieson, Vancouver, BC, Canada.)

Abnormality is often confined to the ileocaecal region and hence may be mistaken for Crohn's disease. Other portions of the intestine are involved less commonly. Radiological findings are very similar to Crohn's disease, although there is disproportionate caecal involvement (Figure 10.14.23). Longstanding disease may produce strictures, a rigid appearing terminal ileum with a patulous ileocaecal valve. Occasionally, the terminal ileum may appear to empty directly into the stenotic ascending colon with lack of opacification of a scarred, contracted caecum (Stierlin's sign). Separation of loops may represent mass effect from enlarged lymph nodes or peritoneal fluid collections. Lymphatic obstruction may produce a malabsorption pattern. Imaging with ultrasound or CT often shows evidence of lymph node disease, peritoneal disease and involvement of other organs.

FURTHER READING

Balthazar EJ, Gordon R, Hulnick D. Ileocecal tuberculosis: CT and radiologic evaluation. American Journal of Roentgenology 1990; 154:499–503.

Bargallo N, Nicolau C, Luburich P et al. Intestinal tuberculosis in AIDS. Gastrointestinal Radiology 1992; 17:115–118.

Cremin BJ. Tuberculosis: the resurgence of our most lethal infectious disease – a review. Pediatric Radiology 1995; 25:620–626.

Makanjuola D, al Orainy I, al Rashid R et al. Radiological evaluation of complications of intestinal tuberculosis. European Journal of Radiology 1998; 26:261–268.

CRYPTOSPORIDIUM

Cryptosporidium may cause non-specific proximal small bowel wall thickening in children with AIDS. The predominant symptom is diarrhoea.

FURTHER READING

Haller JO, Cohen HL. Gastrointestinal manifestations of AIDS in children. American Journal of Roentgenology 1994; 162:387–393.

Lumadue JA, Manabe YC, Moore RD et al. A clinicopathologic analysis of AIDS-related cryptosporidiosis. AIDS 1998; 12:2459–2466.

CANDIDA

Candidal infection within the bowel is usually seen in patients who are immunocompromised due to AIDS or malignancy and their treatment. The colon may also be involved. The predominant symptom is diarrhoea, which may be severe. Non-specific fold thickening will be seen on barium studies.

FURTHER READING

Radin DR, Fong TL, Halls JM et al. Monilial enteritis in acquired immunodeficiency syndrome. American Journal of Roentgenology 1983; 141: 1289–1290.

GIARDIASIS

Giardiasis is the most common parasitic disease of the small bowel in northern climates and developed countries. It is also seen commonly in temperate climates. *Giardia lamblia* is a flagellated protozoan. The organism is acquired by ingestion of cysts, which mature into trophozoites in the small bowel. In North America, a history is often obtained of the ingestion of contaminated water, for instance from a stream. Outbreaks of disease are common. Children with certain immunodeficiencies are more prone to develop the infection, particularly dysgammaglobulinaemia. Symptoms include abdominal pain and diarrhoea. More severe disease causes malabsorption. With mild infection, radiological studies may be normal. On imaging, fold thickening is seen in the distal duodenum and jejunum (Figure 10.14.24). Findings may be seen on small bowel studies or CT (Figure 10.14.25). Secretions may be increased and motility may be disordered. Transient small bowel intussusceptions may be seen on CT. Diagnosis is made by the demonstration of cysts in faeces.

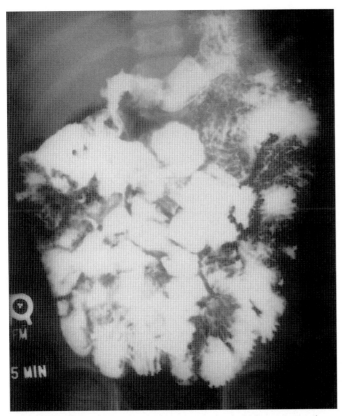

Figure 10.14.24 Giardiasis with secondary protein-losing enteropathy and hypogammaglobulinaemia. Findings include fold thickening, which is diffuse, but more prominent proximally, mild dilation and segmentation.

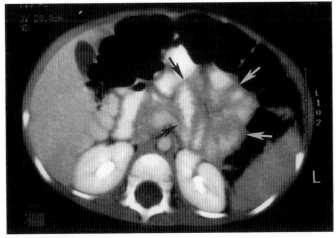

Figure 10.14.25 Giardiasis. CT shows thickening of proximal small bowel wall (arrows).

FURTHER READING

Farthing MJ. Giardiasis. Gastroenterology Clinics of North America 1996; 25:493–515.

Marshak RH, Ruoff M, Lindner AE. Roentgen manifestations of giardiasis. American Journal of Roentgenology, Radium Therapy and Nuclear Medicine 1968; 104:557–560.

HELMINTHS

Parasitic infection with helminths is uncommon in developed countries; however, intestinal parasites do constitute a major public health problem in underdeveloped parts of the world. With travel and immigration, the diseases may occasionally present in non-endemic environments.

FURTHER READING

Barrett-Connor E, Connor JD, Beck JW. Common parasitic infections of the intestinal tract. Pediatric Clinics of North America 1967; 14:235–254.

Thomas AM. Radiological manifestations of parasitic disease. British Journal of Hospital Medicine 1986; 35:303–311.

TAPEWORM

Tapeworm (*Hymenolepis nana*) is rare in developed northern countries but is seen elsewhere. The most common symptom is abdominal pain. Filling defects may be seen on barium studies.

ROUNDWORM

Roundworm (*Ascaris lumbricoides*) is common throughout the world and may be seen in moderately temperate climates. Young children are predisposed as exposure usually occurs due to oral intake of contaminated soil. The ingested eggs hatch at the duodenum. Larvae enter the portal venous system and migrate to the lungs. A transient eosinophilic pneumonia may be seen. Larvae then migrate up the airway and are swallowed, then lodging and maturing in the proximal small bowel. The adult worms are quite large, growing up to several millimetres in diameter and 20–30 cm in length.

Symptoms are usually related to intestinal obstruction, with pain being the most common clinical manifestation. Systemic symptoms include fever and general malaise. A peripheral eosinophilia is seen. Malnutrition may be seen in severe cases. Rarely, the worms may cause perforation and an acute abdomen. Occasionally, the worms may enter and obstruct the biliary tree, pancreatic duct or appendix.

On imaging, the diagnosis is suggested by the demonstration of the worms as filling defects within enteric contrast (Figure 10.14.26). Occasionally, the worm may digest barium itself, producing a thread-like linear opacity within the centre of the worm. Worms may appear solitary or as a tangled mass of several. Rarely, worms are outlined by air and seen on plain radiographs (Figure 10.14.27). Diagnosis of ascariasis is confirmed by recovery of ova or the worms themselves from stools.

FURTHER READING

Beitia AO, Haller JO, Kantor A. CT findings in pediatric gastrointestinal ascariasis. Computerized Medical Imaging and Graphics 1997; 21:47–49.

Khuroo MS. Ascariasis. Gastroenterology Clinics of North America 1996; 25:553–557.

Louw JH. Abdominal complications of ascaris lumbricoides infestation in children. British Journal of Surgery 1966; 53:510–521.

O'Lorcain P, Holland CV. The public health importance of Ascaris lumbricoides. Parasitology 2000; 121:S51–S71.

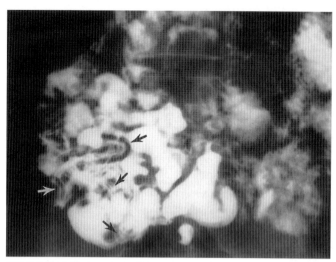

Figure 10.14.26 Ascariasis. Tubular filling defects are seen in distal ileum due to the worms. Note barium centrally within the worms opacifying the intestinal tract (arrows). (Courtesy of A. L. Franklin and B. H. Adler, Columbus, OH, USA.)

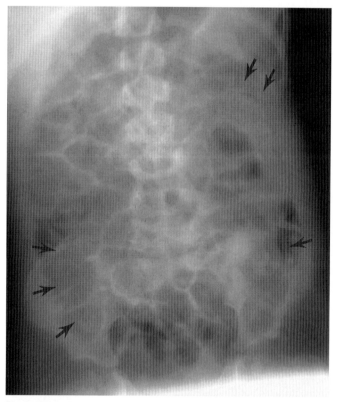

Figure 10.14.27 Ascariasis. Tubular opacities (worms) are seen within bowel (arrows).

Singh PA, Gupta SC, Agrawal R. Ascaris lumbricoides appendicitis in the tropics. Tropical Doctor 1997; 27:241.

Villamizar E, Mendez M, Bonilla E et al. Ascaris lumbricoides infestation as a cause of intestinal obstruction in children: experience with 87 cases. Journal of Pediatric Surgery 1996; 31:201–204.

WHIPWORM

Whipworm (trichuriasis) is seen only in warm climates. Like ascariasis, whipworm is acquired by oral consumption of contaminated soil or food. The swallowed eggs hatch within small bowel but mature worms pass to the colon and attach. Although the disease is thus predominantly colonic, the terminal ileum may be involved. Symptoms, if present, relate to colonic disease. A granular mucosal pattern is seen on barium studies.

FURTHER READING

Manzano C, Thomas MA, Valenzuela C. Trichuriasis. Roentgenographic features and differential diagnosis with lymphoid hyperplasia. Pediatric Radiology 1979; 8:76–78.

Stephenson LS, Holland CV, Cooper ES. The public health significance of Trichuris trichiura. Parasitology 2000; 121:S73–S95.

HOOKWORM

Hookworms (ankylostomiasis) are associated with villous atrophy in the small bowel. Flattening or thickening of mucosal folds may be seen in the proximal small bowel; however, the radiographic abnormality is usually subtle, at best. There is some debate as to whether the villous atrophy is a direct effect of the hookworms or a secondary effect of the associated anaemia and malnutrition.

STRONGYLOIDIASIS

Strongyloidiasis is more common in warmer climates but may be seen in the colder north. Immunocompromised children are predisposed. Exposure is through the skin, with migration of larvae to the lungs and then to the bowel. The proximal small bowel is most affected. Patients present with pain, nausea and vomiting, diarrhoea and malnutrition. Acutely, inflammatory changes with fold thickening and dilatation may be seen. Later, loss of the normal fold pattern and strictures may be seen. Diagnosis can be made by identification of larvae in the stool, vomitus or a duodenal aspirate.

FURTHER READING

Berkmen YM, Rabinowitz J. Gastrointestinal manifestations of the strongyloidiasis. American Journal of Roentgenology, Radium Therapy and Nuclear Medicine 1972; 115:306–311.

Dallemand S, Waxman M, Farman J. Radiological manifestations of Strongyloides stercoralis. Gastrointestinal Radiology 1983; 8:45–51.

Hizawa K, Iida M, Eguchi K et al. Comparative features of double-contrast barium studies in patients with isosporiasis and strongyloidiasis. Clinical Radiology 1998; 53:764–767.

SCHISTOSOMIASIS

Schistosomiasis (trematodes, flukes) is more common in warmer climates. Infection is acquired from contaminated water via the skin. A few of the organisms will pass via the portal vein and lodge in the bowel wall. The infestation may produce anaemia, diarrhoea and protein-losing enteropathy. An inflammatory response to shed ova may be seen in the bowel, leading eventually to stricture formation. Although most species of schistosomiasis predominantly affect the colon, *Schistosoma japonicum* may predominantly affect the small bowel. Schistosomiasis produces granulomatous disease and fibrosis in the liver.

FURTHER READING

Lee RC, Chiang JH, Cou YH et al. Intestinal schistosomiasis japonica: CT-pathologic correlation. Radiology 1994; 193:539–542.
Monzawa S, Uchiyama G, Ohtomo K et al. Schistosomiasis japonica of the liver: contrast-enhanced CT findings in 113 patients. American Journal of Roentgenology 1993; 161:323–327.

EOSINOPHILIC GASTROENTERITIS

Eosinophilic gastroenteritis may occur in relation to a food allergy, such as to milk allergy, or on idiopathic basis. Idiopathic eosinophilic gastroenteritis is an uncommon disorder manifest by infiltration of the bowel wall with eosinophils and an increased number of eosinophils in the circulating blood. Children frequently have a history of other immune disorders including reactive airway disease, atopic dermatitis and atopy. A family history of such disorders is also common. Symptoms of abdominal pain, diarrhoea and vomiting may be prolonged but may wax and wane. With long-standing disease the patient may manifest failure to thrive, weight loss, protein-losing enteropathy or anaemia. The proximal small bowel is commonly involved. There often is concomitant stomach involvement. Non-specific thickening of small bowel and gastric folds is seen. Thickened small bowel folds may appear nodular. The diagnosis is strongly suggested when gastric and proximal bowel fold thickening is seen together with peripheral eosinophilia. The patients respond to treatment with steroids.

The most common allergic gastroenteritis is cows' milk protein allergy. This disorder is relatively common, occurring in 1–5% of children. Children present with diarrhoea. With prolonged exposure, other signs and symptoms may develop including vomiting, failure to thrive, anaemia, blood in stools and protein-losing enteropathy. The diagnosis is usually made by removing the offending agent, usually cows' milk. Imaging studies are often normal; however, small bowel studies may show fold thickening, most prominent in the jejunum (Figure 10.14.28). The radiographic abnormality is usually mild. The abnormality may resolve after the offending agent is removed.

FURTHER READING

Liu HY, Whitehouse WM, Giday Z. Proximal small bowel transit pattern in patients with malabsorption induced by bovine milk protein ingestion. Radiology 1975; 115:415–420.
MacCarty RL, Talley NJ. Barium studies in diffuse eosinophilic gastroenteritis. Gastrointestinal Radiology 1990; 15:183–187.
Teele RL, Katz AJ, Goldman H et al. Radiographic features of eosinophilic gastroenteritis (allergic gastroenteropathy) of childhood. American Journal of Roentgenology 1979; 132:575–580.

RADIATION ENTERITIS

With advancements in the field of radiation oncology and changes in therapy, radiation injury to small bowel in children is now an uncommon problem. Permanent small bowel injury is unlikely in doses under 5000 rad (50 Gy). Acute radiation enteritis produces

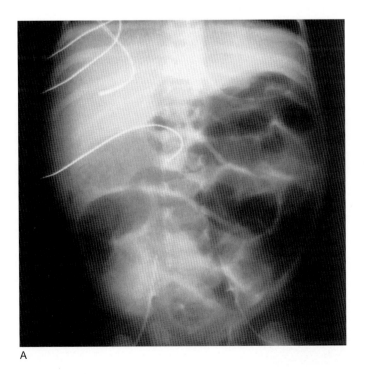

A

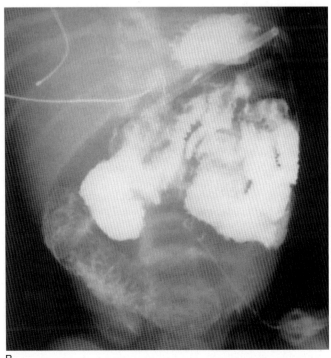

B

Figure 10.14.28 Eosinophilic gastroenteritis – milk allergy. (A) Diffuse dilatation of bowel is seen on radiography. (B) Mild, diffuse irregularity and thickening of small bowel folds is seen in small bowel in the left upper quadrant.

symptoms of pain and diarrhoea. If a small bowel study is performed it may show non-specific fold thickening to bowel localized to the radiation portal. Malabsorption may occur. The delayed finding of stricture may not occur until months or years later.

FURTHER READING

Donaldson SS, Jundt S, Ricour C et al. Radiation enteritis in children. A retrospective review, clinicopathologic correlation, and dietary management. Cancer 1975; 35:1167–1178.

Parisi MT, Fahmy JL, Kaminsky CK et al. Complications of cancer therapy in children: a radiologist's guide. Radiographics 1999; 19:283–297.

CROHN'S DISEASE

Crohn's disease, or regional enteritis, is the most common inflammatory disease of the small bowel in children. Crohn's disease presents throughout childhood. It is very rare in infancy but relatively common in adolescence. Approximately 15–20% of cases present in childhood. Although extensively sought, the cause of Crohn's disease remains unknown. The disease is more common in Caucasians. There is a mild familial predisposition.

In children, as in adults, the terminal ileum is the predominant site of disease. Approximately 75% of children have disease at the terminal ileum at the time of diagnosis. Colonic involvement is common. The majority of patients with colonic disease have concomitant terminal ileal disease. Proximal skip lesions in association with terminal ileal disease are common; however, isolated disease in the jejunum or proximal ileum without terminal ileum disease is uncommon. Involvement of the oesophagus, stomach or duodenum without the terminal ileum involved is distinctly uncommon but can occur (see Figure 10.13.17).

On histology, Crohn's disease is characterized by the presence of non-caseating granulomas. The involvement of small bowel loops is characterized as transmural and often asymmetrical. Transmural involvement of involved bowel loops may contribute to the formation of fistulas. Segments with longstanding disease may become fibrotic and strictured.

The clinical manifestations of Crohn's disease in childhood are myriad; however, abdominal pain is, by far, the most common clinical manifestation. The pain is non-specific but occasionally localized to the right lower quadrant. Although the onset of symptoms is usually gradual, occasionally Crohn's disease presents acutely and may be clinically mistaken for appendicitis. In fact, Crohn's disease may cause appendicitis. Diarrhoea is common and blood is frequently found in the stools. Perianal disease, namely anal fissures and perirectal fistulas, is common. Extensive small bowel involvement may produce malabsorption. Gallstones are common due to disordered enterohepatic circulation. Renal stones are common due to increased oxalate absorption and resultant hyperoxaluria. Systemic, extraintestinal manifestations include fever, arthritis, uveitis, failure to thrive, delayed maturation, anorexia, erythema nodosum and, rarely, even psychiatric changes. In general, the extraintestinal manifestation of sclerosing cholangitis is less common in children than adults. Although there is an increased risk of gastrointestinal malignancy, it is very, very rare to manifest in childhood. The risk for malignancy is substantially less than that of ulcerative colitis.

Findings of Crohn's disease in the oesophagus and stomach are non-specific and rarely identified in children. On careful examination with double-contrast technique, small ulcers (apthae) may be seen. With duodenal involvement, thickened irregular folds are seen with occasional ulceration. Diagnosis of Crohn's disease in the oesophagus, stomach and duodenum is now usually made via endoscopy. Small bowel follow-through is commonly used to identify or monitor small bowel disease. Careful attention to serial films and intermittent fluoroscopy are necessary. Enteroclysis may rarely be utilized in problematic cases, but, in general, is not well tolerated by children. Colonic disease is now usually diagnosed by endoscopy.

Findings of Crohn's disease within the small bowel vary depending on the chronicity of involvement. Separation from adjacent loops may in part represent wall thickening; however, it is also due to increased deposition of mesenteric fat. Small ulcers (apthae) are seen early (Figure 10.14.29). Acutely inflamed mucosa will have cobblestone appearance with ulceration, linear clefts and sinuses (Figures 10.14.30 and 10.14.31). The lumen will appear rigid and narrow due to the bowel wall thickening and spasm. The abnormality is fixed and changes little with palpation. With proximal small bowel involvement, the abnormality may be limited to non-specific nodularity and fold thickening (Figure 10.14.32, see also Fig. 10.13.17). With more longstanding disease, involved segments are strictured due to fibrosis and the mucosa becomes featureless (Figure 10.14.33). The 'string sign' is indicative of a longer segment of stricture. Dilatation may be seen proximal to strictures, and pseudosacculation and kinking may result

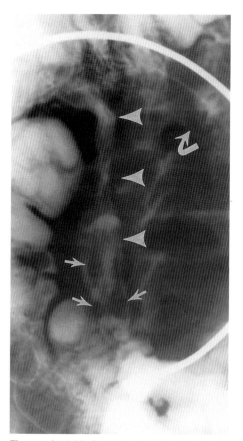

Figure 10.14.29 Crohn's disease. The distal ileum (arrowheads) is narrowed and irregular. Small ulcers (aphthae) are seen (arrows). Curved arrow, suture line from prior partial colectomy. A compression paddle is being applied. (Courtesy of L. Paul Sonda, Ann Arbor, MI, USA.)

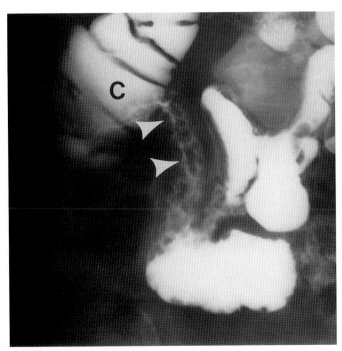

Figure 10.14.30 Crohn's disease. Small bowel follow-through shows cobblestone pattern of terminal ileum with linear ulceration (arrowheads). C, caecum.

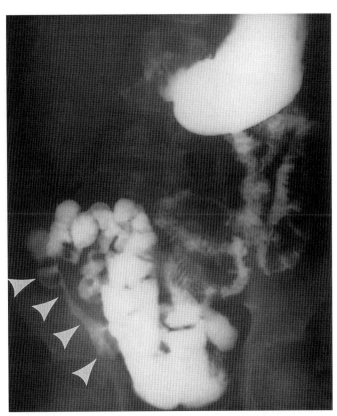

Figure 10.14.32 Crohn's disease. Small bowel follow-through shows skip lesions. Irregular fold thickening is seen throughout jejunum in left upper quadrant. The terminal ileum is strictured with pseudosacculation (arrowheads).

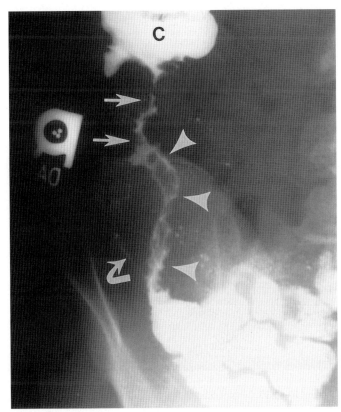

Figure 10.14.31 Crohn's disease. Small bowel follow-through shows inflammatory narrowing of the terminal ileum (arrowheads), caecum and ascending colon (arrows) with an abrupt transition to normal colon (C). Note double tract in terminal ileum and faintly visualized ileocaecal fistula (curved arrow).

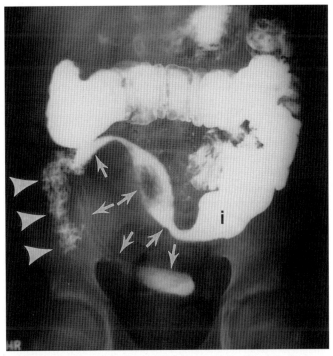

Figure 10.14.33 Crohn's disease. Small bowel follow-through shows narrowing and irregular, spiculated mucosa within an extensive length of distal ileum (arrows). Proximal ileum (i) is mildly dilated. The caecum and proximal ascending colon (arrowheads) appear irregular but are poorly distended.

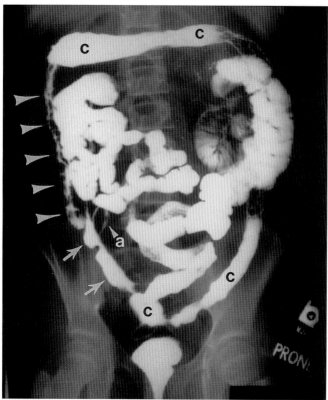

Figure 10.14.34 Crohn's disease. Small bowel follow-through shows diffuse abnormality of terminal ileum including loss of the normal fold pattern, stricture (arrows) and pseudosacculation. The colon (C) is diffusely abnormal with loss of haustra, narrowing of calibre and diffuse nodularity of the ascending colon (arrowheads). a, appendix.

from eccentric fibrosis and stricturing derived from asymmetrical involvement of the bowel wall (Figure 10.14.32 and 10.14.34).

Fistulas may be seen within the bowel wall paralleling the lumen or extending to adjacent small bowel loops or colon (Figure 10.14.35). Most fistulas are seen at the ileocaecal region. Fistulas may occasionally form to the bladder or vagina. Abscesses may cause mass effect on the adjacent bowel. Psoas abscesses are occasionally seen (Figure 10.14.35).

CT, ultrasound and even MRI have been used to diagnose and follow patients with Crohn's disease. The advantage of cross-sectional imaging is being able to image beyond the mucosa. Bowel wall thickening is better appreciated by cross-sectional imaging than on barium studies (Figure 10.14.36). On ultrasound, the thickened bowel wall produces a 'target' lesion. The wall may approach a centimetre in thickness. The inflamed ileum of Crohn's disease is easily distinguished from an inflamed appendix by its size and the degree of wall thickening. Increased blood flow on Doppler interrogation is indicative of active inflammation. Extraintestinal abscesses and inflammatory changes (phlegmon) are well seen by CT (Figure 10.14.35). Fistulas are poorly demonstrated but may be inferred by extraluminal gas or intravesicular gas. Although CT is usually not preferred as the initial mode of imaging, overlap in presenting signs and symptoms with other disorders commonly imaged by CT, namely appendicitis, means many patients are often first diagnosed by CT. CT does play a substantial role in the surveillance for complications, namely abscess.

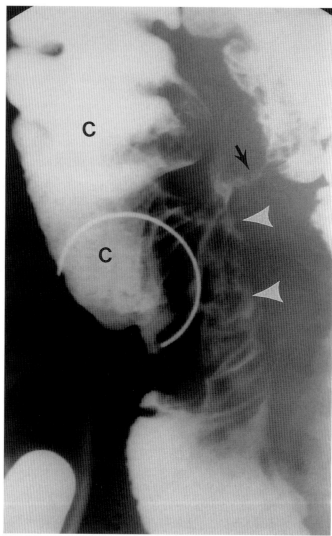

A

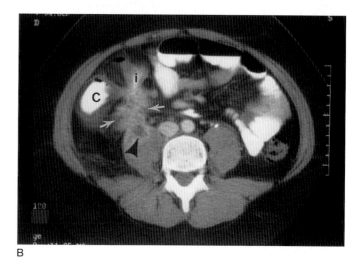

B

Figure 10.14.35 Crohn's disease. (A) Small bowel follow-through shows an irregular terminal ileum (arrowheads), fold thickening in caecum (C), and a fistula from terminal ileum to more proximal ileum (arrow). (B) CT shows an inflammatory mass (arrows) involving caecum (C) and terminal ileum (i). The inflammatory mass extends to the adjacent psoas muscle where a small abscess (arrowhead) is seen.

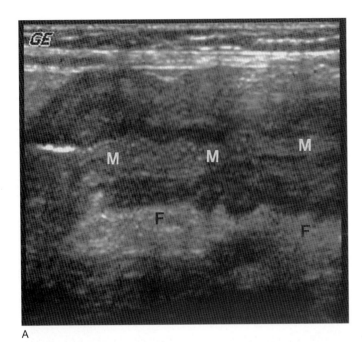

A

B

Figure 10.14.36 Crohn's disease. Longitudinal (A) and transverse (B) ultrasound images show marked thickening of the wall of the terminal ileum. M, mucosa. Note prominent adjacent echogenic fat (F).

MR imaging for Crohn's disease is still under investigation but gadolinium-enhanced fat saturation T1-weighted images have shown promise in delineating active sites of inflammation. [111]Indium-labelled leucocytes and [99m]technetium HM-PAO (hexamethyl propyleneamine-oxime) labelled leucocytes are occasionally used to identify active sites of inflammation.

Medical management of Crohn's disease is preferred if at all possible. The regimen includes steroids. Nevertheless, many patients ultimately do undergo surgery, usually to remove obstructing strictured segments or localized disease recalcitrant to medical management.

The differential diagnosis for Crohn's disease is extensive. Clinical, and even histological, differentiation from ulcerative colitis may be difficult. Backwash ileitis due to ulcerative colitis may mimic Crohn's disease of the terminal ileum, although usually the proper diagnosis is suggested by the concomitant colonic findings. Infections, including *Yersinia enterocolitica*, tuberculosis and fungal disease, may mimic Crohn's disease. Disorders affecting the small bowel mucosal pattern, including neoplasia, malabsorption, parasites, immune deficiency and haemorrhage (Henoch–Schönlein purpura) also may produce abnormality similar to Crohn's disease. Normal lymphoid hyperplasia of the terminal ileum may occasionally be mistaken for Crohn's disease.

FURTHER READING

Aideyan UO, Smith WL. Inflammatory bowel disease in children. Radiologic Clinics of North America 1996; 34:885–902.

Ali ST, Carty HM. Paediatric Crohn's disease: a radiological review. European Radiology 2000; 10:1085–1094.

Charron M, del Rosairo JF, Kocoshis S. Use of technetium-tagged white blood cells in patients with Crohn's disease and ulcerative colitis: is differential diagnosis possible? Pediatric Radiology 1998; 28:871–877.

Charron M, Del Rosario F, Kocoshis S. Assessment of terminal ileal and colonic inflammation in Crohn's disease with 99mTc-WBC. Acta Paediatrica 1999; 88:193–198.

Gryboski JD. Crohn's disease in children 10 years old and younger: comparison with ulcerative colitis. Journal of Pediatric Gastroenterology and Nutrition 1994; 18:174–182.

Halligan S, Nicholls S, Bartram CI et al. The distribution of small bowel Crohn's disease in children compared to adults. Clinical Radiology 1994; 49:314–316.

Halligan S, Nicholls S, Beattie RM et al. The role of small bowel radiology in the diagnosis and management of Crohn's disease. Acta Paediatrica 1995; 84:1375–1378.

Jabra AA, Fishman EK, Taylor GA. Crohn disease in the pediatric patient: CT evaluation. Radiology 1991; 179:495–498.

Jabra AA, Fishman EK, Taylor GA. CT findings in inflammatory bowel disease in children. American Journal of Roentgenology 1992; 162:975–979.

Low RN, Sebrechts CP, Politoske DA et al. Crohn disease endoscopic correlation: single shot fast spin-echo and gadolinium-enhanced spoiled gradient-echo MR imaging. Radiology 2002; 222:652–660.

Munkholm P, Langholz E, Davidson M et al. Intestinal cancer risk and mortality with Crohn's disease. Gastroenterology 1993; 105:1716–1723.

Stringer DA, Sherman P, Liu P et al. Value of the peroral pneumocolon in children. American Journal of Roentgenology 1986; 146:763–766.

Stringer DA. Imaging inflammatory bowel disease in the pediatric patient. Radiologic Clinics of North America 1987; 25:93–113.

BACKWASH ILEITIS (ULCERATIVE COLITIS)

Backwash ileitis is seen in approximately 10% of patients with ulcerative colitis. Backwash ileitis is usually seen with caecal involvement producing a patulous ileocaecal valve and free reflux into the terminal ileum. Usually, the involved segment of terminal ileum is relatively smooth and featureless (Figure 10.14.37). Occasionally, the terminal ileum appears more inflamed, mimicking Crohn's disease.

GRAFT-VERSUS-HOST DISEASE

Graft-versus-host disease (GVHD) is seen in bone marrow transplant recipients. The donor graft cells trigger an immune-mediated

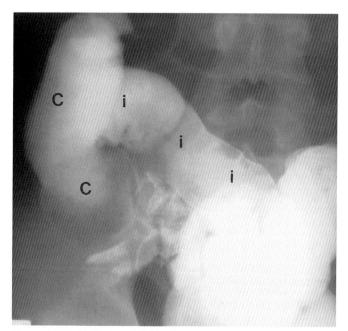

Figure 10.14.37 Backwash ileitis. The ileum (i) is dilated and featureless. The caecum (C) is also featureless.

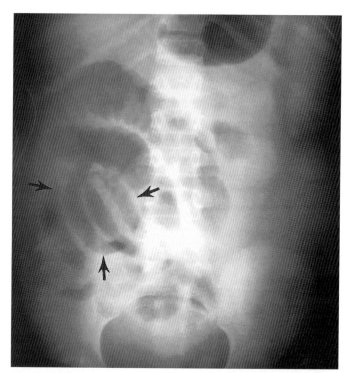

Figure 10.14.38 Graft-versus-host disease. Tubular bowel loops in the right lower abdomen are separated due to wall thickening (arrows). Other bowel loops more cephalad and over midline are dilated with thickened folds.

reaction to the patient's native skin, gastrointestinal tracts, lungs and liver. The diagnosis is often suspected based on clinical examination and confirmed by skin biopsy. When bowel is involved the patient may develop diarrhoea. Plain films often show tubular, featureless gas-filled small bowel loops (Figure 10.14.38). Non-specific radiographic findings include air–fluid levels, dilatation and intramural gas. Barium studies will demonstrate thickened bowel wall with effacement or loss of the normal fold pattern. A rapid transit time and increased secretions may be noted. A layered appearance or marked enhancement of the bowel wall may be seen on CT (Figure 10.14.39). Recovery of involved bowel varies, with most returning to normal, but some strictures may occur. As patients prone to GVHD are immunocompromised, infectious processes may potentially mimic the findings of GVHD or concomitantly affect the small bowel.

FURTHER READING

Donnelly LF. CT imaging of immunocompromised children with acute symptoms. American Journal of Roentgenology 1996; 167:909–913.

Donnelly LF, Morris CL 1996 Acute graft-versus-host disease in children: abdominal CT findings. Radiology 199:265–268

Maile CW, Frick MP, Crass JR et al. The plain abdominal radiograph in acute gastrointestinal graft-vs.-host disease. American Journal of Roentgenology 1985; 145:289–292.

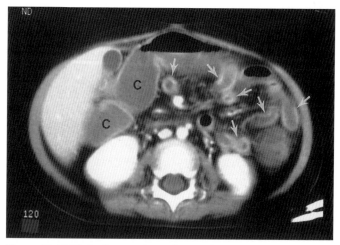

Figure 10.14.39 Graft-versus-host disease. Fluid-filled small bowel loops are seen with densely enhancing walls (arrows). C, colon, filled with fluid.

CHRONIC GRANULOMATOUS DISEASE

Chronic granulomatous disease (CGD) may rarely affect the small bowel. Non-specific fold thickening is noted in the proximal small bowel. Radiographic findings are more evident in the stomach and oesophagus.

FURTHER READING

Ament ME, Ochs HD. Gastrointestinal manifestations of chronic granulomatous disease. New England Journal of Medicine 1973; 288:382–387.

Issacs D, Wright VM, Shaw DG et al. Chronic granulomatous disease mimicking Crohn's disease. Journal of Pediatric Gastroenterology and Nutrition 1985; 4:498–501.

COLLAGEN VASCULAR DISEASES

Small bowel abnormality due to collagen vascular disease is uncommon in childhood as the abnormalities usually occur with longstanding disease. With longstanding scleroderma or dermatomyositis, small bowel motility may be diminished, associated with dilatation, pseudodiverticula and fold thickening. Rarely, the necrotizing vasculitis of dermatomyositis leads to acute small bowel abnormality, including perforation.

FURTHER READING

Magill HL, Hixson SD, Whitington G et al. Duodenal perforation in childhood dermatomyositis. Pediatric Radiology 1984; 14:28–30.

BEHÇET'S DISEASE

Behçet's disease is characterized by the triad of recurrent stomatitis, genital ulceration and ocular symptoms. The disease is rare in children. Small bowel involvement is usually in the terminal ileum and usually with concomitant colonic disease. Any part of the gastrointestinal tract may be involved. Disease most commonly involves the distal small bowel and may clinically and radiologically mimic Crohn's disease. Identification of the extraintestinal symptoms may suggest the diagnosis.

FURTHER READING

Stringer DA, Cleghorn GJ, Durie PR et al. Behcet's syndrome involving the gastrointestinal tract – a diagnostic dilemma in childhood. Pediatric Radiology 1986; 16:131–134.

NEOPLASM

Benign neoplasms of the small bowel are uncommon in children. Presenting signs and symptoms include haemorrhage, anaemia and pain. Lesions may act as a lead point for a small bowel intussusception, producing obstruction. Many lesions are associated with underlying syndromes.

Peutz–Jeghers syndrome is probably the most common syndrome to produce small bowel lesions in children. Patients with Peutz–Jeghers syndrome develop hamartomatous polyps. The polyps may be sessile or pedunculated and are most numerous in the mid- and distal small bowel (Figure 10.14.40). Polyps may act as lead points for intussusceptions, which are usually transient, but may cause symptoms and may occasionally persist necessitating urgent treatment. Peutz–Jeghers syndrome is inherited in an autosomal dominant fashion. Patients with Peutz–Jeghers syndrome have a characteristic mucocutaneous pigmentation, primarily affecting the lips and mouth. The hands and feet are also affected. There is an increased risk of adenocarcinoma of the intestine, although not necessarily due to malignant transformation of a hamartomatous polyp. Patients with Peutz–Jeghers syndrome are at considerably increased risk of developing an extraintestinal malignancy, usually in adulthood.

Patients with familial adenomatous polyposis or Gardner's syndrome may develop adenomatous polyps in the small bowel;

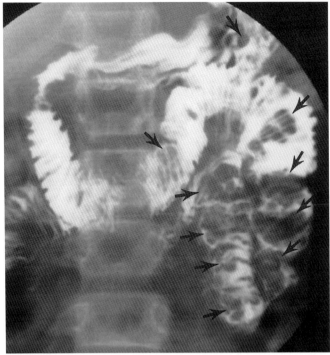

A

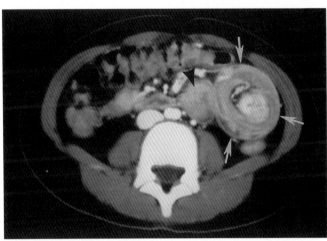

B

Figure 10.14.40 Peutz–Jeghers syndrome. (A) Multiple polyps are seen as filling defects in stomach, distal duodenum and proximal jejunum (arrows). (B) Small bowel intussusception (arrows) due to polyp. Note mesenteric fat and blood vessels within the mass. Adjacent mass (arrowhead) is also part of the intussusception. (Courtesy of E.-L. H. J. Teo, Singapore, Singapore.)

however, the extent and number of small bowel lesions is considerably less than that in the colon. Patients with Gardner's syndrome may develop desmoid tumours within the mesentery, which may secondarily affect the small bowel (see Figure 10.14.67).

Haemangiomas within the retroperitoneum may involve the small bowel. Patients with multiple haemangiomatous lesions, particularly neonates, or syndromes such as Klippel–Trenaunay syndrome or Maffucci syndrome are more likely to have involvement of the bowel. Patients may have one or multiple lesions. Plain films may show phleboliths in larger lesions. Findings on barium study or CT are usually non-specific, although dense enhancement of the lesion or involved bowel may be seen on CT with contrast. Multiple gastrointestinal tract haemangiomas may be seen in blue rubber nevus syndrome. Haemangioma is a rare cause of a false-positive Meckel's scan due to pooling of tracer in the lesion. Lymphangiomatous malformations may also involve the small bowel.

Patients with neurofibromatosis may develop neurofibromas affecting the small bowel. The lesions are submucosal but may produce a polypoid filling defect. Extrinsic mass effect from retroperitoneal or mesenteric neurofibromas is more common (see Figure 10.14.68).

Other benign small bowel lesions, including leiomyoma, lipoma and fibroma, are rare in children. Findings on small bowel studies are non-specific. Identification of fat within a bowel lesion on CT suggests lipoma.

Primary malignant tumours of the small bowel are exceedingly rare in childhood. Adenocarcinoma of the small bowel does not present in childhood. Carcinoid tumour may rarely present in the distal ileum in childhood; however, appendiceal lesions are more common.

Lymphoma is the most common malignant lesion of the small bowel in children. In general, involvement of the bowel in children with lymphoma is uncommon. If the bowel is involved, it is likely that the child has non-Hodgkin's lymphoma, probably the Burkitt subtype. Bowel involvement by lymphoma is most common in children under 8 years of age. Most children with small bowel involvement show evidence of disease at other sites. Focal involvement of the small bowel, primary small bowel lymphoma, can occur but is uncommon. Lymphoma most commonly involves the terminal ileum. At the terminal ileum, the differential diagnosis includes Crohn's disease and infection. Usually, the degree of wall thickening and the presence of extraintestinal manifestations, most notably lymph node disease, will suggest lymphoma.

Patients with small bowel lymphoma may present with gastrointestinal bleeding, anaemia or pain, often resulting from intussusception. Extraintestinal sites of disease or systemic manifestations may also bring the patient to medical attention. Most commonly, small bowel lymphoma is seen as marked thickening of the bowel wall. This may be well demonstrated on ultrasound or CT (Figure 10.14.41). Large masses may cause aneurysmal dilatation of the bowel lumen, which may be suggested on CT but is better demonstrated by a barium study (Figure 10.14.42). Mucosal detail is obliterated in the dilated segment. Lymphoma may also cause diffuse fold thickening, polypoid lesions and large annular lesions (Figure 10.14.43). Lymphoma may act as the lead point for an intussusception. Bowel abnormalities due to lymphoma may be demonstrated on barium studies, which will also show separation of bowel loops due to wall thickening or mesenteric disease. Small bowel may be encased by mesenteric or intraperitoneal disease. Leukaemia can involve the small bowel but this is rare.

Post-transplant lymphoproliferative disease (PTLD) is a neoplastic process occurring in transplant recipients that is linked to the Epstein–Barr virus. It usually represents a B-cell proliferation, ranging from a benign mononucleosis-like illness, easily treated, to fulminant lymphoma, resistant to treatment. In most patients, PTLD is most likely to be seen within or adjacent to the transplanted organ. Patients with intra-abdominal transplanted organs or with fulminant PTLD are therefore more likely to have small

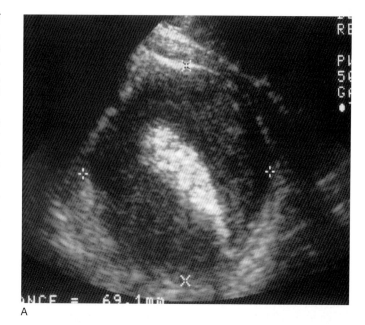

A

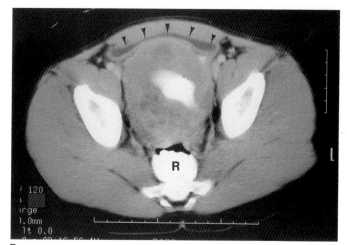

B

Figure 10.14.41 Burkitt's lymphoma. (A) On ultrasound, echogenic bowel lumen is seen centrally with markedly thickened bowel wall (cursors). Echogenic mucosa and bowel contents are seen centrally. (B) On CT, a large soft tissue mass encases a distorted bowel lumen. The bladder (arrowheads) is compressed anteriorly. R, rectum.

bowel involvement. Radiological findings of PTLD are similar to those seen in other patients with lymphoma (Figure 10.14.44).

Secondary involvement of the small bowel by extraintestinal malignancies is very rare. Extrinsic mass effect from large intra-abdominal tumours is common. Actual metastasis to the small bowel is exceedingly rare in children.

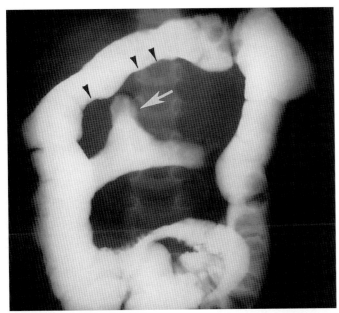

Figure 10.14.42 Lymphoma. Barium refluxed into distal small bowel shows a featureless loop with focal aneurysm (arrow). Mass effect is noted on the inferior margin of the transverse colon (arrowheads).

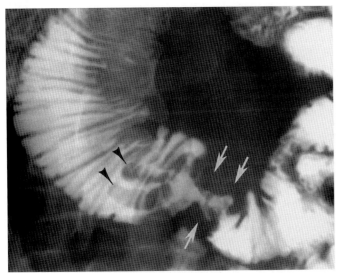

Figure 10.14.43 Partial small bowel obstruction due to lymphoma. The lumen is markedly narrowed and irregular (arrows) and the bowel is dilated proximally. Filling defects (arrowheads) are intestinal contents, retained proximal to the obstruction. (Courtesy of L. Paul Sonda, Ann Arbor, MI, USA.)

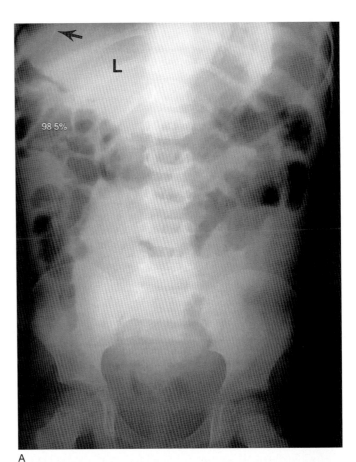

A

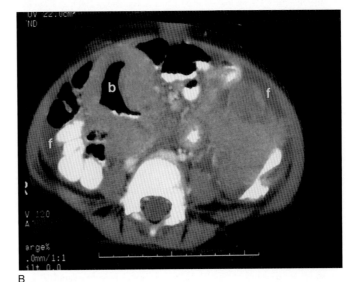

B

Figure 10.14.44 Post-transplant lymphoproliferative disorder. (A) Mass effect is seen in the lower abdomen. Note abnormal liver shadow (L) and surgical sutures (arrow) due to partial liver transplant. (B) CT shows large masses in the mesentery (left) and encasing bowel (b, right). f, fluid.

FURTHER READING

Bank ER, Hernandez RJ, Byrne WJ. Gastrointestinal hemangiomatosis in children: demonstration with CT. Radiology 1987; 165:657–658.

Basaklar AC. Haemangiomas of the gastrointestinal tract in children. Zeitschrift fur Kinderchirurgie 1990; 45:114–116.

Buck JL, Harned RK, Lichtenstein JE et al. Peutz–Jeghers syndrome. Radiographics 1992; 12:365–378.

Buck JL, Sobin LH. Carcinoids of the gastrointestinal tract. Radiographics 1990; 10:1081–1095.

Chow CW, Sane S, Campbell PE et al. Malignant carcinoid tumors in children. Cancer 1982; 49:802–811.

Corredor J, Wambach J, Barnard J. Gastrointestinal polyps in children: advances in molecular genetics, diagnosis, and management. Journal of Pediatrics 2001; 138:621–628.

Davis GB, Berk RN. Intestinal neurofibromas in von Recklinghausen's disease. American Journal of Gastroenterology 1973; 60:410–414.

Donnelly LF, Frush DP, Marshall KW. Lymphoproliferative disorders: CT findings in immunocompromised children. American Journal of Roentgenology 1998; 171:725–731.

Golding RL, Perri G. The radiology of gastrointestinal Burkitt's lymphoma in children. Clinical Radiology 1977; 28:465–468.

Gupta AK, Berry M, Mitra DK. Gastrointestinal smooth muscle tumors in children: report of three cases. Pediatric Radiology 1994; 24:498–499.

Harned RK, Buck JL, Sobin LH. The hamartomatous polyposis syndromes: clinical and radiologic features. American Journal of Roentgenology 1995; 164:565–571.

Harris JP, Mundnen MM, Minifee PK. Sonographic diagnosis of multiple small-bowel intussusceptions in Peutz-Jeghers syndrome: a case report. Pediatric Radiology 2002; 32:681–683.

Mako EK. Small-bowel hemangiomatosis in a patient with Maffucci's and blue-rubber-bleb-nevus syndromes. American Journal of Roentgenology 1996; 166:1499–1500.

Pickhardt PJ, Siegel MJ. Abdominal manifestations of posttransplantation lymphoproliferative disorder. American Journal of Roentgenology 1998; 171:1007–1013.

Pickhardt PJ, Siegel MJ. Posttransplantation lymphoproliferative disorder of the abdomen: CT evaluation in 51 patients. Radiology 1999; 213:73–78.

Scafidi DE, McLeary MS, Young LW. Diffuse neonatal gastrointestinal hemangiomatosis: CT findings. Pediatric Radiology 1998; 28:512–514.

Vessal K, Dutz W, Kohout E et al. Immunoproliferative small intestinal disease with duodenojejunal lymphoma: radiologic changes. American Journal of Roentgenology 1980; 135:491–497.

MALABSORPTION

Malabsorption represents a failure of the small bowel to properly digest food and absorb nutrients. Children with malabsorption present with failure to thrive, abdominal distension and abnormal stools. Stools may be steatorrhoeic, watery or even normal depending on the underlying disorder. Steatorrhoea is due to increased fat in the stools and is characterized by bulky, smelly stools, which float. There are numerous causes for malabsorption, some of which may be clinically obvious, others of which may be more challenging to diagnose. Small bowel biopsy is occasionally performed. Imaging is not usually the primary mode of diagnosis; however, some patients are imaged for various reasons. Abdominal radiographs are usually normal but occasionally may show small bowel dilatation with air–fluid levels. Barium studies will show small bowel fold thickening, dilatation, dilution of barium, segmentation and fragmentation of the barium column, and flocculation (Figure 10.14.45). Flocculation refers to the coarsened, particulate appearance that barium may acquire from mixing with increased intestinal secretions. Flocculation is less common

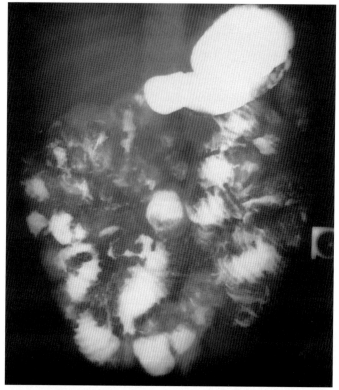

Figure 10.14.45 Malabsorption due to lymphangiectasia. Findings include fold thickening, dilatation, segmentation, flocculation and dilution of barium.

with modern barium preparations. Causes of malabsorption are myriad.

FURTHER READING

Ament ME. Malabsorption syndromes in infancy and childhood. II. Journal of Pediatrics 1972; 81:867–884.

Herlinger H. Radiology in malabsorption. Clinical Radiology 1992; 45:73–78.

Rubesin SE, Rubin RA, Herlinger H. Small bowel malabsorption: clinical and radiologic perspectives. How we see it. Radiology 1992; 184:297–305.

Weizman Z, Stringer DA, Durie PR. Radiologic manifestations of malabsorption: a nonspecific finding. Pediatrics 1984; 74:530–533.

PROTEIN-LOSING ENTEROPATHY

Protein-losing enteropathy (PLE) produces non-specific findings of fold thickening and decreased motility (Figures 10.14.46 and 10.14.47). Identified aetiologies for PLE include abetalipoproteinaemia, allergic gastroenteritis, coeliac disease (sprue), chronic hepatic dysfunction, collagen vascular disease, constrictive pericarditis, cows' milk protein allergy, Crohn's disease, cystic fibrosis, giardiasis, graft-versus-host disease, hereditary angioneurotic oedema, immunodeficiency syndromes, infectious mononucleosis, intestinal lymphangiectasia, lymphoma, mastocytosis, Ménétrier's disease, neuroblastoma, polyarteritis nodosa, progressive systemic sclerosis, structural abnormalities including chronic malrotation, systemic lupus erythematosus, tropical sprue, ulcerative colitis, Whipple's disease and Zollinger–Ellison syndrome.

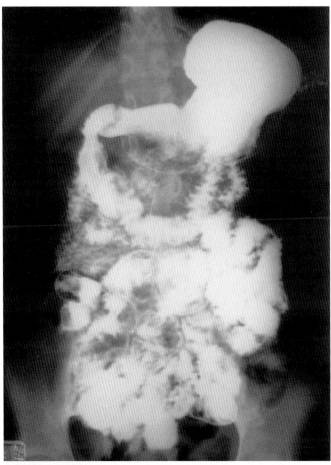

Figure 10.14.46 Protein-losing enteropathy. Small bowel folds are thickened. The small bowel has a granular, 'smudgy' appearance due to dilution of barium and mucosal abnormality.

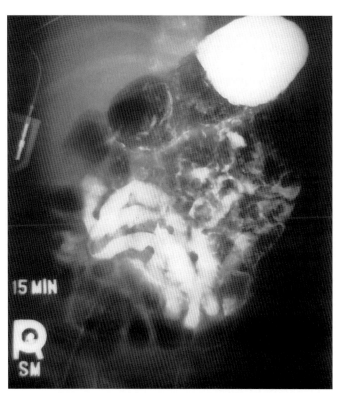

Figure 10.14.47 Protein-losing enteropathy. One-year-old with postinfectious protein-losing enteropathy. Fold thickening, flocculation and dilution of barium are noted.

Many of these disorders are uncommon in children. Recently, patients with a Fontan operation for congenital heart disease have been identified as at increased risk for developing PLE. This may relate to altered hepatic venous drainage related to the haemodynamics of the Fontan circuit. Cirrhosis and nephrotic syndrome result in hypoproteinaemia and secondary thickening of small bowel folds; however, the hypoproteinaemia is not due to loss in the gut.

FURTHER READING

Farthing MJ, McLean AM, Bartram CI et al. Radiologic features of the jejunum in hypoalbuminemia. American Journal of Roentgenology 1981; 136:883–886.

Gorske K, Winchester P, Grossman H. Unusual protein-losing enteropathies in children. Radiology 1969; 92:739–744.

INTESTINAL LYMPHANGIECTASIA

Intestinal lymphangiectasia is the result of maldevelopment of the intestinal lymphatic drainage system. There is resultant dilatation of lymphatic channels in the bowel wall and loss of lymph fluid

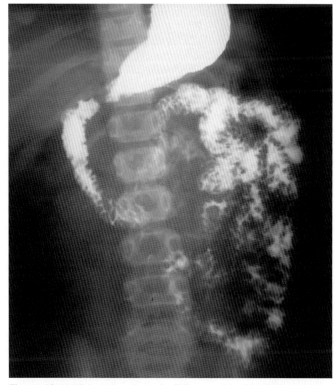

Figure 10.14.48 Lymphangiectasia. Diffuse nodular fold thickening is seen in proximal small bowel.

into the bowel. Excessive protein is lost. There is also resultant disruption of fat absorption leading to steatorrhoeic stools. Symptoms usually present in early childhood, with a poorer prognosis associated with a younger age at presentation. Symptoms include failure to thrive, peripheral oedema, recurrent infection, diarrhoea and vomiting. Peripheral oedema is due to hypoproteinaemia due to protein loss. Recurrent infections are perhaps due to immunoglobulin loss in the gut and associated lymphocytopenia. Concomitant lymphatic malformations may affect the extremities or the lungs. Chylous ascites and chylous pleural effusions may be present.

On barium studies, diffuse small bowel fold thickening is evident (Figure 10.14.48). Increased secretions may dilute the barium. Intestinal calibre is relatively normal. In milder cases, the small bowel study may be normal. Nuclear medicine studies performed with radiolabelled albumin may be used to document intestinal protein loss. The diagnosis is supported by laboratory analysis showing decreased serum albumin, decreased immunoglobulins and lymphocytopenia. Small bowel biopsies will show dilated lymphatic channels in the submucosa with distorted villi.

FURTHER READING

Olmsted WW, Madewell JE. Lymphangiectasia of the small bowel: description and pathophysiology of the roentgenographic signs. Gastrointestinal Radiology 1976; 1:241–243.
Shimkin PM, Waldmann TA, Krugman RL. Intestinal lymphangiectasia. American Journal of Roentgenology, Radium Therapy and Nuclear Medicine 1970; 110:827–841.

ABETALIPOPROTEINAEMIA

Abetalipoproteinaemia (Bassen–Kornzweig syndrome) is an autosomal recessive inherited disorder characterized by retinitis pigmentosa, acanthocytosis and progressive neurological impairment. Steatorrhoea occurs due to impaired fat transport through intestinal mucosal cells. There is resultant deficiency of certain serum lipids and lipoproteins. Radiographically, marked thickening of small bowel folds is noted, which is more severe proximally. The bowel may be mildly dilated. Small bowel biopsy is diagnostic by showing accumulation of lipid within mucosal cells.

FURTHER READING

Weinstein MA, Pearson KS, Agus SG. Abetalipoproteinemia. Radiology 1973; 108:269–273.

HEREDITARY ANGIONEUROTIC OEDEMA

Hereditary angioneurotic oedema is an autosomal recessive disorder characterized by episodes of diffuse oedema affecting the skin, mucous membranes and some internal organs. Laryngeal oedema may be life threatening. Abdominal pain is often present during symptomatic episodes and barium studies performed at such times may show fold thickening and separation of loops due to bowel wall oedema.

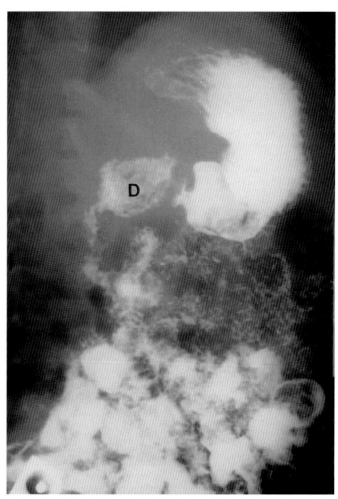

Figure 10.14.49 Immunoglobulin deficiency. Diffuse, nodular lymphoid hyperplasia is present throughout the small bowel, particularly evident in duodenum (D) on this projection. The colon was similarly affected.

FURTHER READING

De Backer AI, De Schepper AM, Vandevenne JE et al. CT of angioedema of the small bowel. American Journal of Roentgenology 2001; 176:649–652.
Pearson KD, Buchignani JS, Shimkin PM et al. Hereditary angioneurotic edema of the gastrointestinal tract. American Journal of Roentgenology, Radium Therapy and Nuclear Medicine 1972; 116:256–261.

IMMUNOGLOBULIN DEFICIENCIES

A variety of immune deficiency disorders are associated with bowel malfunction including Bruton's agammaglobulinaemia, common variable immunodeficiency, dysgammaglobulinaemia and isolated IgA deficiency. Conversely, protein-losing enteropathy can lead to immunoglobulin loss and resultant immune deficiency. Patients with immunoglobulin deficiencies frequently show prominent small bowel lymphoid hyperplasia (Figure 10.14.49). Diffuse fold thickening may be seen (Figure 10.14.50). Patients with immunoglobulin deficiencies are particularly prone to develop infection with giardiasis (see Figure 10.14.24). This is particularly true of patients with IgA deficiency and dysgammaglobulinaemia.

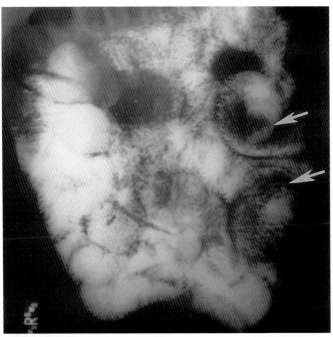

Figure 10.14.50 Immunoglobulin deficiency. The patient had chronic steatorrhoea, iron deficiency anaemia and failure to thrive. She had had one episode of giardia enteritis. The small bowel shows diffuse, slightly nodular fold thickening. Two transient intussusceptions are seen (arrows). The patient was subsequently diagnosed with common variable immunodeficiency. (Courtesy of L. Paul Sonda, Ann Arbor, MI, USA.)

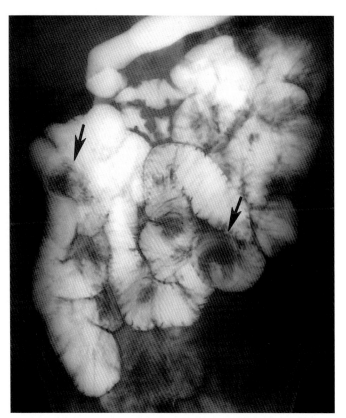

Figure 10.14.51 Coeliac disease. Jejunal folds (upper left) are reduced. Ileal folds (lower right) are increased. Two small bowel intussusceptions (arrows) are seen. (Courtesy of L. Paul Sonda, Ann Arbor, MI, USA.)

FURTHER READING

Marshak RH, Hazzi C, Lindner AE et al. Small bowel in immunoglobulin deficiency syndromes. American Journal of Roentgenology, Radium Therapy and Nuclear Medicine 1974; 122:227–240.
Marshak RH, Lindner AE, Maklansky D. Immunoglobulin disorders of the small bowel. Radiologic Clinics of North America 1976; 14:477–491.
Winchester P, Brill P. Roentgenographic feature of primary immunodeficiency diseases. Pediatric Annals 1976; 5:84–102.

ZOLLINGER–ELLISON SYNDROME

Zollinger–Ellison syndrome is the result of a gastrin-secreting pancreatic endocrine tumour. Gastrin leads to increased acid secretion from the stomach. Inadequately buffered gastric secretions disturb the small bowel mucosa, potentially producing a protein-losing enteropathy. Small bowel fold thickening is seen, which is more prominent proximally. Intestinal secretions are increased. Concomitant ulcers and gastric fold thickening support the diagnosis. The ulcers may be multiple and at unusual locations. CT, MRI or selective venous sampling by angiography may be necessary to localize the primary tumour, which is often subtle.

FURTHER READING

Christoforidis AJ, Nelson SW. Radiological manifestations of ulcerogenic tumors of the pancreas. The Zoillinger–Ellison syndrome. Journal of the American Medical Association 1966; 198:511–516.
Ragins H, Braylan RC. Zollinger–Ellison tumor associated with malabsorption syndrome. With abdominal distention resembling large bowel obstruction. American Journal of Surgery 1966; 112:441–446.

MASTOCYTOSIS

Mastocytosis is rare in children. Small bowel fold thickening is seen and presumably represents small bowel urticaria related to histamine hypersecretion.

FURTHER READING

Clemett AR, Fishbone G, Levine RJ et al. Gastrointestinal lesions in mastocytosis. American Journal of Roentgenology, Radium Therapy and Nuclear Medicine 1968; 103:405–412.

COELIAC DISEASE

Coeliac disease (sprue, gluten enteropathy) is a relatively common cause of malabsorption in childhood. The aetiology is an intolerance to gluten found in foods made from certain grains, including wheat. A familial predisposition does exist. Most patients present early in childhood. Patients present with failure to thrive and diarrhoea. Stools may be steatorrhoeic. Intestinal dilatation may produce abdominal distension. Inadequate resorption of fat-soluble vitamins may produce anaemia. Patients may have a protein-losing enteropathy. Severity of symptoms ranges from mild to severe and life threatening. The diagnosis is often made based on clinical findings, with biopsies performed for confirmation. Often, a repeat biopsy is performed after removal of dietary gluten for further confirmation. Imaging studies are usually not performed for the diagnosis but may occasionally be performed before the diagnosis is realized or for other reasons.

The degree of radiological abnormality varies in coeliac disease. Radiographs may show small bowel dilatation, which is more prominent proximally. Transient small bowel intussusceptions are common. Segmentation of the barium column is seen. Hypersecretion may produce flocculation of barium due to mixing. Segmentation and flocculation are less prominent with modern barium preparations. Folds may be enlarged or effaced. Dilatation of small bowel with effacement of folds produces the 'moulage' sign. Reversal of the normal jejunoileal fold pattern may occasionally be seen with a relatively featureless jejunum and increased ileal folds (Figure 10.14.51). Transit time is often increased.

Treatment of coeliac disease is removal of products containing gluten from the diet. Symptoms and radiological and histological abnormalities will resolve. There is an association of coeliac disease with lymphoma and carcinoma. This is relatively uncommon and rarely manifest in childhood.

FURTHER READING

Barlow JM, Johnson CD, Stephens DH. Celiac disease: how common is jejunoileal fold pattern reversal found at small-bowel follow-through? American Journal of Roentgenology 1996; 166:575–577.

Bova JG, Friedman AC, Weser E et al. Adaptation of the ileum in nontropical sprue: reversal of the jejunoileal fold pattern. American Journal of Roentgenology 1985; 144:299–302.

Haworth EM, Hodson CJ, Pringle EM et al. The value of radiological investigations of the alimentary tract in children with the coeliac syndrome. Clinical Radiology 1968; 19:65–76.

Rubesin SE, Herlinger H, Saul SH et al. Adult celiac disease and its complications. Radiographics 1989; 9:1045–1066.

TROPICAL SPRUE

Tropical sprue is probably an infection-related disorder and is seen only in certain parts of the world. Clinical features simulate sprue; however, there is no response to a gluten-free diet. Rather, patients respond to treatment with folic acid and tetracycline. Radiographic findings of tropical sprue are similar to those seen with sprue.

FURTHER READING

Enat R, Pollack S, Joffe B et al. Antibiotic-responsive malabsorption: a tropical sprue-like syndrome in countries with temperate climates. Israel Journal of Medical Sciences 1981; 17:367–369.

Glynn J. Tropical sprue – its aetiology and pathogenesis. Journal of the Royal Society of Medicine 1986; 79:599–606.

CYSTIC FIBROSIS

Cystic fibrosis is the most common genetic disease affecting the bowel and liver that may be lethal in childhood. It is autosomal recessive in inheritance. Patients are predominantly of Caucasian descent. Many genotypes exist accounting for great variability in presentation and severity of disease. The organs most affected are

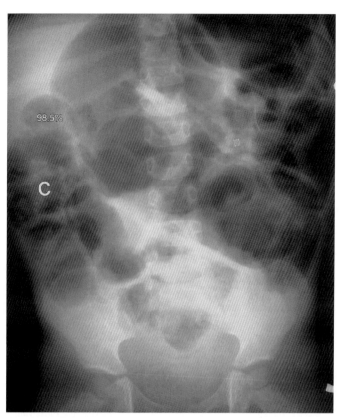

Figure 10.14.52 Distal intestinal obstruction syndrome. Four-year-old with cystic fibrosis and repeated impaction in the ileocaecal region. Faecal debris is present in the caecum (C). Multiple dilated small bowel loops are seen.

the lungs, pancreas, liver and bowel. Approximately 5–10% of patients with cystic fibrosis present in the neonatal period with small bowel abnormality; these disorders are covered in Chapter 10.7. Abnormalities pertaining to the bowel after the neonatal period are addressed here. Abnormalities in the gastrointestinal tract in cystic fibrosis are the consequence of disordered mucus production within the bowel and the secondary effects of pancreatic exocrine insufficiency.

The intestinal contents of a child with cystic fibrosis are often thick and tenacious, disturbing normal propulsion through the bowel. Faecal material can become impacted within the proximal colon or within the terminal ileum. Normally, intestinal contents in this region are liquid in consistency. Although this has been called 'meconium ileus equivalent' in the past, distal intestinal obstruction syndrome (DIOS) is now the preferred term. Patients with poor dietary control or inadequate pancreatic enzyme supplements are predisposed. Patients present with pain, bloating, constipation and often a palpable mass, which is the impacted stool. Plain films may show evidence of faecal impaction in the proximal colon or distal small bowel. The bowel may appear dilated proximal to the obstruction (Figure 10.14.52). Surgery is rarely needed, as enemas are usually effective in therapy. Occasionally, enemas are performed under fluoroscopic guidance using water-soluble contrast media. The contrast is warmed or diluted with warm water. It is important to reflux the contrast into the terminal ileum as faeces commonly impact at this site.

Patients with cystic fibrosis may have malabsorption due to pancreatic exocrine insufficiency. These children often have substantial failure to thrive, a distended abdomen and steatorrhoeic stools. There is improper absorption of fat from the gut. Deficiency of the fat-soluble vitamins is common. Radiographic findings on small bowel study tend to be mild compared to other forms of malabsorption. Mild non-specific fold thickening may be seen. Currently, malabsorption is relatively uncommon in children with cystic fibrosis due to improved control of diet and the use of pancreatic supplements.

Mucosal abnormalities may be seen in children with cystic fibrosis; these are most prominent in the duodenum but occasionally extend further into the small bowel. Duodenal folds may be thick and nodular (See Fig. 10.13.16). The aetiology for duodenal fold thickening is unknown and the severity of the radiographic finding seems unrelated to other clinical parameters.

FURTHER READING

Abramson SJ, Baker DH, Amodio JB et al. Gastrointestinal manifestations of cystic fibrosis. Seminars in Roentgenology 1987; 22:97–113.

Agrons GA, Corse WR, Markowitz RI et al. Gastrointestinal manifestations of cystic fibrosis: radiologic-pathologic correlation. Radiographics 1996; 16:871–893.

Carty H. Abdominal radiology in cystic fibrosis. Journal of the Royal Society of Medicine 1995; 88:18–23.

Cleghorn GJ, Stringer DA, Forstner GG et al. Treatment of distal intestinal obstruction syndrome in cystic fibrosis with a balanced intestinal lavage solution. Lancet i 1986; 8471:8–11.

Djurhuus MJ, Lykkegaard E, Pock-Steen OC. Gastrointestinal radiological findings in cystic fibrosis. Pediatric Radiology 1973; 1:113–118.

Eggermont E, De Boeck K. Small-intestinal abnormalities in cystic fibrosis patients. European Journal of Pediatrics 1991; 150:824–828.

Grossman H, Berdon WE, Baker DH. Gastrointestinal findings in cystic fibrosis. American Journal of Roentgenology, Radium Therapy and Nuclear Medicine 1966; 97:227–238.

Koletzko S, Stringer DA, Cleghorn GJ et al. Lavage treatment of distal intestinal obstruction syndrome in children with cystic fibrosis. Pediatrics 1989; 83:727–733.

Phelan MS, Fine DR, Zentler-Munro PL et al. Radiographic abnormalities of the duodenum in cystic fibrosis. Clinical Radiology 1983; 34:573–577.

Pilling DW, Steiner GM. The radiology of meconium ileus equivalent. British Journal of Radiology 1981; 54:562–565.

SCHWACHMAN–DIAMOND SYNDROME

Pancreatic insufficiency with neutropenia (Schwachman–Diamond syndrome) is occasionally mistaken for cystic fibrosis. As with cystic fibrosis, fatty replacement of the pancreas is seen and there is pancreatic exocrine insufficiency. Routine sweat tests for cystic fibrosis are negative and haematological abnormalities, most prominently neutropenia, are seen that are not typical of cystic fibrosis. Patients may have a mild form of metaphyseal chondrodysplasia. Patients present with failure to thrive and diarrhoea, often steatorrhoea. Radiographic findings in the bowel are non-specific and minimal. Mild fold thickening, dilatation, flocculation and segmentation may be seen.

KWASHIORKOR

Kwashiorkor is due to severe dietary protein deficiency. As it is rare in developed countries and diagnosed clinically, imaging is rarely performed. Barium studies show findings of malabsorption including dilatation, segmentation and flocculation.

FURTHER READING

Kowalski R. Roentgenologic studies of the alimentary tract in kwashiorkor. American Journal of Roentgenology, Radium Therapy and Nuclear Medicine 1967; 100:100–112.

Lagundoye SB. Abdominal X-ray changes in kwashiorkor before and after barium. Journal of Tropical Pediatrics and Environmental Child Health 1975; 21:55–58.

WHIPPLE'S DISEASE

It is very rare for Whipple's disease to present in childhood. Patients present with weight loss, abdominal pain and steatorrhoea. Concomitant arthritic complaints are often noted. Diffuse small bowel fold thickening may be seen on a small bowel study. If CT is performed, enlarged mesenteric lymph nodes may be seen with low attenuation centres. The disease is probably infectious in aetiology. The small bowel biopsy finding of PAS-positive lipid-laden macrophages is characteristic. Patients are treated with antibiotics.

FURTHER READING

Rijke AM, Falke TH, de Vries RR. Computed tomography in Whipple disease. Journal of Computer Assisted Tomography 1983; 7:1101–1102.

MICROVILLOUS INCLUSION DISEASE

Patients with microvillous inclusion disease fall into two categories: those with congenital microvillous atrophy and those with autoimmune (acquired) villous atrophy. Patients with the congenital form present with intractable diarrhoea from birth and failure

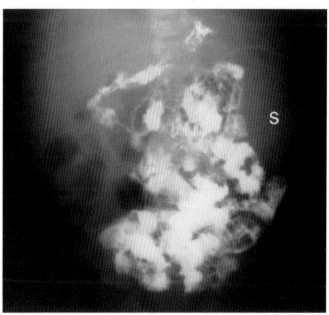

Figure 10.14.53 Microvillous inclusion disease (congenital). Small bowel loops are irregular in calibre with irregular folds. Note mass effect from an enlarged spleen (S).

to thrive. Diagnosis is made by examination of small bowel villi with electron microscopy. Patients with the acquired form present later in life. Presentation may mimic sprue but is unresponsive to removal of gluten from the diet. Radiographic findings are non-specific with loss of the normal jejunal fold pattern, dilatation and segmentation of barium seen (Figure 10.14.53).

FURTHER READING

Croft NM, Howatson AG, Ling SC et al. Microvillous inclusion disease: an evolving condition. Journal of Pediatric Gastroenterology and Nutrition 2000; 31:185–189.

Wilson W, Scott RB, Pinto A et al. Intractable diarrhea in a newborn infant: microvillous inclusion disease. Canadian Journal of Gastroenterology 2001; 15:61–64.

BACTERIAL OVERGROWTH/BLIND LOOP SYNDROME

Blind loop syndrome is the consequence of stasis and bacterial overgrowth occurring in an excluded or dilated loop of small bowel. Vitamin B_{12} deficiency is produced by bacteria interfering with its absorption. In a true 'blind loop', a segment of small bowel is excluded from the normal path through the small bowel. The abnormality may be acquired through surgery, as an intended anatomical result or an incorrect surgical connection, or as a consequence of fistulas. Blind loop syndrome is also produced by bacterial overgrowth within a persistently dilated segment, such as bowel proximal to a partially obstructing stricture or band or dilated bowel due to a congenital atresia persisting proximal to an anastomosis (Figure 10.14.54, also see Figure 10.14.15). Lastly, blind loop syndrome can be due to a large diverticulum. Excluded loops may be difficult to show on small bowel studies but may be inferred by the presence of fistulas or may be demonstrated on CT. Dilated loops in series with normal bowel are manifest on small bowel studies by stasis of barium in the loop and partial obstruction seen distally. Although antibiotics may temporarily alleviate symptoms, bacterial overgrowth often recurs when the antibiotics are stopped. Surgical management is usually required.

FURTHER READING

Bayes BJ, Hamilton JR. Blind loop syndrome in children. Malabsorption secondary to intestinal stasis. Archives of Disease in Childhood 1969; 44:76–81.

Savino JA. Malabsorption secondary to Meckel's diverticulum. American Journal of Surgery 1982; 144:588–592.

Stewart BA, Karrer FM, Hall RJ et al. The blind loop syndrome in children. Journal of Pediatric Surgery 1990; 25:905–908.

DISACCHARIDE INTOLERANCE

Disaccharidase deficiency may either be due to a congenital inborn error in metabolism or the result of an acquired abnormality of the small bowel mucosa. An increased incidence of disaccharidase intolerance is reported in children with HIV infection. Lactase deficiency is the most common form; it may not present until adulthood and usually presents in individuals without underlying disease. Symptoms of disaccharidase deficiency are bloating, dis-

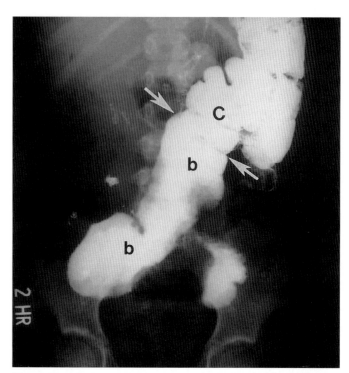

Figure 10.14.54 Bacterial overgrowth syndrome. Seven-year-old with bacterial overgrowth, responsive to antibiotics but recurrent when antibiotics were stopped. The small bowel (b) proximal to the enterocolonic anastomosis (arrows) is dilated. C, colon.

tension and diarrhoea, occurring within a few hours after ingestion of the offending disaccharide. Diagnosis is often made by removal and introduction of the offending substance, with resolution and recurrence of symptoms. Small bowel biopsy or enzyme assay of intestinal contents may be performed. Radiographic imaging is seldom performed. If the diagnosis is suspected, the small bowel is studied using barium with and without the offending substance added. If there is a corresponding enzyme deficiency, addition of the offending substance will produce dilatation of bowel and dilution of barium (Figure 10.14.55). Patient symptoms will also be exacerbated.

FURTHER READING

Thompson JR, Sanders I. Lactose-barium small bowel study. Efficacy as a screening method. American Journal of Roentgenology, Radium Therapy and Nuclear Medicine 1971; 113:255–257.

Yolken RH, Hart W, Oung I et al. Gastrointestinal dysfunction and disaccharide intolerance in children infected with human immunodeficiency virus. Journal of Pediatrics 1991; 118:359–363.

OBSTRUCTION

SMALL BOWEL OBSTRUCTION

Obstruction is a failure of intestinal contents to pass beyond the point of obstruction, causing proximal distension of bowel. Numerous causes for small bowel obstruction exist in children. A

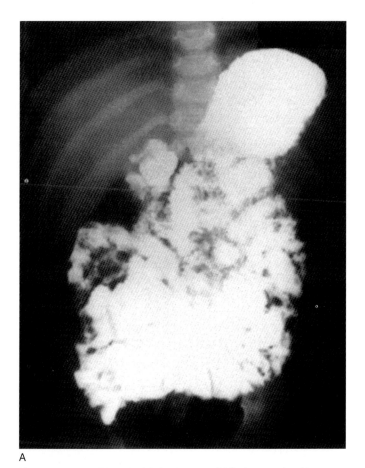
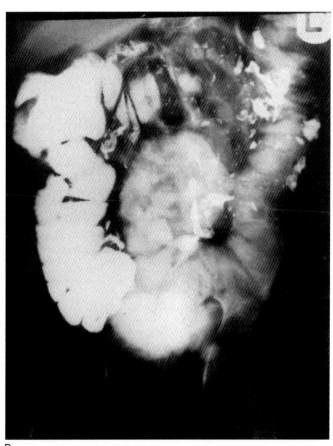

A

B

Figure 10.14.55 Disaccharide intolerance. (A) Barium study without sucrose is normal. (B) Sucrose added to barium. Note the dilution of the barium and retention of flocculated barium in the small bowel with failure of normal clearing. These are typical features of malabsorption.

differential diagnosis for obstruction is included in Chapter 10.7. Many of these processes are distinct clinical processes, which are discussed in detail elsewhere. Adhesions are the most common cause for small bowel obstruction in children who have had prior abdominal surgery. Adhesions may directly occlude the bowel lumen or act as a nidus for a focal small bowel volvulus. Other causes for small bowel obstruction in children include intussusception, incarcerated hernia, complicated appendicitis, complications of a Meckel's diverticulum, duplication, neoplasms, haematoma, Crohn's disease, severe constipation, malrotation, omphalomesenteric duct remnants or masses, bezoars, parasites and foreign bodies.

Presenting symptoms relate to the level and degree of obstruction. Pain, distension and vomiting are common. The pain fluctuates, often recurring acutely with intensity. Vomiting is greater with more proximal obstructions. Marked distension or torsion of obstructed bowel may compromise blood supply, potentially leading to bowel infarction and perforation and potentially dire consequences.

Radiographic findings also relate to the level and degree of obstruction. The hallmark of an obstruction is a differential calibre of bowel proximal to and distal to the point of obstruction. Dilatation is seen proximally with the number of dilated loops offering a clue as to the site of obstruction (Figure 10.14.56). The degree of dilatation is dependent on the degree of obstruction and also on

the chronicity of the obstruction. With mild partial obstruction only slight dilation of a short length of bowel may be seen near the point of obstruction. With more severe and longstanding obstruction, more dilated loops are present. A stair-step appearance of air-filled loops may be seen with distal small bowel obstructions. If the obstructed bowel is fluid filled, findings may be more subtle. The 'string of pearls' sign is due to small bubbles of gas between the folds of a dilated, predominantly fluid-filled loop of bowel. Characteristically, air–fluid levels are seen on upright films. Radiographs may bear clues as to the aetiology of the obstruction including appendicoliths, surgical clips, asymmetric inguinal folds or gas within a hernia (Figure 10.14.57). Care should be taken to look for intramural gas and free intraperitoneal air, which may be indicative of ischaemia and perforation, respectively.

Small bowel studies are of variable value in the delineation of small bowel obstruction. Small bowel follow-through for obstruction is performed with barium. Water-soluble contrast may be ineffective because of dilution by intestinal fluid. In the young child, non-ionic water-soluble contrast may be used. In cases of partial or early obstruction, contrast may delineate the site and degree of obstruction very well. Careful examination under fluoroscopy with palpation is often necessary. With more severe obstruction, passage of contrast may be very slow, if at all, and dilution of contrast with the fluid trapped upstream from an obstruction often renders the study useless in showing the point of obstruction. CT is increas-

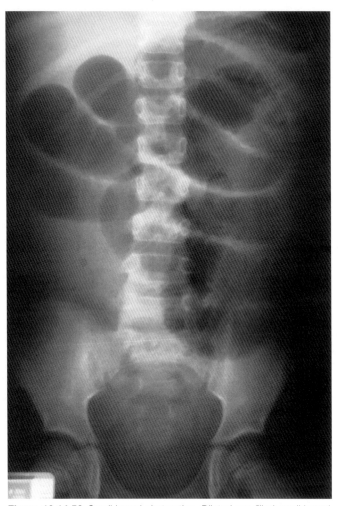

Figure 10.14.56 Small bowel obstruction. Dilated gas-filled small bowel is seen in the upper abdomen with a paucity of gas in the right lower quadrant and pelvis and absent colonic gas. The aetiology for the obstruction was a small bowel intussusception with a Meckel's diverticulum as lead point.

ingly used in studying patients with small bowel obstruction. Oral contrast is of limited utility as it does not reach the point of obstruction and in dilated, obstructed bowel, intraluminal fluid is present (Figure 10.14.58). With careful study, the point of obstruction is usually identified. The cause of obstruction may often be evident. CT may also show intramural gas or sloughed mucosa suggesting ischaemic compromise of the obstructed gut.

FURTHER READING

Ikeda H, Matsuyama S, Suzuki N et al. Small bowel obstruction in children: review of 10 years experience. Acta Paediatrica Japan 1993; 35:504–507.
Jabra AA, Eng J, Zaleski CG et al. CT of small-bowel obstruction in children: sensitivity and specificity. American Journal of Roentgenology 2001; 177:431–436.
Megibow AJ, Balthazar EJ, Cho KC et al. Bowel obstruction evaluation with CT. Radiology 1991; 180:313–318.
Peck JJ, Milleson T, Phelan J. The role of computed tomography with contrast and small bowel follow-through in management of small bowel obstruction. American Journal of Surgery 1999; 177:375–378.

CLOSED LOOP OBSTRUCTION

In closed loop obstruction, a single loop of bowel is fixed and obstructed at its proximal and distal ends. The dilated loop of bowel may twist upon itself and is prone to ischaemia. Often the loop is filled with fluid and produces some mass effect. Findings are best seen on CT, where a focal, fluid-filled dilated loop of bowel emanates from a single point in a circular or horseshoe configuration. Sloughed mucosa or intramural gas within the loop may be indicative of ischaemic damage. A variable degree of dilatation is seen upstream from the closed loop, depending on the chronicity of the obstruction.

FURTHER READING

Balthazar EJ, Birnbaum BA, Megibow AJ et al. Closed-loop and strangulating intestinal obstruction: CT signs. Radiology 1992; 185:769–775.
Ha HK, Rha SE, Kim JH et al. CT diagnosis of strangulation in patients with small-bowel obstruction: current status and future direction. Emergency Radiology 2000; 7:47–55.

SMALL BOWEL VOLVULUS WITHOUT MIDGUT MALROTATION

Although small bowel volvulus is most commonly the result of midgut malrotation and malfixation of the gut, focal distal small bowel volvulus can occur. In these instances, there is usually an underlying lesion tethering the bowel, such as an adhesion or remnant omphalomesenteric band or a mass precipitating volvulus. Deficient mesenteric fixation may contribute. Although radiologic studies will show evidence of small bowel obstruction or delineate the mass, it is unusual to diagnose the volvulus preoperatively (Figure 10.14.59). Occasionally, a whorled appearance in the mesentery or of bowel loops on CT suggests volvulus. Barium studies may show an obstruction.

FURTHER READING3

Fenton LZ, Buonomo C, Share JC et al. Small intestinal obstruction by remnants of the omphalomesenteric duct: findings on contrast enema. Pediatric Radiology 2000; 30:165–167.
Gaisie G, Curnes JT, Scatliff JH et al. Neonatal intestinal obstruction from omphalomesenteric duct remnants. American Journal of Roentgenology 1985; 144:109–112.
Kitano Y, Hashizume K, Ohkura M. Segmental small-bowel volvulus not associated with malrotation in childhood. Pediatric Surgery International 1995; 10:335–338.
Traubici J, Daneman A, Wales P et al. Mesenteric lymphatic malformation associated with small-bowel volvulus – two cases and a review of the literature. Pediatric Radiology 1995; 32:362–365.

HERNIA

INDIRECT INGUINAL HERNIA

During fetal development, the parietal peritoneum protrudes through the inguinal canal and into the scrotum as the processus vaginalis. In girls, the processus vaginalis extends into the labia majora. In most infants, this communication is patent; however, it usually closes in the first few years of life. Hydroceles may form

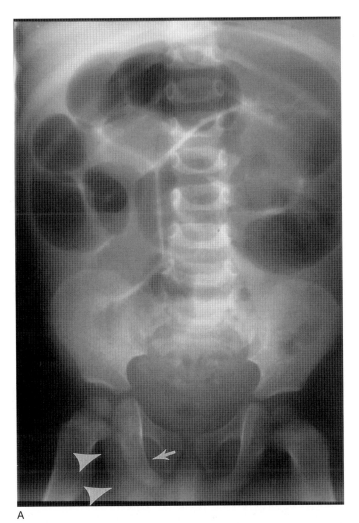

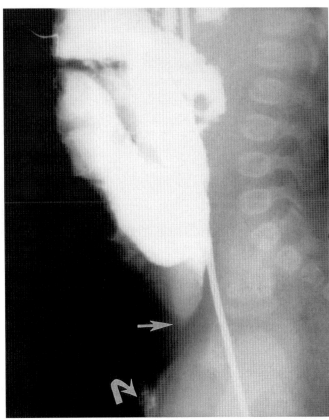

Figure 10.14.57 Incarcerated inguinal hernia with small bowel obstruction. (A) Radiograph shows small bowel dilatation. Note asymmetrical prominence of right inguinal fold (arrowheads). A small bubble of gas is faintly seen within the hernia (arrow). (B) Delayed lateral view from small bowel follow-through shows a beaked obstruction entering the hernia (arrow). Some barium is within bowel in the hernia (curved arrow).

in boys within an unobliterated processus vaginalis. A hernia is present when bowel enters the patent process vaginalis. The hernia may be partial or, if complete, extend all the way into the scrotum. Intestine within the hernia may become incarcerated or obstructed, potentially leading to bowel ischaemia. The diagnosis is usually clinical. Patients present with abdominal pain and vomiting. A palpable mass at the expected location suggests the proper diagnosis. Presentation with a hernia is most common in infants. In fact, an incarcerated inguinal hernia is the most common cause for small bowel obstruction in the young infant after the neonatal period to 6 months of age. Hernias are much more common in boys than girls and are of increased incidence in premature infants. Eighty per cent occur on the right side.

Radiographs may be normal or show obstruction. Bowel gas may be seen within the hernia or asymmetry of the inguinal creases may be noted, suggesting the diagnosis (see Figure 10.14.57). Gonadal shields may obscure the findings. Small bowel obstruction may be seen. Sonography may be employed to confirm bowel within the hernia (Figure 10.14.60). Herniography is no longer performed.

OTHER HERNIAS RESULTING IN A TRAPPED BOWEL

Other abdominal and pelvic hernias can also result in the bowel being entrapped. Apart from umbilical and indirect inguinal hernias, which are common, other types of hernias are rare in children. Umbilical hernias are common, rarely produce problems or symptoms, and usually spontaneously regress. Direct inguinal hernias do not pass through the inguinal ring but rather extend through a weak area in the transversalis fascia bounded by the inguinal ligament, the inferior epigastric vessels and lateral margin of the rectus abdominus muscle tendon. Direct hernias are much less common than indirect hernias in children and when they occur are less likely to produce symptoms. Femoral hernias extend through the femoral ring and appear at the saphenous opening. Sciatic hernias extend through the sciatic foramina. Obturator hernias extend through the obturator canal adjacent to the obturator nerve and vessels. Spigelian hernias extend into the anterior abdominal wall lateral to the rectus muscle. Richter's hernia is a partial hernia in which one side of the bowel wall is entrapped; strangulation can occur without obstruction. Incisional hernias are

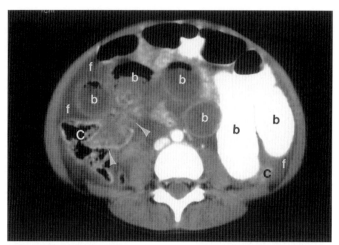

Figure 10.14.58 Small bowel obstruction. CT shows contrast and fluid-filled dilated small bowel loops (b), proximal to the obstruction. Non-dilated distal ileum (arrowheads) and colon (C) is indicative of a distal small bowel obstruction. Obstruction was due to torsion around an omphalomesenteric band. f, fluid.

relatively uncommon in children but may occur if there has been prior surgery.

FURTHER READING

Currarino G. Incarcerated inguinal hernia in infants: plain films and barium enema. Pediatric Radiology 1974; 2:247–250.

Miller PA, Mezwa DG, Feczko PJ et al. Imaging of abdominal hernias. Radiographics 1995; 15:333–347.

Shadbolt CL, Heinze SBJ, Dietrich RB. Imaging of groin masses: inguinal anatomy and pathologic conditions revisited. Radiographics 2001; 21:S261–S271.

Walker J, Carty H. A radiological feature to assist in the diagnosis of intestinal obstruction. British Journal of Radiology 1989; 62:1105–1106.

Zarvan NP, Lee FT, Yandow DR et al. Abdominal hernias: CT findings. American Journal of Roentgenology 1995; 164:1391–1395.

INTERNAL HERNIA

Internal hernias may form in conjunction with malrotation or due to a defect in the mesentery. Paraduodenal hernias are probably the

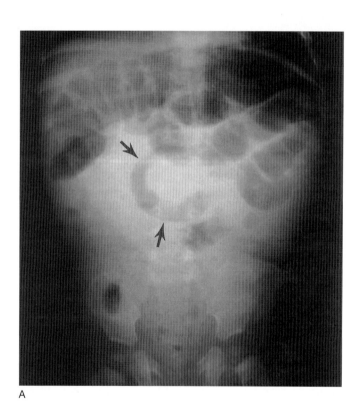

A

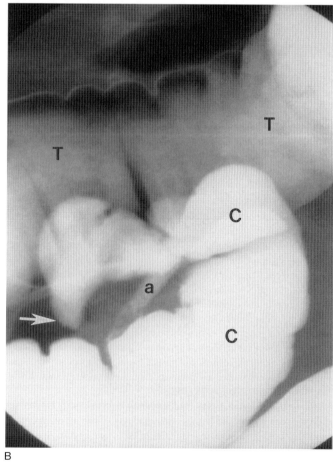

B

Figure 10.14.59 Small bowel obstruction due to volvulus around a mesenteric cyst. (A) Dilated small bowel is seen in the left upper quadrant. A circular loop of bowel (arrows) is seen in the mid-abdomen, suggesting volvulus. Paucity of bowel gas in the right lower quadrant is due to the cyst and fluid-filled loops of obstructed bowel. (B) Beaked obstruction of the distal ileum (arrow) is seen on barium enema. a, appendix; C, malpositioned caecum; T, transverse colon.

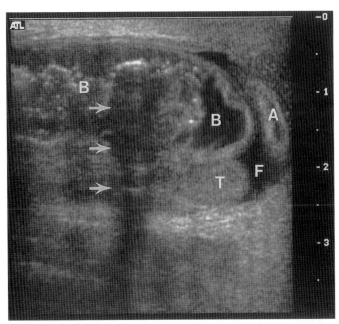

Figure 10.14.60 Inguinal hernia. Bowel (B) and appendix (A) are seen in the scrotum. Gas within bowel causes a posterior acoustic shadow (arrows). T, testicle. F, fluid.

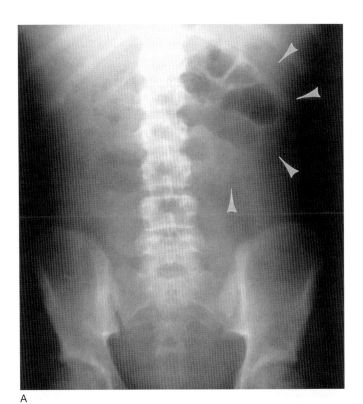

A

manifestation of a less common form of malrotation, with the duodenum rotating anterior to the superior mesenteric artery rather than posterior. With rotation of the caecum, small bowel becomes encased by its mesentery. Mesenteric hernias are usually located at the ileum, less commonly at the jejunum or, rarely, related to the mesentery of a Meckel's diverticulum.

The clinical severity and onset of symptoms in a patient with an internal hernia is dependent on the degree of obstruction. Symptoms relate to intermittent partial obstruction or incarceration of bowel within the hernia. Patients may present acutely or with chronic complaints of crampy pain and vomiting. Plain films are usually unrevealing, although in rare cases an unusual, localized rounded collection of bowel gas may be noted (Figure 10.14.61). With obstruction, barium may fail to reach bowel within the hernia. With lesser degrees of obstruction, barium may opacify a fixed collection of bowel loops confined to the hernia. Careful examination of serial films and direct examination under fluoroscopy may be necessary to show the abnormality, which may be very subtle.

FURTHER READING

Blachar A, Federle MP, Brancatelli G et al. Radiologists performance in the diagnosis of internal hernia by using specific CT findings with emphasis on transmesenteric hernia. Radiology 2001; 221:422–428.

Donnelly LF, Rencken IO, deLorimier AA et al. Left paraduodenal hernia leading to ileal obstruction. Pediatric Radiology 1996; 26:534–536.

Lough JO, Estrada RL, Wiglesworth FW. Internal hernia into Treves' field pouch. Journal of Pediatric Surgery 1969; 4:198–207.

Miller PA, Mezwa DG, Feczko PJ et al. Imaging of abdominal hernias. Radiographics 1995; 15:333–347.

Zarvan NP, Lee FT, Yandow DR et al. Abdominal hernias: CT findings. American Journal of Roentgenology 1995; 164:1391–1395.

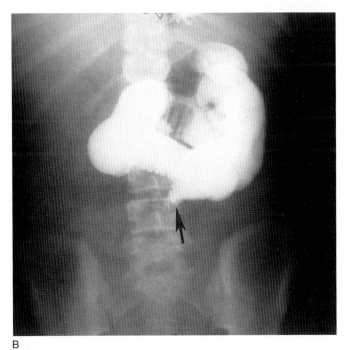

B

Figure 10.14.61 Internal hernia. (A) A focal collection of air-filled small bowel loops in the medial left upper quadrant persisted on multiple films. The margin of the hernia sac is faintly seen (arrowheads). (B) Barium opacifies dilated small bowel in the hernia. A complete obstruction was noted distally where there is a beaked appearance (arrow). (Courtesy of K. A. Garver, MI, Ann Arbor, USA.)

ENTEROENTERIC INTUSSUSCEPTION

Intussusception extending into the colon (ileocolic or ileoileocolic) is discussed in detail in Chapter 10.15. Intrinsic small bowel intussusceptions also occur (ileoileal or enteroenteric). These intussusceptions may be transient and clinically insignificant or persistent and symptom producing, necessitating treatment. Transient small bowel intussusceptions are occasionally seen on CT studies of the abdomen. Resolution of the finding on repeat images or follow-up ultrasound and lack of symptoms referable to the abnormality helps to define the transient nature of the CT abnormality. Transient small bowel intussusceptions may be seen with some mucosal disorders including immunoglobulin deficiency, sprue and giardiasis (see Figures 10.14.50 and 10.14.51). Persistent small bowel intussusceptions produce clinical symptoms and radiographic findings of intussusception. An underlying lesion such as a polyp or Meckel's diverticulum may be the lead point (see Figure 10.14.40). Intramural haemorrhage from Henoch–Schönlein purpura may produce small bowel intussusception. Small bowel intussusception may also be seen after abdominal surgery, although the aetiology of such intussusceptions is unclear. Retrograde intussusceptions can be seen at sites of stricture or anastomoses where there is a calibre change. Small bowel intussusceptions can also occur due to adherent feeding tubes.

Plain films of patients with small bowel intussusception are usually negative, except in the case of a persistent small bowel intussusception causing an obstruction. On CT, the small bowel intussusception is seen as a round, layered filling defect nearly filling the bowel lumen. Fat within the lesion may show continuity with adjacent mesenteric fat. With careful technique, persistent small bowel intussusceptions can be seen with sonography.

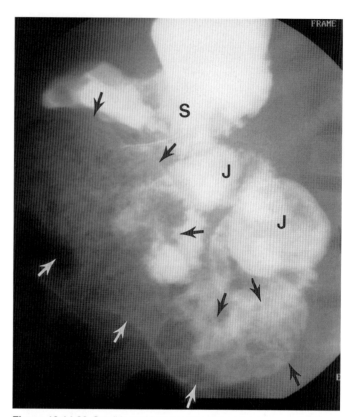

Figure 10.14.62 Small bowel bezoar. The patient is status-post liver transplant and gastrojejunostomy. Mottled lucency with dilated jejunum (arrows) is due to bezoar. The bezoar was chiefly composed of chewing gum. J, jejunum proximal to bezoar; S, stomach.

FURTHER READING

Daneman A, Reilly BJ, de Silva M et al. Intussusception on small bowel examinations in children. American Journal of Roentgenology 1982; 139:299–304.

Kaste SC, Willimas J, Rao BN. Postoperative small-bowel intussusception in children with cancer. Pediatric Radiology 1995; 25:21–23.

Navarro O, Dugougeat F, Kornecki A et al. The impact of imaging in the management of intussusception owing to pathologic lead points in children. A review of 43 cases. Pediatric Radiology 2000; 30:594–603.

Tiao MM, Wan YL, Ng SH et al. Sonographic features of small-bowel intussusception in pediatric patients. Academic Emergency Medicine 2001; 8:368–373.

SMALL BOWEL BEZOAR

Bezoars most commonly affect the stomach. In Rapunzel syndrome, the tail of a gastric trichobezoar extends into the duodenum. Intrinsic small bowel bezoars are less common. We have seen a case of a chewing gum bezoar in the proximal jejunum of a child status-post gastrojejunostomy surgery (Figure 10.14.62).

FURTHER READING

Billaud Y, Pilleul F, Valette PJ. Mechanical small bowel obstruction due to bezoars: correlation between CT and surgical findings. Journal of Radiology 2002; 83:641–646.

West WM, Duncan ND. CT appearances of the Rapunzel syndrome: an unusual form of bezoar and gastrointestinal obstruction. Pediatric Radiology 1998; 28:315–316.

FOREIGN BODIES

It is unusual for foreign bodies entering the small bowel to cause problems. Retention of foreign bodies in the duodenum usually indicates an underlying congenital obstruction, elsewhere it may indicate a Meckel's diverticulum. Most foreign bodies in the intestine pass readily. Longer objects may impact in the duodenum. Intestinal perforation or fistula formation are rare complications.

FURTHER READING

Honzumi M, Shigemori C, Ito H et al. An intestinal fistula in a 3-year-old child caused by the ingestion of magnets: report of a case. Surgery Today 1995; 25:552–553.

O'Gorman MA, Boyer RS, Jackson WD. Toothpick foreign body perforation and migration mimicking Crohn's disease in a child. Journal of Pediatric Gastroenterology and Nutrition 1996; 23:628–630.

Stack LB, Munter DW. Foreign bodies in the gastrointestinal tract. Emergency Medicine Clinics of North America 1996; 14:493–521.

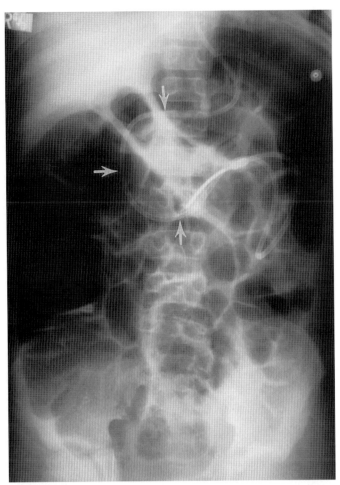

Figure 10.14.63 Ileus. Diffuse gaseous distension of small and large bowel is seen. Note feeding tube outlining the normal duodenal course (arrows).

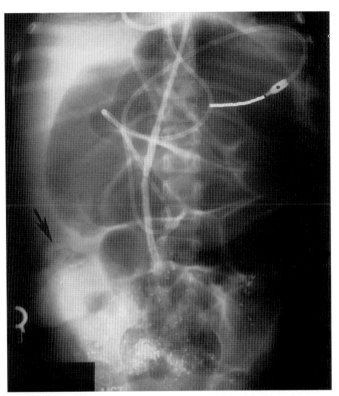

Figure 10.14.64 Idiopathic pseudo-obstruction. Four-year-old with a long history of severe small and large bowel dilatation and no anatomical obstruction by imaging or surgery. Small bowel is markedly dilated. Gas is not seen in colon due to ileostomy (arrow). Barium in distal ileum was administered during feeding tube placement 5 days previously. The feeding tube is malpositioned, looping back on itself in the duodenum with its tip in the stomach.

ILEUS

Strictly speaking, the definition of 'ileus' includes the mechanical obstructions, as have been previously described. In modern usage, 'ileus' is usually used to describe an adynamic or paralytic ileus. In these patients, there is no mechanical lesion blocking the small bowel, rather the small bowel (and colon) are inactive or inefficient in their peristaltic activity. The process is usually transient. Ileus can be seen with infectious or inflammatory disease, postoperatively or due to trauma, and occasionally can be related to metabolic causes, vasculitis or nervous system disorders. Peritonitis causes ileus. Pneumonia or sepsis may occasionally cause ileus. A differential diagnosis for ileus is provided in Chapter 10.7. Symptoms of ileus include distension, pain, and nausea and vomiting. Pain and vomiting may not be as prominent as with a complete obstruction. Bowel sounds are absent.

The hallmark of ileus on radiography is distension of both large and small bowel with gas and fluid (Figure 10.14.63). Positional views show gas–fluid levels. No calibre change will be evident. Positional views may aid in differentiating colon from small bowel, and hence ileus from obstruction. When performed, small bowel studies show slow, but eventual, passage of barium to colon without a point of obstruction. Ultrasound examination shows paucity or absence of peristalsis.

FURTHER READING

Frager DH, Baer JW, Rothpearl A et al. Distinction between postoperative ileus and mechanical small-bowel obstruction: value of CT compared with clinical and other radiographic findings. American Journal of Roentgenology 1995; 164:891–894.

INTESTINAL PSEUDO-OBSTRUCTION

'Pseudo-obstruction' is often used to describe the findings of chronic obstruction-like bowel dilatation in the absence of an identifiable mechanical cause for obstruction. Patients with pseudo-obstruction can be categorized into two main groups. Some patients seem to have an underlying bowel neuropathy and/or myopathy disturbing motility and are considered to have primary pseudo-obstruction (intestinal neuronal dysplasia). The precise aetiology is obscure. These children present with failure to thrive, abdominal distension and pain, which may be punctuated with acute episodes. There may be associated bladder dysfunction. Prognosis is poor. Parenteral nutrition may be required.

The other group of patients with pseudo-obstruction is those patients with severe neurological compromise. These children often have persistent diffuse dilatation of bowel. Knowledge of this history and comparison with old films often helps to alleviate the anxiety produced by diffuse bowel dilation seen on abdominal radiographs.

Patients with pseudo-obstruction will show diffuse gaseous dilation of bowel on radiographs (Figure 10.14.64). Both small and large bowel is involved. If a small bowel study is performed, passage of barium is slow, at times seemingly interminable; however, eventually the barium will pass and no point of mechanical obstruction is seen.

FURTHER READING

Heneyke S, Smith VV, Spitz L et al. Chronic intestinal pseudo-obstruction: treatment and long term follow up of 44 patients. Archives of Disease in Childhood 1999; 81:21–27.
Moore SW, Schneider JW, Kaschula RO. Unusual variations of gastrointestinal smooth muscle abnormalities associated with chronic intestinal pseudo-obstruction. Pediatric Surgery International 2002; 18:13–20.
Rudolph CD, Hyman PE, Altschuler SM et al. Diagnosis and treatment of chronic intestinal pseudo-obstruction in children: report of consensus workshop. Journal of Pediatric Gastroenterology and Nutrition 1997; 24:102–112.

METEORISM

Meteorism (aerophagia) is the swallowing of large quantities of air. Transient bowel distension may result when imaging an infant who has been crying. Usually, the distension abates quickly. Patients with mental retardation may swallow large quantities of air, perhaps contributing to the pseudo-obstruction pattern seen on radiographs.

FURTHER READING

van der Kolk MB, Bender MH, Goris RJ. Acute abdomen in mentally retarded patients: role of aerophagia. Report of nine cases. European Journal of Surgery 1999; 165:507–511.

MESENTERY

EMBRYOGENESIS AND ANATOMY

Development of the mesentery is closely tied to development and rotation of the small bowel. The mesentery is actually a double layer of peritoneum, suspending the bowel. The normal small bowel mesentery has a broad attachment from left upper quadrant to right lower quadrant. The mesentery contains fat, blood vessels, lymph nodes, lymphatic vessels and nerves. The amount of fat present increases with age. Small mesenteric lymph nodes (<1 cm short axis diameter) are frequently seen on CT as a normal finding.

FURTHER READING

Ruess L, Frazier AA, Sivit CJ. CT of the mesentery, omentum, and peritoneum in children. Radiographics 1995; 15:89–104.
Sivit CJ. CT scan of mesentery-omentum peritoneum. Radiologic Clinics of North America 1996; 34:863–884.

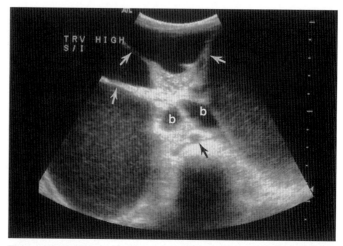

Figure 10.14.65 Lymphangioma (mesenteric cyst). Five-year-old with a protuberant abdomen. A massive tumour occupies most of the abdomen. Large septations (white arrows) are seen. Black arrow, aorta; b, bowel.

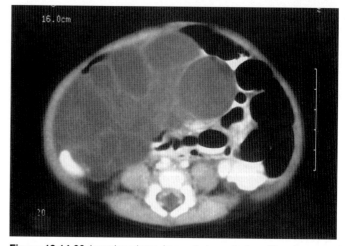

Figure 10.14.66 Lymphangioma (mesenteric cyst). A multilocular mass occupies much of the abdomen, displacing bowel.

Zarewych ZM, Donnelly LF, Frush DP et al. Imaging of pediatric mesenteric abnormalities. Pediatric Radiology 1999; 29:711–719.

MESENTERIC CYST/OMENTAL CYST

Cysts of lymphatic origin (lymphangiomas) can develop in the mesentery or, less commonly, in the omentum or retroperitoneum. These lesions probably arise from maldevelopment and/or obstruction of lymphatic drainage. The lesions are usually asymptomatic, unless large enough to cause abdominal distension. The lesions may fill most of the abdomen. Even so, they are difficult to detect on physical examination due to their soft consistency. Rarely, the cysts may cause a local small bowel volvulus, become infected, have haemorrhage into them or rupture. Mesenteric cysts most often involve the mesentery of the small bowel. The masses may

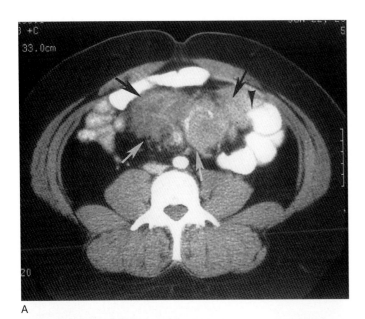

A

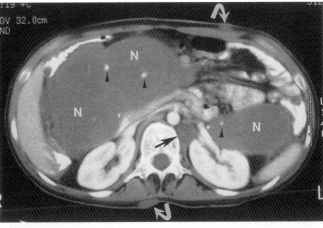

Figure 10.14.68 Neurofibromatosis. Two large neurofibromas (N) are seen in the mesentery. Note enhancing encased vessels (arrowheads), skin lesions (curved arrows) and para-aortic neurofibroma (arrow).

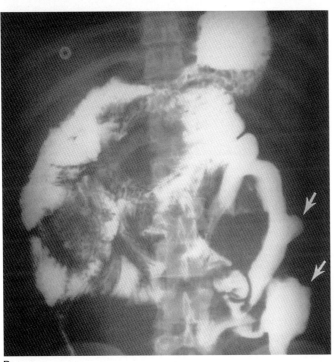

B

Figure 10.14.67 Gardner's syndrome with mesenteric desmoid tumour. (A) A poorly defined mass (arrows) is seen in the mesentery, partially encasing small bowel (arrowhead). (B) Small bowel follow-through shows distortion and separation of bowel loops. Note areas of pseudoaneurysm of bowel (arrows). The patient had had prior colectomy, at which time no desmoid tumour was present.

be unilocular or multilocular. With larger cysts, radiographs show displacement of bowel by the mass. Barium studies will show displacement of bowel; however, obstruction is rarely, if ever, evident. On sonography, the cysts are predominantly anechoic, although debris is frequently present within the fluid. Septations are readily evident on sonography (Figure 10.14.65). On CT, a round or multilobular fluid attenuation mass is seen (Figure

10.14.66). Septations are less well delineated on CT than with sonography. If the lesion is not completely excised, it may recur, hence follow-up imaging is often performed after surgical resection. If MRI is performed, the cysts may appear of higher signal than simple fluid due to high protein content.

FURTHER READING

Lugo-Olivieri CH, Taylor GA. CT differentiation of large abdominal lymphangioma from ascites. Pediatric Radiology 1993; 23:129–130.
Ros PR, Olmsted WW, Moser RP Jr et al. Mesenteric and omental cysts: histologic classification with imaging correlation. Radiology 1987; 164:327–332.
Sato M, Ishida H, Konno K et al. Mesenteric cyst: sonographic findings. Abdominal Imaging 2000; 25:306–310.

DESMOID TUMOURS AND OTHER MESENTERIC TUMOURS

Apart from mesenteric cysts, haematomas and lymph node masses, other mesenteric masses are rare in children. Desmoid tumours may be seen in patients with Gardner's syndrome (Figure 10.14.67). These lesions often do not develop until after colectomy (for polyposis). Desmoid tumours may necrose, forming fistulas and sinus tracts to the adjacent bowel. Mesenteric neurofibromas may be seen in patients with neurofibromatosis (Figure 10.14.68). Mesenteric desmoid tumours and neurofibromas are seen as soft tissue masses, displacing adjacent bowel. Rare mesenteric tumours include rhabdomyosarcoma and infantile myofibroblastic tumour (inflammatory pseudotumour).

FURTHER READING

Brooks AP, Reznek RH, Nugent K et al. CT appearances of desmoid tumours in familial adenomatous polyposis: further observations. Clinical Radiology 1994; 49:601–607.
Clark SK, Neale KF, Landgrebe JC et al. Desmoid tumours complicating familial adenomatous polyposis. British Journal of Surgery 1999; 86:1185–1189.

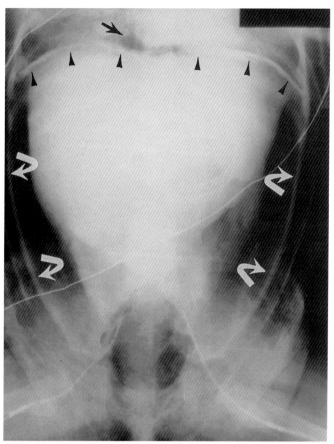

Figure 10.14.69 Extraperitoneal, intra-abdominal free air. Air is seen beneath the diaphragm (arrowheads) in the abdomen; however, it does to delineate the intraperitoneal contents. The gas dissected down from the chest, where a pneumomediastinum (arrow) is noted. Abundant subcutaneous gas is also present. Curved arrows indicate the abdominal wall, separating extraperitoneal, intra-abdominal gas from subcutaneous gas.

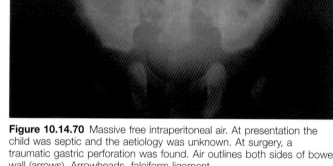

Figure 10.14.70 Massive free intraperitoneal air. At presentation the child was septic and the aetiology was unknown. At surgery, a traumatic gastric perforation was found. Air outlines both sides of bowel wall (arrows). Arrowheads, falciform ligament.

Day DL, Sane S, Dehner LP. Inflammatory pseudotumor of the mesentery and small bowel. Pediatric Radiology 1986; 16:210–215.

Maldjian C, Mitty H, Garten A et al. Abscess formation in desmoid tumors of Gardner's syndrome and percutaneous drainage: a report of three cases. Cardiovascular and Interventional Radiology 1995; 18:168–171.

Sato M, Ishida H, Konno K et al. Abdominal involvement in neurofibromatosis 1: sonographic findings. Abdominal Imaging 2000; 25:517–522.

PERITONEUM

EMBRYOGENESIS AND ANATOMY

The peritoneum initially forms due to degeneration of the embryonic ventral mesentery producing a large cavity inferior to the heart, extending to the pelvis. Parietal peritoneum originates from somatic mesoderm. Visceral peritoneum originates from splanchnic mesoderm. Ligaments represent folds of peritoneum, suspending organs. An omentum is a ligament connecting the stomach to another structure. The ligaments, omenta and mesenteries divide the large peritoneal cavity into smaller subcompartments.

PNEUMOPERITONEUM

Free intraperitoneal air (pneumoperitoneum) has many causes, some benign, others more ominous. Intraperitoneal air is seen after abdominal surgery. Normally, postsurgical intraperitoneal air clears within a few days; however, it may persist for weeks. An increase in the amount of intraperitoneal air suggests a source, such as an anastomotic leak. Rarely, gas may dissect into the peritoneum from a pneumomediastinum, probably via the retroperitoneum and mesentery. Radiographic evidence of pneumomediastinum and lack of abdominal signs and symptoms suggests this benign cause of pneumoperitoneum. Extraperitoneal, intra-abdominal gas may also be seen from extension of a pneumomediastinum and may erroneously be identified as intraperitoneal. Lack of air delineating the margins of bowel, other organs or falciform ligament is a clue to the extraperitoneal location (Figure 10.14.69).

In the absence of recent surgery, preceding peritoneal lavage, peritoneal dialysis or pneumomediastinum, pneumoperitoneum is likely to be due to a perforated viscus and thus an indication for surgery. Overall, the most common cause of pneumoperitoneum in

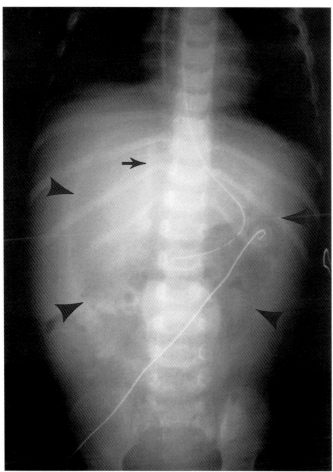

Figure 10.14.71 Supine pneumoperitoneum. A rounded lucency (arrowheads) projects centrally. Arrow, falciform ligament. Perforation was a complication of haemolytic uraemic syndrome.

childhood is necrotizing enterocolitis with perforation. This is covered in the neonatal gastrointestinal tract chapters. Other surgical causes for pneumoperitoneum are bowel trauma including iatrogenic injury, intraperitoneal bladder rupture with subsequent bladder catheterization, perforated ulcer, perforation due to obstruction, ischaemic bowel and other causes, and inflammatory conditions with perforation such as inflammatory bowel disease, ulceration, appendicitis or Meckel's diverticulitis. Free air from perforated Crohn's disease or perforated appendicitis is uncommon because the inflammatory process tends to wall itself off in the right lower quadrant. Rarely, a pneumoperitoneum is seen with benign cases of pneumatosis, thus correlation with clinical findings is important.

Small quantities of pneumoperitoneum are subtle or undetectable on supine films. Upright, decubitus or cross-table lateral views are necessary. Ideally, the patient is positioned for several minutes prior to the radiography to allow air to reach its non-dependent location. With larger quantities of free air, the finding may be obvious on supine films (Figure 10.14.70); however, even with a fairly large quantity of air the only finding on a supine film may be a subtle lucency in the abdomen (Figure 10.14.71). Radiographic signs of pneumoperitoneum include the 'triangle'

sign (air between three loops of bowel or between two loops of bowel and another structure), Rigler's sign (air on both sides of the bowel wall) (Figure 10.14.72), air outlining the falciform ligament, the umbilical ligaments (obliterated umbilical arteries) or urachus, air outlining liver and gallbladder margins, air outlining the inferior surface of the diaphragm and the 'football' sign (peritoneum markedly distended by air bisected by the falciform ligament, questionably resembling an American football). Stomach or bowel underneath the diaphragm and subdiaphragmatic or properitoneal fat can simulate intraperitoneal air. Positional views aid in differentiation.

Occasionally, a contrast study is requested to delineate a potential cause for pneumoperitoneum. Such studies should be performed with water-soluble contrast rather than barium, as barium spill into the peritoneum is not desirable. Cross-sectional imaging is not usually necessary to confirm radiographically identified pneumoperitoneum but may be utilized to delineate the causal process or associated abnormalities. Particularly in the setting of trauma, pneumoperitoneum is often first identified on CT.

FURTHER READING

Kleinman PK, Brill PW, Whalen JP. Anterior pathway for transiaphragmatic extension of pneumomediastinum. American Journal of Roentgenology 1978; 131:271–275.

Rice RP, Thompson WM, Gegauda RK. The diagnosis and significance of extraluminal gas in the abdomen. Radiologic Clinics of North America 1982; 20:819–837.

Wiot JF, Benton C, McAlister WH. Postoperative pneumoperitoneum in children. Radiology 1967; 89:285–288.

INTRAPERITONEAL FLUID

Intraperitoneal fluid (ascites) may originate from many sources. Fluid within the peritoneum may be blood, urine, bile, chyle, intestinal contents or lymph. Sources of ascites may be divided into transudative and exudative aetiologies. Exudative causes include infection, neoplasm, pseudomyxoma peritonei and lymphangiectasia. Transudative causes include portal hypertension, hypoalbuminaemia, congestive heart failure, fluid overload, pancreatitis, renal disease, biliary ascites and urinary ascites. A very small amount of free fluid may be physiological, particularly in girls beyond puberty. Pelvic pathology is a frequent source of free fluid in the adolescent girl, including ruptured ovarian cysts, pelvic inflammatory disease and ectopic pregnancy. A differential diagnosis for intraperitoneal fluid is included in Chapter 10.7.

Small quantities of intraperitoneal fluid are not evident on radiographs. Signs of intraperitoneal fluid on radiographs are medial displacement of colonic gas by fluid in the paracolic gutters, obscuration of the liver margin, fluid in the lateral recesses of the pouch of Douglas in the pelvis producing 'dog ears', centralization of air-filled bowel, and generalized increased opacity of a distended abdomen (Figure 10.14.73).

Sonography is an excellent method of identifying and delineating intraperitoneal fluid. Simple fluid is seen as anechoic areas between the abdominal wall, bowel and other structures. Free fluid settles in dependent areas such as the pelvis, paracolic gutters and hepatorenal fossa (Morison's pouch). Free fluid will change in shape and position with peristalsis of adjacent bowel or change in

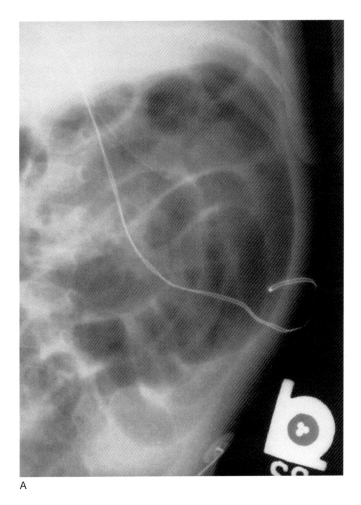

A

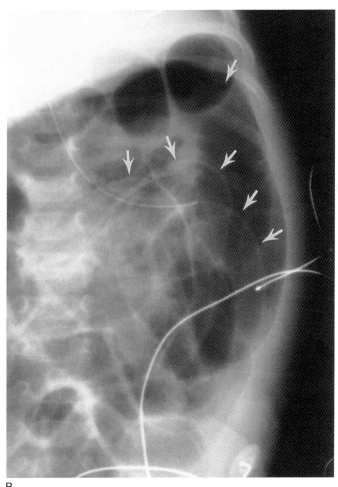

B

Figure 10.14.72 Pneumoperitoneum. Sequential films obtained before (A) and after (B) perforation. The outer surface of bowel wall (arrows) is seen after perforation due to pneumoperitoneum. Perforation was due to infarcted bowel. The child had recently had surgery for congenital heart disease.

patient position. Debris within the fluid may be due to haemorrhage, infection or spill of intestinal contents. Loculation of the fluid suggests a complication process. CT delineates the location and quantity of intraperitoneal fluid (Figure 10.14.74). Although increased density or fluid–fluid levels might suggest haemorrhage as a source, usually the attenuation of the fluid on CT does not serve to identify its source. CT also is effective at differentiating free fluid from loculated fluid. Free fluid insinuates between other structures with little mass effect, has no wall and tends to distribute dependently (compare Figure 10.14.74 to Figure 10.14.75). Loculated collections exhibit mass effect, are often contained by a wall and may be located anywhere within the abdomen. Occasionally, repeat scanning with a change in patient position may be necessary. Both sonography and CT can be used to guide percutaneous access for fluid aspiration.

Chylous ascites occurs due to obstruction of lymphatic drainage of the mesentery. Causes include trauma including by iatrogenic means, neoplasm, infection, congenital lymphatic malformation and central venous occlusion. Patients may have concomitant chylous pleural effusion. Chylous ascites may be lower in attenuation than other forms of ascites.

FURTHER READING

Franken EA JR. Ascites in infants and children. Roentgen diagnosis. Radiology 1972; 102:393–398.
Griscom NT, Colodny AH, Rosenberg HK et al. Diagnostic aspects of neonatal ascites: report of 27 cases. American Journal of Roentgenology 1977; 128:961–969.
Sanchez RE, Mahour GH, Brennen LP et al. Chylous ascites in children. Surgery 1971; 69:183–188.

PERITONITIS

Aetiologies for bacterial peritonitis are bowel perforation, including perforated appendicitis and Meckel's diverticulitis, and other infectious processes, including pelvic inflammatory disease, penetrating trauma and spontaneous bacterial peritonitis. In spontaneous bacterial peritonitis, pre-existing ascitic fluid is infected from an unknown source, probably blood or lymphatics. Patients present with abdominal distention, fever and pain. Diffuse tenderness with guarding and rebound is evident on physical examination. An ileus may be evident on radiographs, which also may

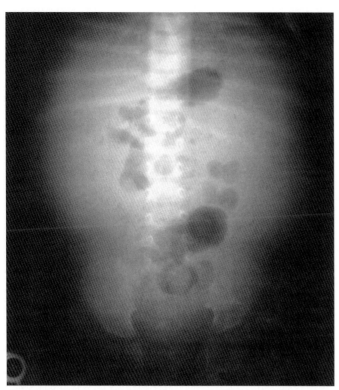

Figure 10.14.73 Ascites. Gas-filled bowel loops are centralized in the abdomen.

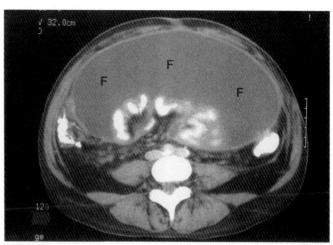

Figure 10.14.75 Peritonitis. 17-year-old peritoneal dialysis patient with recurrent bacterial peritonitis. A large loculated fluid collection (F) has a thick wall. Bowel loops are compressed centrally and have thick walls.

suggest the presence of intraperitoneal fluid. Sonography will confirm the presence of fluid. Debris is often seen in the fluid. On CT, non-specific intraperitoneal fluid is often seen; however, evidence of loculation, septation or thickening or increased enhancement of the peritoneum may suggest peritonitis (Figure 10.14.75). Increased density of the mesenteric fat is also seen.

Non-infectious causes of peritonitis include meconium leak (meconium peritonitis, discussed in Chapter 10.7) and bile leak (bile peritonitis).

TUBERCULOUS PERITONITIS

Tuberculous peritonitis occurs due to spread of mycobacteria into the peritoneal space, usually from an infected lymph node. Findings vary from non-specific, uncomplicated free intraperitoneal fluid to complex peritoneal disease with fibrous thickening of the peritoneum and loculated fluid collections, so-called 'plastic peritonitis'. The high protein content of tuberculous ascites may increase its opacity on CT. Peritoneal thickening may be apparent on sonography or CT. Enhancement of the thickened peritoneum is seen with administration of intravenous contrast.

FURTHER READING

Andronikou S, Welman CJ, Kader E. The CT features of abdominal tuberculosis in children. Pediatric Radiology 2002; 32:75–81.

Demirkazik FB, Akhan O, Ozmen MN et al. US and CT findings in the diagnosis of tuberculous peritonitis. Acta Radiologica 1996; 37:517–520.

Gurkan F, Ozates M, Bosnak M, Dikici B et al. Tuberculous peritonitis in 11 children: clinical features and diagnostic approach. Pediatrics International 1999; 41:510–513.

Hiller N, Lioubashevsky N. Tuberculous peritonitis: a diagnostic challenge. Abdominal Imaging 2001; 26:319–322.

Lee DH, Lim JH, Ko YT et al. Sonographic findings in tuberculous peritonitis of wet-ascitic type. Clinical Radiology 1991; 44:306–310.

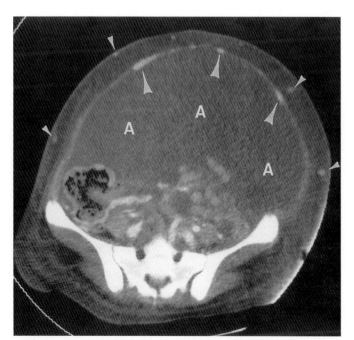

Figure 10.14.74 Massive ascites. A 16-year-old with liver dysfunction and portal vein and inferior vena cava obstruction due to a massive hepatic tumour. A, ascites. Bowel is centralized and dependent. Note venous collaterals from inferior epigastric veins (large arrowheads) and in the oedematous subcutaneous tissues (small arrowheads).

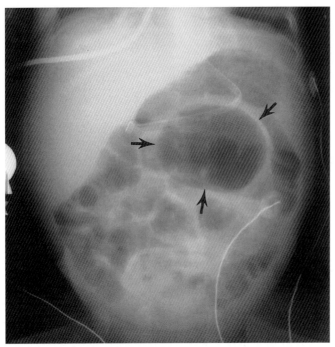

Figure 10.14.76 Abscess. A large, non-anatomical gas collection (arrows) is seen in the left mid-abdomen. This 3-month-old with a history of necrotizing enterocolitis was 8 days status-post surgery (ileostomy takedown).

INTRAPERITONEAL ABSCESS

Abscesses may form anywhere within the peritoneal cavity. The location of an abscess is often indicative of its source. The most frequent cause for intraperitoneal abscess in childhood is perforated appendicitis. Hence, abscesses are most commonly found in the right lower quadrant or right iliac fossa. Other common causes for intraperitoneal abscess in children are postoperative infection and abdominal trauma with bowel perforation. Other common sites for abscesses are the pelvis, and the subphrenic and subhepatic spaces. Patients present with pain and fever. A persistent elevated white blood cell count is noted. Pelvic abscesses may cause secondary inflammation of the rectosigmoid colon and resultant diarrhoea. Subphrenic abscesses may have pain referred to the shoulder.

Plain radiographs usually show evidence of adynamic ileus or occasionally obstruction. Larger abscesses may produce mass effect on bowel. Occasionally, extraluminal gas is evident in the abscess (Figures 10.14.76 and 10.14.77). Sonography can be used to identify abscesses but is limited by bowel gas or skeletal structures, which obscure underlying structures, and by dependence on the ability of the operator. On sonography, an abscess is seen as a hypoechoic fluid collection that appears loculated and may produce mass effect. Debris is usually seen within the fluid. Abscesses containing a large quantity of gas may be difficult to identify by sonography. CT is the most definitive method to identify and delineate intra-abdominal abscesses. A good oral contrast preparation and intravenous contrast administration aid in delineating abscesses. Abscesses are seen as loculated fluid collections, often containing gas (Figures 10.14.77 and 10.14.78). An enhanc-

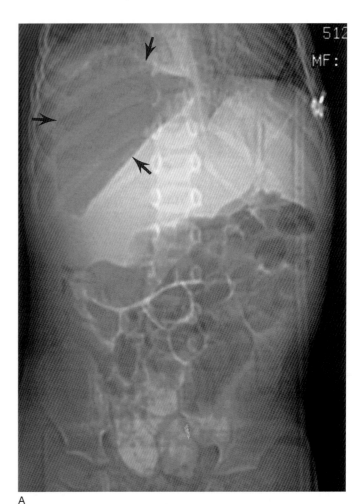

A

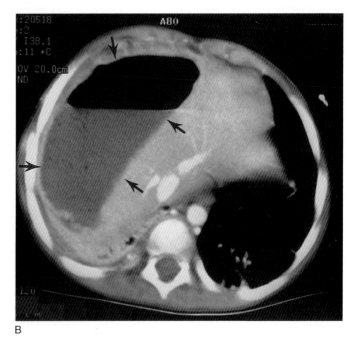

B

Figure 10.14.77 Subphrenic abscess at presentation with perforated appendicitis. (A) CT scout image shows a large, non-anatomical gas collection (arrows) under the right hemidiaphragm. (B) Axial CT image shows a large abscess (arrows) containing gas and fluid, distorting the adjacent liver. A percutaneous drain was subsequently placed under sonographic guidance.

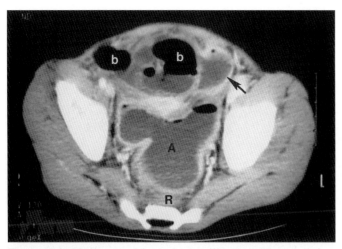

Figure 10.14.78 Abscess. A large abscess (A) is seen dependently in the pelvis. Some gas is present in the abscess. The rectum (R) is compressed posteriorly. Additional extraluminal fluid is seen anteriorly with enhancing peritoneum (arrow) due to peritonitis. b, bowel.

ing wall is often noted. Both sonography and CT can be used to guide percutaneous drainage of abscesses.

FURTHER READING

Jamieson DH, Chait PG, Filler R. Interventional drainage of appendiceal abscesses in children. American Journal of Roentgenology 1997; 169:1619–1622.

Meyers MA, Oliphant M, Berne AS et al. The peritoneal ligaments and mesenteries: pathways of intraabdominal spread of disease. Radiology 1987; 163:593–604.

INTRAPERITONEAL TUMOURS

Primary tumours of the peritoneum are exceedingly rare in childhood. Nonetheless, both benign and malignant peritoneal mesotheliomas have been reported. Secondary or metastatic disease involving the peritoneum is more common. Tumours that may spread to the peritoneal space include lymphoma, rhabdomyosarcoma, neuroblastoma, Wilm's tumour and ovarian germ cell tumour. On sonography or CT, intraperitoneal fluid is invariably present and peritoneal implants or masses may be scattered throughout the peritoneal space. The pelvis is a common site for masses to develop, presumably due to its dependent location (Figure 10.14.79). With advanced disease an 'omental cake' may be evident and encasement of bowel or other structures is seen (Figure 10.14.79).

FURTHER READING

Chung CJ, Bui V, Fordham LA et al. Malignant intraperitoneal neoplasms of childhood. Pediatric Radiology 1998; 28:317–321.

Chung CJ, Fordham L, Little S et al. Intraperitoneal rhabdomyosarcoma in children: incidence and imaging characteristics on CT. American Journal of Roentgenology 1998; 170:1385–1387.

Grenier N, Filiatrault D, Garel L et al. CT features of peritoneal and mesenteric involvement in pediatric malignancies. Experience from thirteen cases. Annals of Radiology 1986; 29:275–285.

Kaste SC, Marina N, Fryrear R et al. Peritoneal metastases in children with cancer. Cancer 1998; 83:385–390.

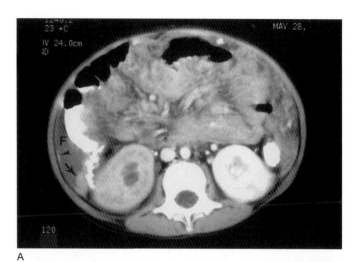

A

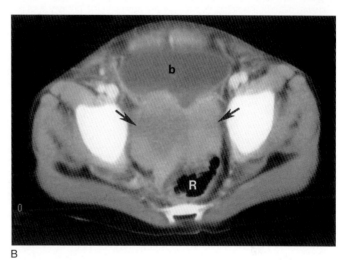

B

Figure 10.14.79 Intraperitoneal lymphoma. (A) CT image at the level of the kidneys shows diffuse mesenteric/omental tumour. Note implants in the right paracolic gutter (arrow) and thickening of the peritoneum (arrowhead). Decreased enhancement of the right kidney is due to ureteral obstruction by pelvic tumour. F, fluid. (B) Large masses are seen in the rectovesicular space (arrows). b, bladder; R, rectum.

Kim Y, Cho O, Song S et al. Peritoneal lymphomatosis: CT findings. Abdominal Imaging 1998; 23:87–90.

McCullagh M, Keen C, Dykes E. Cystic mesothelioma of the peritonieum: a rare cause of 'ascites' in children. Journal of Pediatric Surgery 1994; 29:1205–1207.

Slasky BS, Bar-Ziv J, Freeman AI et al. CT appearances of involvement of the peritoneum, mesentery and omentum in Wilm's tumor. Pediatric Radiology 1997; 27:14–17.

ABDOMINAL LYMPH NODES

INTRA-ABDOMINAL LYMPH NODE ENLARGEMENT

No fixed criteria for intra-abdominal lymph node enlargement exists for children. In general, any lymph nodes over 10 mm in short axis diameter should raise concern for pathology. Normal

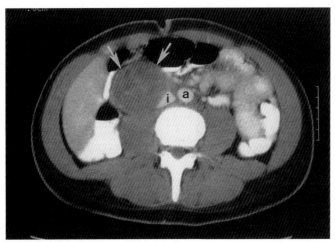

Figure 10.14.80 Retroperitoneal lymph node metastasis. The mass (arrows) distorts the adjacent inferior vena cava (v). The primary was a germ cell tumour of the testicle. a, aorta.

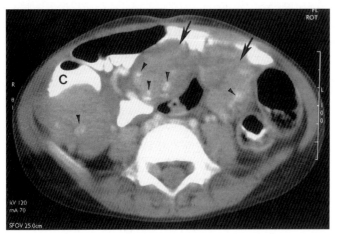

Figure 10.14.81 Lymphoma. The patient is a 7-year-old with congenital HIV infection. A large lymphomatous mass is seen at the posterior aspect of the caecum (c). Conglomerate mesenteric lymph node masses due to lymphoma are seen centrally (arrows). Scattered calcifications are from prior tuberculosis infection (arrowheads).

lymph nodes measuring a few millimetres in size are frequently seen in the para-aortic location, in the mesentery and in the inguinal region. A small collection of borderline enlarged lymph nodes may offer equivocal evidence for pathology. Although enlarged lymph nodes are occasionally identified by sonography, CT offers a more global assessment. Analysis of CT images should include a systematic search for lymph node enlargement including these locations: cardiophrenic, retrocrural, greater curve of stomach, lesser curve of stomach, gastrohepatic, gastrosplenic, coeliac, superior mesenteric, renal hila, portocaval, paracaval, para-aortic, mesenteric, iliac, femoral and inguinal.

Lymph node enlargement is usually due to neoplastic, infectious or inflammatory conditions. Intra-abdominal lymph node enlargement in children is most commonly due to lymphoma or intra-abdominal malignancies including neuroblastoma and Wilm's tumour. Often a malignancy is known or suspected prior to CT. Identification of retroperitoneal lymph node enlargement in a boy

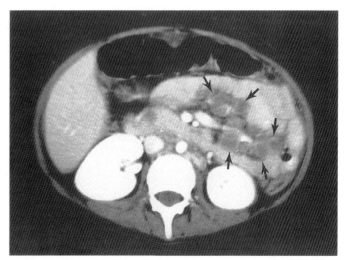

Figure 10.14.82 Tuberculous lymph node enlargement. Multiple enlarged mesenteric lymph nodes are seen (arrows). Low attenuation of the involved lymph nodes is characteristic of tuberculosis. (Courtesy of D. H. Jamieson, Vancouver, BC, Canada.)

in the absence of a known tumour should prompt examination of the testes for tumour (Figure 10.14.80). Post-transplant lympho-proliferative disorder is a cause for lymph node disease in transplant patients and varies in aggressiveness. Massive mesenteric lymph node enlargement may be seen in patients with AIDS, representing lymphoma and/or mycobacterial disease (mycobacterium avium intracellulare or mycobacterium tuberculosis) (Figure 10.14.81).

FURTHER READING

Dorfman RE, Alpern MV, Gross BH et al. Upper abdominal lymph nodes: criteria for normal size determined with CT. Radiology 1991; 180:319–322.

TUBERCULOUS LYMPH NODE ENLARGEMENT

Lymph node enlargement is a characteristic finding of abdominal tuberculosis. Malabsorption may occur due to lymphatic obstruction. Enlarged lymph nodes may be seen without evidence of gut or other organ involvement. Lymph node enlargement from tuberculosis is most frequently in the mesentery, secondarily spreading to the retroperitoneum. Low attenuation of lymph node centres are characteristic (Figure 10.14.82). Calcification is commonly seen and persists after treatment (see Figure 10.14.81).

FURTHER READING

Andronikou S, Welman CJ, Kader E. The CT features of abdominal tuberculosis in children. Pediatric Radiology 2002; 32:75–71.
Pombo F, Rodriguez E, Mato J et al. Patterns of contrast enhancement of tuberculous lymph nodes demonstrated by computed tomography. Clinical Radiology 1992; 46:13–17.

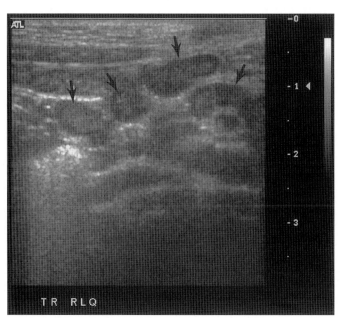

Figure 10.14.83 Mesenteric adenitis. Ultrasound shows multiple mildly enlarged right lower quadrant mesenteric lymph nodes (arrows).

MYCOBACTERIUM AVIUM INTRACELLULARE

Mycobacterium avium intracellulare (MAI) commonly causes massive intra-abdominal lymph node enlargement in patients with AIDS. Low density centres are frequently seen; however, the finding may also be seen in some patients with lymphoma, the chief differential diagnosis.

FURTHER READING

Haller JO, Cohen HL. Gastrointestinal manifestations of AIDS in children. American Journal of Roentgenology 1994; 162:387–393.

Vincent ME, Robbins AH. Mycobacterium avium-intracellulare complex enteritis: pseudo-Whipple disease in AIDS. American Journal of Roentgenology 1985; 144:921–922.

CASTLEMAN'S DISEASE

Castleman's disease (angiofollicular lymph node hyperplasia) is a disease of unknown aetiology. It may be familial but is rarely identified in children. Densely enhancing lymph node masses are seen on CT. The masses may calcify.

FURTHER READING

Ferreiros J, Gomez-Leon N, Mata MI et al. Computed tomography in abdominal Castleman's disease. Journal of Computer Assisted Tomography 1989; 13:433–436.

MESENTERIC ADENITIS

Identification of mildly prominent lymph nodes is common. The finding is non-specific and of questionable significance. Children may exhibit tenderness to palpation in the area of the lymph nodes. In such cases, with the absence of other pathology, the diagnosis of mesenteric adenitis is often assigned. Mesenteric adenitis is largely a diagnosis of exclusion. In primary mesenteric adenitis, no other inflammatory process is identified and there may be mild thickening of the wall of terminal ileum (Figure 10.14.83). With secondary mesenteric adenitis, the findings are associated with an identified intra-abdominal inflammatory process. *Yersinia enterocolitica* may present in this manner.

FURTHER READING

Jelloul L, Fremond B, Dyon JF et al. Mesenteric adenitis caused by Yersinia pseudotuberculosis presenting as an abdominal mass. European Journal of Pediatric Surgery 1997; 7:180–183.

Macari M, Hines J, Balthazar E et al. Mesenteric adenitis: CT diagnosis of primary versus secondary causes, incidence, and clinical significance in pediatric and adult patients. American Journal of Roentgenology 2002; 178:853–858.

Sivit CJ, Newman KD, Chandra RS. Visualization of enlarged mesenteric lymph nodes at US examination. Pediatric Radiology 1993; 23:471–475.

The Colon

Louise E Sweeney, Joanna Turner

GENERAL CONSIDERATIONS

The hindgut extends from the distal third of the transverse colon to the anus. In the sixth week of gestation, the hindgut herniates into the umbilical cord. The embryonic distal bowel grows more slowly than the proximal bowel, therefore it is shorter when the bowel returns to the abdomen at 19 weeks. The calibre of large bowel is larger than the small bowel and decreases progressively from the caecum distally until the rectum, which is larger in diameter. The length, diameter and calibre of the colon is variable. The taenia coli are three longitudinal bands of muscle that extend distally from the caecum at the base of the appendix. One of the three muscles terminates at the splenic flexure and the other two extend as far as the sigmoid or rectum. The colonic wall is sacculated because it is longer than the taenia coli. The haustral markings can be obliterated by excessive pressures, which lengthen the taenia coli. The appendices epiploicae are small fat-containing peritoneal sacs attached to the colon. The mucosal surface of the colon is smooth except for the semilunar fold between haustral sacculations.

The position and size of the ileocaecal valve is variable. It is usually located on the medial wall of the colon and can project 1–2 cm into the colonic lumen. It may be visible on contrast studies and must not be mistaken for an ileocolic intussusception or tumour. The appendix usually projects mediocaudally from the base of the caecum. It is mobile and can be retrocaecal in position.

Innominate grooves may occasionally be seen in the colon in older children on barium enema. They are thought to represent lines between rows of lymphoid collections. Rarely, the glands of Lieberkuhn fill with barium, especially after defaecation, producing a spiculated pattern indistinguishable from fine superficial mucosal ulceration.

LYMPHOID HYPERPLASIA

Lymphoid follicles are distributed throughout the gastrointestinal tract and are a normal finding in children. Normal follicles measure less than 2 mm in diameter and appear as nodular defects that are often most pronounced in the rectosigmoid colon on barium examinations.

Nodular lymphoid hyperplasia is present when follicles measure greater than 3–4 mm and these may be pedunculated simulating a hamartomatous polyp. Lymphoid hyperplasia represents a spectrum of lymphoproliferative activity (Figure 10.15.1) and may be a normal finding; however, occasionally, inflammatory bowel disease and rarely lymphoma are the cause.

FURTHER READING

Byrne WJ, Jimenez JF, Euler AR, Golladay ES. Lymphoid polyps (focal lymphoid hyperplasia) of the colon. Pediatrics 1982; 69:598–600.
Kenney PJ, Koehler RE, Shackelford GD. The clinical significance of large lymphoid follicles of the colon. Radiology 1982; 142:41–46.
Vinton NE. Gastrointestinal bleeding in infancy and childhood. Gastroenterology Clinics of North America 1994; 23:93–122.

ABDOMINAL PAIN

Abdominal pain is a common presenting complaint in children and is caused by a variety of surgical and non-surgical conditions. Plain radiographs of the abdomen are required for suspected bowel obstruction, perforation, trauma and calculi. It is important that the radiographs are reviewed in an ordered way. A suggested approach is to answer the following questions: (1) is the gas distribution ordered and can you see the caecum in the right iliac fossa (RIF); (2) is there air in both the large and small bowel (remember that the haustra are not visible until about 2 months of age and the sigmoid colon is intra-abdominal in the first few years of life, and often lies in the right abdomen); (3) is the bowel of normal calibre throughout; (4) is there any localized ileus to suggest focal pathology (an example would be localized RIF ileus in appendicitis); (5) is there any organomegaly and if so in which organs; (6) is there a mass lesion and if so does it contain calcification or any other identifying density such as fat or a tooth; (7) do the hernial orifices contain gas; (8) are the diaphragms visible or is there any lung base consolidation that might cause referred abdominal pain; (9) is the intraluminal content normal faeces and of normal distribution; (10) are the flank stripes distended, which would indicate ascites; (11) are the bones of spine and pelvis normal and are the disc spaces normal; and (12) are there any stones in the renal tracts or gallbladder.

Plain radiographs of the abdomen can be insensitive if the clinical findings are vague or non-specific. Ultrasound is helpful in making specific diagnoses in a number of conditions including appendicitis and intussusception. Computed tomography (CT) can quickly and accurately diagnose acute appendicitis when the

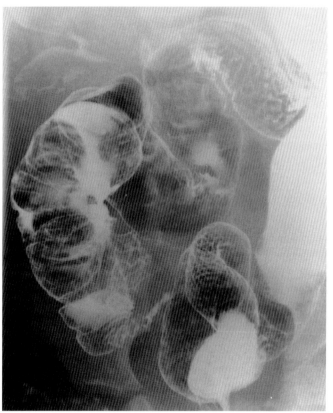

Figure 10.15.1 Lymphoid hyperplasia. Note the umbilicated nodular defects in the rectum. Film taken postreduction of intussusception, hence the caecal oedema.

clinical findings are difficult or atypical and is the method of choice for imaging abdominal trauma.

INTUSSUSCEPTION

Intussusception is a common cause of an acute abdomen in infancy. It occurs when a segment of bowel, the intussusceptum, becomes telescoped into the bowel distally, the intussuscipiens. Intussusception usually occurs in children under 2 years of age and is most frequently seen in infants under 1 year. The majority of intussusceptions are ileocolic or ileoileocolic. Ileoileal and colocolic intussusceptions are much less common. Most cases of intussusception are idiopathic and do not have a lead point other than lymphoid hypertrophy. Pathological leadpoints occur in 1.5–12% of patients and are more common in older children. They include Meckel's diverticulum, duplication cyst of the bowel, lymphoma, polyps, Henoch–Schönlein purpura syndrome and inspissated bowel content in children with cystic fibrosis.

The clinical presentation is characterized by intermittent colicky abdominal pain with drawing up of the legs, vomiting, 'red currant jelly' stools (present in about one-third of patients) and a palpable abdominal mass. Clinical examination may be difficult and the mass not felt. Drowsiness and lethargy may also occur. If diagnosis is delayed the disease may progress to mechanical bowel obstruction causing vascular compromise and bowel infarction,

which may present clinically as shock. The initial diagnostic approach to intussusception is plain radiography of the abdomen and ultrasonography. Subsequent management is based on the ultrasound (US) findings. A supine abdominal radiograph may demonstrate signs of intussusception such as a soft tissue mass, most often seen in the right upper quadrant and sometimes containing concentric circular lucencies due to mesenteric fat trapped in the intussusception (Figure 10.15.2). The apex of the intussusceptum may be outlined by gas in the colon, the meniscus sign (Figure 10.15.3). Other findings include a sparse amount of bowel gas, bowel obstruction and perforation. The plain abdominal radiograph is normal in 50% of cases of intussusception and can be useful in helping diagnose other causes of abdominal pain.

Ultrasonography is highly sensitive in the diagnosis of intussusception. Ideally, a linear array 5–7 mHz transducer should be used. Characteristic appearances include the multiple concentric rings sign on axial scans and the sandwich sign on longitudinal scans (Figure 10.15.4). The pseudokidney sign occurs when the intussusception is imaged obliquely or it is curved. A crescent in doughnut appearance refers to the identification of the apex of the intussusception and its trailing mesentery, which causes a crescentic echogenicity on the transverse scan (Figure 10.15.5). The mesenteric crescent may contain hypoechoic areas representing lymph nodes (Figure 10.15.6). Enlarged Peyer's patches may be

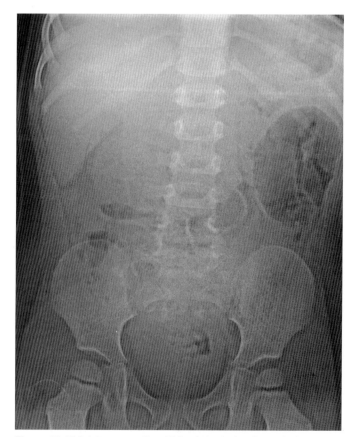

Figure 10.15.2 Intussusception. Plain abdominal radiograph showing a round soft tissue mass in the right hypochondrium, containing concentric circular areas of lucency.

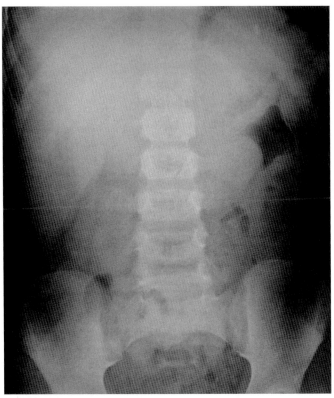

Figure 10.15.3 Intussusception. Plain abdominal radiograph showing a round soft tissue mass protruding into the gas-filled transverse colon: the meniscus sign.

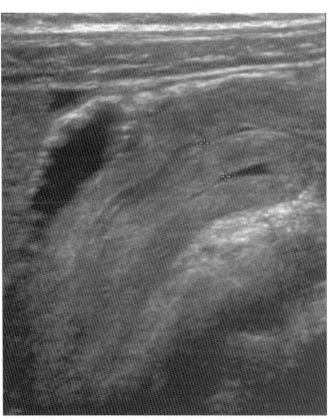

Figure 10.15.4 Intussusception. Ultrasound scan in the longitudinal plane shows the multilayered appearance with the outer hypoechoic layer formed by the intussuscipiens and the everted returning limb of the intussusceptum. The hyperechoic area represents the mesentery.

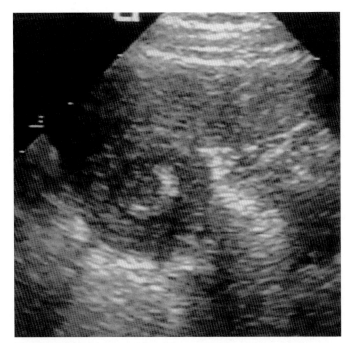

Figure 10.15.5 Intussusception. Transverse US scan showing the crescent-shaped hyperechoic centre due to the mesentery.

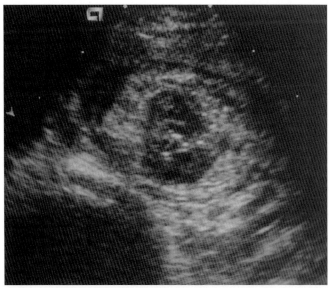

Figure 10.15.6 Intussusception containing oval hypoechoic mesenteric lymph nodes.

seen in the bowel wall. The presence of fluid trapped between the intussusceptum and intussuscipiens is uncommon but is associated with vascular compromise and irreducibility of the intussusception (Figure 10.15.7). The presence of small amounts of free intraperitoneal fluid is common and is not a predictor of irreducibility. Visualization of blood flow in the intussusception on Doppler US is a good prognostic factor and suggests reduction is likely to be successful. Spontaneous reduction is sometimes observed on US. Lead points in intussusception occur in 1.5–12% of cases and are best shown by US. These include Meckel's diverticulum, polyp, duplication cyst and lymphoma.

Enema reduction is the standard non-operative method of treatment of intussusception. This may be hydrostatic reduction using water-soluble contrast or barium, or pneumatic using air. Absolute contraindications to attempted reduction by enema are peritonism, pneumoperitoneum or persistent signs of shock that have not been corrected following initial resuscitation. Reduction of intussusception should not be attempted before consultation with surgical colleagues. Analgesic sedation prior to the enema is thought to improve the reduction rate although sedation may prevent the patient from performing the Valsalva manoeuvre and increasing the intraluminal pressure during straining.

Air enema reduction of intussusception has largely replaced the barium enema. Pneumatic reduction of intussusception using oxygen or carbon dioxide has also been described. The air enema is quick, clean and has a higher reduction rate than barium enema. A large Foley catheter (14G) is inserted into the rectum. An adequate anal seal is essential in order to maintain intracolonic pressure. The air or gas can be delivered using a hand-held bulb of an adapted sphygmomanometer or electric pump or from a wall supply. Inclusion of a commercially available safety valve in the system for instantaneous colonic decompression is recommended. The maximum pressure used is 120 mmHg. A trochar must be immediately available to relieve a pneumoperitoneum if one occurs during reduction. Pressure is sustained as long as the intussusception is moving retrogradely. Successful reduction is indicated when gas is observed entering the distal small bowel (Figure 10.15.8). The ileocaecal valve may be oedematous and look like an unreduced intussusception preventing gas entering the terminal ileum even though complete reduction has been achieved. Some centres will repeat the enema after a period in these circumstances but clinical monitoring will equally confirm successful reduction as symptoms disappear. In a small group of children, failure of initial reduction may be followed by a successful reduction after a wait of 30 min or so. Policy must be agreed in each centre. Sonography may be helpful in confirming absence of residual intussusception and showing a swollen ileocaecal valve when there is not too much gas in the bowel.

Hydrostatic reduction of intussusception using water-soluble contrast material is well described but as yet has not gained widespread popularity. It has the advantage of no radiation to the patient, low perforation rate and reported success rates of up to 95%. The process is operator dependent and can be time-consuming.

Reduction is less likely to be successful if the duration of symptoms is over 48 h, there is rectal bleeding, small bowel obstruction or the dissection sign during the enema. The dissection sign occurs when contrast material passes between or 'dissects' the intussusceptum and the intussuscipiens. Perforation may occur in ischaemic or normal bowel and is a more common occurrence during therapeutic air enema than barium enema, although the perforation tends to be smaller with air enema and is associated with less faecal spillage or peritoneal contamination. If perforation does occur during air enema it may lead to respiratory compromise due to a pneumoperitoneum. Emergency decompression using a large bore needle may be necessary.

Approximately 5–10% of intussusceptions recur after operative or non-operative reduction. A pathological lead point may not be apparent at the time of reduction, particularly with air enema, and should be suspected after three episodes of intussusception. Intussusceptions with pathological lead points may be safely reduced. Further management depends on the clinical findings in each case.

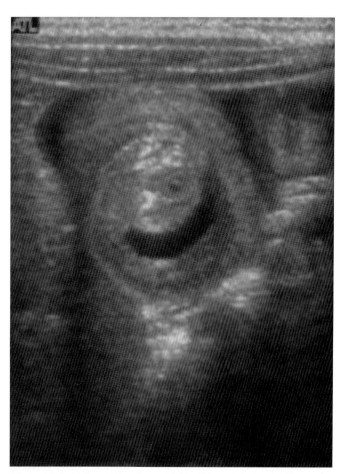

Figure 10.15.7 Trapped peritoneal fluid within an intussusception and free peritoneal fluid.

FURTHER READING

Britton I, Wilkinson A. Ultrasound features of intussusception predicting outcome of air enema. Pediatric Radiology 1999; 29:705–710.

Crystal C, Hertzanu Y, Farber B, Shabshin N, Barki Y. Sonographically guided hydrostatic reduction of intussusception in children. Journal of Clinical Ultrasound 2002; 30:343–348.

del-Pozo G, Albillos J, Tejedor D et al. Intussusception in children: Current concepts in diagnosis and enema reduction. Radiographics 1999; 19:299–319.

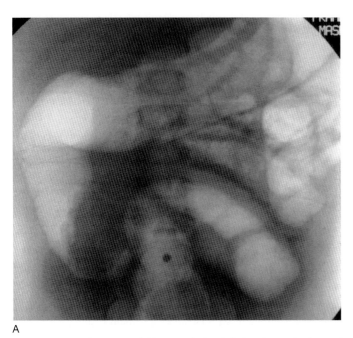

A

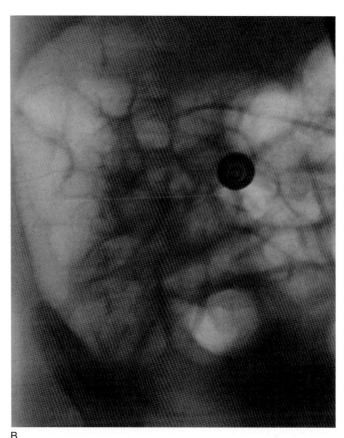

B

Figure 10.15.8 Air enema. (A) Image obtained during the study shows the intussusceptum outlined by air in the caecum. (B) Following complete reduction gas has entered the small bowel. A residual soft tissue mass in the caecum represents a swollen ileocaecal valve.

Gu L, Zhu H, Wang Set al. Sonographic guidance of air enema reduction in children. Pediatric Radiology 2000; 30:339–342.

Hanquinet S, Anooshiravani M, Vunda A, Le Coultre C, Bugmann P. Reliability of color and power Doppler sonography in the evaluation of intussuscepted bowel viability. Pediatric Surgery International 1998; 13:360–362.

Harrington L, Connolly B, Wesson D, Babyn P, Schuh S. Ultrasonographic and clinical predictors of intussusception. Journal of Pediatrics 1998; 132:836–839.

Kornecki A, Daneman A, Navarro O et al. Spontaneous reduction of intussusception clinical spectrum, management and outcome. Pediatric Radiology 2000; 30:58–63.

Koumanidou C, Vakaki M, Pitsoulakis G, Kakavakis K, Mirilas P. Sonographic detection of lymph nodes in the intussusception of infants and young children: Clinical evaluation and hydrostatic reduction. American Journal of Roentgenology 2002; 178:445–450.

McAlister W. Intussusception; Even Hipprocates did not standardise his technique of enema reduction. Radiology 1998; 206:595–598.

Meradji M, Hussain S, Robben S, Hop W. Plain film diagnosis in intussusception. British Journal of Radiology 1994; 67:147–149.

Navarro O, Dugougeat F, Shuckett B, Alton D, Daneman A. The impact of imaging in the management of intussusception owing to pathologic lead points in children. Pediatric Radiology 2000; 30:594–603.

Rohrschneider W, Tröger J. Hydrostatic reduction of intussusception under US guidance. Pediatric Radiology 1995; 25:530–534.

APPENDICITIS

Acute appendicitis is the most common indication for emergency abdominal surgery in children. Clinical findings include crampy periumbilical or right lower quadrant pain, nausea, vomiting, tenderness in the right iliac fossa and rebound tenderness. Approximately one-third of children with acute appendicitis have atypical clinical findings and the diagnosis is difficult. Diagnosis is also difficult in young children unable to describe their symptoms clearly. Delay in diagnosis may lead to perforation of the appendix, abscess formation, sepsis and even death. Other complications of perforation include wound infection, adhesions, possible infertility in females and bowel obstruction. It has been considered safer to perform a negative laparotomy than risk the complications of perforation. A negative laparotomy rate of approximately 25% is considered acceptable. Many non-surgical conditions may mimic the signs and symptoms of acute appendicitis.

The frequency of radiological investigations for children with appendicitis has a wide variation. In the UK, in most centres, imaging is reserved for causes of clinical doubt and a negative laparotomy is accepted. Imaging is more frequently used in the USA, including plain radiographs, US and CT. The aim of imaging is to assist in early diagnosis of acute appendicitis when the clinical suspicion is low or the clinical findings are vague, or to make an alternative diagnosis and reduce the negative laparotomy rate and perforation rate in acute appendicitis. The plain abdominal radiograph may demonstrate an appendicolith in 15% of cases (Figure 10.15.9) and will show perforation or bowel obstruction, although it is relatively insensitive and non-specific for acute appendicitis. Other plain film signs of appendicitis are a localized RIF ileus, distension of the flank stripe on the right or abscess gas

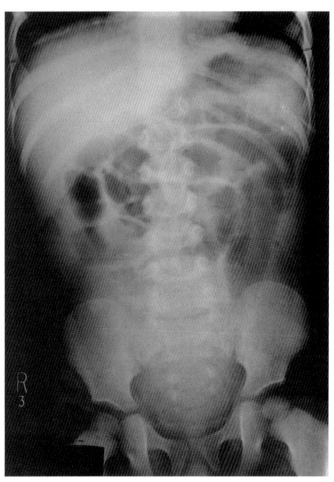

Figure 10.15.9 Plain abdominal radiograph showing an appendicolith in the right iliac fossa and distal small bowel obstruction in a child subsequently proven to have a perforated appendix.

which, when there is peritonitis, may be distant from the RIF. Appendicitis with peritonitis is probably the most frequent cause of a subphrenic abscess in children. Unless bowel obstruction or perforation is suspected, routine use of the plain abdominal radiograph is not recommended.

The graded compression technique of ultrasonography is of value mainly in children who have equivocal clinical findings to diagnose acute appendicitis or other conditions that can cause abdominal pain. A high frequency linear array transducer is used and gentle gradual compression applied to the anterior abdominal wall in the right lower quadrant causing displacement and compression of normal bowel loops. Adequate compression is achieved when the iliac vessels and psoas muscle are visualized and there is near apposition of the anterior and posterior abdominal walls. Scanning is performed in the longitudinal and transverse planes. Technical failure may occur due to severe pain or patient obesity. Scanning in the coronal plane can overcome the presence of intestinal gas interposed between the appendix and the transducer.

The inflamed appendix is a fluid-filled, non-compressible, blind-ending tubular structure with a maximum transverse diameter of greater than 6 mm. In a non-perforated appendix, the inner echogenic submucosa can be identified. On transverse view, the fluid-filled lumen of the appendix is surrounded by the echogenic mucosa and hypoechoic muscularis (Figure 10.15.10). An echogenic focus with acoustic shadowing representing an appendicolith may be seen. Additional findings include a periappendicular collection of fluid, which occurs with early perforation, increased periappendiceal echogenicity representing fat infiltration and enlarged reactive mesenteric lymph nodes. When perforation of the appendix occurs there is loss of the echogenic submucosal layer. Other features include a loculated periappendicular collection of fluid (Figure 10.15.11), abscess formation (Figure 10.15.12) or pelvic fluid collection. The appendix is visible in 40–60% of patients with appendiceal perforation. A normal appendix is visible in up to 50% of children allowing confident exclusion of acute appendicitis. Colour Doppler US does not increase sensitivity in acute appendicitis but it will increase the confidence in diagnosis. In the non-perforated appendix, colour Doppler will show hyperperfusion, which in the early stages of acute appendicitis may be limited to the tip of the appendix. The vascularity of the appendix decreases with necrosis and perforation. Appendiceal perforation leads to hyperaemia of the surrounding tissue although this is a non-specific sign and can be due to other conditions. The normal appendix has no demonstrable flow on colour Doppler and does not have adjacent inflammatory changes. Portal pyaemia is a rare and often lethal complication of appendicitis. Portal vein gas is seen on US as echogenic bubbles.

Computed tomography is highly sensitive and specific for diagnosing acute appendicitis and is superior to US. It is also useful for evaluating complications such as phlegmon and abscess formation or suggesting an alternative diagnosis, e.g. Crohn's disease, renal colic, mesenteric adenitis, ovarian torsion. There are several techniques for CT of the appendix, which include CT of the abdomen and pelvis or CT limited to the pelvis only, with various combinations of oral, rectal and intravenous contrast material or no contrast material at all. The simplest technique is probably to use intravenous contrast without rectal contrast. This is well tolerated by children. CT techniques that use colon contrast material and intravenous contrast have higher sensitivity and accuracy. If a limited CT scan is normal the examination can be extended to include the rest of the abdomen.

Computed tomography signs of acute appendicitis include an enlarged appendix (transverse diameter greater than 7 mm), a non-opacified appendiceal lumen, appendiceal wall enhancement after intravenous contrast material administration, periappendiceal fat stranding (in younger children there may be too little fat), circumferential or focal caecal wall thickening, appendicolith (which may be obscured by oral or rectal contrast), free peritoneal fluid, phlegmon, abscess and adjacent bowel wall thickening (Figures 10.15.13 and 10.15.14). The most specific CT findings are an enlarged appendix (diameter greater than 6 mm) and caecal apical thickening. Potential pitfalls in the CT diagnosis of acute appendicitis include difficulty in differentiating retained oral contrast in the appendix from an appendicolith or mistaking an inflamed appendix for an unopacified loop of bowel. It is important to identify the entire appendix as inflammation may be limited to the tip.

Magnetic resonance imaging (MRI) has been used in the evaluation of acute appendicitis, particularly in patients who have atypical symptoms, are obese or have a retrocaecal appendix and where US has been limited. It has a sensitivity equivalent to that of CT

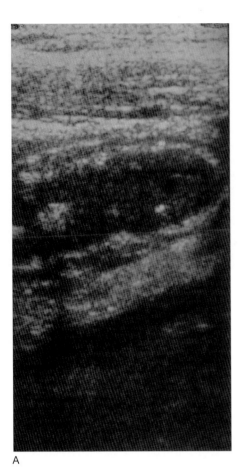

A

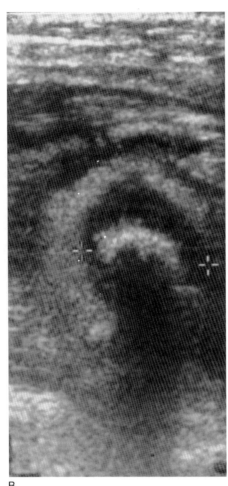

B

Figure 10.15.10 Acute appendicitis. (A) Longitudinal and (B) transverse US scans show the enlarged appendix and the hyperechoic mucosa. The lumen contains fluid and an appendicolith. Periappendicular increased echogenicity represents infiltration of mesenteric fat.

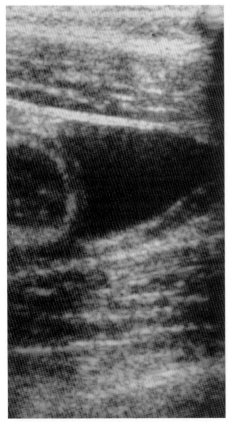

Figure 10.15.11 Acute appendicitis. Ultrasound scan showing periappendicular fluid collection.

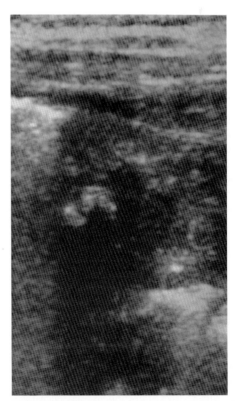

Figure 10.15.12 Perforated appendix. Ultrasound scan shows a complex mass containing an appendicolith.

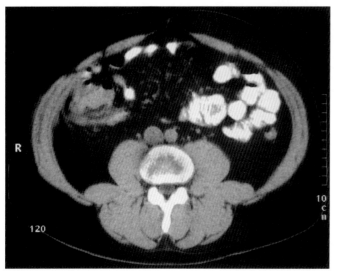

Figure 10.15.13 Acute appendicitis. CT scan shows thickening of the caecal wall, fat stranding, pericaecal fluid, thickening of the abdominal wall musculature laterally on the right and subcutaneous oedema. (Courtesy of Dr Mark Love, Royal Victoria Hospital, Belfast, Northern Ireland.)

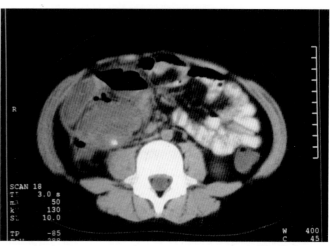

Figure 10.15.14 Acute appendicitis. CT scan shows an appendix abscess containing an appendicolith. There is also some adjacent fat stranding. (Courtesy of Dr Mark Love, Royal Victoria Hospital, Belfast, Northern Ireland.)

and is more accurate than US. The appearance of acute appendicitis on MR images consists of a fluid-filled, tubular structure with a thickened enhancing wall. Calcified faecoliths are not routinely seen, nor is a normal appendix. The disadvantages of MRI are lack of scanner availability leading to a delay in performing the examination and subsequent management, high cost and the requirement for sedation in younger children.

INTRA-ABDOMINAL AND SUBPHRENIC ABSCESS

Intra-abdominal abscesses may occur at many sites in the abdomen. The most frequent are the pelvis, the subphrenic space and the paracolic gutters. The subhepatic space and the mesentery are also sometimes involved depending on the cause. The most frequent causes of abdominal abscesses in children are perforation of the appendix, a Meckel's diverticulum and peritonitis following abdominal trauma or postsurgery. Less frequent are abscesses secondary to infected peritoneal dialysis catheters and ventriculo-peritoneal shunt tubing. The spread of infection within the peritoneum is influenced by the location of the peritoneal ligaments and the mesentery. Pelvic or subphrenic abscesses may be the presenting feature of a perforated appendix. Swelling of the abdominal wall is a clinical presentation of intra-abdominal sepsis in young children and may be the presentation of a perforated Meckel's diverticulum.

Symptoms of an abdominal abscess depend on the location of the collection and the degree of peritoneal inflammation. Most children have pain and fever. Diarrhoea may be the presentation of a pelvic abscess. Shoulder tip pain may reflect a subphrenic collection. Urinary tract infection is an occasional presentation.

Once the clinical suspicion of an abscess is raised, initial imaging should be an erect chest x-ray and a supine abdomen. The yield from the latter is low. Signs to look for are: (1) a mass lesion with displaced bowel loops; (2) bubbles of gas outside the bowel lumen; (3) localized dilated loops of bowel indicating ileus; and (4) air–fluid levels in the subphrenic spaces. These are easy to see on the right but care is needed on the left so as not to confuse them with the colon. If there is doubt the examination can be repeated following the administration of oral contrast and waiting for it to reach the colon.

Abdominal US with a full bladder should be performed. An abscess is seen as a fluid collection that may contain debris and gas bubbles. The wall will be thick if it is of some days duration. There may be a localized ileus and mesenteric oedema. Associated peritonitis will result in free fluid in the peritoneum. In many children, US is unsatisfactory due to a combination of pain and bowel gas distension. Abdominal CT is indicated in these circumstances to confirm or refute the diagnosis. It should be performed with intravenous contrast enhancement using a low-dose technique and covering the abdomen from diaphragm to pubis. Abscess collections are seen as fluid collections with enhancing walls. Air–fluid levels may be observed.

Percutaneous drainage is often the treatment of choice and is best performed under US or CT control depending on the location and complexity of the collection.

FURTHER READING

Ang A, Chong N, Daneman A. Pediatric appendicitis in "real-time": The value of sonography in diagnosis and treatment. Pediatric Emergency Care 2001; 17:334–340.

Applegate K, Sivit C, Myers M, Pschesang B. Using helical CT to diagnose acute appendicitis in children: Spectrum of findings. American Journal of Roentgenology 2001; 176:501–505.

Callaghan M, Rodriguez D, Taylor G. CT of appendicitis in children. Radiology 2003; 224:325–332.

Hörmann M, Paya K, Eibenberger K et al. MR imaging in children with nonperforated acute appendicitis: Value of unenhanced MR imaging in sonographically selected cases. American Journal of Roentgenology 1998; 171:467–470.

Hörmann M, Puig S, Peokesch S, Partik B, Helbich T. MR imaging of the normal appendix in children. European Journal of Radiology 2002; 12:2313–2316.

Kaiser S, Frenckner B, Jorulf H. Suspected appendicitis in children: US and CT – A prospective randomised study. Radiology 2002; 223:633–638.

Lane M, Mindelzun R. Appendicitis and its mimickers. Seminars in Ultrasound, CT and MRI 1999; 20:77–85.

Lowe L, Draud K, Hernanz-Schulman M et al. Nonenhanced limited CT in children suspected of having appendicitis: Prospective comparison and resident interpretations. Radiology 2001; 221:755–759.

Lowe L, Perez R, Scheker L et al. Appendicitis and alternate diagnoses in children: findings on unenhanced limited helical CT. Pediatric Radiology 2001; 31:569–577.

Meyers M, Oliphant M, Berne A, Feldberg M. The peritoneal ligaments and the mesentries: pathways of intraabdominal spread of disease. Radiology 1987; 163:593–604.

Mullins M, Kirchner M, Ryan D et al. Evaluation of suspected appendicitis in children using limited helical CT and colonic contrast material. American Journal of Roentgenology 2001; 176:37–41.

Peña B, Taylor G, Fishman S, Mandl K. Costs and effectiveness of ultra-sonography and limited computed tomography for diagnosing appendicitis in children. Pediatrics 2000; 106:672–676.

Quillan S, Siegal M. Appendicitis: Efficacy of color Doppler sonography. Pediatric Radiology 1994; 191:557–560.

Quillan S, Siegal M. Diagnosis of appendiceal abscess in children with acute appendicitis; Value of Color Doppler sonography. American Journal of Roentgenology 1995; 164:1251–1254.

Rao P, Rhea J, Noveline R, Mostafavi A, McCabe C. Effect of computed tomography of the appendix on treatment of patients and use of hospital resources. New England Journal of Medicine 1998; 338:141–146.

Sivit C, Dudgeon D, Applegate K et al. Evalution of suspected appendicitis in children and young adults: Helical CT. Radiology 2000; 216:430–433.

Sivit C, Siegal M, Applegate K, Newman K. When appendicitis is suspected in children. Radiographics 2001; 21:247–262.

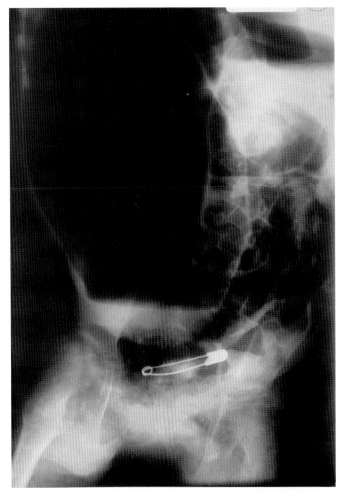

Figure 10.15.15 Volvulus. Mentally subnormal girl with a 48-h history of abdominal distension. The huge gas-filled bowel loop is the trapped sigmoid colon, which has undergone volvulus (note safety pin fastens her nappy).

VOLVULUS AND MALROTATION

Large bowel volvulus can be divided into caecal, transverse colonic, sigmoid colonic and ileosigmoid knotting. It is usually due to congenitally anomalous or absent ligamentous fixation of the large bowel with an abnormal mesocolon or common ileocolomesentery, resulting in twisting of the mesentery at the base of a redundant loop. Volvulus is more frequent in patients who are mentally ill or have a neurological disorder, as these children often have a bowel that is distended due to excess swallowed air. Volvulus can occur at any age, even in the neonatal period.

The major clinical manifestation is acute abdominal pain. Initial investigation is with a plain supine radiograph, which is often inconclusive, as the findings will depend on the site of volvulus. These findings include air–fluid levels with distension of proximal colon with a 'coffee bean' sign sometimes present in sigmoid volvulus (Figure 10.15.15). A water-soluble contrast enema is advised when there is discrepancy between the clinical picture and the plain radiographic findings and leads to the correct diagnosis being made in greater than 60% of cases. On contrast enema, a bird's beak appearance is considered pathognomonic but a rounded termination at the site of obstruction may also be present. Although the enema may be therapeutic, resulting in hydrostatic reduction,

surgical therapy is more definitive. Ultrasound may be helpful by detecting the site of colonic obstruction by showing a fluid-filled colon when the plain abdominal radiograph is inconclusive. It is particularly useful in critically ill patients in whom a contrast enema is not possible.

The findings encountered in small bowel malrotation have been covered in other sections. Almost all children with abnormalities of colonic fixation have associated abnormal duodenal rotation. Isolated colonic malrotation is rare but will be normal upper gastrointestinal (GI) tract contrast examination. Malrotation is diagnosed using upper GI tract contrast studies but a follow-through or enema may be helpful in problem patients. The highest prevalence of volvulus due to short mesentery occurs when the caecum lies in the left or right upper quadrant. When the caecum is located in the left lower quadrant (complete non-rotation) there is usually little risk of volvulus but it has been reported. Dependence on clinical features is particularly important in this instance. Caution must also be exercised regarding interpretation of caecal position, as a mobile caecum occurs in 16% and hence may appear abnormally high in children.

FURTHER READING

Chirdan LB, Ameh EA. Sigmoid volvulus and ileosigmoid knotting in children. Pediatric Surgery International 2001;17:636–637.

Houshian S, Sorensen JS, Jensen KE. Volvulus of the transverse colon in children. Journal of Pediatric Surgery 1998; 33:1399–1401.

Ismail A. Recurrent colonic volvulus in children. Journal of Pediatric Surgery 1997; 32:1739–1742.

Mellor MF, Drake DG. Colonic volvulus in children: value of barium enema for diagnosis and treatment in 14 children. American Journal of Roentgenology 1994; 162:1157–1159.

Samuel M, Boddy SA, Nicholls E, Capps S. Large bowel volvulus in childhood. Australian and New Zealand Journal of Surgery 2000; 70:258–262.

EPIPLOIC APPENDAGITIS AND SEGMENTAL OMENTAL INFARCTION (SOI)

The epiploic appendages are small pockets of fat, which arise from the serosal surface of the colon and contain blood vessels. They vary in size, being larger in obese individuals, and are more numerous in the descending and sigmoid colon. Epiploic appendagitis and segmental omental infarction result from torsion or venous thrombosis. This gives rise to surrounding inflammation resulting in abdominal pain. Presentation typically is with severe acute focal pain, which may mimic appendicitis, ureteric colic or Meckel's diverticulitis. The white cell count is usually normal.

Ultrasound will show an avascular, hyperechoic non-compressible mass deep to the region of maximal surface tenderness. Findings of epiploic appendagitis at CT are typically of a 1–4 cm fat density (approximately -60 Hounsfield units) oval and usually left-sided pericolic lesion with surrounding mesenteric inflammation resulting in a ring sign. SOI has a similar appearance on US but on CT the mass appears more heterogeneous and can be larger and right sided. Treatment is conservative for both epiploic appendagitis and SOI.

FURTHER READING

Horton KM, Corl FM, Fishman EK. CT evaluation of the colon: inflammatory disease. Radiographics 2000; 20:399–418.

McClure MJ, Khalili K, Sarrazin J, Hanbidge A. Radiological features of epiploic appendagitis and segmental omental infarction. Clinical Radiology 2001; 56:819–827.

TRAUMA AND NON-ACCIDENTAL INJURY

Due to the mobility of the colon within the abdominal cavity in childhood, colonic injuries due to non-accidental injury are uncommon in children. Abdominal injuries may be classed as blunt or penetrating, blunt trauma typically occurring in motor vehicle accidents. Distal colonic and anal injuries may be due to iatrogenic instrumentation (e.g. rectal thermometers) but are more commonly found following sexual abuse and imaging is seldom required.

Initial radiological assessment following trauma is with a supine AXR and an erect CXR or left lateral decubitus AXR if perforation is suspected. Large volumes of 'free' intraperitoneal gas are common following colonic perforation. Prompt surgical intervention is required. If the plain film series is inconclusive, intravenous contrast-enhanced CT is required, especially if bowel injury is suspected. The role of oral contrast remains controversial and although useful in assessment of other gastrointestinal injuries is unlikely to aid in evaluation of the colon. CT is more sensitive in detecting free fluid or gas within the abdomen than plain film series. A bowel wall defect, bowel wall thickening (>3 mm) or a focal haematoma may be apparent on CT images.

FURTHER READING

Canty TG Sr, Canty TG Jr, Brown C. Injuries of the gastrointestinal tract from blunt trauma in children: a 12-year experience at a designated pediatric trauma center. Journal of Trauma 1999; 46:234–240.

Carty H. Non-accidental injury: a review of the radiology. European Radiology 1997; 7:1365–1376.

Kleinman PK. Diagnostic imaging of child abuse, 2nd edn. St Louis: Mosby; 1998:261.

Shankar KR, Lloyd DA, Kitteringham L, Carty HM. Oral contrast with computed tomography in the evaluation of blunt abdominal trauma in children. British Journal of Surgery 1999; 86:1073–1077.

Strouse PJ, Close BJ, Marshall KW, Cywes R. CT of bowel and mesenteric trauma in children. Radiographics 1999; 19:1237–1250.

COLONIC CAUSES OF GI BLEEDING

Colonic causes of GI bleeding are legion. In many cases, endoscopy has superseded radiological imaging, particularly barium enema examinations. Our role as radiologists is often to define the extent of disease and monitor treatment in addition to providing a diagnosis. Imaging the large bowel by nuclear medicine, CT and US is now more useful than ever before. As in all clinical scenarios the modality used must be tailored to the suspected diagnosis whilst adhering to the ALARA (as low as reasonably achievable) principle.

ULCERATIVE COLITIS

Ulcerative colitis (UC) is uncommon in young children, with most paediatric cases occurring in the second decade of life. Presentation is usually with diarrhoea which may be bloody and growth failure but an acute onset with rectal bleeding and toxic megacolon is more common in children than in adults. After 10 years there is a 20% risk per decade of developing carcinoma. The timing of colectomy with stoma or ileal pouch formation is a clinical decision.

The aetiology of UC remains unknown but the condition has been related to immunological hypersensitivity, childhood infection and genetic predisposition. Extra-colonic manifestations are less common than with Crohn's disease. Arthritis and spondylitis are not related to the severity of the bowel disease and are more common in boys. Biochemical evidence of liver disturbance is common but radiological evidence is rare in children. Erythema nodosum occurs in 10% of cases but pyoderma gangrenosum is rare.

Ulcerative colitis is confined to the mucosa and submucosa of the colon with continuous inflammation extending from the rectum proximally. There may be distal sparing if treatment per rectum has been utilized. In children, it is uncommon to see isolated proctitis (15%). A pancolitis is present in 60–65% of cases at diagnosis. Histology reveals distortion of crypt architecture, crypt abscesses and goblet cell depletion.

A plain abdominal radiograph is the initial investigation when onset of symptoms is acute or if there is clinical concern that a surgical complication is present. Irregularity of the mucosa, colonic wall thickening, haustral thickening and absence of faecal residue may be apparent. The plain film can be helpful and indicate the extent of disease, as faeces are absent in areas of bowel with active colitis. Absence of faeces in the caecum indicates a pancolitis. The plain film is not always a reliable guide of disease severity but is particularly helpful if toxic megacolon (Figure 10.15.16) and/or perforation is suspected.

Colonoscopy has largely replaced barium enema in the diagnosis of UC. However, if a barium enema study is needed, and for it to be diagnostic, proper complete bowel preparation is required for a double-contrast technique, which is often difficult in children. A barium enema is contraindicated if there are severe symptoms or clinical evidence of toxicity. Mucosal granularity, loss of haustration and collar stud ulcers (due to submucosal tracking of barium) are typical findings (Figure 10.15.17). In the late stages, the colon becomes shortened and rigid with widening of the postrectal space. The ileocaecal valve is often patulous, which can give rise to backwash ileitis (Figure 10.15.18). Postinflammatory or filiform polyps can be present in the healing phase (Figure 10.15.19).

The instant barium enema, i.e. a modified enema not requiring bowel preparation due to the inflamed colon being devoid of faecal residue, is rarely if ever used in children and is completely contraindicated when plain films indicate toxic megacolon.

Ultrasound is generally not used in the assessment of inflammatory bowel disease unless perforation and abscess are suspected. Differentiation of Crohn's disease and UC is not possible although some authors suggest that loss of normal bowel wall stratification is more common in Crohn's disease. Other non-specific findings of inflammatory bowel disease include bowel wall thickening, reduced bowel compressibility and increased Doppler flow in both the superior mesenteric artery and the bowel wall.

Nuclear medicine using technetium 99m HMPAO-labelled white cells is far more useful in defining the extent of disease at a lower radiation dose than a barium enema examination (Figure 10.15.20). Early inflammation is occasionally scintigraphically negative. Scans are judged as abnormal if bowel activity is present on 30-min and 1-h images. Bowel activity is normally present on 3-h images. Using anterior and posterior images helps differentiation of intrapelvic small bowel from rectum. Although nuclear medicine may be diagnostic its major role in UC is assessing

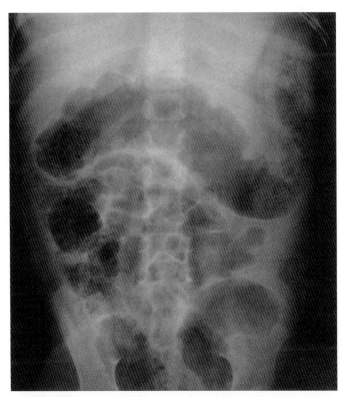

Figure 10.15.16 Toxic megacolon in a child with UC. Plain abdominal radiograph shows gaseous distension of the large bowel and pneumatosis coli.

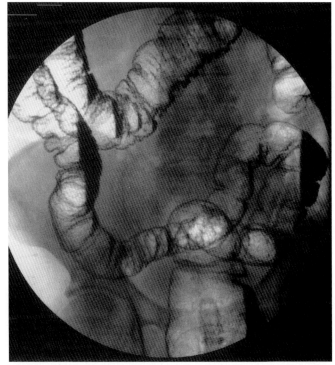

Figure 10.15.17 Ulcerative colitis. Barium enema showing involvement of the entire colon. There is extensive mucosal ulceration, loss of haustration and shallow ulceration.

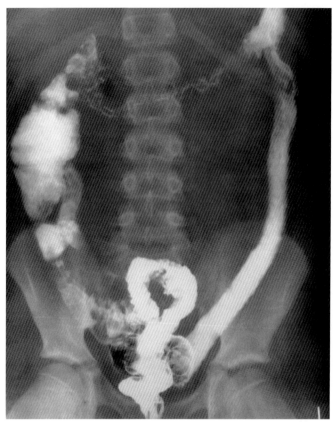

Figure 10.15.18 Total colonic involvement with UC. Note the loss of haustration, patulous ileocaecal valve and reflux ileitis (courtesy of Dr P. Rice, Craigavon Area Hospital, Northern Ireland).

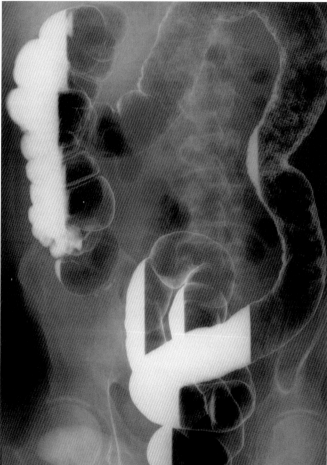

Figure 10.15.19 Filiform mucosal polyps in UC, best seen in the descending colon.

response to treatment or in differentiation from Crohn's disease when histology is non-specific. Pancolitis occurs in both Crohn's disease and UC but if uptake is continuous and left sided UC is much more likely. Abnormal activity that is irregular, non-continuous, involves the small bowel or spares the rectum favours Crohn's disease.

Computed tomography is not usually required in UC but may be helpful when patients do not respond to medical management. Signs of a severe colitis include thickened bowel wall, pericolic stranding and ascites. If there is associated colonic dilatation then developing toxic megacolon is likely and patient management can be altered. Associated pyophlebitis, a major cause of morbidity and mortality, can be identified if intravenous contrast is administered. The use of rectal contrast is usually contraindicated. Submucosal deposition of fat occurs in longstanding UC (Figure 10.15.21).

CROHN'S COLITIS

Colonic Crohn's disease is relatively uncommon in children. When it occurs it is usually in the second decade of life. Crohn's disease

is usually associated with small bowel (especially terminal ileal) disease. Presentation depends on the regions of the gastrointestinal tract involved, colonic disease usually presenting with bloody diarrhoea. Approximately 15% of cases present with acute abdominal pain mimicking appendicitis and, in this instance where there is clinical doubt, an US can be very helpful in differentiating and hence preventing an unnecessary laparotomy. Failure to thrive and erythema nodosum are more common in Crohn's disease than UC and perianal disease is a distinguishing feature.

Radiological imaging is aimed at the region of gastrointestinal tract in which disease is suspected. Nuclear medicine (see above) will define the extent and distribution of disease. The large bowel and upper gastrointestinal tract are best examined by endoscopy but, if indicated, a double-contrast barium enema can determine the extent of colonic disease. Radiological imaging of the small bowel (barium follow-through) is most useful for demonstration of extent of disease, especially fistulas and strictures. Enteroclysis is unnecessary in children and gives no more information of any clinical value. A per-oral pneumocolon can give excellent visualization of the terminal ileum if it is poorly seen on the follow-through study. Associated abscesses can be demonstrated on both

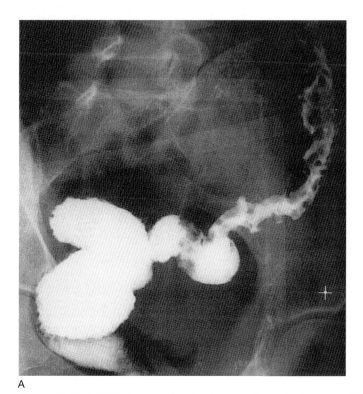

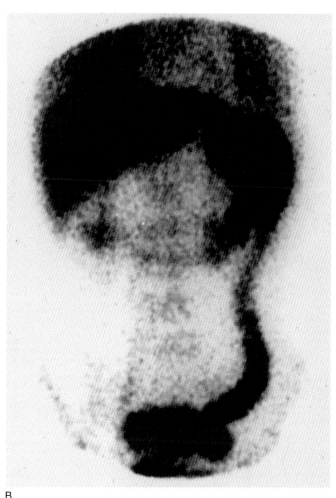

A   B

Figure 10.15.20 (A) Water-soluble contrast enema demonstrating acute UC extending from the rectum showing collar stud ulcers. The procedure was abandoned due to patient discomfort. (B) Technetium 99m HMPAO white cell scan in the same patient shows the true extent of colonic involvement.

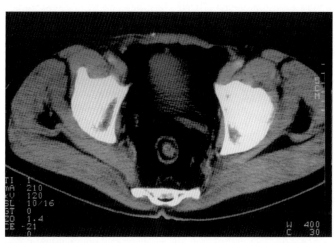

Figure 10.15.21 Axial CT scan showing submucosal deposition of fat in the rectum in longstanding UC (courtesy of Dr P. Rice, Craigavon Area Hospital, Northern Ireland).

CT and US. Crohn's disease will also appear as a thickened bowel on CT. When colonic disease is extensive, Crohn's disease may be indistinguishable from UC and even pseudomembranous colitis. Differentiating features include right-sided colonic involvement, asymmetrical ulceration, skip lesions and deep 'rose thorn' ulceration (Figure 10.15.22). Fibrosis in longstanding disease will result in strictures and antimesenteric pseudodiverticula.

FURTHER READING

Aideyan UO, Smith WL. Inflammatory bowel disease in children. Radiologic Clinics of North America 1996; 34:885–902.

Ali SI, Carty HM. Paediatric Crohn's disease: a radiological review. European Radiology 2000; 10:1085–1094.

Charron M, del Rosario FJ, Kocoshis SA. Pediatric inflammatory bowel disease: assessment with scintigraphy with 99mTc white blood cells. Radiology 1999; 212:507–513.

Cucchiara S, Celentano L, de Magistris TM et al. Colonoscopy and technetium-99m white cell scan in children with suspected inflammatory bowel disease. Journal of Pediatrics 1999; 135:727–732.

Faure C, Belarbi N, Mougenot JF et al. CT evaluation of the colon: inflammatory disease. Radiographics 2000; 20:399–418.

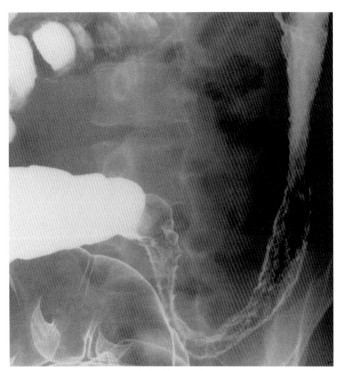

Figure 10.15.22 Crohn's colitis. Deep ulcers are visible in the sigmoid and descending colon.

Imbriaco M, Balthazar EJ. Toxic megacolon: role of CT in evaluation and detection of complications. Clinical Imaging 2001; 25:349–354.

Stringer DA. Imaging inflammatory bowel disease in the pediatric patient. Radiologic Clinics of North America 1987; 25:93–113.

Stringer MD, Randall T, Rutter DP, Picton SV, Puntis JW. Appropriate investigation of inflammatory bowel disease in children. Journal of the Royal Society of Medicine 1998; 91:589–591.

POLYPOSIS SYNDROMES

POLYPS

Colonic polyps may be hamartomatous, adenomatous or postinflammatory. Multiple adenomatous polyps occur in the familial adenomatous polyposis syndrome of which Gardner's syndrome and Turcot's syndrome can be considered variants. Multiple hamartomatous polyps occur in the Peutz–Jegher's syndrome, Cowden's disease and Cronkhite–Canada syndrome. The histology of juvenile polyps and juvenile polyposis syndromes is controversial with some pathologists classifying them as hamartomas.

SOLITARY POLYPS

Juvenile polyps are the most common colonic tumours of childhood. Most are found in the rectosigmoid and 45% are multiple. When multiple polyps are present the diagnosis of one of the juvenile polyposis syndromes should be considered. Presentation is most commonly painless rectal bleeding in an otherwise well

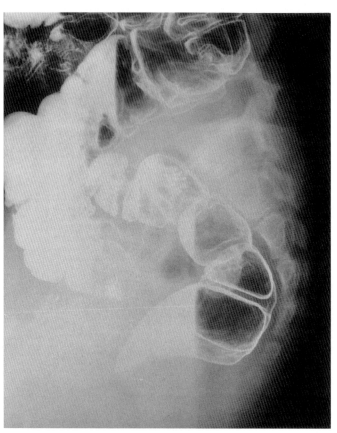

Figure 10.15.23 Solitary polyp on the anterior wall of the rectum in an 8-year-old boy with rectal bleeding.

child. Intussusception and prolapses may also occur. Solitary polyps are benign and the risk of malignant change is practically negligible.

The diagnosis is usually made by colonoscopy. A double-contrast barium enema (DCBE) will demonstrate 70% of polyps (Figure 10.15.23). Most are small and pedunculated. The average age of onset is 5 years and DCBE is likely to be technically difficult. Graded compression sonography may also detect colonic polyps. If a polyp is discovered (even incidentally), complete colonoscopy should be performed and a relevant family history sought.

JUVENILE POLYPOSIS SYNDROME

There are a number of juvenile polyposis syndromes with a wide range of pathological and radiological features and variable geographical locations. One form of juvenile polyposis syndrome (JPS) is a condition characterized by multiple polyps of the gastrointestinal tract that predominantly affects the colon. Twenty-five per cent of cases are inherited as an autosomal dominant trait. The remainder are the result of new mutations. Other morphological abnormalities, such as macrocephaly, cleft lip or congenital heart diseases are often present. The minimum number of polyps required for diagnosis is a controversial issue with figures of between three and six suggested in various sources. JPS may occur in infancy when the prognosis is poor. Most present in the second decade with rectal bleeding. JPS is a premalignant condition with adenomatous change seen as young as 3 years. Surveillance colonoscopy is advised when polyp numbers are small but colectomy should be considered when numerous polyps are present. First-degree relatives should be screened.

HAMARTOMATOUS POLYPOSIS SYNDROMES

Peutz–Jegher's syndrome is an autosomal dominant condition of multiple hamartomatous GI polyps and mucosal and cutaneous macular melanin pigmentation. Although the small intestine is primarily involved, gastric and colonic polyps also occur. Diagnosis is usually made by enteroscopy or small bowel barium studies. The risk of developing malignancy in the GI tract and elsewhere is greater than in the general population. Cowden's disease (named after the first patient) is the association of colonic and other GI polyps with macrocephaly, breast cancer or fibrocystic disease and thyroid carcinoma. Cronkhite–Canada syndrome (Figure 10.15.24) is characterized by the association of anorexia, protein-losing enteropathy, macrocephaly, clubbing and nail atrophy. This is usually a condition of adults, with JPS sometimes considered its paediatric form.

FAMILIAL ADENOMATOUS POLYPOSIS

Familial adenomatous polyposis (FAP) is an AD condition with a high degree of penetrance in which multiple GI adenomatous polyps are present, primarily in the colon. A family history is usually present and screening is important, as colorectal carcinoma is inevitable by the fifth decade of life. There is an association with other tumours, namely duodenal, pancreatic and thyroid carcinomas, hepatoblastomas and desmoid tumours. Turcot's syndrome is the association of multiple colorectal adenomatous polyps with a primary brain tumour and can be considered a variant of FAP. Gardner's syndrome in which there are osteomata and desmoplastic tumours in association with GI polyps is another variant. Although most children have a positive family history or colorectal symptoms a minority present with extracolonic manifestations and hence unusual and rare tumours in children should raise the possibility of FAP, especially if a sibling is affected.

Radiologically, FAP appears as multiple small filling defects that can carpet the entire colon on a barium enema (Figure 10.15.25). Colonoscopy is the diagnostic and surveillance investigation of choice. Colectomy is the only treatment and close follow-up by endoscopy is important from time of diagnosis until colectomy is to be performed. Hence, colectomy can usually be deferred until teenage years if colonoscopy has shown no dysplasia.

FURTHER READING

Cynamon HA, Milov DE, Andres JM. Diagnosis and management of colonic polyps in children. Journal of Pediatrics 1989; 114:593–596.

Hyer W. Polyposis syndromes: pediatric implications. Gastrointestinal Endoscopy Clinics of North America 2001; 11:659–682, vi–vii.

Kucukaydin M, Patiroglu TE, Okur H, Icer M. Infantile Cronkhite-Canada syndrome? – Case report. European Journal of Pediatric Surgery 1992; 2:295–297.

Lehmann CU, Elitsur Y. Juvenile polyps and their distribution in pediatric patients with gastrointestinal bleeding. West Virginia Medical Journal 1996; 92:133–135.

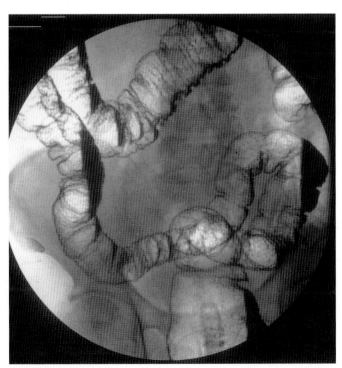

Figure 10.15.24 Cronkhite–Canada syndrome. Numerous very small polyps throughout the large bowel (courtesy of Dr P. Rice).

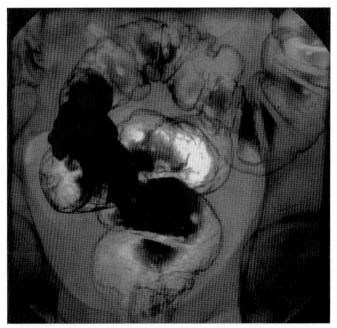

Figure 10.15.25 Familial polyposis coli. Multiple small polyps are present throughout the colon (courtesy of Dr P. Rice).

VASCULAR MALFORMATIONS

Haemangiomata may occur as isolated benign mesenchymal tumours but vascular malformations of the large bowel are generally rare and when present are often associated with a generalized syndrome.

Klippel–Trenaunay syndrome, a rare congenital multifactorial disorder characterized by skeletal or soft tissue hypertrophy, multiple haemangiomata and venous malformation, affects the large bowel in 13% of cases. Extensive colonic haemangiomata may be present or more commonly multiple anorectal lesions. Imaging can be difficult. Double-contrast barium enema will demonstrate submucosal lesions, which may be indistinguishable from polyps. CT can be useful as phleboliths are more readily demonstrated and haemangiomata have a characteristic enhancement pattern, filling in from the peripheries. This is much easier to appreciate in a solid organ than in the colon. MRI may be helpful if haemangiomata are large but this is often not the case in the colon. Endoscopy is usually the investigation of choice, with angiography if surgery or embolization is contemplated.

Blue rubber bleb naevus syndrome, which consists of cutaneous and visceral haemangiomata, may also affect the colon. Again barium studies may simulate polyposis syndromes and colonoscopy is the investigation of choice to demonstrate colonic lesions. Primary varices of the colon have been described and may be familial. The imaging findings are similar to those described above.

FURTHER READING

Samuel H, Spitz L. Klippel-Trenaunay syndrome: Clinical features, complications and management in children. British Jounal of Surgery 1995; 82:757–761.

Wong YC, Li YW, Chang MH. Gastrointestinal bleeding and paraparesis in blue rubber bleb nevus syndrome. Pediatric Radiology 1994; 24:600–601.

BEHÇET'S DISEASE

Behçet's disease is a multisystem inflammatory disease characterized by a triad of recurrent genital and oral ulceration with ocular inflammation. Although involvement of any part of the gastrointestinal tract can occur, colonic involvement is frequent and may be life threatening. The caecum and ascending colon are most frequently involved usually with ileal disease. Classically, barium studies show large discrete ulcers with normal intervening mucosa. The disease is often radiologically indistinguishable from Crohn's disease.

FURTHER READING

Aideyan UO, Smith WL. Inflammatory bowel disease in children. Radiologic Clinics of North America 1996; 34:885–902.

Stringer DA. Imaging inflammatory bowel disease in the pediatric patient. Radiologic Clinics of North America 1987; 25:93–113.

Stringer DA, Cleghorn GJ, Durie PR, Daneman A, Hamilton JR. Behcet's syndrome involving the gastrointestinal tract – a diagnostic dilemma in childhood. Pediatric Radiology 1986; 16:131–134.

COWS' MILK PROTEIN INTOLERANCE

Cows' milk protein intolerance is a cause of lower GI bleeding in both infancy and childhood. It may occur in exclusively breast-fed infants due to antigens in breast milk. Often there is a coincidental intolerance to soya bean proteins. The diagnosis is usually a clinical one but as presentation in childhood may mimic inflammatory bowel disease, diagnostic imaging may be requested.

Plain films are not helpful diagnostically. Ultrasound findings described include non-specific thickening of the colon predominately affecting the mucosa of the colon. Irregular narrowing of the rectum with a calibre change to normal sigmoid colon similar to Hirschsprung's disease may be demonstrated by barium enema. Radiology is rarely required to make this diagnosis but it can be used to monitor improvement.

FURTHER READING

Machida HM, Catto Smith AG, Gall DG, Trevenen C, Scott RB. Allergic colitis in infancy: clinical and pathologic aspects. Journal of Pediatric Gastroenterology and Nutrition 1994; 19:22–26.

Patenaude Y, Bernard C, Schreiber R, Sinsky AB. Cow's-milk-induced allergic colitis in an exclusively breast-fed infant: diagnosed with ultrasound. Pediatric Radiology 2000; 30:379–382.

Stringer DA. Imaging inflammatory bowel disease in the pediatric patient. Radiologic Clinics of North America 1987; 25:93–113.

LIPOMATA

Lipomata are rare in the paediatric population. Most are asymptomatic but rectal bleeding may occur. Barium enema will demonstrate a polypoid lesion, usually on the right side of the colon. CT findings of a round, smooth, well-defined mass of fat density are characteristic and provide the definitive diagnosis.

FURTHER READING

Franc-Law JM, Begin LR, Vasilevsky CA, Gordon PH. The dramatic presentation of colonic lipomata: report of two cases and review of the literature. The American Surgeon 2001; 67:491–494.

COLITIS CYSTICA PROFUNDA

Colitis cystica profunda (CCP) is a rare benign lesion of the colon. It is more commonly seen in adults but cases in children have been described. Presentation is typically with rectal bleeding and diarrhoea.

Radiologically, CCP resembles a mucin-producing adenocarcinoma. Most lesions are found in the rectum but all areas of the colon and small intestine may be affected. Coexisting colonic disease is uncommon but diffuse involvement may occur with chronic colitis. Transrectal US demonstrates the typical feature of a mass containing submucosal cysts that do not extend beyond the submucosa.

FURTHER READING

Heusinkveld DC, Barnard JA 3rd. Colitis cystica profunda in a pediatric patient. Journal of Pediatric Gastroenterology and Nutrition 1994; 18:395–398.

ISCHAEMIC COLITIS

Ischaemic colitis may be due to arterial or venous occlusion or a low flow state following hypovolaemic shock. The latter is more common in children because it usually occurs following trauma. The 'watershed' areas of the splenic flexure and rectosigmoid are affected and the ischaemia is usually confined to the mucosa and submucosa. Isolated right-sided colonic involvement has also been described. Plain radiographs of the abdomen may be normal or demonstrate a non-specific bowel dilatation indicating a degree of paralytic ileus. Thumb printing and pneumatosis are more specific, the latter being an ominous sign.

Barium enema is rarely performed in this situation. Findings evolve over time especially if the ischaemia is transmural. Initially, thumb printing, ulceration and transverse ridging are present. Healing can result in stricture formation as early as 1 month following injury.

Ultrasound with duplex and colour flow Doppler study may show bowel thickening and reduced or absent intramural blood flow. CT scanning is the radiological investigation most frequently indicated following trauma given the need to evaluate the other intra-abdominal organs. Unenhanced images can show a high density of acute mucosal or submucosal haemorrhage but since the examination is usually performed in a trauma setting, intravenous contrast is recommended. Water is the most useful oral contrast medium. CT will demonstrate circumferential bowel thickening, bowel dilatation, intense persistent enhancement of bowel wall and a narrow calibre vena cava or aorta.

FURTHER READING

Horton KM, Fishman EK. Computed tomography evaluation of intestinal ischemia. Seminars in Roentgenology 2001; 36:118–125.
Teefey SA, Roarke MC, Brink JA et al. Bowel wall thickening: differentiation of inflammation from ischemia with color Doppler and duplex US. Radiology 1996; 198:547–551.
Wiesner W, Willi UV. Nonocclusive ischemic colitis in a 12-year-old girl: value of unenhanced spiral computed tomography. International Journal of Colorectal Disease 2001; 16:55–57.

VASCULITIS

The vasculitic bowel diseases such as Henoch–Schönlein purpura (HSP) and haemolytic uraemic syndrome are described in Chapter 10.7. Both are multisystem diseases. GI involvement may affect both the large and small bowel. Children present with colicky abdominal pain, GI bleeding and blood per rectum.

If the symptoms antedate the rash in HSP, the initial diagnosis is usually intussusception. The appearances on abdominal radiographs are those of bowel wall oedema with thumbprinting as seen in ischaemic colitis. Thickened bowel is also seen at US.

DIARRHOEA

PNEUMATOSIS COLI

This is a condition rarely seen in children. There are multiple gas-filled cysts in the colonic wall in the submucosa. This gives a characteristic appearance on abdominal radiographs, the cysts being seen as radiolucent blebs, which gives a bubbly appearance to the colon as the cysts affect it circumferentially. In adults, there is an association of the condition with obstructive airways disease. It is occasionally seen in adolescent children with severe cystic fibrosis.

INFECTIOUS COLITIS

Diarrhoea has many causes that may also present with lower GI tract bleeding. Of these, infectious colitides are the commonest but rarely require imaging, unless presentation is atypical. Many pathogens can affect the colon. *Escherichia coli*, salmonella and shigella types, campylobacter fetus and *Yersinia enterocolitica* may all affect the colon, usually as a generalized enterocolitis.

If imaging is performed the findings are that of a non-specific paralytic ileus or colitis with mucosal oedema and occasionally toxic dilatation. Salmonella colitis may mimic Hirschsprung's disease due to rectal spasm. Haemolytic uraemic syndrome has been described following infection by *E. coli* and shigella organisms and is a triad of microangiopathic haemolytic anaemia, renal failure and thrombocytopenia.

Invasive amoebiasis of the colon is due to infection by the protozoan *Entamoeba histolytica*, which is endemic in many parts of the world. Four manifestations have been described: ulcerative rectocolitis, typhloappendicitis, amoebomata and a fulminating colitis. Ulcerative rectocolitis is best demonstrated by double-contrast barium enema but is rarely indicated. Findings include mucosal oedema and ulceration with intervening normal mucosa usually in the rectosigmoid and right side of the colon. Typhloappendicitis is often accompanied by hepatic abscesses and the imaging findings are similar to other forms of typhlitis. Amoebomata are segmental lesions of the colon causing concentric narrowing with lack of shouldering on barium enemas. They are frequently multiple. Fulminating colitis, although rare, is more common in children than in adults and is radiologically indistinguishable from other causes of toxic megacolon.

FURTHER READING

Bhatt R, Rickett A. Salmonella colitis: a mimic of Hirschsprung disease. Paediatric Radiology 2000; 30:379–382.

Cardoso JM, Kimura K, Stoopen M et al. Radiology of invasive amebiasis of the colon. American Journal of Roentgenology 1997; 128:935–941.

Stringer DA. Imaging inflammatory bowel disease in the pediatric patient. Radiologic Clinics of North America 1987; 25:93–113.

PSEUDOMEMBRANOUS COLITIS (PMC)

Pseudomembranous colitis (PMC) is a necrotizing enteropathy, histologically similar to neonatal necrotizing enterocolitis and neutropenic enterocolitis, that occurs following antibiotic therapy. There is overgrowth of toxin producing *Clostridium difficile* resulting in profuse watery diarrhoea. It is usually related to administration of oral rather than intravenous antibiotics. However, virtually all antibiotics and routes of administration have been implicated. PMC is occasionally non-antibiotic related, occurring in ischaemic colitis and other conditions that cause mucosal ischaemia. Classically, a pancolitis is seen with formation of pseudomembranes. Isolated segmental disease has been reported. The diagnosis is usually confirmed in the laboratory when the toxin is identified.

Imaging findings reflect the severity of the disease. Plain films may be diagnostic if nodular mucosal thickening is present; however, this is only found in severe cases. Less specific but more commonly, colonic ileus is present which may progress to a toxic megacolon. Barium examination is rarely if ever indicated and is completely contraindicated in severe disease. If performed it typically shows thickened haustra with raised mucosal nodules.

In children, US is the imaging modality of choice. The triad of marked colonic wall thickening (up to 3 cm), ascites and lack of intraluminal gas is characteristic. Thickening of the bowel wall in PMC is greater than in any condition other than Crohn's disease and ascites is uncommon in the latter.

Computed tomography is excellent for documenting PMC. The major findings are again colonic wall thickening but with disproportionate lack of pericolic inflammation. The accordion sign (Figure 10.15.26), which describes the strips of oral contrast trapped between swollen haustra, was initially described in PMC and may also occur in Crohn's disease.

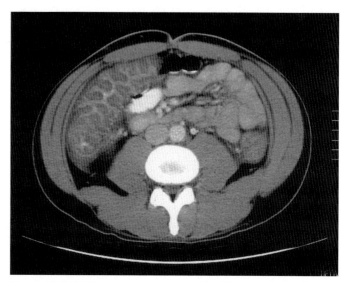

Figure 10.15.26 Pseudomembranous colitis. CT scan showing the 'accordion sign' due to mucosal oedema (courtesy of Dr S. Gillespie, Royal Victoria Hospital, Belfast, Northern Ireland).

centration is not usually sufficient to be corrosive. When concentrations are high the result is a severe colitis, particularly if alkaline detergents or soap enemas are used. The effect may be likened to the oesophagitis caused by ingestion of corrosives. Initially, there is oedema followed by ulceration and ultimately stricture formation. Radiological findings vary depending on the timing of the examination and include toxic dilatation, ulceration, perforation and strictures.

FURTHER READING

Kirchner SG, Buckspan GS, O'Neill JA, Page DL, Burko H. Detergent enema: a cause of caustic colitis. Pediatric Radiology 1997; 28:6:141–146.

Stringer DA. Imaging inflammatory bowel disease in the pediatric patient. Radiologic Clinics of North America 1987; 25:93–113.

EOSINOPHILIC GASTROENTERITIS

Eosinophilic gastroenteritis (EGE) is a rare disorder characterized by eosinophilic infiltration of the mucosa of the gastrointestinal tract. Any part of the gastrointestinal tract may be affected but large bowel involvement is relatively uncommon. The disease has been reported in all age groups. The clinical presentation is variable – abdominal pain, atopy, growth retardation and protein-losing enteropathy have all been reported. Radiologically, there is no pathognomonic appearance of EGE and it may be indistinguishable from Crohn's disease. A generalized or focal colitis and a caecal mass have been described. Sonographically, thickening of all layers of the bowel wall is present and a pseudokidney appearance of dense central echoes with a hypoechoic periphery may be present mimicking intussusception.

FURTHER READING

Gillett PM, Russell RK, Wilson DC, Thomas AE. *C. difficile* induced pneumatosis intestinalis in a neutropenic child. Archives of Disease in Childhood 2002; 87:85.

Horton KM, Corl FM, Fishman EK. CT evaluation of the colon: inflammatory disease. Radiographics 2000; 20:399–418.

Ros PR, Buetow PC, Pantograg-Brown L, Forsmark CE, Sobin LH. Pseudomembranous colitis. Radiology 1996; 198:1–9.

CAUSTIC COLITIS

A number of substances have been implicated as causes of caustic colitis of which detergents and herb enemas are the most frequent. A transient colitis is more common following an enema, as the con-

The diagnosis is usually made following biopsy of the affected portion, which will demonstrate eosinophilic infiltration. Whether eosinophilic infiltration is a primary phenomenon or secondary to the presence of an unknown antigen remains unclear and it is likely that EGE represents a spectrum of disorders of differing aetiologies.

FURTHER READING

Huang FC, Ko SF, Huang SC, Lee SY. Eosinophilic gastroenteritis with perforation mimicking intussusception. Journal of Pediatric Gastroenterology and Nutrition 2001; 21:613–615.

Kelly KJ. Eosinophilic gastroenteritis. Journal of Pediatric Gastroenterology and Nutrition 2000; 30(Suppl):S28–S35.

Shweiki E, West JC, Klena JW et al. Eosinophilic gastroenteritis presenting as an obstructing cecal mass – a case report and review of the literature. American Journal of Gastroenterology 1999; 94:3644–3645.

Stringer DA. Imaging inflammatory bowel disease in the pediatric patient. Radiologic Clinics of North America 1987; 25:93–113.

CONSTIPATION

Constipation is common in children accounting for 3% of referrals to general paediatricians. Clinical features include difficulty, pain or delay in defaecation that may be associated with abdominal pain, faecal soiling or encopresis. Rarely, the presenting feature is anuria with bladder outlet obstruction secondary to compression by the faecal mass. Faecal soiling can present as diarrhoea. Chronic constipation generally follows an inadequately managed acute episode. There is no definition of the normal passage of stool per diem. Most children have at least one bowel motion but diet plays a significant role in determining the number and texture of stool.

The majority of children have a functional constipation that is not associated with an organic aetiology and many have psychological disorders. Constipation is particularly common in children who are sedentary, or who have cerebral palsy, disorders of the spinal cord or an endocrine disease such as hypothyroidism. The diagnosis of constipation is usually made from history and clinical examination. Investigations such as anorectal manometry and imaging may be required to exclude an organic aetiology in cases where there is diagnostic difficulty, the constipation is severe or persists despite treatment.

The plain abdominal radiograph is not routinely used in the diagnosis of constipation. It will demonstrate the amount of faecal loading of the large bowel (Figure 10.15.27). This may cause huge enlargement of the rectum and sigmoid colon in idiopathic constipation. By contrast, children with a delayed diagnosis of Hirschsprung's disease tend to have a more even distribution of faeces. Scoring systems have been used to assess faecal loading from the plain radiograph but are of dubious merit. Evidence of intestinal obstruction in Hirschsprung's disease, neuronal intestinal dysplasia and chronic intestinal pseudo-obstruction may also be demonstrated on a plain abdominal radiograph. Spinal anomalies such as partial sacral agenesis can also be shown. Colonic transit time can be assessed using solid radiopaque markers. The radiopaque markers are ingested on three consecutive days and on the 4th or 5th day, depending on the method used, a plain abdominal radiograph is taken and the number of residual markers counted and their distribution noted (Figure 10.15.28). Oral 131 In DTPA has also been used in the assessment of colonic transit but is now abandoned. A single contrast unprepared barium enema may be required to exclude Hirschsprung's disease if biopsy is not to be performed. This enema should be limited to showing the relationship of the anus and level of faecal loading. Defecating proctography is occasionally helpful in children with chronic constipation and defecation disorders. Lesions demonstrated include rectoceles and rectal intussusception in older children, similar to adults, reflecting the chronic nature of the problem. In younger children, one may see an apparent elongation of the anal canal. This is due to dyskinetic contraction of the levator ani and puborectalis muscles (Figure 10.15.29).

FURTHER READING

Bautista Casasnovas A, Varela Cives R, Villaneuva Jeremias A et al. Measurement of colonic transit time in children. Journal of Pediatric Gastroenterology and Nutrition 1991; 13:42–45.

Fotter R. Imaging of constipation in children. European Journal of Radiology 1998; 8:248–258.

Leech S, McHugh K, Sullivan P. Evaluation of a method of assessing faecal loading on plain abdominal radiographs in children. Pediatric Radiology 1999; 29:255–258.

Rockney R, McQuade W, Days A. The plain abdominal roentgenogram in the management of encopresis. Archives of Pediatric Medicine 1995; 149:623-637.

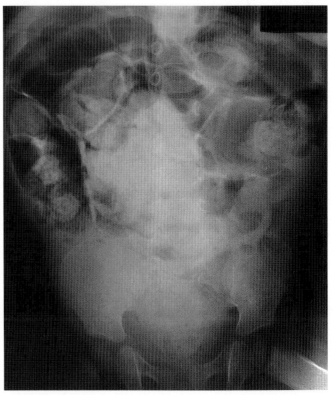

Figure 10.15.27 Plain radiograph of a child with acquired megacolon.

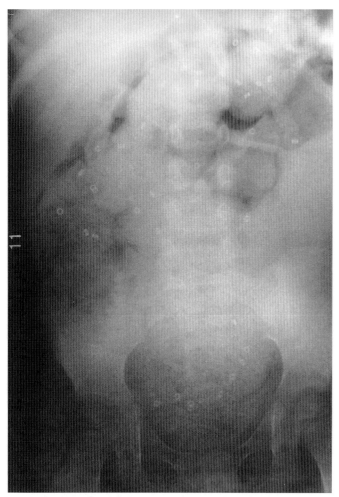

Figure 10.15.28 Colonic transit study using radiopaque markers.

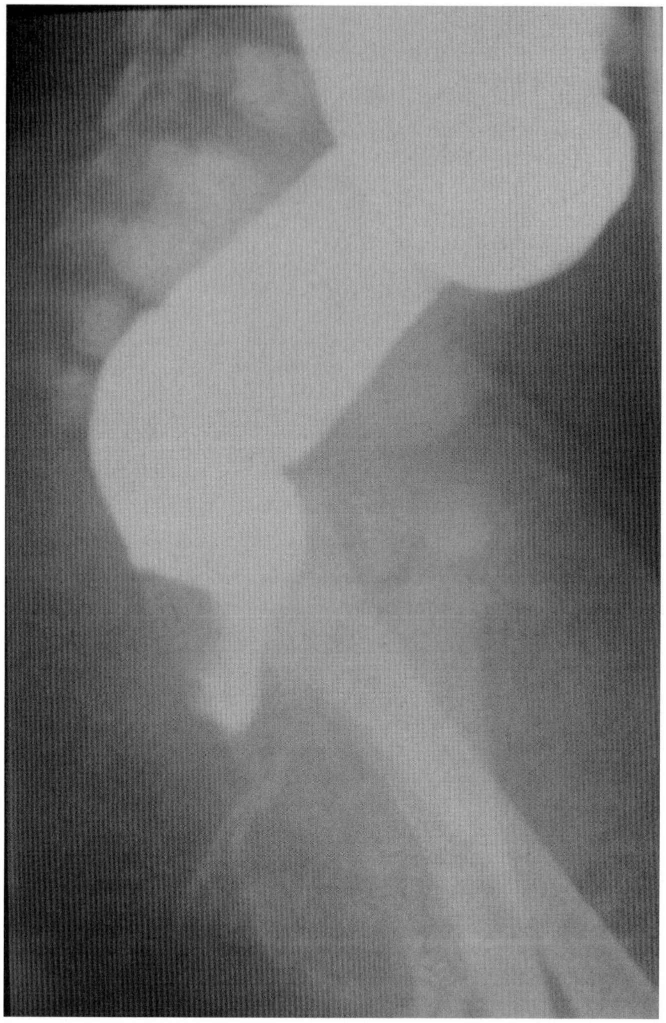

Figure 10.15.29 Child with constipation. Note the elongated anorectal canal secondary to dysynergic contraction of the levator ani and puborectalis muscles.

HIRSCHSPRUNG'S DISEASE

Hirschsprung's disease is due to a failure of caudal migration of the neurones of the neural crest, resulting in an absence of the ganglion cells in more distal bowel from the point of neuronal arrest to the anus. This results in a functional obstruction. In the majority of cases, the aganglionic segment is limited to the rectosigmoid region. Total colonic aganglionosis involves the entire colon and part of the terminal ileum. Rarely, the aganglionosis can affect all of the small bowel as well as the large, a condition incompatible with life. At the other end of the spectrum, ultrashort segment Hirschsprung's disease is also rare with the aganglionic segment confined to the internal anal sphincter. Hirschsprung's disease may be associated with several congenital anomalies that include Down's syndrome, intestinal atresia, malrotation, pigmented ocular defects and neuroblastoma (a form of neurocristopathy).

Presentation of Hirschsprung's disease is most often in the neonatal period with abdominal distension, vomiting and failure to pass meconium. Children who present later than the neonatal period have a history of constipation. The definitive diagnosis of Hirschsprung's disease is made by a suction or full thickness rectal biopsy.

Single-contrast unprepared barium enema examination is reserved for children where the diagnosis is uncertain or biopsy is not going to be performed; often, this is in older children. No cleansing enemas are performed or digital examination or preparatory laxatives are given prior to the procedure. The catheter tip is placed just proximal to the anus and the barium is introduced slowly. Balloon catheters are not used to avoid expanding a narrow segment of aganglionic bowel. As the bowel is filled with barium, irregular contractions may be seen, which is a sensitive indicator of aganglionosis. Otherwise, bowel is filled as far as the transition zone from undilated aganglionic bowel to dilated ganglionic bowel (Figure 10.15.30). Sometimes, a transition zone is not present, especially in all cases of the rarer total colonic aganglionosis. There is a risk of barium impaction proximally if too much is introduced. The rectum should have a diameter greater than that of the colon and a rectosigmoid index of less than 1, and retention of barium for over 24 h suggests Hirschsprung's disease. However, the diagnosis has to be confirmed by biopsy, which is also an accurate way in which to find the transition zone intraoperatively.

Enterocolitis is a serious complication of Hirschsprung's disease pre- and postoperatively (Figure 10.15.31). Postoperatively, it has an incidence of approximately 33%. Clinical presentation is with severe bloody diarrhoea, sepsis and shock.

Surgical treatment of Hirschsprung's disease is initially by colostomy to relieve the intestinal obstruction and then by a second surgical procedure to remove the aganglionic bowel and anastomose normally innervated bowel to the distal rectum. The various surgical procedures include:

1. The Svenson's proctocolectomy with an end-to-end anastomosis between normal colon and the rectum.
2. The Duhamel procedure – a pull-through with end-to-side anastomosis to aganglionic rectum (Figure 10.15.32).
3. The Soave operation – a pull-through of ganglionated bowel submucosally through a sleeve of rectum to the anus.

There is also a trend towards J-type and S-type pull-through operations to give a larger reservoir for faeces above the anus.

Postoperative complications include anastomotic stricture, rectourethral fistula (Figure10.15.33), anastomotic leaks, enterocolitis, persistent constipation and anal incontinence. In the past,

following the second stage surgery, it was usual to leave a colostomy to allow healing of the anastomosis. There is a recent trend of performing a one stage pull-through procedure without colostomy. Prior to closure of a colostomy a contrast study of the distal bowel is performed to exclude leaks or stricture formation using water-soluble contrast material.

FURTHER READING

Becmeur F, Moog R, De Luca G, Christmann D, Sauvage P. Radiological evaluation of Duhamel's operation in Hirschsprung's disease. European Journal of Pediatric Surgery 2000; 10:182–185.

Das K, Alladi A, Kini U, Babu M, Cruz A. Hirschsprung disease, associated rare congenital anomalies. Indian Journal of Pediatrics 2001; 68:835–837.

Elhalaby E , Coran A, Blane C, Hirschl R, Teitelbaum D. Enterocolitis associated with Hirschsprung disease: A clinical-radiological characterization based on 168 patients. Journal of Pediatric Surgery 1995; 30:76–83.

Harjai M. Hirschsprung disease: Revisited. Journal of Postgraduate Medicine 2000; 46:52–54.

Reding R, de Ville de Goyet J, Gosseye S et al. Hirschsprung disease: A 20 year experience. Journal of Pediatric Surgery 1997; 32:1221–1225.

Reid J, Buonomo C, Moreira C, Kozakevich H, Nurko S. The barium enema in constipation: comparison with rectal manometry and biopsy to exclude Hirschsprung disease after the neonatal period. Pediatric Radiology 2000; 30:681–684.

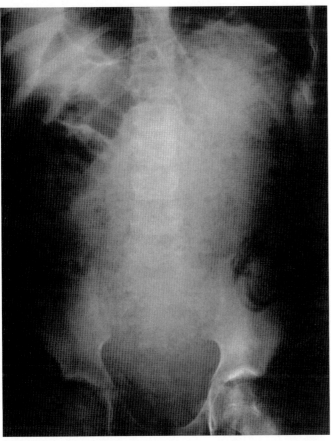

A

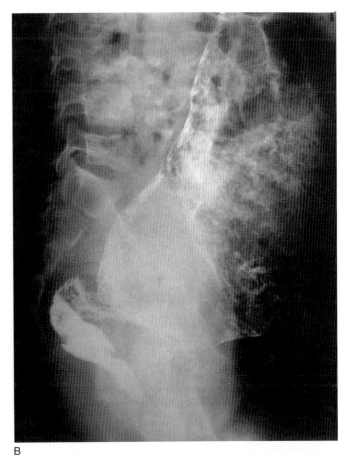

B

Figure 10.15.30 (A) Plain radiograph of a 1-year-old child with Hirschsprung's disease showing gross distension of the colon with faeces. (B) Barium enema in the same child shows the zone of transition in the rectosigmoid junction of the colon.

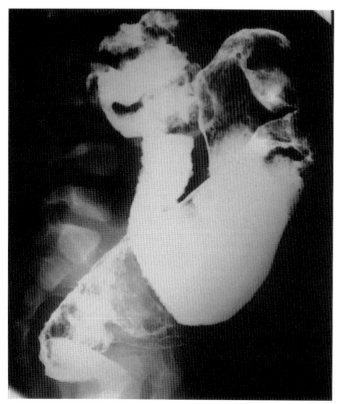

Figure 10.15.31 Barium enema in a child with Hirschsprung's disease showing enterocolitis and a zone of transition at the rectosigmoid junction and mucosal ulceration.

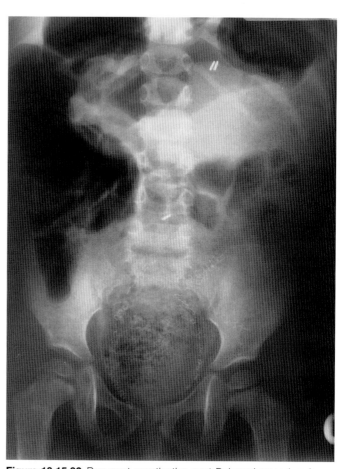

Figure 10.15.32 Recurrent constipation post-Duhamel procedure for Hirschsprung's disease. The staples outlining the resection are characteristic.

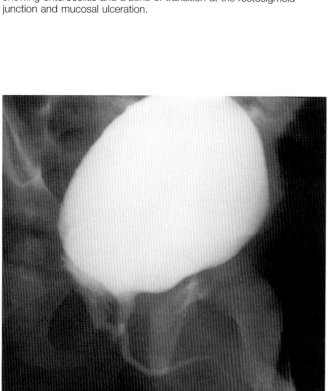

Figure 10.15.33 Hirschsprung's disease with failed pull-through. Micturating cystourethrogram shows a rectourethral fistula.

NEURONAL INTESTINAL DYSPLASIA

Neuronal intestinal dysplasia (NID) is characterized by decreased intestinal motility. There is absent or rudimentary sympathetic ganglion innervation of the gut (type A) or hyperplasia of the cholinergic nerve fibres and neuronal bodies (type B). Type A typically presents with bloody stools and symptoms of functional obstruction and type B, which is more common, presents with severe constipation. NID often presents as longstanding constipation after a pull-through operation in patients with Hirschsprung's disease. The incidence in Hirschsprung's disease is 50%. Type B NID usually shows a slow spontaneous recovery of colon motility. If there is no response to conservative treatment surgery may be required. The imaging features can be similar to those of Hirschsprung's disease (Figure 10.15.34).

FURTHER READING

Fotter R. Imaging of constipation in infants and children. European Journal of Radiology 1998; 8:248–258.

Simpser E, Kahn E, Kenigsberg K et al. Neuronal intestinal dysplasia: quantitative diagnostic criteria and clinical management. Journal of Pediatric Gastroenterology and Nutrition 1991; 12:61–64.

CHRONIC INTESTINAL PSEUDO-OBSTRUCTION

Chronic intestinal pseudo-obstruction (CIP) syndrome is a rare condition that is defined as the existence of permanent or recurrent signs of intestinal obstruction in the absence of identifiable organic obstruction. It is an intestinal motility disorder usually caused by a visceral neuropathy or myopathy. It can involve small segments or the entire gastrointestinal tract. CIP is a spectrum of disorders that vary in severity and have been described under a variety of names that include chronic adynamic ileus, pseudo-Hirschsprung's disease, adynamic bowel syndrome, colonic neuronal dysplasia, hollow visceral myopathy and megacystis–microcolon–intestinal hypoperistalsis syndrome. The latter is the most severe form of CIP and is usually fatal in the first year of life. CIP can be familial and there is also a high incidence of associated anomalies that include midgut malrotation.

Presentation of symptoms is usually in the first month of life but can occur at any age. In neonates, the clinical features include abdominal distension and bilious vomiting. Beyond the neonatal period chronic constipation, abdominal distension and vomiting are the most common presenting findings. The purpose of imaging in CIP is to exclude mechanical obstruction. Abdominal radiographs will show dilated loops of bowel and air–fluid levels. Contrast studies of the entire gastrointestinal tract are generally required to exclude a mechanical obstruction and show associated anomalies such as malrotation or short bowel.

FURTHER READING

Berdon W, Baker D, Blanc W et al. Megacystis-microcolon-intestinal hypoperistalsis syndrome: A new cause of intestinal obstruction in the newborn: Report of radiologic findings in five newborn girls. American Journal of Roentgenology 1976; 126:957–964.

Cucchiara S. Chronic intestinal pseudo-obstruction: The clinical perspective. Journal of Pediatric Gastroenterology and Nutrition 2001; 32:S21–S22.

Goulet O, Jobert-Giraud A, Michel J-L et al. Chronic intestinal pseudo-obstruction syndrome in pediatric patients. European Journal of Pediatric Surgery 1999; 9:83–90.

Heneyke S, Smith V, Spitz L, Milla P. Chronic intestinal pseudo-obstruction: treatment and long term follow up of 44 patients. Archives of Disease in Childhood 1999; 81:21–27.

Moore S, Schneider J, Kaschula R. Non-familial visceral myopathy: clinical and pathologic features of degenerative leiomyopathy. Pediatric Surgery International 2002; 18:6–12.

CHAGAS' DISEASE

Chagas' disease is caused by chronic infection with the protozoan parasite *Trypanosoma cruzi* and is a major health problem in Latin America. The infection has an acute self-limiting phase followed by an initially asymptomatic chronic phase. Clinical manifestations occur after 5–20 years involving the heart and GI tract. Colonic involvement presents with slowly progressive constipation. Autopsy studies have shown megacolon to be more common than megaoesophagus. Due to the long latent phase of the illness, the disease is uncommon in childhood.

Plain films show markedly dilated loops of large bowel and constipation, which is often severe. The diagnosis can be made with a barium enema, which will demonstrate a dilated and elongated sigmoid colon in nearly all cases and rectal involvement in 80%. The proximal large bowel is rarely affected.

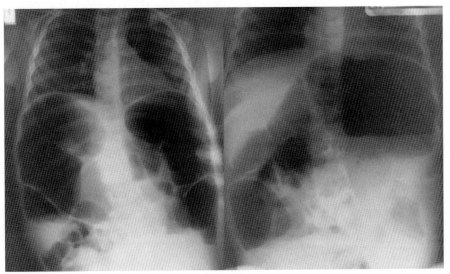

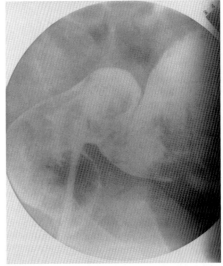

A

B

Figure 10.15.34 A 3-year-old boy with neuronal dysplasia. (A) Erect and supine abdomen. He complained of recurrent attacks of abdominal pain and chronic constipation. Note the marked dilation of the colon without small bowel distension. The colonic appearance is similar to that seen in pseudo-obstruction. (B) Barium enema. There is an apparent transition zone between at the rectosigmoid junction. All biopsies showed normal ganglia but more detailed examination showed histological features of neuronal dysplasia.

FURTHER READING

Corbett CE, Ribeiro U Jr, Prianti MG et al. Cell-mediated immune response in megacolon from patients with chronic Chagas' disease. Diseases of the Colon and Rectum 2001; 44:993–998.

de Oliveira RB, Troncon LE, Dantas RO, Menghelli UG. Gastrointestinal manifestations of Chagas' disease. American Journal of Gastroenterology 1998; 93:884–889.

NEUROFIBROMATOSIS

Gastrointestinal involvement occurs in 25% of cases of neurofibromatosis, usually affecting the stomach and jejenum. Colonic involvement is rare. Subserosal neurofibromas, megacolon with a pseudo-Hirschsprung's appearance and polypoid masses have been described. There is an association with lymphoma and familial polyposis. Adenocarcinoma has been reported. Given the differing manifestations, presentation of colonic involvement is varied but constipation and occult bleeding are the most common. Imaging should be tailored to the clinical presentation.

FURTHER READING

Kim HR, Kim YJ. Neurofibromatosis of the colon and rectum combined with other manifestations of von Recklinghausen's disease: report of a case. Diseases of the Colon and Rectum 1998; 41:1187–1192.

Shearer P, Parham D, Kovnar E et al. Neurofibromatosis type I and malignancy: review of 32 pediatric cases treated at a single institution. Medical and Pediatric Oncology 1994; 22:78–83.

Stone MM, Weinberg B, Beck AR, Grishman E, Gertner M. Colonic obstruction in a child with von Recklinghausen's neurofibromatosis. Journal of Pediatric Surgery 1986; 21:741–743.

COLONIC DUPLICATION CYSTS

Duplication cysts are less common in the colon than in the small bowel. Caecal and appendiceal are the most frequent origins of large bowel duplication cysts. The presentation depends on location, size and presence of ectopic mucosa. Right-sided duplications typically present with pain, a palpable mass or bleeding. Left-sided duplications usually present with constipation.

Morphologically, duplications can be spherical or tubular and have the same features as duplication cysts elsewhere in the GI tract, namely adherence to a part of the GI tract, presence of a well-developed smooth muscle wall and an internal lining of alimentary epithelium. They can be saccular or, less commonly, tubular. Tubular duplications may be a distinct entity and in 80% of cases exist with other anomalies, particularly those of the genitourinary tract, and communication with the bowel is common, occurring in 50% of cases.

Plain radiographs can reveal a faecal mass, occasionally with calcification. In tubular duplications, US is often difficult due to the frequent communication with normal bowel. Contrast studies will give the best anatomical detail (Figure 10.15.35). When two ani are present, opacification of each colon with different densities of contrast following appropriate catheter placement is a useful technique. In male patients with a rectoureteric fistula, micturating cystourethrography or retrograde urethrogram may demonstrate the duplicated colon more clearly.

Spherical duplication cysts are best demonstrated by US as a mass of varying echogenicity, with an inner echogenic rim and a surrounding hypoechoic muscle layer (Figure 10.15.36). Peristaltic activity in the wall of the cyst provides further supportive evidence. If ulceration has occurred the inner echogenic rim will often be interrupted or absent. CT and MRI can confirm the relationship of the duplication to bowel but are usually unnecessary.

Technetium 99m pertechnetate scintigraphy is less useful for identifying duplication cysts of the colon as ectopic gastric mucosa is infrequently found; however, if scintigraphy is positive it will provide definitive evidence.

FURTHER READING

Macpherson RI. Gastrointestinal tract duplications: clinical, pathologic, etiologic, and radiologic considerations. Radiographics 1993; 13:1063–1080.

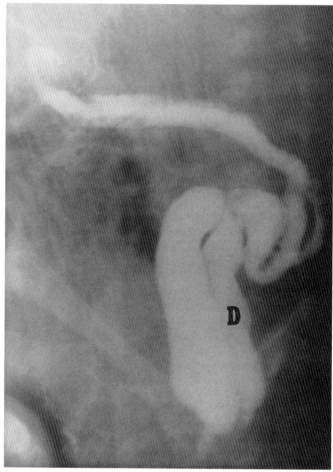

Figure 10.15.35 Colonic duplication in a 1-month-old infant. Barium enema done for investigation of bloody stools. There is a colonic duplication, which is communicating with the normal channel at the rectosigmoid junction and filling retrogradely to the rectum. D = duplication.

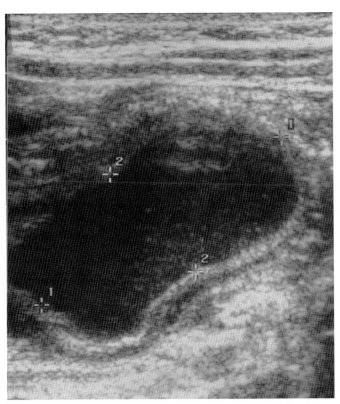

Figure 10.15.36 Spherical duplication cyst. Echogenic inner rim of mucosa with surrounding hypoechoic muscle wall in a child presenting with a history of constipation.

Segal SR, Sherman NH, Rosenberg HK et al. Ultrasonographic features of gastrointestinal duplications. Journal of Ultrasound Medicine 1994; 13:863–870.

Spottswood SE. Peristalsis in duplication cyst: a new diagnostic sonographic finding. Pediatric Radiology 1994; 24:344–345.

Yousefzadeh DK, Bickers GH, Jackson JH Jr, Benton C. Tubular colonic duplication – review of 1876–1981 literature. Pediatric Radiology 1983; 13:65–71.

FAECAL INCONTINENCE

This is a frequent problem in children with mental subnormality and sometimes in neurologically impaired children, although in these conditions, constipation is more frequent, without underlying organic pathology. Overflow incontinence is a feature of gross constipation. Incontinence may follow surgery for repair of anorectal malformations or Hirschsprung's disease. A contrast enema may be helpful in demonstrating the site and configuration of the anastomosis, and continence during straining. During normal defaecation there is relaxation descent of the pelvic floor muscles, and straightening and widening of the anorectal canal. Failure of these movements is often found in both constipation and in incontinence. Endorectal US is an excellent method of assessing the sphincteric muscles in children who are old enough to cooperate and in whom a suitable probe size is available. Pelvic floor musculature and the location of any surgically fashioned neo-

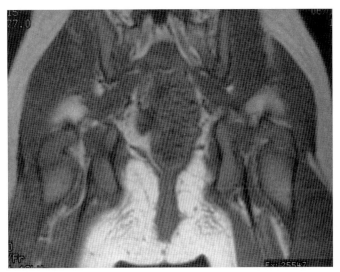

Figure 10.15.37 Coronal MRI showing hypoplastic left levator ani muscle.

rectum is also well demonstrated by coronal and axial MRI (Figure 10.15.37).

COLONIC DISORDERS IN CYSTIC FIBROSIS

Cystic fibrosis is not uncommon in Caucasians but is very rare in the Chinese and is uncommon in children from the Indian subcontinent. Advances in the management of children with cystic fibrosis have increased their life expectancy. This has also been associated with an increased prevalence of various colonic disorders and the appearance of others that were previously unrecognized, e.g. fibrosing colonopathy. Similarities in the clinical presentation of these conditions in cystic fibrosis can result in delayed diagnosis and management.

DISTAL INTESTINAL OBSTRUCTION SYNDROME

Distal intestinal obstruction syndrome (DIOS) is due to impaction of mucofaeculent material in the terminal ileum and right colon that leads to complete obstruction. It is secondary to dilatory or incorrect taking of pancreatic replacement enzymes. It occurs in 10–15% of older children and young adults with cystic fibrosis and its prevalence increases with age. Characteristic features include abdominal pain, constipation and a palpable mass in the right lower quadrant. Abdominal distension, nausea and vomiting are also common. The differential diagnosis includes acute appendicitis, intussusception, subacute obstruction of bowel due to strictures, adhesions or volvulus, fibrosing colonopathy and Crohn's disease.

A plain abdominal radiograph will demonstrate dilated small bowel and the impacted faecal mass (Figure 10.15.38). The obstruction is relieved by softening and mobilizing the faeces with oral balanced electrolyte solutions, such as Golytely®. It is very rare for enemas to be required.

INTUSSUSCEPTION IN CYSTIC FIBROSIS

Intussusception can occur as a complication of cystic fibrosis. The average age of presentation is about 10 years, far older than in idiopathic intussusception. The aetiology is related to either the thick tenacious faeces or DIOS or a chronically distended appendix, all of which can act as a lead point. The intussusception is usually ileocolic. The clinical symptoms include abdominal pain and vomiting, which can be similar to DIOS. The passage of bloody stools is uncommon. The intussusception may be reduced by hydrostatic or air enema. The imaging findings and enema techniques are similar to those described above in 'Intussusception'.

FIBROSING COLONOPATHY IN CYSTIC FIBROSIS

The cause of colonic stricture in cystic fibrosis has not been firmly established but may be related to high strength pancreatic enzyme supplements. The methacrylic acid copolymer of the enteric coating of microencapsulated enzyme preparations may be a causal factor. Clinical presentation is with abdominal pain and signs of intestinal obstruction and may mimic DIOS. Symptoms of colitis with bloody diarrhoea can occur. The right colon is most frequently involved. A plain radiograph of the abdomen may show thickening of the colon wall.

Ultrasound can demonstrate a stricture and thickening of the colonic wall. The typical features on contrast enema are narrowing of the colonic lumen, (Figure 10.15.39) loss of haustration and shortening of the colon. Treatment is surgical resection of the affected segment of colon. The diagnosis is confirmed by the histological findings that include submucosal fibrosis and fatty infiltration.

ACUTE APPENDICITIS IN CYSTIC FIBROSIS

This is an uncommon complication of cystic fibrosis. The appendiceal lumen becomes obstructed by inspissated secretions. The clinical presentation may mimic DIOS, intussusception or Crohn's

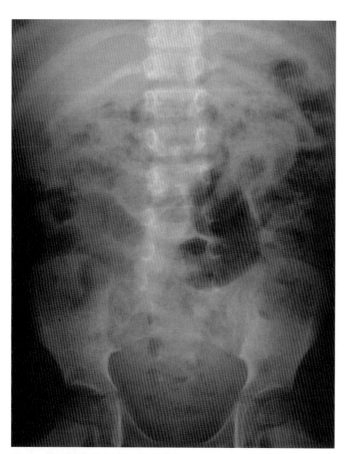

Figure 10.15.38 Distal intestinal obstruction syndrome. Plain radiograph showing faecal loading of the colon and dilated loops of small bowel.

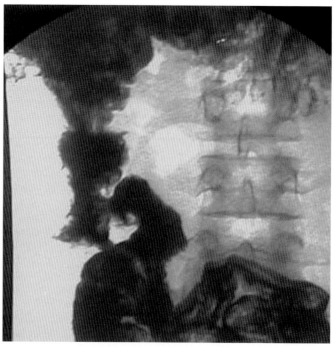

Figure 10.15.39 Fibrosing colonopathy. Child with cystic fibrosis who complained of abdominal pain and had lost weight. Barium enema shows narrowing of the caecum and ascending colon.

disease leading to a delay in diagnosis. This can result in serious complications, such as perforation and appendix abscess. Antibiotic therapy for pulmonary disease may mask the usual clinical features of acute appendicitis. The swollen appendix can act as a lead point for intussusception. Imaging with US or CT is helpful if the clinical findings are atypical.

CARCINOMA IN CYSTIC FIBROSIS

There is an increased risk of cancers in the GI tract in adults with cystic fibrosis. It has been postulated that the differential expression of the cystic fibrosis transmembrane regulator gene may be a factor in the increased risk of cancer in the GI tract. The presentation of colonic carcinoma can be with anaemia (but this is common in cystic fibrosis), or it may mimic DIOS, which can lead to a delay in diagnosis.

FURTHER READING

Ablin D, Ziegler M. Ulcerative type of colitis associated with the use of high strength pancreatic enzyme supplements in cystic fibrosis. Pediatric Radiology 1995; 25:113–116.

Agrons G, Corse W, Markowitz R, Suarez E, Perry D. Gastrointestinal manifestations of cystic fibrosis: Radiologic-pathologic correlation. Radiographics 1996; 16:871–893.

Brown J, Mason A, Cooperberg P. Gastrointestinal manifestations of cystic fibrosis in adults: pictorial essay. Canadian Association of Radiologists Journal 1999; 50:165–169.

Carty H. Abdominal radiology in cystic fibrosis. Journal of the Royal Society of Medicine 1995; 88:18–23.

Chaun H. Colonic disorders in adult cystic fibrosis. Canadian Journal of Gastroenterology 2001; 15:586–589.

Haber H, Benda N, Fitke G et al. Colonic wall thickness measured by ultrasound: striking differences in patients with cystic fibrosis versus healthy controls. Gut 1997; 40:406–411.

Jones R, Franklin K, Spicer R, Berry J. Colonic strictures in children with cystic fibrosis on low strength pancreatic enzymes (letter). Lancet 1995; 346:499.

MacSweeney E, Oades P, Buchdahl R, Rosenthal M, Bush A. Relation of thickening of colon wall to pancreatic-enzyme treatment in cystic fibrosis. Lancet 1995; 345:752–756.

Neglia J, Fitzsimmons S, Maisonneuve P et al. and Cystic Fibrosis and Cancer Study Group. The risk of cancer among patients with cystic fibrosis. New England Journal of Medicine 1995; 332:494–499.

Pohl M, Krackhart B, Posselt H, Lembcke B. Ultrasound studies of the intestinal wall in patients with cystic fibrosis. Journal of Pediatric Gastroenterology and Nutrition 1997; 25:317–320.

Ramsden W, Moya E, Littlewood J. Colonic wall thickness, pancreatic enzyme dose and type of preparation in cystic fibrosis. Archives of Diseases in Childhood 1998; 79:339–343.

vanVelzen D. Colonic strictures in children with cystic fibrosis on low-strength pancreatic enzymes (letter). Lancet 1995; 346:499–500.

MALIGNANT TUMOURS

Colorectal malignancies in children are rare. The diagnosis tends to be made at surgery in the majority of children. Endoscopy and double-contrast barium enema can be used to diagnose tumours of the large bowel, as in adults. Ultrasound and CT can demonstrate the primary tumour and show metastases if present.

CARCINOID TUMOUR

Carcinoid tumours of the appendix or large bowel are rare in childhood. They are neuroendocrine neoplasms and are classified as APUDomas (amine precursor uptake and decarboxylation tumours). Although carcinoid tumours are usually slow growing, they have the potential to become malignant. The appendix is the most common location for carcinoid tumours and most present clinically mimicking acute appendicitis and are found incidentally at appendicectomy. Therefore, they may not be imaged. Carcinoid tumours of the large bowel may also present as obstruction or intussusception. Malignant carcinoid tumour can metastasize to the liver and cause carcinoid syndrome. This is due to serotonin produced by the metastases and is characterized by flushing attacks, diarrhoea, abdominal cramps, asthma and cardiac failure.

Computed tomography may show a primary mass infiltrating the caecum and mesentery or a polypoid or mural mass in the colon. Hepatic metastases are best demonstrated on CT during the arterial phase of the intravenous contrast injection. I123MIBG and somatostatin receptor scintigraphy can also be used to detect metastases.

FURTHER READING

D'Aleo C, Lazzareschi I, Ruggerio A, Riccardi R. Carcinoid tumors of the appendix in children: Two case reports and review of the literature. Pediatric Hematology and Oncology 2001; 18:347–351.

Davey M, Cohen M. Imaging of gastrointestinal malignancy in childhood. Radiologic Clinics of North America 1996; 34:717–742.

Doede T, Foss H, Waldschmidt J. Carcinoid tumors of the appendix in children – Epidemiology, clinical aspects and procedure. European Journal of Pediatric Surgery 2000; 10:372–377.

Hanson M, Feldman J, Blinder R, Moore J, Coleman R. Carcinoid tumors: Iodine-131 MIBG scintigraphy. Radiology 1989; 172:699–703.

Pelage J-P, Soyer P, Brocheriou-Spelle L et al. Carcinoid tumors of the abdomen: CT features. Abdominal Imaging 1999; 24:240–245.

CARCINOMA

Carcinoma of the colon and rectum is extremely rare in children and the incidence increases with age. All parts of the colon are equally affected and the most common histological type is the mucin-secreting adenocarcinoma. There is an increased incidence risk of colorectal carcinoma in children with predisposing diseases such as UC, Crohn's disease or the polyposis syndromes. However, the majority of cases occur in previously healthy children.

The most common presenting symptom is abdominal pain, which is often recurrent and may mimic acute appendicitis. Weight loss, rectal bleeding or a change in bowel habit, usually constipation, are less common presentations. Bowel obstruction or perforation can also occur. The diagnosis is usually delayed because it is unsuspected and rarely considered in children.

A combination of endoscopy and imaging by double-contrast barium enema are the most important diagnostic tests. The radiological appearances are similar to those in adults with stricture and mucosal irregularity. Ultrasound and CT can also demonstrate the primary tumour as well as identifying extracolonic spread and metastases. The poor prognosis of colorectal carcinoma in children is due to the delay in diagnosis resulting in more advanced disease at presentation and to the predominant histological type of mucin-producing adenocarcinoma.

FURTHER READING

Bethel C, Bhattacharyya N, Hutchinson C, Ruymann F, Cooney D. Alimentary tract malignancies in children. Journal of Pediatric Surgery 1997; 32:1004–1009.

Brown R, Rode A, Millar A, Sinclair-Smith, Cywes S. Colorectal carcinoma in children. Journal of Pediatric Surgery 1992; 27:919–921.

Sebbag G, Lantsberg L, Arish A, Levi I, Hoda J. Colon carcinoma in the adolescent. Pediatric Surgery International 1997; 12:446–448.

Vastyan A, Walker J, Pintér A, Gerrard M, Kajtar P. Colorectal carcinoma in children and adolescents – A report of seven cases. European Journal of Pediatric Surgery 2001; 11:338–341.

LYMPHOMA

Lymphoma is the most common primary bowel malignancy in childhood and is less common in large bowel than small bowel. The lymphoma is most commonly non-Hodgkin's type. There is an increased risk of colonic lymphoma in longstanding UC, following immunosuppressive therapy or in AIDS. Presentation is usually with abdominal pain, weight loss, constipation, bowel obstruction, intussusception or abdominal mass. A primary form with a polypoid mass in the caecum, or less commonly in the rectum, can occur, although secondary involvement with diffuse nodular infiltration is more frequent. The nodules are smooth and sessile but may ulcerate. Para-aortic and mesenteric lymphadenopathy usually coexist.

Abdominal radiographs often have non-specific findings that include displacement of bowel loops by a mass or signs of bowel obstruction. Double-contrast barium enema may show obstruction or narrowing of the large bowel, mucosal irregularity or ulceration. On sonography the tumour mass in the thickened bowel wall is usually hypoechoic but can appear anechoic (Figure 10.15.40). CT and sonography may show bowel wall thickening or a mass and identify mesenteric lymphadenopathy or associated disease in the liver, spleen, kidneys, pancreas or chest. CT is routinely performed for staging and follow-up of lymphoma to assess response to chemotherapy. F-18 fluorodeoxyglucose (FDG) positron emission tomography combined with CT has been used to stage lymphoma and evaluate response to treatment in adults. Its place in the management of childhood lymphoma has still to be evaluated.

FURTHER READING

Bar-Shalom R, Mor M, Yekremov N, Goldsmith S. The value of Ga-67 scintigraphy and F-18 fluorodeoxyglucose positron emission tomography in staging and monitoring the response of lymphoma to treatment. Seminars in Nuclear Medicine 2001; 311:177–190.

Cohen M. Imaging of children with cancer. St Louis: Mosby Year Book; 1992:89–126.

Crump M, Gospodarowicz M, Shepherd FA. Lymphoma of the gastrointestinal tract. Seminars in Oncology 1999; 26:324–337.

Dodd GD. Lymphoma of the hollow abdominal viscera. Radiologic Clinics of North America 1990; 28:771–783.

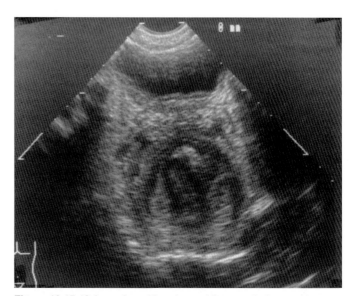

Figure 10.15.40 Large bowel lymphoma. Ultrasound of rectum in a 9-year-old boy presenting with a 1-week history of constipation. There is eccentric narrowing of the rectal lumen by the large lymphomatous mass.

Hwang K, Park C, Kim H et al. Imaging of malignant lymphomas with F-18 FDG coincidence detection positron emission tomography. Clinical Nuclear Medicine 2000; 25:789–795.

Lee H, Han J, Kim T et al. Primary colorectal lymphoma: spectrum of imaging findings with pathologic correlation. European Radiology 2002; 12:2242–2249.

INFLAMMATORY PSEUDOTUMOUR OF THE ABDOMEN

Inflammatory pseudotumours are recorded at all sites in the abdomen in children but compared with neoplastic masses are very rare. The most frequent sites in the abdomen are the stomach and the ileocaecal region, seen mostly in young girls. They are also seen in the retroperitoneum, the liver and the pancreas. Hepatic inflammatory pseudotumour is increasingly seen in Asia. Most of these occur in children and young adults.

Clinical presentation is with abdominal pain, a palpable mass and anaemia. The imaging appearances are those of an aggressive tumour and the initial imaging diagnosis is usually a malignant lesion. On CT the mass is of intermediate density, may contain calcification, is poorly defined and has heterogeneous enhancement. Central necrosis may be present in large lesions. On MRI they are hypointense to muscle on T1-weighted and have high signal on T2-weighted images. Involvement of the gastrointestinal tract includes ulceration of the mucosa and infiltration of the wall with extramural extension. Surgical excision is curative.

FURTHER READING

Das Narla L, Newman B, Spottswood S, Narla S, Kolli R. Inflammatory pseudotumour. Radiographics 2003; 23:719–729.

THE IMMUNOCOMPROMISED CHILD

AIDS

The colon is frequently involved with infectious and neoplastic conditions in AIDS affected patients. Pseudomembranous colitis and typhlitis may also occur. The most devastating of the infectious agents is cytomegalovirus. Plain films demonstrate thumb printing and toxic megacolon in severe cases. Barium enema abnormalities are variable and include spasm, aphthous and deep ulceration, and occasionally large discrete ulcers. CT and US may reveal a typhlitis-type picture with bowel wall thickening and pericolic inflammation.

Bacterial enteropathogens are generally similar to those affecting other immunocompetent individuals with the exception of *Mycobacterium avium intracellulare* (MAI) but this rarely involves the large bowel. Intra-abdominal MAI usually results in lymphadenopathy, although a frank colitis may occur. Fungal infections due to histoplasmosis are described and this can be radiologically indistinguishable from Crohn's disease. Documentation of systemic infection with a chest radiograph is helpful to confirm the diagnosis.

Gastrointestinal tract involvement by Kaposi's sarcoma is uncommon in children and the colonic manifestations are variable. Double-contrast barium enema findings include loss of the haustral pattern and fine mucosal ulceration similar to longstanding inflammatory bowel disease. Submucosal nodules may also be present but are more common in the small bowel.

Direct infection of the colonic mucosa by HIV may result in colitis with ulceration and is most commonly found in homosexual men. The diagnosis is made after exclusion of other infections, notably cytomegalovirus.

also used by many to more specifically indicate neutropenic enterocolitis (ileocaecal syndrome). Neutropenic enterocolitis is a necrotizing inflammatory enteropathy of the colon and ileum, which is similar histologically to neonatal necrotizing enterocolitis and pseudomembranous enterocolitis. The condition usually occurs in neutropenic patients as a result of chemotherapy. However, it may also occur prior to chemotherapy in leukaemia and in other conditions such as cyclical neutropenia, in AIDS and following organ transplantation. The caecum is thought to have a predilection for inflammation due to the relative stasis of bowel contents allowing overgrowth of bacteria. Chemotherapy-induced mucosal damage may also play a part.

Clinically, the patient presents with right-sided abdominal pain, fever and diarrhoea. Although these findings are non-specific, in the correct clinical setting neutropenic enterocolitis must be considered. It should be remembered that appendicitis and intussusception may coexist.

Plain films are often inconclusive in assessment of neutropenic enterocolitis but may show a variety of signs including paucity of bowel gas in the right lower quadrant, a dilated fluid-filled ascending colon, caecal intramural gas and/or small bowel obstruction. Due to its portability and the lack of ionizing radiation, US is usually the modality of choice in the paediatric population. US will show a thickened caecal wall with echogenic mucosa (Figure 10.15.41). An inflammatory mass, pericaecal fluid and ascites may also be present (Figure 10.15.42). Doppler study can also show increased blood flow to the bowel wall. Lack of blood flow is seen in the most severe cases when the bowel has become necrotic. CT is particularly useful for surgical evaluation as pneumoperitoneum, pneumatosis and abscesses are more easily demonstrated. Mucosal oedema and intramural inflammatory masses have been described on contrast enemas but these are rarely if ever indicated due to the poor clinical condition of the patients.

FURTHER READING

Grattan-Smith D, Harrison LF, Singleton EB. Radiology of AIDS in the pediatric patient. Current Problems in Diagnostic Radiology 1992; 21:79–109.

Haller JO, Cohen HL. Gastrointestinal manifestations of AIDS in children. American Journal of Roentgenology 1994; 162:387–993.

Monkemuller KE, Wilcox CM. Diagnosis and treatment of colonic disease in AIDS. Gastrointestinal Endoscopy Clinics of North America 1998; 168:889–911.

Solomon JA, Levine MS, O'Brien C, Jacobs JE. HIV colitis: clinical and radiographic findings. American Journal of Roentgenology 1997; 168:681–682.

NEUTROPENIC ENTEROCOLITIS (TYPHLITIS)

The term 'typhlitis' comes from the Greek (*typhlon*) meaning caecum. Hence 'typhlitis' is a non-specific term meaning inflammation of the caecum or caecitis. However, the term typhlitis is

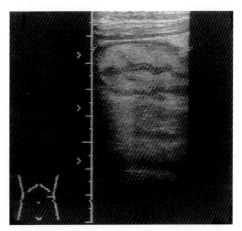

Figure 10.15.41 Typhlitis in a child with neutropenia. Ultrasound scan shows thickened bowel wall.

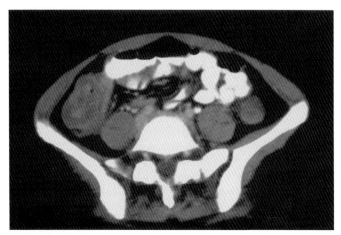

Figure 10.15.42 Contrast-enhanced CT scan in a child with typhlitis showing thickened bowel wall in the caecum and descending colon with pericolic fluid.

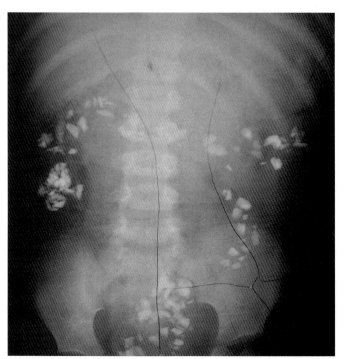

Figure 10.15.43 Pica. Plain abdominal radiograph showing a 2-year-old child with multiple dense particles scattered throughout the large bowel following ingestion of stones.

FURTHER READING

Horton KM, Corl FM, Fishman EK. CT evaluation of the colon: inflammatory disease. Radiographics 2000; 20:399–418.

Kamal M, Wilkinson AG, Gibson B. Radiological features of fungal typhlitis complicating acute lymphoblastic leukaemia. Pediatric Radiology 1997; 27:18–19.

McNamara MJ, Chalmers AG, Morgan M, Smith SEW. Typhlitis in acute childhood leukaemia: Radiological features. Clinical Radiology 1986; 37:83–86.

Monkemuller KE, Wilcox CM. Diagnosis and treatment of colonic disease in AIDS. Gastrointestinal Endoscopy Clinics of North America 1998; 8:889–911.

Ojala AE, Lanning FP, Lanning BM. Abdominal ultrasound findings during and after treatment of childhood acute lymphoblastic leukemia. Medical and Pediatric Oncology 1997; 29:266–271.

MALAKOPLAKIA

Malakoplakia is a very rare chronic granulomatous disease, which is most often found in the urinary tract of middle-aged individuals without systemic disease. In children, however, colonic involvement is more common and may be regarded as an opportunistic bacterial infection in an immunocompromised host. Boys are more commonly affected with a peak age in both sexes of 13 years. The presenting symptoms are non-specific and include rectal bleeding, diarrhoea, abdominal pain and fever.

Double-contrast barium enema findings are variable. Non-specific colitis with ulceration, multiple nodular lesions and single large polypoid masses have been described.

FURTHER READING

Boudny P, Kurrer MO, Stamm B, Laeng RH. Malakoplakia of the colon in an infant with severe combined immunodeficiency (SCID) and CHARGE association. Pathology Research and Practice 2000; 196:577–582.

Cipolletta L, Bianco MA, Fumo F, Orabona P, Piccinino F. Malacoplakia of the colon. Gastrointestinal Endoscopy 1995; 41:255–258.

Radin DR, Chandrasoma P, Halls JM. Colonic malacoplakia. Gastrointestinal Radiology 1984; 9:359–361.

PICA

Pica is the ingestion of non-food substances whereas geophagia refers to the ingestion of clay or dirt and is endemic in certain parts of India and the southern states of the USA. Children, especially toddlers, may ingest a wide variety of foreign materials but geophagia can be considered a cultural phenomenon in certain circumstances. Mixed pica (paper, plastic bags, cloth, string) is more likely to present acutely with intestinal obstruction as the most common complication.

The plain abdominal x-ray is a valuable examination in the investigation of suspected pica, especially when a low kilovolt technique is used (Figure 10.15.43). Radiological findings depend on the radiopacity and volume of the ingested material. Lead in paint chips, and the silicon and calcium found in clay are readily visible due to the high atomic number of these minerals. Therefore, geophagia can be suspected when there is opacification of large bowel. The large bowel frequently appears atonic in configuration. Bizarre opaque particles from impure clay may be another clue. Other radiological evidence of pica may also be present. Because pica may cause replacement of nutritious substances in the diet, increased haemapoietic activity due to iron deficiency anaemia can occur and this may result in a delayed bone age. Dense metaphyseal bands due to lead poisoning are occasionally seen.

FURTHER READING

Anderson JE, Akmal M, Kittur DS. Surgical complications of pica: report of a case of intestinal obstruction and a review of the literature. American Surgery 1991; 57:663–667.

Maravilla AM, Berk RN. The radiology corner. The radiographic diagnosis of pica. American Journal of Gastroenterology 1978; 70:94–99.

Vessal K, Ronaghy HA, Zarabi M. Radiological changes in pica. American Journal of Clinical Nutrition 1975; 28:1095–1098.

CHILAIDITI'S SYNDROME

The interposition of colon between the liver and the right hemidiaphragm is known as Chilaiditi's syndrome. It is of no clinical significance. It is often transient and is seen on one chest film but not the next. It may mimic a loculated pneumoperitoneum but the child is asymptomatic.

ASCITES

The term ascites describes free fluid in the peritoneal cavity. This may be a transudate and due to pancreatitis, hypoproteinaemia, intestinal lymphangiectasia, urinary ascites due to a ruptured bladder, and chyle. Chylous ascites in children may result from trauma to or obstruction of the cisterna chyli. Exudative ascites is associated with peritonitis and tumours. Free fluid is also seen with intraperitoneal implants such as ventriculoperitoneal (VP) shunt tubing and peritoneal dialysis catheters.

Trauma

Osnat Konen-Cohen, Paul S Babyn

INTRODUCTION

Injury to the bowel can be caused by a wide variety of agents including chemical agents, foreign bodies, iatrogenic and other physical trauma, radiation therapy and medications.

This chapter reviews the various aetiologies of bowel injury and their common manifestations and evaluation.

CHEMICAL INJURY

CORROSIVE OESOPHAGITIS

Oesophagitis secondary to ingestion of corrosive material is becoming less common due to increased public awareness. Severe oesophageal burns can be caused by ingestion of alkaline chemicals found in a number of household detergents, e.g. lye, which contains 95% sodium, and potassium hydroxide.

The type, amount, concentration, viscosity and duration of contact between the caustic agent and the oesophageal mucosa influence the severity and location of the injury. While acids tend to cause limited coagulation necrosis, alkaline chemicals cause liquefactive necrosis that progresses by direct extension and produces extensive transmural tissue necrosis. Swallowed liquids burn the whole oesophagus, while ingested crystals are expectorated after ingestion and cause localized burns in the mouth and pharynx. The burns may involve only the mucosal layer causing superficial ulcerations or involve the whole wall thickness causing complete wall necrosis.

Initial evaluation typically proceeds with chest radiography. Mediastinal widening, pneumomediastinum, widening of the paraspinal lines and pleural effusions are suggestive of extensive damage with perioesophageal inflammation and perforation. Although oesophagoscopy is an accurate procedure to evaluate the extent of the damage, it may lead to perforation.

Upper gastrointestinal tract contrast studies are performed to evaluate the extent of the damage and to rule out perforation, which is the most common acute complication of chemical oesophagitis. A non-ionic water-soluble contrast should be used first to assess for perforation. This may be followed by barium studies once perforation has been excluded to better delineate the oesophageal pathology. Early changes include an air-filled aperistaltic oesophagus, irregular peristalsis, mucosal oedema and ulcerations.

Focal, corrosive oesophageal burns can occur following ingestion of alkaline disc batteries, Clinitest tablets that are used by diabetic patients to test the urine or by tetracycline tablets.

Strictures complicate up to one-third of the cases of corrosive oesophagitis. The length of the stricture is variable and will require supine contrast studies to delineate it properly. Chronic findings on barium swallow include areas of oesophageal narrowing, diminished oesophageal peristalsis, pseudodiverticulae and shortening of the oesophagus with hiatal hernia formation (Figure 10.16.1). Oesophageal strictures may be treated with repetitive dilatations. Oesophageal bypass is performed if no satisfactory lumen can be established, preferably with a retrosternally placed colonic segment.

CORROSIVE GASTRITIS

Acid corrosives cause less destruction to the oesophagus than alkali agents, and tend to cause severe injury to the stomach, especially to the gastric antrum. The location of the gastric injury is related to the position of the patient while ingesting the corrosive agent, the nature of the ingested material, and to whether the stomach was full or empty prior to the ingestion of the corrosive agent.

Ingestion of caustic agents can cause acute pylorospasm retaining the chemical agent in the stomach, worsening mucosal ulceration and muscle necrosis. This may result in perforation and peritonitis. Late sequelae include pyloric scarring and antral fibrosis with consequent gastric outlet obstruction.

FURTHER READING

Biller JA, Flores A, Buie T, et al. Tetracycline-induced esophagitis in adolescent patients. Journal of Pediatrics 1992;120:144–145.

Burrington JD. Clinitest burns of the esophagus. Annals of Thoracic Surgery 1975;20:400–404.

Franken EA Jr. Caustic damage of the gastrointestinal tract: roentgen features. American Journal of Roentgenology and Radium Therapeutic Nuclear Medicine 1973;118:77–85.

Kost KM, Shapiro RS. Button battery ingestion: a case report and review of the literature. Journal of Otolaryngology 1987;16:252–257.

Leape LL, Ashcraft KW, Scarpelli DG, et al. Hazard to health-liquid lye. New England Journal of Medicine 1971;284:578–581.

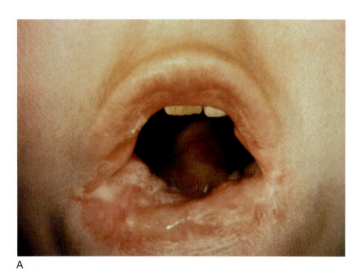

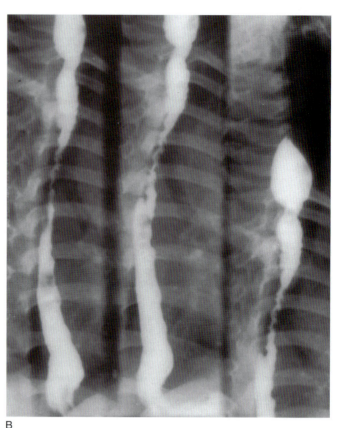

A   B

Figure 10.16.1 Six weeks following lye ingestion scarring of the mouth is present (A). Oesophageal strictures are demonstrated on upper GI series (B). Note the typical long segment, irregular stenosis.

Lowe JE, Graham DY, Boisaubin EV Jr, et al. Corrosive injury to the stomach: the natural history and role of fiberoptic endoscopy. American Journal of Surgery 1979;137:803–806.

Muhletaler CA, Gerlock AJ Jr, de Soto L, et al. Acid corrosive esophagitis: radiographic findings. American Journal of Roentgenology 1980;134:1137–1140.

Muhletaler CA, Gerlock AJ Jr, de Soto L, et al. Gastroduodenal lesions of ingested acids: radiographic findings. American Journal of Roentgenology 1980;135:1247–1252.

Ragheb MI, Ramadan AA, Khalil MA. Corrosive gastritis. American Journal of Surgery 1977;134:343–345.

Stannard MW. Corrosive esophagitis in children. Assessment by the esophagogram. American Journal of Diseases in Children 1978;132:596–599.

Symbas PN, Vlasis SE, Hatcher CR Jr. Esophagitis secondary to ingestion of caustic material. Annals of Thoracic Surgery 1983;36:73–77.

FOREIGN BODIES

Swallowed foreign bodies are commonly encountered in the paediatric population. Infants and young children accidentally ingest foreign bodies, while older children may deliberately do so either as an attempt to seek attention or as part of a suicidal attempt.

The foreign bodies ingested by children are of wide variety. Coins are the most frequent ingested foreign body in children. In many cases the child gives the history of foreign body ingestion, but some cases may be unsuspected and present with gastrointestinal or even respiratory symptoms (Figure 10.16.2). Many patients are asymptomatic at presentation; however, gastrointestinal symptoms such as dysphagia, salivation, increased secretions, drooling, gagging, vomiting and poor feeding may be noted. Respiratory symptoms may be present in young children when the foreign body in the oesophagus compresses the trachea causing wheezing and stridor. In other cases, foreign bodies may cause chronic respiratory symptoms sometimes mistaken for asthma, recurrent pneumonias and failure to thrive.

Most of the foreign bodies pass through the gastrointestinal tract without complication. The passage usually occurs within 2 to 6 days but may take up to 4 weeks. However, some ingested foreign bodies may cause obstruction typically at levels of anatomic narrowing such as the cricopharyngeus muscle, aortic knob, or gastroesophageal junction (Figure 10.16.3). Foreign bodies lodged at other sites along the oesophagus suggest that there may be an underlying abnormality such as congenital strictures, webs, extrinsic mass compressing the oesophagus, e.g. vascular ring, or acquired strictures due to oesophagitis or surgical repair of tracheoesophageal fistula. Most foreign bodies that pass into the stomach tend to pass spontaneously unless there are congenital anomalies such as antral web, duodenal stenosis, windsock duodenum or annular pancreas. In these cases the foreign body is retained for longer periods, thus raising the suspicion of anatomical narrowing.

A foreign body impacted in the oesophagus is unlikely to pass spontaneously. When not removed promptly, surrounding

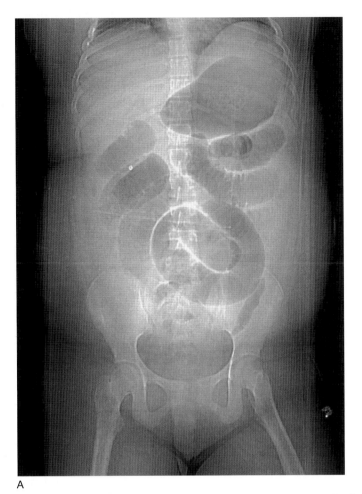

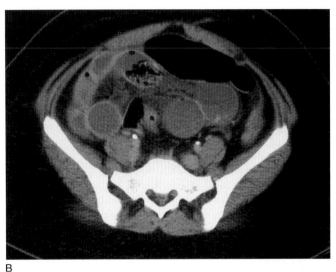

A   B

Figure 10.16.2 CT survey image and axial scan of a 6-year-old girl with developmental delay presenting with abdominal pain and distention. Asymmetric dilatation of small bowel loop representing small bowel obstruction is seen (A,B). At operation an ingested glove was found as the cause of the small bowel obstruction.

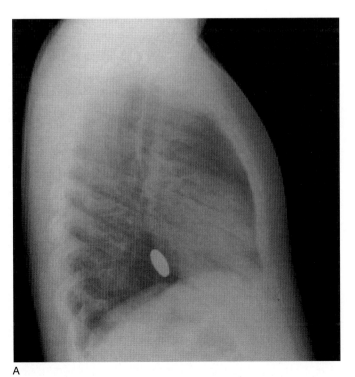

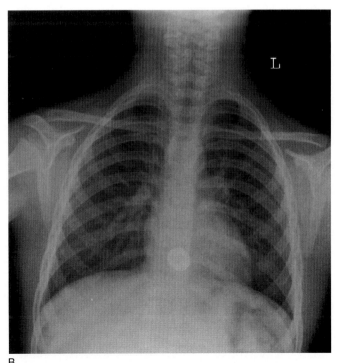

A   B

Figure 10.16.3 A 7-year-old boy who accidentally swallowed a coin. Lateral (A) and PA (B) views of chest radiograph demonstrate the coin's location. On follow-up radiographs the coin did not advance beyond the gastroesophageal junction for 24 hours. The coin was then removed endoscopically.

inflammatory reaction may be incited and lead to ulceration, stenosis, perforation, mediastinitis, abscess formation and respiratory compromise (Figure 10.16.4). Rare complications include formation of tracheoesophageal fistula, oesophagoaortic fistula, false oesophageal diverticula and extraluminal migration.

Radiologic investigation initially consists of a combination lateral neck radiograph and frontal thoracoabdominal radiograph. A lateral chest radiograph may also be needed to localize the foreign body. Ingested foreign bodies can be demonstrated on radiographs if they are radio-opaque. If they are not radio-opaque then a contrast swallow is necessary. A non-ionic low-osmolar water-soluble contrast medium is routinely used due to the possibility of occult perforation.

Ultrasound can be used to follow-up gastric foreign bodies. To avoid the limitations of the intestinal gas, the stomach may be distended by an anechoic liquid. The foreign body will appear as hyperechoic lesion with an acoustic shadow inside the stomach.

Prompt endoscopic removal is recommended for sharp foreign bodies and disc batteries to prevent perforation and caustic erosion. Smooth-surfaced foreign bodies present for less than 24 hours may be removed by either a Foley catheter under fluoroscopic guidance or by using a basket wire. Others prefer to use bougienage of the coins down into the stomach if the coin is lodged in the distal two-thirds of the oesophagus. Some authors recommend endoscopic removal under anaesthesia as the preferred method to extract coins, especially if the coin has been lodged in the oesophagus for longer than 24 hours. Medications causing dilatation of the oesophagus or carbonated beverages may aid in passing the foreign body to the stomach.

Metallic foreign bodies may be removed by using a magnetic orogastric tube. Complications may occur during removal, including oesophageal or gastric perforation by instrumentation, aspiration of stomach content or even aspiration of the foreign body itself.

FURTHER READING

Alexander AA, Hayden CK Jr, Swischuk LE. Catheter removal of esophageal foreign bodies: push or pull? American Journal of Roentgenology 8;151:835.

Beer S, Avidan G, Viure E, Starinsky R. A foreign body in the oesophagus as a cause of respiratory distress. Pediatric Radiology 1982;12:41–42.

Bonadio WA, Emslander H, Milner D, Johnson L. Esophageal mucosal changes in children with an acutely ingested coin lodged in the esophagus. Pediatric Emergency Care 1994;10:333–334.

Campbell JB, Davis WS. Catheter technique for extraction of blunt esophageal foreign bodies. Radiology 1973;108:438–440.

Campbell JB, Quattromani FL, Foley LC. Foley catheter removal of blunt esophageal foreign bodies. Experience with 100 consecutive children. Pediatric Radiology 1983;13:116–118.

Carlson DH. Removal of coins in the esophagus using a foley catheter. Pediatrics 1972;50:475–476.

Currarino G, Nikaidoh H. Esophageal foreign bodies in children with vascular ring or aberrant right subclavian artery: coincidence or causation? Pediatric Radiology 1991;21:406–408.

Kassner EG, Rose JS, Kottmeier PK, et al. Retention of small foreign objects in the stomach and duodenum. A sign of partial obstruction caused by duodenal anomalies. Radiology 1975;114:683–686.

Kelley JE, Leech MH, Carr MG. A safe and cost-effective protocol for the management of esophageal coins in children. Journal of Pediatric Surgery 1993;28:898–900.

Kerschner JE, Beste DJ, Conley SF, et al. Mediastinitis associated with foreign body erosion of the esophagus in children. International Journal of Pediatric Otorhinolaryngology 2001;59:89–97.

Macpherson RI, Hill JG, Othersen HB, et al. Esophageal foreign bodies in children: diagnosis, treatment, and complications. American Journal of Roentgenology 1996;166:919–924.

Myer CM 3rd. Potential hazards of esophageal foreign body extraction. Pediatric Radiology 1991;21:97–98.

Namasivayam S. Button battery ingestion: a solution to a management dilemma. Pediatric Surgery International 1999;15:383–384.

Nandi P, Ong GB. Foreign body in the oesophagus: review of 2394 cases. British Journal of Surgery 1978;65:5–9.

Newman DE. The radiolucent esophageal foreign body: an often-forgotten cause of respiratory symptoms. Journal of Pediatrics 1978;92:60–63.

O'Hara SM. Acute gastrointestinal bleeding. Radiology Clinics of North America 1997;35:879–895.

Paulson EK, Jaffe RB. Metallic foreign bodies in the stomach: fluoroscopic removal with a magnetic orogastric tube. Radiology 1990;174:191–194.

Smith PC, Swischuk LE, Fagan CJ. An elusive and often unsuspected cause of stridor or pneumonia (the esophageal foreign body). American Journal of Roentgenology and Radium Therapeutic Nuclear Medicine 1974;122:80–89.

Spina P, Minniti S, Bragheri R. Usefulness of ultrasonography in gastric foreign body retention. Pediatric Radiology 2000;30:840–841.

Toyonaga T, Shinohara M, Miyatake E, et al. Penetration of the duodenum by an ingested needle with migration to the pancreas: report of a case. Surgery Today 2001;31:68–71.

IATROGENIC INJURY

Iatrogenic trauma may complicate endoscopy, passage of nasogastric or other tubes, dilatation procedures, enemas or operative procedures. The symptoms, evaluation and treatment differ according to the site and nature of the insult.

OESOPHAGEAL TRAUMA

Perforation of the oesophagus can complicate endoscopic procedures, balloon dilatation or bouginage treatment of oesophageal strictures or follow nasogastric tube insertion. This latter more frequently occurs at pharyngeal level. The perforation is usually noted at the time of injury. The patients demonstrate clinical signs of discomfort, respiratory distress, tachycardia, tachypnoea, grunting, use of accessory respiratory muscles and subcutaneous emphysema. Late-presenting symptoms may include fever, dysphagia and chest pain. The mortality rate of children postoesophageal perforation is significantly lower than reported in adults, and is estimated at 4%. In most instances operation can be avoided and conservative treatment with broad-spectrum antibiotics and parenteral nutrition are sufficient. Thoracotomy may be indicated if there is clinical deterioration and signs of mediastinitis.

Radiologic finding of oesophageal rupture include subcutaneous emphysema, pneumomediastinum, mediastinal widening and hydropneumothorax. Contrast studies using water-soluble contrast media will demonstrate the site and extent of the perforation. Extra luminal contrast in the mediastinum has an irregular appearance and fails to clear. Silent perforation may present later with mediastinitis and abscess formation best evaluated with CT examination.

Intramural oesophageal haematomas may also occur following instrumentation of the oesophagus or even after minor trauma such as rapid ingestion of effervescent drinks. These children present with dysphagia and epigastric pain. Contrast studies will demonstrate luminal compression on the barium filled oesophagogram.

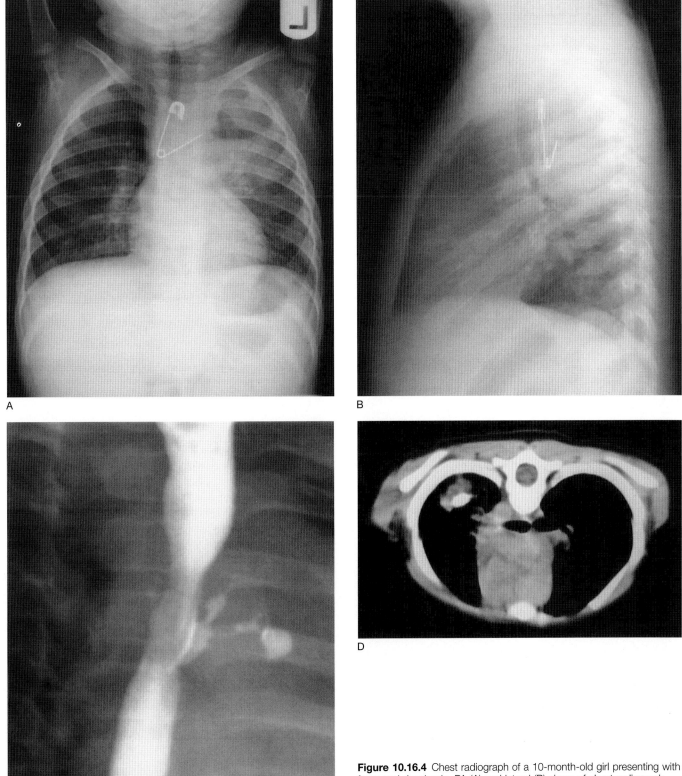

Figure 10.16.4 Chest radiograph of a 10-month-old girl presenting with fever and dysphagia. PA (A) and lateral (B) views of chest radiograph demonstrate a safety pin lodged in the oesophagus and a left upper lobe lung abscess. Following surgical removal of the pin, an upper GI series demonstrated fistulous tract from the oesophagus to the lung abscess (C). Contrast in the cavity is demonstrated on the CT scan (D).

GASTRIC PERFORATION

Neonatal gastric perforation may occur with gastric dilatation from mechanical ventilation, especially in premature babies. It may complicate nasogastric tube insertion or any other gastric instrumentation. Indomethacin therapy for ductal closure in preterm babies has been associated with gastric perforation. The first clinical sign of gastric perforation may be abdominal distention. Other symptoms include acute abdominal pain, vomiting, respiratory distress, peritonitis and shock. Gastric perforation is associated with the highest mortality rate in perforations of the gastrointestinal tract. Plain films of the abdomen will show a large pneumoperitoneum and absence of a gastric air–fluid level on erect abdominal radiograph with normal or decreased gas in small and large bowel (Figure 10.16.5).

SMALL BOWEL PERFORATION

Insertion of nasogastric tubes, feeding tubes or endoscopic procedures may be complicated by duodenal or small bowel perforation. Free intraperitoneal gas may be noted on decubitus or erect radiographs.

COLONIC PERFORATION

Iatrogenic colonic injury can occur during colonoscopy or barium enema (Figure 10.16.6). The risk of colonic perforation following barium enema examination is 0.04%. Colonic perforation has also been reported during therapeutic enemas for intussusception reduction. Rectal perforation may occur during insertion of rectal thermometers in babies or it may even complicate physical examination of the rectum (Fig 10.16.7).

Rectal perforation can be either intraperitoneal and cause pneumoperitoneum, or occur below the peritoneal reflection leading to retroperitoneal air with outlining of the kidneys and adrenal glands.

Clinical symptoms include abdominal pain, rebound, tenderness and guarding, but these patients may be initially asymptomatic. Colorectal perforation generally carries the lowest risk of mortality of all gastrointestinal perforations.

Plain radiographs may show free air on erect films or decubitus films; however, small amounts of free air or extravasated contrast may only be disclosed by CT.

FURTHER READING

Akel SR, Haddad FF, Hashim HA, et al. Traumatic injuries of the alimentary tract in children. Pediatric Surgery International 1998;13:104–107.

Bruce J, Bianchi A, Doig CM, et al. Gastric perforation in the neonate. Pediatric Surgery International 1993;8:17–19.

Fonkalsrud EW, Clatworthy HW. Accidental perforation of the colon and rectum in newborn infants. New England Journal of Medicine 1965; 272:1097–1100.

Humphry A, Ein SH, Mok PM. Perforation of the intussuscepted colon. American Journal of Roentgenology 1981;137:1135–1138.

Nagaraj HS, Sandhu AS, Cook LN, et al. Gastrointestinal perforation following indomethacin therapy in very low birth weight infants. Journal of Pediatric Surgery 1981;16:1003–1007.

Panieri E, Millar AJ, Rode H, et al. Iatrogenic esophageal perforation in children: patterns of injury, presentation, management, and outcome. Journal of Pediatric Surgery 1996;31:890–895.

Pochaczevsky R, Bryk D. New roentgenographic signs of neonatal gastric perforation. Radiology 1972;102:145–147.

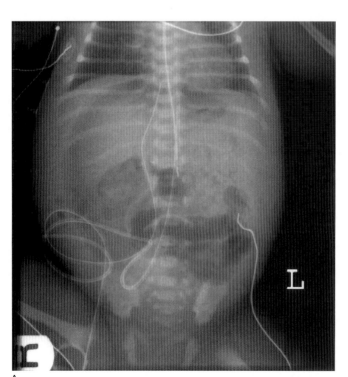

A

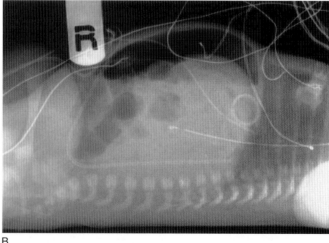

B

Figure 10.16.5 Supine (A) and cross-table (B) abdominal radiographs of neonate with abdominal distension and upper gastrointestinal bleed demonstrates extensive pneumoperitoneum seen on the supine views as 'football sign'. There is no identifiable gastric bubble and the NG tube position is abnormal. At surgery, gastric perforation was found.

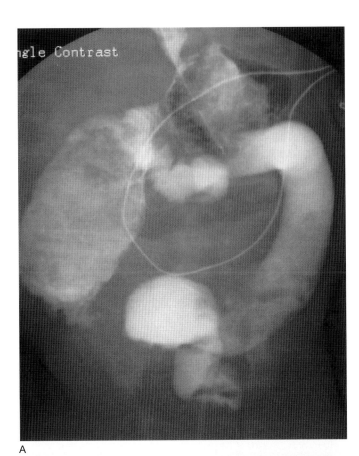

A

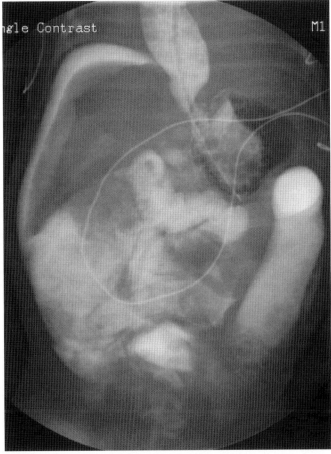

B

Figure 10.16.6 A 7-month-old child referred to rule out intestinal malrotation. After performing an upper GI examination, a contrast enema was performed. A caecal perforation with small amount of contrast leak is seen (A) followed by immediate spread of contrast within the peritoneal cavity (B).

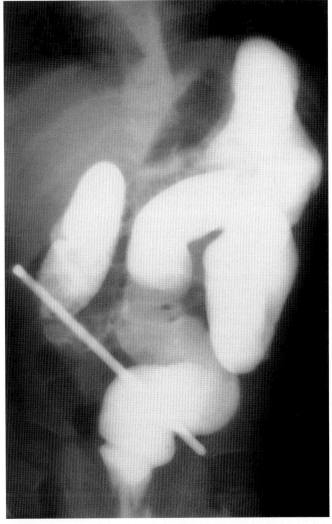

Figure 10.16.7 A thermometer free in intraperitoneal cavity demonstrated on barium enema examination.

Tan CE, Kiely EM, Agrawal M, et al. Neonatal gastrointestinal perforation. Journal of Pediatric Surgery 1989;24:888–892.

RADIATION AND CHEMOTHERAPY-INDUCED INJURY

Children who are treated with radiation or chemotherapy are often subject to gastrointestinal complications. Radiotherapy may cause an acute inflammatory response early after exposure. This causes alterations in intestinal fluid and electrolyte transport, resulting in radiation-induced diarrhoea. The severity of the acute response to radiation correlates with the incidence of chronic radiation enteritis that arises months to years following radiation exposure.

Chronic graft-versus-host disease (GVHD) is an immunologic disorder that may occur after bone marrow transplantation for severe aplastic anaemia, in immunodeficiency disorders and in certain malignancies. The donor lymphocytes damage host tissue, including the intestinal tract. Children with GVHD can present in the acute phase with symptoms of abdominal pain, fever and diarrhoea. Abdominal films may disclose signs of bowel wall thickening, distended fluid-filled bowel loops, pneumatosis intestinalis and free air. On contrast imaging small bowel wall thickening or small bowel wall effacement 'ribbon bowel' can be demonstrated. The most common site involved is the jejunum, but it may affect the whole gastrointestinal tract. Chronic symptoms of small bowel obstruction may ensue due to stricture formation. During the acute phase of GVHD, contrast studies of the colon demonstrate mucosal irregularity and ulcerations throughout the colon, loss of haustral folds, luminal narrowing and mural thickening.

The oesophagus can also be involved in chronic GVHD with resulting dysphagia, painful swallowing, chest pain, regurgitations and weight loss. These symptoms may develop months to years after successful bone marrow transplantation. Strictures in the mid and upper oesophagus, oesophageal webs or ring-like strictures may be seen (Figure 10.16.8).

Typhlitis (neutropenic colitis) is a necrotizing inflammation of the caecum, appendix and terminal ileum encountered in neutropenic patients. It most commonly occurs in patients with leukaemia, but it may also develop in lymphoma, aplastic anaemia, AIDS and after transplantation. The incidence of typhlitis has increased most probably as a consequence of the usage of more aggressive chemotherapies. Fortunately the survival rate has increased significantly due to early recognition and appropriate treatment. The symptoms can be variable and include fever, abdominal pain, abdominal distention, vomiting, diarrhoea and bloody stools. In many instances these symptoms mimic symptoms of acute appendicitis, pseudomembranous colitis, ischaemic colitis, intussusception, and small bowel obstruction.

Histopathologic findings include mucosal and submucosal necrosis, intramural oedema, bacterial invasion and haemorrhage. Plain films may demonstrate gasless right lower quadrant, right sided abdominal mass, bowel wall thickening, pneumatosis intestinalis, small bowel obstruction or ileus. Contrast studies are not advisable due to high risk of perforation. Contrast enema may demonstrate a contracted, rigid caecum, caecal mass and thickened mucosal folds with thumbprinting of the bowel wall. Ultrasound

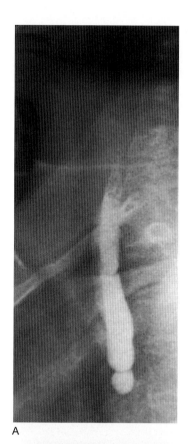

A

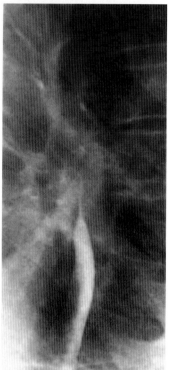

B

Figure 10.16.8 Barium swallow in a 16-year-old girl with Hodgkin's lymphoma treated with chemotherapy complaining of dysphagia. Oesophageal web in the proximal oesophagus (A) with tapered stricture and a string of contrast extending distally (B) are seen.

and CT offer a rapid and non-invasive means of diagnosing typhlitis and for evaluation of complications such as perforation, peritonitis and abscess formation (Figure 10.16.9). On ultrasound a target pattern is seen. It is described as a rounded hypoechoic periphery with highly echogenic, markedly thickened, pseudopolypoid mucosa. This appearance is not specific. On CT examination diffuse thickening of the caecal wall is seen. Sometimes there are areas of low attenuation within the bowel wall consistent with oedema, haemorrhage or necrosis. Conservative medical management and supportive treatments are generally used, while surgical intervention is reserved for patients with severe bleeding or perforation.

FURTHER READING

Abramson SJ, Berdon WE, Baker DH. Childhood typhlitis: its increasing association with acute myelogenous leukemia. Report of five cases. Radiology 1983;146:61–64.

Alexander JE, Williamson SL, Seibert JJ, et al. The ultrasonographic diagnosis of typhlitis (neutropenic colitis). Pediatric Radiology 1988;18:200–204.

Fisk JD, Shulman HM, Greening RR, et al. Gastrointestinal radiographic features of human graft-vs.-host disease. American Journal of Roentgenology 1981;136:329–336.

Frick MP, Maile CW, Crass JR, et al. Computed tomography of neutropenic colitis. American Journal of Roentgenology 1984;143:763–765.

Katz JA, Wagner ML, Gresik MV, et al. Typhlitis. An 18-year experience and postmortem review. Cancer 1990;65:1041–1047.

McDonald GB, Sullivan KM, Plumley TF. Radiographic features of esophageal involvement in chronic graft-vs.-host disease. American Journal of Roentgenology 1984;142:501–506.

McNamara MJ, Chalmers AG, Morgan M, et al. Typhlitis in acute childhood leukaemia: radiological features. Clinical Radiology 1986;37:83–86.

Thomson AB, Keelan M, Thiesen A, et al. Small bowel review: diseases of the small intestine. Digestive Diseases and Sciences 2001;46:2555–2566.

Wagner ML, Rosenberg HS, Fernbach DJ, et al. Typhlitis: a complication of leukemia in childhood. American Journal of Roentgenology Radium Therapy and Nuclear Medicine 1970;109:341–350.

ACCIDENTAL BOWEL TRAUMA

Blunt trauma is much more common than penetrating injury as a cause of bowel injuries. Two different mechanisms may cause injury in blunt abdominal trauma: compressive forces (external compression against fixed object such as the spine) and deceleration forces (stretching of the involved bowel with a burst or shearing injury). The majority of post-traumatic bowel rupture occurs in restrained children involved in motor vehicle accidents. In the child, lap belts typically course over the mid-abdomen, overlying their relatively underdeveloped abdominal wall musculature. Following a high velocity frontal collision, the child moves forward and the lap belt can injure the abdominal wall, underlying bowel and mesentery. Associated bowel rupture should strongly be suspected whenever lap-belt ecchymoses are present across the lower abdomen and flank in restrained children who are involved in motor vehicle crashes. Other associated injuries include lumbar compression fractures, Chance fractures of the second and third lumbar vertebrae, and injuries to the abdominal aorta (Figure 10.16.10). Another well-known mechanism causing bowel injuries in paediatric patients is handle-bar injuries from bicycle accidents.

Despite the frequency of abdominal trauma, bowel rupture is relatively uncommon following trauma in children. Clinical findings suggestive of bowel rupture include rebound tenderness, rigidity, guarding and absent bowel sounds; however they are present in only 30% of the patients and may have delayed presentation. If there is a strong clinical suspicion of bowel perforation and the patient is clinically unstable, surgery is required. If the patient is stable then imaging evaluation may proceed for determination of the location and extent of injury. Plain films and CT are the primary imaging modalities for assessing gastrointestinal perforation in blunt trauma patients.

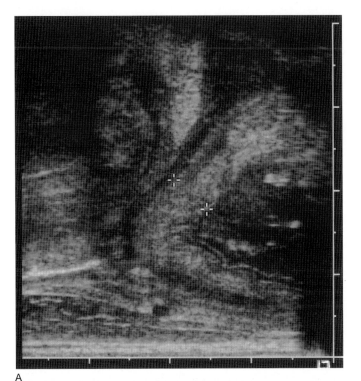

A

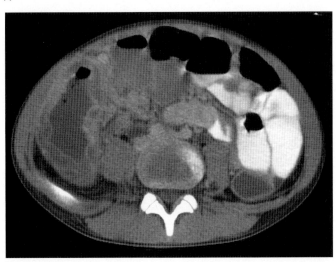

B

Figure 10.16.9 Ultrasound of the right iliac fossa in a 10-year-old boy with leukaemia. There is circumferential caecal wall thickening and free intraperitoneal fluid consistent with neutropenic colitis (A). On CT, diffuse thickening of the caecal wall is seen accompanied by a moderate amount of free peritoneal fluid (B).

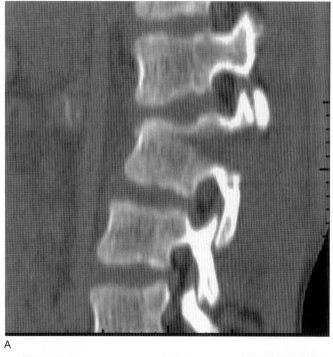

A

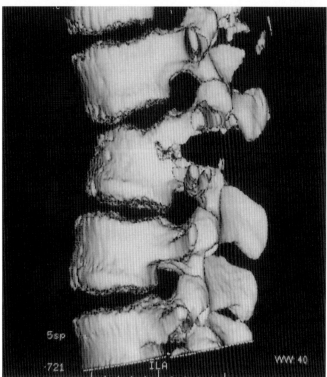

B

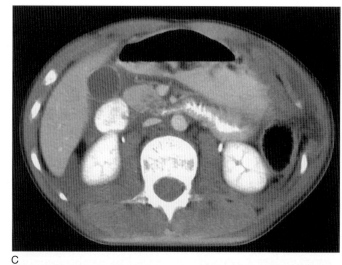

C

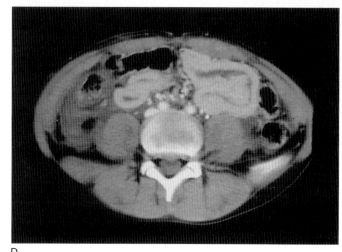

D

Figure 10.16.10 Sagittal reconstructions (A) and 3D reformats (B) of a Chance fracture of L3 with comminuted fracture of L2 spinous process in a child with lap-belt injury. CT of the abdomen shows duodenal wall thickening from duodenal haematoma (C) as well as thick hyperdense small bowel loops representing bowel wall injury (D).

Hollow viscus injury may result in perforation and pneumoperitoneum. Conventional plain film signs of pneumoperitoneum include subdiaphragmatic free air, gas outlining both sides of the intestinal wall, a small amount of air trapped in between three adjoining bowel loops, outlining of the falciform ligament with air, accumulation of air anterior to the liver resulting in

characteristic appearance or large anterior mid-abdominal air collection.

CT is highly sensitive for detection of pneumoperitoneum, and even small air bubbles can be diagnosed accurately. To increase the diagnosis rate the use of 'lung windows' with wide window widths and low window levels is advised.

STOMACH

Gastric injury is rare and reported in less than 2% of patients with blunt trauma. It occurs more often in children than in adults, and occurs frequently after a recent meal with a full stomach. The anterior wall is the most common site of perforation, followed by the greater curvature and least frequently the posterior wall. Grossly, bloody aspirates may be obtained from the nasogastric tube. Pneumoperitoneum is more commonly seen in gastric perforations than in small bowel injuries and it is seen on 50%–60% of the plain films obtained. With stomach perforation the degree of pneumoperitoneum may be large and extravasation of gastric content as well as oral contrast material may be seen on CT examination.

DUODENUM

The duodenum is the most common site of bowel injury in blunt abdominal trauma and accounts for 25% of these injuries. Blunt trauma to the upper abdomen can cause duodenal compression against the spine resulting in duodenal haematomas or tear. Duodenal haematomas and perforation occur most commonly in the second and third duodenal segments and are frequently accompanied by pancreatic injury (Figure 10.16.11). These are serious injuries, and any delay in diagnosis of duodenal injury can increase the mortality significantly from 5% to 60%. Since these injuries are difficult to diagnose, one must maintain a high index of suspicion. The most frequent presentation is vomiting due to partial obstruction of the duodenum. Sometimes it may be accompanied by minimal pain. Occasionally, the patient presents with a mass from the haematoma that will be demonstrated on US examination as a complex mass. On contrast examination it may be documented as an intraluminal-filling defect with contrast curving around the mass (Figure 10.16.12). If the haematoma is large, it can cause mass effect on the adjacent stomach or colon.

Duodenal perforation may be intraperitoneal and associated with signs of pneumoperitoneum on plain films, or it may perforate posteriorly resulting in retroperitoneal air outlining the psoas or kidneys.

The distinction between duodenal haematomas and duodenal perforation is important, since most duodenal haematomas without perforation are treated conservatively and resolve spontaneously, while duodenal perforation is an acute surgical emergency. CT is the most accurate diagnostic modality to assess duodenal injury. Duodenal haematomas will be seen as a mass within the duodenal wall compressing the duodenal lumen. In duodenal rupture, extravasated oral contrast material and extraluminal gas will be seen in the right anterior pararenal space or may spread to other retroperitoneal compartments. Perforation near the ligament of Treitz will result in intraperitoneal extravasation of contrast and gas.

JEJUNAL AND ILEAL INJURY

Small bowel injury occurs in 5–15% of patients with abdominal injuries from blunt abdominal trauma. The most common site of

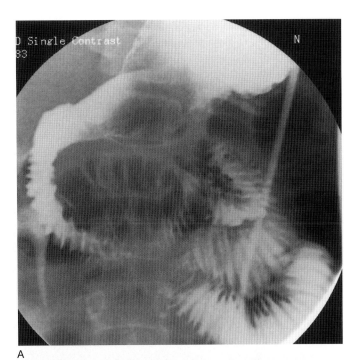

A

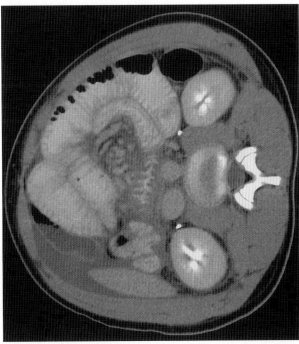

B

Figure 10.16.11 Handle-bar injury resulting in duodenal haematoma. Upper GI (A) and correlative CT of the abdomen obtained in right decubitus position (B), demonstrating thick mucosal folds in the horizontal part of the duodenum.

bowel rupture is the jejunum or ileum. The small bowel is usually injured at the site of fixation such as the ligament of Treitz or the ileocaecal valve. Clinical symptoms of small bowel perforation develop slowly because of the neutral pH and low bacterial count of the small bowel.

Pneumoperitoneum resulting from small bowel perforation is infrequently noted on plain radiographs since the small intestine contains little air. In the presence of dissecting pneumomedi-

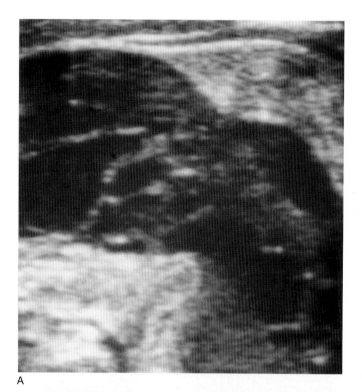

A

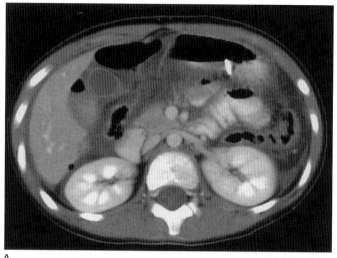

A

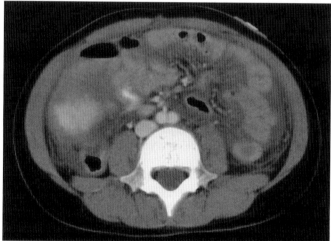

B

Figure 10.16.13 CT of the abdomen of a 7-year-old boy involved in motor vehicle accident demonstrates a moderate amount of free intraperitoneal fluid with no evidence of solid organ injury. A small intraperitoneal air bubble is present in Morrison's pouch (A) along with bowel wall thickening of several small bowel loops in the left upper abdomen, and mesenteric infiltration (B). At surgery, jejunal perforation was disclosed.

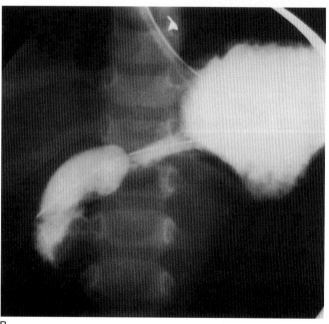

B

Figure 10.16.12 A 2-year-old boy who fell from his bicycle presented two days later with bilious vomiting and abdominal pain. On US a complex epigastric mass was demonstrated (A). On upper GI series, a large duodenal haematoma causing complete obstruction is seen (B).

astinum and chest barotraumas the source of the peritoneal air may be from that origin and not from bowel injury. Sonography is not sensitive in the diagnosis of bowel perforation and CT is recommended. The two pathognomonic findings for bowel rupture on CT are free peritoneal air and extraluminal contrast leak confirming the presence of bowel rupture. Pneumoperitoneum is not a sensitive sign for bowel rupture since it is present in less than one-half of all patients with bowel disruption. The size of the pneumoperitoneum does not correlate with the degree of bowel injury. Large tears may seal quickly and cause little or no free air. The prevalence of contrast extravasation is even lower (0–25%).

The most frequent findings include the presence of peritoneal fluid without evidence of associated pelvic fracture or solid organ injury and abnormal intense enhancement of bowel wall. These two findings are highly sensitive and specific for detection of bowel rupture. Other less specific findings include bowel dilatation, bowel wall thickening, focal haematomas surrounding a bowel loop (sentinel clot), intramural air, focal intense bowel wall enhancement, fluid or haemorrhage between bowel loops and infiltration of the mesenteric fat (Figure 10.16.13).

Mesenteric infiltration and free intraperitoneal fluid are the most frequent CT findings associated with bowel trauma. Free fluid without an obvious source is an important clue to assist in recognizing bowel or mesenteric injury. Continued active mesenteric haemorrhage makes surgical intervention necessary because of the potential for vascular compromise of the bowel and the potential associated bowel wall injury.

Bowel wall haematomas may be caused by blunt abdominal trauma. Plain films can be normal or demonstrate variable signs, including: distended, isolated loop of bowel representing localized ileus, thickened valvulae or thumbprinting representing mucosal oedema or haemorrhage. On US examination a mass-like lesion can be demonstrated. At CT, intramural haematomas appear as focal bowel wall thickening of more then 3 mm. The CT appearance depends on the age of the haematoma. It can be isodense to circulating blood in the acute phase and become hyperdense to blood subacutely and show decreased density as the clot lyses. Large haematomas can result in obstruction.

Mesenteric injuries can be suspected when focal mesenteric haematomas or mesenteric fluid is detected. The presence of a moderate amount of free peritoneal fluid without solid organ laceration should raise the suspicion of mesenteric or bowel injury.

A delayed presentation of small bowel obstruction can be seen related to post-traumatic ischaemic intestinal strictures with children developing late signs and symptoms of partial small bowel obstruction. Small bowel contrast studies (enteroclysis) may be necessary to delineate the site of stenosis. CT evaluation may be helpful in defining the level and aetiology of the small bowel obstruction. In patients with history of remote abdominal trauma the diagnosis of traumatic ischaemic stricture should be considered whenever a narrowed and thickened segment of bowel is identified.

COLONIC INJURY

Colonic trauma due to blunt abdominal injury is much rarer than trauma to the duodenum or small bowel. Perforation of the colon is rarer than trauma to the duodenum and usually results from severe traumatic forces and thus often will be accompanied by other organ injury. It can complicate flank or back penetrating injury in patients with pelvic fractures. Haematochezia may be encountered. The perforation site will usually be in a relatively fixed location, usually the hepatic flexure, sigmoid colon or caecum. Colonic perforation may lead to faecal contamination of the peritoneum. Plain radiographs may show free air in large or small amount on the erect or decubitus films. CT findings include focal wall thickening, intraperitoneal or extraperitoneal air collections and haemoperitoneum.

Rectal trauma may result in extraperitoneal perforation (Figure 10.16.14).

Injuries to the colon may result in intramural haematomas without perforation. Long-term sequelae of mesenteric and vascular injuries include colonic strictures.

HYPOPERFUSION COMPLEX

The hypovolaemic or hypoperfusion complex, is seen in children with severe CNS and/or abdominal injury. These patients have

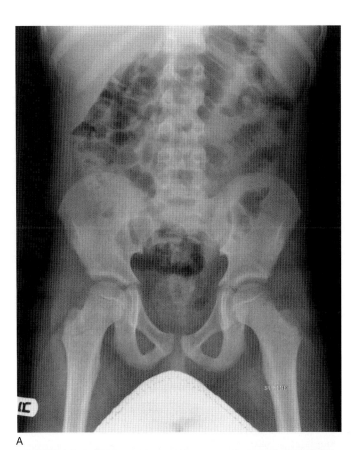

A

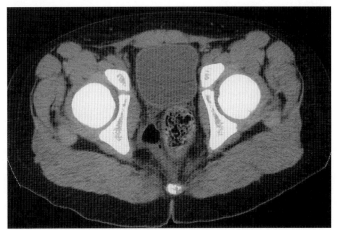

B

Figure 10.16.14 Plain abdominal film (A) and CT of the pelvis (B) of an 8-year-old boy who accidentally fell on a bottle while wrestling with his brother. He presented with rectal bleeding. An extraluminal air bubble is seen just to the left of the rectum with perirectal soft tissue infiltration consistent with rectal perforation.

histories of shock initially responding to resuscitation and they may appear haemodynamically stable. They actually have clinically occult hypovolaemia with large third space volume loss to the peritoneum and the gastrointestinal tract. They respond with vasoconstriction. The typical CT findings include decreased aortic, inferior vena cava and mesenteric vessels calibre, free intraperitoneal fluid, dilatation of fluid-filled intestine and abnormally intense contrast enhancement of bowel wall, mesentery, pancreas

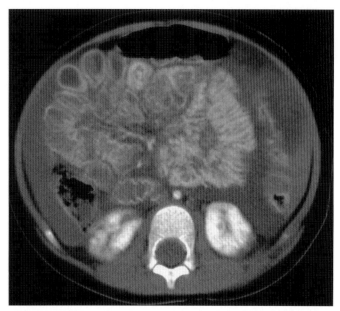

Figure 10.16.15 CT of a 3-year-old girl who was involved in a high speed motor vehicle accident. Diffuse intestinal dilatation, abnormal increased enhancement of bowel wall, and kidneys, small aortic and inferior vena cava calibre are consistent with hypoperfusion complex. Resuscitation efforts failed and the patient subsequently died.

and kidneys (Figure 10.16.15). This complex is associated with poor clinical outcome and a high mortality rate.

FURTHER READING

Akgur FM, Aktug T, Olguner M, et al. Prospective study investigating routine usage of ultrasonography as the initial diagnostic modality for the evaluation of children sustaining blunt abdominal trauma. Journal of Trauma 1997;42:626–628.

Albanese CT, Meza MP, Gardner MJ, et al. Is computed tomography a useful adjunct to the clinical examination for the diagnosis of pediatric gastrointestinal perforation from blunt abdominal trauma in children? Journal of Trauma 1996;40:417–421.

Basile KE, Sivit CJ, O'Riordan MA, et al. Acute hemoperitoneum in children: prevalence of low-attenuation fluid. Pediatric Radiology 2000;30:168–170.

Bensard DD, Beaver BL, Besner GE, et al. Small bowel injury in children after blunt abdominal trauma: is diagnostic delay important? Journal of Trauma 1996;41:476–483.

Benya EC, Lim-Dunham JE, Landrum O, et al. Abdominal sonography in examination of children with blunt abdominal trauma. American Journal of Roentgenology 2000;174:1613–1616.

Brody JM, Leighton DB, Murphy BL, et al. CT of blunt trauma bowel and mesenteric injury: typical findings and pitfalls in diagnosis. Radiographics 2000;20:1525–1536.

Butela ST, Federle MP, Chang PJ, et al. Performance of CT in detection of bowel injury. American Journal Roentgenology 2001;176:129–135.

Cho KC, Baker SR. Extraluminal air. Diagnosis and significance. Radiology Clinics of North America 1994;32:829–844.

Clancy TV, Ragozzino MW, Ramshaw D, et al. Oral contrast is not necessary in the evaluation of blunt abdominal trauma by computed tomography. American Journal of Surgery 1993;166:680–684.

Coley BD, Mutabagani KH, Martin LC, et al. Focused abdominal sonography for trauma (FAST) in children with blunt abdominal trauma. Journal of Trauma 2000;48:902–906.

Cox TD, Kuhn JP. CT scan of bowel trauma in the pediatric patient. Radiology Clinics of North America 1996;34:807–818.

Espinoza R, Rodriguez A. Traumatic and nontraumatic perforation of hollow viscera. The Surgical Clinics of North America 1997;77:1291–1304.

Federle MP, Yagan N, Peitzman AB, et al. Abdominal trauma: use of oral contrast material for CT is safe. Radiology 1997;205:91–93.

Filiatrault D, Garel L. Commentary: pediatric blunt abdominal trauma—to sound or not to sound? Pediatric Radiology 1995;25:329–331.

Frick EJ Jr, Pasquale MD, Cipolle MD. Small-bowel and mesentery injuries in blunt trauma. Journal of Trauma 1999;46:920–926.

Hara H, Babyn PS, Bourgeois D. Significance of bowel wall enhancement on CT following blunt abdominal trauma in childhood. Journal of Computer Assisted Tomography 1992;16:94–98.

Hardacre JM 2nd, West KW, Rescorla FR, et al. Delayed onset of intestinal obstruction in children after unrecognized seat belt injury. Journal Pediatric Surgery 1990;25:967–968.

Jamieson DH, Babyn PS, Pearl R. Imaging gastrointestinal perforation in pediatric blunt abdominal trauma. Pediatric Radiology 1996;26:188–194.

Kaufman RA, Babcock DS. An approach to imaging the upper abdomen in the injured child. Seminars in Roentgenology 1984;19:308–320.

Killeen KL, Shanmuganathan K, Poletti PA, et al. Helical computed tomography of bowel and mesenteric injuries. Journal of Trauma 2001;51:26–36.

Kunin JR, Korobkin M, Ellis JH, et al. Duodenal injuries caused by blunt abdominal trauma: value of CT in differentiating perforation from hematoma. American Journal of Roentgenology 1993;160:1221–1223.

Lim-Dunham JE, Narra J, Benya EC, et al. Aspiration after administration of oral contrast material in children undergoing abdominal CT for trauma. American Journal of Roentgenology 1997;169:1015–1018.

Lingawi SS, Buckley AR. Focused abdominal US in patients with trauma. Radiology 2000;217:426–429.

McGahan JP, Richards JR. Blunt abdominal trauma: the role of emergent sonography and a review of the literature. American Journal of Roentgenology 1999;172:897–903.

McGahan JP, Wang L, Richards JR. From the RSNA refresher courses: focused abdominal US for trauma. Radiographics 2001;21 Spec No:S191–S199.

Novelline RA, Rhea JT, Bell T. Helical CT of abdominal trauma. Radiology Clinics of North America 1999;37:591–612, vi–vii.

Novelline RA, Rhea JT, Rao PM, Stuk JL. Helical CT in emergency radiology. Radiology 1999;213:321–339.

Plancq MC, Villamizar J, Ricard J, et al. Management of pancreatic and duodenal injuries in pediatric patients. Pediatric Surgery International 2000;16:35–39.

Raptopoulos V. Abdominal trauma. Emphasis on computed tomography. Radiology Clinics of North America 1994;32:969–987.

Richards JR, Knopf NA, Wang L, et al. Blunt abdominal trauma in children: evaluation with emergency US. Radiology 2002;222:749–754.

Ruess L, Sivit CJ, Eichelberger MR, et al. Blunt abdominal trauma in children: impact of CT on operative and nonoperative management. American Journal of Roentgenology 1997;169:1011–1014.

Shanmuganathan K, Mirvis SE, Reaney SM. Pictorial review: CT appearances of contrast medium extravasations associated with injury sustained from blunt abdominal trauma. Clinical Radiology 1995;50:182–187.

Shuman WP, Ralls PW, Balfe DM, et al. Imaging of blunt abdominal trauma. American College of Radiology. ACR Appropriateness Criteria. Radiology 2000;215(Suppl):143–151.

Shuman WP. CT of blunt abdominal trauma in adults. Radiology 1997;205:297–306.

Sivit CJ. Gastrointestinal emergencies in older infants and children. Radiology Clinics of North America 1997;35:865–877.

Sivit CJ. Detection of active intraabdominal hemorrhage after blunt trauma: value of delayed CT scanning. Pediatric Radiology 2000;30:99–100.

Sivit CJ, Kaufman RA. Commentary: sonography in the evaluation of children following blunt trauma: is it to be or not to be? Pediatric Radiology 1995;25:326–328.

Sivit CJ, Eichelberger MR, Taylor GA. CT in children with rupture of the bowel caused by blunt trauma: diagnostic efficacy and comparison with hypoperfusion complex. American Journal Roentgenology 1994;163:1195–1198.

Sivit CJ, Taylor GA, Bulas DI, et al. Blunt trauma in children: significance of peritoneal fluid. Radiology 1991;178:185–188.

Sivit CJ, Taylor GA, Bulas DI, et al. Posttraumatic shock in children: CT findings associated with hemodynamic instability. Radiology 1992;182:723–726.

Sivit CJ, Taylor GA, Newman KD, et al. Safety-belt injuries in children with lap-belt ecchymosis: CT findings in 61 patients. American Journal of Roentgenology 1991;157:111–114.

Strouse PJ, Close BJ, Marshall KW, et al. CT of bowel and mesenteric trauma in children. Radiographics 1999;19:1237–1250.

Taylor GA. Imaging of pediatric blunt abdominal trauma: what have we learned in the past decade? Radiology 1995;195:600–601.

Wotherspoon S, Chu K, Brown AF. Abdominal injury and the seat-belt sign. Emergency Medicine (Fremantle) 2001;13:61–65.

Zahran M, Eklof O, Thomasson B. Blunt abdominal trauma and hollow viscus injury in children: the diagnostic value of plain radiography. Pediatric Radiology 1984;14:304–309.

GASTROINTESTINAL TRACT TRAUMA IN CHILD ABUSE

The incidence of non-accidental injury and neglect continues to increase. Although head injuries are responsible for the majority of fatalities in non-accidental injuries, beyond infancy, intra-abdominal injuries become increasingly important with the overall mortality rate as high as 45%. This high mortality rate is generally attributed to the delay in seeking medical care. Injuries that are associated with fatal outcome often involve the hollow viscera with death resulting from massive haemorrhage or peritonitis due to small intestinal perforation. Although the precise description of the mechanism that led to the visceral trauma is rarely provided the injuries may be caused by either a blunt blow to the abdomen (clenched fist, kick, hit with an object) or by sudden deceleration when the child is thrown. The radiologist is sometimes the one that raises the possibility of abuse when the extent of the visceral or hollow viscus injury is not explained by the mechanism of injury provided. Other described mechanisms of child abuse are intentional childhood poisoning and foreign body insertion.

THE PHARYNX, HYPOPHARYNX AND OESOPHAGUS

The mouth is a well-known target for physical and sexual abuse. Injuries include intraoral lacerations, erosions and dental fractures. Radiology plays no role in evaluation of the oral cavity, but oral injuries may imply other remote injuries to the gastrointestinal tract. The history of the insult is usually withheld. Careful questioning may help find features suggestive of child abuse. A history of frequent respiratory illness, feeding problems, unusual cry, and irritability can be encountered. Clinical findings may include respiratory difficulties, inspiratory stridor, bloody sputum, swelling and crepitus in the neck. Perforations are usually encountered in the posterior pharynx, hypopharynx or cervical oesophagus. The most common abnormality detected on plain films is abnormal accumulation of air within the neck. Non-ionic water-soluble contrast examinations assist in defining the site of perforation. Some perforation will extend to the mediastinum causing mediastinal emphysema and abscess; these are best demonstrated by CT.

THE STOMACH

Gastric perforation from non-accidental injury is rare and accounts for 0.9–1.7% of all hollow viscus rupture involving the stomach. A history of injury after ingestion of a meal is often elicited. The rupture usually causes a massive pneumoperitoneum. The rupture may be associated with other abdominal injuries. If unrecognized; gastric perforation may lead to sepsis, shock and death.

Intramural haematoma of the stomach is probably a more common injury than described in the literature. Haematomas may cause luminal narrowing on upper GI series, or on CT demonstrate gastric wall thickening.

One should be aware that marked acute gastric distention can occur in neglected children. These patients are usually below the third percentile in weight. The pathogenesis of the acute gastric atony in the deprived child is thought to be related to structural and functional changes in the stomach. These children have voracious appetites. On abdominal radiographs a huge stomach is seen mimicking on supine views an intra-abdominal mass and an air–fluid level within the stomach on upright or decubitus films.

THE SMALL INTESTINE

Small intestine perforation is a well-recognized injury in child abuse. It is usually caused by a blow to the abdomen or when a child is thrown onto a solid object. Approximately 60% occur in the jejunum just distal to the ligament of Treitz, with 30% in the duodenum and 10% in the ileum. Intraperitoneal perforations are usually associated with abdominal pain, distention, leukocytosis and fever. Retroperitoneal duodenal perforations may not display peritoneal signs.

CT is an ideal method to identify intestinal perforation as was discussed in accidental intestinal perforation (Figure 10.16.16). Perforation should lead to immediate exploration.

Small intestine haematomas are among the more classic intra-abdominal injuries encountered in child abuse. In contrast to intestinal perforation that can have a variety of causes, intestinal haematomas, unless there is a known history of bleeding diathesis, are caused by previous trauma.

Most duodenal haematomas are encountered in the transverse part of the duodenum and in the lateral aspect of the descending part of the duodenum, while small intestinal haematomas are found in the mesenteric side and bleeding within the small bowel mesentery may be an associated finding.

Clinical symptoms are characteristic and include abdominal pain and vomiting. It may be accompanied by signs of blood loss, inflammation or perforation. Associated pancreatic injury is frequent. Intramural haematomas are generally treated conservatively.

Plain films may be normal or may demonstrate bowel obstruction. The characteristic pattern on upper GI series is of a smooth, rounded intramural mass displacing the intestinal lumen. It may cause complete obstruction or may let small amount of contrast to pass between the mass and the mucosa causing a 'coiled spring' appearance. The adjacent mucosal folds are crowded.

Sonography is ideal for evaluation of duodenal haematomas. The sonographic appearance depends on the extent and age of the haematoma. At presentation, haematomas appear as well-defined hyperechoic masses. Over time they developed decreased echogenicity, ultimately becoming an anechoic cystic mass. CT is mandatory to assess for other associated injuries and for complications. On CT, intramural haematomas appear as a large discrete mass or as focal bowel wall thickening. Initially the blood is of

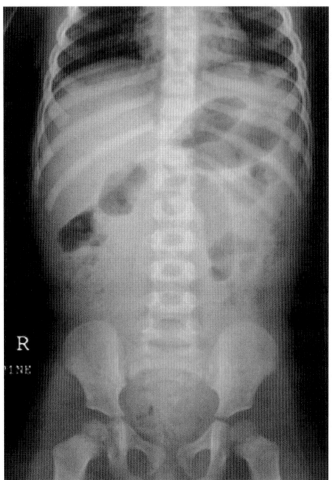

A

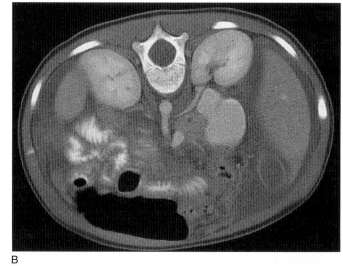

B

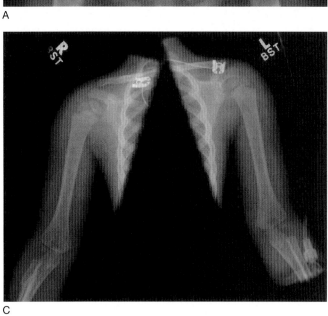

C

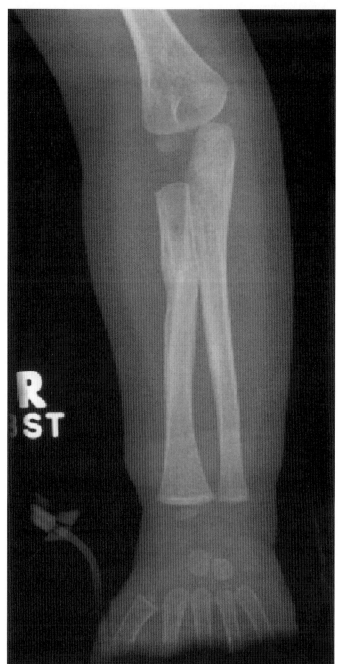

D

Figure 10.16.16 An 18-month-old girl with a four day history of vomiting and lethargy. An abnormal gas pattern with one distended small bowel loop is seen on the frontal radiograph (A). US showed unexplained free intraperitoneal fluid. Subsequent CT of the abdomen documented pancreatic laceration, diffuse bowel wall thickening and large amount of free fluid (B). On surgery ileal perforation was found. The type of injury raised suspicion of battered child. Skeletal survey revealed bilateral proximal humeral metaphyseal fractures (C) and healing right radial fracture (D).

high attenuation, but with time decreases in attenuation as the haematomas liquefies and resolves.

Late complications of intestinal haematomas include intestinal strictures. The children present with vague abdominal complaints and vomiting. Radiographic signs of small bowel obstruction may be seen from strictures that can be confirmed with contrast studies.

MISCELLANEOUS LESIONS

Pneumatosis intestinalis and portal gas may occur in child abuse. A mucosal break allows gas to dissect into the bowel wall. This appears as linear or cystic intramural gas collections. The gas may pass to the portal system resulting in branching pattern of intrahepatic gas.

Intussusception is a rare manifestation of abuse.

THE COLON

Colonic injuries due to blunt injuries are rare in abused children, resulting in intramural haematomas that can be diagnosed with barium enema, endoscopy and CT. Distal colonic and anal injuries are more common with sexual abuse and are rarely documented radiographically.

FURTHER READING

Ablin DS, Reinhart MA. Esophageal perforation with mediastinal abscess in child abuse. Pediatric Radiology 1990;20:524–525.

Cooper A, Floyd T, Barlow B, et al. Major blunt abdominal trauma due to child abuse. Journal of Trauma 1988;28:1483–1487.

Eisenstein EM, Delta BG, Clifford JH. Jejunal hematoma: an unusual manifestation of the battered-child syndrome. Clinical Pediatrics 1965;4:436–440.

Felsom B, Levin EJ. Intramural hematoma of the duodenum. A diagnostic roentgen sign. Radiology 1954;63:823–829.

Franken EA Jr, Fox M, Smith JA, et al. Acute gastric dilatation in neglected children. American Journal of Roentgenology 1978;130:297–299.

Fulcher AS, Das Narla L, Brewer WH. Gastric hematoma and pneumatosis in child abuse. American Journal of Roentgenology 1990;155:1283–1284.

Gornall P, Ahmed S, Jolleys A, et al. Intra-abdominal injuries in the battered baby syndrome. Archives of Diseases in Childhood 1972;47:211–214.

Kirks DR. Radiological evaluation of visceral injuries in the battered child syndrome. Pediatric Annals 1983;12:888–893.

Kleinman PK. Diagnostic imaging of child abuse. 2nd edn. St. Louis: Mosby: 1998: 248–284.

Kleinman PK, Brill PW, Winchester P. Resolving duodenal-jejunal hematoma in abused children. Radiology 1986;160:747–750.

Ledbetter DJ, Hatch EI Jr, Feldman KW, et al. Diagnostic and surgical implications of child abuse. Archives of Surgery 1988;123:1101–1105.

Mahour GH, Woolley MM, Gans SL, et al. Duodenal hematoma in infancy and childhood. Journal of Pediatric Surgery 1971;6:153–160.

McDowell HP, Fielding DW. Traumatic perforation of the hypopharynx—an unusual form of abuse. Archives of Diseases in Childhood 1984; 59:888–889.

Merten DF, Carpenter BL. Radiologic imaging of inflicted injury in the child abuse syndrome. Pediatric Clinics of North America 1990;37:815–837.

Ng CS, Hall CM, Shaw DG. The range of visceral manifestations of non-accidental injury. Archive of Diseases in Childhood 1997;77:167–174.

Schechner SA, Ehrlich FE. Case reports. Gastric perforation and child abuse. Journal of Trauma 1974;14:723–725.

Shah P, Applegate KE, Buonomo C. Stricture of the duodenum and jejunum in an abused child. Pediatric Radiology 1997;27:281–283.

Sivit CJ, Taylor GA, Eichelberger MR. Visceral injury in battered children: a changing perspective. Radiology 1989;173:659–661.

Wu JW, Chen MY, Auringer ST. Portal venous gas: an unusual finding in child abuse. Journal of Emergency Medicine 2000;18:105–107.

SECTION | 11

THE LIVER, BILIARY TRACT, SPLEEN AND PANCREAS

Introduction

David A Stringer

Following careful clinical history and examination, radiological investigation is often required to investigate the solid intra-abdominal organs. Those included in this chapter are the liver, biliary tree, pancreas and spleen.

Plain films and contrast examinations are rarely helpful in the investigation of these organs. Because children tend to be smaller and have less fat than adults this makes ultrasound a superb imaging technique for children and is usually the initial radiological examination of choice, forming the basis for decisions about further radiological evaluation.

Following on from ultrasound, computed tomography (CT) and magnetic resonance imaging (MRI) are increasingly being used. When CT is utilized low-dose CT techniques should be used (see Chapter 1.4). When CT is considered, the value of MRI should also be analyzed, as it holds great interest for the future, having the advantage of not using ionizing radiation and being able to visualize the duct structures by magnetic resonance cholangio-pancreatography (MRCP).

FURTHER READING

Dobranowski J, Stringer DA, Somers S, Stevenson GW. Procedures in gastrointestinal radiology. New York: Springer-Verlag; 1990.

Stringer DA and Babyn P. Paediatric gastrointestinal imaging and intervention, 2nd edn. Hamilton: B.C. Decker Inc.; 2000.

Various authors. Imaging of the paediatric gastrointestinal tract. In: Walker WA, Durie PR, Hamilton JR, Walker-Smith JA, Watkins JB (eds). Paediatric gastrointestinal disease, 3rd edn. Hamilton: Decker Inc.; 2000:1538-1682.

Techniques of Imaging the Liver

11.2

Helen R Nadel, David A Stringer

Following careful clinical history and examination radiological investigation is often required to investigate the solid intra-abdominal organs. Plain films and contrast examinations are rarely helpful but ultrasound, nuclear medicine studies, computed tomography (CT), magnetic resonance imaging (MRI) and angiographic and interventional studies all play a role in the investigation of childhood disorders of the liver, biliary tree, pancreas and spleen.

Each of the techniques will be discussed briefly in turn.

ULTRASOUND

Ultrasound has changed the investigation of paediatric solid intra-abdominal organs. Ultrasound is a rapid non-invasive test that does not require sedation. It enables evaluation of organ size, shape and echogenicity. Doppler studies can evaluate the vascular flow patterns.

To properly evaluate these organs the ultrasound unit needs to be 'state of the art' with a range of high frequency transducers to enable adequate evaluation of different size and shape of patients. The biliary tree is easily seen with ultrasound, and gallstones and choledochal cysts are readily diagnosable. Hence, cholangiography has been replaced by ultrasound. Ultrasound can be very useful to guide biopsy or other interventional procedures. Solid tumours can also be well seen and differentiation made to a high degree between benign and malignant lesions.

The radiologists involved should be familiar with the full spectrum of paediatric diseases as they are so different from adults. This is essential in order to avoid some of the common paediatric pitfalls. For example, a very echogenic structure in the spleen, more echogenic than surrounding splenic tissue, may represent a congenital splenic cyst filled with cholesterol crystals, whereas the inexperienced radiologist may well suspect that it is a solid and malignant lesion.

Doppler studies using spectral, colour and power Doppler are all useful in the evaluation of more complex diseases. It can help distinguish haemangioendothelioma from hepatoblastoma. Doppler studies are especially helpful in those who have had, or are about to undergo, liver transplantation. In this regard, the most useful evaluating tool is colour Doppler; however, spectral measurements can also give valuable information.

NUCLEAR MEDICINE (NM) TECHNIQUES

Radionuclide liver/spleen scanning will assess both congenital and acquired disease. Technetium 99m (Tc 99m) sulphur colloid is phagocytosed by Kupfer cells in the reticuloendothelial system and so can be used to image the spleen and liver. With the increased use of ultrasound and other non-invasive anatomical imaging studies, liver/spleen scintigraphy is now used mainly in the assessment of visceral heterotaxy and functional hyposplenism.

Visceral heterotaxy syndromes include asplenia and polysplenia. Children with asplenia are at risk for overwhelming bacterial infections. Prompt identification of asplenia can ensure the patient will obtain the necessary prophylaxis to prevent sepsis. In infants with suspected visceral heterotaxy who have equivocal ultrasound examinations, liver spleen scintigraphy with Tc-99m colloid alone or combined with heat-damaged red blood cell scintigraphy can demonstrate position of the liver and the presence or absence of the spleen.

Functional hyposplenism may be clinically manifested by the presence of circulating Howell–Jolly bodies. In children with polysplenia, the multiple spleens may not have adequate reticuloendothelial cell function. Other causes of functional asplenia include vascular occlusion, haemoglobinopathies, infiltrative disorders (including tumour and amyloid), coeliac sprue, systemic lupus erythematosis, previous radiotherapy or chemotherapy, and immunodeficiency syndromes. In children who are noted by other anatomical imaging to have a spleen, the non-visualization of splenic activity on a Tc-99m colloid liver/spleen scan based on RES phagocytosis will confirm significant functional asplenia.

Selective spleen scintigraphy visualizes the spleen alone without interfering activity from the liver. This is most useful in suspected asplenia or when a midline centrally placed liver is present, which could obscure an abnormally sited spleen. Functional asplenia and suspected splenic hypoplasia may also be indications, although assessment by Tc 99m sulphur colloid based on RES phagocytosis is usually adequate. By damaging the patient's red blood cells with heat and reinjecting them labelled with technetium 99m, the spleen alone can be visualized. Normally, the spleen avidly sequesters damaged red blood cells and appears hot on scan with only faint hepatic visualization. If no functioning spleen is present, there will be marked liver localization secondary to RES phago-cytosis and some excretion of free pertechnetate by the kidneys.

BILIARY SCAN

Imaging of the patency and function of the biliary tree is possible using one of the iminodiacetic (IDA) derivatives, which is actively taken up by the hepatocytes and excreted into the bile canaliculi. Hepatobiliary scintigraphy using IDA radiopharmaceuticals pro-vides clinically useful information on function of the biliary tract in a variety of pathological processes in children, including neona-tal jaundice, gallbladder dysfunction, trauma and liver transplan-tation. In children, the commonest iminodiacetic compounds used are diisopropyliminodiacetic acid (DISIDA) and methyltri-broiminodiacetic acid (mebrofenin). These agents have the great-est hepatocyte uptake and lowest renal excretion.

A minimum fast of 4h in young infants and children and 6–8 hours in older children is required for patient preparation. Prolonged fasting for more than 24h is to be avoided, as should hyperalimentation, as this may cause non-visualization of the gall-bladder due to the presence of viscous bile in the gallbladder.

If the indication for the examination is to distinguish between neonatal hepatitis and atresia, the patient is premedicated with phe-nobarbitol orally in a dose of 5mg/kg daily given in divided doses each day for 5 days prior to the scan. This is to enhance enzymatic excretion of bile and therefore reduce false positive interpretations of biliary obstruction when cholestasis is present. The end point of the examination is the visualization of excretion of activity into the gastrointestinal tract. Imaging is continued after the initial 30min of dynamic imaging intermittently for up to 24h if no excretion of activity is seen in the gastrointestinal tract.

One of the common specific indications is to distinguish between neonatal hepatitis and biliary atresia as a cause of neona-tal jaundice by assessing hepatocyte clearance and biliary excre-tion into the intestine. Biliary atresia can be ruled out in an infant if a patent biliary tree is demonstrated with passage of activity into the bowel. If no radiopharmaceutical is seen in the bowel on imaging for up to 24h, distinction between severe hepatocellular disease and biliary atresia cannot be made. A sensitivity and speci-ficity of 97% and 82%, respectively, has been achieved for hepa-tobiliary imaging in the diagnosis of biliary atresia. However, the study is less accurate in infants older than 3 months in whom hepatic parenchymal damage has developed secondary to biliary atresia. Following Kasai procedure for biliary atresia, hepatobil-iary scanning is useful to assess the patency of the hepatic/enteric anastomosis. Bile leak following this procedure and in liver trans-plantation and trauma is also readily identified. Cholescintigraphy in suspected bile leak provides information generally not available with other techniques except for direct cholangiography.

Biliary scintigraphy readily establishes the diagnosis of chole-dochal cyst in all age groups and differentiates this from other causes of cystic masses in the right upper quadrant. In this respect, it is complimentary to sonography and CT. The impairment of both intra- and extrahepatic biliary drainage is an important cause of liver disease in cystic fibrosis. More than 50% of patients with cystic fibrosis have sonographic and scintigraphic abnormalities of the gallbladder and cystic duct. Hepatobiliary scintigraphy in cystic fibrosis has shown characteristic patterns of dilatation of mainly the left hepatic duct, narrowing of the distal common bile duct, gallbladder dysfunction and delayed bowel transit.

Cholecystitis in children may be acalculous and a complication of prolonged illness, infection or trauma. The combination of ultra-sonography and hepatobiliary scintigraphy findings are helpful in establishing the diagnosis. Hepatobiliary scintigraphy may show the characteristic scintigraphic pattern described in adults of non-visualization of the gallbladder. The gallbladder can, however, be visualized in the presence of acalculous cholecystitis and toxic cholecystitis. Hepatobiliary imaging in children who have under-gone liver transplantation can assess graft vascularity, parenchy-mal function, biliary drainage, presence of a leak and obstruction.

COMPUTED TOMOGRAPHY

Computed tomography can beautifully delineate liver, pancreatic and splenic abnormalities. Lesions, such as liver tumours, detected by ultrasound can be further evaluated with CT which gives addi-tional useful information, such as the involvement of vessels and presence of spread to other regions. The technique used should be meticulous using fast scan techniques and low dose. Multidetec-tor scans are particularly useful in the evaluation of vascular supply with 3D reconstruction techniques (CT angiography, (CTA)), however, they do have a higher radiation dose than con-ventional CT scanners.

CONTRAST MEDIA IN CT

Intravenous contrast media are nearly always required for CT. Often, oral contrast material is also given and occasionally con-trast may be given per rectum. Fast scanning techniques can be very helpful in evaluating children and repeating the scan at various phases of contrast enhancement can be extremely useful in the liver. These should be done on an individual basis, to answer specific questions and not performed routinely. This approach limits the radiation dose. Three-dimensional reconstruction and multiplanar reconstruction of vascular structures can also be helpful, especially in the evaluation of liver transplant patients.

No CT evaluation of the abdomen for abdominal trauma is com-plete without using lung windows settings to ensure that there is no free intraperitoneal gas. Intravenous contrast should always be used in the evaluation of trauma but the value of oral contrast is more debatable.

MAGNETIC RESONANCE IMAGING

More experience with MRI in the abdominal solid organs is showing it to be of increasing value. It is now routinely employed in all tumours. In addition to an evaluation similar to CT, the advantages include no radiation and evaluation of the biliary tree and pancreatic ducts using long T1-weighted techniques. Magnetic resonance cholangiopancreatography (MRCP) is increasingly replacing diagnostic endoscopic retrograde cholangiopancreatography (ERCP) in children.

MRI can also evaluate the vascular supply with 3D reconstruction techniques (MR angiography, (MRA)).

The disadvantages include the length of examination and cost, need for sedation in younger children, artifacts from movement, primarily respiratory, and difficulty of monitoring very sick infants and children.

ANGIOGRAPHY

With the new CTA and MRA techniques, digital angiography is now rarely indicated. One of the few remaining indications is pre-liver transplantation if CTA and MRA have failed to delineate the anatomy.

FURTHER READING

Dobranowski J, Stringer DA, Somers S, Stevenson GW. Procedures in gastrointestinal radiology. New York: Springer-Verlag; 1990.

Nadel HR. Hepatobiliary scintigraphy in children. Seminars in Nuclear Medicine 1996; 26:25-42.

Stringer DA and Babyn P. Paediatric gastrointestinal imaging and intervention, 2nd edn. Hamilton: B.C. Decker Inc.; 2000.

Various authors. Imaging of the paediatric gastrointestinal tract. In: Walker WA, Durie PR, Hamilton JR et al. (eds). Paediatric gastrointestinal disease, 3rd edn. Hamilton: B.C. Decker Inc.; 2000:1538-1682.

Interventional Techniques

Peter G Chait, Devon Jacobson

Areas that will be discussed in this chapter include biopsy of the liver, spleen and pancreas, aspiration and drainage of the liver, spleen and pancreas and a separate section on drainage and intervention of the biliary tract.

PERCUTANEOUS BIOPSY

Image-guided percutaneous biopsy techniques have improved with better imaging technology and needle choices to become the method of choice in the biopsy of most solid organs. Image-guided ultrasound is the imaging tool of choice for most biopsies of the liver, pancreas and spleen. Fluoroscopy is generally not helpful. Computed tomography (CT) is used when lesions are not visualized on ultrasound or are deep and close to vital structures.

High-resolution real-time linear and curvilinear probes are generally used for biopsies. Most experienced interventionalists prefer a free-hand technique, especially where lesions are smaller and deeply situated, when the needle and ultrasound probe are distant from each other or when the ultrasonic window is very small. It is essential in either technique to maintain a perpendicular relationship between the needle and transducer (to increase reverberation artifact and therefore improve needle visualization) and to keep both target and needle in the imaging plane on the transducer. The movement of the needle is thus observed throughout its course. It is also important as a rule not to move the transducer and needle at the same time.

CT offers good tissue differentiation for abdominal biopsies. Helical CTs and CT fluoroscopy have improved the diagnostic accuracy; however, one always has to be aware of the high radiation exposure to the patient and the operator. During CT-guidance, it is important to orientate the needle perpendicular to the skin and to tilt the gantry to see the entire course of the needle.

Positron emission tomography (PET) and single photon emission computed tomography (SPECT) and magnetic resonance imaging (MRI) assist to differentiate pathophysiological tissue from normal tissue and may yield improvements in specificity. At the present time, these technologies are not in common use for biopsies of solid organs.

BIOPSY NEEDLES

The ideal needle should provide as much tissue as possible without causing undue artifact or complications. Fine needle aspiration maximizes safety; however, in most paediatric situations, fine needle aspiration of solid masses is not sufficient for pathological diagnosis. Thin-walled, small-gauge core biopsy needles with a variety of tips provide sufficient tissue for diagnosis, depending on the underlying pathology. Coaxial systems, i.e. a larger needle, are used to access the organ and several core biopsies are performed through an inner needle, which allows for more yield and a single puncture to the capsule and also allows one to embolize the tract. A variety of needles have been used for tissue acquisition. They can be divided into non-cutting and cutting needles and into manual and automated needles. Non-cutting (manual aspiration) needles (Chiba or spinal) allow for sampling of cells for cytopathology and microbiology analysis. Manual cutting needles include endcutting needles, such as a Mangini, Turner, Jam Shidi and Surecut, and side-cutting needles, such as True Cut. Automated systems include endcutting (Angiomed Autovac) and side-cutting devices (Biopty, Monopty). Both of these automated needles allow a variety of lengths for biopsies.

Unless aspiration cytology is needed, automated cutting needles are the needles of choice.

The Angiomed Autovac Needle (18–21 gauge) is used primarily for solid masses and organs. Automated side-cutting needles are used where there is gelatinous tissue or mobile tissue that does not allow acquisition of good endcutting core sample. In the solid organs of the abdomen, we do not use a needle larger than 18 gauge.

Special needles are manufactured for specific applications, including needles designed for easy visualization with ultrasound and non-ferrous needles for MRI procedures, kits for transjugular biopsies and flexible needle holders designed to protect the operator's hands in the CT gantry.

FURTHER READING

Gazelle GS, Haaga JR. Guided percutaneous biopsy of intraabdominal lesions. American Journal of Roentgenology 1989; 153:929–935.

Jaeger HJ, MacFie J, Mitchell CJ et al. Diagnosis of abdominal masses with percutaneous biopsy guided by ultrasound. British Medical Journal 1990; 301:1188–1191.

Katada K, Anno H, Takeshita G et al. [Development of real-time CT fluoroscopy]. Nippon Igaku Hoshasen Gakkai Zasshi 1994; 54:1172–1174.

Reading CC, Charboneau JW, James EM, Hurt MR. Sonographically guided percutaneous biopsy of small (3 cm or less) masses. American Journal of Roentgenology 1988; 151:189–192.

Reddy VB, Gattuso P, Abraham KP et al. Computed tomography-guided fine needle aspiration biopsy of deep-seated lesions. A four-year experience. Acta Cytologica 1991; 35:753–756.

Sawhney S, Berry M, Bhargava S. Percutaneous real-time ultrasonic guided biopsy in the diagnosis of deep-seated, non-palpable intra-abdominal masses (initial experience). Australasian Radiology 1987; 31:295–299.

PATIENT PREPARATION

Prior to the biopsy procedure, the patient's imaging studies should be reviewed with the referring physicians and surgeons to determine a clinical radiological diagnosis and discuss potential risks and benefits of a percutaneous approach. Close consultation with a pathologist is essential and the desired transport medium and handling procedures for the biopsy material clarified. Patient preparation is otherwise the same as any other interventional procedure. When sampling small lesions or those next to vital structures, general anaesthesia with controlled respiration may be necessary to reduce the risk and improve the success rate.

FURTHER READING

Dabbs DJ, Wang X. Immunocytochemistry on cytologic specimens of limited quantity. Diagnostic Cytopathology 1998; 18:166–169.
Zardawi IM. Fine needle aspiration cytology in a rural setting. Acta Cytologica 1998; 42:899–906.

CONTRAINDICATION TO BIOPSY

There are no absolute contraindications to percutaneous biopsy. The decision to obtain a biopsy should be made with consideration of risks and benefits to each patient. However, biopsy should not be undertaken where the result would not influence the management or when surgical excision is planned regardless of the percutaneous result. Relative contraindications include coagulation abnormalities that increase the risk of postprocedure bleeding (alternative methods such as transjugular biopsy or embolization of the tract may be considered), and absence of a safe pathway from skin to target site.

PERCUTANEOUS LIVER BIOPSY

Liver biopsy is performed to diagnose suspected benign or malignant lesions or suspected inflammatory lesions. It is also used to characterize diffuse hepatocellular disease. Our technique of performing a standard liver biopsy is to use a midline subcostal approach using ultrasound guidance. This procedure is usually performed under sedation with the administration of local anaesthetic. The biopsies of diffuse or focal lesions are usually performed with an Angiomed Autovac 18-gauge needle that gives good quality and size of tissue samples.

For small lesions, ultrasound again is used and, depending on the size of the lesion, the same needle is used, either 18- or 21-gauge. It is preferable to go through normal liver tissue into the biopsy site. In cases where there is a higher risk of bleeding, the tract can be embolized using a coaxial technique with a gel foam slurry (gel foam mixed with contrast).

Transluminal biopsies can be performed for central fibrotic lesions (Figure 11.3.1).

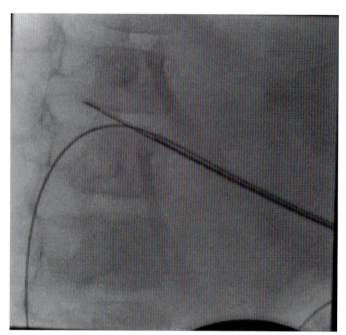

Figure 11.3.1 Percutaneous transductal biopsy under ultrasound and fluoroscopy guidance with the wire down the common bile duct.

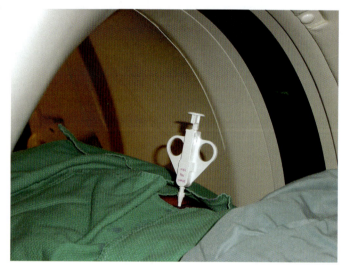

Figure 11.3.2 CT-fluoroscopic guided biopsy of a small liver lesion.

Very seldom is CT required for liver biopsies but it may be necessary where ultrasound does not visualize the lesion (Figure 11.3.2).

TRANSJUGULAR LIVER BIOPSY

Since 1994, 80 transjugular liver biopsies have been performed at Hospital for Sick Children, Toronto, mainly on children with uncorrectable coagulopathies or in children suspected of having portal hypertension. The incidence of minor complications was 12%, with one death due to ventricular arrhythmia following the

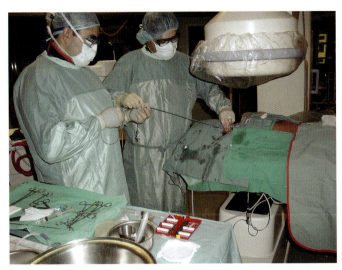

Figure 11.3.3 Transjugular liver biopsy: patient set up with combined fluoroscopy and ultrasound guidance.

procedure. This procedure is performed under general anaesthetic with paralysis used to control respiration, and under ultrasound guidance, usually the right internal jugular vein. Occasionally, when this vein is thrombosed, the left jugular vein can be used. A quick core transjugular set (labs 100 Cook Inc. Bloomington, Indiana) is our system of choice for all patients (Figure 11.3.3).

The catheter is introduced into the sheath and the directional catheter is advanced over a hydrophilic wire. Pressure measurements are taken from the inferior vena cava (IVC) and hepatic vein, both free and wedged. The corrected wedge pressure (portosystemic gradient) is calculated as the difference between the IVC pressure and the portal pressure (wedge pressure). A normal portosystemic gradient is 2–4 mm of mercury, a gradient higher than or equal to 6 mm of mercury is evidence of portal hypertension, and greater than 15 mm constitutes severe portal hypertension. A normal free hepatic venogram confirms patency of the main hepatic veins. A wedge hepatic venogram is also performed, which results in filling of the portal venous structures and allows visualization of the portal venous anatomy and directional flow. Retrograde venous filling during wedge hepatic venography indicates reversal of portal flow and suggests portal hypertension. The biopsy needle is introduced through an 8 French cannula with an internal stiffener, and the needle tip is advanced to the tip of the catheter. We use ultrasound guidance to examine the liver with the needle in position and avoid vital structures. Ultrasound control also allows one to do biopsies from the middle and left hepatic veins as well as biopsies in transplant and segmental transplant of the liver.

In patients with periductal obstructing masses, it is possible to do a transductal biliary dilatation. This is performed after access is obtained to the biliary ducts and a sheath is introduced. Biopsy can then be performed under ultrasound or fluoroscopic guidance, using a cutting needle.

FURTHER READING

Chait PG, Shlomovitz E, Connolly BL et al. Percutaneous cecostomy: updates in technique and patient care. Radiology 2003; 227:246–250.

PERCUTANEOUS SPLENIC BIOPSY

Splenomegaly and focal splenic lesions are commonly seen in immunocompromised or immunosuppressed patients. The nature of these splenic lesions is often of primary and diagnostic importance and defines the course of therapy. In the past, fine needle aspirations were done on many of these patients. Many of these patients required further investigation with the pathological diagnosis being made on the excised spleen. Ultrasound-guided core biopsy of the spleen is performed under ultrasound guidance using an 18-gauge end- or side-cutting needle with a coaxial 17-gauge needle used, depending on whether embolization of the tract or numerous cores are needed. This is normally done under general anaesthetic as the splenic lesion may be obscured between ribs and difficult to visualize.

FURTHER READING

Zeppa P, Vetrani A, Luciano L et al. Fine needle aspiration biopsy of the spleen. A useful procedure in the diagnosis of splenomegaly. Acta Cytologica 1994; 38:299–309.

PANCREATIC BIOPSIES

Primary pancreatic tumours are relatively rare in the paediatric population. Principles of biopsy are similar to other solid mass biopsies. A decision to do a percutaneous biopsy depends on the extent of the primary lesion, the presence of secondary lesions and the other surgical alternatives. Visualization on ultrasound is usually good, depending on the size of the lesion. It is important to exclude vascular tumours that are not suitable for percutaneous biopsy (Figures 11.3.4 and 11.3.5).

Pancreatitis, bleeding and seeding of the biopsy tract are primary risks of this procedure. A window should be sought that

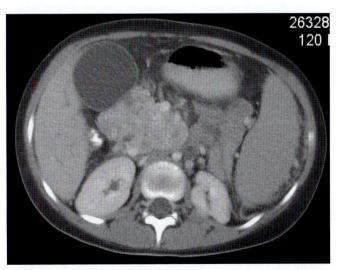

Figure 11.3.4 CT demonstrating a large mass in the head of the pancreas with a request for a percutaneous biopsy.

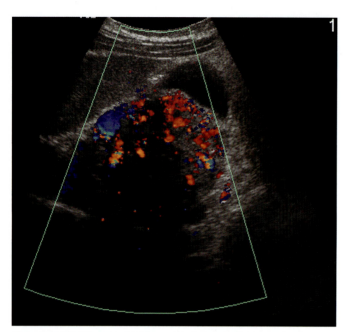

Figure 11.3.5 Ultrasound of the mass demonstrating extensive vascularity, which is a contraindication to the biopsy.

allows one to not transverse bowel and preferably do it directly percutaneously, from a retroperitoneal approach or even through the liver.

FURTHER READING

Murakami T, Veki K, Kawakami H et al. Pancreatoblastoma: case report and review of treatment in the literature. Medical and Pediatric Oncology 1996; 27:193–197.

Schwartz M.Z. Unusual peptide-secreting tumors in adolescents and children. Seminars in Pediatric Surgery 1997; 6:141–146.

Synn AY, Mulvihill SJ, Fonkalsrud EW. Surgical disorders of the pancreas in infancy and childhood. American Journal of Surgery 1988; 156:201–205.

Willnow U, Willberg B, Schwamborn D et al. Pancreatoblastoma in children. Case report and review of the literature. European Journal of Pediatric Surgery 1996; 6:369–372.

Yagi M, Shiraiwa K, Abiko M et al. A solid and cystic tumor of the pancreas in a 10-year-old girl: report of a case and review of the literature. Surgery Today 1994; 24:826–828.

PERCUTANEOUS ASPIRATION AND DRAINAGE

INDICATIONS AND CONTRAINDICATIONS

Percutaneous aspiration drainage has been performed for many years and has become the procedure of choice in most visualized collections. Absolute contraindications to abscess drainage include uncorrectable bleeding problems and an unsafe route for drainage. Suspected fungal abscesses, which can be quite invasive, may be considered a relative contraindication to percutaneous drainage unless local antifungal therapy with anti-fungal agent that can be injected directly is anticipated.

LIVER ABSCESSES

Hepatic abscesses are uncommon in the paediatric population. Pyogenic abscesses are most commonly seen in abdominal trauma and in immunocompromised patients, or those with chronic granulomatous disease. Pyogenic abscesses may complicate appendicitis, portal vein thrombosis or liver infarction. Depending on their size, pyogenic abscesses may be aspirated or drained. Smaller abscesses would be drained with a Chiba needle under ultrasound guidance. Larger abscesses are drained using ultrasound guidance followed by contrast, wire, then dilatation and drainage catheter placement under fluoroscopy. Just as for liver biopsies, a choice of access routes through interposed normal liver, between the capsule and the collection, is helpful to prevent haemorrhage and intraperitoneal contamination (Figures 11.3.6, 11.3.7).

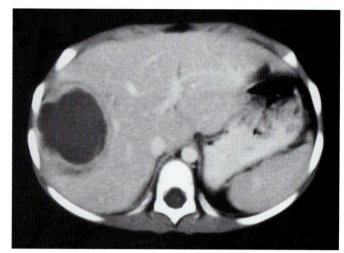

Figure 11.3.6 CT demonstrating a liver abscess.

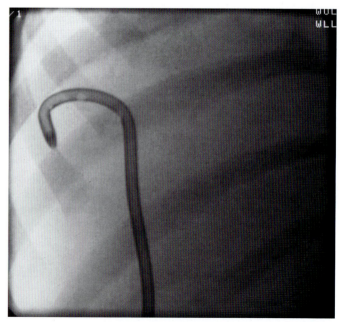

Figure 11.3.7 Drainage catheter in position.

Percutaneous drainage plays an important role in the management of patients with infected collections related to liver transplantation. Retransplantation has been avoided in some children. In the immunocompromised patient, focal micro abscesses are often seen as the presenting feature of fungal infections and diagnostic aspirations are important.

Multiloculated cysts seen in *Echinococcus granulosa* infections are preferentially treated with antibiotics (albendizol) alone. These abscesses can be drained with ultrasound guidance and replacing the cyst fluid with hypotonic saline. The replacement technique avoids interperitoneal spillage of infected fluid. Treatment with alcohol or silver nitrate solution may be used in some cases.

Patients from underdeveloped areas are at risk of having amoebic liver abscesses. Most cases present as an abscess and usually in the right lobe. Percutaneous drainage for failed antibiotic therapy or imminent rupture is indicated.

CHOLECYSTOSTOMY AND PERICHOLECYSTIC COLLECTIONS

Drainage of pyogenic cholecystitis or a calculus cholecystitis is also performed using a standard technique of ultrasound guidance followed by catheter placement. These catheters are usually left in place for 4–6 weeks prior to removal (Figure 11.3.8).

FURTHER READING

Montoya F, Alam M, Couture A et al. [Liver abscess in a newborn infant. Cure following percutaneous puncture under echographic control]. Pediatrie 1983; 38:547–551.

Ni YH, Chang M, Hsu H et al. Ultrasound-guided percutaneous drainage of liver abscess in children. Zhonghua Min Guo Xiao Er Ke Yi Xue Hui Za Zhi 1995; 36:336–341.

Okoye BO, Rampersad B, Marantos A et al. Abscess after appendicectomy in children: the role of conservative management. British Journal of Surgery 1998; 85:1111–1113.

Wang DS, Chen DS, Wang YZ et al. Bacterial liver abscess in children. Journal of the Singapore Paediatric Society 1989; 31:75–78.

SPLENIC ABSCESSES

The optimal approach to splenic abscesses is controversial. There are concerns about the safety of transplenic percutaneous intervention. Abscesses have been drained adequately percutaneously. Percutaneous drainage offers the advantage of preserving splenic function and the associated host immunity. Aspiration can be performed in any size lesion. Drainage with a catheter should be considered in a significantly sized lesion that is not close to vascular structures or the periphery.

FURTHER READING

Quinn SF, van Sonnenberg E, Casola G et al. Interventional radiology in the spleen. Radiology 1986; 161:289–291.

Tikkakoski T, Siniluoto T, Paivansalo M et al. Splenic abscess. Imaging and intervention. Acta Radiologica 1992; 33:561–565.

PANCREATIC COLLECTIONS

Percutanous drainage of pancreatic fluid collections is indicated in cases of infected symptomatic or persistent pseudocysts. Pancreatic phlegmon, pancreatic necrosis and pseudoaneurysm or varices are relative contraindications to percutaneous management. Abscesses are rare but have been seen in immunocompromised children. Depending on their size and position, they may be drained with a thin needle or with a catheter. Pseudocysts are usually drained transgastrically if possible, using a combination of ultrasound and fluoroscopy and, if necessary, CT guidance (Figure 11.3.9). The transgastric approach utilizes the percutaneous gastrostomy access and then once access is obtained to the stomach the needle is advanced into the pseudocyst through which the wire and dilator are placed. The catheter is left in situ for 6 weeks or more, to allow the tract to mature. Catheter checks are performed to see if there is communication with the pancreatic duct.

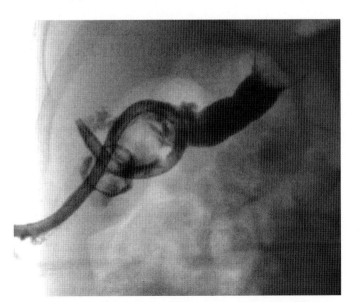

Figure 11.3.8 Cholecystostomy with a calculus at the neck of the gallbladder.

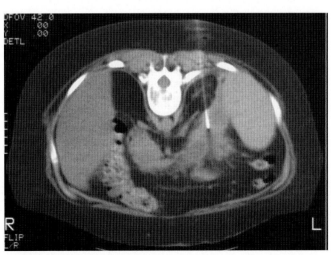

Figure 11.3.9 Prone CT aspiration and drainage of pancreatic collections.

FURTHER READING

Amundson GM, Towbin RB, Mueller DL et al. Percutaneous transgastric drainage of the lesser sac in children. Pediatric Radiology 1990; 20:590–593.

Burnweit C, Wesson D, Strunger D et al. Percutaneous drainage of traumatic pancreatic pseudocysts in children. Journal of Trauma 1990; 30:1273–1277.

Jaffe RB, Arata JA Jr, Matlak ME. Percutaneous drainage of traumatic pancreatic pseudocysts in children. American Journal of Roentgenology 1989; 152:591–595.

vanSonnenberg E, Wittich GR, Casola G et al. Complicated pancreatic inflammatory disease: diagnostic and therapeutic role of interventional radiology. Radiology 1985; 155:335–340.

BILIARY INTERVENTION

Percutaneous transhepatic cholangiography (PTC) and percutaneous transhepatic transcholecystic cholangiography (PTTC), percutaneous biliary drainage, dilation of biliary strictures and stenting are well-established techniques in the biliary system. The need for these has increased significantly since the advent of liver transplantation in the paediatric population.

FURTHER READING

Bhatnagar V, Dhawan A, Chaer M et al. The incidence and management of biliary complications following liver transplantation in children. Transplant International 1995; 8:388–391.

Burhenne HJ. The history of interventional radiology of the biliary tract. Radiologic Clinics of North America 1990; 28:1139–1144.

Burke DR. Biliary and other gastrointestinal interventions. Current Opinion in Radiology 1991; 3:151–159.

Coons H. Biliary intervention – technique and devices: a commentary. Cardiovascular Interventional Radiology 1990; 13:211–216.

Ring EJ, Kerlan RK Jr. Interventional biliary radiology. American Journal of Roentgenology 1984; 142:31–34.

Venbrux AC. Interventional radiology in the biliary tract. Current Opinion in Radiology 1992; 4:83–92.

PERCUTANEOUS TRANSHEPATIC BILIARY DRAINAGE

All percutaneous biliary procedures begin with needle access to the biliary tree under image guidance. These procedures are performed under strict sterile conditions. Most of the procedures are performed under general anaesthesia with patients intubated and suspended respiration as necessary. Prior imaging is reviewed and an ultrasound is done to identify position of ducts. Preprocedure antibiotics are used, usually triple antibiotics including gentamicin, ampicillin and metronidazole. Ultrasound is the guidance of choice and is used to identify dilated ducts or the position of undilated ducts. Colour Doppler is used to identify vessels and help with the needle placement. A right-sided or left-sided approach can be used. When a right-sided approach is used, the approach should be as low as possible to avoid a haemo- or pneumothorax.

Once access is obtained, a slipring T connector is attached to the syringe and contrast injected. If specimen is needed for culture,

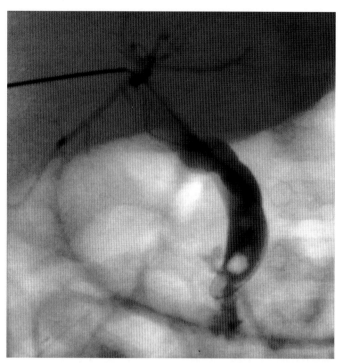

Figure 11.3.10 Percutaneous transhepatic cholangiography (PTC) with a distal filling defect and a wire in the duct.

this is aspirated prior to injection. With injection of contrast, other ducts will be visualized and, depending on the type of intervention, further access may be needed to facilitate intervention (Figure 11.3.10). The investigation of injury or obstruction in the biliary tree following liver transplant is the most common indication for cholangiography at our institution. Other indications are obstruction due to biliary atresia, choledochal cyst infection and inflammatory conditions like sclerosing cholangitis or ascending cholangitis.

PERCUTANEOUS TRANSHEPATIC TRANSCHOLECYSTIC CHOLANGIOGRAPHY

When the bile ducts are undilated and repeated attempts at ERCP or transhepatic access to the ducts is unsuccessful, a transcholecystic approach may be the best route for cholangiography. This procedure is performed under general anaesthetic with antibiotic coverage. Access is obtained to the gallbladder with a transhepatic approach using a 25-gauge spinal needle. Once the gallbladder is entered, bile is aspirated. Diluted contrast is injected and the filling of the ducts observed. If necessary, the patient can be placed in the Tredelenburg position to fill the intrahepatic ducts and morphine can be given to paralyze the sphincter of Oddi to encourage intrahepatic filling (Figure 11.3.11). Leakage is the main risk of this procedure and at the end, it is important to aspirate the gallbladder until it is empty and to keep the patient NPO overnight.

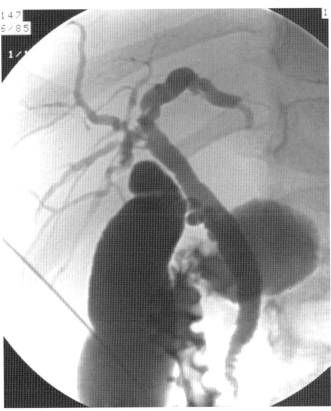

Figure 11.3.11 Percutaneous transhepatic transcholecystic cholangiography (PTTC) demonstrating primary sclerosing cholangitis.

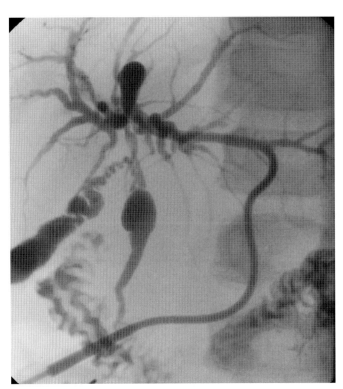

Figure 11.3.12 Left-sided biliary drainage with a common hepatic duct stenosis and common bile duct dilatation.

FURTHER READING

Garel LA, Belli D, Grignon A et al. Percutaneous cholecystography in children. Radiology 1987; 165:639–641.

Giorgio A, Amorosa P, de Stefano G et al. Ultrasonically-guided percutaneous transcholecystic cholangiography – an alternative approach in cases of biliary obstruction and failure of percutaneous transhepatic cholangiography. Hepatogastroenterology 1988; 35:268–270.

BILIARY DRAINAGE AND DILATATION

Indications for biliary drainage include any cause for obstruction with associated cholangitis and symptoms. The most common cause in the paediatric patient group is biliary strictures post-transplant. Percutaneous drainage may avoid the need for surgical re-exploration and preserve the graph or avoid retransplantation. After access is obtained with a 22-gauge Chiba needle, a wire is then introduced and preferably placed across the area of stricture. The access is dilated with a Neff introducer system and a 035 wire is introduced. The system can then be dilated and stented. Because of the different sizes of paediatric patients, catheters are usually made with side holes cut to accommodate the different size of patients and livers. After the catheter has been placed, the patient is returned to the ward and the catheter is flushed with saline twice daily. Once drainage is clear, the catheter is capped so that the bile drains internally (Figure 11.3.12).

FURTHER READING

Chardot C, Candinas D, Mirza D et al. Biliary complications after paediatric liver transplantation: Birmingham's experience. Transplant International 1995; 8:133–140.

Hoffer FA, Teele RL, Lillehei CW et al. Infected bilomas and hepatic artery thrombosis in infant recipients of liver transplants. Interventional radiology and medical therapy as an alternative to retransplantation. Radiology 1988; 169:435–438.

BILIARY DILATATION

Biliary dilatation is performed with an angioplasty-type balloon. The size of the balloon and diameter of the duct proximal to the stricture is measured. Several dilatations are performed for about 15–30 s (Figure 11.3.13). After dilatation, a biliary drain is left across the area of stricture with side holes made above and below the stricture (Figure 11.3.14).

FURTHER READING

Hancock BJ, Wiseman NE, Rusnak BW. Bile duct stricture in an infant with gastroschisis treated by percutaneous transhepatic drainage, biliary stenting, and balloon dilation. Journal of Pediatric Surgery 1989; 24:1071–1073.

Morrison MC, Lee MJ, Saini S et al. Percutaneous balloon dilatation of benign biliary strictures. Radiologic Clinics of North America 1990; 28:1191–1201.

Ward EM, Kiely MJ, Maus TP et al. Hilar biliary strictures after liver transplantation: cholangiography and percutaneous treatment. Radiology 1990; 177:259–263.

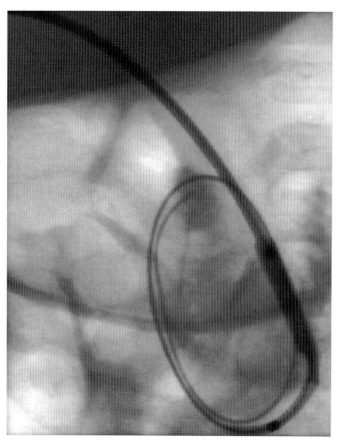

Figure 11.3.13 Balloon dilatation of a distal biliary stricture.

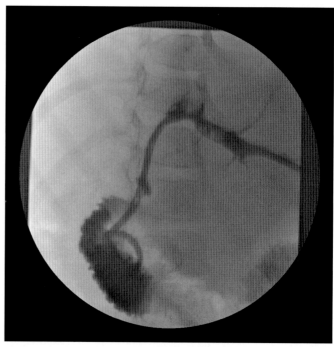

Figure 11.3.14 Internal external biliary drainage.

TRANSHEPATIC REMOVAL OF BILIARY CALCULI

Biliary calculi are rare; however, they can be removed with a basket and sheath, using a combination of snares.

FURTHER READING

Chiang HJ, Shan TY, Chen CJ. Percutaneous biliary stone removal under fluoroscopy. Zhonghua Yi Xue Za Zhi (Taipei) 1994; 54:343–348.

Park JH, Choi BI, Han MC. Percutaneous removal of residual intrahepatic stones. Radiology 1987; 163:619–623.

Portal Hypertension

Helen Carty

Portal hypertension exists when the portal venous pressure rises. The pressure difference between the wedged hepatic vein and the inferior vena cava (IVC) is normally no higher than 8 mmHg. Higher pressure differences than this indicate portal hypertension. It is classified as prehepatic, hepatic or posthepatic depending on the anatomical level at which the obstruction occurs. Causes of portal hypertension in children are shown in Table 11.4.1.

Clinical presentation is usually insidious, with gastrointestinal bleeding, either haematemesis, melaena or anaemia being the symptoms. Splenomegaly is clinically as well as radiologically evident. As the disease progresses, ascites occurs.

IMAGING

RADIOGRAPHS

Radiographs normally do not play a part in the diagnosis of portal hypertension; however, an incidental finding of splenomegaly (Figure 11.4.1) or ascites on a radiograph taken for some other purpose may first indicate the problem. Splenic enlargement is present if the tip of the spleen is visible below the 12th rib unless the lungs are hyperinflated. The spleen enlarges caudally and medially. It displaces the stomach bubble medially and the splenic flexure inferiorly.

Ascites has to be significant before it is seen on x-ray. When it is evident it is identified by lateral displacement of the flank stripes and central displacement of the bowel gas. As volumes increase, the abdomen becomes increasingly featureless.

Very rarely, one may see gastric varices in the fundus of the stomach.

ULTRASOUND

Ulrasound (US) is the simplest way of confirming a suspected diagnosis of portal hypertension (Figure 11.4.2). The patency or otherwise, the size and the direction of flow in the portal vein is easily demonstrated with colour flow Doppler imaging. Although flow measurements are obtainable, the main measurement of value is the peak velocity in the main portal vein. Values of less than 10 cm are abnormal. With progression of disease the flow in the portal vein oscillates with a to and fro pattern (Figure 11.4.2B),

then becomes stationary before it reverses to hepatofugal flow. Increased hepatic arterial flow may be seen in some patients. The positive diagnosis of portal hypertension relies on the demonstration of a hepatofugal collateral circulation. Ultrasound is also the initial imaging diagnostic tool in the demonstration of occlusion of the portal vein, cavernomatous transformation and the varying congenital malformations and fistulae. Hepatic and IVC patency are easily assessed in suspected cases of Budd–Chiari syndrome. Splenorenal shunts when present are easily shown. Varices at the lower oesophagus and in the gastric fundus, and gastroesophageal shunts in the lesser omentum may be visualized. The thickness of the omentum at the level of origin of the coeliac axis should be a maximum of one and a half times the size of the aortic diameter (Figure 11.4.3); in portal hypertension, due to stasis of lymphatic flow and the presence of omental varices, it is greater than this and may be up to three or four times thicker.

The presence of a patent paraumbilical vein in the ligamentum teres is also a sign of portal hypertension (Figure 11.4.4).

COMPUTED TOMOGRAPHY

Computed tomography (CT), though used less frequently in children than in adults in the investigation of portal hypertension

Table 11.4.1 Causes of portal hypertension in children

Prehepatic
1. Portal vein thrombosis – neonatal umbilical vein catheterization
2. Malformations – congenital portosystemic shunts sometimes associated with congenital heart disease
3. Infection – omphalitis, portal pyaemia and hepatic abscess or helminth infection
4. Tumour – liver, pancreatic or bile duct tumours

Hepatic
1. Biliary cirrhosis – biliary atresia, Byler's disease, congenital paucity of intrahepatic bile ducts, cystic fibrosis, choledochal cyst, sclerosing cholangitis, alpha-1 antitrypsin deficiency
2. Posthepatitis cirrhosis
3. Metabolic disease – e.g. Wilson's disease, tyrosinaemia
4. Congenital hepatic fibrosis

Posthepatic
1. Veno-occlusive disease – centrilobular
2. Budd–Chiari syndrome – hepatic vein or suprahepatic IVC thrombosis
3. Cardiac causes – constrictive pericarditis, chronic cardiac failure and rarely cortriatriatum

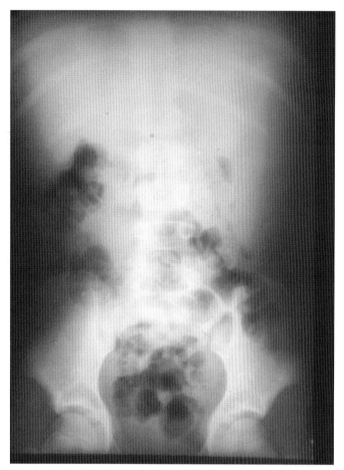

Figure 11.4.1 Abdominal radiograph showing an enlarged spleen. Note the displacement of the intestinal shadows away from it.

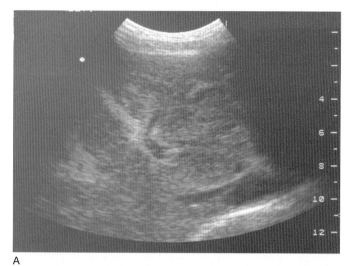

A

B

Figure 11.4.2 (A) Ultrasound of the liver in a girl with portal hypertension. Note fibrotic strands within the liver, seen as echodense structures, due to obliteration of the portal radicles. (B) Doppler study from the main portal vein showing a to and fro flow pattern.

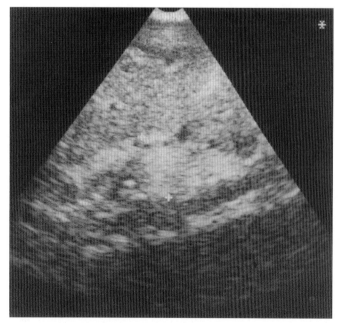

Figure 11.4.3 There is a thickened lesser omentum measured on the longitudinal scan between the posterior aspect of the left lobe of the liver and the aorta (cross).

because of the improved resolution of US in children, can be of value in the demonstration of cirrhosis (Figure 11.4.5) and of omental, gastric fundal and oesophageal varices in obese children and those with gassy abdomens or skeletal deformity, which makes US difficult. Ascites is easily detected. Extrahepatic changes of portal hypertension such as omental oedema, gastric and small bowel wall oedema and portosystemic shunts are shown, the latter comparing pre- and postcontrast scans.

MAGNETIC RESONANCE IMAGING (MRI)

There is little experience published to date on the value of MRI in portal hypertension. As the sophistication of MR angiographic techniques develops it may be a way of mapping the

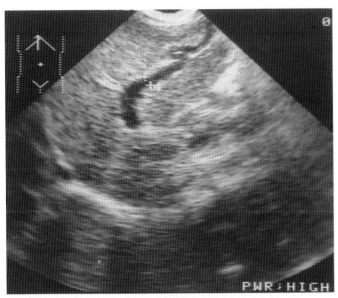

Figure 11.4.4 There is a patent paraumbilical vein in the ligamentum teres continuing into the left portal vein.

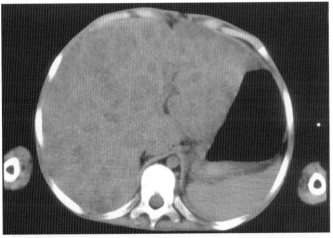

Figure 11.4.5 CT of a cystic fibrosis patient with gross macronodular cirrhosis of the liver and portal hypertension.

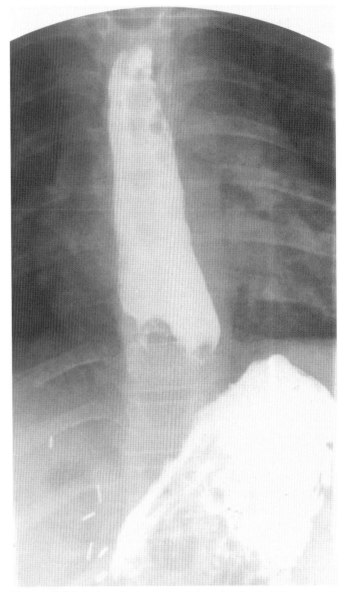

Figure 11.4.6 A view of an oesophagogram showing typical appearances of oesophageal varices. Note the serpiginous filling defects and the baggy oesophagus. Previous surgical clips relate to a nephrectomy for a Wilms' tumour. This child's portal hypertension is secondary to radiation injury to the liver.

abnormalities without invasive techniques. They are currently used in adults in difficult cases where US is not possible.

FLUOROSCOPY

Oesophageal and gastric varices may be demonstrated on contrast swallows. This as a diagnostic technique has been replaced by endoscopy but varices may be discovered incidentally during a study and radiologists should recognize them and know how to distinguish them from the rare lymphomatous infiltration of the oesophagus that may mimic varices. Both appear as irregular filling defects in the oesophageal mucosa (Figure 11.4.6). Varices alter in calibre in the supine position and with a Valsalva manoeuvre, getting bigger while lymphomatous deposits are not affected. The oesophagus with varices is often baggy and atonic.

ANGIOGRAPHY AND SPLENOPORTOGRAPHY

Both of these techniques have been replaced by non-invasive US and, where indicated, CT or MRI. When used today they are used selectively to show patency of the portal veins or shunts when other techniques have failed or are equivocal, or before surgery. Coeliac and mesenteric angiography with delayed images to show the portal venous phase are in general the preferred choice.

PREHEPATIC CAUSES OF PORTAL HYPERTENSION

PORTAL VEIN THROMBOSIS

Portal vein thrombosis is the most frequent cause of portal hypertension in children. It may occur without an identifiable cause. The liver, both clinically and on US, is usually normal in size. The portal vein is replaced by tortuous vessels (Figure 11.4.7), which are hepatopetal collateral veins and are known as a cavernoma. The main portal vein is not patent and is replaced by an echogenic strand (Figure 11.4.7). Sometimes, one of the collateral veins is large enough to simulate the portal vein (Figure 11.4.8) itself but this collateral vein is less straight than the portal vein and it is surrounded by other collateral veins. Varices in the lower oesophagus

and gastric fundus are usually present. Hepatopetal veins may be present in a thickened gallbladder wall.

The cavernoma may enlarge sufficiently to compress the bile ducts and lead to bile duct dilatation, which reverses after a portosystemic shunt. Management of children with portal vein thrombosis is initially conservative with prophylactic sclerotherapy of the varices but intervention is usually ultimately required to decrease the portal venous pressure by the creation of a portosystemic shunt or a porto-rex shunt. This latter procedure consists of joining the superior mesenteric vein or the splenic vein to the left portal vein when it is patent via the ligamentum teres. It is preferred to all the porto-systemic shunts because it is more physiological and it avoids the complications which are secondary to the diversion of the portal flow away from the liver: hepato-pulmonary syndrome (hypoxia due to pulmonary arterio-venous shunting), pulmonary hypertension and development of liver tumours. Full mapping of the entire portal venous system is then required. These children are managed in specialized children's liver units.

INTRAHEPATIC PORTOSYSTEMIC SHUNTS

These may arise congenitally but do not usually present until late childhood or in adult life. Clinical presentation may be with hepatic encephalopathy. There are multiple small portovenous shunts in the periphery of an otherwise normal liver.

ARTERIOVENOUS SHUNTS

These are very rare in children but may result from trauma or be congenital. They also occur with hereditary haemorrhagic telangiectasia, (Osler–Weber–Rendu disease) but clinical presentation in childhood is excessively rare (see Chapter 11.10).

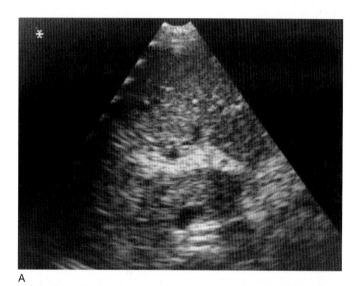

A

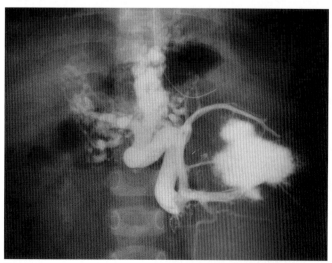

B

Figure 11.4.7 (A) Child with portal hypertension. The normal portal vein is replaced by fibrotic hyperechoic tissue. There are small tortuous vessels around it indicating a small cavernoma. (B) Splenoportogram showing typical appearances of a cavernoma. Note the enlarged tortuous splenic vein and multiple tortuous hepatopetal veins.

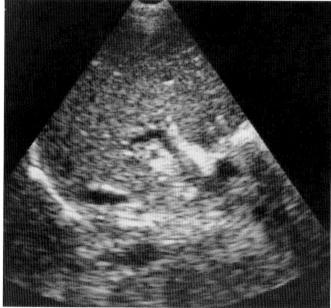

Figure 11.4.8 Oblique scan through the liver showing a large collateral hepatopetal vein, which could be mistaken for the main portal vein. Note the echogenic thrombosed portal vein adjacent to it.

HEPATIC CAUSES OF PORTAL HYPERTENSION

The main hepatic causes of portal hypertension are listed in Table 11.4.1. These can be summed up in two words – cirrhosis and fibrosis. Although there are many causes of cirrhosis, the ultrasonic appearance is broadly similar. Initially, the liver has a normal echotexture, which gradually progresses to an irregular texture (Figure 11.4.9) with either a micronodular or macronodular (Figure 11.4.5) appearance. The portal venous system is patent. In biliary cirrhosis, there may be dilatation of the bile ducts. Fatty replacement of the liver, which shows as diffuse increase in echogenicity, may progress to cirrhosis. A diffuse alteration in the attenuation of the liver may be seen on CT (Figure 11.4.10).

CONGENITAL HEPATIC FIBROSIS

This is a rare autosomal recessive disorder in which the children have both liver and renal disease (Figure 11.4.11). The renal disease is of the infantile polycystic kidney variety with slightly enlarged hyperechoic kidneys. This hyperechogenicity may be generalized or limited to the renal medulla, similar to that seen in medullary sponge kidneys. If an intravenous urography (IVU) is done there is streaky opacification of the dilated tubules. An IVU is not routinely indicated but the appearance may cause confusion if the examination is done for some other reason. The liver disease dominates the renal disease.

Clinical presentation is usually at around 12 years and may be the incidental finding of an enlarged spleen or with haematemesis from a bleeding oesophageal varix. Episodes of severe cholangitis are well-recognized complications. Disease severity is variable. The hepatic abnormalities on US include bright echoes from the portal radicles due to the fibrosis and sometimes cystic dilatation of the bile ducts. Hepatic cysts are seen with autosomal dominant polycystic renal disease but not with congenital hepatic fibrosis.

On angiography, duplication of the intrahepatic portal branches has been described as having hepatopetal collateral veins parallel to the normal patent portal vein, which may simulate a cavernoma. These are thought to be secondary to thrombosis or hypoplasia of the portal venous radicles, which has been described on liver biopsy.

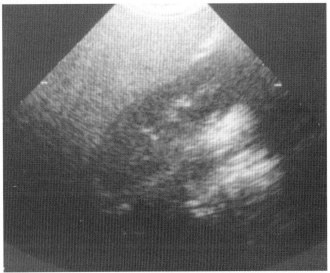

A

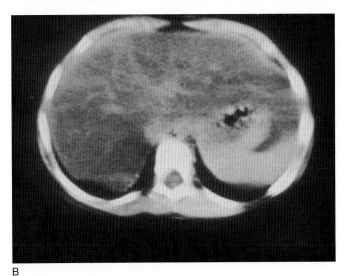

B

Figure 11.4.10 (A) US and (B) CT images of a girl with fatty replacement of the liver secondary to drug toxicity. Note the hyperechoic featureless liver on US and the low attenuation liver parenchyma on CT.

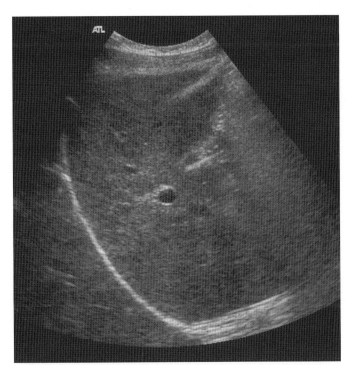

Figure 11.4.9 Longitudinal scan through the liver in a patient with cirrhosis. Note the irregular echotexture of the liver.

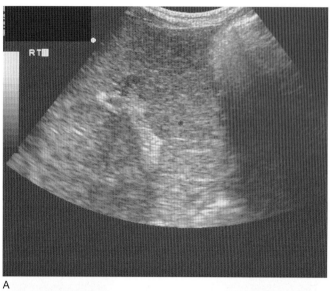

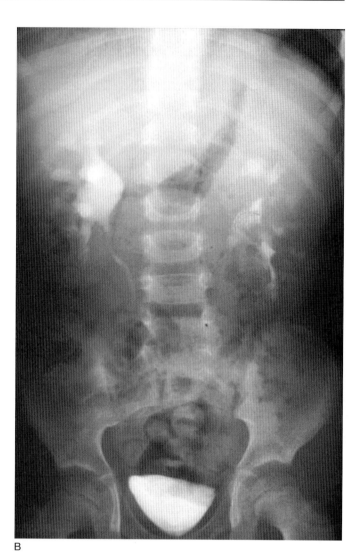

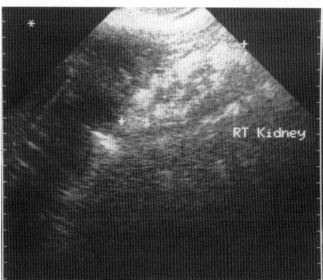

Figure 11.4.11 Ultrasound of the liver and an IVU film in a boy with congenital hepatic fibrosis. Note the replacement of the portal vein by the hyperechoic thrombosed portal vein (A). (B) IVU film of the same boy showing the enlarged kidneys with distortion of the pelvicalyceal system on the left and a blush at the renal papillae on the right due to the tubular filling. (C) Ultrasound image of another boy showing a hyperechoic kidney with the hyperechogenic areas in the renal medulla simulating nephrocalcinosis.

POSTHEPATIC CAUSES OF PORTAL HYPERTENSION

BUDD–CHIARI SYNDROME

Obstruction of the hepatic veins is usually secondary to IVC obstruction by thrombus, such as may occur with tumour or very rarely in children who have a thrombophilia or thrombotic tendency, such as occurs with antiphospholipid syndrome or Factor 5 Leiden deficiency. Occlusion of the major hepatic vein branches is termed the Budd–Chiari syndrome. Other described causes are oral contraceptive use, trauma to the hepatic veins, either accidental or at surgery, and congenital webs in the IVC. It is a rare occurrence in children and frequently the cause of the problem is not identified. In most patients, there is relative preservation of the caudate lobe of the liver, which may massively enlarge. This lobe drains directly into the IVC below the confluence of the hepatic veins and therefore may not be affected. This is reflected in sulphur colloid scintigraphy, when diminished activity is shown in most of the liver compared with the relatively normal activity in the caudate lobe. Clinical presentation may be acute and abrupt with

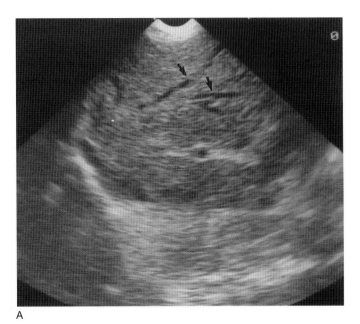

A

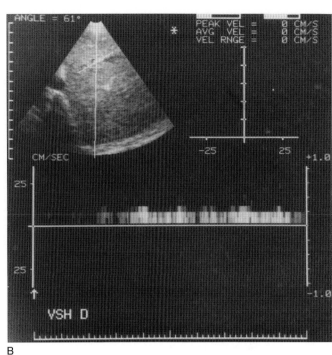

B

Figure 11.4.12 Two images from an 8-year-old child with Budd–Chiari syndrome who presented with hepatomegaly and ascites. (A) Ultrasound. The right hepatic vein is tortuous and there are collaterals (arrows). (B) Duplex Doppler study demonstrating inverted flow in the right hepatic vein.

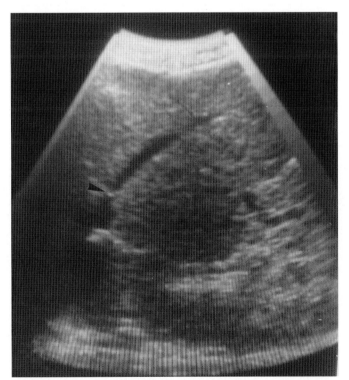

Figure 11.4.13 Ultrasound. Another child with Budd–Chiari syndrome showing narrowing of the ostium of the right hepatic vein with proximal dilatation.

abdominal pain, ascites and hepatomegaly but in children it is usually more insidious and presentation is mostly with the features of portal hypertension.

Ultrasound shows the occluded hepatic veins and if the IVC is involved thrombus or occlusion of it. The occluded veins are replaced by echogenic strands, dilatation behind the occlusions and variably tortuous collateral veins (Figures 11.4.12 and 11.4.13). Pulsed Doppler shows flow reversal in patent radicles. The hepatic veins are normally visible. The absence of any hepatic vein demonstration or flow is very suspicious of Budd–Chiari but this may also occur in cirrhosis and some caution is needed in the presence of this.

CT shows decreased attenuation and patchy enhancement in the enlarged congested liver with relative preservation of the caudate lobe (Figure 11.4.14).

Surgical management is by the creation of a portocaval shunt but, before this is done, mapping of the caval and hepatic vein anatomy by cavography is required. The venographic appearance is described as a spider's web (Figure 11.4.15). Hepatic vein opacification may be demonstrated by retrograde venography via the inferior or superior vena cava or, if this is impossible, via a transhepatic approach. If suitable lesions are found, transluminal angioplasty may be performed to dilate limited stenoses.

VENO-OCCLUSIVE DISEASE

Veno-occlusive disease is seen in two groups of patients. It was originally reported in Caribbean children who ingested bush tea that contained pyrolizidine alkaloids but is now more frequently seen in children who have had bone marrow transplants. The hepa-

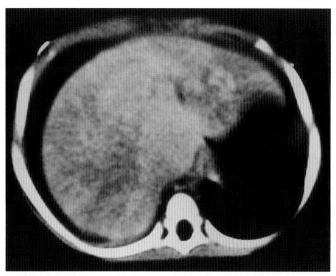

Figure 11.4.14 CT image of a 3-year-old with Budd–Chiari syndrome. There is heterogeneous contrast enhancement of the right and left lobes of the liver with normal contrast enhancement of the caudate lobe, typical of Budd–Chiari syndrome.

totoxins cause oedema, which slows blood flow in the portal and hepatic venules to the point at which thrombosis occurs. It may also result from radiation and chemotherapy. In some cases, it appears to be idiopathic. There is obliteration of the central draining veins of the hepatic lobules by an inflammatory fibrotic process. The main portal and hepatic veins are patent. As pressures rise, reversal of normal portal venous flow occurs so that it becomes hepatofugal. There is decreased hepatic arterial flow and an increased hepatic artery resistive index. Oedema of the gallbladder wall, ascites and liver enlargement are seen. Recognition is important as anticoagulation may halt the process.

CARDIAC CAUSES OF PORTAL HYPERTENSION

These are usually obvious clinically but occasionally constrictive pericarditis may not be diagnosed before US. Ultrasonic clues are the demonstration of the thickened pericardium, enlargement of the IVC with dampening of the variation with respiration and engorgement of the hepatic veins.

DEMONSTRATION OF SURGICAL PORTOSYSTEMIC SHUNTS

Most children who have undergone surgery for relief of their portal hypertension are followed up in specialized centres for children's liver disease. Before embarking on US, which is the main investigation for assessing shunt patency, it is important to know what kind of surgery took place and what type of shunt has been fashioned. Shunt patency is established in the early postoperative period and then monitored. Indirect signs of shunt patency are: a decrease in the number and size of collateral veins around the oesophagus and a decrease in size of omental thickness, a decrease of the portal flow and a return to hepatofugal flow on Doppler studies, and an increase in the diameter of the IVC with dampening of the variation of the size of the IVC with respiration.

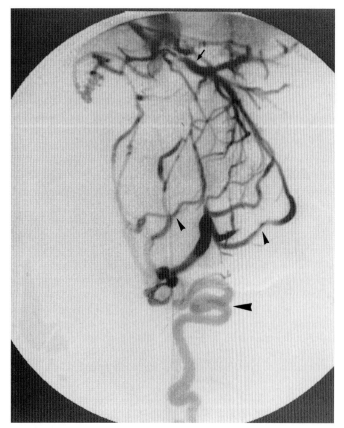

Figure 11.4.15 Budd–Chiari syndrome. Retrograde phlebography showing a spider web network of intrahepatic vein collaterals. The arrowheads demonstrate obstruction of the hepatic vein ostium. The catheter is in the left hepatic vein (small arrow). Contrast drains by a tortuous extrahepatic parietal vein (large arrowhead). Figure courtesy of Dr Daniele Pariente.

FURTHER READING

Agrons GA, Corse WR, Markowitz RI, Suarez ES, Perry DR. Gastrointestinal manifestations of cystic fibrosis: radiologic-pathologic correlation. Radiographics 1996; 16:871–893.

Barakat M. Doppler sonographic findings in children with idiopathic portal vein cavernous deformity and variceal hemorrhage. Journal of Ultrasound Medicine 2002; 21:825–830.

Bayraktar Y, Balkanci F, Kayhan B, et al. Congenital hepatic fibrosis associated with cavernous transformation of the portal vein. Hespatogastroenterology 1997; 44:1588–1594.

Brown JJ, Naylor MJ, Yagan N. Imaging of hepatic cirrhosis. Radiology 1997; 202:1–16.

Day DL, Carpenter BLM. Abdominal complications in paediatric bone marrow transplantation recipients. Radiographics 1993; 13:1101–1112.

Herbetko J, Grigg AP, Buckley AR et al. Venoocclusive liver disease after bone marrow transplantation: findings at duplex sonography. American Journal of Roentgenology 1992; 158:1001–1005.

Lenthall R, Kane PA, Heaton ND, Karani JB. Segmental portal hypertension due to splenic vein obstruction: imaging findings and diagnostic pitfalls in four cases. Clinical Radiology 1999; 54:540–544.

Lomas DJ. The liver. In: Grainger R, Allison D, Adam A et al., eds. Grainger & Allison's Diagostic Radiology, 4th edn; London: Harcourt Publishers; 2001; 1237–1376.

Patriquin H, Lenaerts C, Smith L et al. Liver disease in children with cystic fibrosis: US-biochemical comparison in 195 patients. Radiology 1999; 211:229–232.

Shapir R, Stancato-Pasik A, Glajchen N et al. Color Doppler applications in hepatic imaging. Clinical Imaging 1998; 22:272–279.

Shun A, Delaney DP, Martin HC, Henry GM, Stephen M. Portosystemic shunting for paediatric portal hypertension. Journal of Pediatric Surgery 1997; 32:489–493.

Siegel MJ. Pediatric sonography, 3rd edn. Philadelphia: Lippincott, Williams & Wilkins; 2002.

Stringer D, Babyn P. Pediatric gastrointestinal imaging and intervention, 2nd edn. Hamilton, Ontario: Decker; 2000.

Uno A, Ishida H, Konno K et al. Portal hypertension in children and young adults: sonographic and color Doppler findings. Abdominal Imaging 1997; 22:72–78.

Vocke AK, Kardorff R, Ehrich JH. Sonographic measurements of the portal vein and its intrahepatic branches in children. European Journal of Ultrasound 1998; 7:121–127.

Westra S, Zaninovic A, Vargas J et al. The value of portal vein pulsatility on duplex sonograms as a sign of portal hypertension in children with liver disease. American Journal of Roentgenology 1995; 165:167–172.

Liver Infections

Danièle Pariente

LIVER ABSCESS

Liver abscess is an uncommon condition in childhood. Early diagnosis with ultrasound (US) and aspiration, and treatment with appropriate antibiotic therapy and percutaneous drainage have dramatically improved the prognosis. Although mainly reported in immunocompromised children with chronic granulomatous disease, underlying malignancy and immunosuppression, liver abscess can occur without any identifiable predisposing disease. Liver abscesses have been encountered in all age groups. In the neonatal period, it may be secondary to umbilical vein catheterization, omphalitis, septicaemia or abdominal surgery (Figure 11.5.1). In older children, it may be secondary to other intra-abdominal sites of infection, e.g. appendicitis, or to systemic bacteraemia.

The clinical presentation is non-specific but hepatomegaly with tenderness, fever and biological signs of infection are present in most children. A raised hemidiaphragm with basal pneumonia, atelectasis or pleural effusion are frequently seen on chest films. US is the screening modality of choice but it shows a broad spectrum of patterns, ranging from an anechoic to a highly echogenic mass (Figure 11.5.2). The lesion may have thick walls or ill-defined borders, a fluid-filled centre or contain gas. It may be isolated in one lobe or be multiple and involve both lobes. Computed tomography (CT) scanning (Figure 11.5.3) may suggest the diagnosis when it shows a fluid-filled centre and peripheral enhancement but these signs are not constant. The diagnosis is made by percutaneous aspiration under imaging guidance, which yields purulent material from which the infecting organism may be identified. If the aspiration is negative, a percutaneous needle biopsy has to be performed so that a tumour with necrosis, which may mimic an abscess, is not missed.

The imaging appearance is similar irrespective of the infective organism, which may include *Staphylococcus*, *Streptococcus*, *Escherichia coli*, *Klebsiella*, *Pseudomonas*, *Proteus*, *Candida* and amoebiasis. The management of all liver abscesses, irrespective of aetiology, that require drainage is percutaneous drainage using a pigtail catheter inserted under US or CT guidance. Surgery is reserved for those cases that do not resolve.

Complications include a biliary fistula but this is rare unless associated with trauma. Neonates are at risk for the development of portal vein thrombosis and subsequent cavernoma.

Amoebic abscess of the liver may occur in the absence of amoebic colitis. About half of the cases have a history of diarrhoea.

It is most prevalent in children younger than 3 years with a peak incidence in the first year of life (Figure 11.5.4). Delayed or absent seropositivity, which are frequent in children, may delay the diagnosis and increase the risk of extension or rupture to adjacent organs or spaces, pleura, lungs, pericardial sac, intra-abdominal or abdominal wall.

Hepatic candidiasis is a rare though serious complication seen in immunocompromised children. Diffuse micronodules involving the liver and also the spleen may be seen on US, CT or magnetic resonance imaging (MRI) (Figure 11.5.5). In some cases, a typical pattern of 'wheels within wheels' is demonstrated by US.

The early identification of the infecting organism and prompt institution of treatment with appropriate antibiotics are mandatory. If blood cultures or serological tests are negative, needle aspiration of the abscess under US guidance has to be performed as soon as possible. Percutaneous drainage is recommended if the abscess is large, if there is failure to respond to medical therapy and if there are signs of impending rupture into adjacent organs such as the pleural space or the pericardium. Surgery is only reserved for the very uncommon cases that fail to respond to percutaneous drainage.

Resolution of the abscess cavity can be monitored by US and careful follow-up is especially recommended in neonates who seem to be more at risk of developing portal vein thrombosis and cavernoma.

FURTHER READING

Chusid MJ. Pyogenic liver abscess in infancy and childhood. Pediatrics 1978; 62:554–559.

Garel LA, Pariente DM, Nezeloff C et al. Liver involvement in chronic granulomatous disease: the role of US in diagnosis and treatment. Radiology 1984; 153:117–121.

Johannsen EC, Sifri CD, Madoff LC. Pyogenic liver abscesses. Infectious Disease Clinics of North America 2000; 14:547–563.

Merten DF, Kirks DR. Amebic liver abscess in children: the role of diagnostic imaging. American Journal of Roentgenology 1984; 143:1325–1329.

Moore S, Millar AJW, Cywes S. Liver abscess in chilhood: a 13-year review. Pediatric Surgery International 1988; 3:27–32.

Moss TJ, Pysher TJ. Hepatic abscess in neonates. American Journal of Disease in Childhood 1981; 135:726–728.

Pastakia B, Shawker TH, Thaler M, O'Leary T, Pizzo PA. Hepatosplenic candidiasis: wheels within wheels. Radiology 1988; 166:417–421.

Rajak CL, Gupta S, Jain S et al. Percutaneous treatment of liver abscesses: needle aspiration versus catheter drainage. American Journal of Roentgenology 1998; 170:1035–1039.

Vachon L, Diament MJ, Stanley P. Percutaneous drainage of hepatic abscesses in children. Journal of Pediatric Surgery 1986; 21:366–368.

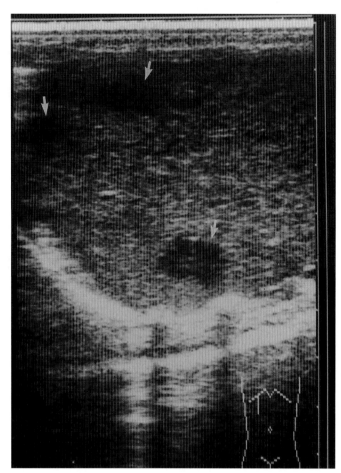

Figure 11.5.1 Multiple pyogenic abscesses in a newborn baby girl with staphylococcus sepsis secondary to umbilical venous catheterization. There are multiple hypoechoic nodules consistent with abscesses (arrows). With antibiotic treatment, the abscesses resolved but portal cavernoma developed following portal vein thrombosis.

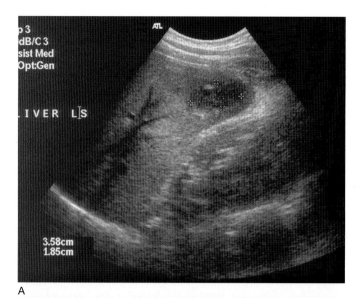

A

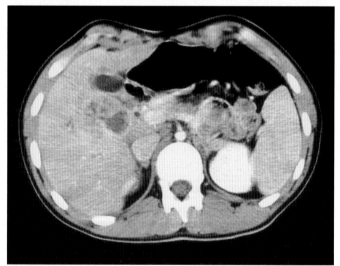

B

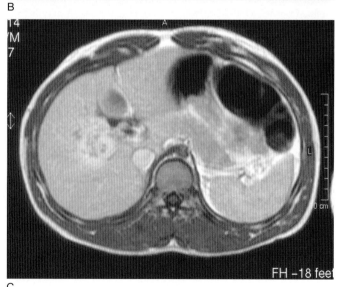

C

Figure 11.5.2 (A) Ultrasound, (B) contrast-enhanced CT and (C) contrast-enhanced T1-weighted MRI of a boy with immunodeficiency and liver abscesses. Note, on US (A) the hypoechoic and poorly defined abscess. On both CT and MRI, the abscesses are seen to better effect.

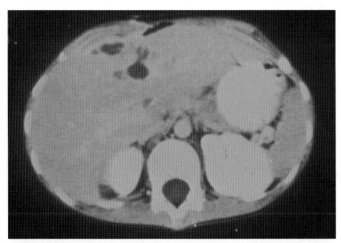

Figure 11.5.3 CT of a child with post-traumatic liver abscess. Note the fluid-filled cavities with peripheral enhancement. The air-filled lesion anteriorly is the tracker of a drain.

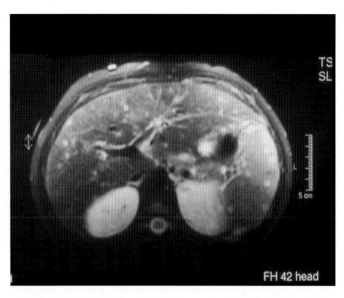

Figure 11.5.5 T2-weighted MRI of liver showing the typical nodular appearances of candidiasis.

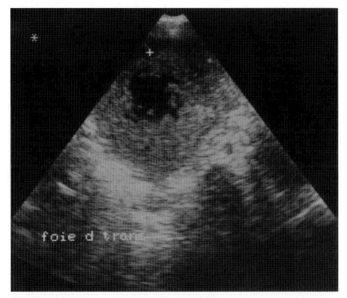

Figure 11.5.4 Amoebic abscess in an 18-month-old boy visible as a 7-cm mass with central liquefaction. Percutaneous drainage was performed (foie d trans = right transverse liver).

and on a specific serological test. Spontaneous resolution generally occurs. Normally, the granulomas disappear within 1–5 months; in some cases, there are residual hepatic and/or splenic calcifications. Cases of associated portal vein thrombosis and severe ascites have been reported.

FURTHER READING

Danon O, Duval-Arnould M, Osman Z et al. Hepatic and splenic involvement in cat-scratch disease: imaging features. Abdominal Imaging 2000; 25:182–183.

Hopkins KL, Simoneaux SF, Patrick LE et al. Imaging manifestations of cat-scratch disease. American Journal of Roentgenology 1996; 166:435–438.

Ruess M, Sander A, Brandis M, Berner R. Portal vein and bone involvement in disseminated cat-scratch disease: report of 2 cases. Clinical Infectious Diseases 2000; 31:818–821.

Talenti E, Cesaro S, Scapinello A, Perale R, Zanesco L. Disseminated hepatic and splenic calcifications following cat-scratch disease. Pediatric Radiology 1994; 24:342–343.

Windsor JJ. Cat-scratch disease: epidemiology, aetiology and treatment. British Journal of Biomedical Sciences 2001; 58:101–110.

CAT-SCRATCH DISEASE

This is a clinical syndrome that usually presents as a lymphadenopathy associated with a cat scratch or bite. Atypical presentation is seen in up to 25% of cases including hepatic or hepatosplenic lesions. It has a worldwide distribution and is probably underdiagnosed. The organism responsible is *Bartonella henselae*, a Gram-negative bacillus. Radiological features of US, CT and MRI are not specific, consisting of multinodular hypoechoic and hypodense lesions throughout the liver and spleen, sometimes associated with hepatic pedicle adenopathy (Figure 11.5.6). The key to the diagnosis relies on a history of cat contact

HEPATIC TUBERCULOSIS

Although the last decade has seen a resurgence in the incidence of tuberculosis, abdominal involvement is uncommon in children, complicating pulmonary tuberculosis in 1% to 5% of cases. Liver involvement consists of single or multiple low-density lesions with calcification and sometimes ring enhancement with contrast. Splenic lesions are often associated. The other findings of abdominal tuberculosis mainly include lymphadenopathy with a low-density centre and a contrast-enhancing rim, and sometimes calcification, high-density ascites, omental and mesenteric involvement, and thickening of bowel loop walls. Calcification is seen frequently with healing of the infection.

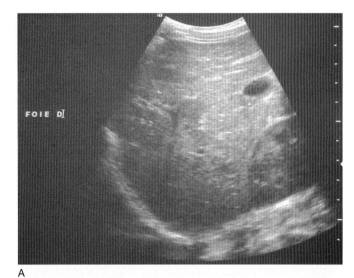

A

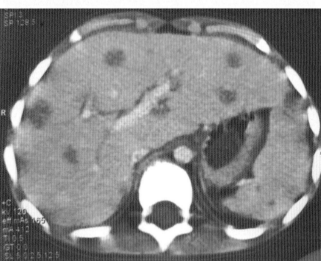

B

Figure 11.5.6 Cat-scratch disease. A 7-year-old child presenting with prolonged fever. History of cat scratches. (A) US examination showed multiple hypoechoic nodules (→) and adenopathies in the liver hilum. (B) Contrast-enhanced CT confirms the multiple hypodense nodules consistent with cat-scratch disease. Without any treatment, a follow-up US examination 1 month later demonstrated complete resolution of the nodules.

FURTHER READING

Andronikou S, Welman CJ, Kader E. The CT features of abdominal tuberculosis in children. Pediatric Radiology 2002; 32:75–81.

HYDATID DISEASE

Hydatid disease is common in sheep-grazing countries such as those of Southern Europe and particularly in the Mediterranean basin. Man is infected by contact with the excreta of dogs when it contains the ova of tapeworms of the genus *Echinococcus*. The ova are ingested and then hatch into larvae, which burrow through the intestinal mucosa and are carried in the portal vein to the liver

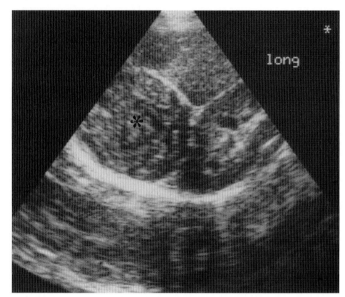

Figure 11.5.7 Heterogeneous hydatid cyst presenting as a solid mass in a 4-year-old Algerian boy (*). Diagnosis was made at surgery.

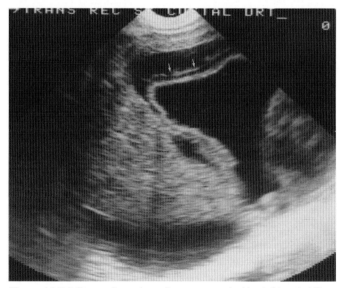

Figure 11.5.8 Traumatic rupture of an unsuspected hydatid cyst. US shows fluid in the pouch of Douglas and a large cystic intrahepatic mass with a double wall corresponding to the germinative membrane (arrows).

where they develop into adult cysts. Cysts may also occur in the lungs, spleen, peritoneum, bones, brain, orbit, heart and soft tissues.

Most cysts are clinically silent but pain, abdominal distension and a palpable mass may be present. The hydatid cysts are easily seen with US, which is the method of choice for the diagnosis of the disease in the liver. There is a spectrum of findings depending on the stage of the lesion, which range from a simple anechoic cyst to a double-walled cyst with visibility of the germinative membrane, or a cyst with septations and internal heterogeneous echoes (Figure 11.5.7 and 11.5.8). The diagnosis may be confirmed by serological tests but these are only positive in 80% of cases. CT is useful to define the precise extent of the disease before treatment (Figure 11.5.9 and 11.5.10). Complications include intraperitoneal rupture of an intrahepatic cyst, rupture into the biliary tract with, in a few cases, biliary obstruction and dissemination to other abdominal organs. Ultrasound-guided percutaneous sclerotherapy has been developed and reported by Turkish teams and seems to represent an alternative to surgery when the cysts are multiple and large.

FURTHER READING

Andronikou S, Welman CJ, Kader E. Classic and unusual appearances of hydatid disease in children. Pediatric Radiology 2002; 32:817–828.

Kabaalioglu A, Karaali K, Apaydin A et al. Ultrasound-guided percutaneous sclerotherapy of hydatid liver cysts in children. Pediatric Surgery International 2000; 16:346–350.

Lewall DB, Mc Corkell SJ. Hepatic echinococcal cysts: sonographic appearance and classification. Radiology 1985; 155:773–775.

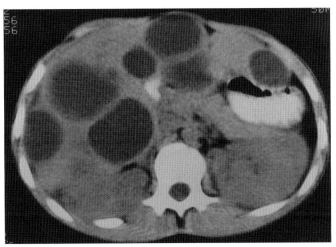

Figure 11.5.9 Hydatid disease. Multiple hypodense hydatid cysts involve the whole liver: 16 cysts could be identified on CT.

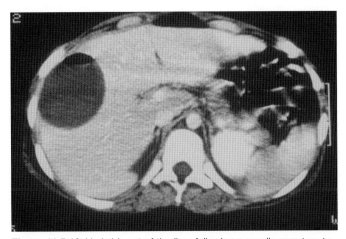

Figure 11.5.10 Hydatid cyst of the liver following a needle puncture to obtain material for diagnosis.

ASCARIASIS

The normal habitat of the adult parasite *Ascaris lumbricoides* is the small intestine of humans. The worms may migrate into the biliary system and cause one of the most severe complications of ascariasis, which is much greater in children than in adults.

The clinical manifestations vary in severity depending upon the number of parasites in the biliary system: these include jaundice, fever, rupture of the hepatic or common bile duct with biliary peritonitis and abscess. Two severe complications are infective phlebitis and embolization from the inferior vena cava (IVC) to the pulmonary artery.

The diagnosis is made by finding ova in the faeces or the adult worm in the digestive tract. The worm may be seen in the gallbladder or dilated bile duct on US examination and also in the bowel loops. The worm may also be seen by endoscopy in the intestine or on retrograde cholangiopancreatography, during which procedure the worms may be removed from the biliary duct.

FURTHER READING

Bahu Mda G, Baldisseroto M, Custodio CM, Grahla CZ, Mangili AR. Hepatobiliary and pancreatic complications of ascariasis in children: a study of seven cases. Journal of Pediatric Gastroenterology and Nutrition 2001; 33:271–275.

Danaci M, Belet U, Selcuk MB, Akan H, Bastemir M. Ascariasis of the gallbladder: radiological evaluation and follow-up. Pediatric Radiology 1999; 29:80.

FASCIOLASIS

This is due to infection by the large leaf-shaped trematode, *Fasciola hepatica*, common in Europe. Man acquires the infection by ingestion of aquatic plants, particularly watercress, or by drinking water containing the metacercariae (cystic form of the parasite). It migrates through the duodenum, enters the peritoneal cavity and reaches the capsule of the liver. The acute phase of the disease corresponds to migration through the liver: there is hepatomegaly, abdominal pain, fever and leucocytosis with a characteristic marked eosinophilia. US and CT may show superficial granulomas previously seen only on laparoscopy or at surgery. These lesions may be arranged in a track-like fashion (burrow tract), which is characteristic.

During the chronic phase, the parasite resides in the biliary tract. Patients may be asymptomatic or present with biliary obstruction or cholangitis. US may display the parasite in the gallbladder or in the common bile duct as an echogenic lesion or as multiple conglomerate lesions, without acoustic shadowing and sometimes mobile.

FURTHER READING

Cauquil P, Pariente D, Loyer E, Lallemand D. Unusual sonographic appearance of a case of hepatic fasciolasis. Journal of Radiology 1986; 67:715–717.

Han JK, Choi BI, Cho JM et al. Radiological findings of human fascioliasis. Abdominal Imaging 1993; 18:261–264.

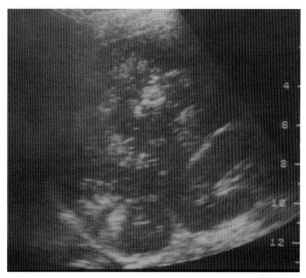

Figure 11.5.11 Ultrasound of the liver showing typical appearances of gas in the distribution of the portal veins. The gas is seen as bright echogenic lesions. This boy had portal pyaemia from appendicitis.

PORTAL PYAEMIA

Septicaemia arising from gastrointestinal tract infection may result in portal pyaemia. The two most frequent causes are necrotizing enterocolitis, seen in neonates, and an appendix abscess in older children. Bubbles of gas are seen within the portal venous radicles on US (Figure 11.5.11). In severe cases, the portal vein gas, with its typical branching pattern, is seen on abdominal radiographs.

Liver Tumours

Ganesh Krishnamurthy, E L Harvey J Teo

Primary paediatric hepatic neoplasms are the most common primary malignancies of the gastrointestinal tract in children and these constitute only 0.5–2% of all paediatric malignancies. Hepatic masses in general constitute 5–6% of all intra-abdominal masses in children. Among the primary tumours, hepatoblastomas are the third most common abdominal malignancy, after Wilm's tumour and neuroblastoma.

MODALITIES AND TECHNIQUES

With the rapidly improving technology used in diagnostic imaging, the diagnosis and characterization of lesions have improved significantly. Diagnostic imaging techniques help to characterize lesions, distinguish benign from malignant lesions and define the precise anatomical location of the lesions. Because surgical resection remains the mainstay of treatment of many of the liver lesions, definition of the extent of the mass lesion and its relationship to hepatic segmental anatomy is essential.

The usual presentation of a benign malignant liver tumour in children is a palpable mass. Other presentations include anorexia, vomiting, pain, jaundice, haemorrhage, congestive heart failure, paraneoplastic syndromes and symptoms related to metastases.

There are many imaging modalities available for imaging paediatric hepatic masses, including plain radiography, ultrasonography (US), computed tomography (CT), magnetic resonance imaging (MRI), angiography and radionuclide techniques. The choice and sequence of the imaging modalities depends upon the availability, the institution's protocol and the physician's or radiologist's preference. Plain films in most cases show nonspecific findings such as calcifications, lung or bony metastasis, and bowel obstruction. US is the most commonly used initial imaging technique used to evaluate a suspected hepatic mass in a child. US accurately identifies or excludes a mass and identifies the organ of origin, and characterizes it as cystic or solid. US findings help the radiologist to determine the remainder of the child's imaging work-up. Intraoperative US using high frequency transducers is very helpful in detecting focal hepatic lesions.

Frequency shifts and peak systolic velocity identified by Doppler studies have been used to differentiate benign from malignant lesions. Contrast agents help to evaluate the lesion's vascularity. Nevertheless, Doppler findings are usually non-specific in distinguishing benign from malignant liver lesions.

Whether CT scans or MRI is the imaging modality of choice for the evaluation of liver masses in children is still a controversial issue. New generation multislice CT scanners are fast and provide excellent information when evaluating a hepatic mass. Multislice fast scanners are particularly useful in hypervascular tumours and for multiplanar reconstruction. CT arterial portography (CTAP) and lipiodol CT, which increase the sensitivity and specificity of characterizing liver lesions, are rarely if ever done in children.

The newer MRI sequences that use shorter scan times result in fewer motion artifacts and also provide better spatial resolution. These sequences can image the entire liver in a single breath-hold of as little as 10 s, using echo-planar and gradient-echo imaging. The use of intravenous gadolinium has been shown to increase the detection of hepatic lesions. Simultaneous magnetic resonance angiography (MRA) demonstrates the hepatic vasculature, which is required for surgical planning. MRI, which gives maximum characterization of anatomical detail of the lesion, makes it a preferred imaging technique to CT.

Radionuclide scintigraphy still plays a useful role in evaluating certain focal liver lesions like haemangioma by distinguishing regenerating nodules from hepatocellular carcinoma and by characterizing certain tumour-like conditions, particularly focal nodular hyperplasia. Interventional techniques such as tumour embolization and percutaneous biopsy are performed in specialized institutions.

The age of the child, presentation, level of alpha fetoprotein (AFP) and whether the lesion is solitary or multiple also help prebiopsy diagnosis. The types of liver tumour vary among young and older children. Under 5 years of age, the common hepatic tumours include infantile haemangioendothelioma, mesenchymal hamartoma and metastasis from neuroblastoma or Wilm's tumour. In children over 5 years, hepatocellular carcinoma, undifferentiated embryonal sarcoma, hepatocellular adenoma and metastasis are more frequent. A raised serum AFP usually indicates hepatoblastoma or hepatocellular carcinoma or, very rarely, infantile haemangioendothelioma (less than 3%). Other hepatic tumours are not associated with a rise in serum AFP. The presence of multiple lesions in the liver usually indicates a metastatic disease or a lymphoproliferative disorder. A history of immunocompromise suggests a lymphoproliferative disorder and a history of congestive heart failure with liver mass usually suggests infantile haemangioendothelioma.

FURTHER READING

Baron RL. Detection of liver neoplasms: techniques and outcomes. Abdominal Imaging 1994; 19:320–324.

Blakeborough A, Ward J, Wilson D et al. Hepatic lesion detection at MR imaging: A comparative study with four sequences. Radiology 1997; 203:79–82.

Bluemke DA, Soyer PA, Chan BW et al. Spiral CT during arterial portography: technique and applications. Radiographics 1995; 15:623–626.

Blumke DA, Soyer P, Fishman EK. Helical (spiral) CT of the liver. Radiologic Clinics of North America 1995; 33:863–867.

Butts K, Riederer SJ, Ehman RL et al. Echo-planar imaging of the liver with a standard MR imaging system. Radiology 1993; 189:259–262.

Davey MS, Cohen MD. Imaging of gastrointestinal malignancy in childhood. Radiologic Clinics of North America 1996; 34:717–742.

de Lange EE, Mugler JPR, Bosworth JE et al. MR imaging of the liver: Breath-hold T1-weighter MPGRE compared with conventional T2-weighter SE imaging – lesion detection, localization, and characterisation. Radiology 1994; 190:727–730.

Drane WE. Nuclear medicine techniques for the liver and biliary system: update for the 1990s. Radiologic Clinics of North America 1991; 29:1129–1150.

Earls JP, Rofsky NM, DeCorato DR et al. Hepatic arterial phase dynamic gadolinium-enhanced MR imaging: optimization with a test examination and a power injector. Radiology 1997; 202:268–271.

Fujita M, Kuroda C, Kumatani T et al. Comparison between conventional and spiral CT in patients with hypervascular hepatocellular carcinoma. European Journal of Radiology 1994; 18:134–138.

Gazelle GS, Haaga JR. Hepatic neoplasms: surgically relevant segmental anatomy and imaging techniques. American Journal of Roentgenology 1992; 158:1015–1018.

Hamm B, Mahfouz AE, Taupitz M et al. Liver metastases: improved detection with dynamic gadolinium-enhanced MR imaging. Radiology 1997; 202:677–680.

Larson RE, Semelka RC, Bagley AS et al. Hypervascular malignant liver lesions: comparison of various MR imaging pulse sequences and dynamic CT. Radiology 1994; 192:393–399.

Lencioni R, Pinto F, Armillotta N et al. Intrahepatic metastatic nodules of hepatocellular carcinoma detected at Lipiodo-CT: Imaging-pathologic correlation. Abdominal Imaging 1997; 22:253–257.

Lupetin AR, Cammisa BA, Beckman I et al. Spiral CT during arterial portography. Radiographics 1996; 16:723–726.

Nelson RC. Techniques for computed tomography of the liver. Radiologic Clinics of North America 1991; 29:1199–1201.

Numata K, Tanaka K, Mitsui K et al. Flow characteristics of hepatic tumours at color Doppler sonography: correlation with arteriographic findings. American Journal of Roentgenology 1993; 160:515–521.

Pobeil RS, Bisset GS III. Pictorial essay: Imaging of liver tumours in infant and child. Pediatric Radiology 1995; 25:495–506.

Polacin A, Kalender WA, Marchal G. Evaluation of section sensitivity profiles and image noise in spiral CT. Radiology 1992; 185:29–35.

Reinhold C, Hammers L, Taylor CR et al. Characterisation of focal hepatic lesions with duplex sonography: findings in 198 patients. American Journal of Roentgenology 1995; 164:1131–1135.

Shirkoda A, Konez O, Shetty AN et al. Mesenteric circulation: Three dimensional MR angiography with gadolinium enhanced multi echo gradient echo technique. Radiology 1997; 202:257–262.

Shuckett BM, Chee H, Williams T et al. The Liver. In: Stringer DA, Babyn P, eds. Paediatric gastrointestinal imaging and intervention, 2nd edn. Hamilton: B.C. Decker Inc.; 2000: 611–699.

Teo ELHJ, Strouse PJ, Prince MR. Applications of magnetic resonance imaging and magnetic resonance angiography to evaluate the hepatic vasculature in the pediatric patient. Pediatric Radiology 1999; 29:238–243.

MALIGNANT TUMOURS OF THE LIVER

PRIMARY TUMOURS

The important primary malignant hepatic tumours in children include hepatocellular carcinoma (including fibrolamellar hepatocellular carcinoma), rhabdomyosarcoma and undifferentiated embryonal sarcoma.

There are no pathognomonic imaging features for hepatic malignancies. Though the age of presentation, clinical features and biochemistry may suggest the diagnosis, radiography is required for definitive diagnosis. The primary role of imaging is to define accurately the extent of the lesion in relation to the lobar anatomy of the liver, vascular and biliary anatomy. This is essential for surgical resection. Tumour confined to the left or right lobe or the right lobe plus the medial segment of the left lobe can be considered surgically resectable. If the tumour is deemed non-resectable at initial imaging, the line of management changes to chemotherapy with or without radiation, following biopsy.

FURTHER READING

Davey MS, Cohen MD. Imaging of gastrointestinal malignancy in childhood. Radiologic Clinics of North America 1996; 34:717–742.

Finn JP, Hall-Craggs MA, dicks-Mireaux C et al. Primary malignant liver tumours in childhood: Assessment of respectability with high-field MR and comparison with CT. Pediatric Radiology 1990; 21:34–38.

Pobeil RS, Bisset GS III. Pictorial essay: Imaging of liver tumours in infant and child. Pediatric Radiology 1995; 25:495–506.

Reinhold C, Hammers L, Taylor CR et al. Characterisation of focal hepatic lesions with duplex sonography: findings in 198 patients. American Journal of Roentgenology 1995; 164:1131–1135.

HEPATOBLASTOMA

Hepatoblastoma is the most common primary liver tumour in children under the age of 3 years, comprising 43% of total liver masses. The median age of occurrence is 1 year. The tumour is seen more commonly in boys than in girls with a 2:1 incidence ratio. Over the age of 5 years, the gender difference is no longer seen. There are a number of well-known predisposing factors and associations. The two most important genetic conditions associated with hepatoblastoma are Beckwith–Wiedemann syndrome and familial adenomatous polyposis. The incidence of hepatoblastoma is 200–800 times greater in familial adenomatous polyposis kindreds than in the general population. Hepatoblastoma has a reported association with dysplastic kidneys, Meckel's diverticulum, prematurity with a very low birth weight and prolonged hospitalization, maternal oral contraceptive exposure, fetal alcohol syndrome and gestational exposure to gonadotrophins. The most common clinical presentation is a painless abdominal mass (90%). Other features include anorexia, weight loss, pain, jaundice and precocious puberty.

Pathologically, hepatoblastoma occurs as a single pseudo-encapsulating large mass in more than 80% of cases. The right lobe is involved in approximately 58% of cases (Fig. 11.6.1), the left in 15% and the remaining 27% present either as a single mass extending across the midline or as multiple lesions in both the lobes. A diffuse type has also been described. Metastases occur in 10–20% of children, pulmonary lesions being the most common; bone, brain, eye and ovaries follow in that order.

More than 90% of children with hepatoblastoma show elevated levels of serum AFP. Extreme levels of AFP are associated with a poor outcome. Very low AFP levels or absence is seen in hepatoblastoma with poor differentiation (small cell undifferentiated tumours). Tumours with wide extension and metastasis show very high levels of serum AFP. The overall survival rate for hepatoblastoma is 63–65%.

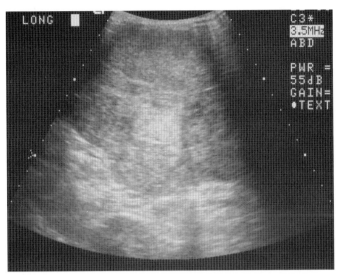

Figure 11.6.1 Hepatoblastoma in a 3-year-old boy. US showing a large heterogeneous mass lesion in the right lobe.

Abdominal radiography may show hepatomegaly as evidenced by elevation of the right hemidiaphragm and displacement of bowel gas. Hepatic calcifications may be seen, although they are not diagnostically specific. Pulmonary metastases are rare on chest x-rays. On US, hepatoblastoma may appear as a solitary mass, a dominant mass with smaller satellite lesions or multiple nodules throughout the liver. Rarely, hepatoblastoma may infiltrate the entire liver. Most tumours have some hyperechoic areas relative to normal liver, often with some inhomogeneity resulting from the presence of mesenchymal elements. Calcifications may be present and appear as brightly echogenic punctate or linear foci with acoustic shadowing. Portal vein invasion can be seen as echogenic intraluminal thrombus. Areas of necrosis and haemorrhage appear as anechoic foci. Doppler sonography may detect neovascularity around the rim of the neoplasm and may demonstrate increased hepatic arterial flow with frequency shifts over 5 kHz, which are much higher than in haemangioendothelioma or haemangioma.

On Tc 99m sulphur colloid liver scintigraphy, hepatoblastomas usually demonstrate hypervascularity, with prominent tracer avidity at the site of the tumour within a few seconds of the appearance of the bolus in the abdominal aorta. This increased activity persists into the venous phase. Delayed images typically demonstrate a photopenic defect at the tumour site from replacement of Kupffer cells by the tumour. Less commonly, in tumours containing large foci of necrosis, a photopenic defect is seen on both the static and dynamic portions of the examination. Rarely, hepatoblastomas may demonstrate increased uptake on delayed imaging, mimicking focal nodular hyperplasia.

The appearance of hepatoblastoma on CT varies greatly. Prior to contrast administration, an epithelial-type tumour appears as a homogeneous hypodense mass, while a mixed mesenchymal-epithelial tumour demonstrates a more heterogeneous appearance. Calcifications may be present in either type: small and fine in the epithelial type and coarse and extensive in the mixed type (Fig. 11.6.2). Following the injection of intravenous contrast, some enhancement of the tumour is seen but this is usually less than in normal liver tissue. The enhancement pattern typically is inhomogeneous and a peripheral rim of enhancement may be observed if

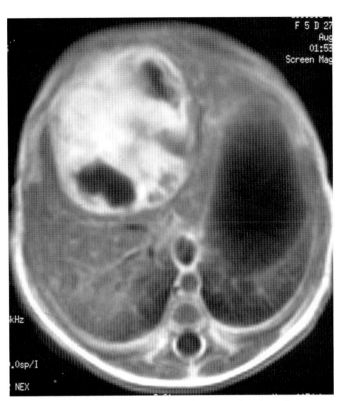

Figure 11.6.2 Contrast-enhanced axial CT image showing a large heterogeneous mass. Specks of calcification are also seen – hepatoblastoma.

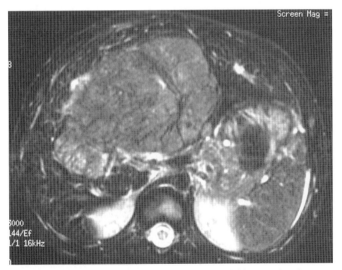

Figure 11.6.3 Hepatoblastoma – T2-weighted axial image showing a large hyperintense mass lesion.

imaging is performed during the early arterial phase. The tumour may involve one, two or three segments or may diffusely involve the entire liver.

Similar to CT, the MRI appearance of hepatoblastoma varies with its histological nature. The epithelial type has a homogeneous appearance and is hypointense on T1-weighted images and hyperintense on T2-weighted images (Fig. 11.6.3), while the mixed type is more heterogeneous, depending on the presence of necrosis, haemorrhage, fibrosis, calcification, cartilage and septa. Septations appear as hypointense bands on both T1- and T2-weighted images. Vascular invasion is demonstrated best by gradient echo MRI or contrast-enhanced MR angiography. The combination of CT or MRI and CT angiography or contrast-enhanced MR angiography provides the surgeon with complete information for operative planning of partial hepatectomy or orthotopic liver transplantation.

FURTHER READING

Al-qabandi W, Jenkinson HC, Buckels JA et al. Orthotopic liver transplantation for unresectable hepatoblastoma: A single center's experience. Journal of Pediatric Surgery 1999; 31:1563–1567.

Endo EG, Walton DS, Albert DM. Neonatal hepatoblastoma metastatic to the choroids and iris. Archives of Ophthalmology 1996; 114:757–761.

Helmberger TK, Ros PR, Mergo PG. Pediatric liver neoplasms: Radiologic-pathologic correlation. European Journal of Radiology 1999; 9:1339–1347.

Ishak K, Goodman Z, Stocker J. Tumours of the liver and intrahepatic bile ducts. Washington DC: Armed Forces Institute of Pathology; 2000.

King SJ, Babyn PS, Greenberg MLS. Value of CT in determining the resectability of hepatoblastoma before and after chemotherapy. American Journal of Roentgenology 1993; 164:793–798.

Kurahashi H, Takami K, Oue T et al. Biallelic inactivation of APC gene in hepatoblastoma. Cancer Research 1995; 55:5007–5011.

Oda H, Imai Y, Nakatsuru Y et al. Somatic mutations of the APC gene in sporadic hepatoblastomas. Cancer Research 1996; 56:3320–3323.

Pobeil RS, Bisset GS III. Pictorial essay: Imaging of liver tumours in infant and child. Pediatric Radiology 1995; 25:495–506.

Reynolds M. Conversion of unresectable hepatoblastoma and long-term follow-up study. World Journal of Surgery 1995; 19:814–816.

Robertson PL, Muraszko KM, Axtell RA. Hepatoblastoma metastatic to brain. Prolonged survival after multiple surgical resection of a solitary brain lesion. Journal of Pediatric Hematology and Oncology 1997; 19:168–171.

Ross JA, Gurney JG. Hepatoblastoma incidence in the United States from 1973 to 1992. Medical and Pediatric Oncology 1998; 30:141–142.

von Schweinitz D, Wischmeyer P, Leuschner I et al. Clinico-pathological criteria with prognostic relevance in hepatoblastoma. European Journal of Cancer 1994; 30A:1052–1058.

HEPATOCELLULAR CARCINOMA

Hepatocellular carcinoma is the most common primary malignant tumour of children over 4 years of age. It is the second most common paediatric liver tumour after hepatoblastoma and accounts for 23% of childhood liver masses. The peak age of occurrence is bimodal, with peaks at 4–5 years and more commonly at 12–14 years. In adults, it is the most common primary malignant hepatic neoplasm. Hepatocellular carcinoma is a malignant tumour of hepatocellular origin that develops in patients with risk factors that include alcohol abuse, viral hepatitis (hepatitis B and C), and pre-existing liver diseases like glycogen storage disease, tyrosinaemia, haemochromatosis and alpha-1-antitrypsin deficiency. Other predisposing factors include hepatocarcinogens such as aflatoxin, the toxin produced by *Aspergillus flavus* that grows on improperly stored corn, grains and peanuts. Usually the child presents with an abdominal mass, fever of unknown origin, abdominal pain, weight loss, malaise and symptoms related to paraneoplastic syndrome.

Pathologically, the lesions are multifocal, solitary, diffuse or infiltrative. The diffusely infiltrative type of tumour may be difficult to detect in an end-stage cirrhotic liver. Hepatocellular carcinoma can undergo haemorrhage and necrosis because of a lack of fibrous stroma. Vascular invasion, particularly of the portal system,

is common (44%). Less commonly, invasion into the hepatic venous system and inferior vena cava can be seen (4–6%). Invasion of the biliary system is less common than vascular invasion. The encapsulated form of hepatocellular carcinoma has a better prognosis because it does not invade the portal system and is more readily resectable. Large hepatocellular carcinomas greater than 3 cm in diameter have a tendency to necrose and haemorrhage centrally. Aggressive hepatocellular carcinoma can cause hepatic rupture and haemoperitoneum. Metastases are usually present in up to 50% of cases at the time of diagnosis and the overall survival rate is approximately 0–29%. Most of the cases show an increase in the serum AFP levels.

Plain film findings are non-specific. Calcification is very rare in hepatocellular carcinomas. The US appearance of hepatocellular carcinoma is variable. Small hepatocellular carcinomas can be homogeneously hyperechoic and can mimic haemangioma. This can result when a large proportion of fat is present in the tumour. Small hepatocellular carcinomas can appear hypoechoic with larger hepatocellular carcinomas frequently mixed in echogenicity. Lesions less than 5 cm in diameter sometimes can show a peripheral hyperechoic halo. Vascular invasion can be evaluated adequately using colour Doppler imaging with conventional greyscale ultrasound. Colour Doppler has been reported to be highly sensitive and specific in detecting blood flow in tumour thrombus and hence can distinguish tumour thrombus from bland thrombus. Portal venous invasion is more common in hepatocellular carcinoma but hepatic vein invasion is more specific for hepatocellular carcinoma. On both colour Doppler and angiography, a basket pattern of a fine blood flow network around the hepatocellular carcinoma nodule has been described as a characteristic appearance.

CT imaging in the hepatic-arterial and portal-venous phases, as well as delayed-contrast images, is important in detecting hepatocellular carcinomas. Lesions may be missed if early vascular imaging is not performed. It is important to use high injection rates and appropriate bolus timing. Sensitivity of good-quality dual- or triple-phase CT for the detection of patients with tumours is 60–70%.

The CT appearance of hepatocellular carcinomas varies depending on tumour size and the imaging phase. The most common attenuation pattern is isoattenuation on precontrast scan, hyperattenuation on arterial phase followed by isoattenuation on venous phase. However, this pattern is shared by other hepatocellular nodules, including regenerative and dysplastic nodules. Unenhanced CT typically reveals an iso-hypodense mass. If the mass is large, central areas of necrosis may be seen. Calcification can sometimes be seen. In the hepatic-arterial phase, lesions typically are hyperdense (relative to hepatic parenchyma) as a result of hepatic-arterial supply. Larger tumours may have necrotic central regions that typically are hypodense during this imaging phase. Sometimes the presence of neovascularity can indicate the presence of inconspicuous lesions. In the portal-venous phase, small lesions may be isodense or hypodense and difficult to see since the remainder of the liver increases in attenuation. Larger lesions with necrotic regions remain hypodense. In the delayed postcontrast phase, small lesions may be inconspicuous. Delayed phase scans may show a tumour capsule, one of the more specific signs indicating hepatocellular carcinomas.

CT can also evaluate complications such as portal-venous or hepatic-venous invasion. A tumour thrombus produces an enhancing expanding filling defect in the portal or hepatic veins. The enhancement pattern may resemble the neovascular 'thread and streak sign' described on selective arteriography. Portal vein tumour thrombus can extend into the splenic or superior mesenteric veins and can be associated with significant varices. Hepatic vein tumour thrombus can result in inferior vena caval obstruction and pulmonary tumour emboli. Spontaneous intraperitoneal tumour rupture with haemoperitoneum can occur. Infiltrating hepatocellular carcinoma can produce biliary obstruction.

Hepatocellular carcinoma appearance varies on MRI depending on multiple factors, such as haemorrhage, degree of fibrosis, histological pattern, degree of necrosis and the amount of fatty change. Hepatocellular carcinoma on T1-weighted images may be isointense, hypointense or hyperintense relative to the liver. On T2-weighted images, hepatocellular carcinoma usually is hyperintense. Pre- and postcontrast MRI has a 70–85% chance of detecting a solitary mass of hepatocellular carcinoma. MRI can help differentiate cirrhotic nodules from hepatocellular carcinoma. If the mass is bright on T2-weighted images, it is hepatocellular carcinoma until proven otherwise, whereas, if the mass is dark on T1- and T2-weighted images, it is a siderotic regenerative nodule or siderotic dysplastic nodule, and if the mass is bright on T1-weighted images and dark or isointense on T2-weighted images, it is a dysplastic nodule or low-grade hepatocellular carcinoma.

Gadolinium-enhanced MRI typically demonstrates that hepatocellular carcinomas densely enhance, usually in the arterial phase and particularly if they are small. A lesion showing arterial enhancement is most likely hepatocellular carcinoma. The degree of enhancement varies, particularly with the degree of necrosis in larger tumours. Studies have also shown that the degree of tumour enhancement correlates well with the degree of histological differentiation of the tumour. Administration of superparamagnetic iron oxide may demonstrate hepatocellular carcinoma since most hepatocellular carcinomas contain fewer or no Kupffer cells. The contrast agent mangafodipir trisodium can evaluate questionable lesions in the liver. Mangafodipir trisodium is taken up by normal hepatocytes and masses that contain hepatocytes, causing increased signal on T1-weighted images. This agent may help differentiate a tumour of hepatocellular origin, such as hepatocellular carcinoma, from secondary hepatic masses. Complications (e.g. vascular invasion) are evaluated well by MRI.

Gallium may help distinguish regenerating nodules of cirrhosis from hepatocellular carcinoma since regenerating nodules typically do not label with gallium. On a liver/spleen scan, a sulphur colloid study typically demonstrates an area of decreased labelling in hepatocellular carcinomas.

Positron emission tomography with fluorodeoxyglucose (FDG PET) is primarily useful in assessing the degree of differentiation and in staging moderately and poorly differentiated tumours rather than in primary lesion detection. Sensitivities of FDG PET for the detection of hepatocellular carcinoma range from 50% to 70%. This limited sensitivity is due to the low level of FDG uptake in well-differentiated tumours. However, FDG PET may be superior to CT in detecting extrahepatic spread.

Ethanol injection, acetic acid injection, interstitial laser hyperthermia and microwave therapy have been used to treat hepatocellular carcinoma in adults but are rarely employed in children. Percutaneous radiofrequency ablation has also been advocated recently for the treatment of small hepatocellular carcinomas. Percutaneous radiofrequency ablation appears to be effective in achieving tumour necrosis in hepatocellular carcinoma.

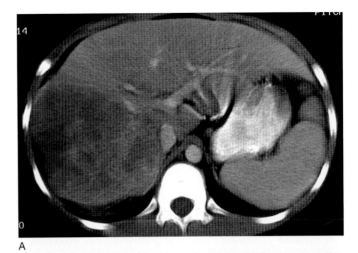

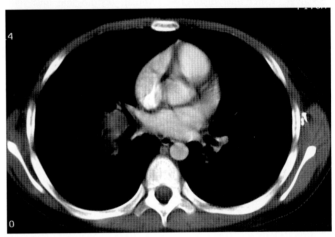

Figure 11.6.4 (A) Hepatocellular carcinoma in a 12-year-old boy, a known case of hepatitis B. Contrast-enhanced axial CT image showing a large heterogeneous mass lesion in the right lobe. (B) Axial section through the thorax showing lung metastasis.

FURTHER READING

Crawford JM. The liver and biliary tract. In: Cotran R, Kumar V, Robbins S, eds. Pathologic basis of disease. Philadelphia: W.B. Saunders; 1994: 831–895.

Donnelly LF, Bisset GS. Pediatric hepatic imaging. Radiologic Clinics of North America 1998; 36:413–427.

Fernandez MDP, Redvanly RD. Primary hepatic malignant neoplasms. Radiologic Clinics of North America 1998; 36:333–348.

Huang WS, Liu YC, Yu CY, Chou JM, Jen TK. Unusual presentation of hepatocellular carcinoma and assisted diagnosis by liver scan. Clinical Nuclear Medicine 2000; 25:563–564.

Murakami T, Baron RL, Peterson MS et al. Hepatocellular carcinoma: MR imaging with mangafodipir trisodium (Mn-DPDP). Radiology 1996; 200:69–77.

Ni Y-H, Chang M-H, Hsu H-Y et al. Hepatocellular carcinoma in childhood: Clinical manifestations and prognosis. Cancer 1991; 68:1737–1741.

O'Brien MO, Gottlieb L. The liver and biliary tract. In: Robbins S, Cotran RS, eds. Pathologic basis of disease. Philadelphia: W.B. Saunders; 1979:1009–1191.

Ros PR, Murphy EJ, Buck JL et al. Encapsulated hepatocellular carcinoma: Radiological findings and pathological correlation. Gastrointestinal Radiology 1990; 15:233–237.

Rossi S, Buscarini E, Garbagnati F. Percutaneous treatment of small hepatic tumours by an expandable RF needle electrode. American Journal of Roentgenology 1998; 170:1015–1022.

Sironi S, Livraghi T, Meloni F. Small hepatocellular carcinoma treated with percutaneous RF ablation: MR imaging follow-up. American Journal of Roentgenology 1999; 173:1225–1229.

Tanaka S, Kitamura T, Fugita M et al. Color Doppler flow imaging of liver tumours. American Journal of Roentgenology 1990; 154:509–514.

Wang LY, Lin ZY, Change WY et al. Duplex pulse Doppler sonography of portal vein thrombosis in hepatocellular carcinoma. Journal of Ultrasound Medicine 1991; 10:265–269.

Yamashita Y, Mitsuzaki K, Yi T et al. Small hepatocellular carcinoma in patient with chronic liver damage: prospective comparison of detection with dynamic MR imaging and helical CT of the whole liver. Radiology 1996; 200:79–85.

FIBROLAMELLAR CARCINOMA

Fibrolamellar carcinoma is an uncommon malignant neoplasm of the liver, which has distinctive clinical, histological and radiographic features that distinguish it from the relatively more common hepatocellular carcinoma. Compared to hepatocellular carcinoma, fibrolamellar carcinoma has no known predisposing factors, is typically not associated with elevated serum AFP levels and it is seen in a younger age group ranging from 5 to 35 years, with a mean age of approximately 20 years. There is no sex predilection and 5-year survival is approximately 60%. Symptoms are usually abdominal mass, pain, nausea and vomiting.

Pathologically, fibrolamellar carcinoma is most commonly seen as a solitary large intrahepatic mass with well-defined margins and a lobulated contour. The tumour is typically large at the time of diagnosis, with a mean diameter of 10–20 cm. Regional lymph node metastases are found in more than half of the patients at the time of initial diagnosis. Portal or hepatic venous invasion is not common. The tumour has a central stellate scar or fibrotic bands. Central calcification is present in 35–60% of patients. Haemorrhage and necrosis are uncommon.

On US, the primary tumour can be seen as a solitary, well-defined hepatic mass with a heterogeneous echotexture. The scar of the tumour may be seen as a central hyperechoic structure and calcification may be represented by an echogenic focus with shadowing. US is less sensitive than CT in depicting tumoural characteristics, such as scars and calcifications, which aid in the differentiation of fibrolamellar carcinoma from other intrahepatic tumours. After initial detection of the intrahepatic mass with US, further evaluation with CT or MRI is usually necessary for the definitive diagnosis and staging of fibrolamellar carcinoma.

Abdominal CT is the preferred imaging method for the diagnosis, staging and follow-up surveillance of fibrolamellar carcinoma. CT has high sensitivity in the detection of intrahepatic tumours and regional lymph node metastases. On non-enhanced scans, the primary fibrolamellar tumour typically appears as a large, solitary, hypoattenuating mass with well-circumscribed and lobulated margins. During the arterial enhancing phase, the tumour is heterogeneously enhancing and becomes generally hyperattenuating with respect to the relatively less strongly enhancing surrounding liver. During the portal and delayed phases, the tumour remains enhanced and becomes more homogeneous in appearance, with its density more closely matching that of the liver as equilibrium is achieved. Central scars are present in 50–70% of fibrolamellar carcinomas and appear on CT scans as a central stellate hypoattenuating and hypoenhancing region in the mass. The scars may not enhance at all or may show mild enhancement on delayed enhanced scans. Calcifications occur in 30–60% of fibrolamellar

tumours and they can be best identified as hyperattenuating foci on non-enhanced CT images. Metastatic lymphadenopathy is present at the time of initial diagnosis of fibrolamellar carcinoma in 50–70% of patients and the lymph nodes are frequent sites for recurrent disease after surgical resection of the primary lesions. Lymph node metastases are found most often in the porta hepatis and they can have a CT appearance similar to that of intrahepatic lesions.

Fibrolamellar carcinoma of the liver is typically identified on MRI as a large, well-defined, lobulated mass. On T1-weighted images, the tumour tends to be mostly homogeneous and hypointense relative to the liver. A minority of tumours may be heterogeneous and isointense. On T2-weighted images, the tumour is commonly heterogeneous and, most often, hyperintense with respect to the liver.

The central scar usually appears hypointense on all images obtained with all sequences. The appearance of the scar on MRI can be useful in differentiating fibrolamellar carcinomas from focal nodular hyperplasia. Fibrolamellar carcinomas typically do not contain intracellular fat; therefore, the presence of fat on fat-saturated, in-phase and out-of-phase MRI images suggests adenoma or hepatocellular carcinoma. On gadolinium-enhanced MRI, the enhancement patterns seen in fibrolamellar carcinomas are similar to those seen on contrast-enhanced CT scans. Early heterogeneous enhancement occurs during the arterial phase and progresses to more homogeneous enhancement during delayed phases. The central scar does not enhance during the arterial phase but it may demonstrate mild enhancement in the later portal or equilibrium phases.

FURTHER READING

Fernandez MDP, Redvanly RD. Primary hepatic malignant neoplasms. Radiologic Clinics of North America 1998; 36:333–348.

McLarney JK, Rucker PT, Bender GN et al. Fibrolamellar carcinoma of the liver: radiologic-pathologic correlation. Radiographics 1999; 19:453–471.

Soyer P, Roche A, Levesque M, Legmann P. CT of fibrolamellar hepatocellular carcinoma. Journal of Computer Assisted Tomography 1991; 15:533–538.

Stevens WR, Johnson CD, Stephens DH, Nagorney DM. Fibrolamellar hepatocellular carcinoma: stage at presentation and results of aggressive surgical management. American Journal of Roentgenology 1995; 164:1153–1158.

UNDIFFERENTIATED EMBRYONAL SARCOMA

Undifferentiated embryonal sarcoma is a highly malignant tumour. It is also known as malignant mesenchymoma or hepatic mesenchymal sarcoma and is the fourth commonest hepatic tumour in the paediatric age group after hepatoblastoma, haemangioendothelioma and hepatocellular carcinoma, with the majority of cases occurring between 6 and 10 years of age. There is no sex predominance. Abdominal pain or an abdominal mass is seen at presentation in the majority of cases. Other symptoms include anorexia, vomiting, lethargy and malaise. Unusual presentations include cardiac murmur caused by the extension of the tumour along the inferior vena cava into the right atrium. Undifferentiated embryonal sarcoma can sometimes be difficult to differentiate from mesenchymal hamartoma. In both the tumours, the serum AFP levels are normal. Undifferentiated embryonal sarcoma tends to be more solid and usually occurs after the age of 5 years, whereas mesenchymal hamartoma occurs between 4 months and 2 years of age. As mentioned above, undifferentiated embryonal sarcoma presents with abdominal pain or an abdominal mass, compared to mesenchymal hamartoma, which is usually asymptomatic.

Pathologically, the mass usually arises from the right lobe of the liver (69%), less commonly from the left lobe (14%) and both the lobes (17%). Undifferentiated embryonal sarcoma is usually very large at presentation, ranging from 7 to 18 cm in size. The tumour appears solid and gelatinous, with cystic areas and large areas of haemorrhage and necrosis. Even though this tumour is considered highly malignant, long-term survival has been achieved in many cases with complete resection and adjuvant chemotherapy.

US reveals a very large predominately echogenic mass with few anechoic areas representing areas of cystic necrosis. A CT scan demonstrates a well-circumscribed low-attenuation mass lesion and on contrast studies, enhancing solid portions of the tumour, peripheral enhancement and enhancement of the septae can be seen. Very rarely, punctuate calcifications can be demonstrated. On MRI, the tumour appears hypointense on T1-weighted images, with few high signal areas representing haemorrhage. On T2-weighted images, undifferentiated embryonal sarcoma appears hyperintense with hypointense septae.

FURTHER READING

Marti-Bonmati L, Ferrer D, Menor F et al. Hepatic mesenchymal sarcoma: MRI findings. Abdominal Imaging 1993; 18:176–179.
Moon WK, Kim WS, Kim IO et al. Undifferentiated embryonal sarcoma of the liver: US and CT findings. Pediatric Radiology 1994; 24:500–503.
Newman KD, Schilsgall R, Reaman G et al. Malignant mesenchymoma of the liver in children. Journal of Pediatric Surgery 1989; 24:781–783.

RHABDOMYOSARCOMA OF THE BILIARY TREE

Rhabdomyosarcoma of the biliary tree accounts for 1% of all the liver tumours and 0.8% of all rhabdomyosarcomas. It usually occurs in children under 5 years of age (75% of cases) and rarely in those over 15 years. Jaundice is the presenting symptom in more than 80% of cases and is accompanied by hyperbilirubinaemia, pale stools and hepatomegaly and hence may be confused with infectious hepatitis. Other symptoms include fever, abdominal distension, nausea and vomiting.

Pathologically, the tumour is seen as a gelatinous mass occluding the lumen of the right and left or common bile duct. The ducts proximal to the lesion are frequently dilated and the walls of the duct containing the lesion are thickened. The tumour may extend into the liver as a soft lobulated mass.

US shows the dilatation of the proximal biliary tree and a non-homogeneous echogenic mass. The mass is often in the porta hepatis. The presence of fluid (bile) around the tumour in the porta is the most specific but differentiation from hepatic tumours is difficult.

CT shows an ill-defined or a well-outlined relatively low-attenuating mass with some enhancement. The CT scan is the best

at showing the anatomy and the relationship of the portal vein, and bile ducts are better depicted. MR appearances are usually non-specific with the mass appearing hypointense on T1-weighted images and hyperintense on T2-weighted images. The dilated biliary tree is very well shown by magnetic resonance cholangiopancreatography (MRCP).

FURTHER READING

Arnand O, Boscq M, Asquier E et al. Embryonal rhabdomyosarcoma of the biliary tree in children: a case report. Pediatric Radiology 1987; 17:250–251.
Geoffray A, Couanet D, Montagne JP et al. Ultrasonography and computed tomography for diagnosis and followup of biliary duct rhabdomyosarcomas in children. Pediatric Radiology 1987; 17:127–131.

SECONDARY HEPATIC MALIGNANCIES AND LYMPHOPROLIFERATIVE DISORDERS

Common childhood malignancies that metastasize to liver include neuroblastoma, Wilm's tumour and lymphoma. Diffuse involvement of the liver by leukaemia can also occur but additional loci of disease at extrahepatic sites are usually evident. Stage IV-S neuroblastoma often shows diffuse, heterogeneous involvement of the entire liver. Hepatic metastasis occurs late in the disease. This is especially true for Wilm's tumour, renal cell carcinoma, non-infantile neuroblastoma and other tumours.

The increasing incidence of immunocompromised children, related to increased use of bone marrow transplantation, organ transplantation and HIV infection, has led to an increased incidence of lymphoproliferative disorders affecting the liver. Lymphoproliferative disorders consist of a spectrum of diseases ranging from polyclonal B-cell hyperplasia to monoclonal B-cell lymphoma. The disease is secondary to proliferation of Epstein–Barr-infected B-cells. Infected cells proliferate and cause lymphoma-like diseases. Hepatic involvement is common in children and can appear as focal liver masses. Often, lymphoproliferative disorders resolve when the patients' immunosuppressive therapy is reduced.

US shows the metastatic lesions usually as multiple hypoechoic foci and the sensitivity of the ultrasound in detecting the metastatic lesions approximates to 54%. The CT scan is more sensitive for detection of liver metastasis. Sometimes it is easy to miss a metastatic lesion, since more than 40% of patients with hypervascular liver metastases have lesions that become isointense to liver parenchyma if imaging is not performed in the arterial phase.

Magnetic resonance imaging is emerging as the best modality to detect hepatic metastasis. The use of contrast is shown to further increase the sensitivity in detecting liver metastasis.

FURTHER READING

Green B, Bree RL, Goldstein HM et al. Grey scale ultrasound evaluation of hepatic neoplasms: patterns and correlations. Radiology 1997; 124:203–208.

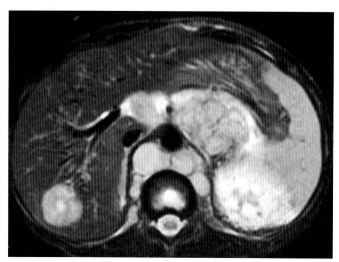

Figure 11.6.5 T2-weighted MR image showing a hyperintense metastatic lesion in the right lobe of the liver from neuroblastoma.

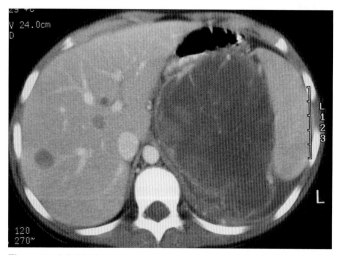

Figure 11.6.6 Multiple hypodense non-enhancing metastatic lesions in the liver.

Scheible W, Gosink BB, Leopold GR. Grey scale echographic patterns of hepatic metastatic disease. American Journal of Roentgenology 1997; 129:983–987.

Soyer P, Van Beers B, Teillet-Thiebaud F et al. Hodgkin's and non-Hodgkin's hepatic lymphoma: sonographic findings. Abdominal Imaging 1993; 18:339–343.

BENIGN LESIONS

Benign lesions of the liver are rare in children. They include:

- tumour-like epithelial lesions (focal nodular hyperplasia)
- epithelial tumours (adenoma)
- cysts and tumour-like mesenchymal lesions (cystic mesenchymal hamartoma)
- mesenchymal tumours (haemangioma, haemangioendothelioma)
- benign teratoma.

FURTHER READING

Mergo PJ, Ros PR. Benign lesions of the liver. Radiologic Clinics of North America 1998a; 36:319–331.

FOCAL NODULAR HYPERPLASIA

Focal nodular hyperplasia is uncommon in children; most cases are seen in women in the third to fifth decade of life. It is the second most common benign liver tumour, second only to haemangioma. Though oral contraceptives are a known association, studies have shown that oral contraceptives act only to promote the growth of focal nodular hyperplasia, not to induce its formation.

Pathologically, focal nodular hyperplasia occurs as a solitary lesion that is usually less than 5 cm. Generally, the tumour does not have internal haemorrhage or necrosis. Most focal nodular hyperplasia lesions are well defined but lack the presence of a true capsule. The most important distinguishing and prevalent feature is the presence of a central fibrous scar. This scar is vascular, with vessels extending outward via fibrous septae to the periphery of the tumour. Although bile ducts are present, they do not communicate with the normal biliary radicals.

Ultrasonography shows a well-defined mass that is either hyper- or isoechoic with the liver. The scar is usually hypoechoic and demonstration of arterial flow in the central scar is highly suggestive of the diagnosis. On unenhanced CT, the lesion looks hypo- or isodense compared to the rest of the liver. When seen, the central scar is relatively hypodense. Calcification is seen in only 1% of patients, thus, its presence should suggest another diagnosis. The lesion tends to be hyperdense compared to the rest of the liver parenchyma in the arterial phase because of its rich hepatic arterial supply. In the portovenous phase, the lesion becomes isodense to liver. However, with the diffusion of contrast into the central scar, the scar becomes hyperdense compared to the remainder of the lesion and the normal liver. On MRI, focal nodular hyperplasia is iso- to hypointense, with the central scar being more hypointense on T1-weighted images. On T2-weighted images, the lesion appears mildly hyperintense, with the scar being more hyperintense. On contrast studies using gadolinium, focal nodular hyperplasia is hyperintense compared to the normal liver. With delay, focal nodular hyperplasia becomes more isointense and the central scar becomes more hyperintense compared to the normal liver. Because needle biopsies can overlap with those of well-differentiated hepatocellular adenoma or carcinoma, open biopsy or surgical resection is often required.

FURTHER READING

Mergo PJ, Ros PR. Benign lesions of the liver. Radiologic Clinics of North America 1998a; 36:319–331.

Schiebler MLS, Kressel HY, Saul SH et al. MR imaging of focal nodular hyperplasia of the liver. Journal of Computer Assisted Tomography 1987; 11:651–654.

HEPATIC ADENOMAS

Hepatic adenoma is a rare benign tumour of the liver. Two types of hepatic adenomas have been described, including tumours of

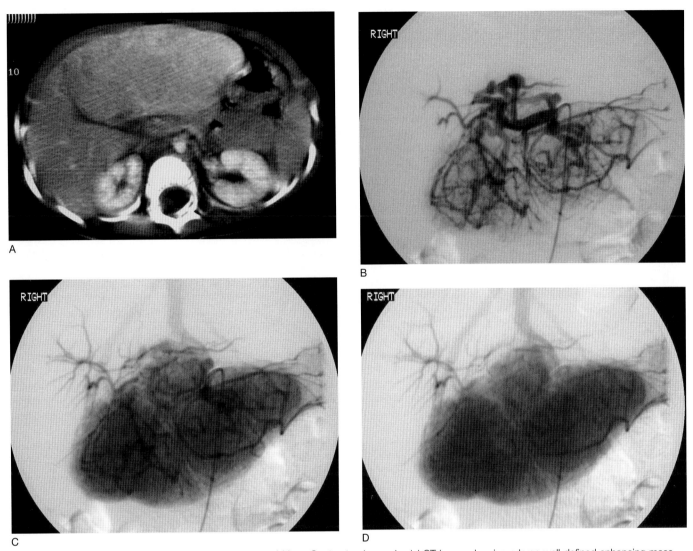

Figure 11.6.7 (A) Focal nodular hyperplasia in a 10-year-old boy. Contrast-enhanced axial CT image showing a large well-defined enhancing mass. (B–D) Preoperative angiogram showing the hypervascular mass.

bile duct origin and tumours of liver cell origin. Oral contraceptives and androgen steroids have been identified as the causative agents of hepatic adenomas. Hepatic adenomas can also occur spontaneously or can be associated with type I glycogen storage disease and diabetes mellitus.

Pathologically, sheets of well-differentiated hepatocytes characterize hepatic adenomas. The hepatocytes contain fat and glycogen and can produce bile; however, no bile ducts are present. A characteristic lack of portal venous tracts and terminal hepatic veins are noted. Approximately 80% of adenomas are solitary and 20% are multiple. Most hepatic adenomas do not contain Kupffer cells. Although benign, hepatic adenomas can present a diagnostic challenge since lesions can be difficult to distinguish from other benign or malignant hepatic tumours. Clinically, patients with hepatic adenomas may be asymptomatic and lesions may be found incidentally during laparotomy or when radiological studies are performed. As a result of their size (often 8–15 cm) the patient or physician may notice a right upper quadrant mass or hepatomegaly, resulting in a referral for imaging. Hepatic adenomas can

rupture and bleed, causing right upper quadrant pain, which may be mistaken clinically for acute cholecystitis. On rare occasions, rupture may lead to haemorrhagic shock.

Rarely, hepatic adenomas undergo malignant transformation to hepatocellular carcinoma. Serum AFP levels are helpful in differentiating hepatic adenoma from hepatocellular carcinoma.

On US, hepatic adenomas demonstrate variable echogenicity. They may be hypoechoic, isoechoic or hyperechoic to liver parenchyma. Usually, differentiating hepatic adenomas from other liver lesions such as focal nodular hyperplasia or hepatocellular carcinoma is not possible based on either grey-scale or Doppler characteristics. The primary role of ultrasound is to screen patients with hepatic masses that are discovered incidentally or who have a clinical history of abnormal liver function test results. Further imaging is then indicated using MRI, CT and/or nuclear medicine.

Hepatic adenomas are often discovered incidentally on CT scans performed for other reasons. Once identified, a multiphasic CT scan should be performed to better characterize most hepatic tumours. Protocols differ between institutions.

Typically, helical CT scans are obtained, first of the unenhanced liver. Then, images are obtained in the hepatic arterial phase using intravenous injection of approximately 120–150 ml of non-ionic contrast at a rate of 3–5 ml/s with a 25–30-s delay. Images are then acquired in the portal venous phase after a scanning delay of 60–80 s. On CT, the most consistent finding in hepatic adenomas is the enhancement pattern. Most lesions (90% according to Ichikawa et al.) show homogeneous enhancement in the hepatic arterial phase. Unfortunately, this feature is not specific to hepatic adenomas, since hepatocellular carcinomas, hypervascular metastases and focal nodular hyperplasia can demonstrate similar enhancement in the hepatic arterial phase. Since hepatic adenomas are composed histologically of uniform hepatocytes, most are isoattenuating to healthy liver tissue. In a fatty liver, hepatic adenomas usually are hyperattenuating. The finding of haemorrhage as an area of high attenuation can be seen in as many as 40% of patients. Fat deposition within adenomas is identified on CT in only approximately 7% of patients. Typically, hepatic adenomas have well-defined borders and do not have lobulated contours. A low-attenuation pseudocapsule can be seen in as many as 25% of patients. Coarse calcifications are seen in only 5% of patients.

MRI findings are similar to CT findings. However, MRI is usually more sensitive in detecting fat and haemorrhage. Hepatic adenomas tend to be hyperintense or isointense to liver tissue on T1-weighted images (up to 93%). High signal on T1-weighted images probably relates to the presence of fat or, less commonly, to haemorrhage within the lesion. Chemical-shift imaging showing loss of signal on out-of-phase images can confirm the presence of fat. Unfortunately, hepatocellular carcinoma is known to contain fat in as many as 40% of lesions; therefore, the presence of fat does not help differentiate the lesions. Other hepatic lesions can be hyperintense on T1-weighted images, such as melanoma metastases and cavities containing proteinaceous material. On T2-weighted images, hepatic adenomas most often are slightly hyperintense to liver tissue. This finding is not specific since many hepatic lesions, including hepatocellular carcinoma and metastases, are hyperintense on T2-weighted images.

Heterogeneity, defined as any difference of signal within a lesion on T1-weighted or T2-weighted images, is seen in approximately one-half of patients. Heterogeneity relates to the presence of either haemorrhage or necrosis. This finding is not specific since hepatocellular carcinoma and metastases can bleed and become necrotic. Although uncommon, focal nodular hyperplasia also can be haemorrhagic. A peripheral rim corresponding histologically to a pseudocapsule is seen in 17–31% of patients. Signal characteristics of the rim are variable. Most often, the peripheral rim, when seen, is of low signal intensity on T1-weighted images, variable intensity on T2-weighted images and usually does not enhance. After gadolinium administration, the pattern of enhancement is similar to that of CT. Most hepatic adenomas show intense enhancement in the arterial phase and are isointense to liver tissue on delayed imaging. Hepatic adenomas, unlike focal nodular hyperplasia, do not have a central scar. If a low signal intensity scar is seen on T1-weighted images and the scar enhances after gadolinium is administered, the diagnosis of focal nodular hyperplasia is strongly favoured. A central scar has never been reported in a hepatic adenoma.

On routine MRI of the liver consisting of T1-weighted and T2-weighted images, chemical-shift imaging, and dynamic gadolinium-enhanced imaging, distinguishing between hepatic adenomas, hepatocellular carcinoma and hypervascular metastases usually is not possible. Recent studies performed to determine if MRI using ferumoxides (superparamagnetic iron oxides) shows enhancement pattern may help to improve the distinction of focal nodular hyperplasia from hepatic adenoma and hepatocellular carcinoma in indeterminate cases.

Mangafodipir trisodium (formerly termed Mn-DPDP) is a hepatobiliary MRI contrast agent. It is taken up by hepatocytes and excreted into bile. Because hepatic adenoma, focal nodular hyperplasia and hepatocellular carcinoma all contain hepatocytes, they may demonstrate enhancement with this agent. Metastases and haemangiomas do not contain hepatocytes and do not enhance; therefore, this agent can help differentiate hepatic adenoma, which enhances, from metastases, which do not enhance.

A combination of radiotracers may help make the diagnosis of hepatic adenomas in equivocal cases. On gallium-67 (Ga-67) scans, hepatic adenomas demonstrate decreased uptake compared to healthy liver tissue, which can be explained by the benign nature of the cells. In contrast, HCC often demonstrates equivocal or greater Ga-67 uptake than liver, with studies reporting that 90–95% of hepatocellular carcinomas demonstrate uptake or equivocal uptake of Ga-67.

Since hepatic adenomas usually have few or absent Kupffer cells, they show focal defects on sulphur-colloid liver/spleen scans. However, occasional hepatic adenomas contain enough Kupffer cells to demonstrate normal uptake of sulphur colloid. Hepatocellular carcinomas almost always appear as defects on sulphur-colloid scintigraphy because they lack Kupffer cells. Focal nodular hyperplasia contains Kupffer cells and usually demonstrates uptake of sulphur colloid. In summary, sulphur-colloid uptake strongly favours a diagnosis of focal nodular hyperplasia. Lack of sulphur-colloid uptake is not specific and can be attributed to many other hepatic lesions, including hepatocellular carcinoma, hepatic adenomas and metastases.

Using hepatobiliary agents, hepatic adenomas usually demonstrate early uptake with subsequent retention of the radiotracer because hepatic adenomas do not contain bile ducts; thus, the radiotracer is not excreted by the lesion, which remains hot on delayed images. This is in contrast to hepatocellular carcinoma, which shows focal defects on early scans. Avid uptake becomes detectable only after 2–5 h.

When hepatic adenoma is indistinguishable from hepatocellular carcinoma and focal nodular hyperplasia radiologically, a combination of radionuclide imaging including sulphur-colloid, gallium-67 and technetium 99m pyridoxyl-5-methyltryptophan (PMT) uptake may help establish the correct diagnosis. Most hepatic adenomas demonstrate decreased gallium uptake, decreased sulphur-colloid uptake, and early and retained uptake of hepatobiliary agents.

FURTHER READING

Arrive L, Flejou JF, Vilgrain V et al. Hepatic adenoma: MR findings in 51 pathologically proved lesions. Radiology 1994; 193:507–512.

Herman P, Pugliese V, Machado MA et al. Hepatic adenoma and focal nodular hyperplasia: differential diagnosis and treatment. World Journal of Surgery 2000; 24:372–376.

Ichikawa T, Federle MP, Grazioli L, Nalesnik M. Hepatocellular adenoma: multiphasic CT and histopathologic findings in 25 patients. Radiology 2000; 214:861–868.

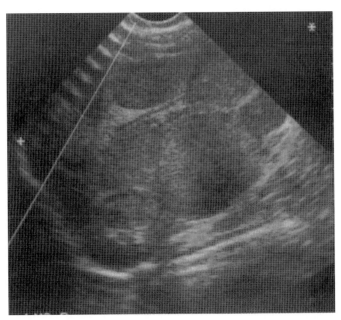

Figure 11.6.8 Adenomas. 15-year-old girl with type I glycogen storage disease. US examination showing homogeneous isoechoic nodules.

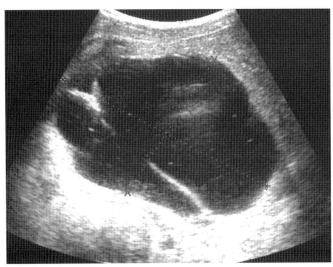

Figure 11.6.9 Mesenchymal hamartoma in a 3-year-old girl. US examination showing a large lobulated cystic mass lesion with septae within.

Kume N, Suga K, Nishigauchi K et al. Characterisation of hepatic adenoma with atypical appearance on CT and MRI by radionuclide imaging. Clinical Nuclear Medicine 1997; 22:825–831.

Paley MR, Mergo PJ, Torres GM, Ros PR. Characterisation of focal hepatic lesions with ferumoxide-enhanced T2-weighted MR imaging. American Journal of Roentgenology 2000; 175:159–163.

Paulson EK, McClellan JS, Washington K et al. Hepatic adenoma: MR characteristics and correlation with pathologic findings. American Journal of Roentgenology 1994; 163:113–116.

MESENCHYMAL HAMARTOMA

These are primary benign tumours that occur exclusively during infancy and childhood, although a few cases do occur in the older age group. The mean age of presentation is 16 months, the range being from newborn to 5 years. Many consider mesenchymal hamartoma as a developmental anomaly rather than a true tumour. Boys are affected slightly more than girls (3:2).

Most of the cases are asymptomatic while other cases are detected incidentally when patients present with right upper quadrant mass, fever and dyspnoea. Rapid accumulation of fluid within the lesion often leads to observations by the parent of an enlarging abdominal mass in the infant. Conditions reported in association with mesenchymal hamartoma include small bowel malrotation, neonatal hyperbilirubinaemia, hydrops fetalis, endocardial fibroelastosis, idiopathic thrombocytopenic purpura and diffuse endocrinopathy. Liver function tests usually remain within normal limits.

Pathologically, mesenchymal hamartoma consists of gelatinous serous fluid in cystic spaces with bile duct and connective tissue matrix.

On US, mesenchymal hamartomas appear as large cystic lesions with echogenic septae within. Mesenchymal hamartomas may be detected as hypoechoic lesions on prenatal ultrasound. On CT the

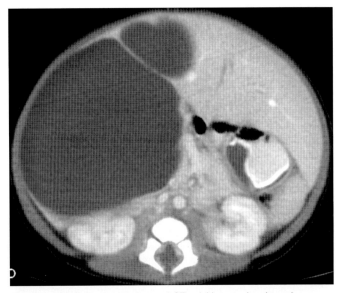

Figure 11.6.10 Contrast-enhanced CT axial image showing a large cystic mass lesion with septa – mesenchymal hamartoma.

lesion appears cystic and the septae might show enhancement on contrast studies. MRI findings are similar to CT, lesion being hypointense on T1-weighted images and hyperintense on T2-weighted images. The septae appear hypointense on T2-weighted images. Provided they are in a favourable position, primary resection is the treatment.

FURTHER READING

De Maioribus CA, Lally KP, Kenneth S. Mesenchymal hamartomas of the liver. A 35-years review. Archives of Surgery 1990; 125:598–600.

Siegel MJ, Luker GD. MR imaging of the liver in children. MRI Clinics of North America 1996; 4:637–656.

CAVERNOUS HAEMANGIOMA

Cavernous haemangioma is the most common benign tumour in adults but is not so common in children. These tumours are usually asymptomatic but on rare occasions can cause abdominal pain, nausea or vomiting as a result of compression of adjacent structures, rupture, haemorrhage or thrombosis.

Pathologically, two types of haemangiomas have been described: the capillary and the cavernous type. The capillary type refers to the growth phase of the haemangioma and the cavernous type refers to the involutional phase. (Note: Cavernous haemangiomas and infantile haemangioendotheliomas are mesenchymal tumours that demonstrate growth and involution phases that differentiate them from arteriovenous malformations that grow with the child.) Haemangiomas are well-circumscribed, blood-filled masses of variable size. Lesions that are larger than 6–10 cm are called giant haemangiomas. Haemangiomas may be multiple in up to 10% of cases.

The typical appearance on US is a small hyperechoic mass in the right lobe of the liver that is well circumscribed and homogeneous. This appearance is noted in 70–80% of cases. These hyperechoic masses never have a hypoechoic halo around them. Some of the lesions may exhibit central hypoechogenicity representing either fibrosis or necrosis. Occasionally, cavernous haemangiomas demonstrate acoustic enhancement but this is not thought to be a uniformly helpful sign for separating haemangiomas from other hyperechoic lesions. Variations in the typical appearance include hypoechoic haemangiomas, which are seen in 15–20% of patients. If a haemangioma is seen on a background of fatty infiltration, it may appear hypoechoic because of the increased echogenicity of the background liver.

On CT, haemangiomas are vascular lesions with relatively static circulation. Definitive findings are a well-defined hypoattenuating mass on precontrast study, rim enhancement in the early phase after contrast injection and progressive uniform centripetal enhancement on delayed scans. The enhancing rim, which is often nodular and the central region of the haemangioma, remains isoattenuating with the vascular compartment. Both the vascular compartment and haemangioma progressively decrease in attenuation and become isoattenuating with the liver. The rate of uniform centripetal enhancement has no direct relationship to lesion size. In 45% of hepatic haemangiomas, enhancement characteristics on bolus enhanced incremental dynamic CT studies are not very characteristic. In these cases, there is either patchy peripheral or central enhancement in the early phase simulating a vascular primary lesion or metastasis. In lesions less than 2 cm, the CT enhancement pattern cannot be defined primarily due to variability of a suspended respiration during sequential imaging at a single level. This results in variable degrees of partial volume averaging of normal hepatic parenchyma and haemangioma, which interferes with the delineation of early rim and delayed centripetal enhancement.

Magnetic resonance imaging is more specific and sensitive for the diagnosis of haemangiomas. Diagnosing haemangiomas with MRI relies on the use of morphological features and signal characteristics. Haemangiomas tend to be well-marginated, peripherally located lesions with lobulated contours. They tend to be homogeneously hypointense on T1-weighted images and significantly hyperintense on T2-weighted images relative to liver and other hepatic lesions. Even at late echoes on a multiecho sequence, the haemangioma retains its marked hyperintense signal. The degree of hyperintensity on T2-weighted sequences visually compares with and is similar to that of the gallbladder or cerebrospinal fluid. Simple hepatic cysts may have similar hyperintensity on T2-weighted images but can usually be distinguished by their relative greater hypointensity on T1-weighted images. Imaging using single breath-hold dynamic imaging after administration of gadolinium shows an enhancement pattern similar to that on CT. Early peripheral enhancement occurs, followed by filling in of the central portion of the lesion. Persistence of enhancement on delayed images can be seen in contradistinction to metastasis, which equilibrates quickly with surrounding liver parenchyma.

The gold standard for the diagnosis of hepatic cavernous haemangiomas is red blood cell-labelled single photon emission CT (RBC-SPECT). For lesions greater than 2.5 cm, radionuclide study is the preferred investigation because it has close to 100% specificity and is lower in cost. Studies have shown that MRI has greater sensitivity and is more accurate than labelled RBC-SPECT for lesions less than 2 cm. More recently, the introduction of the multiheaded gamma camera with rapid three-dimensional reconstruction has reduced the size limitations for accurate diagnosis with SPECT, and haemangiomas as small as 1.4 cm can be accurately assessed.

FURTHER READING

Birnbaum BA, Weinreb JC, Megibow AJ et al. Definitive diagnosis of hepatic hemangiomas: MR imaging versus Tc-99m-labeled red blood cell SPECT. Radiology 1990; 176:95–98.

Choi BI, Han MC, Kim CW. Small hepatocellular carcinoma versus small cavernous hemangioma: differentiation with MR imaging at 2.0 T. Radiology 1990; 176:103–108.

Gibney RG, Hendin AP, Cooperberg PL. Sonographically detected hepatic hemangiomas: Absence of change over time. American Journal of Roentgenology 1987; 149:953–957.

Hamm B, Fischer E, Taupitz M. Differentiation of hepatic hemangiomas from metastases by dynamic contrast-enhanced MR imaging. Journal of Computer Assisted Tomography 1990; 14:205–216.

Kudo M, Ikekubo K, Yamamoto K et al. Distinction between hemangioma of the liver and hepatocellular carcinoma: value of labeled RBC SPECT scanning. American Journal of Roentgenology 1989; 152:977–980.

Leslie DF, Johnson CD, Johnson CM et al. Distinction between cavernous hemangiomas of the liver and hepatic metastases on CT: value of contrast enhancement patterns. American Journal of Roentgenology 1995; 164: 625–629.

INFANTILE HAEMANGIOENDOTHELIOMA

Infantile haemangioendothelioma is the most common benign tumour of the liver in children. It is almost exclusively (86%) seen in the first 6 months of life (86%), with about one-third presenting in the first month. Very rarely, it is seen in children over 3 years of age. This tumour is more commonly seen in girls with a 2:1 incidence ratio. Clinical presentation usually involves an enlarging abdomen noted by a parent, although about 10–15% of children present with features of congestive heart failure including high cardiac output, elevated right and left end diastolic pressure, and small systolic pressure gradient across the pulmonary outflow

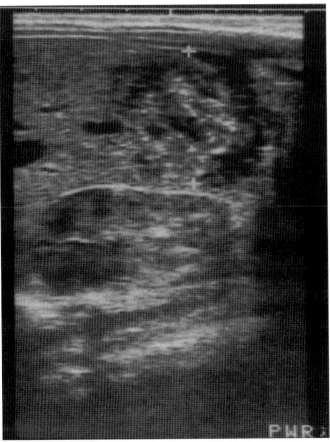

Figure 11.6.11 Solitary haemangioma in a 1-month-old baby girl presenting with hepatomegaly. US shows a 3-cm heterogeneous mass with central calcification.

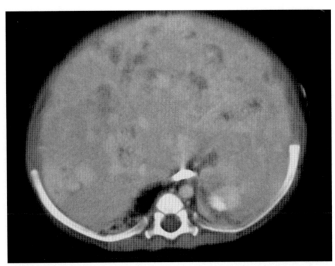

Figure 11.6.12 Diffuse haemangioma in a 1-year-old baby girl. Contrast-enhanced axial CT image showing enhancement of multiple nodules.

tract and mild elevated artery pressure. Less frequently, symptoms include jaundice, failure to thrive and, rarely, liver failure or tumour rupture. Haemangiomas at other sites, including skin, lung, lymph nodes, pancreas, retroperitoneum and bone are seen in 10–15% of children. The most frequently involved site is the skin. A variety of anomalies and associations are associated with infantile haemangioendothelioma. These include Kasabach–Merritt syndrome, deletion of chromosome 6q, diaphragmatic hernia, trisomy 21, extranumery digits, hydrocele, congenital heart disease and angiosarcoma of liver.

On plain film radiography, hepatomegaly or abdominal mass may be noted. Fine speckled calcifications may be seen in 16% of patients. Findings of congestive heart failure may be seen.

On US, lesions are complex or predominately hypoechoic, usually with well-defined margins. Although hyperechoic lesions typical of adult haemangiomas may be seen, this is unusual in haemangioendothelioma. On Doppler studies, the hepatic artery and proximal aorta appear enlarged with tapering of the aorta distal to the coeliac axis. Higher flow velocities than that seen in cavernous haemangiomas can be seen. The hepatic veins may also be enlarged due to increased flow.

A CT scan most commonly demonstrates a hypodense mass lesion with or without calcification. Multifocal lesions are less likely to calcify. Following contrast administration, there is early enhancement of the periphery of the tumour with a variable degree of central enhancement. Delayed scans may show filling of the central low-attenuating area but the centre may often remain hypoattenuating, particularly in large solitary lesions. Large lesions contain areas of infarction or haemorrhage that do not enhance. Small multifocal lesions may enhance completely as they often lack haemorrhage or necrosis.

On MRI, haemangioendothelioma tends to be heterogeneously hypointense on T1-weighted images. Smaller lesions appear homogeneously hypointense on T1-weighted images. Occasionally, a few hyperintense areas can be seen on T1-weighted images, which represent areas of haemorrhage. Similarly, on T2-weighted images, small lesions appear uniformly hyperintense, whereas the larger ones exhibit some degree of heterogeneity. The proximal abdominal aorta, coeliac axis and the main hepatic artery tend to be enlarged in patients with congestive heart failure. In many cases, the descending aorta superior to the level of the coeliac artery may appear abnormally enlarged as compared with the infrahepatic aorta; this is related to increased blood flow due to intratumoural bleeding.

On angiography, the abrupt decrease in the calibre of the aorta beyond the coeliac axis can be seen, with enlargement and tortuosity of the hepatic artery and extrahepatic feeding vessels. The portal vein may also supply the lesions. Persistent pooling of contrast material within some or all of the lesions may be seen. Arterial venous shunting with early draining veins may also be appreciated, distinguishing infantile haemangioendothelioma from the adult cavernous haemangioma, in which such shunting is essentially never seen.

On scintigraphy, both technetium 99m sulphur colloid and tagged red blood cells demonstrate increased flow to the viable parts of the lesions during the angiographic phase, which is distinct from the appearance in the adult cavernous haemangioma, which is typically photopenic in the early phase. On delayed images with sulphur colloid, after clearing of the agent, the lesions appear photopenic. On delayed red blood cell images there is

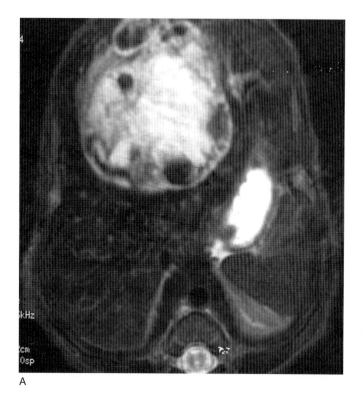

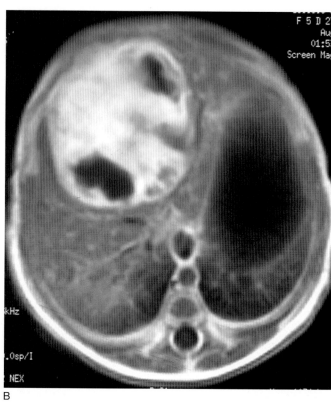

Figure 11.6.13 (A) Axial T2-weighted MR image in a 6-month-old baby showing a large heterogeneous predominately hyperintense mass lesion in the left lobe – infantile haemangioendothelioma. (B) Contrast-enhanced axial T1-weighted MR image showing intense enhancement of the mass lesion.

usually increased activity, which is typically seen unless large areas of haemorrhage, necrosis or fibrosis are present.

FURTHER READING

Daller JA, Bueno J, Gutierrez J et al. Hepatic hemangioendothelioma: Clinical experience and management strategy. Journal of Pediatric Surgery 1999; 34:98–105.

Gianni W, De Vincentis G, Graziano P et al. Scintigraphic imaging of hepatic epithelioid hemangioendothelioma. Digestion 1997;58:498–500.

Hase T, Kodama M, Kishida A et al. Successful management of infantile hepatic hilar hemangioendothelioma with obstructive jaundice and consumption coagulopathy. Journal of Pediatric Surgery 1995; 30:1485–1487.

Robbins RC, Chin C, Yun KL et al. Arterial switch and resection of hepatic hemangioendothelioma. Annals of Thoracic Surgery 1995; 59:1575–1577.

Selby DM, Stocker JT, Waclawiw MA et al. Infantile hemangioendothelioma of the liver. Hepatology 1994; 20:39–45.

Stover B, Laubenberger J, Niemeyer C et al. Haemangiomatosis in children: value of MRI during therapy. Pediatric Radiology 1995; 25:123–126.

LIPOMATOUS BENIGN TUMOURS

These are mesenchymal tumours and they are classified according to their major histological components. These components vary and may show a mixture of fat, muscle, vascular and haemopoietic tissue.

Hepatic angiomyolipoma is rare, occurring only in about 5–10% of cases of tuberous sclerosis and very rarely occurring spontaneously. The lesions tend to be multiple and range from almost entirely lipomatous to completely solid masses of soft tissue density on CT scan.

Pure lipomas are very rare. They are seen as highly echogenic and well-defined lesions on ultrasound. On CT scan, they classically show low-density lesions with attenuation values less than –20 Hounsfield units and lack of contrast enhancement. With MRI, the lesions are homogeneous and hyperintense on T1-weighted images, less hyperintense on T2-weighted images and show loss of signal on fat suppression sequences.

Focal fatty infiltration may simulate a focal tumour. Focal fatty infiltration is not well circumscribed and is usually located at the periphery of liver or its segments. Blood vessels may be seen coursing through the focal fatty infiltration.

FURTHER READING

Cheung H, Ambrose RE, Lee PO. Liver hamartomas in tuberous sclerosis. Clinical Radiology 1993; 47:421–423.

Ros PR. Hepatic angiomyolipoma: is fat in the liver friend or foe? Abdominal Imaging 1994; 19:552–553.

Liver Trauma

Oscar M Navarro, Mónica Epelman

In children with blunt abdominal trauma, the liver is the most commonly injured organ. The liver can also be injured as a result of penetrating trauma, gunshot wounds and stabbings, and although these are uncommon mechanisms of liver trauma in the paediatric population, their incidence is increasing.

Liver trauma can also be the result of child abuse. In a series of 328 cases of paediatric liver injuries, 5% were secondary to child abuse. In this group of children, the diagnosis of liver injury can be delayed, as sometimes there are no clinical findings to suggest this pathology. Elevated transaminase levels should arouse suspicion for liver injury, which can be confirmed with imaging. In this clinical setting, the documentation of liver injury by imaging is imperative for the determination of abuse.

Most liver injuries after blunt abdominal trauma affect the right lobe, particularly the posterior segments. This has been attributed not only to the larger volume of the right lobe compared to the left, but also to the fixation of the liver by the coronary ligaments in this region and the fact that the right lobe of the liver is surrounded by relatively fixed structures such as the ribs and the spine against which the liver can be compressed. Injuries to the right lobe tend to be simpler and more superficial, whereas injuries to the left lobe tend to be deeper, complex and more commonly associated with significant complications. In child abuse, in contrast to accidental injury, hepatic injuries are more common in the left lobe.

The majority of children with liver injury who are haemodynamically stable can be successfully managed non-operatively. This conservative management has been facilitated by the continuous improvement of imaging techniques, especially computed tomography (CT). CT can accurately assess the extent of hepatic injury, document the presence of active haemorrhage and identify associated injuries. Different CT grading systems of liver injury have been proposed. These grading systems, including that recommended by the American Association for the Surgery of Trauma, have proven to be poor predictors of clinical outcome or the need for surgery in these patients and are generally not of clinical value.

In most centres of North America, intravenously enhanced contrast CT is the preferred imaging modality for assessment of paediatric abdominal trauma. On CT, a variety of types of hepatic injury can be outlined (Table 11.7.1). Parenchymal hepatic injuries can be divided into lacerations and haematomas. Lacerations appear as linear or stellate-shaped, hypodense lesions, while intraparenchymal haematomas appear as round, ellipsoid or irregular lesions, mainly hypodense with possible intermixed hyperdense blood (Figure 11.7.1). Subcapsular haematomas appear as lenticular, peripheral, hypodense lesions that cause compression of the

underlying hepatic parenchyma, a sign that is useful in their differentiation from perihepatic intraperitoneal fluid (Figure 11.7.2). Juxtahepatic vascular injuries, that is, injuries of the retrohepatic vena cava and/or major hepatic veins should be suspected when liver lacerations extend towards major hepatic veins or inferior vena cava in association with profuse haemoperitoneum (Figure 11.7.3). Wedge-shaped unenhanced areas that extend to the periphery of the liver may represent areas of hepatic devascularization. Devascularization can occur with lacerations involving perihilar vessels or from complete or partial hepatic avulsion. Peripheral and diffuse periportal low attenuation in the absence of parenchymal disruption is not considered to represent liver injury but rather distension of periportal lymphatic vessels and lymphoedema

Table 11.7.1 Types of traumatic liver injury

Parenchymal laceration
Parenchymal haematoma
Subcapsular haematoma
Juxtahepatic venous injuries
Hepatic vascular avulsion
Parenchymal devascularization
Active haemorrhage
Bile duct injuries

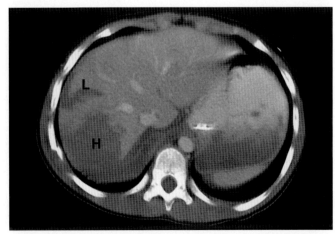

Figure 11.7.1 Contrast-enhanced CT of the liver in a 7-year-old boy struck by a truck. A linear hypodense laceration (L) is seen anteriorly in the right lobe of the liver extending towards the liver capsule. More posteriorly in the right lobe there is a somewhat rounded hypodense parenchymal haematoma (H) with irregular borders.

secondary to vigorous intravenous fluid administration during resuscitation.

Intraabdominal pooling of intravenous contrast on CT indicates extravasation of blood. Pooling that occurs within the liver parenchyma, without associated haemoperitoneum, is often the result of a self-limited haemorrhage. If pooling occurs within the liver associated with haemoperitoneum or there is pooling in the peritoneal cavity in association with parenchymal injury, active bleeding must be suspected (Figures 11.7.3 and 11.7.4).

Ultrasonography (US) is also used in some centres for the primary evaluation of paediatric blunt abdominal trauma, although its use has been restricted due to the higher accuracy of CT in the detection of injury to other abdominal organs. Initially, liver haematomas appear as hyperechoic ill-defined intraparenchymal lesions that become progressively hypoechoic and smaller with time (Figure 11.7.5). Some lacerations may appear slightly hyperechoic but may be difficult to identify initially, becoming easier to recognize days after the initial injury when they become hypoechoic. Subcapsular haematomas appear as peripheral hepatic fluid collections and may be hyper- or hypoechoic.

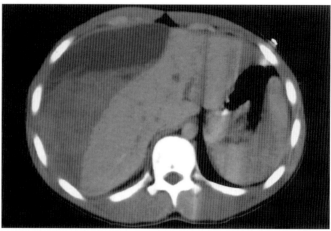

Figure 11.7.2 Contrast-enhanced CT of the liver in a 16-year-old boy two days after blunt abdominal trauma. There is a peripheral subcapsular haematoma that causes compression on the underlying parenchyma of the right lobe of the liver. The haematoma demonstrates a fluid–fluid level in its dependent aspect from settling of blood.

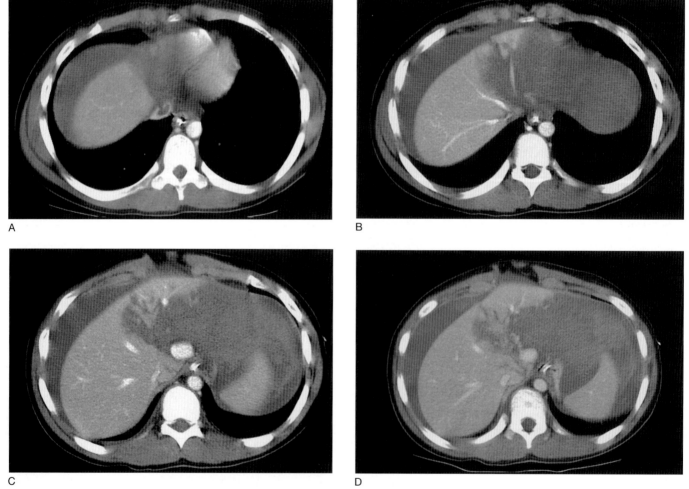

Figure 11.7.3 Contrast-enhanced CT images at different levels of the upper abdomen in a 13-year-old boy after severe abdominal trauma. There is extensive haematoma of the left lobe of the liver extending towards the region of the inferior vena cava (IVC) associated with profuse haemoperitoneum. There is a filling defect in the lumen of the IVC compatible with a thrombus (A). The haematoma is noted to surround the left hepatic vein without opacification of the IVC (B). Pooling of contrast in the posterior aspect of the haematoma indicates active bleeding (C, D). The more distal retrohepatic IVC appears opacified (D). In addition, there is disruption of the anterior abdominal wall (C, D). Surgery confirmed laceration of the IVC and left hepatic vein.

Magnetic resonance imaging (MRI) has not been used in the evaluation of children with liver trauma. There are few reports of its use in the adult population, which have shown that gadolinium-enhanced MRI is at least as reliable as intravenously contrast enhanced CT in the detection of traumatic hepatic lesions. Currently, its use in the acute setting of liver trauma is only considered in cases of allergy to iodinated contrast material or the rare instances that CT imaging might be unavailable.

US and CT are frequently used to assess stability and healing of hepatic injuries. However, in most asymptomatic children with blunt hepatic trauma initially managed non-operatively, routine follow-up imaging studies are of limited value since generally they do not provide information that affects their management. Repeat imaging is only justified when clinical findings reappear or persist, which may suggest the development of a complication.

Complications such as persistent or delayed haemorrhage, haemobilia, biliary leaks and abscess formation can occur in children managed operatively and non-operatively (Table 11.7.2). These usually have a delayed presentation, occurring often 2 weeks or longer after the initial trauma. Repeat imaging evaluation with US or CT will usually demonstrate these complications but their appearance are frequently not specific and correla-

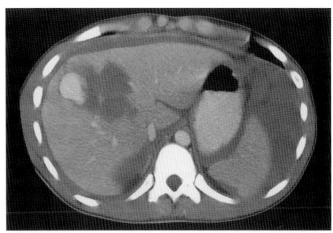

Figure 11.7.4 Contrast-enhanced CT performed 10 days after blunt abdominal trauma in a 16-year-old boy who returned to the hospital with pain, hypotension and haemoglobin drop. There is pooling of intravenous contrast in the right lobe of the liver associated with a parenchymal haematoma. A large haemoperitoneum is visible around the liver and spleen. Surgery confirmed active bleeding from portal vein branch injury. (Reproduced from Navarro et al. (2000) with permission of Springer-Verlag.)

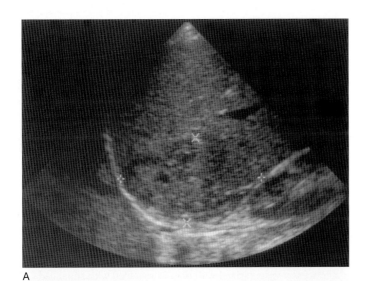

A

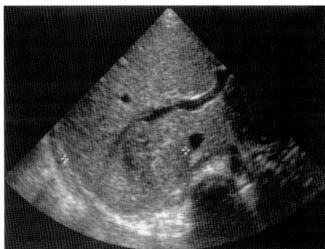

B

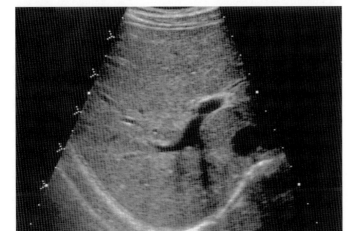

C

Figure 11.7.5 US images of the liver in a 6-year-old boy after blunt abdominal trauma. (A, B) Longitudinal and transverse images obtained 3 days after injury show it is an ill-defined parenchymal haematoma of mixed echogenicity in the right lobe of the liver (outlined by cursors). (C) Transverse image obtained at a similar level as (B) 5 weeks later shows interval decrease in size and echogenicity of the parenchymal haematoma.

Table 11.7.2 Complications of traumatic liver injury

Delayed haemorrhage
Haemobilia
Arterial pseudoaneurysm
Biloma/bile peritonitis
Abscess

tion with the clinical findings is needed to guide appropriate management.

Delayed bleeding is reported to occur in 1–3% of patients after blunt hepatic injury. Persistence or increase in the volume of peritoneal fluid, enlargement of a liver haematoma, new appearance of perihepatic collections and pooling of intravenous contrast on CT can be signs of ongoing bleeding (Figure 11.7.4). On occasion, delayed bleeding may present with haemobilia as a result of a traumatic communication between the hepatic arterial and biliary systems. A non-specific finding of haemobilia is the detection of high attenuation blood within the gallbladder lumen and dilated bile ducts. However, high-density material within the gallbladder can also be seen with calculi, gallbladder wall haematomas, vicarious excretion of intravenous contrast, biliary sludge and milk of calcium bile. Hepatic arterial pseudoaneurysms can rarely develop after liver trauma. A pseudoaneurysm is a pulsatile haematoma that results from leakage of blood through a disruption of the arterial wall; thus the blood is contained only by hepatic parenchyma or surrounding haematoma. Although pseudoaneurysms can present with bleeding, many of them are discovered on evaluation for other reasons. On US, a pseudoaneurysm appears as an intraparenchymal hypoechoic area that fills with a jet or turbulent flow on colour or power Doppler interrogation (Figure 11.7.6). CT depicts a pseudoaneurysm as a focal, rounded area of avid enhancement of density similar to the aorta (Figure 11.7.7A). Arteriography demonstrates a pseudoaneurysm as an extravasation from the arterial lumen that communicates with a perivascular collection of contrast media that persists into the venous phase (Figure 11.7.7B). Transcatheter embolization can be used with success in the treatment of haemorrhagic complications associated with traumatic hepatic arterial injuries in the vast majority of patients. Some cases of vascular injury require emergency surgical treatment.

Biliary duct injuries are difficult to diagnose on CT in the acute phase. Repeat US or CT can demonstrate the presence of localized fluid collections or increasing peritoneal fluid. When a bile leak is suspected clinically, a HIDA scan or image-guided aspiration of the suspected collection can confirm the biloma. MRI has been proven to be useful in differentiating intrahepatic biloma from subacute intrahepatic haematoma. Endoscopic retrograde cholangiopancreatography allows localization of the site of injury and may be used for endobiliary stenting. Magnetic resonance cholangiopancreatography in one adult has recently been reported to be useful in identifying the site of injury in blunt extrahepatic bile duct disruption. Bilomas can be drained percutaneously under imaging guidance while ongoing bile leaks or biliary-peritoneal communications can be managed by diverting the flow of bile via percutaneous biliary drainage, including external drainage, as well as internal-external biliary drainage.

Abscess formation may occur when a liver haematoma is superinfected. US or CT can demonstrate a focal collection of fluid that occasionally may contain bubbles of gas. Depending on the age of

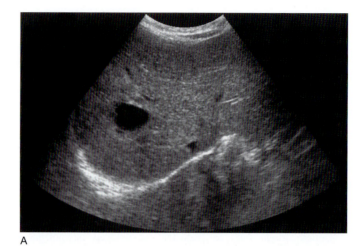

A

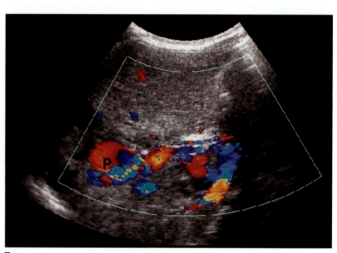

B

Figure 11.7.6 Five-year-old boy or girl with blunt liver trauma after being struck by a car. Follow-up US obtained 10 days after injury. (A) Transverse US image of the liver shows an arterial pseudoaneurysm as a well-defined, anechoic, ovoid area in the right lobe. (B) On colour Doppler interrogation the pseudoaneurysm (P) fills with turbulent flow.

the abscess a vascularized wall may be revealed with enhanced CT or colour/power Doppler US. Abscesses can be drained percutaneously under imaging guidance.

FURTHER READING

Basile KE, Sivit CJ, Sachs PB et al. Hepatic arterial pseudoaneurysm: a rare complication of blunt abdominal trauma in children. Pediatric Radiology 1999; 29:306–308.

Brick SH, Taylor GA, Potter BM et al. Hepatic and splenic injury in children: role of CT in the decision for laparotomy. Radiology 1987; 165:643–646.

Christensen R. Invasive radiology for pediatric trauma. Seminars in Pediatric Surgery 2001;10:7–11.

Coant PN, Kornberg AE, Brody AS et al. Markers for occult liver injury in cases of physical abuse in children. Pediatrics 1992; 89:274–278.

Cooper A. Liver injuries in children: treatments tried, lessons learned. Seminars in Pediatric Surgery 1992; 1:152–161.

Fang JF, Chen RJ, Wong YC et al. Classification and treatment of pooling of contrast material on computed tomographic scan of blunt hepatic trauma. Journal of Trauma 2000; 49:1083–1088.

Filiatrault D, Garel L. Commentary: pediatric blunt abdominal trauma – to sound or not to sound? Pediatric Radiology 1995; 25:329–331.

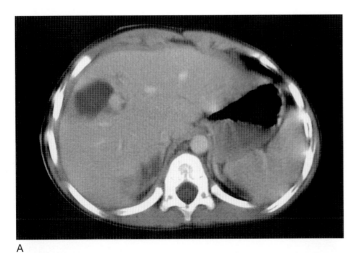

A

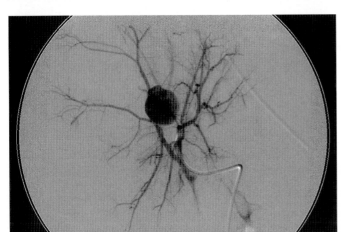

B

Figure 11.7.7 Nine-year-old boy with blunt liver trauma after motor vehicle accident. (A) Contrast enhanced CT performed 15 days after initial injury due to gastrointestinal bleeding and concern for haemobilia. There is a focal rounded collection of contrast identified in the right lobe of the liver adjacent to a hypodense parenchymal haematoma. (B) Selective hepatic arteriography depicts a pseudoaneurysm arising from a posterior branch of the right hepatic artery. A focal region of decreased perfusion in the superior aspect of the right hepatic lobe is seen due to the parenchymal haematoma. This pseudoaneurysm was successfully embolized under angiographic guidance.

Gross M, Lynch F, Canty T Sr et al. Management of pediatric liver injuries: a 13-year experience at a pediatric trauma center. Journal of Pediatric Surgery 1999; 34:811–817.

Hackam DJ, Potoka D, Meza M et al. Utility of radiographic hepatic injury grade in predicting outcome for children after blunt abdominal trauma. Journal of Pediatric Surgery 2002; 37:386–389.

Kleinman PK. Visceral trauma. In: Kleinman PK, ed. Diagnostic imaging of child abuse, 2nd edn. St. Louis: Mosby; 1998:248–284.

Lam AH, Shulman L. Ultrasonography in the management of liver trauma in children. Journal of Ultrasound in Medicine 1984; 3:199–203.

McGahan JP, Wang L, Richards JR. Focused abdominal US for trauma. Radiographics 2001; 21:S191–S199.

McGillivray DC, Valentine RJ. Nonoperative management of blunt pediatric liver injury – late complications: case report. Journal of Trauma 1989; 29:251–254.

Navarro O, Babyn PS, Pearl RH. The value of routine follow-up imaging in pediatric blunt liver trauma. Pediatric Radiology 2000; 30:546–550.

Poli ML, Lefebvre F, Ludot H et al. Nonoperative management of biliary tract fistulas after blunt abdominal trauma in a child. Journal of Pediatric Surgery 1995; 30:1719–1721.

Ruess L, Sivit CJ, Eichelberger MR et al. Blunt hepatic and splenic trauma in children: correlation of a CT injury severity scale with clinical outcome. Pediatric Radiology 1995; 25:321–325.

Sanders DW, Andrews DA. Conservative management of hepatic duct injury after blunt trauma: a case report. Journal of Pediatric Surgery 2000; 35:1503–1505.

Shanmuganathan K, Mirvis SE, Amoroso M. Periportal low density on CT in patients with blunt trauma: association with elevated venous pressure. American Journal of Roentgenology 1993; 160:279–283.

Shanmuganathan K, Mirvis SE. CT evaluation of the liver with acute blunt trauma. Critical Reviews in Diagnostic Imaging 1995; 36:73–113.

Shigemura T, Yamamoto F, Shilpakar SK et al. MRI differential diagnosis of intrahepatic biloma from subacute hematoma. Abdominal Imaging 1995; 20:211–213.

Shilyansky J, Navarro O, Superina R et al. Delayed haemorrhage after nonoperative management of blunt hepatic trauma in children: a rare but significant event. Journal of Pediatric Surgery 1999; 34:60–64.

Sidhu MK, Shaw DWW, Daly CP. Post-traumatic hepatic pseudoaneurysms in children. Pediatric Radiology 1999; 29:46–52.

Stalker HP, Kaufman RA, Towbin R. Patterns of liver injury in childhood: CT analysis. American Journal of Roentgenology 1986; 147:1199–1205.

Taylor GA, O'Donnell R, Sivit CJ et al. Abdominal injury score: a clinical score for the assignment of risk in children following blunt trauma. Radiology 1994; 190:689–694.

Terk MR, Rozenberg D. Gadolinium-enhanced MR imaging of traumatic hepatic injury. American Journal of Roentgenology 1998; 171:665–669.

Vock P, Kehrer B, Tschaeppeler H. Blunt liver trauma in children: the role of computed tomography in diagnosis and treatment. Journal of Pediatric Surgery 1986; 21:413–418.

Wong YC, Wang LJ, Chen RJ et al. Magnetic resonance imaging of extrahepatic bile duct disruption. European Radiology 2002; 12:2488–2490.

The Biliary Tract

Danièle Pariente

Imaging has a major role to play in biliary tract diseases. The clinical presentation with most biliary tract lesions in childhood is with jaundice or pain. Jaundice may be due to obstruction to excretion of bile, hepatic parenchymal disease or prehepatic causes. The aim of imaging is to establish the cause of the disease. The aetiology to consider differs according to the age of the child (Tables 11.8.1 and 11.8.2). In the neonatal period, the leading cause is biliary atresia, which requires urgent surgical treatment to reduce the need for early liver transplantation. In childhood, when there is bile duct dilatation the main problem is to differentiate a choledochal cyst from cholelithiasis.

Imaging begins with ultrasound (US) to determine whether the biliary system is dilated or non-dilated and whether the gallbladder or gallstones are visible. If the biliary system is dilated, some form of cholangiography is then undertaken to determine the cause of obstruction. If the system is non-dilated, radionuclide studies to demonstrate excretion of the pharmaceutical into the gastrointestinal (GI) tract excludes an obstructive jaundice. In some cases a percutaneous liver biopsy is often required to establish the cause of jaundice. This chapter discusses the major causes of biliary disease in infants and children and their imaging findings. The reader is referred to larger textbooks of paediatric liver disease for a description of the other conditions. The diagnosis is made on clinical features, biochemistry and often biopsy.

NEONATAL CHOLESTASIS

BILIARY ATRESIA

DEFINITION, PATHOGENESIS AND ANATOMICAL FORMS

This is the single most common cause of neonatal cholestasis, accounting for approximately half of all cases and more than 90% of the extrahepatic causes. The diagnosis should be established as soon as possible, as it has been proved that early surgical treatment improves the prognosis.

Biliary atresia is a congenital anomaly, consisting of the obliteration of the extrahepatic bile duct. Its pathogenesis is unknown but it is currently thought to be an acquired progressive inflammatory disease of the biliary tract. The atresia of the extrahepatic bile duct may be complete or partial but the intrahepatic bile ducts have been shown to be always abnormal with a plexiform and moniliform appearance on preoperative or postoperative cholangiography.

Multiple anatomical types of biliary atresia are described depending on the extent of the sclerotic process (Figure 11.8.1). The whole extrahepatic bile duct may be atretic (60%). The gallbladder may be preserved, isolated (filled by epithelium secretion) or associated with a patent choledochus or more rarely with a patent common hepatic duct. In about 10% of cases, a cyst may be found on the remnant of the extrahepatic bile duct. Its size is variable, ranging from 2 mm to 4 cm. It may or may not communicate with a patent gallbadder and with the abnormal intrahepatic bile ducts but it does not communicate with the distal choledochus and the duodenum. When this cyst is large, the prognosis following surgery seems to be better.

In about 10% of cases, biliary atresia is associated with a malformation syndrome, which has been called the 'non-cardiac polysplenia syndrome'. This syndrome may include some of the following elements: polysplenia or rarely asplenia, abdominal and/or thoracic situs inversus, preduodenal portal vein, anomaly of the inferior vena cava (azygous or hemiazygous continuation or left inferior vena cava), multiple and/or aberrant hepatic arteries, and malrotation of the intestine.

CLINICAL PRESENTATION

In up to 80% of patients with biliary atresia, the clinical presentation of persistent white acholic stools with an enlarged and firm liver strongly suggests the diagnosis. In the remaining patients, these clinical findings are not as evident and further investigation is indicated to establish the diagnosis as soon as possible. This includes ultrasonography, percutaneous liver biopsy, percutaneous cholangiography in some selected cases and even exploratory laparotomy. The place of radionuclide studies, magnetic resonance imaging and also endoscopic retrograde cholangiography will be discussed in this chapter.

US FINDINGS

US in these infants must be carried out with high-frequency transducers (7–14 MHz). The diagnosis of biliary atresia cannot be made on the basis of absence of visibility of the extrahepatic bile duct because of the multiple anatomical forms of biliary atresia

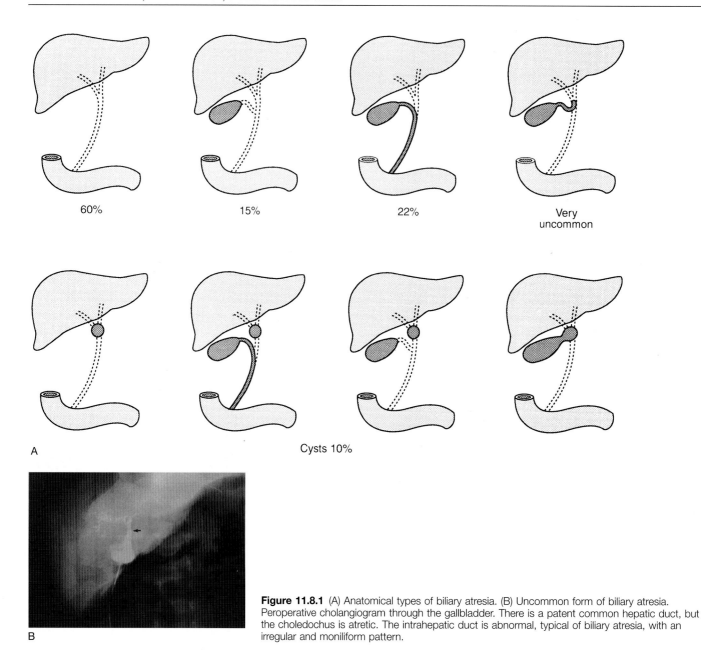

A

Cysts 10%

B

Figure 11.8.1 (A) Anatomical types of biliary atresia. (B) Uncommon form of biliary atresia. Peroperative cholangiogram through the gallbladder. There is a patent common hepatic duct, but the choledochus is atretic. The intrahepatic duct is abnormal, typical of biliary atresia, with an irregular and moniliform pattern.

and because the normal common bile duct of the newborn is rarely totally visible, unless it is dilated, measuring less than 1 mm in diameter. It must not be confused with the hepatic artery, which is often prominent (measuring 2–3 mm) and sometimes multiple. The hepatic artery is well identified with colour Doppler imaging. The abnormality of the intrahepatic bile ducts, which seems to be constant in biliary atresia, cannot be demonstrated by ultrasonography in neonates.

The 'triangular cord sign' has been reported to be a highly reliable finding of biliary atresia. It corresponds to the visualization of the fibrotic remnant of the hepatic ducts junction seen as a triangular or band-like echogenic mass at the porta hepatis, cranial to the portal vein (Figure 11.8.2). However, in practice, this sign does not seem to be constant, is often difficult to differentiate from the echogenic tissue surrounding the termination of the hepatic artery, and may be encountered in other causes of neonatal cholestasis in which liver fibrosis is present (Figure 11.8.3).

The presence or absence of the gallbladder is not a completely reliable diagnostic finding. A large gallbladder, even emptying after a meal may be found in biliary atresia. Failure to demonstrate the gallbladder is not completely specific to biliary atresia and may be found in other types of intrahepatic cholestasis, such as Alagille's syndrome, cystic fibrosis or transient neonatal cholestasis.

Table 11.8.1 Causes of neonatal cholestasis

Type of lesion	Cause	Type of cause
Extrahepatic bile duct lesions (about 5%)	Cholelithiasis Choledochal cyst Perforation Duodenal duplication Pancreatic haemangioma . . .	Surgical causes
Extra- and intrahepatic bile duct lesions (40%)	**Biliary atresia**	Surgical cause

Intrahepatic bile duct lesions (55%)	Sclerosing cholangitis
	Transient neonatal
	    cholestasis
	Paucity of interlobular
	    bile duct (Alagille's
	    syndrome and the
	    non-syndromic form)
	Byler's disease
	Alpha 1 antitrypsin
	    deficiency
	Infections
	Cystic fibrosis
	Parenteral nutrition
	Niemann–Pick disease
	Tyrosinaemia
	Galactosaemia
	Mitochondrial respiratory
	    chain disorders . . .
		Medical causes

Table 11.8.2 Causes of childhood cholestasis

Type of lesion	Cause	Type of cause
Extrahepatic bile duct lesions	Cholelithiasis Choledochal cyst Tumoral compression Portal vein obstruction Postsurgical stenosis Liver trauma	Surgical causes
Extra- and intrahepatic bile duct lesions	Sclerosing cholangitis	Medical cause

Intrahepatic bile duct lesions	Viral hepatitis
	Drug-induced hepatitis
	Benign recurrent
	    cholestasis
	Alpha 1 antitrypsin
	    deficiency
	Cystic fibrosis
	Byler's disease
	Alagille's syndrome
		Medical causes

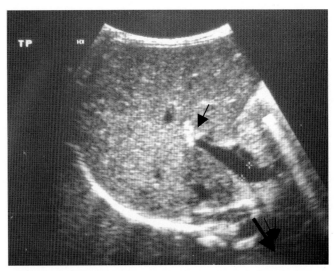

Figure 11.8.2 Biliary atresia. Two-month-old infant with severe cholestasis. Longitudinal scan through the portal vein showing a triangular hyperechoic area (arrows) just in front of the termination of the portal vein. This corresponds to the fibrotic remnant of the obliterated extrahepatic bile duct. This finding is suggestive of the diagnosis of biliary atresia but is not completely reliable.

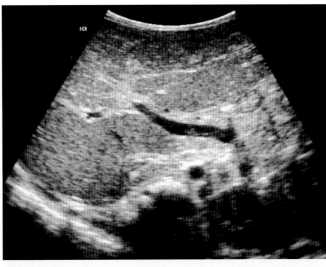

Figure 11.8.3 Intrahepatic medical cause of neonatal cholestasis. One-month-old baby presenting with cholestasis and hepatosplenomegaly. US examination showing marked hyperechogenicity at the vicinity of the portal vein was suggestive of biliary atresia. However, the final diagnosis was Niemann–Pick disease.

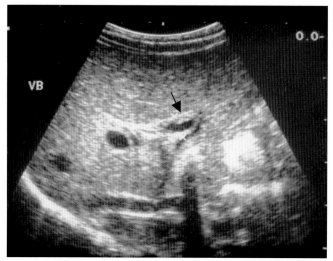

Figure 11.8.4 Biliary atresia. Six-week-old infant with cholestasis. Transverse scan through the gallbladder (arrow) showing that it is small with marked hyperechogenicity of the walls. This finding is very suggestive of the diagnosis of biliary atresia.

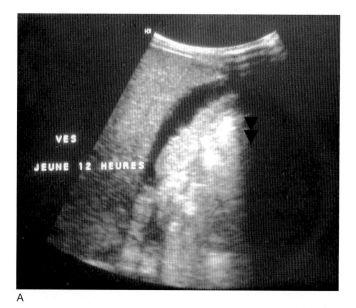

A

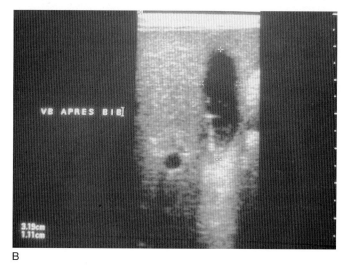

B

Figure 11.8.5 Biliary atresia. Three-week-old baby with cholestasis. (A) After 12 h of fasting, US showed a large gallbladder but with slightly irregular and hyperechoic walls. (B) After feeding, the gallbladder did not empty. At surgery, there was obliteration of the choledochus and of the common hepatic duct and the gallbladder was excluded or blind, filled with colourless fluid.

However, some findings, together with the clinical presentation, are suggestive of biliary atresia: an absent or very small gallbladder following a 6-h fast, a gallbladder with irregular and echogenic walls (Figure 11.8.4) or a large gallbladder that does not empty after a meal (Figure 11.8.5).

The diagnosis of biliary atresia can be made on ultrasonography if there is a cyst at the porta hepatis. It may be a large cyst, sometimes seen antenatally, which can be differentiated from a choledochal cyst by the absence of intrahepatic bile duct dilatation in a cholestatic neonate (Figure 11.8.6 and 11.8.7). It may be a tiny cyst of 2–5 mm only seen with a high-frequency transducer and colour Doppler (Figure 11.8.8).

The elements of the polysplenia syndrome also have to be searched for because they are diagnostic (Figures 11.8.9 to Figure 11.8.11) but they are not always evident at first glance.

Finally, biliary atresia can only be ruled out with certitude when there is dilatation of the bile duct, which is a rare event in neonatal cholestasis (only 5% of the cases in our series).

OTHER IMAGING FINDINGS

RADIONUCLIDE STUDIES

Radionuclide studies are used where facilities are available. They are not 100% reliable but are helpful in distinguishing cholestasis from biliary atresia. In normal patients, IDA compounds labelled with technetium are rapidly cleared from the bloodstream and bind to biliary radicles following intravenous (IV) injection. Excretion commences within 5 min with clearance from the liver by about 30 min. In biliary atresia, before cirrhosis is established, there is rapid clearance of the radionuclide from the bloodstream but there is failure of excretion of the compound into the GI tract (Figure 11.8.12). In infants with cholestatic jaundice, there is more liver damage and thus poor clearance of the compound from the bloodstream, with associated poorer liver definition (Figure 11.8.13). Excretion of the compound into the GI tract may not be demonstrated if there is severe cholestasis and thus biliary atresia cannot be excluded. To maximize biliary uptake and excretion, the infant is premedicated with phenobarbitone (5 mg/kg for 3 days). The examination is always performed fasting.

ENDOSCOPIC RETROGRADE CHOLANGIOPANCREATOGRAPHY

This technique is used by a few experts to make the diagnosis. However, it is difficult to perform and the diagnosis of biliary

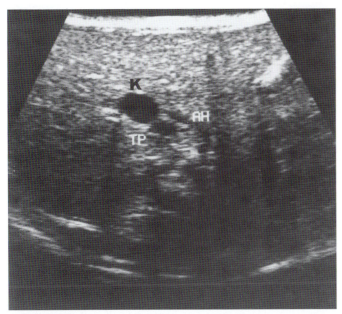

Figure 11.8.6 Pedicular cyst of biliary atresia. There is a 1.5 cm cyst (K) located in the porta hepatis between the hepatic artery (AH) and the portal vein (TP).

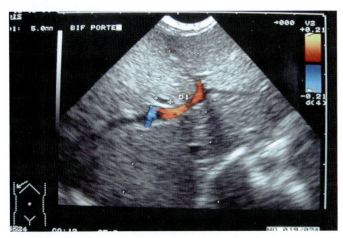

Figure 11.8.8 Biliary atresia. One-month-old infant with cholestasis. US examination with colour Doppler showed a small cyst (cross marks) at the porta hepatis, just in front of the right portal vein. This finding is diagnostic of biliary atresia.

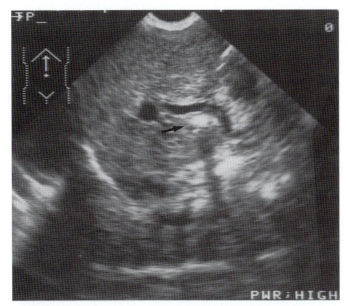

Figure 11.8.10 Preduodenal portal vein. Abnormal course of the portal vein in front of the duodenal shadow (arrow) in biliary atresia with associated malformation complex.

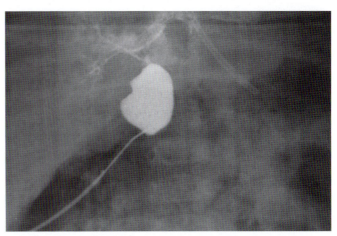

Figure 11.8.7 Preoperative opacification of another case of biliary atresia with a cyst. This large cyst communicates with intrahepatic abnormal bile ducts. There is no communication with the duodenum.

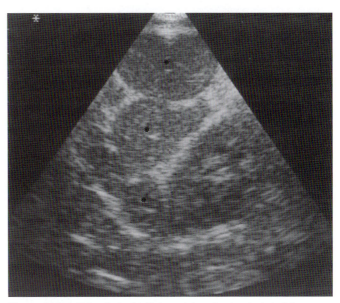

Figure 11.8.9 Polysplenia. Multiple nodules of polysplenia in biliary atresia with malformation complex (•).

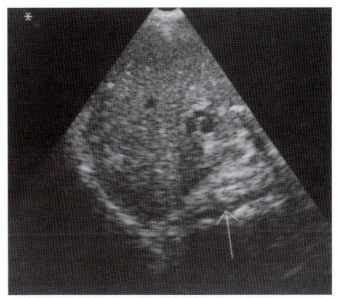

Figure 11.8.11 Azygos continuation of IVC. This retrohepatic vessel corresponds to the azygos vein and does not join the inferior aspect of the right atrium.

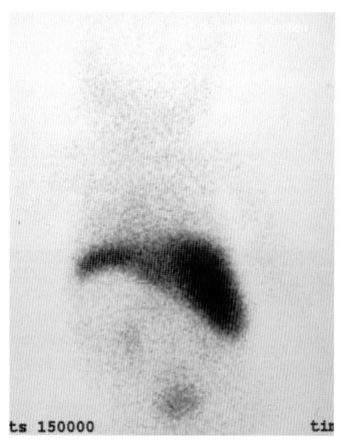

ts 150000   tin

Figure 11.8.12 Technetium HIDA scan in an infant with biliary atresia. Image taken 5 h postinjection. There has been good clearance from the bloodstream but there is no excretion. The activity seen outside the liver in the abdomen is in the kidney and bladder.

atresia is based on a negative sign, which is the absence of catheterization of the choledochus.

MAGNETIC RESONANCE IMAGING

This is being increasingly used to demonstrate the biliary tree and is likely to become the modality of choice in the future. It is a very satisfactory technique in older children but in infants the results are still equivocal, with false-positive and false-negative results.

PERCUTANEOUS TRANSHEPATIC CHOLECYSTOGRAPHY

If the gallbladder is present and large enough, percutaneous transhepatic cholecystography (PTC), under US guidance, can be performed to demonstrate the atretic common hepatic duct (Figure 11.8.14), or to make the diagnosis of sclerosing cholangitis or normal bile duct (Figure 11.8.15).

SURGERY

The spontaneous evolution of biliary atresia is poor, with death occurring at the age of 2 years with the complications of biliary cirrhosis. However, liver transplantation is not considered as the first treatment of biliary atresia, except in patients with missed diagnosis and advanced liver disease. The current opinion is that the Kasai procedure has to be undertaken ideally before 45 days

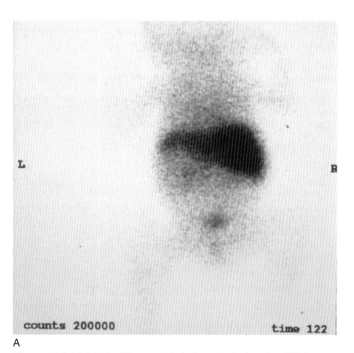

L   R

counts 200000   time 122

A

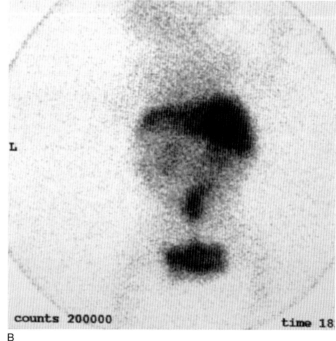

L

counts 200000   time 18

B

Figure 11.8.13 Infant with neonatal cholestasis. Technetium HIDA scan: at 45 min (A) and at 23 h (B). Note the retention of radiopharmaceutical in the liver but on the 23-h image some is in the rectum. There is still radionuclide not fixed in the liver. This is a common finding in neonatal cholestasis. The radionuclide in the colon at 23 h demonstrates that the biliary tree is patent.

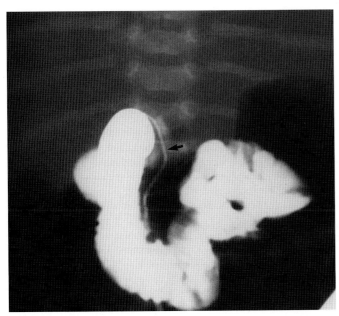

Figure 11.8.14 Biliary atresia. A large gallbladder (3 cm in length) punctured under US guidance: there is a patent choledochus (arrow) but an atretic common hepatic duct.

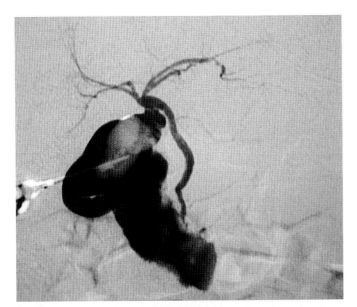

Figure 11.8.15 Two-month-old infant presenting with severe cholestasis and a history of perinatal distress. US examination was unremarkable and MRI unconclusive. Percutaneous transhepatic cholangiogram by puncture of the gallbladder shows a normal biliary tree. The final diagnosis is transient benign neonatal cholestasis.

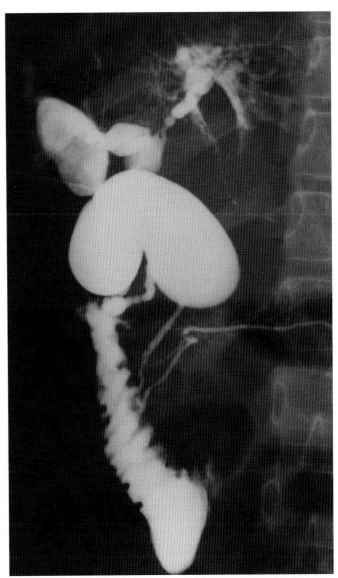

Figure 11.8.16 Postoperative cholangiography. Fourteen-year-old girl with a history of biliary atresia and portocholecystostomy, presenting with episodes of cholangitis. PTC via the gallbladder shows a very small calibre of the choledochus with tiny intraluminal filling defects. Large intrahepatic cystic cavities are opacified corresponding to parenchymal nectrotic areas filled with bile. She underwent liver transplantation a few months later.

of life to provide the best chance (up to 80%) of clearing the jaundice and survival with a good quality of life and reducing the need for liver transplantation.

The operative procedure depends on the anatomical type of biliary atresia. It consists of a hepatoporto-enterostomy (Kasai procedure), that is resection of the fibrous remnant of the extrahepatic bile duct and jejunal anastomosis at the porta hepatis. The fundus of the gallbladder may be used for this anastomosis if the gall-bladder is large enough and the choledochus is patent (hepatoportocholecystostomy) (Figure 11.8.16). A complication of the latter procedure is anastomotic leakage with bile peritonitis, which requires surgical repair.

COMPLICATIONS

Cholangitis, portal hypertension and biliary cirrhosis are the main complications following surgery. Biliary atresia accounts for 50% of the indications for liver transplantation in childhood. Acute deterioration is also possible, probably secondary to ischaemic damage of the liver, and liver transplantation must be performed as an emergency in these cases.

Ultrasound plays an important role in the follow-up of these patients. It may demonstrate intrahepatic cystic cavities, often filled with echogenic material, and corresponding to bile-filled parenchymal necrotic areas. If there is clinical evidence of cholangitis, these cavities may be punctured under US guidance to obtain aspirate for culture and to identify the correct antibiotic treatment. If the cholangitis is resistant to medical treatment and the cavities are large, external drainage may be useful.

The degree of portal hypertension and development of cirrhosis can be monitored by US. Pretransplantation work-up is also based on US.

Pulmonary arteriovenous shunting is a known complication of cirrhosis and occurs very early in patients with biliary atresia and polysplenia syndrome. It is detected by pulmonary scintigraphy with technetium (Tc) 99m microaggregated albumin. Pulmonary artery hypertension is more rare and may be detected by echocardiography.

Hypertrophic osteoarthropathy has also been reported. It is characterized by periosteal reaction involving the shaft of the long bones, soft tissue swelling about the joints and digital clubbing. The pathogenesis is unknown.

FURTHER READING

Barbe T, Losay J, Grimon G et al. Pulmonary arteriovenous shunting in children with liver disease. Journal of Pediatrics 1995; 126:571–579.

Chardot C, Carton M, Spire-Bendelac N et al. Prognosis of biliary atresia in the era of liver transplantation: French national study from 1986 to 1996. Hepatology 1999; 30:808–810.

Chardot C, Carton M, Spire-Bendelac N et al. Is the Kasai operation still indicated in children older than 3 months diagnosed with biliary atresia? Journal of Pediatrics 2001; 138:224–228.

Choi SO, Park WH, Lee HJ. Ultrasonographic 'triangular cord': the most definitive finding for noninvasive diagnosis of extrahepatic biliary atresia. European Journal of Surgery 1998; 8:12–16.

Farrant P, Meire HB, Mieli-Vergani G. Improved diagnosis of extrahepatic biliary atresia by high frequency ultrasound of the gallbladder. British Journal of Radiology 2001; 74:952–954.

Gubernick JA, Rosenberg HK, Ilaslan H, Kessler A. US approach to jaundice in infants and children. Radiographics 2000; 20:173–195.

Kim MJ, Park YN, Han SJ et al. Biliary atresia in neonates and infants: triangular area of high signal intensity in the porta hepatis at T2-weighted MR cholangiography with US and histopathologic correlation. Radiology 2000; 215:395–401.

Norton KI, Glass RB, Kogan D et al. MR cholangiography in the evaluation of neonatal cholestasis: initial results. Radiology 2002; 222:687–691.

Park WH, Choi SO, Lee HJ et al. A new diagnostic approach to biliary atresia with emphasis on the ultrasonographic triangular cord sign: comparison of ultrasonography, hepatobiliary scintigraphy, and needle biopsy in the evaluation of infantile cholestasis. Journal of Pediatric Surgery 1997; 32:1555–1559.

Tanano H, Hasegawa T, Kawahara H, Sasaki T, Okada A. Biliary atresia associated with congenital structural anomalies. Journal of Pediatric Surgery 1999; 34:1687–1690.

OTHER CAUSES OF NEONATAL CHOLESTASIS

INTRAHEPATIC CAUSES OF NEONATAL CHOLESTASIS

Intrahepatic causes of neonatal cholestasis are diverse and are listed in Table 11.8.1. The term 'neonatal hepatitis', which is frequently used in the literature, has been replaced by all the medical causes that can now be identified. Imaging with US and radionuclide studies is performed to exclude obstructive causes of jaundice and to define normal anatomy. The diagnosis of these entities is mainly based on biological and histological findings. However, a few characteristic imaging findings have to be known. The diagnosis of sclerosing cholangitis with neonatal onset is made by percutaneous cholecystography when moniliform intrahepatic bile ducts and a patent extrahepatic bile duct are identified. Several elements of Alagille's syndrome (syndromic paucity of the interlobular bile duct) may also be found on radiological examinations. They include mainly the 'butterfly vertebrae', pulmonary artery branch stenoses and on cholangiography (best performed via the gallbladder), paucity and attenuation of intrahepatic bile ducts (Figure 11.8.17 to 11.8.19). Other skeletal findings have also been reported: narrow lumbar spine, shortness of the ulna and radioulnar synostosis. The clinical features include a peculiar facies and posterior embryotoxon on slit lamp examination of the eyes. Some genetic mutations have been identified.

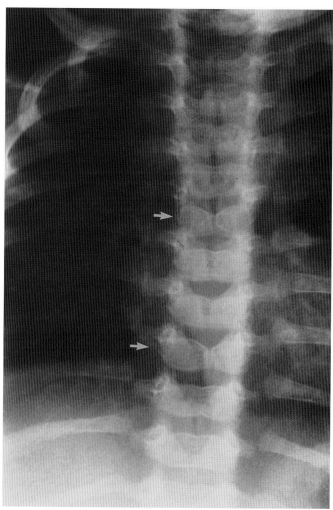

Figure 11.8.17 'Butterfly' vertebrae (arrows) in cholestatic newborn with cholestatic jaundice. The diagnosis is that of syndromic paucity of interlobular bile ducts (Alagille's syndrome).

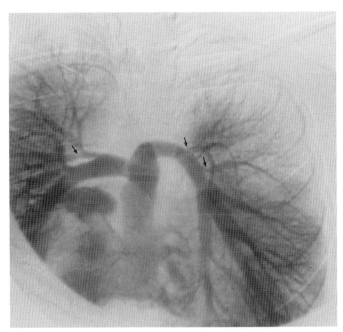

Figure 11.8.18 Pulmonary branches stenoses. Seven-year-old boy with syndromic paucity of bile duct and cardiac murmur. Digital venous subtraction angiography shows multiple discrete stenoses with pulmonary hypoperfusion (arrows).

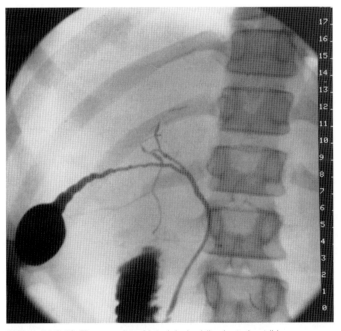

Figure 11.8.19 The paucity of interlobular bile ducts is striking on percutaneous cholecystography performed in this 14-year-old boy with Alagille's syndrome.

EXTRAHEPATIC CAUSES OF NEONATAL CHOLESTASIS

Besides biliary atresia, extrahepatic causes of neonatal cholestasis are rare, representing 5% of the cases in our series. They include cholelithiasis, choledochal cyst, spontaneous perforation of the biliary tract and rare cases of extrinsic compression by duodenal duplication or pancreatic haemangioma or other tumours. In all these cases, the diagnosis is based on imaging.

CHOLELITHIASIS IN INFANCY

This is a rare entity, first described as the 'bile plug syndrome'. The aetiology is still unclear. The calculi are pigment stones confirmed by morphology (blackish and crumbly at extraction) and by biochemical analysis. The following causative factors have been reported: haemolysis, prematurity, dehydration, infection, parenteral nutrition, furosemide treatment and gastrointestinal dysfunction. This entity is probably due to a transient bile disturbance resulting from deficient glucurono-conjugation. The clinical presentation is non-specific with fluctuating jaundice and hepatomegaly. The biliary tract is normal and there is no recurrence after treatment. Mild and even dilatation of the extra- and intrahepatic bile ducts is usually present at US examination (Figure 11.8.20) but in some cases the dilatation may be marked. Sludge or calculi may be found in the gallbladder and sometimes antenatally. The obstructive calculus may be depicted in the distal end of the choledochus as an echogenic ball, with or without acoustic shadowing; however, it may be obscured by the overlying bowel gas of the duodenum. Spontaneous resolution has been documented on US, probably secondary to passage of the calculus into the duodenum. However, cholangitis and even liver abscesses may complicate this entity and thus the presence of fever or the persistence of severe cholestasis is an indication for treatment (Figure 11.8.21). Percutaneous cholangiography or cholecystography with flushing of the biliary tree with saline and contrast in order to push the stone into the duodenum is the treatment of choice and has been successful in about 75% of our cases (Figure 11.8.22). The placement of an external drain is recommended to permit repeat lavage. If this fails, the infant will require surgery.

SPONTANEOUS PERFORATION OF THE BILIARY TRACT IN INFANCY

This is a rare disorder that has been reported at ages of from 1 week to 4 years, with a higher rate between 1 and 3 months. The pathogenesis is unknown. The perforation is often located at the junction of the cystic and common hepatic duct and it has been suggested that there is an area of weakness in the bile duct wall at this point. Other recorded sites of perforation are the gallbladder, the cystic duct, the common hepatic duct and the common bile duct. The clinical presentation is variable, ranging from an acute surgical emergency to, more commonly, a chronic illness. Abdominal distension, ascites, hernia and fluctuating mild jaundice are the main findings. At US examination there is diffuse ascites or, in some cases, a loculated fluid collection in and around the porta hepatis. Bile duct dilatation is not constant. Hepatobiliary scintigraphy is diagnostic, showing free spillage of the radionuclide into the peritoneal cavity (Figure 11.8.23). Treatment is surgical and should not be delayed to avoid the complication of infection. Spontaneous healing of the perforation with stenosis, bile duct dilatation and accumulation of stones has also been described.

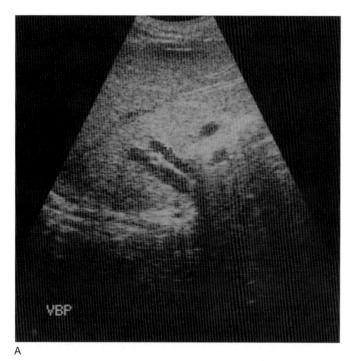

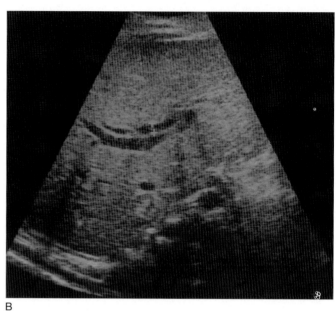

A   B

Figure 11.8.20 Common bile duct lithiasis. One-month-old baby boy with fluctuating cholestasis. US shows mild and regular extrahepatic (A) and intrahepatic (B) bile duct dilatation. The distal choledochal lithiasis is not seen because of overlying duodenal gas.

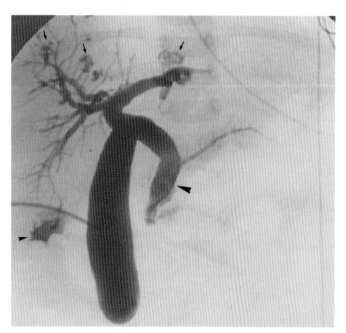

Figure 11.8.21 Common bile duct lithiasis in a 3-week-old baby girl with *E.coli* septicaemia and multiple hepatic abscesses. PTC obtained via gallbladder: there is obstruction of the common bile duct with a large intraluminal defect (large arrowhead). There is opacification of parenchymal cavities (arrows) and subcapsular leakage (small arrowhead). Clearing of the common bile duct and resolution of the abscesses were easily achieved by washing with saline.

OTHER CAUSES

The choledochal cyst is another cause of extrahepatic neonatal cholestasis and is described in the next section.

Duplication of the second portion of the duodenum can cause compression of the distal choledochus with dilatation of the biliary tract (Figure 11.8.24). This diagnosis may be made by US.

FURTHER READING

Alagille D. Intrahepatic cholestasis with morphological changes of intrahepatic bile ducts. In: Roy CC, Silverman A, Alagille D, eds. Pediatric clinical gastroenterology. St Louis: CV Mosby; 1995:672–678.

Chardot C, Iskandarani F, De Dreuzy O et al. Spontaneous perforation of the biliary tract in infancy: a series of 11 cases. European Journal of Pediatric Surgery 1996; 6:341–346.

Debray D, Pariente D, Gauthier F, Bernard O. Cholelithiasis in infancy: a study of 40 cases. Journal of Pediatrics 1993; 122:385–391.

Hadchouel M. Alagille syndrome. Indian Journal of Pediatrics 2002; 69:815–818.

Holgersen LO, Stolar C, Berdon WE, Hilfer C, Levy JS. Therapeutic and diagnostic implications of acquired choledochal obstruction in infancy: spontaneous resolution in three infants. Journal of Pediatric Surgery 1990; 25:1027–1029.

Jacquemin E, Lykavieris P, Chaoui N, Hadchouel M, Bernard O. Transient neonatal cholestasis: origin and outcome. Journal of Pediatrics 1998; 133:563–567.

Pariente D, Bernard O, Gauthier F, Brunelle F, Chaumont P. Radiological treatment of common bile duct lithiasis in infancy. Pediatric Radiology 1989; 19:104–107.

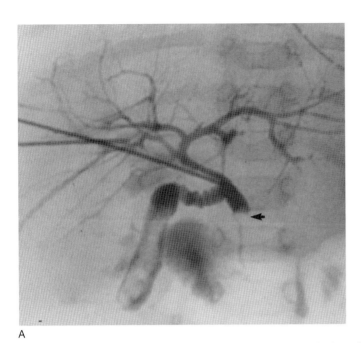
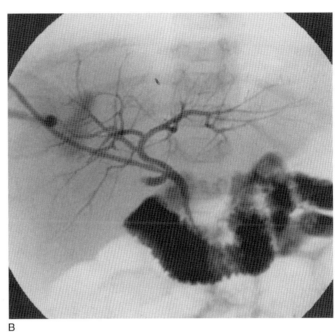

A

B

Figure 11.8.22 (A) Common bile duct lithiasis (arrow) and sludge in the gallbladder in a 4-week-old baby boy with mild intraheptic bile duct dilatation. Placement of external drainage and washing with saline. (B) Two days later the stones have disappeared and the duct size has returned to normal.

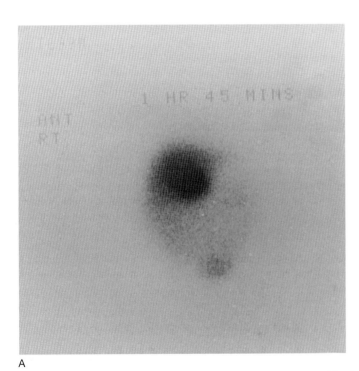
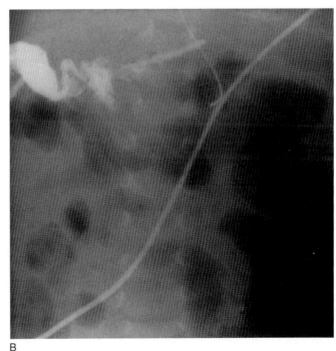

A

B

Figure 11.8.23 Infant with spontaneous perforation of the common bile duct who presented with ascites that was bile stained. (A) Hepatobiliary iminodiacetic acid (HIDA) scan showing circulation of HIDA in the peritoneum. (B) Operative cholangiogram showing leak at the junction of the cystic and common bile duct.

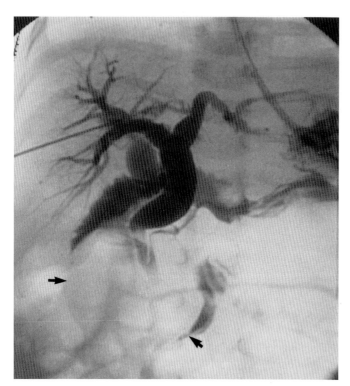

Figure 11.8.24 Duodenal duplication. Two-month-old baby girl with mild cholestasis. On US there is bile duct dilatation and a large cystic mass that appears distinct from the common bile duct. PTC shows the compression of the common bile duct by the duodenal duplication (arrows).

CHILDHOOD CHOLESTASIS

(TABLE 11.8.2)

CHOLEDOCHAL CYST

PATHOGENESIS

This congenital entity represents the most frequent cause of extra-hepatic cholestasis in childhood. It should be named congenital dilatation of the common bile duct as it is not a true cyst. The precise aetiology is unknown but the most commonly accepted theory of pathogenesis is the presence of an anomalous junction of the biliary and pancreatic channel with a long common duct allowing reflux of the pancreatic juice into the common bile duct. Pancreatic enzymes have been found in the bile and raised levels have been demonstrated after IV cholecystokinin during percutaneous cholangiography. However, antenatal diagnosis has been reported as early as in the 15th week of gestation, when the secretion of active pancreatic enzymes does not yet seem to be established. Various classifications have been proposed but practically all of the cysts are fusiform. The pedunculated type is rare and a choledochocele is exceptional, and probably is closer to a duplication cyst of the duodenum in aetiology. The size of the cystic dilatation of the common bile duct is variable, as is the associated dilatation of the intrahepatic bile duct. The degree of dilatation is not related to the age of the child.

CLINICAL PRESENTATION

Half of the cases are discovered in the first 10 years of life. The classical triad of features suggesting the diagnosis of choledochal cyst (abdominal pain, right upper quadrant mass and intermittent obstructive jaundice) is nowadays rarely complete. There is increasing frequency of discovery by sonography antenatally or in asymptomatic children or in the work-up of chronic abdominal pain. Single or recurrent episodes of pancreatitis may also be a presentation.

Complications of choledochal cyst include cholangitis, lithiasis, traumatic or spontaneous rupture with biliary peritonitis, which may be the presenting event, biliary cirrhosis and degeneration in late childhood. Cholangiocarcinoma is a recognized complication but is usually seen in adults.

DIAGNOSIS

The diagnosis is suspected on US examination, which demonstrates the cystic dilatation of the choledochus often associated with intrahepatic bile duct dilatation (Figure 11.8.25). This affects the main left and right hepatic ducts but not the smaller ducts. In most other cases of obstructive jaundice, the dilatation is more even. Pre- or peroperative cholangiography is usually performed to identify the precise anatomy of the lesion and to provide the surgeons with the anatomical map of the pancreaticobiliary ductal union and also variations of the biliary tree (Figure 11.8.26). The results of MR cholangiopancreatography are improving and this technique could avoid more invasive cholangiography in many cases in the future (Figure 11.8.27).

SURGERY

Surgery consists of complete resection of the cyst and hepaticojejunostomy in order to deconnect the biliary and pancreatic ducts and to prevent degeneration. In most cases, the prognosis is good with regression of liver fibrosis if present at diagnosis and a return to normal calibre of the intrahepatic bile ducts. Complications may include stenosis of the biliary-jejunal anastomosis, which is accessible to percutaneous transluminal dilatation. In very few cases, there is persistent cystic dilatation of the intrahepatic bile ducts with episodes of cholangitis and formation of stones, which raises the possibility of associated Caroli's disease. Complete excision is important as there is an increased risk of cholangiocarcinoma if cystic remnants remain.

DIFFERENTIAL DIAGNOSIS

In the neonatal period, the main differential diagnosis is biliary atresia with a cyst on the remnant of the atretic extrahepatic bile duct. The clinical presentation of biliary atresia is quite different with complete cholestasis and US fails to show communication of the cyst with dilated bile ducts.

In childhood, when the dilatation of the choledochus is mild, the differential diagnosis is cholelithiasis without anomaly of the bile duct. Primary cholelithiasis must be diagnosed preoperatively as surgery is different, including only cholecystectomy, usually performed under laparoscopy, and not hepaticojejunostomy.

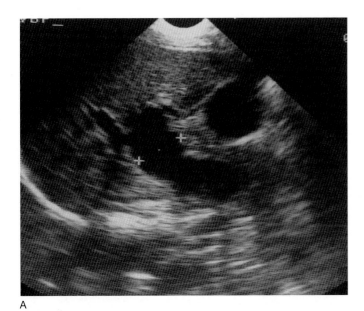
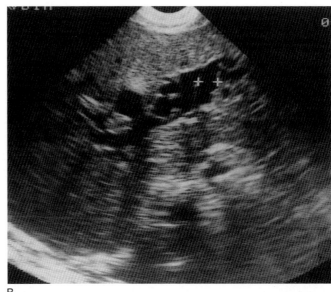

A

B

Figure 11.8.25 Choledochal cyst. Three-year-old girl presenting with an acute episode of abdominal pain and increased level of pancreatic enzymes. US demonstrates marked dilatation of the common bile duct (2 cm) (A) and intrahepatic bile ducts (B). No abnormality of the pancreas is found. PTC confirmed diagnosis.

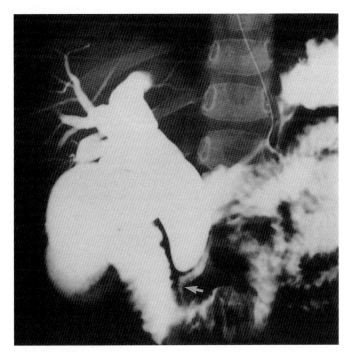

Figure 11.8.26 Choledochal cyst in a 6-year-old boy with abdominal pain and mild jaundice. PTC shows a choledochal cyst with intrahepatic bile duct dilatation. An abnormal choledocho-pancreatic common channel is evident (arrow).

FURTHER READING

Imazu M, Iwai N, Tokiwa K et al. Factors of biliary carcinogenesis in choledochal cysts. European Journal of Pediatric Surgery 2001; 11:24–27.

Kim MJ, Han SJ, Yoon CS et al. Using MR cholangiopancreatography to reveal anomalous pancreaticobiliary ductal union in infants and children with choledochal cysts. American Journal of Roentgenology 2002; 179:209–214.

Levy AD, Rohrmann CA Jr, Murakata LA, Lonergan GJ. Caroli's disease: radiologic spectrum with pathologic correlation. American Journal of Roentgenology 2002; 179:1053–1057.

Mackenzie TC, Howell LJ, Flake AW, Adzick NS. The management of prenatally diagnosed choledochal cysts. Journal of Pediatric Surgery 2001; 36:1241–1243.

GALLSTONES AND CHOLELITHIASIS

Although gallstones occur much more commonly in adult life, the frequency of the diagnosis in children has been increasing since the extensive use of US, and fetal and neonatal gallstones have even been documented. Spontaneous resolution does occur and surgical treatment is only recommended in cases of symptomatic migration of the stones into the bile duct with persistent jaundice or signs of cholangitis. The main causes of gallstones in children are shown in Table 11.8.3.

The diagnosis is made by US. The stones are seen as mobile, echogenic foci in the gallbladder (Figure 11.8.28). Clinical presentation may be asymptomatic, with the stones detected on an US carried out for another reason. Symptomatic stones present with pain in the RUQ and jaundice if there is migration into the common bile duct.

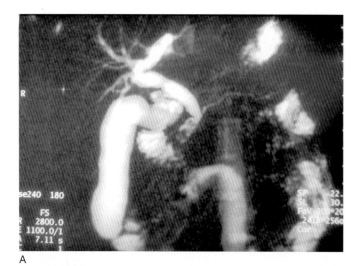

A

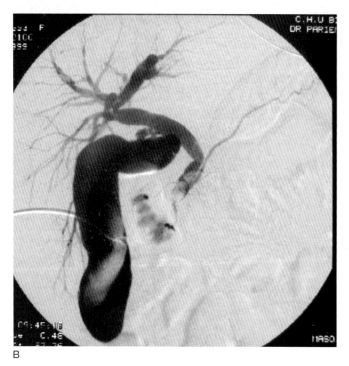

B

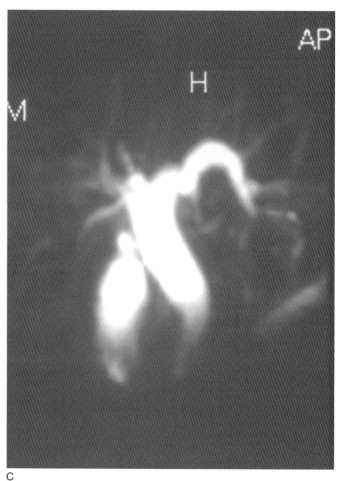

C

Figure 11.8.27 Choledochal cyst. Five-year-old girl presenting with episodes of abdominal pain and mild cholestasis. US examination showed fusiform dilatation of the bile duct. (A) On MR cholangiogram, there was suspicion of an abnormally long common bilio-pancreatic channel, containing calculus. (B) Preoperative percutaneous cholangiogram confirmed this finding, with very good correlation. (C) MR cholangiopancreatography in another child with a more extensive fusiform dilatation of the common duct and dilatation of the left hepatic duct, typical appearances of a choledochal cyst.

Table 11.8.3 Causes of gallstones in childhood

Haemolytic anaemia (spherocytosis, sickle-cell disease, thalassaemia)
Cirrhosis
Cystic fibrosis
Wilson's disease
Crohn's disease or ileal resection
Parenteral nutrition
Drugs: furosemide, ceftriaxone
Biliary tract obstruction (choledochal cyst, sclerosing cholangitis)
Caroli's disease
Obesity
Familial history
Metachromatic leukodystrophy

BILE SLUDGE

Bile sludge is echogenic debris that does not cast an acoustic shadow and is detected in the gallbladder during sonography (Figure 11.8.29). This moves with alteration in the patient's position. Bile sludge is most often due to biliary stasis.

LIMEY BILE

Though more common in adults, in children, one occasionally encounters bile debris in the gallbladder that is dense enough to cause a shadow on x-ray; this is more commonly seen as a high attenuation fluid in the gallbladder on CT. This is called limey bile and is thought to represent bile stasis.

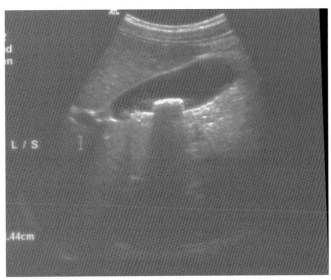

Figure 11.8.28 Ultrasound of gallbladder containing a large stone that shows acoustic shadowing.

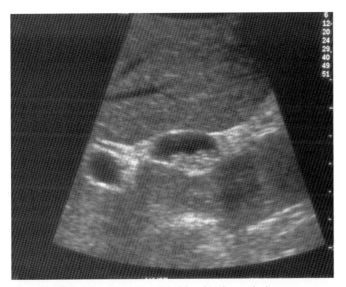

Figure 11.8.29 Ultrasound of gallbladder showing typical appearances of bile sludge as echogenic debris at the base of the gallbladder.

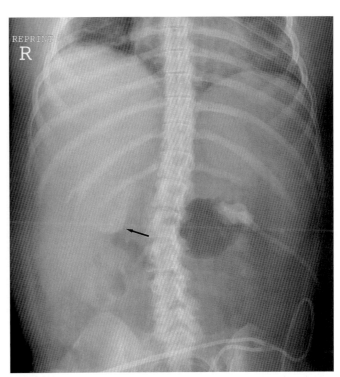

Figure 11.8.30 Note calcified 'porcelain' gallbladder in RUQ. This child is neurologically disabled and it is presumed that this appearance has been caused by chronic inflammation of the gallbladder.

PORCELAIN GALLBLADDER

Occasionally, the gallbladder wall calcifies and is seen on abdominal radiographs as an opacity to the RUQ (Figure 11.8.30). It is related to chronic low-grade inflammation.

ADENOMYOMATOSIS OF THE GALLBLADDER

This condition is rarely seen in childhood. There is proliferation of the surface epithelium of the gallbladder with glandular formation and Rokitansky–Aschoff sinuses. This may be seen diffusely throughout the gallbladder or, when seen in childhood, more commonly as a focal segment of abnormality. Ultrasonically, this appearance is identified as thickening and irregularity of the mucosa and gallbladder wall. There may be endoluminal narrowing of the gallbladder, which may have a septum across it, and this must be differentiated from the normal variant, a Phrygian cap. Gallstones may be associated with adenomyomatosis.

PHRYGIAN CAP

This is a normal congenital variant and is an infolding of the gallbladder wall near the fundus, giving the appearance of a septum across it.

DUPLICATION OF THE GALLBLADDER

This is a rare congenital anomaly, usually only described in case reports, in which part or the whole of the gallbladder is duplicated but the rest of the biliary tree is normal. The most frequent variant is a junction at the cystic duct level. There is stasis within the accessory gallbladder, which may present as cholecystitis.

SCLEROSING CHOLANGITIS

This is a rare cause of chronic progressive liver disease in children, characterized by an inflammatory obliterative fibrosis affecting the intra- and extrahepatic biliary tree. The pathogenesis remains unknown, but the disorder has an association with a variety of other diseases, including chronic inflammatory bowel disease, Langerhans' cell histiocytosis, immunodeficiency disorders (Figure 11.8.31) and autoimmune hepatitis. Some cases are isolated and neonatal onset (Figure 11.8.32) has been noted in some of these idiopathic cases. Clinical findings include

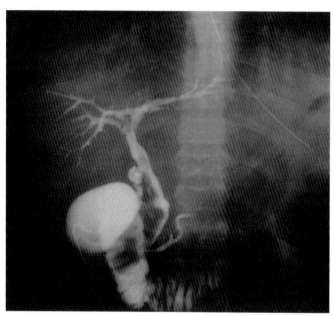

Figure 11.8.31 Sclerosing cholangitis. Fourteen-year-old boy with severe congenital immunodeficiency and abnormal liver function. Percutaneous cholecystography: there is moderate bile duct dilatation with irregularities of peripheral bile duct and filling defect in the common bile duct corresponding to thick bile.

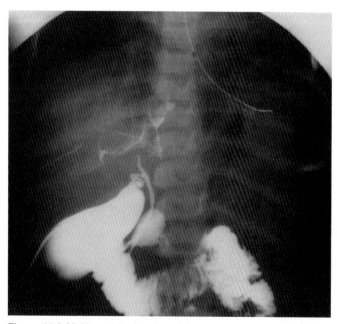

Figure 11.8.32 Neonatal sclerosing cholangitis. Four-year-old boy with biliary cirrhosis and a history of neonatal cholestasis. Percutaneous cholecystography shows multiple stenoses of intrahepatic bile ducts interposed with dilated segments. There is also a pruned-tree appearance of the biliary tract.

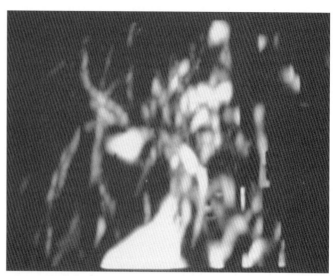

Figure 11.8.33 Sclerosing cholangitis. Six-year-old child presenting with Langerhans' cell histiocytosis and hepatosplenomegaly. MR cholangiogram shows diffuse irregularities of intrahepatic bile ducts, diagnostic of sclerosing cholangitis.

hepatomegaly and jaundice. Liver function tests and histological changes are often non-specific. Imaging of the biliary tree is essential to establish the diagnosis. Typical anomalies include strictures in multiple segments of the bile ducts with intervening dilated segments. Amputation of some segmental bile ducts is frequent. The disease may be limited to the intrahepatic bile duct at the time of diagnosis. In some cases, irregular dilatation of the bile ducts and thickening of bile duct wall can be demonstrated by US. MR cholangiopancreatography can be proposed as the first non-invasive imaging modality for this diagnosis as it can demonstrate the typical abnormalities with a high specificity (Figure 11.8.33). In cases of negative or inconclusive findings, a more invasive study such as ERCP or percutaneous transhepatic cholangiography or cholecystography should be attempted.

The prognosis is poor with progressive evolution to biliary cirrhosis. Liver transplantation is then required. No recurrence in the transplanted liver has been observed at more than 10 years follow-up.

FURTHER READING

Debray D, Pariente D, Urvoas E, Hadchouel M, Bernard O. Sclerosing cholangitis in children. Journal of Pediatrics 1994; 124:49–56.
Ferrara C, Valeri G, Salvolini L, Giovagnoni A. Magnetic resonance cholangiopancreatography in primary sclerosing cholangitis in children. Pediatric Radiology 2002; 32:413–417.

MISCELLANEOUS

CAROLI'S DISEASE

Caroli's disease is a complicated spectrum of diseases, characterized by cystic, non-obstructive dilatation of the intrahepatic bile ducts:

- Most of the cases in children are diffuse and associated with congenital hepatic fibrosis and recessive polycystic kidney disease of variable severity.
- A few cases are associated with a choledochal cyst. The cystic dilatation of the intrahepatic ducts may be segmental and require surgery.
- Very rare paediatric cases have been described as the only hepatic lesion without portal fibrosis. Some authors believe that the term Caroli's disease should be restricted to those rare cases.

HYDROPS OF THE GALLBLADDER

This is a rare disorder in which there is acute distension of the gallbladder without any mechanical obstruction of the cystic duct. The pathogenesis is unknown. It may be associated with various diseases and sometimes is the initial presenting feature. These include: scarlet fever and *Streptococcus* infection, Kawasaki disease, leptospirosis, *Salmonella* and *Shigella* infection, extensive burning, polyarteritis nodosa, familial paroxysmal polyseritis and prolonged parenteral nutrition. The age range is large with cases reported in the newborn period. Spontaneous resolution is the usual outcome. Perforation is rare and surgery is usually not necessary.

THICKENING OF THE GALLBLADDER WALL

Thickening of the gallbladder wall is seen in the following conditions: ascites, hypoalbuminaemia, cholecystitis (infectious and calculous), portal hypertension, viral hepatitis (Figure 11.8.34), cardiac failure and partial emptying of the gallbladder.

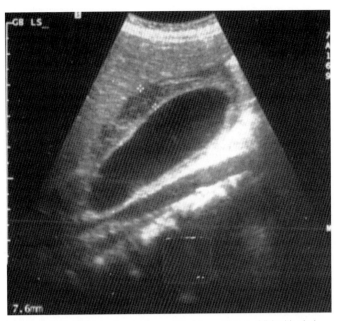

Figure 11.8.34 Thickening of the gallbladder wall in a child with viral hepatitis.

FURTHER READING

Levy AD, Rohrmann CA Jr, Murakata LA, Lonergan GJ. Caroli's disease: radiologic spectrum with pathologic correlation. American Journal of Roentgenology 2002; 179:1053–1057.

Liver Transplantation

Gabriel BH Lau, David A Stringer

Over the past few years, the remarkable results of liver transplantation have changed the management and prognosis of children with liver diseases.

In children, the main indication for transplantation is biliary atresia. Less common indications include Alagille syndrome, Byler's disease, alpha-1-antitrypsin deficiency, chronic hepatitis, fulminant hepatitis, tyrosinaemia, glycogen storage disease type I with adenomas and metabolic disorders.

In most series, the rate of survival is approximately 80%, with a better prognosis when transplant is carried out electively than as an emergency.

Liver transplantation requires extensive use of many imaging modalities and heavily involves the radiological team in the preoperative as well as in the postoperative work-up. Cadaveric transplant may be difficult to arrange and so in many children a living related transplant might be used with the donor giving left or right lobe, or part thereof. These living related donors also need to have a similar very thorough work-up.

PREOPERATIVE RADIOLOGICAL WORK-UP OF RECIPIENT

Preoperative work-up includes evaluation of cardiac and pulmonary status because increased cardiac output, hypoxia due to pulmonary shunts and pulmonary arterial hypertension are well known but unexplained complications of cirrhosis and portal hypertension. Their presence may hasten the need for transplantation or even preclude it (Figure 11.9.1).

It is essential to evaluate the patency and anatomy of the inferior vena cava and the hepatic veins, portal vein and hepatic artery and biliary tree, all of which represent critical anatomical information for surgical planning. Although this is often adequately obtained with ultrasound (US) and pulsed (Figure 11.9.2) or colour Doppler in many patients, surgeons require more detailed information for surgical planning and computed tomography (CT; Figure 11.9.3) or magnetic resonance angiography (MRA; Figure 11.9.4) have been useful in these situations. Angiography is performed if information is still incomplete (Figure 11.9.5). The biliary tree can be assessed by MRCP (Figure 11.9.6).

It should be remembered that sometimes other abnormalities are associated with biliary atresia such as the following malformation complex, the so-called non-cardiac polysplenia syndrome. This includes one or several of the following anomalies:

- polysplenia;
- thoracic or abdominal situs inversus with gastrointestinal malrotation (Fig11.9.7);
- preduodenal portal vein;
- azygos continuation of the inferior vena cava. In this case, hepatic veins directly enter the right atrium; and
- anomalous origin of the hepatic artery.

All these anomalies may be depicted on US; however, vascular anatomy may be very complex and CTA or MRA and maybe angiography will be indicated. Multiplanar reconstructions are particularly helpful in this regard.

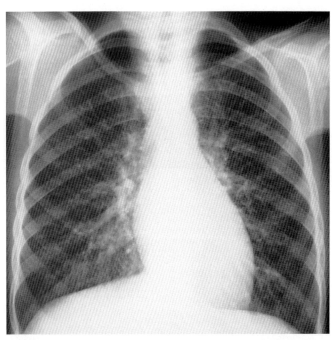

Figure 11.9.1 Chest film of a 14 year-old girl with Budd–Chiari syndrome treated by mesocaval anastomosis. Secondary appearance of hypoxia. There is a spidery network mimicking an interstitial pattern: multiple arteriovenous shunts were demonstrated on scintigraphy. Liver transplantation was planned.

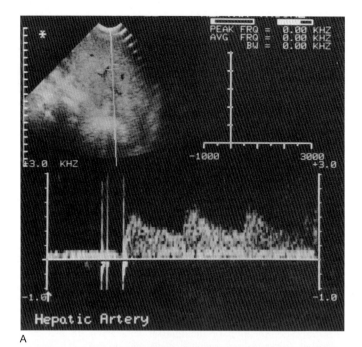

A

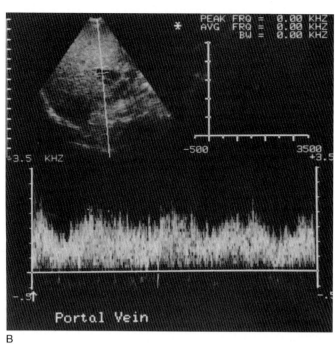

B

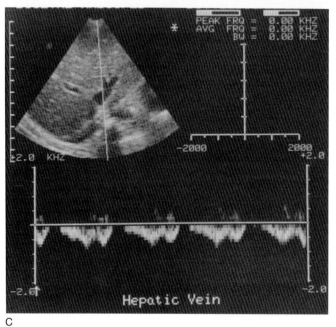

C

Figure 11.9.2 The ultrasound and Doppler sonography appearances are the same pre- and post-transplant in the most successful patients, as in this case. In this post-transplant patient, the vascular anastomoses are patent. (A) Normal intrahepatic signal of the hepatic artery. Because of respiratory movement there is successive recording of venous and arterial flow, a common phenomenon. (B) Normal portal venous flow. (C) Normal triphasic hepatic vein flow.

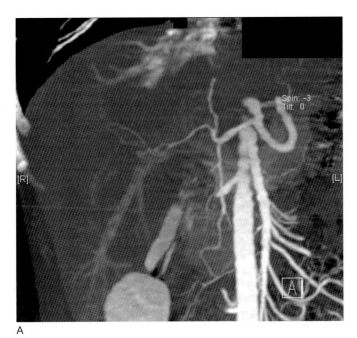

A

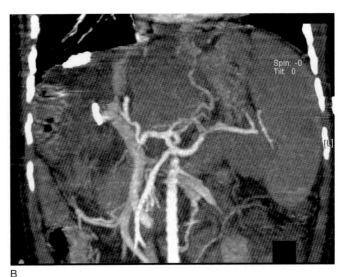

B

Figure 11.9.3 CTA demonstrates the anatomy precisely: (A) preoperatively and (B) postoperatively. Note the central location of liver and vessels in (B) postoperatively.

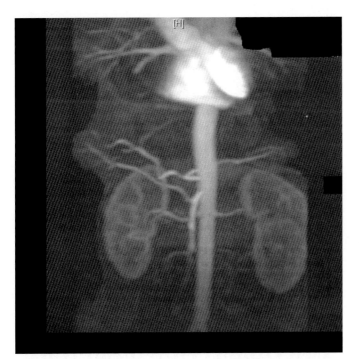

Figure 11.9.4 Preoperative MRA shows the right hepatic artery is arising from the superior mesenteric artery, a normal variant.

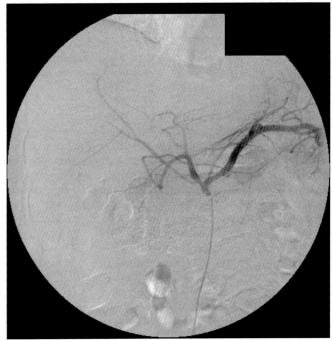

Figure 11.9.5 Preoperative angiography via the coeliac axis shows the hepatic artery and splenic artery.

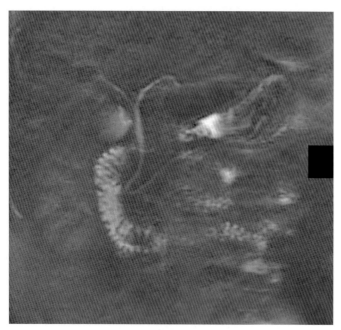

Figure 11.9.6 Preoperative MRCP shows the biliary tree anatomy.

PREOPERATIVE RADIOLOGICAL WORK-UP OF LIVING RELATED DONOR

Living related donors are common in paediatric transplantation as the size of the child relative to the adult donor is disparate, enabling part of the donor liver to be sufficient for the transplant to be successful.

When working up the living related donor, safety has to be of prime consideration. It is essential that nothing untoward happens to this healthy person and it has to be remembered that there is a small but significant risk of death or morbidity in those donating part of their liver. This behoves the physicians, surgeons and radiologists to ensure that the donor and recipient are a sufficient surgical and medical match. This requires as rigorous a work-up for the donor as for the recipient, which includes a detailed analysis of vascular and biliary anatomy using CTA, MRA and/or angiography (see Figures 11.9.2 to 11.9.6).

In addition, the size and fat content of the liver segments and lobes has to be assessed to ensure there is sufficient tissue for success to be possible. This requires that the non-fatty component of the transplanted liver is at least 20% of the recipient's body weight (Figure 11.9.8). CT can best assess this by using a surface rendered technique. If the liver appears fatty then a biopsy is arranged to test for extent of fatty change and this is used to calculate the proportional increase in size of liver that needs to be taken from the donor.

FURTHER READING

Cardella JF, Amplate K. Preoperative angiographic evaluation of prospective liver recipients. Radiologic Clinics of North America 1987; 25:299–308.

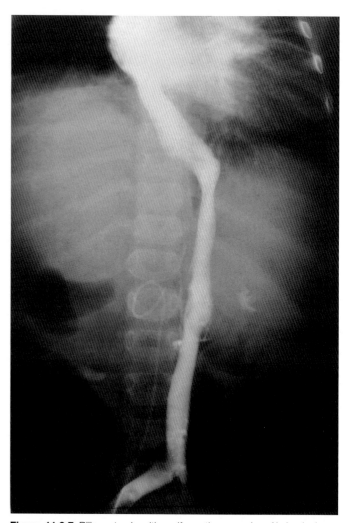

Figure 11.9.7 Biliary atresia with malformation complex. Abdominal situs inversus and a left-sided inferior vena cava are present.

Cheng YF, Huang TL, Lee TY, Chen TY, Chen CL. Overview of imaging in living related donor hepatic transplantation. Transplantation Proceedings 1996; 28:2412–2414.
Claus D, Clapuyt PH. Liver transplantation in children: role of the radiologist in the preoperative assessment and the post-operative follow-up. Transplantation Proceedings 1987; 19:3344–3357.
Day DL, Letourneau JG, Allan BT, Ascher NL, Hund G. MR evaluation of the portal vein in pediatric liver transplant candidates. American Journal of Roentgenology 1986; 147:1027–1030.
Zajko AH, Campbell WI, Bron KM et al. Diagnostic and interventional radiology in liver transplantation. Gastroenterology Clinics of North America 1988; 17:105–143.

INTRAOPERATIVE WORK-UP

The practice of intraoperative US and Doppler assessment varies from centre to centre. In some centres, Doppler is used to demarcate the vessels in the living related donor prior to resection and/or assess the anastomosis prior to the abdominal wound being closed. This is often followed by an examination after wound closure before taking the patient off the operating table. Occasionally,

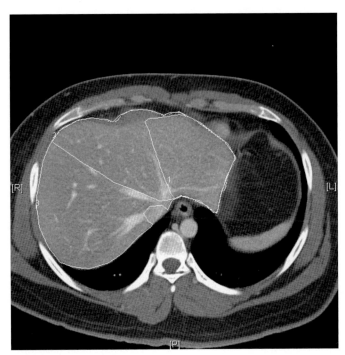

Figure 11.9.8 Preoperative CT can divide the liver into different volumes for preoperative assessment.

when this often large organ is inserted into the abdomen there may be kinking or compression of the blood vessels necessitating immediate re-opening of the abdomen. In severe cases, primary abdominal wall closure may not be possible and a temporary Teflon graft may need to be used, with complete closure at a later date.

FURTHER READING

Cheng YF, Huang TL, Chen CL et al. Intraoperative Doppler ultrasound in liver transplantation. Clinical Transplantation 1998; 12:292–299.

POSTOPERATIVE WORK-UP

After transplantation, US with pulsed or colour Doppler is the initial method of choice for detection of the main complications. It can be performed as a portable examination at the bedside in the early postoperative period in these critical patients. This is particularly useful as the clinical and biochemical findings are non-specific in the diagnosis of most of the complications.

VASCULAR COMPLICATIONS

The flow velocity and waveform of the hepatic veins, hepatic artery and portal vein should all be assessed by pulsed and colour Doppler, which can also accurately depict the patency of vascular anastomoses.

HEPATIC ARTERY THROMBOSIS

This is a frequent complication of paediatric liver transplantation, reported in approximately 10% of cases. It mainly occurs with infant donors or recipients. It can be a devastating condition, although less so than in adults. Its clinical presentation is highly variable and includes fulminant necrosis and septicaemia necessitating retransplantation on an emergency basis, or delayed biliary complications due to ischaemia of the biliary tract, or relapsing fever and bacteraemia.

The diagnosis is based on the absence of an intrahepatic arterial Doppler signal. Colour Doppler may facilitate this diagnosis. It has to be confirmed by CTA or MRA but the use of Doppler avoids unnecessary studies. Contrast-enhanced CT can evaluate the extension of parenchymal ischaemia, which is variable, often predominant in the left lobe and is important in the prognosis (Figure 11.9.9).

Bile duct necrosis may occur at any portion of the biliary tract or at the anastomosis with the appearance of intra- or extrahepatic bilomas and of bile duct dilatation and stenosis. These complications are well depicted on US if one is aware of the frequent echogenic appearance of the dilated bile ducts filled with sludge and epithelial debris (Figure 11.9.10).

Cholangiography via an indwelling surgical drain or by a percutaneous approach may have to be performed, to identify the precise extension of the lesions and to plan the treatment by percutaneous drainage, dilatation or surgery. Long-term drainage has proved useful in most cases as a treatment for the cholangitis and prior to retransplantation. Arterial collateral circulation occurs in many children with hepatic artery thrombosis, 3 weeks to 1 month later on Doppler studies and on CTA/MRA or angiography (Figure 11.9.11). This collateral circulation carries a risk of massive haemorrhage during surgery and it does not seem to prevent delayed biliary complications, as these occur even with delayed hepatic artery thrombosis. Because dreadful complications

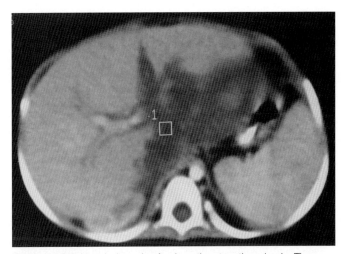

Figure 11.9.9 Liver ischaemia after hepatic artery thrombosis. There is a large hypodensity in the left lobe of the liver without contrast enhancement corresponding to liver infarction, which is well demonstrated by CT.

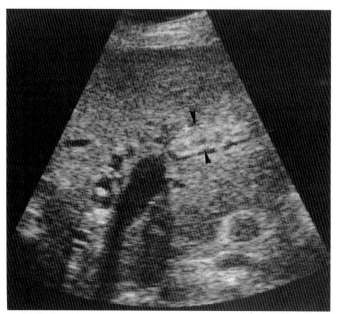

Figure 11.9.10 There is bile duct dilatation filled with echogenic material; this represents sludge and epithelial debris after hepatic artery thrombosis.

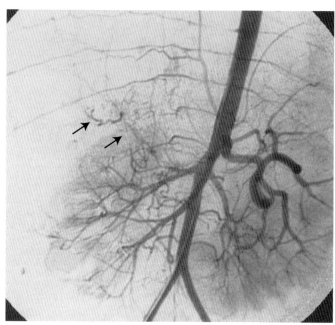

Figure 11.9.11 Collateral arterial vascularization of liver (arrows), 2 months after hepatic artery thrombosis, is shown on this arteriogram.

seem to occur in all cases of hepatic artery thrombosis it is important to diagnose it as soon as possible and to perform surgical arterial recanalization to save the graft.

The protocol of post-transplant work-up consists of a routine regular Doppler US examination during the first 2 weeks when the risk of hepatic artery thrombosis is at its greatest. Later on, US may be performed as clinically indicated.

OTHER VASCULAR COMPLICATIONS

Hepatic artery stenosis may be asymptomatic or may be complicated by biliary problems. Portal vein thrombosis is fortunately a more rare problem than hepatic artery thrombosis, however it is a major complication. Pulsed or colour Doppler are diagnostic and prompt surgery can give quick relief. Portal vein stenosis is uncommon and is secondary to a mechanical problem at the anastomotic site. It presents with the appearance of the clinical and radiological signs of portal hypertension. It should be remembered that the portal anastomosis is often prominent on US, with an echogenic area of narrowing and sometimes with the impression of kink, so to make a correct diagnosis of portal vein stenosis the flow has to be significantly abnormal (Figure 11.9.12).

Inferior vena cava thrombosis in its retrohepatic portion may be encountered, especially with an adult reduced size graft and an incongruous large inferior vena cava. However, in most cases, hepatic vein drainage is preserved and no complication occurs. Generally, less attention has been given to the drainage of hepatic veins but these need to be carefully assessed at every US examination. This is because the hepatic veins can become compressed secondary to post-transplant swelling of the liver, which may precipitate liver transplant failure.

A few cases of secondary Budd–Chiari syndrome have been reported, which can be successfully treated by percutaneous angioplasty.

Arterial aneurysms are a very serious complication as they carry a risk of dissection with intractable haemorrhage. They may be secondary or associated with chronic infection ('mycotic aneurysms') or with severe rejection. They are very difficult to depict with US and CTA or MRA is required if arterial aneurysms are suspected.

FURTHER READING

Flint KW, Sumkin JH, Zajku AB, Bowen AD. Duplex sonography of hepatic artery thrombosis after liver transplantation. American Journal of Roentgenology 1988; 151:481–483.

Parieute D, Riou JY, Schmit P et al. Variability of clinical presentation of hepatic artery thrombosis in pediatric liver transplantation: role of imaging modalities. Pediatric Radiology 1990; 20:253–257.

Stringer MD, Marshall MM, Muisen P et al. Survival and outcome after hepatic artery thrombosis complicating paediatric liver transplantation. Journal of Paediatric Surgery 2001; 36:888–891.

Zajko AB, Calus D, Clapuyt P et al. Obstruction to hepatic venous drainage after LT: treatment with balloon angioplasty. Radiology 1989; 170:763–765.

BILIARY COMPLICATIONS

These are frequent and occur in about 15% of cases. Their severity is a function of the aetiology. The main cause of biliary complication is hepatic artery thrombosis or stenosis and is due to necrosis of the biliary tract because it is only vascularized by the

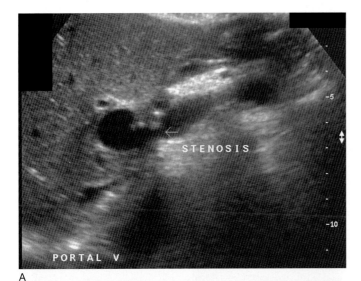

A

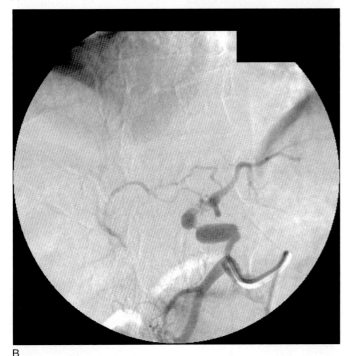

B

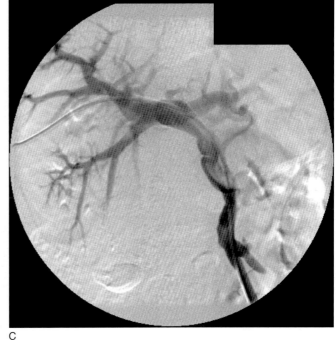

C

Figure 11.9.12 Portal vein stenosis was discovered on ultrasound study (A) with high-frequency shifts on Doppler confirming the grey scale impression. Stenosis was confirmed on angiography (B) and stent inserted (C) with decrease in patients' symptoms and return of liver enzymes to normal.

hepatic artery in the transplanted liver; the pretransplant collaterals arising from the gastroduodenal artery are interrupted during surgery. Necrosis may occur at any portion of the biliary tract leading to bile lakes (Figure 11.9.13), leakage (Figure 11.9.14), stenosis and dilatation. The prognosis is often poor, even with multiple surgical procedures, percutaneous drainage (Figure 11.9.15), and/or balloon dilatation, and retransplantation may be required. Biliary anastomotic stenosis may occur in isolation. It has been observed with choledochocholedochostomy or choledochojejunostomy. The diagnosis is made on US, as biochemical findings are often non-specific. Percutaneous dilatation may be successful and may avoid surgery. In some cases, this anastomotic stenosis may be due to a kink or plication during surgery and reoperation

is necessary, although this should have been detected on the pre-closure scan.

A few cases of obstructing bile sludge have been reported without a mechanical obstruction. These cases can be treated with cholangiography and lavage.

Formation of a mucocoele of the cystic duct remnant is an uncommon event, which may compress the common bile duct and cause bile duct dilatation. The treatment is surgical. Cholangiography either by an indwelling surgical drain or by percutaneous approach has to be performed under antibiotic cover, as it carries a serious risk of cholangitis and septicaemia in these immuno-compromised children. External drainage or immediate surgery is recommended if a significant obstruction is discovered.

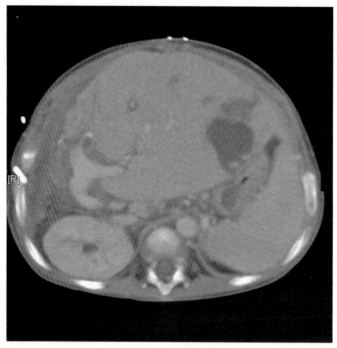

Figure 11.9.13 Bilomas are not uncommon, especially if there is ischaemia from hepatic artery thrombosis, as in this case demonstrated by CT.

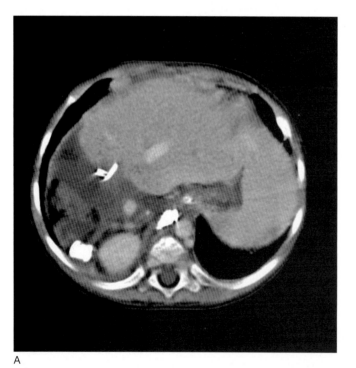

A

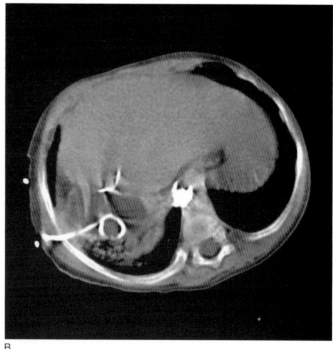

B

Figure 11.9.14 A biloma seen on CT (A) was drained by the only route available, i.e. transpulmonary (B), with good results. Note adjacent biliary stent visible on both images that had been inserted at time of transplantation.

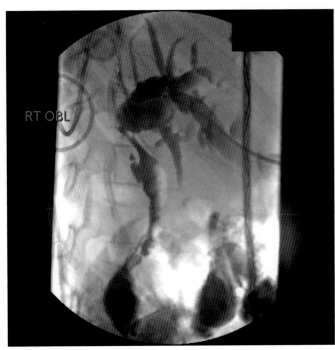

Figure 11.9.15 A percutaneous transhepatic cholangiogram can show a bile duct stenosis if this is not seen well on MRCP, or as part of a stenting procedure.

FLUID COLLECTIONS

Right pleural effusions and ascites are common after liver transplantation. Collections around the ligamentum teres and the ligamentum venosus are nearly always present and represent transient lymphatic stasis. Intraperitoneal fluid collections are easily demonstrated on US but their nature is often difficult to predict without aspiration (see Figure 11.9.14). They may represent abscess, haematoma, biloma or just loculated ascites in these multioperated patients.

FURTHER READING

Hoffer FA, Teele RL, Lillchei CW, Vacanti JP. Infected bilomas and hepatic artery thrombosis in infant recipients of liver transplants. Radiology 1988; 169:435–438.

Letourneau JC, Hunter DW, Ascher NL et al. Biliary complications after liver transplantation in children. Radiology 1989; 170:1095–1099.

Pariente D, Hibet MH, Tammam S et al. Biliary complications after transplantation in children: role of imaging modalities. Pediatric Radiology 1991; 21:175–178.

REJECTION

This is one of the most common complications of liver transplantation, which has to be recognized early to be effectively treated. Unfortunately, no imaging modality appears to be really reliable in making this diagnosis. A high resistive index on duplex Doppler can be highly suggestive of rejection but unfortunately is not specific or reliably diagnostic. Percutaneous liver biopsy has to be performed to demonstrate its presence. US is useful to guide the needle, especially in the reduced size livers with disturbed anatomy, as most paediatric transplants are much more midline, or even left sided, than a normal liver.

FURTHER READING

Marden DM, De Marino GB, Sumkin JH, Sheahan DG. Liver transplant rejection: value of the resistive index in Doppler US of hepatic arteries. Radiology 1989; 173:127–129.

Miscellaneous Liver Diseases

Danièle Pariente

PELIOSIS HEPATIS

This is a rare condition characterized by multiple cystic blood-filled spaces of varying size in the liver. It has been mainly reported in adults in association with various wasting diseases and after the administration of anabolic and corticosteroid therapy, azothioprine and contraceptives. Only a few cases have been described in children, in association with *Escherichia coli* pyelonephritis and with myopathy. Depending on the size and extent of the lesions, the clinical spectrum of peliosis hepatis ranges from subclinical disease diagnosed incidentally on liver biopsy to an acute diffuse form with hepatic failure, rupture and haemoperitoneum. The pathogenesis remains unclear and treatment is still debatable.

Angiography was the first reported imaging modality, demonstrating multiple collections of contrast material during the parenchymal and venous phases of hepatic angiography and wedge-hepatic venography. The ultrasound (US) appearances are rarely mentioned in the literature. Hypo- or hyperechoic areas are found depending on the size and the age of the cavities (Figure 11.10.1). The appearance is non-specific but together with the clinical presentation it is suggestive of the diagnosis. Computed tomography (CT) shows multiple low-attenuation areas without contrast enhancement. Magnetic resonance imaging (MRI) findings with mutiple foci of brighter signal in all sequences have been reported.

FURTHER READING

Cragg A, Castaneda-Zuniga W, Lund G, Salomonowi E, Amplatz K. Infantile peliosis hepatis. Pediatric Radiology 1984; 14:340–342.

Jacquemin E, Pariente D, Fabre M et al. Peliosis hepatis with initial presentation as acute hepatic failure and intraperitoneal hemorrhage in children. Journal of Hepatology 1999; 30:1146–1150.

Saatci I, Coskun M, Boyvat F, Cila A, Gurgey A. MR findings in peliosis hepatis. Pediatric Radiology 1995; 25:31–33.

Wang SY, Ruggles S, Vade A, Newman BM, Borge MA. Hepatic rupture caused by peliosis hepatis. Journal of Pediatric Surgery 2001; 36: 1456–1459.

CONGENITAL HEPATIC FISTULAS

These are rare disorders with variable severity and clinical presentation depending on the type of abnormal vascular communication. US and Doppler studies can demonstrate these vascular malformations with accuracy.

CONGENITAL PORTACAVAL FISTULA

This rare anomaly is often called congenital absence of the portal vein, because of the absence of visibility of the intrahepatic portal branches. It may be isolated or associated with a malformation complex such as Goldenhar's, Down's or Noonan's syndromes. The communication between the portal vein and the inferior vena cava may be extrahepatic or intrahepatic, sometimes by the ductus venosus.

Complications are related to the diversion of the portal vein flow, which does not pass through the liver. These include hypoxia due to pulmonary arteriovenous shunting, pulmonary arterial hypertension and also liver tumours such as regenerative nodular hyperplasia, adenoma and hepatocellular carcinoma (Figure 11.10.2). These complications may be the presenting sign and one has to search for portacaval fistula on imaging. Pulmonary complications and benign tumours can regress with treatment of the fistula, which may be occluded by surgery and/or embolization.

CONGENITAL INTRAHEPATIC PORTOHEPATIC VENOUS SHUNT

This is an abnormal communication between a portal vein branch and a hepatic vein, most often located in the periphery of the liver (Figure 11.10.3). In most cases, it is fortuitously discovered by US or on neonatal screening for hypergalactosaemia. Spontaneous closure occurs in most before 2 years of age. Clinical signs have

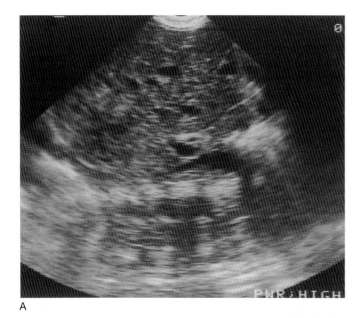

A

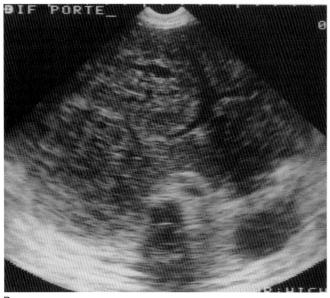

B

Figure 11.10.1 Peliosis hepatis. Two-year-old girl referred for sudden onset of fever, hepatomegaly, anaemia, thombocytopenia, increased serum transaminase values and liver failure. US demonstrates multiple hypoechoic lesions in the whole liver with fluid in the pouch of Douglas. (A) Longitudinal scan. (B) Transverse scan. Surgical liver biopsy: peliosis hepatis. Slow recovery with supportive and antibiotic treatment. An associated *E. coli* urinary tract infection was found.

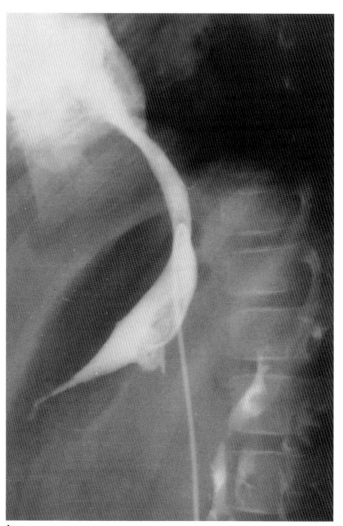

A

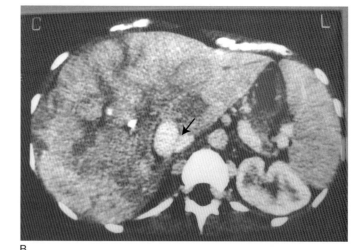

B

Figure 11.10.2 (A) Congenital portacaval fistula. Lateral view of cavogram. The catheter has been introduced into the communication between portal vein and IVC. In this 5-year-old girl this was associated with Budd–Chiari syndrome and gallstones. (B) At the age of 19, she came back with abdominal pain. Diffuse hepatocellular carcinoma was diagnosed on CT and she died a few weeks later. Note the portacaval fistula, well seen on this slice (arrow).

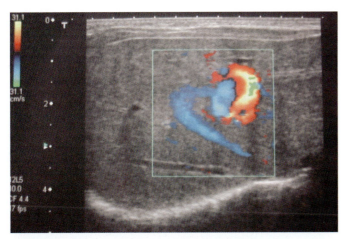

Figure 11.10.3 Newborn baby with antenatal diagnosis of an intrahepatic fistula joining the left portal vein branch and the middle hepatic vein. In the control study, there was evident decrease in the size of the fistula 1 month later.

been mainly reported in adult patients who present with encephalopathy and hypoglycaemia.

CONGENITAL ARTERIOPORTAL FISTULA

This vascular malformation may present with gastrointestinal bleeding, anaemia, ascites, diarrhoea or heart failure. The diagnosis is made by US showing the communication between an enlarged hepatic artery and a dilated portal vein branch. In a few cases, the communication may be diffuse. In most cases, there is inversion of flow in the portal vein, which is well seen on Doppler study. The prognosis is poor. Treatment may be achieved by single or multiple interventional radiological procedures using arterial or venous approaches but recurrence or portal vein thrombosis have been reported and surgery (resection or even transplantation) may be indicated (Figure 11.10.4).

FURTHER READING

Alvarez AE, Ribeiro AF, Hessel G, Baracat J, Ribeiro JD. Abernethy malformation: one of the etiologies of hepatopulmonary syndrome. Pediatric Pulmonology 2002; 34:391–394.

Heaton ND, Davenport M, Karani J, Mowat A, Howard ER. Congenital hepatoportal arteriovenous fistula. Surgery 1995; 117:170–174.

Khoda E, Saeki M, Nakano M et al. Congenital absence of the portal vein in a boy. Pediatric Radiology 1999; 29:235–237.

Kumar N, De Ville De Goyet J, Sharif K, Mc Kiernan P, John P. Congenital, solitary, large, intrahepatic arterioportal fistula in a child: management and review of the literature. Pediatric Radiology 2003; 33:20–23.

Lewis AM, Aquino NM. Congenital portohepatic vein fistula that resolved spontaneously in a neonate. American Journal of Roentgenology 1992; 159:837–838.

Marchand V, Uflacker R, Baker SS, Baker RD. Congenital hepatic arterioportal fistula in a 3-year-old child. Journal of Pediatric Gastroenterology and Nutrition 1999; 28:435–441.

Uchino T, Matsuda I, Endo F. The long-term prognosis of congenital portosystemic venous shunt. Journal of Pediatrics 1999; 135:254–256.

Vauthey JN, Tomczak RJ, Helmberger T et al. The arterioportal fistula syndrome: clinicopathologic features, diagnosis and therapy. Gastroenterology 1997; 113:1390–1401.

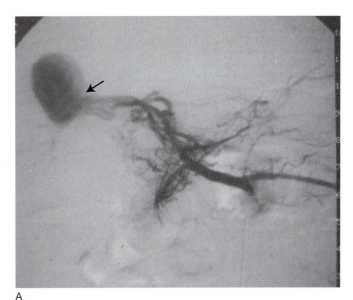

A

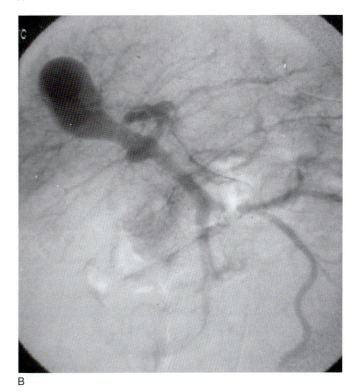

B

Figure 11.10.4 Six-month-old infant presenting with gastrointestinal bleeding. US examination with Doppler imaging made the diagnosis of arterioportal fistula. Arteriography showed that the fistula (arrow) was fed by multiple arterial branches coming from the hepatic artery (A) and also from the superior mesenteric artery. In the late phase (B) of the hepatic artery injection, there was massive opacification of the whole portal vein system through the fistula. Despite embolization of two arterial pedicles coming from the hepatic artery, the fistula remains patent. At first, the child underwent a partial hepatic resection including the fistula and then a splenorenal shunt. He is cured with a follow-up of 10 years.

Table 11.10.1 Causes of calcification in the liver

Infections: tuberculosis, brucellosis, cytomegalovirus, toxoplasmosis, herpes virus, syphilis, hydatid disease, cat-scratch disease, chronic granulomatous disease.
Tumours: all malignant types, haemangioma, adenoma
Post-trauma
Cystic fibrosis
Vascular calcification: umbilical vein catheterization, arterial or venous thromboembolism
Calculus in dilated intrahepatic bile duct
Capsular in meconium peritonitis

LIVER CALCIFICATIONS

The cause of the calcification may be obvious (tumour or infection) but the calcification is often discovered fortuitously on plain films or by US examination, even antenatally. The main causes of calcification are shown in Table 11.10.1.

The type of calcification and its distribution may help in identifying the cause. Tumour calcification is disorganized and irregular. Granulomas tend to be dense and multiple. Vascular calcification may be tubular or punctate. If it is in the major vessels, it obviously correlates with their location. Infective granulomatous calcification may also be present in the spleen. There are patients in whom, in spite of extensive investigation, the cause is not identified. When discovered incidentally, the main concern is to exclude a liver tumour. Initial assessment is with US, to be followed by cross-sectional imaging, as appropriate.

FURTHER READING

Hawass ND, El Badawi MG, Fatani JA et al. Foetal hepatic calcification. Pediatric Radiology 1990; 20:528–535.
Herman TE. Extensive hepatic calcification secondary to fulminant neonatal syphilitic hepatitis. Pediatric Radiology 1995; 25:120–122.
Lykavieris P, Guillot M, Pariente D, Bernard O, Hadchouel M. Liver calcifications in cystic fibrosis. Journal of Pediatric Gastroenterology and Nutrition 1996; 23:565–567.

FATTY INFILTRATION OF THE LIVER

Fatty infiltration of the liver has a variety of causes. These include metabolic disorders, such as glycogen storage disease, diabetes, fructose intolerance and tyrosinaemia, Reye's syndrome, acute starvation or severe malnutrition states, obesity, parenteral nutrition, malabsorption syndromes, cystic fibrosis and steroid therapy. Idiopathic cases have also been reported.

At US the liver is unusually bright compared to the right kidney.

On unenhanced CT scans there is diffuse decrease in attenuation of the liver parenchyma, which may be marked enough to produce spontaneous hyperdensity of the vessels (Figure 11.10.5). Less commonly, the fatty infiltration may be uneven and focal, mimicking tumour. But there is no mass effect and no displacement of vessels. MRI with fat suppression sequences has proved very reliable in making the diagnosis.

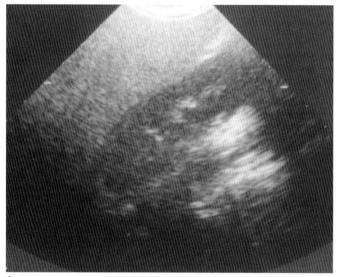

A

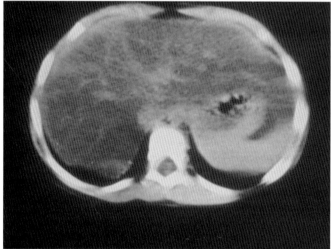

B

Figure 11.10.5 (A) Ultrasound and (B) CT in a child with severe hepatitis who developed a fatty liver. Note the increased echogenicity on US and low density of the liver parenchyma on CT, with the vessels outlined against this low-density parenchyma.

FURTHER READING

Kammen BF, Pacharn P, Thoeni RF et al. Focal fatty infiltration of the liver: analysis of prevalence and CT findings in children and young adults. American Journal of Roentgenology 2001; 177:1035–1039.
Labuski MR, Eggli KD, Boal DK et al. Focal fatty infiltration of the liver in a healthy child. Pediatric Radiology 1992; 22:281–282.

WILSON'S DISEASE

Wilson's disease or hepatolenticular degeneration is an inborn error of copper metabolism, characterized by defective biliary copper excretion and the accumulation of toxic amounts of copper in the liver, brain, kidney and cornea. It is inherited as an autosomal recessive trait. Clinical features include cirrhosis of the liver, sometimes with an acute and fulminant presentation, renal tubular injury, episodes of haemolytic anaemia and degeneration in the central nervous system. The diagnosis is made on the presence of Kayser–Fleischer rings at the corneal limbus, or on serum caeruloplasmin, urinary copper, or determination of the copper content on liver biopsy. Cerebral CT findings consist of low density in the basal ganglia and variable white matter atrophy. MRI findings consist of bilateral and symmetrical T2-weighted hyperintensity in the basal ganglia.

NEONATAL HAEMOCHROMATOSIS

This is a rare disease, also known as perinatal haemochromatosis, that is characterized by siderosis of hepatocytes and of extrahepatic parenchymal cells at a variety of sites (pancreas, myocardium, thyroid gland, oral mucosa) with sparing of the reticuloendothelial cells in the spleen, lymph nodes and bone marrow. Neonatal haemochromatosis is not a variant of hereditary haemochromatosis, which has an adult onset.

It presents with severe and usually fatal fulminant hepatic failure of antenatal onset. It may occur in siblings. The only effective treatment seems to be liver transplantation.

The diagnosis of neonatal haemochromatosis is based on MRI, which may demonstrate the presence of iron overload in the pancreas and liver, and the absence of siderosis of the spleen. On T2-weighted images the signal intensity of the liver and of the pancreas is markedly diminished compared to the paravertebral muscles, whereas it is normal in the spleen. In the absence of extrahepatic siderosis (pancreas or myocardium), the diagnosis of neonatal haemochromatosis should not be made, because marked siderosis is physiological in the perinatal period.

Antenatal diagnosis has been reported in the fetus of a mother who had previously had an infant with neonatal haemochromatosis.

FURTHER READING

Hayes AM, Jaramillo D, Levy HL, Knisely AS. Neonatal hemochromatosis: diagnosis with MR imaging. American Journal of Roentgenology 1992; 159:623–625.
Liet JM, Urtin-Hostein C, Joubert M et al. Hémochromatose néonatale. Archives of Pediatrics 2000; 7:40–44.
Oddone M, Bellini C, Bonacci W et al. Diagnosis of neonatal hemochromatosis with MR imaging and duplex doppler sonography. European Journal of Radiology 1999; 9:1882–1885.

RADIATION INJURY TO THE LIVER

Since the decrease in the use of abdominal irradiation for childhood tumours, the incidence of radiation injury has greatly diminished. Described changes include decreased CT attenuation similar to that of fat, to be followed by increased attenuation. A sharp line of demarcation separating the normal from the irradiated liver may be seen on scintigraphy.

Table 11.10.2 Main causes of cirrhosis in childhood (adapted from Pediatric Clinical Gastroenterology, Roy C, Silverman A, Alagille D, Mosby-Year Book, Inc 1995)

Biliary cirrhosis
  Biliary atresia
  Paucity of interlobular bile ducts
  Choledochal cyst
  Sclerosing cholangitis
  Byler's disease
Postnecrotic cirrhosis
  Neonatal hepatitis (TORCH infections)
  Postviral hepatitis
  Autoimmune hepatitis
Inborn errors of metabolism
  Wilson's disease
  Alpha 1 antitrypsine deficiency
  Cystic fibrosis
  Tyrosinemia
  Gaucher's
  Nieman-Pick type C
  Sickle cell and thalassemia
Passive venous congestion
  Veno occlusive disease
  Budd-Chiari syndrome
  Constrictive pericarditis
  Pulmonary hypertension
Toxic cirrhosis
  Drugs, toxins, poisons
  Radiation therapy
Cirrhosis of unknown etiology

CIRRHOSIS OF THE LIVER

Diffuse liver disease that progresses to cirrhosis is rare in childhood compared with adults. Cirrhosis is the end stage of many diseases that lead to hepatocellular death and regeneration. In adults, alcoholism and chronic hepatitis are the main causes. Causes in children are listed in Table 11.10.2. All are rare. Even children with cystic fibrosis liver disease rarely develop symptomatic cirrhosis in childhood. Early cirrhosis cannot be detected with imaging and is a histological diagnosis. With disease progression, there is alteration in the liver echotexture, with patchy echogenicity and loss of normal liver parenchymal architecture (Figure 11.10.6). Portal hypertension may follow and can be detected by Doppler studies and the identification of varices around the oesophagus and stomach. In severe cases, there may be alteration in liver texture on both CT and MRI and varices may be identified.

FURTHER READING

Akata D, Adhan O, Ozcelik U et al. Hepatobiliary manifestations of cystic fibrosis in children: correlation of CT and US findings. European Journal of Radiology 2002; 41:26–33.
Bader TR, Beavers K, Semelka R. MR imaging features of primary sclerosing cholangitis: patterns of cirrhosis in relationship to clinical severity of disease. Radiology 2003; 226:675–685.
Semelka R, Chung J, Hussain S, Marcos H, Woosley J. Chronic hepatitis: correlation of early patchy and late linear enhancement patterns on gadolinium-enhanced MR images with histopathology initial experience. Journal of Magnetic Resonance Imaging 2001; 13:385–391.

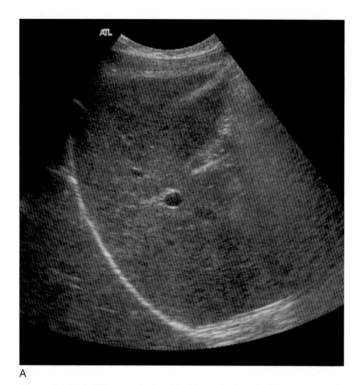

A

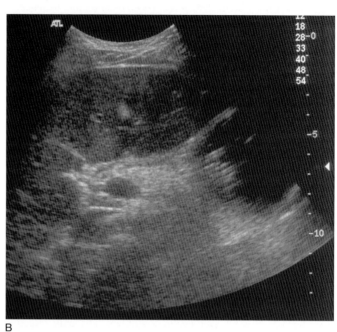

B

Figure 11.10.6 Ultrasound of a girl with cystic fibrosis. (A) Note the diffusely abnormal echotexture of the liver typical of cirrhosis of the liver. (B) Transverse scan showing the dense head of pancreas and altered echotexture in the left lobe.

HEPATOBILIARY DISEASE IN CYSTIC FIBROSIS

Gallstones are found on routine surveillance in up to 10% of children with cystic fibrosis. These stones may form from viscous bile or from interference with the enterohepatic circulation due to previous ileal surgery or distal ileal obstruction syndrome. Cirrhosis may result from impaired bile drainage due to the viscosity of the bile or from focal fibrosis. The liver texture becomes heterogeneous with increased echoes round the portal venous radicles.

Other abdominal manifestations of cystic fibrosis found on US surveillance may include: (1) thickening of the gallbladder wall or a small gallbladder due to chronic cholecystitis; (2) hyperechogenicity of the pancreas with, sometimes, cysts; (3) intussusception – often transient and in the small bowel but may also be of the more typical types; and (4) splenic enlargement due to portal hypertension.

Abdominal pain is frequent in children with cystic fibrosis and US should include both the organs and the bowel. Other bowel manifestations such as DIOS or fibrosing colonopathy are described in Chapter 10.15.

FURTHER READING

Patriquin H, Lenaerts C, Smith L et al. Liver disease in children with cystic fibrosis: US-biochemical comparison in 195 patients. Radiology 1999; 211:229–232.

The Spleen

Kamaldine Oudjhane

The spleen is part of the reticuloendothelial system. It is involved in haematopoiesis, haemolysis and the immune function. It is also connected to the portal venous system. With the advent of modern imaging modalities, a variety of splenic abnormalities can be delineated either as an isolated disease or in systemic disorders. Clinical examination is sensitive in identifying splenomegaly. Cross-sectional imaging methods allow a comprehensive assessment of focal or diffuse splenic lesions with sonography, computed tomography (CT) and magnetic resonance imaging (MRI). Isotopic studies with labelled damaged red blood cells show their sequestration in the spleen. Technetium 99m (Tc 99m) sulphur colloid scanning delivers information about the splenic reticuloendothelial system.

THE NORMAL SPLEEN/IMAGING APPROACH

EMBRYOGENESIS

The spleen develops starting from the fifth gestational week and originates from mesenchymal cells located between the layers of the dorsal mesogastrium. The fetal spleen shows a lobulated configuration. Lymphoid follicles of white pulp are situated between vascular sinuses of red pulp. The white-to-red pulp ratio increases with age and progressive antigenic stimulation.

NORMAL CT APPEARANCE

The splenic architecture may demonstrate anatomical variants on CT or MRI. A heterogeneous splenic enhancement pattern is observed on helical CT studies within the first minute or so after initiation of the contrast medium injection (Figure 11.11.1). This is related to the different rates of blood flow in the red and white pulp. A rapid injection, the increasing age of the child and the absence of splenomegaly are the main factors associated with such an artifact, not to be considered a pathological sign. Three patterns of heterogeneous enhancement are described: arciform, focal or diffuse. CT imaging at the portal venous phase will demonstrate, however, a homogeneous attenuation.

MRI APPEARANCES

The MRI signal intensity of the spleen is related to the white/red pulp ratio. In the neonate, the spleen is hypointense relative to the liver on both T1- and T2-weighted images, because the lymphoid tissue of the white pulp has not matured. Non-thrombotic blood of sinusoids contributes to the signal of the red pulp. Such findings should not be mistaken for haemochromatosis. By 8 months of age, the signal intensity of the spleen resembles that of an adult spleen.

SONOGRAPHY

The splenic tissue is homogeneous in echo texture and is differentiated from the liver. The spleen is less than 6 cm long at birth and grows during childhood in a logarithmic fashion with increasing age. Calculation of splenic volume can be cumbersome. In practice, when the spleen is more than 1.25 times longer than the adjacent kidney, splenomegaly should be suspected.

PATTERN APPROACH TO SPLENIC IMAGING

The spleen has multiple physiological functions and may be involved in a variety of focal or systemic pathological processes. Imaging assessment should review initially the external characteristics of this organ: its number (asplenia, polysplenia), location (situs inversus, wandering spleen), shape (clefts, notches, lobules) and size (atrophy, splenomegaly). This should be followed by analysis of splenic parenchymal involvement: solitary or multiple focal lesions or diffuse disease (Table 11.11.1).

FURTHER READING

Donnelly LF, Emery KH, Bove KE et al. Normal changes in the MR appearance of the spleen during early childhood. American Journal of Roentgenology 1996; 166:635–639.

Donnelly LF, Foss JN, Frush DP et al. Heterogeneous splenic enhancement patterns on spiral CT images in children: minimizing misinterpretation. Radiology 1999; 210:493–497.

Emery KH. Splenic emergencies. Radiology Clinics of North America 1997; 35:831–843.

Paterson A, Frush DP, Donnelly LF et al. A pattern-oriented approach to splenic imaging in infants and children. Radiographics 1999; 19:1465–1485.

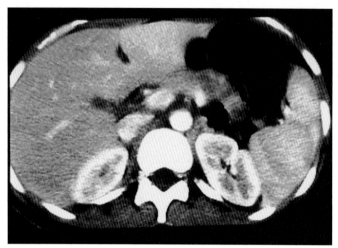

Figure 11.11.1 Normal spleen CT: technical artifact of curvilinear hypodensities in the spleen because of differential enhancement of white versus red pulp on dynamic helical CT imaging.

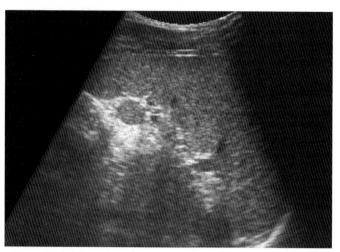

Figure 11.11.2 Accessory spleen, near the hilum, transverse US.

Table 11.11.1 Pattern-oriented approach to spleen imaging

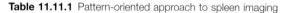

External characteristics
Number (asplenia, polysplenia, accessory)
Location (situs, wandering spleen)
Shape (cleft, notches, lobules)
Size (atrophy, splenomegaly)

Splenic parenchyma involvement
Solitary lesion: cyst, tumour
Multiple focal lesions
Diffuse disease

Rosenberg HK, Markowitz RI, Kolberg H et al. Normal splenic size in infants and children: sonographic measurements. American Journal of Roentgenology 1991; 157:119–121.

Schlesinger AE, Edgar KA, Boxer LA. Volume of the spleen in children as measured on CT scan: normal standards as a function of body weight. American Journal of Roentgenology 1993; 160:1107–1109.

ANOMALIES OF SIZE/SHAPE/NUMBER/LOCATION

ACCESSORY SPLEEN

An accessory spleen or splenule can be seen in about 1.5% of sonographic studies in children. Its prevalence has been reported to reach 16% in a series of paediatric splenectomies. It is of variable size (from a few millimetres to a few centimetres), usually less than 1 cm, and it is of variable number (one to six). It is commonly identified near the splenic hilum (Figure 11.11.2) but can be located along the splenic vessels or within layers of the omentum. Splenogonadal fusion presents as a soft tissue mass in the left lower abdomen. This is due to the close relationship between the left gonadal anlage, the mesonephros and the developing spleen. This is a rare congenital anomaly, with a male/female ratio of 16:1. Two types are identified, the continuous and the discontinuous types, and depend on whether a cord-like structure exists or not between the ectopic splenule and the normal spleen. The clinical issue is not to miss it, otherwise an orchidectomy is performed. Sonography, CT and sulphur colloid scintigraphy help identify the condition.

The splenule may get hypertrophic. If this occurs following a splenectomy, recurrence of disease should be considered. Torsion of an accessory spleen has been reported and its MRI appearance includes a low T1 and T2 signal intensity of the diseased spleen, with subsequent elevation of the T2 signal intensity.

WANDERING SPLEEN

A wandering spleen results from laxity of or lack of ligamentous attachments of the spleen. It may occur in patients with deficient anterior abdominal musculature (prune belly syndrome). Gastric volvulus has been described in association with a wandering spleen. Abdominal pain is the presenting symptom, especially in the case of torsion of the spleen. Sonography identifies the ectopic mass to be a spleen by its splenic echotexture and its ectopic location. On CT, the tortuous splenic pedicle has a characteristic 'whorled' appearance (Figure 11.11.3A,B). Torsion is a major complication, leading to ischaemia and infarction. On CT, the spleen has heterogeneous enhancement with a hypoattenuated portion (Figure 11.11.3C). On US, a splenic artery occlusion may be shown with a heterogeneous splenic echogenicity and lack of Doppler signals in the parenchyma. Chronic torsion of the wandering spleen has misleading clinical features, mimicking intestinal obstruction with an abdominal mass. Radionuclide studies with sulphur colloid demonstrate the absence of splenic uptake or functional asplenia. On CT, the abnormal spleen has an enhancing pseudocapsule. The spleen may be ectopic, intrathoracic in case of congenital diaphragmatic hernia or eventration, or located behind the left kidney.

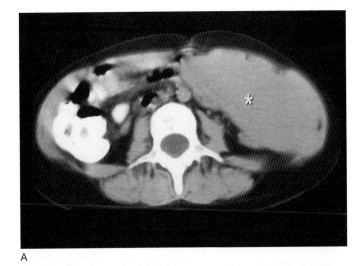

A

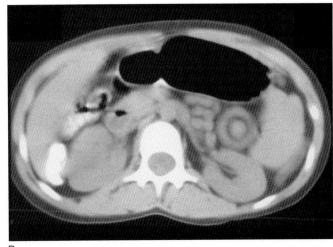

B

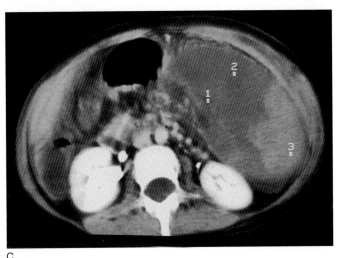

C

Figure 11.11.3 Wandering spleen. (A) CT shows wandering spleen (*) corresponding to the palpated abdominal mass. (B) CT at a higher level: 'whorled' appearance of the splenic vessels. (C) Torsion of the wandering spleen with focal hypodensity in the parenchyma on CT.

SPLENOSIS

Splenosis represents fragments of functionary splenic tissue, scattered along the peritoneal surfaces, following trauma of the spleen. Radionuclide studies using Tc sulphur colloid agents or denatured labelled red cells are best at defining them. It is of clinical importance that splenosis is recognized for multiple reasons. The developing new spleen may mimic masses such as lymphoma or metastatic disease. Its presence may confer protection against infection if splenectomy has been performed in a child. In cases of idiopathic thrombocytopenic purpura, treated with splenectomy, recurrence of the disease may be related to these splenic nodules.

HETEROTAXY SYNDROMES

Asplenia and polysplenia are part of the heterotaxy syndromes, which have an overlapping spectrum of findings. Three clinical features are stressed. Malrotation of the mid-gut is a frequent feature with the risk of volvulus. There is an increased risk of con-

genital heart disease, which is more severe and complex in asplenia. Immunodeficiency is associated with asplenia.

Polysplenia is more common in females. It is characterized by the presence of multiple splenic masses, identified on US (Figure 11.11.4), CT, MRI or sulphur colloid scintigraphy. Associated anomalies may include interruption of infrahepatic portion of the inferior vena cava with azygos continuation, a preduodenal portal vein, a bilateral left-sidedness of lungs and bronchi. The described congenital cardiac disease is commonly non-cyanotic in the form of left-to-right shunts. The gallbladder may be absent. Biliary atresia is also associated with a non-cardiac polysplenia syndrome.

Asplenia is more prevalent in males. Scintigraphy helps confirm the absence of spleen. Heinz or Howel–Jolly bodies are characteristic microscopic features in peripheral red blood cells. There is a bilateral right-sidedness of viscera. The cardiac disease is more complex and of a cyanotic type. Gallbladder duplication has also been described in this syndrome.

FURTHER READING

Applegate KE, Goske MJ, Pierce G et al. Situs revisited: imaging of the heterotaxy syndromes. Radiographics 1999; 19:837–852.

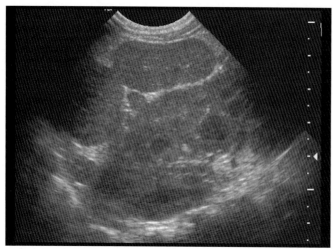

Figure 11.11.4 Polysplenia: longitudinal US in a patient with left atrial isomerism.

Table 11.11.2 Principal causes of splenomegaly

1. **Haematogenous disorders**
   Lymphoma/leukaemia
   Haemolytic anaemias
   Thrombocytopenic purpura
2. **Cardiovascular causes**
   Portal hypertension
   Congestive heart failure
   Budd–Chiari syndrome
   A-V malformation
3. **Metabolic/storage disorder**
   Gaucher disease
   Niemann–Pick disease
   Mucopolysaccharidosis
   Tyrosinosis
4. **Neoplasms/cysts of the spleen**
5. **Infections**
   Infectious mononucleosis
   Tuberculosis
   Typhoid fever
   Kala Azar
   Echinococcosis
   Cytomegalo virus infection
   Malaria

Bakir M, Bilgic A, Özmen M, Caglar M. The value of radionuclide splenic scanning in the evaluation of asplenia in patients with heterotaxy. Pediatric Radiology 1994; 24:25–28.

Ditchfield MR, Hutson TM. Intestinal rotational abnormalities in polysplenia and asplenia syndromes. Pediatric Radiology 1998; 28:303–306.

Kao P, Tzen K, Tsai M et al. 99mTc-sulfur-colloid and heat denaturated 99mTc-labelled red cell scans demonstrating a giant intrapelvic spleen in a girl after splenectomy. Pediatric Radiology 2001; 31:283–285.

Kalomenopoulou M, Katsimba D, Arvaniti M et al. Male splenic-gonadal fusion of the continuous type: sonographic findings. European Radiology 2002; 12:374–377.

Oleszczuk-Raschke K, Set PA, Von Lengerke HJ. Abdominal sonography in the evaluation of heterotaxy in children. Pediatric Radiology 1995; 25:S150–S156.

Sio T, Ivo T, Watanabe Y. Torsion of an accessory spleen presenting as an acute abdomen with inflammatory mass: US, CT and MRI findings. Pediatric Radiology 1994; 24:532–534.

Swischuk LE, Williams JB, John SD. Torsion of the wandering spleen: the whorled appearance of the splenic pedicle on CT. Pediatric Radiology 1993; 23:476–477.

FUNCTIONAL ASPLENIA

Functional asplenia is defined by the absence of splenic uptake of radiotracer and is encountered in patients with splenic tumoural invasion or following bone marrow transplantation. It is also seen in sickle cell disease.

SPLENOMEGALY

Enlargement of the spleen is present in many medical conditions (Table 11.11.2, Figure 11.11.5). Portal hypertension, infection and lymphoma/leukaemia infiltration are the most common causes of splenomegaly. Abdominal sonography should include Doppler assessment. Multiple varieties of collateral circulation of venous

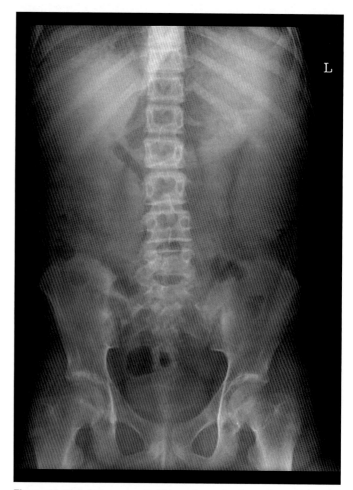

Figure 11.11.5 Splenomegaly. Plain radiograph of a patient with underlying liver cirrhosis of biliary atresia.

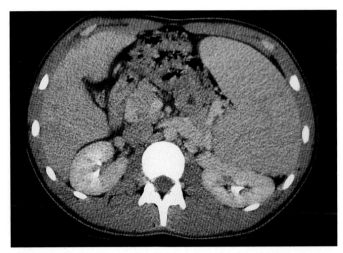

Figure 11.11.6 Splenomegaly. CT depiction of splenorenal shunt in a patient with portal hypertension.

shunting may be seen. CT/MR angiography delineate porto-portal or porto-systemic venous shunts (Figure 11.11.6). Significant gastrointestinal bleeding may be the clinical mode of presentation of rupture of oesophageal varices. Gaucher disease is a typical example of metabolic aetiology of splenomegaly. Sickle cell disease in its homozygous form presents with splenomegaly because of sequestration *in situ* pooling of blood in the spleen in a crisis. A rapid drop of haemoglobin level and platelet counts, and hypovolaemic shock develop rapidly. As it is a clinical emergency it is rarely imaged but if done at CT there is splenomegaly with a hypodense splenic parenchyma either diffusely or in peripheral zones. Sonography depicts hypoechoic areas in an enlarged spleen. Splenic vessels are obvious on Doppler study. MRI may demonstrate a subacute haemorrhage with areas of increased signal intensity on T1- and T2-weighted images. Extramedullary haematopoiesis in haemolytic anaemias or infiltrative marrow disorder may result in diffuse splenomegaly or focal splenic masses. Infants who undergo extracorporeal membrane oxygenation may develop splenomegaly. This is thought to be secondary to the increased load of splenic removal of damaged red cells.

FURTHER READING

Lotfus WK, Metrevelli C. Ultrasound assessment of mild splenomegaly: spleen/kidney ratio. Pediatric Radiology 1998; 28:98–100.

SPLEEN ATROPHY

This is a less common entity. It is usually secondary to recurrent bacterial infection or to sequelae of multiple recurrent infarction as in sickle cell disease. This leads to autosplenectomy. Splenic calcifications are usual.

TRAUMA

The spleen is frequently involved in trauma, especially in motor vehicle accidents. Non-operative management of splenic injuries, if possible, is presently the standard, because of the risk of sepsis (pneumococcal) in postsplenectomy patients. It has greater success in children than in adults, due to a relatively thicker splenic capsule in children containing the bleeding. Varying degrees of splenic injury include laceration, rupture, intraparenchymal and subcapsular haematomas. Contrast enhanced CT is the gold standard for imaging splenic injuries. Sonography underestimates the extent of the lesions (Figure 11.11.7) but usually points out the presence of haemoperitoneum and perisplenic fluid. Grading of splenic injury by CT does not direct clinical management (Figure 11.11.8). The haemodynamics status of the patient is the main factor. Active haemorrhage, defined by a focal high attenuation area (greater than 90 Hounsfield units) is a rare finding in blunt trauma. It may be non-obvious on immediate helical CT scanning after IV injection but will be well identified on a 5-min delayed CT scan. It constitutes an indication for surgical intervention.

Follow-up of splenic injuries is by serial US examinations. A delayed splenic rupture occurring more than 48 h after blunt trauma may be due to rupture of a subcapsular haematoma. Such risk is low and is apparently unaffected by imaging protocols. There is, however, correlation between the initial grade of splenic injury and the rate of healing as identified on sonography. Development of delayed complications such as pseudoaneurysm, haemorrhage or abscess may not preclude a successful non-operative care of the paediatric splenic injury. Splenosis is a possibility following splenic trauma or splenectomy. Patients with splenomegaly are at greater risk of splenic rupture after even a minor trauma. This is seen in the case of infectious mononucleosis, portal hypertension, Gaucher disease and haemoglobinopathies.

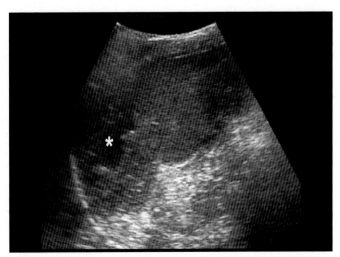

Figure 11.11.7 Spleen trauma, US: parenchymal haematoma (*).

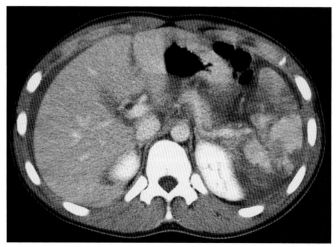

Figure 11.11.8 Spleen trauma, CT: 'fracture' of the spleen. Successful non-operative management.

FURTHER READING

Emery KH, Babcock DS, Borgman AC et al. Splenic injury diagnosed with CT: US follow up and healing rate in children and adolescents. Radiology 1999; 212:515–518.

Frumiento C, Sartorelli K, Vane D. Complications of splenic injuries: expansion of the nonoperative theorem. Journal of Pediatric Surgery 2000; 35:788–791.

Huebner S, Reed MH. Analysis of the value of imaging as part of the follow-up of splenic injury in children. Pediatric Radiology 2001; 31:852–855.

Kluger Y, Paul DB, Raves JJ et al. Delayed rupture of the spleen: myths, facts, and their importance. Case reports and literature review. Journal of Trauma 1994; 36:568–571.

Sivit CJ. Detection of active intra-abdominal hemorrhage after blunt trauma: value of delayed CT scanning. Pediatric Radiology 2000; 30:99–100.

Tran CN, Oudjhane K, Sinsky AB et al. Splenic laceration with pseudoaneurysm of the splenic artery. Canadian Journal of Surgery 1996; 39:450–486.

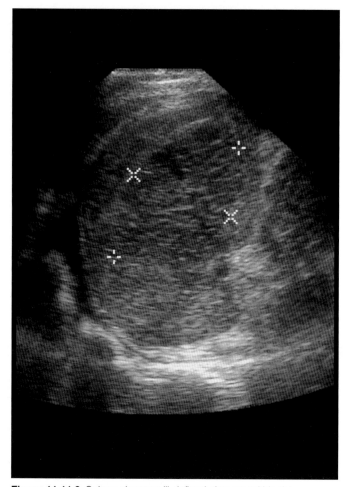

Figure 11.11.9 Spleen abscess: ill-defined abscess within the parenchyma on US.

INFECTION/INFLAMMATION

ABSCESS

Splenic abscesses are rare but occur more frequently in immuno-compromised children. Other predisposing conditions include bacterial endocarditis, splenic trauma, pyogenic infection and sickle cell disease. Haematogenous seeding of infection is the usual mechanism. Pancreatitis may be the source of contiguous extension of infection. Alteration of splenic architecture after infarction or haematoma is the third mechanism. Abscesses manifest as ill-defined hypoechoic lesions with internal septa on US (Figure 11.11.9). Gas bubbles in the purulent collection may be seen at CT. A hypodense area is a typical appearance with a rim enhancement pattern.

FUNGAL INFECTIONS

Fungal infections (candida, aspergillus, cryptococcus) present as small multiple abscesses of a few millimetres in size (Figures 11.11.10 and 11.11.11). Hepatosplenomegaly is usually associated with fungal sepsis. Classical sonographic features are the 'target' or 'bull's eye' sign of central echogenicity with a hypoechoic circle corresponding to peripheral fibrosis. The 'wheel in wheel' appearance represents necrosis and the development of the hyperechogenic nidus. Enhanced CT optimizes the diagnosis of multiple hypodense lesions.

GRANULOMATOUS DISEASE

Granulomatous lesions are commonly seen in cat scratch disease, histoplasmosis and tuberculosis. Residual scars and calcifications may be seen (see Figure 11.11.12). Cat scratch disease is caused by a Gram-negative bacillus, *Bartonella henselae*, following scratching or bites from a cat. It is a common cause of regional subacute or chronic lymphadenopathy. Systemic involvement is possible and splenomegaly with microabscess can develop. On US, well-defined hypoechoic homogeneous lesions are seen. The non-contrast CT appearance is of hypodense granulomata with a variable degree of enhancement.

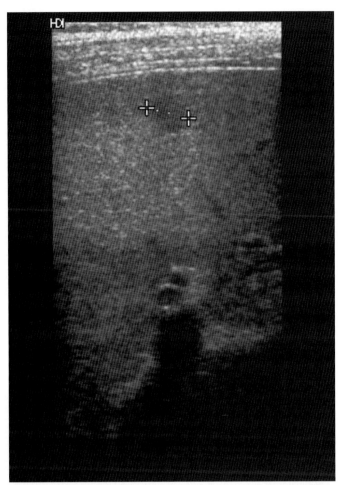

Figure 11.11.10 Fungal infection of the spleen, US: focal hypoechoic lesion in a patient with neutropenia.

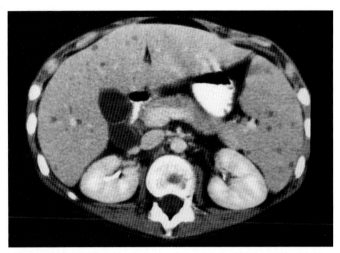

Figure 11.11.11 Fungal infection of the spleen, enhanced CT demonstrating multiple hypodense foci in the spleen and liver of an immunodepressed child.

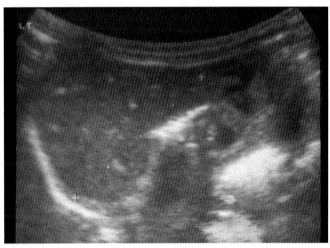

Figure 11.11.12 Granulomas of the spleen; multiple echogenic scars on US.

FURTHER READING

Hopkins KL, Simoneaux SF, Patrick LE et al. Imaging manifestations of cat-scratch disease. American Journal of Roentgenology 1996; 166:435–438.
Larsen CE, Patrick LE. Abdominal (liver, spleen) and bone manifestations of cat-scratch disease. Pediatric Radiology 1992; 22:353–355.

METABOLIC DISORDER

GAUCHER DISEASE

This is a lysosomal storage disorder, due to a deficit in glucocerebrosidase. Glucocerebroside accumulates in the cells of the reticuloendothelial system. Three clinical forms have been described. The most common is the type 1, non-neuropathic form. All cases manifest with massive hepatosplenomegaly, hypersplenism and lung disease. Bone involvement may be symptomatic (avascular necrosis, pathological fracture). On sonograms, the splenomegaly may include clusters of hypoechoic nodules. Echogenic nodules are composed of Gaucher cells and fibrosis. On MRI, T1 signal intensity is decreased, T2 signal is unchanged. Nodular clusters are isointense on T1-weighted and hypointense on T2-weighted images. The spleen is prone to trauma. Splenic infarction and fibrosis results in a multifocal appearance. Splenic volume shows a dramatic response to enzyme replacement therapy as seen on serial US or MRI studies.

HAEMACHROMATOSIS

This can be a primary condition or can occur after transfusion overload. It results in the accumulation of iron in the reticuloendothelial system. MRI signal intensity of the spleen is decreased on T1 and T2 conventional sequences. Dark spleens and livers are also seen on MRI in patients after chemotherapy.

FURTHER READING

Hill SC, Damasca BM, Ling A et al. Gaucher Disease: abdominal MR imaging findings in 46 patients. Radiology 1992; 184: 561–566.

Kornreich L, Horev G, Yaniv I et al 1997. Iron overload following bone marrow transplantation in children: MR findings. Pediatric Radiology 1997; 27:869–872.

Patlas M, Hadas-Halpern I, Abrahamov A et al. Spectrum of abdominal sonographic findings in 103 pediatric patients with Gaucher Disease. European Radiology 2002; 12:397–400.

SPLEEN INFARCTION

Spleen infarction is due to occlusion of terminal branches of the splenic arterial supply, which is of a non-communicating type. It occurs in children with sickle cell anaemia, valvular heart disease, diffuse intravascular coagulation, Gaucher disease and leukaemia. Clinical complications include fever, abscess, splenic pseudocyst and spleen rupture. Splenic infarcts may initially manifest as ill-defined hypoechoic areas due to oedema and necrosis (Figure 11.11.13). They then become well defined with fibrosis and organization (Figure 11.11.14). In sickle cell disease, areas of hypoechogenicity in an echogenic spleen may also represent preserved functioning islands of splenic tissue. The CT features include a mottled appearance at the hyperacute phase. Subsequently, the infarct is better delineated, peripheral and wedge-shaped. The end result is either focal calcification, a focal cortical defect, atrophy or autosplenectomy. A decreased MRI signal on T1- and T2-weighted sequences represents fibrosis, calcification and haemosiderin deposits.

FURTHER READING

Goerg C, Schwerk WB. Splenic infarction: sonographic patterns, diagnosis, follow-up and complications. Radiology 1990; 174: 803–807.

Levin TL, Berdon WE, Haller JO et al. Intrasplenic masses of "preserved" functioning splenic tissue in sickle cell disease: correlation of imaging findings (CT, ultrasound, MRI and nuclear scintigraphy). Pediatric Radiology 1996; 26:646–649.

Sheth S, Ruzal-Shapiro C, Piomelli S et al. CT imaging of splenic sequestration in sickle cell disease. Pediatric Radiology 2000; 30:830–833.

Walker TM, Serjeant GR. Focal echogenic lesions in the spleen in sickle cell disease. Clinical Radiology 1993; 47:114–116.

SPLEEN CALCIFICATIONS

Splenic calcifications are seen in many conditions (Figures 11.11.15 and 11.11.16). When seen early in life they are thought to be related to antenatal vascular insults or to infectious fetopathy. Calcifications are seen in cat scratch disease, histoplasmosis, tuberculosis, brucellosis and chronic granulomatosis disease. Other associations include splenic infarction, focal cysts (echinococcosis) or masses (haemangioma, hamartoma), abscess and haematoma.

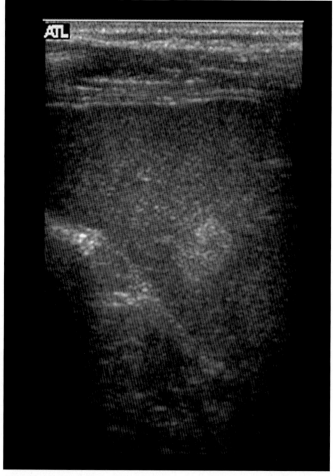

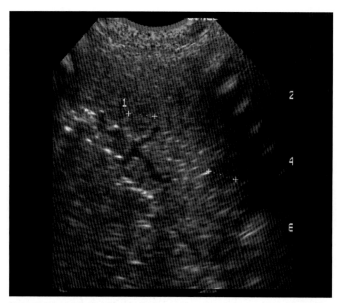

Figure 11.11.13 Sickle cell disease with recent infarcts: US shows few hypoechoic areas.

Figure 11.11.14 Sickle cell disease, US demonstrating echogenic areas of evolving infarcts.

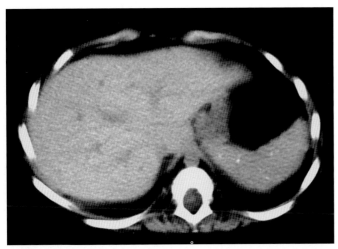

Figure 11.11.15 Splenic calcification: punctiform calcifications of splenic granulomas on CT.

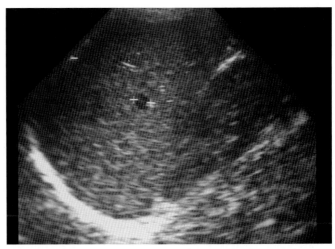

Figure 11.11.17 Lymphoma, US showing a hypoechoic nodule of lymphoma relapse.

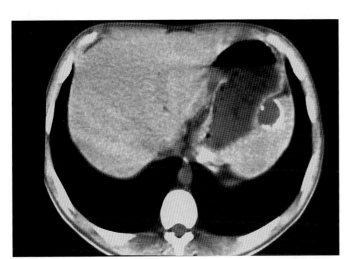

Figure 11.11.16 Splenic calcification, CT: linear calcification in the wall of a splenic cyst in a child with cystic fibrosis and insulin-dependent diabetes.

FURTHER READING

Talenti E, Cesaro S, Scarpinello A et al. Disseminated hepatic and splenic calcifications following cat-scratch disease. Pediatric Radiology 1994; 24:342–343.

HAEMATOLOGICAL DISORDERS

LYMPHOMA/LEUKAEMIA

Splenic malignancies are mostly leukaemia and lymphoma and usually manifest as splenomegaly. Lymphomatous involvement is frequent in children, seen in 30% in Hodgkin's disease and in 15%

in non-Hodgkin's lymphoma. A diffuse pattern is related to infiltration. Focal lesions may be evident, identified on US by hypoechoic zones without acoustic enhancement and on CT as hypodense areas (Figure 11.11.17) and on MR as high signal on T2. Adjacent lymphadenopathy is present at the hilum and along the splenic vessels.

LANGERHANS' CELL HISTIOCYTOSIS (LCH)

LCH is due to proliferation of histiocytes and may be multivisceral, involving the skin, lungs, bone, bone marrow and the reticuloendothelial system. Splenomegaly is usual in the systemic form. Hypoechoic nodules are less frequently encountered on sonography.

FURTHER READING

Goerg C, Weide R, Schwerk WB. Malignant splenic lymphoma: sonographic patterns, diagnosis and follow-up. Clinical Radiology 1997; 52:535–540.
Muwakkit S, Gharagozloo A, Sovid AK et al. The sonographic appearance of lesions of the spleen and pancreas in an infant with Langerhans cell histiocytosis. Pediatric Radiology 1994; 24:222–223.

CYSTS AND TUMOURS

Primary tumours of the spleen are extremely rare. Splenic cysts are the most common benign tumours. The histological classification of cysts is based on the presence of epithelial cells lining true cysts versus none in pseudocysts. Pseudocysts are thought to be post-traumatic or postinfarct. Clinical symptoms are pain and splenomegaly, with an increased risk of infection or rupture. Reliable distinction between true and false splenic cysts does not seem possible by imaging. True cysts include congenital or epidermoid cysts and parasitic cysts (hydatid disease).

EPIDERMOID CYSTS

A strong female preponderance is noted. Such cysts are well-defined, thin-walled, anechoic and stable over time. Linear wall calcification may be seen in 10% of the cases. Increased echogenicity of the cyst fluid due to cholesterol crystals is suggestive. At CT, the cyst is a round, well-delineated, non-enhancing lesion that is isodense to water. If there has been haemorrhage, internal echogenic debris and increased MR signal intensity will be obvious.

ECHINOCOCCAL CYST

Hydatid cyst involves the spleen in 2% of patients. It is usually associated with other visceral involvement. It may occur following systemic spread or intraperitoneal seeding of infection due to *Echinococcus granulosus*. Splenomegaly is common. On US, a well-defined cyst with occasional wall calcification is present. Cysts may be multiple with daughter cysts. It is a well-defined non-enhancing hypodense lesion on CT. If complicated (prerupture or rupture) the cyst may present as a solid lesion with unfolded membranes.

HAEMANGIOMA

Splenic haemangiomas are rare. They may be of the cavernous or capillary type or a combination of the two. They are isolated or associated with skin or skeletal haemangiomas in Klippel–Trenaunay syndrome. They have been described in patients with Turner or Beckwith–Wiedemann syndrome. A haemangioma may be symptomatic with splenomegaly, portal hypertension or present with splenic rupture and haemoperitoneum. With a large haemangioma, thrombocytopenia and consumptive coagulopathy and anaemia may develop as occurs in Kasabach–Merritt syndrome. Sonography shows a lesion of variable echogenicity (Figure 11.11.18) with calcification or cysts, with vascular flow on a Doppler tracing. On CT it is solid, iso- or hypodense to splenic tissue and enhances from the periphery to the centre. The cystic components do not enhance. The MRI appearance is heterogeneous. A haemangioma can be hypo- or isointense to spleen on T1-weighted images and hyperintense on T2 sequences. A subacute haemorrhage causes an increased signal intensity on T1 imaging. Haemangiomas do not take up sulphur colloid. An infantile haemangioendothelioma is a very vascular tumour, which is symptomatic early in life with splenomegaly and congestive heart failure. It is hypoechoic on sonography. High blood flow results in zones of signal void on T1-weighted sequences and increased signal intensity on gradient echo imaging.

LYMPHANGIOMA

This vascular malformation may be simple or multiple. In the latter case, splenic lymphangioma is often an incidental finding in

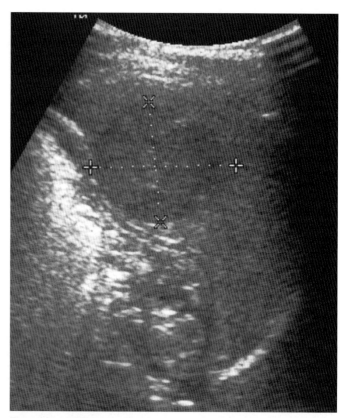

Figure 11.11.18 Splenic haemangioma, US: hypoechoic intraparenchymal lesion.

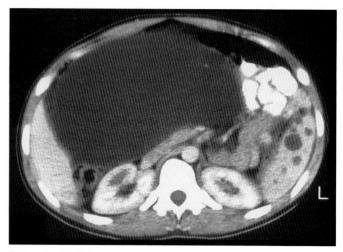

Figure 11.11.19 Lymphangiomatosis, CT: multiple small hypodense lesions in the spleen. The patient has a huge intraperitoneal lymphangioma as well as right renal involvement.

patients with diffused multivisceral lymphangiomatosis (Figure 11.11.19). Cystic lesions, often septated, are found. They do not enhance on CT. Curvilinear calcifications may be present. The cyst contents have increased T2 signal intensity with a high signal intensity on T1 imaging due to the proteinaceous nature of the fluid or to haemorrhage. Multiple lymphangiomata have a 'Swiss cheese' appearance on CT or angiography.

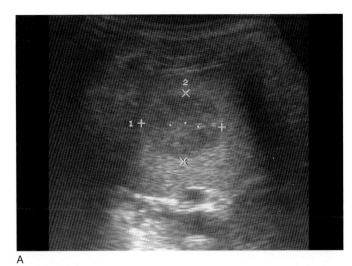

A

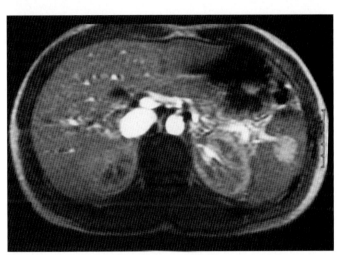

B

Figure 11.11.20 Splenic haemartoma in a boy with skin haemangioma. (A) US: focal hypoechoic heterogeneous splenic lesion. (B) MRI: dynamic spoiled gradient echo (SPGR) image post-IV gadolinium injection showing enhancement of the hamartoma.

HAMARTOMA

This non-tumoural lesion includes a mixture of disorganized splenic components around white and red pulp. It may be simple or associated with other hamartomas as in tuberous sclerosis. The majority of patients are asymptomatic. Systemic symptoms are rarely present. A hamartoma is hypoechoic (Figure 11.11.20A) and on CT the attenuation is similar to that of the spleen. A heterogeneous appearance with calcification has been described. On MRI, it is isointense on T1 imaging and heterogeneously hypointense on T2 sequences. Its enhancement may be prolonged and heterogeneous (Figure 11.11.20B).

FURTHER READING

Dachman AH, Ros PR, Murari PJ et al 1986. Non parasitic splenic cysts: a report of 52 cases with radiologic-pathologic correlation. American Journal of Roentgenology 1986; 147:537–542.

Kassarjian A, Patenaude YG, Bernard C et al. Symptomatic splenic hamartoma with renal, cutaneous and hematological abnormalities. Pediatric Radiology 2001; 31:111–114.

Pandel M, Terrier F, Michel G et al. Splenic hemangioma – report of three pediatric cases with pathologic correlation. Pediatric Radiology 1992; 22:213–216.

Ramani M, Reinhold C, Semelka RC et al. Splenic hemangiomas and hamartomas: MR imaging characteristics of 28 lesions. Radiology 1997; 202:166–172.

Spencer NJ, Arthur RJ, Stringer MD. Ruptured splenic epidermoid cyst: case report and imaging appearances. Pediatric Radiology 1996; 26:871–873.

Wadsworth PT, Newman B, Abramson SJ et al. Splenic lymphangiomatosis in children. Radiology 1997; 202:173–176.

The Pancreas

Douglas Jamieson

EMBRYOLOGY

The pancreas develops from the endoderm of two pancreatic buds. The dorsal bud arises directly from the duodenal region of the foregut. Ventral to this, an hepatic diverticulum develops and from this structure the ventral bud of pancreas arises (Figure 11.12.1). By the fourth week of fetal life, the developing ductal system of the dorsal bud drains directly into the foregut lumen while the ventral bud ducts drain into the distal embryonic biliary tree. In the sixth to eighth weeks of life, rotation and return of the gut to the abdomen occurs. The dorsal and ventral pancreas rotate with duodenal rotation and displacement to the right and then fuse (Figure 11.12.2A,B,C). The ventral bud gives rise to the uncinate process and most of the pancreatic head while the dorsal bud forms the remainder of the head, body and tail of the pancreas. The ventral duct (duct of Wirsung), which drains into the common bile duct, becomes the main drainage pathway. The dorsal duct (duct of Santorini) becomes an accessory duct with a duodenal accessory ampulla (Figure 11.12.3A). In 20% of the population, the accessory duct will atrophy (Figure 11.12.3B) and in 10%, the two ducts may not fuse retaining independent drainage, known as pancreas divisum (Figure 11.12.3C).

FURTHER READING

Moore KL, Persaud TVN. The digestive system. In: The developing human: clinically oriented embryology, 6th edn. Philadelphia: W.B. Saunders; 1998:271–302.
Williams PL, Warwick R. Embryology. In: Gray's Anatomy, 36th edn. Edinburgh: Churchill Livingstone; 1980:72–227.

ANATOMY

The pancreas is a fleshy, lobulated gland composed largely of tubuloacinar structures responsible for exocrine function. The secretory cells of each acinus produce the digestive pancreatic enzymes, which include amylase, trypsin, chymotrypsin and lipase. The endocrine function of the pancreas is performed by small clusters of cells known as the islets of Langerhans. They are located outside the tubuloacinar structures within the pancreatic connective tissues. These cells produce hormones, which include insulin, glucagon, somatostatin, gastrin, pancreatic polypeptide and vasoactive polypeptide.

The pancreas is in the retroperitoneum, positioned in a transverse oblique plane across the anterior pararenal space. The head and uncinate process lie within the curve of the first, second and third parts of the duodenum with the inferior vena cava posterior. The uncinate process extends medially behind the superior mesenteric vessels anterior to the aorta. The neck and body lie across the spine with the splenic–superior mesenteric vein confluence and splenic vein, an intimate posterior relationship. The tail extends up to the splenic hilum where it has a small peritoneal exposure anteriorly. The pancreas is not bound by a capsule, thus pancreatic pathology has ready access to the anterior pararenal space, transverse mesocolon, splenorenal ligament and the mediastinum.

The acinar ductules drain to the main pancreatic duct (duct of Wirsung), which runs the length of the gland to join the common bile duct in, or posterolateral to, the pancreatic head. This empties into the duodenum at the major ampulla (ampulla of Vater), entering the posterior second part of the duodenum. The accessory duct (duct of Santorini), when present, opens at the minor ampulla 1–2 cm above the major ampulla.

The pancreas has a very rich blood supply. The common hepatic artery, off the coeliac trunk, gives rise to the gastroduodenal artery, which supplies the superior pancreatico duodenal arteries. The superior mesenteric artery gives rise to the inferior pancreatico duodenal vessels. These interconnect and supply the head and neck. The splenic artery, off the coeliac trunk, gives rise to the superior pancreatic artery and multiple smaller direct vessels, which supply the body and tail. Venous drainage is to splenic and superior mesenteric vein flowing to portal vein. The rich vasculature and well-developed capillary beds are vital to the complex control mechanisms of both exocrine and endocrine pancreatic function. These functions also utilize autonomic nervous supply, especially vagal cholinergic enervation. Lymphatic drainage is equally abundant with drainage posterior to nodes along the splenic vein progressing towards the coeliac axis. The head and neck lymphatics drain along the pancreatico duodenal supply vessels connecting with gastric and hepatic lymphatics or drain posterior to mesenteric nodes.

FURTHER READING

Williams PL, Warwick R. Splanchnology. In: Gray's Anatomy, 36th edn. Edinburgh: Churchill Livingstone; 1980:1368–1374.

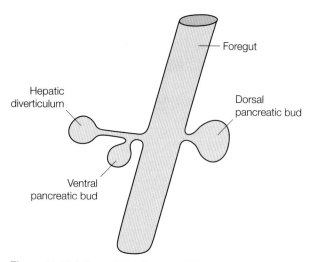

Figure 11.12.1 Foregut development: 4th week fetal life.

IMAGING

The pancreas is relatively large in the first year of life. Antero-posterior (AP) measurements of the head and body should be similar, measuring about 1 cm in the newborn and up to 2 cm by late adolescence. The pancreatic neck is thinner and should not measure in excess of 1.5 cm at any age.

SONOGRAPHY

The pancreas can be well visualized in children. A transverse or transverse oblique plane via an anterior approach provides good acoustic access to the head, neck and body using the left lobe of the liver as a window, or directly if the stomach is empty (Figure 11.12.4A). The tail of the pancreas is usually best seen from the left flank using the spleen as an acoustic window in an oblique coronal plane. Pancreatic tissue should be homogeneous but is

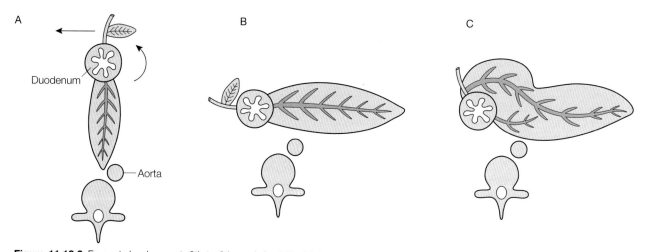

Figure 11.12.2 Foregut development: 6th to 8th week fetal life. (A) Duodenum will rotate and displace to right (arrows). (B) Dorsal pancreatic bud lies across retroperitoneum. (C) Fusion of ventral and dorsal pancreatic buds.

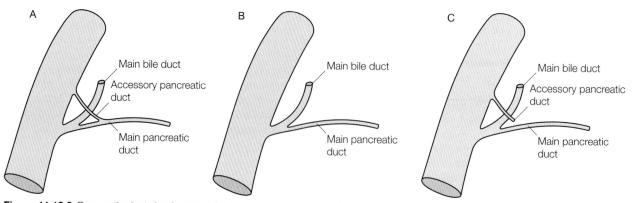

Figure 11.12.3 Pancreatic duct development. (A) Accessory duct opens at minor ampulla in the duodenum and remains connected to the main pancreatic duct. (B) Accessory duct atrophies. (C) Accessory and main pancreatic ducts do not fuse – pancreas divisum.

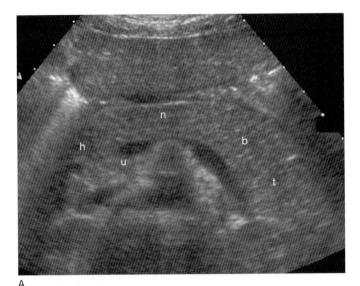

A

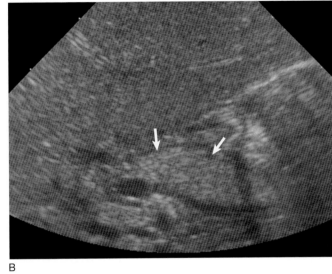

B

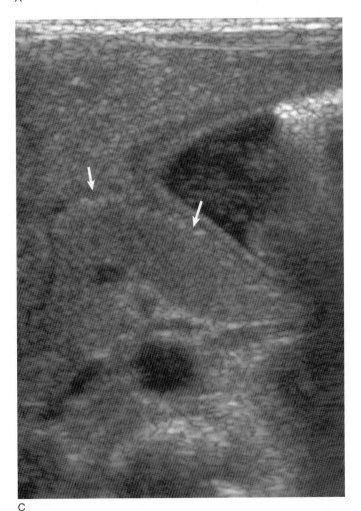

C

Figure 11.12.4 Sonography normal pancreas. (A) 12-year-old male; anterior transverse oblique plane utilizing the left lobe of the liver as an acoustic window. Pancreas is homogeneous, isoechoic to liver demonstrating uncinate process (u), head (h), neck (n), body (b) and tail (t). (B) 1-year-old female; pancreas hyperechoic to liver (arrows) but homogeneous. (C) Newborn male; pancreas well delineated with linear probe, hypoechoic to liver (arrows).

quite variable in its echogenic appearance (Figure 11.12.4B). In neonates, the pancreas is usually hypoechoic compared to liver (Figure 11.12.4C). In most children, the pancreas will become isoechoic or slightly hyperechoic compared to the liver. However, 10% of normal children may have pancreas parenchyma hypoechoic compared to adjacent liver. The pancreatic duct can be seen with high-resolution linear probes. It may be a single echogenic line. The anechoic lumen should not measure in excess of 1–2 mm and the walls should be linear and smooth.

COMPUTED TOMOGRAPHY

The pancreas is well delineated by computed tomography (CT). Modern multidetector scanners and work stations with multiplanar reformatting ability have significantly improved pancreas imaging. The pancreas should be homogeneous, with a density comparable to liver and a uniform contrast enhancement (Figure 11.12.5A,B,C). The outline may be smooth or lobulated but should always be well defined. Precontrast studies may occasionally show calcification to better effect but should not be routine in children. A single portal venous phase study is usually all that is required although arterial phase studies and dedicated thin slice studies may be valuable in specific situations. Oral contrast fluids have been recommended for abdominal CT imaging. However, clear fluids quite adequately distend bowel lumen, create less artifact and allow better evaluation of bowel wall.

MAGNETIC RESONANCE

Magnetic resonance imaging (MRI) is facilitated by high field strength magnets and appropriate coils to allow faster acquisition and breath-hold imaging. Cost, availability and need for sedation

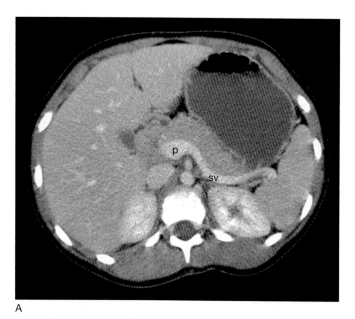

A

C

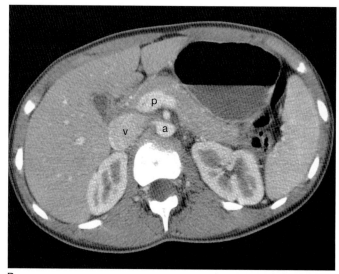

B

Figure 11.12.5 IV enhanced CT, normal pancreas. sv, splenic vein; p, portal confluence; a, aorta; v, IVC; s, superior mesenteric artery; m, superior mesenteric vein; d, duodenum; g, gallbladder; j, jejunum; u, uncinate process; arrow, common bile duct in head of pancreas. (A) 10-year-old male; slight obliquity due to patient position approximates sonography (see Figure 11.12.4A). (B,C) 14-year-old male; upper (B) and lower (C) CT images demonstrate pancreas anatomy and relationships.

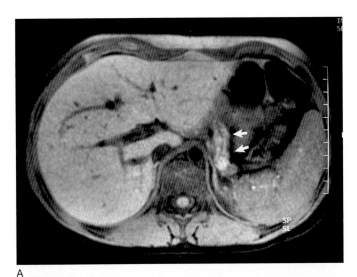

A

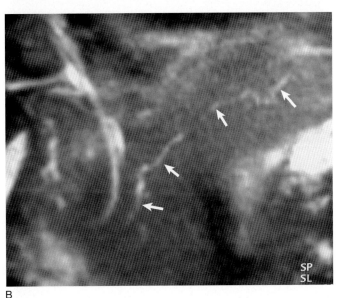

B

Figure 11.12.6 MR normal pancreas. Axial, fat-saturated, T1 effect, spoiled gradient echo image shows pancreas slightly hyperintense compared to liver (arrows). (B) MRCP resolves an undilated pancreatic duct in a 10-year-old female (arrows). (Courtesy of Dr P. Shipman, Princess Margaret Hospital for Children, Perth, Western Australia.)

in young children have restricted its application. Recommended imaging includes breath-hold, spoiled gradient echo, T1-weighted sequences and fat-suppressed, T1-weighted sequences followed by IV gadolinium enhancement. Pancreas parenchyma should be isointense to liver on the spoiled gradient echo T1 images and becomes hyperintense in the fat-suppressed sequences (Figure 11.12.6A). This is attributed to the aqueous proteins produced by the acinar glands. Gadolinium produces early, uniform enhancement, in excess of early hepatic enhancement, which fades within a few minutes. Immediate imaging following the gadolinium bolus and delayed imaging is recommended. T2-weighted sequences are less useful but may show cysts and fluid collections to better advantage (Figure 11.12.19E). Most exciting is the development of heavily T2-weighted breath-hold techniques producing MR cholangiopancreatography (MRCP) (Figure 11.12.6B). Improving resolution allows visualization of pancreatic ducts although in

small children resolving non-dilated ducts remains challenging. Resolution down to 1 mm is reported with half-Fourier RARE (rapid acquisition with relaxation enhancement) MRCP.

ENDOSCOPIC RETROGRADE CHOLANGIOPANCREATOGRAPHY (ERCP)

ERCP remains the 'gold standard' for anatomic duct delineation. In children, it is technically challenging, seldom indicated and carries the risk of inducing pancreatitis. The major indication for ERCP in paediatrics is delineation of ductal damage following trauma or pancreatitis (Figure 11.12.14B).

ANGIOGRAPHY

Angiography and transhepatic portal venous sampling has limited application in evaluating persistent hyperinsulinaemic hypoglycaemia of infancy and functional islet cell tumours. This would only be available at highly specialized centres.

FURTHER READING

Bret PM, Reinhold C, Taourel P et al. Pancreas divisum: evaluation with MR cholangiopancreatography. Radiology 1996; 199:99–103.
Chigot V, De Lonlay P, Nassogne MC et al. Pancreatic arterial calcium stimulation in the diagnosis and localization of persistent hyperinsulinemic hypoglycemia of infancy. Pediatric Radiology 2001;31:155–158.
Dubois J, Brunelle F, Touati G et al. Hyperinsulinism in children: diagnostic value of pancreatic venous sampling correlated with clinical, pathological and surgical outcome in 25 cases. Pediatric Radiology1995;25:512–516.
Fulcher AS, Turner MA, Capps GW et al. Half-Fourier RARE MRCP in 300 subjects. Radiology 1998; 207:21–32.
Herman TH, Siegel MJ. CT of the pancreas in children. American Journal of Roentgenology 1991; 157:375–379.
Hirohashi S, Hirohashi R, Uchida H et al. Pancreatitis: evaluation with MR cholangiopancreatography in children. Radiology 1997; 203:411–415.
Kim M, Han SJ, Yoon CS et al. Using MR cholangiotography to reveal anomalous pancreaticobiliary ductal union in infants and children with choledochal cysts. American Journal of Roentgenology 2002; 179:209–214.
Semelka RC, Ascher SM. MR imaging of the pancreas. Radiology 1993;188: 593–602.
Siegel MJ, Martin KW, Worthington JL. Normal and abnormal pancreas in children: US studies. Radiology 1987; 165:15–18.

CONGENITAL ABNORMALITIES

PANCREAS DIVISUM

Many variations in ductal anatomy occur due to irregularity of ductal fusion. Pancreas divisum has non-union of the dorsal and ventral ducts (Figure 11.12.3C). This occurs in 5–10% of the population. A significant increase in recurrent pancreatitis is reported to be associated with this anomaly. The pancreatitis usually manifests in early adulthood but the initial bouts of inflammation may start in childhood. Up to 25% of patients with recurrent pancreatitis have been reported to have pancreas divisum at ERCP and similar results have been reported in adults undergoing MRCP. Aetiology of the pancreatitis is felt to be impaired drainage of exocrine secretions at the smaller minor ampulla of the dorsal duct (duct of Santorini). An enlarged, lobulated pancreatic head and a cleavage plane between dorsal and ventral components have been reported at sonography and CT, but are not reliable signs for pancreas divisum. MRCP is the only non-invasive imaging likely to identify this condition.

ANNULAR PANCREAS

This results from the ventral bud fusing to the dorsal bud around the duodenum. A ring of pancreatic tissue may surround the duodenum or a component of the ring may be fibrous. Associated congenital anomalies are common, up to 75%, although in many, the annular pancreas will not be clinically obvious. They include duodenal atresia, duodenal stenosis, malrotation, oesophageal atresia, tracheoesophageal fistula, Down's syndrome and anorectal malformation. Symptoms of incomplete obstruction relate to the calibre of the duodenal lumen at the annular pancreas. The proximal duodenum dilates and contrast studies show concentric narrowing of the second part of the duodenum (Figure 11.12.7A). This may be quite subtle in some patients. Sonography may identify a ring of pancreatic tissue but a fibrous band can easily be overlooked. CT can elegantly display the pathology (Figure 11.12.7B). Surgical treatment is a duodeno-duodenostomy.

PARTIAL AGENESIS

Agenesis of the pancreas would not be compatible with life. Partial agenesis, usually involving the dorsal bud, is rarely described. Insulin deficiency causing diabetes mellitus is associated but exocrine function is adequately maintained. This is usually an incidental finding at cross-sectional imaging with deficient pancreatic body and tail. Associated conditions are Shwachman–Diamond syndrome, Johanson–Blizzard syndrome and leprechaunism.

HETEROTOPIC PANCREAS

Heterotopic pancreas is commonly found in the gastrointestinal tract (up to 15% at autopsy). It is mostly asymptomatic and incidentally detected. 70% are found in the upper GI tract although the 2 mm to 4 cm nodules can be found in the small bowel, colon, Meckel's diverticulum, liver, gallbladder, omentum, in duplication cysts and in extra-abdominal sites such as bronchogenic cysts and sequestrations. Reported complications include bleeding, intestinal obstruction and creating lead points for intussusception.

CONGENITAL CYSTS

Isolated congenital cysts are extremely rare and may only be confirmed by pathological confirmation of epithelial wall lining.

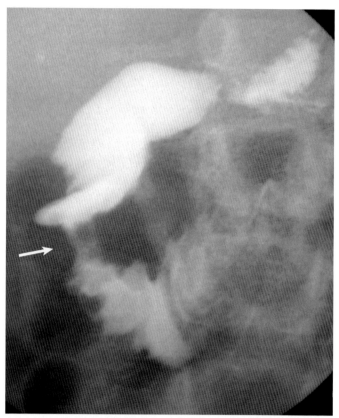

A

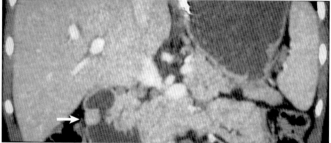

B

Figure 11.12.7 Annular pancreas; 4-year-old male presenting with longstanding but intermittent emesis. (A) Concentric narrowing of the second part of the duodenum (arrow). (B) Coronal reconstruction of an IV contrast enhanced CT delineates collar of pancreatic tissue encircling duodenum (arrow).

FURTHER READING

Berrocal T, Torres I, Gutierrez J et al. Congenital anomalies of the upper gastrointestinal tract. Radiographics 1999; 19:855–872.

Bret PM, Reinhold C, Taourel P et al. Pancreas divisum: evaluation with MR cholangiopancreatography. Radiology 1996; 199:99–103.

Casadei R, Campione O, Greco VM et al. Congenital true pancreatic cysts in young adults: case report and literature review. Pancreas 1996; 12:419–421.

Gold RP. Agenesis and pseudo-agenesis of the dorsal pancreas. Abdominal Imaging 1993; 18:141–144.

Hirohashi S, Hirohashi R, Uchida H et al. Pancreatitis: evaluation with MR cholangiopancreatography in children. Radiology 1997; 203:411–415.

Lai ECS, Tompkins RK. Heterotopic pancreas. Review of 26 years experience. The American Journal of Surgery 1986; 151:697–700.

Lerner A, Branski D, Lebenthal E. Pancreatic Disease in Children. Pediatric Clinics of North America 1996; 43:125–156.

Shah KK, Deridder PH, Schwab RE et al. CT diagnosis of dorsal pancreas agenesis. Journal of Computer Assisted Tomography 1989; 1:140–141.

Vaughn DD, Jabra AA, Fishman EK. Pancreatic disease in children and young adults: evaluation with CT. Radiographics 1998; 18:1171–1187.

PANCREATITIS

ACUTE PANCREATITIS

Non-traumatic, acute pancreatitis is an uncommon cause of abdominal pain in childhood. In adults, most acute pancreatitis is related to alcohol abuse and biliary calculi. In children, the causes of pancreatitis are more varied and often less obvious.

Aetiologies include:

- viral infections (mumps, enterovirus, Epstein–Barr, hepatitis A, cytomegalovirus, coxsackie, influenza);
- drugs (steroids, L-asparaginase, thiazides, sulphonamides, azathioprine, organophosphates);
- congenital ductal anomalies (pancreas divisum, choledochal cyst);
- non congenital biliary obstruction (gallstones, pseudocyst, tumour, ascaris lumbricoides);
- metabolic disease (hypercalcaemia, uraemia, haemochromatosis, hypertriglyceridaemia);
- systemic disease (diabetes mellitus, polyarteritis nodosa, Henoch–Schonlein purpura, systemic lupus erythematosis, Crohn's disease, Kawasaki disease);
- hereditary disorders (cystic fibrosis, familial pancreatitis, hyperlipoproteinaemia, alpha 1 antitrypsin deficiency).

Up to 20% of childhood pancreatitis will still be called idiopathic.

The pathophysiology of pancreatic inflammation is not fully understood. Contributing factors are bile reflux up the ductal system, duct distention, increased permeability of the duct lining and inappropriate activation of exocrine enzymes. The consequences range from localized oedema to haemorrhagic necrosis.

The clinical presentation of epigastric pain, nausea, vomiting and acute abdomen may be quite variable in children. Mild acute pancreatitis may be a short, self-limiting process while severe pancreatitis can have a fulminant course with many complications. Elevated serum amylase and lipase support the diagnosis although false positive and false negative results are not uncommon.

Acute complications include shock, circulatory collapse, disseminated intravascular coagulopathy and multiorgan failure. Renal decompensation is important to evaluate if IV contrast is to be given for CT. Intra- and extrapancreatic fluid collections and pancreatic necrosis develop early. It is interesting that severe disease manifests early and progression from mild to severe disease is unusual.

Late complications include pseudocyst formation, abscess, fat necrosis and vascular thrombosis. Most acute fluid collections resolve but some persist and may enlarge. If, by 2–4 weeks, a well-developed pseudocapsule forms around a fluid collection, it is termed a pseudocyst. Half will resolve spontaneously, often over an extended period. Many will be symptomatic or become infected and require drainage. Image-guided percutaneous drainage can be effective; drainage is often fairly long term. Internal drainage from pseudocyst to gastric lumen can be very successful. Unregulated lipase activity can cause necrosis and saponification of mesenteric fat. Proteolytic enzyme action and inflammation can damage arterial walls causing pseudoaneurysm formation with a potential to rupture. Splenic and pancreatico duodenal arteries are most commonly affected. Venous complication of acute thrombosis is most common in splenic and superior mesenteric veins.

IMAGING

Imaging may identify unsuspected acute pancreatitis but usually supports a clinical diagnosis. Imaging early in the course of disease or in mild pancreatitis may be unremarkable. Often the extra pancreatic effects are more striking than the abnormality in the gland itself.

Plain film findings are usually non-specific. They may show the consequence of inflammation extending down the transverse mesocolon causing the 'colon cut off' or inflammation extending into the peritoneum with a dilated 'sentinal loop' of small bowel.

Sonography will identify focal or diffuse enlargement of the pancreas, often with hypoechoic changes, in 40–60% of patients with acute pancreatitis (Figure 11.12.8A). However, in ill patients, often with overlying bowel ileus, visualization of the retroperitoneum can be difficult. Extrapancreatic fluid collections occur in about 50% of patients, mostly in the anterior pararenal space and may be the only finding (Figure 11.12.8B). Evaluation for biliary calculi is important and sonography may be more sensitive than CT in this regard (Figure 11.12.9A,B,C). Sonography is effectively used to follow up pseudocyst size.

CT findings of acute pancreatitis are diffuse or focal gland enlargement, hypodense change, duct dilatation (Figure 11.12.10) and intra- or extrapancreatic fluid collections. Intrapancreatic fluid collections are seen in 10%, and extrapancreatic collections are present in 50% of children with acute pancreatitis. The lack of a gland capsule allows ready extension of inflammation with collections common in the anterior pararenal space, lesser sac and transverse mesocolon. Attenuation and contrast enhancement of parenchyma may be variable. CT is superior to sonography for delineation of fluid collections and their extent. It is important to note false negative rates for CT detection of acute pancreatitis are reported between 30 and 50%. Adult CT literature indicates that the development and extent of pancreatic necrosis correlates well to disease severity and attendant morbidity increase. Necrosis is inferred by focal or diffuse areas of non-enhancing pancreatic tissue (Figure 11.12.9A,B). Assessment of necrosis is most reliably done 48–72 h after the pancreatitis has clinically declared itself. Pancreatic pseudocysts are well delineated, round, low-density structures usually with a prominent enhancing pseudocapsule (Figure 11.12.11). Haemorrhage or infection can give a variable density to the cyst content and imaging alone cannot exclude abscess development.

MRI can display all of the morphological changes described for CT imaging. Increased sensitivity for detection of subtle changes of peripancreatic inflammation or minor pancreatic tissue abnormality is reported. The value of this information in the context of the mild pancreatitis needs to be weighted against MRI availability, cost and possible anaesthesia requirement. MRCP can delineate biliary anomalies such as choledochal cyst (Figure 11.12.12) and can compete with ERCP for diagnosing pancreas divisum.

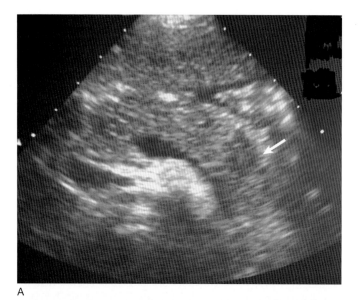

A

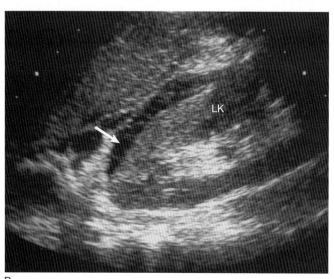

B

Figure 11.12.8 Sonography pancreatitis. (A) Swollen body with ill-defined hypoechoic area (arrow). (B) Left perinephric collection (arrow).

TRAUMATIC PANCREATITIS

Abdominal trauma is a common cause of acute pancreatitis in children. It is usually the result of blunt trauma although penetrating wounds and iatrogenic intraoperative injury can occur. The trauma typically applies compressive force to the upper abdomen impacting the pancreas where it drapes over the vertebral body. There is a high incidence of associated injury involving duodenum, liver, spleen and spine. The traumatic history is usually obvious. Motor vehicle accidents (particularly in the lap-belt complex injury), impalement on bicycle handlebars, crush injury and falls are common mechanisms of injury. In this setting of blunt abdominal trauma, the incidence of pancreatic injury is reported to be between 3 and 12%. Child abuse with a blow to the upper abdomen as a non-accidental injury is a well-described cause of acute

pancreatitis. Regrettably a history may not be forthcoming, which can significantly delay diagnosis.

IMAGING

CT is the most likely investigation a child with suspected blunt abdominal trauma will undergo. Studies have suggested CT may underdiagnose up to a third of patients with traumatic pancreatic injury. However, a paediatric study of 35 patients with retrospective review of CT studies, identified at least some suggestive findings of pancreatic injury in all cases. Multidetector scanners and awareness of associated findings should improve prospective diagnosis of pancreatic injury. A third of children will have an identifiable traumatic cleft, transection or obvious focal parenchymal abnormality. Associated findings are: free intraperitoneal fluid, mesenteric fluid or haematoma, lesser sac fluid, focal peripancreatic fluid, anterior pararenal fluid, thickened gerota's fascia, fluid between splenic vein and pancreas, fluid around superior mesenteric vein and portal vein, and fluid between pancreas and duodenum (Figure 11.12.13). Injury to the pancreatic head has greater morbidity than that to the body or tail and pancreatic duct transection increases the likelihood of persistent pseudocyst complications.

The literature on adults has advocated early ERCP and distal pancreatectomy where ductal transection and leakage is detected (Figure 11.12.14). There is good paediatric literature advocating conservative management of pancreatic injury. Healing of transected pancreatic duct has been documented and percutaneous drainage of pseudocysts and abscesses has been found to be effective, thus restricting pancreatectomy and pancreaticoenterostomy to those who 'earn' their operation. This expectant surgical management does rely on good cross-sectional imaging information. MRCP will have an increasing role in ductal evaluation with the obvious advantages of not inducing additional pancreatitis and the ability to visualize duct distal to a transection.

CHRONIC PANCREATITIS

Progression and recurrence of pancreatitis to the point of permanent structural change and loss of exocrine and endocrine function is extremely rare in children. It does occur in undeveloped countries where malnutrition, worm infestation and childhood infections are rife. Juvenile tropical pancreatitis syndrome is a term that has been applied to this group of patients.

FAMILIAL HEREDITARY PANCREATITIS

This is an autosomal dominant disorder with variable penetrance. Initial presentation of pancreatitis is usually by 10 years of age. Progression to pancreatic atrophy, calcification, duct stricture and duct dilatation depends on recurrence and severity of attacks, which is variable. Other than the complications of acute pancreatitis, exocrine insufficiency may occur. Diabetes mellitus will develop in up to 30% of patients and there is a long-term risk of

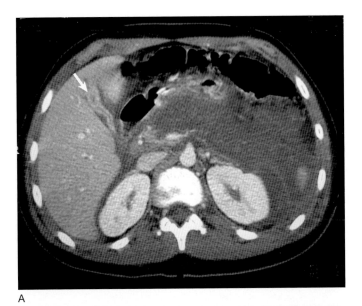

A

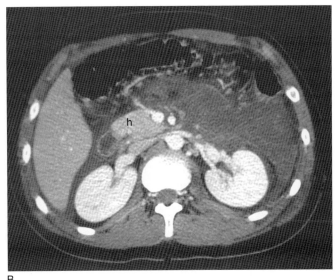

B

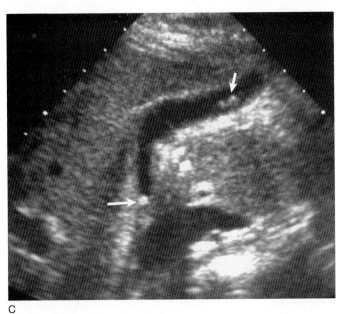

C

Figure 11.12.9 Gallstone pancreatitis in a 13-year-old male. (A,B) IV contrast enhanced CT demonstrates enhancing pancreatic head (h) but necrosis of the neck, body and tail with no parenchymal enhancement. Marked inflammatory change extends into the mesentery. The gallbladder demonstrates no obvious calculi (arrow). (C) Sonography identifies aetiology of the pancreatitis by showing cholilithiasis (arrows).

pancreatic cancer reported to be as high as 20%. Genetic mutations on chromosome 7q35, the gene that codes for cationic trypsinogen, have been identified. It is believed that the mutations allow trypsinogen to be activated to trypsin within the acinar gland leading to autodigestion, inflammation and pancreatitis. The intermittent nature of the disease suggests inhibitory factors secreted by the pancreas have a protective role but may be overwhelmed. This interesting work may finally help elucidate the pathophysiology of acute pancreatitis.

Cross-sectional imaging demonstrates atrophy, calcification, intraductal calculi and duct dilatation. ERCP is recommended to delineate ductal strictures and attempt duct dilatation and calculus extraction. Surgical resection and pancreaticojejunostomy circumventing strictures can provide symptomatic relief. MRI should have an increasing role in evaluation of chronic pancreatitis with the ability to delineate ducts at MRCP, assess gland morphology

with T1 fat-suppressed sequences and assess fibrosis as manifested by poor enhancement on immediate postgadolinium enhancement imaging.

FURTHER READING

Akhrass R, Kim K, Brandt C. Computed tomography: an unreliable indicator of pancreatic trauma. American Surgeon 1996; 62:647–651.

Arkovitz MS, Garcia VF. Spontaneous recanalization of the pancreatic duct: case report and review. Journal of Trauma 1996; 40:1014–1016.

Balthazar EJ. Acute pancreatitis: assessment of severity with clinical and CT evaluation. Radiology 2002; 223:603–613.

Balthazar EJ, Freeny PC, vanSonnenberg E. Imaging and intervention in acute pancreatitis. Radiology 1994; 193:297–306.

Bret PM, Reinhold C, Taourel P et al. Pancreas divisum: evaluation with MR cholangiopancreatography. Radiology 1996; 199:99–103.

Fulcher AS, Turner MA. MR pancreatography: a useful tool for evaluating pancreatic disorders. Radiographics 1999; 19:5–24.

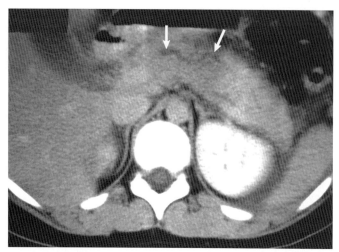

Figure 11.12.10 IV contrast enhanced CT in a 13-year-old female with pancreatitis shows swollen but enhancing parenchyma and a dilated main bile duct (arrows).

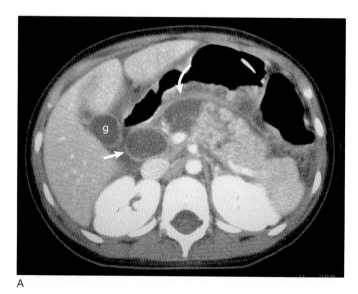

A

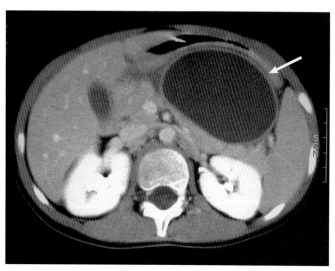

Figure 11.12.11 IV contrast enhanced CT in a 7-year-old male shows a well delineated pseudocyst with enhancing rim (arrow).

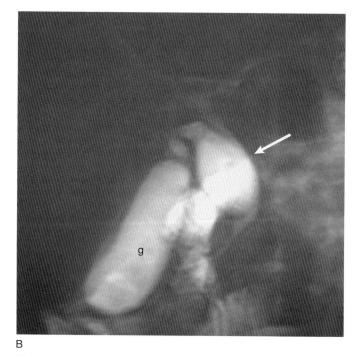

B

Figure 11.12.12 A 6-year-old female with choledochal cyst and pancreatitis. (A) IV contrast enhanced CT confirmed the sonographic findings of cyst at the pancreatic head (arrow), separate from gallbladder (g) and a swollen inhomogeneous pancreas body with non-enhancing head and neck (curved arrow). (B) MRCP shows the choledochal cyst (arrow) involving the distal cystic duct and main bile duct with no intrahepatic duct dilatation.

Herman TH, Siegel MJ. CT of the pancreas in children. American Journal of Roentgenology 1991; 157:375–379.

Hirohashi S, Hirohashi R, Uchida H et al. Pancreatitis: evaluation with MR cholangiopancreatography in children. Radiology 1997; 203:411–415.

Jeffrey RB, Federle MP, Crass RA. Computed tomography of pancreatic trauma. Radiology 1983; 147:491–494.

Kim M, Han SJ, Yoon CS et al. Using MR cholangiotography to reveal anomalous pancreaticobiliary ductal union in infants and children with choledochal cysts. American Journal of Roentgenology 2002; 179:209–214.

King RL, Siegel MJ, Balfe DM. Acute pancreatitis in children: CT findings of intra and extrapancreatic fluid collections. Radiology 1995; 195:196–200.

Kleinman P. Visceral trauma. In: Kleinman P Diagnostic imaging of child abuse, 2nd edn. St Louis: Mosby; 1998:248–284.

Lane MJ, Mindelzun RE, Sandhu JS et al. CT diagnosis of blunt pancreatic trauma: importance of detecting fluid between the pancreas and the splenic vein. American Journal of Roentgenology 1994; 163:833–835.

Lerner A, Branski D, Lebenthal E. Pancreatic disease in children. Pediatric Clinics of North America 1996; 43:125–156.

Rescorla FJ, Plumley DA, Sherman S et al. The efficacy of early ERCP in pediatric pancreatic trauma. Journal of Pediatric Surgery 1995; 30:336–340.

Semelka RC, Ascher SM. MR imaging of the pancreas. Radiology 1993; 188:593–602.

Shilyansky J, Sena LM, Kreller M et al. Nonoperative Management of Pancreatic Injuries in Children. Journal of Pediatric Surgery 1998; 33:343–349.

Sivit CJ, Eichelberger MR, Taylor GA et al. Blunt pancreatic trauma in children: CT diagnosis. American Journal of Roentgenology 1992; 158:1097–1100.

Siegel MJ, Sivit JC. Pancreatic emergencies. Radiology Clinics of North America 1997; 35:815–830.

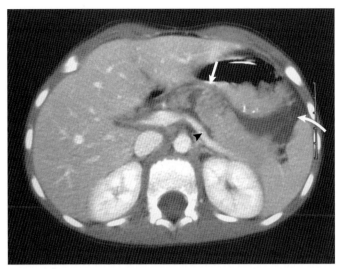

Figure 11.12.13 A 7-year-old male impaled on bicycle handle bars. IV contrast enhanced CT shows a traumatic cleft (arrow), fluid anterior to splenic vein (arrowhead) and a fluid collection in lesser sac (curved arrow).

VanSonnenberg E, Wittich G, Casola G et al. Percutaneous drainage of infected and non infected pancreatic pseudocyst: experience in 101 cases. Radiology 1989; 170:757–761.

Vaughn DD, Jabra AA, Fishman EK. Pancreatic disease in children and young adults: evaluation with CT. Radiographics 1998; 18:1171–1187.

Whitecomb DC. Hereditary pancreatitis: a model for understanding the genetic basis of acute and chronic pancreatitis. Pancreatology 2001; 1:565–570.

Whitcomb DC, Preston RA, Aston CE et al. A gene for hereditary pancreatitis maps to chromosome 7q35. Gastroenterology 1996; 110:1975–1980.

INHERITED DISORDERS

CYSTIC FIBROSIS

Cystic fibrosis is an autosomal recessive condition and the most common form of inherited pancreatic insufficiency. It is common in Caucasians (approximately 1:2000) but rare in African and Asian populations. The cystic fibrosis transmembrane conductance regulator gene was identified in 1989. The delta F508 mutation on the q31 area of chromosome 7 is the most common, appearing in about 70% of cases; however, at least 400 other mutations in cystic fibrosis have been identified. This gene encodes a protein that controls transmembrane chloride and sodium ion exchange with associated water exchange. In the pancreas, it manifests in the secretory cells of the acinar glands. Its malfunction results in abnormal, high-viscosity secretions, which clear poorly and obstruct proximal ductules. This results in underdevelopment and destruction of acinar cells, progressive fibrosis and fatty replacement. Dystrophic calcification, duct calculi and cystic changes can occur. When exocrine function is reduced to below 15%, the patients become pancreatic insufficient. This occurs in 85–90% of cystic fibrosis patients. Management of the exocrine insufficiency is oral replacement of pancreatic enzyme preparations to correct the malabsorption and steatorrhoea. Although 50% of patients will have an abnormal glucose tolerance test, only a small number will mani-

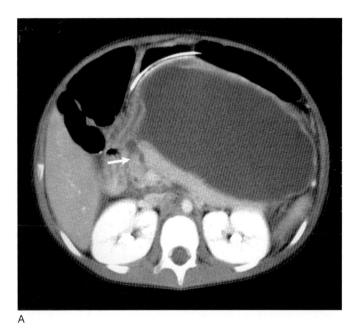

A

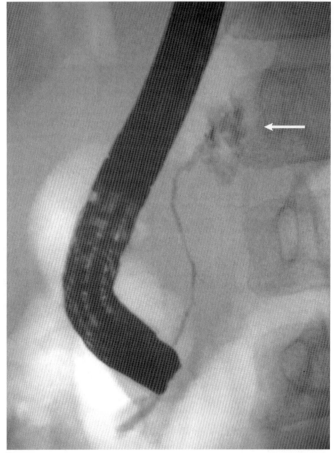

B

Figure 11.12.14 A 6-year-old female with post-traumatic pseudocyst. (A) IV contrast enhanced CT shows large pseudocyst and persistent cleft in the pancreatic head (arrow). (B) ERCP shows main pancreatic duct interrupted and leaking into the pseudocyst (arrow).

fest diabetes mellitus in childhood. With the increased longevity of cystic fibrosis patients, cystic fibrosis related diabetes is an increasing problem, with a 50% incidence by 30 years of age.

IMAGING

Pancreas imaging has no role in the diagnosis of cystic fibrosis, yet it will often be performed during evaluation of abdominal symptoms or liver surveillance.

Abdominal x-ray may show punctate parenchymal calcification or more focal calculi. Sonography may be normal or show minimal changes in the 10–15% of pancreas-sufficient patients. In patients with established pancreas-insufficient disease, the pancreas is usually small and of increased echogenicity (Figure 11.12.15). This is attributed to atrophy, fibrosis and fatty replacement. Pancreatic duct dilatation and calcification may be seen. Cystic changes are common but usually small, under 3 mm. Rarely, larger cysts can develop, occasionally replacing the pancreas. This has been termed pancreatic cystosis (Figure 11.12.16).

CT findings reflect the spectrum of pancreas pathology, ranging from normal to atrophic with fibrous and fatty replacement. The fatty change results in decreased attenuation, which may be focal or diffuse. Fibrous change retains higher soft tissue attenuation. Calcification, duct dilatation and cystic change can be identified.

MR imaging equals CT in its ability to evaluate pancreas morphology but has the advantage of not using ionizing radiation. Fatty change, which can be focal or diffuse, is well delineated with increased signal intensity on T1-weighted sequences. Complete fatty replacement may retain a glandular lobulate appearance or less commonly show loss of this lobulation suggesting destruction of the connective stroma in addition to the acinar structures.

SHWACHMAN–DIAMOND SYNDROME

This is the second most common form of inherited pancreatic insufficiency (approximately 1:10000 to 1:20000). It is likely to be an autosomal recessive disorder but its genetic basis has yet to be determined. The pancreas may be normal or reduced in size and shows marked fatty infiltration with preservation of ductal and lobular anatomy. The disorder is characterized by pancreatic insufficiency, bone marrow dysfunction, stunted growth and metaphyseal chondrodysplasia although phenotypic expression is variable.

Exocrine pancreatic insufficiency presents in infancy with malabsorption and steatorrhoea. Chloride levels in a sweat test remain normal excluding cystic fibrosis. Oral replacement therapy usually controls these symptoms and with increasing age there may be some improvement in pancreatic exocrine function.

The bone marrow dysfunction is most commonly a neutropenia, which is usually cyclical and occurs in 95% of cases. Thrombocytopenia and anaemia are common. If all three cell lines are deficient there is a significant risk for acute myelogenous leukaemia.

Stunted growth and delayed bone age are constant features of the syndrome. Mean height and weight are below the 5th percentile although from 6 months of age growth velocity is maintained.

Up to 15% of cases may display metaphyseal chrondrodysplasia with irregular lucent defects and sclerotic serrations in the metaphyses abutting growth plates. Metaphyseal widening can occur. Changes are most commonly seen at the hips and knees and are symmetrical. Irregular ossification of anterior rib ends, coxa vara, slipped femoral capital epiphysis and genu varus can occur. Long bone tubulation, clinodactaly, phalangeal hypoplasia and

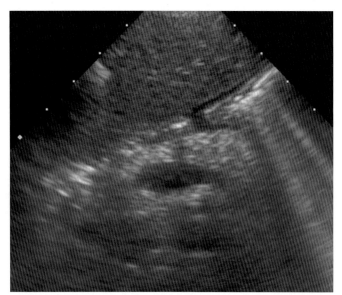

Figure 11.12.15 Sonography of an 8-year-old female with cystic fibrosis showing a small echogenic pancreas.

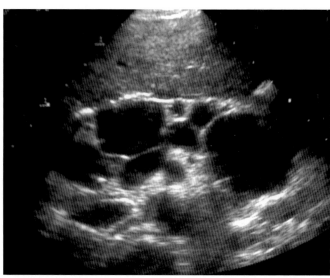

Figure 11.12.16 Sonography of a 12-year-old female with cystic fibrosis and pancreatic cystosis.

narrow sacroiliac notches are described. Other associated problems include hepatomegaly, liver enzyme abnormalities, impaired lung function, renal tubular abnormalities, ichthyosis and developmental or intellectual delays.

IMAGING

Plain radiographs will demonstrate the skeletal abnormalities and evaluate bone age. The fatty pancreas is well demonstrated with increased echogenicity at sonography, low density at CT and increased signal intensity on T1-weighted MRI.

JOHANSON–BLIZZARD SYNDROME

This is a rare autosomal recessive disorder with pancreatic insufficiency, nasal alar hypoplasia, hypothyroidism, congenital deafness, absent permanent teeth, midline ectodermal scalp defects, mental retardation, urogenital anomalies (including double vagina and uterus) and anorectal abnormalities (usually imperforate anus). The genetic defect remains unknown but the pancreatic abnormality is a primary acinar cell defect with normal outflow of fluids and electrolytes but deficient enzyme secretion. The pancreas can show complete fatty replacement with retention of ductal anatomy similar to Shwachman–Diamond syndrome.

PERSISTANT HYPERINSULINAEMIC HYPOGLYCAEMIA OF INFANCY (PHHI)

This rare and heterogeneous disorder seems to be mostly sporadic; however, familial forms are documented with abnormalities mapped to chromosome 11p15. Gene defects related to dysfunction of the inward rectifying potassium-ATP channels and sulfonylurea receptors have been shown to produce unregulated hyperinsulinaemia. PHHI needs to be differentiated from transient neonatal hypoglycaemia seen in infants of diabetic mothers, erythroblastosis fetalis and Beckwith–Wiedemann syndrome. The condition was initially known as nesidioblastosis alluding to the pathologically evident exuberant neoproliferation of functional neuroendocrine islet cells. There are two forms: a focal adenomatous hyperplasia and a diffuse abnormality of islet cells. The distinction is important as the diffuse abnormality requires a near total or 95% pancreatectomy with a high long-term risk for diabetes. The focal form requires partial pancreatectomy with removal of the focus.

Cross-sectional imaging is not helpful in diagnosis or separating focal from diffuse disease. Pancreas venous sampling can detect focal secretion of insulin and identify focal adenomatous hyperplasia. Access to pancreatic veins via the femoral vein and transhepatic access to the portal vein, would only be available in highly specialized interventional radiology centres. Techniques of selective arterial calcium stimulation and venous sampling in hepatic veins are described but not felt to be as accurate as the technically more challenging pancreas venous sampling.

VON HIPPEL LINDAU (VHL) SYNDROME

This genetic disorder usually presents with haemangioblastomas of the retina and CNS, renal cysts, renal cell carcinoma and phaeochromocytoma. Pancreatic cysts also occur. They are benign, epithelial cysts and can get large. They usually present in early adulthood but have been reported in teenagers with VHL. Less common pancreatic pathology in VHL includes islet cell tumours and serous cystic (microcystic) adenomas.

AUTOSOMAL DOMINANT POLYCYSTIC RENAL DISEASE

Cysts may be seen in autosomal dominant polycystic disease along with renal and hepatic cysts, however they usually only manifest in later life.

FURTHER READING

Agrons GA, Corse WR, Markowitz R et al. Gastrointestinal manifestations of cystic fibrosis: radiologic-pathologic correlation. Radiographics 1996; 16:871–893.

Berrocal T, Simon MJ, Al-Assir I et al. Shwachman–Diamond syndrome: clinical, radiological and sonograhic findings. Pediatric Radiology 1995; 25:356–359.

Chigot V, De Lonlay P, Nassogne MC et al. Pancreatic arterial calcium stimulation in the diagnosis and localization of persistant hyperinsulinemic hypoglycemia of infancy. Pediatric Radiology 2001; 31:155–158.

Choyke PL, Glenn GM, Walther MM et al. Von Hippel Lindau disease: genetic, clinical and imaging features. Radiology 1995; 146:629–642.

Daentl DL, Frias JL, Gilbert EF et al. The Johanson–Blizzard syndrome: case report and autopsy findings. American Journal of Medical Genetics 1979; 3:129–135.

Daneman A, Gaskin K, Martin DJ et al. Pancreatic changes in cystic fibrosis: CT and sonographic appearances. American Journal of Roentgenology 1983; 141;653–655.

De Lonlay-Debeney P, Poggi-Travert F, Fournet J-C et al. Clinical features of 52 neonates with hyperinsulinism. The New England Journal of Medicine 1999; 340:1169–1175.

Dubois J, Brunelle F, Touati G et al. Hyperinsulinism in children: diagnostic value of pancreatic venous sampling correlated with clinical, pathological and surgical outcome in 25 cases. Pediatric Radiology1995; 25:512–516.

Ferrozzi F, Bove D, Campodonico F et al. Cystic fibrosis: MR assessment of pancreatic damage. Radiology 1996; 198: 875–879.

Ginzberg H, Shin J, Morrison J et al. Shwachman syndrome: phenotypic manifestations of sibling set and isolated cases in a large patient cohort are similar. Journal of Pediatrics 1999; 135:81–88.

Hernandez-Schulman M, Teele R, Perez-Atayde A et al. Pancreatic cystosis in cystic fibrosis. Radiology 1986; 158: 629–631.

Johanson A, Blizzard R. A syndrome of congenital aplasia of the alae nasi, deafness, hyothyroidism, dwarfism, absent permanent teeth, and malabsorption. Journal of Pediatrics 1971; 79:982–987.

Jones NL, Hofley PM, Durie PR. Pathophysiology of pancreatic defect in Johanson–Blizzard syndrome: a disorder of acinar development. Journal of Pediatrics 1994; 125:406–408.

Lang S. Glucose intolerance in cystic fibrosis patients. Paediatric Respiratory Review 2001; 2:253–259.

Lerner A, Branski D, Lebenthal E. Pancreatic disease in children. Pediatric Clinics of North America 1996; 43:125–156.

Mack DR, Forstner GG, Wilschanski M et al. Shwachman syndrome: exocrine pancreatic dysfunction and variably phenotypic expression. Gastroenterology 1996; 111:1593–1602.

Tham RT, Heyerman HG, Falke TH et al. Cystic fibrosis: MR imaging of the pancreas. Radiology 1991; 179:183–186.

Willi U, Reddish JM, Teele R. Cystic fibrosis: its characteristic appearance on abdominal sonography. American Journal of Roentgenology 1980; 134:1005–1010.

Woods B. Cystic fibrosis: 1997. Radiology 1997; 204:1–10.

NEOPLASM

Pancreatic tumours are rare in childhood with large paediatric centres seeing one, maybe two, a year. The ductal adenocarcinoma, which comprises 90% of adult pancreatic malignancy, is virtually never seen in children. Similarly, cystic neoplasm of the pancreas (less than 5% of all pancreas neoplasia) are not paediatric conditions. The benign, serous cystic (microcystic) neoplasm occurs in middle-aged to elderly females. The mucinous cystic (macrocystic) neoplasm is also mostly seen in females but may present at a slightly earlier age. They have significant potential for progression to cystadenocarcinoma and require complete resection. This tumour has been reported in the late teenage years.

Initial imaging for pancreatic mass lesions is likely to be sonography. CT, utilizing multidetector technology and appropriate contrast enhancement, will provide better evaluation of tumour extent and possible spread. MRI is seeing increased utilization and the reported advantages in the adult literature are detection of small lesions that do not distort pancreas contour and in imaging of cystic neoplasms.

Malignant, epithelial neoplasms of childhood are pancreatoblastoma and solid and papillary epithelial neoplasm. Islet cell tumours are very rare unless associated with the multiple endocrine neoplasia type 1 syndrome. They include insulinoma, gastrinoma, glucagonoma, VIPoma, APUDoma and ACTHoma. Primary non-epithelial tumours localized to the pancreas are very rare and include lymphoma, primitive neuroectodermal tumour and rhabdomyosarcoma. Metastatic non-epithelial tumour such as widespread lymphoma (Figure 11.12.17) or direct extension of neuroblastoma is more common. Ewing's sarcoma and rhabdomyosarcoma metastases are described (Figure 11.12.18). Other mesenchymal tumours such as lymphangioma, teratoma, schwannoma, fibroma and haemangioma are exceedingly rare.

PANCREATOBLASTOMA

Histologically, this tumour resembles early fetal pancreatic acini. They present between 1 and 8 years of age but have been reported in neonates and adults. Incidence is higher in males and patients of Asian origin. Pancreatoblastoma is associated with the Beckwith–Wiedemann syndrome. They often present as a palpable abdominal mass but may have pain, early satiation, vomiting and occasionally obstructive jaundice. Elevated alpha-fetoprotein is found in 50% of patients, and associated Cushing syndrome and inappropriate ADH secretion have been reported.

These tumours are pathologically soft and gelatinous. They are slow-growing and usually present as large, well-circumscribed lesions but they can be lobulated, ill defined and their origin may appear to be hepatic or retroperitoneal. The mass may be hetero-

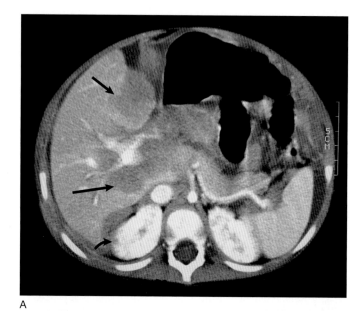

A

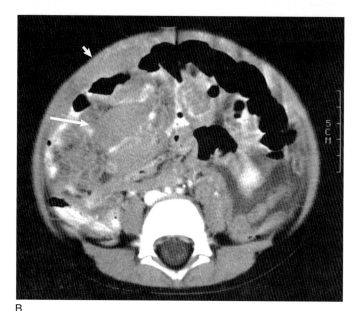

B

Figure 11.12.17 IV contrast enhanced CT in a 4-year-old male with widespread Burkitt's lymphoma. (A) Nodal mass lesions involve pancreatic head (large arrow); liver lesion (small arrow) and renal lesions (curved arrow) are present. (B) Bowel wall disease (arrow) and peritoneal disease (arrowhead) are shown.

geneous due to septae, necrosis, haemorrhage and calcification. Metastases to the liver are most common (30–35%) with omental, duodenal and peritoneal extension well described. The tumour may encase mesenteric vessels and inferior vena cava. Lung metastases can occur and there is a case report of bone metastatic disease. Complete surgical resection offers good prognosis. Metastatic and unresectable disease treated by chemotherapy and radiotherapy have a poor outcome.

There are no pathognomonic imaging features. Sonography will identify a soft tissue mass. CT will delineate a mass largely hypo-

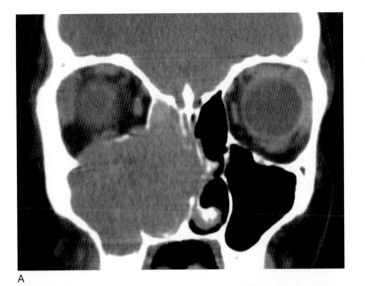

A

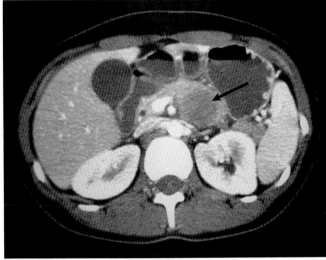

B

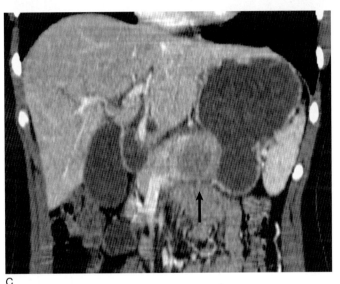

C

Figure 11.12.18 A 15-year-old female with alveolar rhabdomyosarcoma. (A) Coronal CT shows right maxillary antrum mass. (B,C) IV contrast enhanced CT; axial (B) and coronal reconstruction (C) show a pancreatic mass (arrow) confirmed at laparoscopy to be alveolar rhabdomyosarcoma.

dense to liver but heterogeneous. Variable IV contrast enhancement, particularly of septa, may occur. Areas of necrosis with nonenhancing low density may be prominent and 30% will show calcification. MRI findings show similar heterogeneity with the mass usually T1 hypointense and variable IV gadolinium enhancement. T2 hyperintense and hypointense signal is reported. Haemorrhage and necrosis increases heterogeneity especially on gradient echo sequences (Figure 11.12.19).

If the tumour is confidently localized to the pancreas a differential diagnosis includes solid and cystic papillary tumour, nonfunctioning islet cell tumours, lymphoma, primitive neuro ectodermal tumour and sarcoma. When the pancreas origin of the mass is uncertain, neuroblastoma, hepatoblastoma, lymphoma and nephroblastoma enter the differential diagnosis. On occasion, pancreatitis and pseudocyst formation may be misdiagnosed.

SOLID AND PAPILLARY EPITHELIAL NEOPLASM

This rare tumour is of low grade malignancy and occurs mostly in young adult females (mean age 25 years). They present with abdominal pain or a palpable mass. Fifteen per cent will have evidence of local infiltration or liver metastatic disease. Surgical resection is curative.

Pathologically, the tumours are usually large (3–17 cm), with a well-developed fibrous capsule. The solid components are well-vascularized sheets of epithelial cells and papillary regions with a fibrovascular core lined by epithelial cells. Cystic degeneration occurs where cell growth in the papillary regions exceeds vascularization. It is invariably a haemorrhagic degeneration.

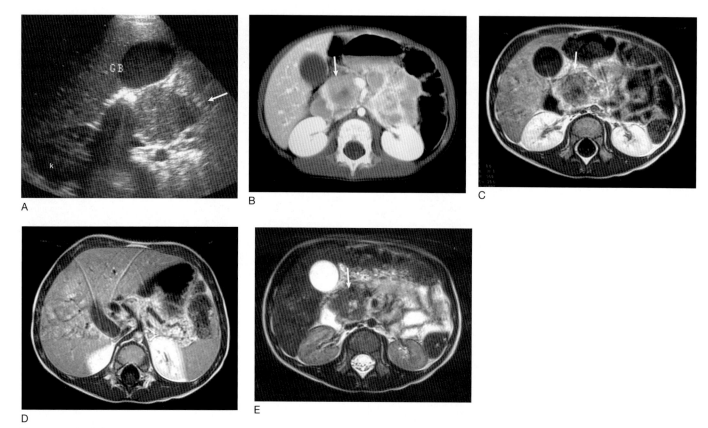

Figure 11.12.19 Pancreatoblastoma in a 4-year-old male. (A) Sonography shows solid mass lesion in the region of the pancreatic head (arrow). (B) IV contrast enhanced CT shows a poorly enhancing pancreatic head mass (arrow) with a central non-enhancing low density. (C) Axial, T1-weighted, spin echo MRI following IV gadolinium shows poor enhancement (arrow) and a hypointense, non-enhancing central area. (D) Axial, T1-weighted, spin echo MRI following IV gadolinium demonstrates normal enhancement of the pancreas body and tail, in excess of the liver. There is dilatation of the main pancreatic duct (arrow). (E) Axial, T2-weighted, spin echo MRI shows the mass to be hypointense (arrow) with a focus of hyperintense signal corresponding to the T1 hypointense, non-enhancing focus. An area of necrosis is suspected.

Imaging identifies the well-circumscribed pancreatic mass, which is heterogeneous, reflecting the pathology. Sonography shows hyperechoic solid and haemorrhagic components. Cystic spaces are hypoechoic with through transmission and fluid–fluid levels may be identified. CT images delineate soft tissue components that enhance with IV contrast. Cystic spaces are hypodense and do not enhance. Recent haemorrhage will affect cyst density and fluid–fluid levels may be discerned. Calcification is seen in 30% and is usually punctate and peripheral. MRI findings reflect the heterogeneous nature of the tumour with blood products causing increased T1 signal intensity. Blood products and cyst fluid can be T2 hyperintense. The fibrous tumour capsule is T2 hypointense and this capsule and the solid components of the tumour will enhance with IV gadolinium (Figure 11.12.20).

The imaging findings are not diagnostic and the main differential diagnosis includes a non-functioning islet cell tumour and pancreatoblastoma, although pancreatoblastoma would tend to occur in younger patients. A pancreatic pseudocyst with some peripheral calcification may mimic this tumour.

ISLET CELL TUMOURS

Functioning islet cell tumours present clinically with endocrine symptoms; symptomatic hypoglycaemia in insulinoma and Zollinger–Ellison syndrome in gastrinoma. These tumours are small and the role of imaging is to locate the tumour. Non-functioning islet cell tumours (15%) present as larger mass lesions with cystic degeneration, haemorrhage and calcification. Insulinomas are the most common and 90% are benign. The other endocrine tumours have a 50% likelihood of malignancy. Metastatic disease is usually hepatic. These tumours are exceedingly rare in childhood and are only likely to be encountered in type 1 multiple endocrine neoplasia syndrome, which is an association of parathyroid adenoma, pituitary adenoma and adrenal cortical tumours.

Imaging becomes problematic with identification of small lesions. Ultrasound may have a role in intraoperative location of non-palpable tumours. Contrast enhanced CT will identify small enhancing mass lesions; hepatic arterial phase, thin slice width, dedicated pancreatic studies are required. MRI demonstrates T1 hypointense lesions, which enhance with IV gadolinium; fat-suppressed imaging is recommended.

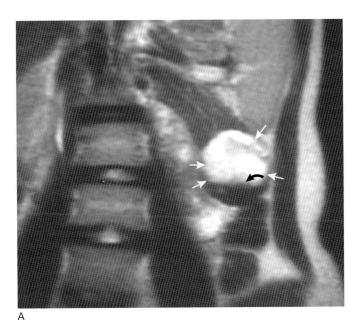

A

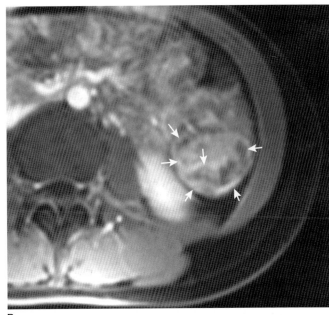

B

Figure 11.12.20 MR imaging of a solid and papillary epithelial neoplasm in a 15-year-old female. (A) Coronal, T2 effect, spoiled gradient echo image showing a mass arising from the pancreas tail. Hypointense capsule tissue (small arrows) and fluid–fluid level suggesting altered blood products (curved arrow) are demonstrated. (B) Axial, fat-saturated, T1 effect, spoiled gradient echo image following IV gadolinium enhancement. Variable enhancement of tumour capsule and solid internal septa (small arrows) is shown. (Courtesy of Dr P. Strouse, C. S. Mott Children's Hospital, University of Michigan Health System.)

FURTHER READING

Buetow PC, Buck JL, Pantongrag-Brown L et al. Solid and papillary epithelial neoplasm of the pancreas: imaging-pathologic correlation in 56 cases. Radiology 1996; 199.707–711.

Buetow PC, Miller DL, Parrino TV et al. Islet cell tumours of the pancreas: clinical, radiologic, and pathologic correlation in diagnosis and localization. Radiographics 1997; 17:453–472.

Ferrozzi F, Zuccoli G, Bova D et al. Mesenchymal tumours of the pancreas: CT findings. Journal of Computer Assisted Tomography 2000; 24:622–627.

Jaksic T, Yaman M, Thorner P et al. A 20 year review of pancreatic tumours. Journal of Pediatric Surgery 1992; 27:1315–1317.

Ky A, Shilyansky J, Gerstle J et al. Experience with papillary and solid epithelial neoplasms of the pancreas in children. Journal of Pediatric Surgery 1998; 33:42–44.

Mergo PJ, Helmberger TK, Buetow PC et al. Pancreatic neoplasms: MR imaging and pathologic correlation. Radiographics 1997; 17:281–301.

Montemarano H, Lonergan GL, Bulas DI et al. Pancreatoblastoma: imaging findings in 10 patients and review of the literature. Radiology 2000; 214:476–482.

Roebuck D, Yuen MK, Wong YC et al. Imaging features of pancreatoblastoma. Pediatric Radiology 2001; 31:501–506.

Vaughn DD, Jabra AA, Fishman EK. Pancreatic disease in children and young adults: evaluation with CT. Radiographics 1998; 18:1171–1187.

SECTION | 12

NEURORADIOLOGY

Congenital Malformations of the Spine and Spinal Cord

Paolo Tortori-Donati, Andrea Rossi

INTRODUCTION

Congenital malformations of the spine and spinal cord are also called spinal dysraphisms. These conditions are usually diagnosed at birth or in early infancy but may sometimes be discovered in older children or adults. Magnetic resonance imaging (MRI) offers a basis for classification and is very helpful for both diagnosis and treatment planning. Classification of spinal dysraphisms is based on a correlation of clinical, neuroradiological and embryological data. This chapter offers basic concepts about normal and abnormal spinal cord development, describes the main malformations and approaches diagnostic and treatment decision-making from a practical perspective.

FURTHER READING

Tortori-Donati P, Rossi A, Cama A. Spinal dysraphism: a review of neuroradiological features with embryological correlations and proposal for a new classification. Neuroradiology 2000; 42:471–491.

EMBRYOLOGY

The basic embryological stages during which the spinal cord is formed are gastrulation (weeks 2–3), primary neurulation (weeks 3–4) and secondary neurulation (weeks 5–6). Spinal dysraphisms originate from abnormalities occurring during one of these periods.

GASTRULATION

At the time of implantation in the uterine wall, changes occurring within the blastocyst result in the formation of the embryonic disc. The embryonic disc is initially bilaminar, being composed of the epiblast (future ectoderm) and hypoblast (future endoderm). Gastrulation involves formation of the intervening mesoderm, resulting in a trilaminar arrangement of the embryonic disc. On day 14 or 15, a stripe of thickened epiblast composed of totipotential cells,

the primitive streak, is formed along the midline of the dorsal surface of the embryo. The cranial extremity of the primitive streak shows a knob-like thickening called the Hensen's node. Formation of the mesoderm occurs by orderly migration of epiblastic cells through the Hensen's node to the epiblast–hypoblast interface. Of particular interest is cell migration along the midline, which eventually results in the formation of the notochord, the foundation of the axial skeleton and the inductor of the neural ectoderm.

PRIMARY NEURULATION

Interaction between the notochord and the overlying ectoderm results in formation of the neuroectoderm, either by direct induction or by preservation of an initial neuroectodermal default state. The neural ectoderm initially is flat, forming a neural plate. The neural plate bends and folds progressively along the midline, until eventually its margins merge with each other to form the neural tube. Neural tube closure is immediately followed by disjunction of the neural ectoderm from the surface endoderm, which forms a continuous coverage that will become the skin and subcutaneous tissues. Migration of mesenchymal tissue between the neural and cutaneous ectoderm will form the posterior vertebral elements, muscles and ligaments. Neural tube closure is traditionally believed to proceed bidirectionally in a zipper-like fashion, starting from the future craniocervical junction. Closure of the two extremities of the neural tube is not simultaneous. The cranial end (rostral neuropore) closes at day 25, whereas the caudal end (caudal neuropore) closes at day 27 or 28, thereby terminating primary neurulation.

SECONDARY NEURULATION

This process begins after completion of primary neurulation and proceeds until gestational day 48. During secondary neurulation, an additional part of the neural tube is produced caudad to the posterior neuropore by the tail bud, a mass of cells deriving from the caudal portion of the primitive streak. The secondary neural tube is initially solid but subsequently becomes cavitated. The secondary neural tube eventually results in the tip of the conus medullaris and the filum terminale through the process of retrogressive differentiation, in which a combination of regression, degeneration and further differentiation occur. The conus medullaris contains the terminal ventricle, representing a remnant of the lumen of the secondary neural tube.

FURTHER READING

Catala M. Genetic control of caudal development. Clinical Genetics 2002; 61:89–96.

Naidich TP, Blaser SI, Delman BN et al. Embryology of the spine and spinal cord. Proceedings of the American Society of Neuroradiology Congress 2002:3–13.

Nievelstein RAJ, Hartwig NG, Vermeji-Keers C, Valk J. Embryonic development of the mammalian caudal neural tube. Teratology 1993; 48:21–31.

Tortori-Donati P, Rossi A, Biancheri R, Cama A. Magnetic resonance imaging of spinal dysraphism. Topics in Magnetic Resonance Imaging 2001; 12:375–409.

Tortori-Donati P, Rossi A, Cama A. Spinal dysraphism: a review of neuroradiological features with embryological correlations and proposal for a new classification. Neuroradiology 2000; 42:471–491.

TERMINOLOGY

OPEN AND CLOSED SPINAL DYSRAPHISMS

Congenital malformations of the spinal cord are categorized into open spinal dysraphisms (OSDs) and closed spinal dysraphisms (CSDs) (Figure 12.1.1). In OSDs, the nervous tissue is exposed to the environment through a congenital skin defect. Conversely, CSDs are covered by skin, although cutaneous birthmarks are present in up to 50% of cases. Therefore, use of the term 'occult spinal dysraphisms' is not encouraged, as it suggests complete absence of any external marker of the underlying abnormality.

SPINA BIFIDA

The term 'spina bifida' is commonly used as a synonym of spinal dysraphism, although it properly refers to defective fusion of posterior spinal bony elements, i.e. schisis of the posterior neural arch. The terms 'spina bifida aperta' or 'cystica' and 'spina bifida occulta' were once used to refer to OSD and CSD, respectively, but have been progressively discarded.

PLACODE

The placode is a segment of flattened, non-neurulated embryonic neural tissue. A placode is found in all OSDs as well as in several varieties of CSDs. It is exposed to air in the former and covered by the integuments in the latter. Placodes may further be categorized into terminal and segmental depending on location. A terminal placode lies at the caudal end of the spinal cord and may in turn be either apical or parietal, depending on whether the defect involves the apex or a longer segment of the cord. A segmental placode lies at an intermediate level along the spinal cord; caudad to the abnormality the cord regains normal morphology and structure.

TETHERED CORD SYNDROME

The tethered cord syndrome (TCS) is not a malformation. Instead, it is a clinical syndrome that may ensue as a complication of myelomeningocele repair or as the clinical presentation of several dysraphic conditions including spinal lipomas, tight filum terminale, diastematomyelia and caudal agenesis. TCS involves traction on a low-lying conus medullaris with progressive neurological deterioration due to metabolic derangement. The clinical picture includes motor and sensory dysfunction, muscle atrophy, decreased or hyperactive reflexes, urinary incontinence, spastic gait and orthopaedic deformities such as scoliosis or foot and hip deformities.

FURTHER READING

Drolet B. Birthmarks to worry about. Cutaneous markers of dysraphism. Dermatologic Clinics 1998; 16:447–453.

French BN. The embryology of spinal dysraphism. Clinical Neurosurgery 1983; 30:295–340.

Sattar MT, Bannister CM, Turnbull IW. Occult spinal dysraphism – The common combination of lesions and the clinical manifestations in 50 patients. European Journal of Pediatric Surgery 1996; 6 (Suppl I):10–14.

Tortori-Donati P, Rossi A, Biancheri R, Cama A. Magnetic resonance imaging of spinal dysraphism. Topics Magnetic Resonance Imaging 2001; 12:375–409.

Tortori-Donati P, Rossi A, Cama A. Spinal dysraphism: a review of neuroradiological features with embryological correlations and proposal for a new classification. Neuroradiology 2000; 42:471–491.

Warder DE. Tethered cord syndrome and occult spinal dysraphism. Neurosurgery Focus (serial online). January 2001; 10:Article 1. Available at http://www.neurosurgery.org/focus/jan01/10-1-1.

Warder DE, Oakes WJ. Tethered cord syndrome and the conus in a normal position. Neurosurgery 1993; 33:374–378.

Warder DE, Oakes WJ. Tethered cord syndrome: the low-lying and normally positioned conus. Neurosurgery 1994; 34:597–600.

CLASSIFICATION

The initial step in a logical approach to classification of spinal dysraphisms (Table 12.1.1) is based on clinical examination and basically involves a categorization into OSDs and CSDs. In the individual case, such categorization is easily performed by simply inspecting the child's back.

OSDs do not usually cause major diagnostic concern. In fact, myelomeningocele accounts for the vast majority of cases. Myelomeningoceles are distinguished from the far less common myeloceles because the neural placode protrudes above the cutaneous surface due to expansion of the underlying subarachnoid

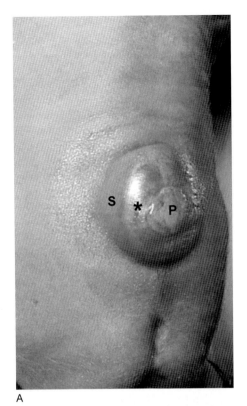

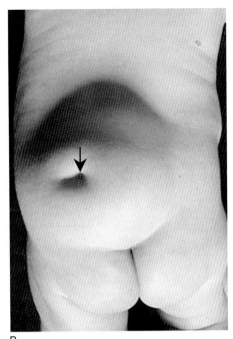

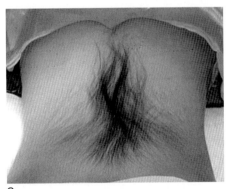

Figure 12.1.1 Clinical features of open and closed spinal dysraphisms. (A) Open spinal dysraphism: myelomeningocele. Low back of 1-hour-old newborn prior to surgery. The placode (P) is directly exposed to the environment and is surrounded by partially epithelized skin (membrano-epithelial zone) (asterisk). More laterally, intact skin (S) is elevated by underlying expanded subarachnoid spaces. (B) Closed spinal dysraphism with subcutaneous mass. Low back of 1-year-old patient with lipomyelocele. A large subcutaneous mass lies above the intergluteal crease. There is a continuous skin coverage to the abnormality. Notice associated dermal sinus (arrow). (C) Closed spinal dysraphism without subcutaneous mass. Back of 3-year-old patient with diastematomyelia. There is marked hirsutism, i.e. a hairy tuft along the midline of the back . Although hairy tufts may belie several varieties of closed spinal dysraphism, diastematomyelia should be suspected when they lie at a relatively cranial level along the child's back.

spaces, whereas in myelocele the placode is flush with the cutaneous surface. More important diagnostic issues include the assessment of the Chiari II malformation, the associated hydrocephalus and the complications of surgical repair.

CSDs are much more heterogeneous than OSDs. A crucial diagnostic element is the presence of a subcutaneous mass on the patient's back, usually at a lumbosacral level. Only four malformations will present with a subcutaneous mass in such a location, i.e. lipomyelocele, lipomyelomeningocele, meningocele and terminal myelocystocele. Lipomyelocele and lipomyelomeningocele are far more common; the mass is represented by a subcutaneous lipoma in both cases. In lipomyeloceles, the lipoma enters the spinal canal through a bony spina bifida and attaches to the neural placode, i.e. the placode–lipoma interface lies within the spinal canal. Conversely, in lipomyelomeningoceles, expansion of the subarachnoid spaces pushes the neural placode out of the spinal canal, i.e. the placode–lipoma interface lies outside the spinal canal. Therefore, assessment of the location of the placode–lipoma interface permits a confident differential diagnosis.

Several birthmarks, other than subcutaneous masses, may indicate underlying dysraphism. Among these, hirsutism is significantly associated with CSDs. When a hairy tuft (usually in the form of a faun tail naevus) lies relatively cephalad along the child's back, diastematomyelia is very likely. Dorsal dimples or ostia indicate a dermal sinus. All dermal sinuses located above the intergluteal crease should be presumed to communicate with the subarachnoid space until proven otherwise. Conversely, skin pits located within the intergluteal crease are related to sacrococcygeal cysts or fistulas and usually do not require further diagnostic investigation. Caudal agenesis may be suggested by a rudimentary tail, lower limb abnormalities or anorectal malformations. Imperforate anus is associated with surgically correctable intradural pathology in at least 10% of patients. A palpable bony gibbus with congenital kyphosis in a paraplegic or paraparetic infant is suggestive of segmental spinal dysgenesis. Although these clinical signs are very important in suggesting the diagnosis and thus restrict the diagnostic investigations, the category of CSD without a subcutaneous mass presents the most significant challenge to the neuroradiologist.

IMAGING OF SPINAL DYSRAPHISM

Initial imaging of spinal dysraphism requires sagittal T1- and T2-weighted sequences of the whole cord with axial T1- and T2-weighted sequences across the area of abnormality. Axial slices are also required across the distal cord to confirm the level of the conus. The brain should also be imaged to identify any congenital malformation, in particular a Chiari malformation, or hydrocephalus.

The normal conus lies normally between the lower border of T12 and upper border of L2. Progression from cord to conus is identified by the 'spider's web' appearance of the filum as compared with the solid normal appearance of the cord.

FURTHER READING

Herman JM, McLone DG, Storrs BB, Dauser RC. Analysis of 153 patients with myelomeningocele or spinal lipoma reoperated upon for a tethered cord. Pediatric Neurosurgery 1993; 19:243–249.

McLone DG, Dias MS. Complications of myelomeningocele closure. Pediatric Neurosurgery 1991–92; 17:267–273.

Scott RM, Wolpert SM, Bartoshesky LF, Zimbler S, Klauber GT. Dermoid tumors occurring at the site of previous myelomeningocele repair. Journal of Neurosurgery 1986; 65:779–783.

Tortori-Donati P, Rossi A, Biancheri R, Cama A. Magnetic resonance imaging of spinal dysraphism. Topics in Magnetic Resonance Imaging 2001; 12:375–409.

Tortori-Donati P, Rossi A, Cama A. Spinal dysraphism: a review of neuroradiological features with embryological correlations and proposal for a new classification. Neuroradiology 2000; 42:471–491.

OPEN SPINAL DYSRAPHISMS

MYELOMENINGOCELE AND MYELOCELE

Myelomeningoceles and myeloceles are characterized by exposure of the placode through a midline defect in the back. In myelomeningoceles, expansion of the underlying subarachnoid space results in elevation of the placode above the cutaneous surface, whereas in myeloceles the placode is flush with the cutaneous surface. Ulceration of the placode and infection cause increased mortality in untreated newborns. Therefore, these patients are operated on soon after birth. The subsequent clinical picture includes sensorimotor deficits of the lower extremities, bowel and bladder incontinence, hindbrain dysfunction, and intellectual and psychological disturbances.

Both myelomeningoceles and myeloceles originate from defective closure of the primary neural tube, with persistence of a segment of non-neurulated placode. Most are located at the lumbosacral level and the placode is terminal. Because neurulation does not occur, the cutaneous ectoderm does not detach from the neural ectoderm and remains in a lateral position. This results in a midline skin defect. Therefore, the external surface of the placode is directly visible on inspection (Figure 12.1.1). Because the mesenchyme does not migrate behind the neural tube, bones, cartilage, muscles and ligaments develop anterolaterally to the neural tissue, and therefore will appear everted. The ventral surface of the placode is in fact the external surface of the spinal cord. The nerve roots originate from this surface and course obliquely through the subarachnoid space to reach their corresponding neural foramina.

Owing to the need for emergency surgery, preoperative MRI studies are not always performed. Nevertheless, we suggest that MRI should be performed whenever possible, in order to obtain: (1) anatomical characterization of the various components of the malformation, i.e. the relationships between the placode and nerve roots; (2) presurgical evaluation of the entity and morphology of the malformation sequence (hydromyelia, Chiari II malformation and associated hydrocephalus); and (3) identification of rare cases with associated cord splitting (hemimyelomeningoceles and hemimyeloceles). MRI of untreated OSDs shows dehiscence of the subcutaneous fat at the level of the spina bifida and a low position of the spinal cord that forms the dorsal wall of the defect. In myelomeningoceles (Figure 12.1.2), the subarachnoid spaces are widely dilated and are crossed by nerve roots arising from the

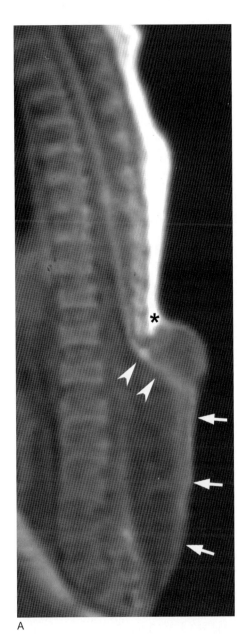

A

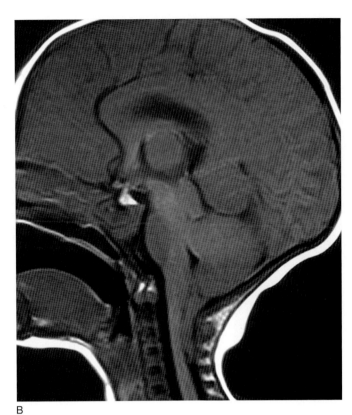

B

Figure 12.1.2 Myelomeningocele, 10-h-old male newborn. Same case as in Figure 12.1.1A. (A) Sagittal T1-weighted image of the lumbosacral spine shows the spinal cord (arrowheads) crosses the meningeal outpouching and ends with an exposed terminal parietal placode (arrows). Notice dehiscent subcutaneous fat (asterisk). (B) Sagittal T1-weighted image of the brain shows Chiari II malformation.

ventral surface of the placode, which is elevated above the skin surface; in myeloceles (Figure 12.1.3), the placode is flush with the skin.

Hydrocephalus may be present at birth but, if not, it usually appears within 2–3 days after surgery. Evaluation of ventricular size is the major reason for postoperative neuroimaging. Subsequent deterioration of previously stable neurological function may be caused by retethering of the spinal cord, dysontogenetic masses and hydromyelia. Retethering by scar is difficult to demonstrate on MRI and is usually an exclusion diagnosis. Dysontogenetic masses may result from inadvertent inclusion of epidermal cells during surgery and are usually located in close vicinity to the surgical site. These masses are usually slightly hyperintense to CSF both in T1- and T2-weighted images, and may enhance with gadolinium administration in case of superimposed infection. Hydromyelia

occurs in as many as 80% of operated patients, and may cause scoliosis if left untreated.

HEMIMYELO(MENINGO)CELE

Myelomeningoceles and myeloceles are associated with diastematomyelia in 8–45% of cases. However, when only one hemicord fails to neurulate the malformation is called hemimyelocele. When there is associated meningeal expansion, the malformation is called hemimyelomeningocele. Clinically, neurological impairment is similar to that seen in patients with diastematomyelia but is markedly asymmetrical. A hairy tuft located along one side of the exposed placode may be strongly suggestive of these rare

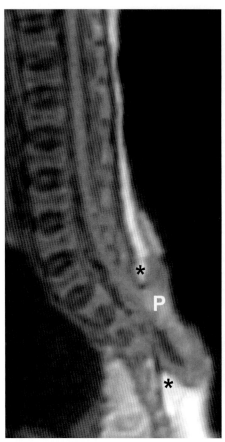

Figure 12.1.3 Myelocele, 12-h-old newborn. Sagittal T1-weighted images shows exposed, slightly funnel-shaped placode (P) lying flush with the skin surface. There is dehiscence of subcutaneous fat (asterisks). The lack of expansion of subarachnoid spaces is the only difference from the much more common myelomeningocele.

malformations. Embryologically, hemimyelo(meningo)celes are related to abnormal gastrulation (see section on diastematomyelia), with superimposed failure of primary neurulation of one hemicord.

CHIARI II MALFORMATION

There is a 100% association between OSDs and the Chiari II malformation, a congenital hindbrain anomaly characterized by a small posterior fossa with caudal displacement of the vermis, brainstem and fourth ventricle (Figure 12.1.2). McLone and Knepper proposed a theory to explain this consistent association. Normally, the medial walls of the primitive central canal of the neural tube ('neurocele') appose and occlude the neurocele transiently during primary neurulation. Failure to occlude the neurocele allows free downward CSF flow. Therefore, CSF leaks freely through the spinal defect into the amniotic sac because the neural tube remains non-neurulated. This results in chronic CSF hypotension within the developing neural tube. Consequently, the rhombencephalic vesicle fails to expand, causing lack of induction of the perineural mesenchyme of the posterior cranial fossa. Both the cerebellum and brainstem are eventually forced to develop

within a smaller than normal posterior fossa, and consequently herniate through both the tentorial groove and the foramen magnum in search of vital space.

FURTHER READING

Breningstall GN, Marker SM, Tubman DE. Hydrosyringomyelia and diastematomyelia detected by MRI in myelomeningocele. Pediatric Neurology 1992; 8:267–271.

Cama A, Tortori-Donati P, Piatelli GL, Fondelli MP, Andreussi L. Chiari complex in children. Neuroradiological diagnosis, neurosurgical treatment and proposal of a new classification (312 cases). European Journal of Pediatric Surgery 1995; 5(Suppl 1):35–38.

Herman JM, McLone DG, Storrs BB, Dauser RC. Analysis of 153 patients with myelomeningocele or spinal lipoma reoperated upon for a tethered cord. Pediatric Neurosurgery 1993; 19:243–249.

McLone DG, Dias MS. Complications of myelomeningocele closure. Pediatric Neurosurgery 1991–92; 17:267–273.

McLone DG, Knepper PA. The cause of Chiari II malformation: a unified theory. Pediatric Neuroscience 1989; 15:1–12.

Naidich TP, Blaser SI, Delman BN et al. Embryology of the spine and spinal cord. Proceedings of the American Society of Neuroradiology Congress 2002:3–13.

Naidich TP, McLone DG, Fulling F. The Chiari II malformation. Part IV. The hindbrain deformity. Neuroradiology 1983; 25:179–197.

Pang D. Split cord malformation. Part II: clinical syndrome. Neurosurgery 1992; 31:481–500.

Pang D, Dias MS, Ahab-Barmada M. Split cord malformation. Part I: a unified theory of embryogenesis for double spinal cord malformations. Neurosurgery 1992; 31:451–480.

Scott RM, Wolpert SM, Bartoshesky LF, Zimbler S, Klauber GT. Dermoid tumors occurring at the site of previous myelomeningocele repair. Journal of Neurosurgery 1986; 65:779–783.

Tortori-Donati P, Cama A, Fondelli MP, Rossi A. Le malformazioni di Chiari. In: Tortori-Donati P, Taccone A, Longo M, eds. Malformazioni cranio-encefaliche. Neuroradiologia. Turin: Minerva Medica; 1996:209–236.

Tortori-Donati P, Rossi A, Cama A. Spinal dysraphism: a review of neuroradiological features with embryological correlations and proposal for a new classification. Neuroradiology 2000; 42:471–491.

CLOSED SPINAL DYSRAPHISMS

CSDs WITH SUBCUTANEOUS MASS

LIPOMAS WITH DURAL DEFECT: LIPOMYELOCELE AND LIPOMYELOMENINGOCELE

Lipomyeloceles and lipomyelomeningoceles are characterized by a subcutaneous fatty mass located above the intergluteal crease (Figure 12.1.1) and usually extending asymmetrically into one buttock. Because the mass is clinically evident at birth, the diagnosis is usually made before neurological deterioration ensues. Histologically, the mass is composed of clusters of mature adipocytes separated by collagenous bands, usually associated with other tissues such as striated muscle, cartilage, bone, nerve cells, ependyma and aberrant neuroglial tissue. Although congenital intraspinal lipomas are anatomically stable, they may grow as part of the normal increase of adipose tissue throughout childhood, other than in particular conditions such as obesity or pregnancy.

Embryologically, spinal lipomas result from defective primary neurulation, involving focal premature disjunction of the cutaneous ectoderm from the neuroectoderm. As a consequence, mesenchyme freely enters the interior of the neural tube and contacts the ependymal lining, which induces it to develop into adipose tissue. Some authors have suggested abnormalities of the dorsal mesoderm that could either be primitive or secondary to defective induction from the neural tube.

In lipomyelocele (synonym: lipomyeloschisis) (Figure 12.1.4), the placode–lipoma interface lies within the spinal canal and may extend over several vertebral levels. There is continuity of the intraspinal lipoma with the subcutaneous fat through a posterior bony spina bifida. The calibre of the spinal canal may be increased depending on the size of the lipoma but the size of the subarachnoid space ventral to the cord is consistently normal.

In lipomyelomeningoceles, the placode–lipoma interface lies outside the anatomical boundaries of the spinal canal because of expansion of the subarachnoid spaces, resulting in a posterior meningocele. The archetypal condition in which the placode–lipoma interface lies exactly along the midline is not the rule but, rather, an exception (Figure 12.1.5). In most instances, the placode is stretched and rotated eccentrically towards the lipoma to one side, whereas the meninges herniate to the opposite side (Figure 12.1.6). Unlike with lipomyeloceles, the spinal canal is dilated due to expansion of ventral subarachnoid spaces.

FURTHER READING

Catala M. Embryogenesis. Why do we need a new explanation for the emergence of spina bifida with lipoma? Childs Nervous System 1997; 13:336–340.

Knittle JL, Timmers K, Ginsberg-Fellner F, Brown RE, Katz DP. The growth of adipose tissue in children and adolescents. Cross-sectional and longitudinal studies of adipose cell number and size. Journal of Clinical Investigation 1979; 63:246–269.

Naidich TP, Blaser SI, Delman BN et al. Embryology of the spine and spinal cord. Proceedings of the American Society of Neuroradiology Congress 2002:3–13.

Naidich TP, McLone DG, Mutleur S. A new understanding of dorsal dysraphism with lipoma (lipomyeloschisis): radiological evaluation and surgical correction. American Journal of Neuroradiology 1983; 4:103–116.

Pierre-Kahn A, Zerah M, Renier D et al. Congenital lumbosacral lipomas. Childs Nervous System 1997; 13:298–334.

Tortori-Donati P, Rossi A, Biancheri R, Cama A. Magnetic resonance imaging of spinal dysraphism. Topics in Magnetic Resonance Imaging 2001; 12:375–409.

MENINGOCELE

Posterior meningoceles are herniations of CSF-filled sacs lined by dura and arachnoid through a posterior bony spina bifida (Figure 12.1.7). Most are lumbar or sacral in location but cervicothoracic

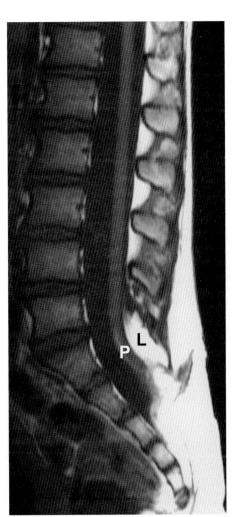

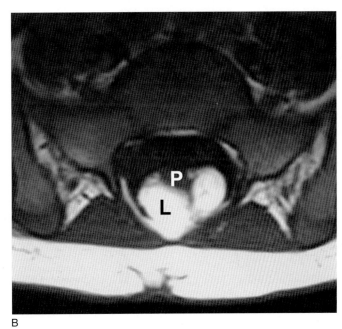

Figure 12.1.4 Lipomyelocele, 6-year-old girl. (A) Sagittal T1-weighted image shows large subcutaneous lipoma with fatty tissue creeping through a wide posterior bony spina bifida into the spinal canal (L) to connect with the placode (P). The size of the subcutaneous lipoma may not seem huge; however, consider that the mass is flattened as the child lies supine. (B) Axial T1-weighted image demonstrates the placode (P)–lipoma (L) interface into the spinal canal.

A

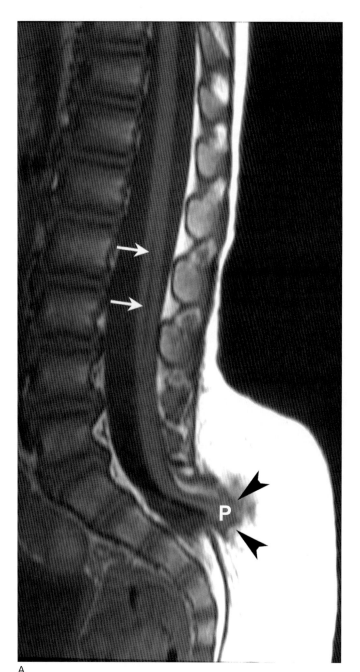

A

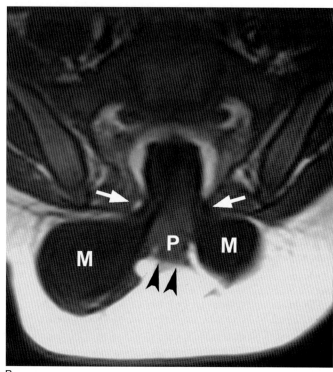

B

Figure 12.1.5 Lipomyelomeningocele, 1-year-old boy. (A) Sagittal T1-weighted image shows large subcutaneous lipoma. The spinal cord exits the spinal canal through a posterior sacral spina bifida and ends in a terminal apical placode (P) that connects to the inner surface of the lipoma (black arrowheads). Notice concurrent hydromyelia (white arrows). (B) Axial T1-weighted image shows terminal apical placode. Expansion of the subarachnoid spaces causes the placode to bulge outside the anatomical boundaries of the spinal canal through a wide posterior spina bifida (white arrows). The meningocele (M) develops symmetrically to both sides of the placode (P). The placode–lipoma interface lies on the midline (black arrowheads).

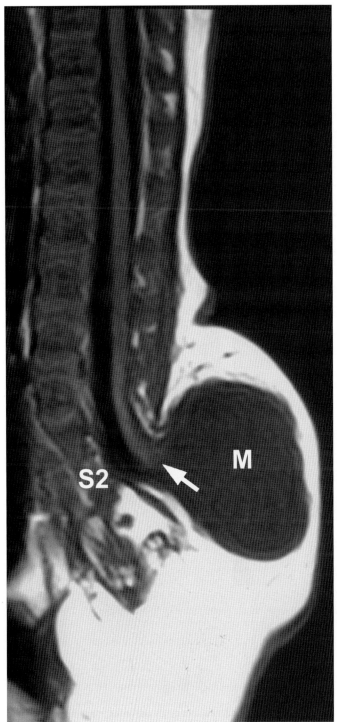

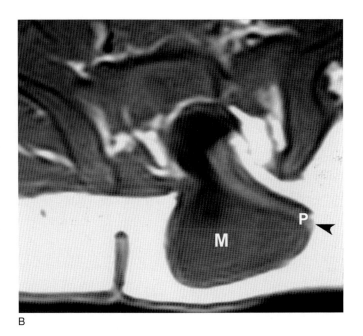

Figure 12.1.6 Lipomyelomeningocele, 40-day-old girl. (A) Sagittal T1-weighted image shows large meningocele (M) contained within a huge subcutaneous lipoma. The spinal cord (white arrow) is seen to approach the neck of the meningocele in this midsagittal view. Notice the last visible vertebra is S2, consistent with an associated picture of caudal agenesis. (B) Axial T1-weighted image shows the spinal cord projects out of the spinal canal and courses along the left side of the meningocele (M) to connect to the lipoma (arrowhead): therefore, the placode (P) is terminal apical and the off-midline placode–lipoma interface lies outside the anatomical boundaries of the spinal canal, consistent with a diagnosis of lipomyelomeningocele.

A

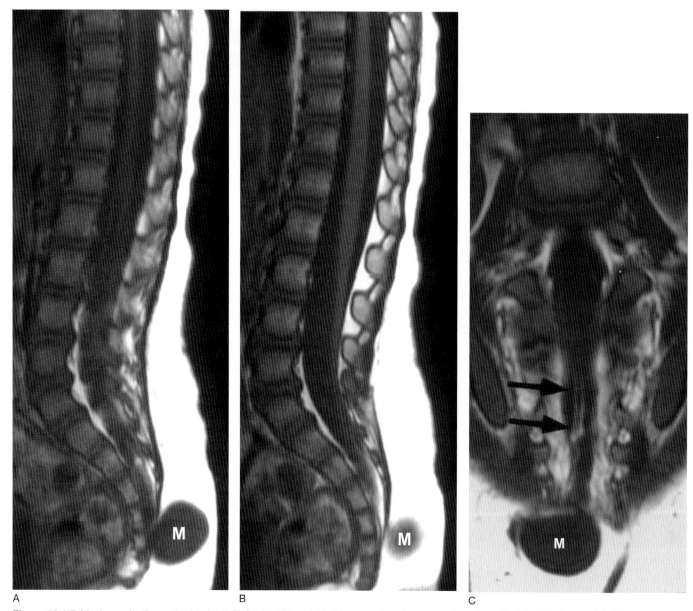

Figure 12.1.7 Meningocele, 7-month-old girl. (A,B) Sagittal T1-weighted images show large sacral cerebrospinal fluid-filled mass (M). The overlying skin is continuous. The conus medullaris is low. (C) T1-weighted images show associated lipomatous filum terminale (arrows).

meningoceles may be found. Their embryogenetic origin is unknown but they might result from ballooning of the meninges through a posterior spina bifida due to relentless CSF pulsations. By definition, the spinal cord is not contained within the meningocele, although it may be tethered to its neck. Conversely, redundant nerve roots or the filum terminale may course within the meningocele.

Anterior meningoceles are typically presacral and are found in patients with caudal agenesis. They are usually discovered in older children or adults complaining of low-back pain, urinary incontinence or constipation. They may be incidentally detected on ante-

rior views of the lumbar spine or an abdomen x-ray as a soft tissue mass lesion in association with displacement laterally of the distal sacrum, or a central defect within the distal sacrum. They may also be found as a transonic mass on ultrasound. The differential diagnosis in girls is an ovarian cyst.

FURTHER READING

Lee KS, Gower DJ, McWhorter JM, Albertson DA. The role of MR imaging in the diagnosis and treatment of anterior sacral meningocele. Report of 2 cases. Journal of Neurosurgery 1988; 69:628–631.

may represent a severe, disruptive variety of persistent terminal ventricle.

FURTHER READING

Byrd SE, Harvey C, Darling CF. MR of terminal myelocystoceles. European Journal of Radiology 1995; 20:215–220.

Carey JC, Greenbaum B, Hall BD. The OEIS complex (omphalocele, exstrophy, imperforate anus, spinal defects). Birth Defects Original Article Series 1978; 14:253–263.

McLone DG, Naidich TP. Terminal myelocystocele. Neurosurgery 1985; 16:36–43.

Peacock WJ, Murovic JA. Magnetic resonance imaging in myelocystoceles. Report of two cases. Journal of Neurosurgery 1989; 70:804–807.

Smith NM, Chambers HM, Furness ME, Haan EA. The OEIS complex omphalocele-exstrophy-imperforate anus-spinal defects: recurrence in sibs. Journal of Medical Genetics 1992; 29:730–732.

Tortori-Donati P, Rossi A, Biancheri R, Cama A. Magnetic resonance imaging of spinal dysraphism. Topics in Magnetic Resonance Imaging 2001; 12:375–409.

Tortori-Donati P, Rossi A, Cama A. Spinal dysraphism: a review of neuroradiological features with embryological correlations and proposal for a new classification. Neuroradiology 2000; 42:471–491.

Warder DE. Tethered cord syndrome and occult spinal dysraphism. Neurosurgery Focus (serial online). January 2001; 10:Article 1. Available at http://www.neurosurgery.org/focus/jan01/10-1-1.

CSDs WITHOUT SUBCUTANEOUS MASS

SIMPLE DYSRAPHIC STATES

This subset of abnormalities is embryologically heterogeneous, since it includes defects of both primary and secondary neurulation. However, they may be grouped clinically, as they represent the most common abnormalities found in relatively older children who usually do not have significant low-back cutaneous stigmata but complain of symptoms of TCS.

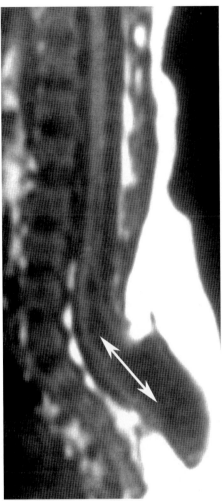

Figure 12.1.8 Terminal myelocystocele. Sagittal T1-weighted image shows large subcutaneous syringocele continuous with hydromyelia (arrow) through a wide spina bifida. (Courtesy of P. D. Barnes, Boston, MA, USA.)

TERMINAL MYELOCYSTOCELE

Terminal myelocystoceles basically involve herniation of a huge terminal syrinx ('syringocele') into a posterior meningocele through a wide posterior bony spina bifida. The terminal syrinx communicates with the ependymal canal (Figure 12.1.8), whereas the meningocele communicates with the subarachnoid space. The syringocele and meningocele usually do not communicate with each other. Terminal myelocystoceles are mainly found in patients with the OEIS association (omphalocele, exstrophy of the cloaca, imperforate anus and spinal anomalies). Affected patients typically have no bowel or bladder control and poor lower extremity function.

Embryologically, a terminal myelocystocele could result from inability of CSF to exit from the neural tube, causing the terminal ventricle to balloon into a cyst that disrupts the overlying mesenchyme. Therefore, the terminal myelocystocele

INTRADURAL AND INTRAMEDULLARY LIPOMA

Intradural and intramedullary lipomas do not differ from lipomas with dural defects both in pathological and embryological terms. However, they are contained within an intact dural sac. Intradural lipomas lie along the midline in the groove formed by the dorsal surface of the unapposed folds of the placode and may bulge posteriorly in the subarachnoid spaces elevating the pia mater. Large lipomas may displace the cord laterally, resulting in an off-midline placode–lipoma interface. In rare instances, lipomas are completely intramedullary. Intradural lipomas are commonly located at lumbosacral level and usually present with TCS, whereas cervicothoracic lipomas generally produce insidious signs of spinal cord compression. On MRI (Figure 12.1.9), lipomas appear as masses that are isointense to subcutaneous fat in all sequences, including those acquired with fat suppression techniques.

FILAR LIPOMA

Filar lipoma is an elementary anomaly of secondary neurulation characterized by a fibrolipomatous thickening of the filum terminale. The occurrence of incidental fat within the filum terminale in the normal adult population is estimated to be 1.5% to 5% in unselected MRI studies. Therefore, it may be considered an anatomical variant if there are no signs of TCS. Impaired canalization of the tail bud and persistence of cells capable of maturing into adipocytes are likely to be involved in the embryogenesis of filar lipomas. MRI detects fatty tissue within a thickened filum terminale as a stripe of increased signal intensity on sagittal T1-weighted images (Figure 12.1.10). As the filum frequently lies slightly off the midline, axial and coronal T1-weighted images are also helpful.

TIGHT FILUM TERMINALE

The tight filum terminale is characterized by a short, hypertrophic filum terminale that produces tethering and impaired ascent of the conus medullaris. Isolated cases are uncommon, whereas the abnormality is more frequent in patients with other malformations, such as diastematomyelia (Figure 12.1.11; see also Figure 12.1.17) or dermal sinuses. In 86% of the patients, the tip of the conus medullaris lies inferior to L2.

Embryologically, the tight filum terminale is due to abnormal retrogressive differentiation of the secondary neural tube, producing a thicker filum. The filum terminale is not >2 mm in diameter in normal individuals but the exact thickness of the filum terminale may be difficult to measure on MRI.

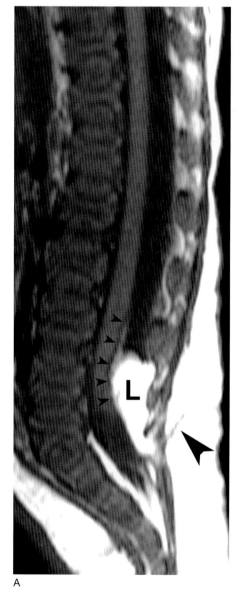

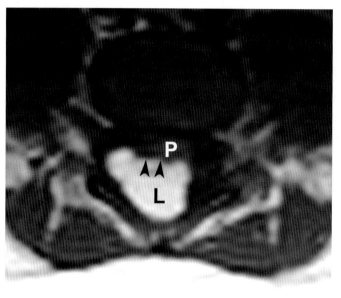

Figure 12.1.9 Intradural lipoma, 2-month-old girl. (A) Sagittal T1-weighted image shows low-lying spinal cord tethered (small arrowheads) to the anterior surface of a lumbosacral lipoma (L). The lipoma is not continuous with the subcutaneous fat. Notice concurrent dermal sinus (large arrowhead). (B) Axial T1-weighted image shows the placode (P)–lipoma (L) interface (arrowheads). The lipoma is intradural and clearly separated from the subcutaneous fat.

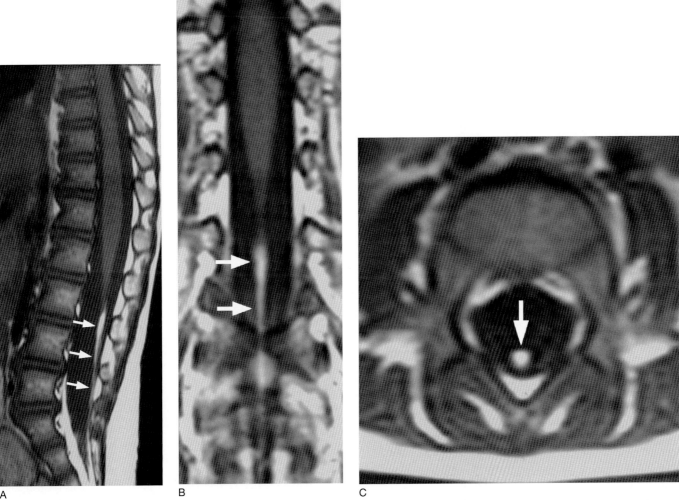

Figure 12.1.10 Filar lipoma, 2-year-old boy. (A,B) Sagittal and coronal T1-weighted images show that the filum terminale is largely replaced by fat (arrows). The spinal cord is tethered and low. (C) Axial T1-weighted image shows that the hyperintense fatty filum (arrow) clearly stands out against the hypointense cerebrospinal fluid.

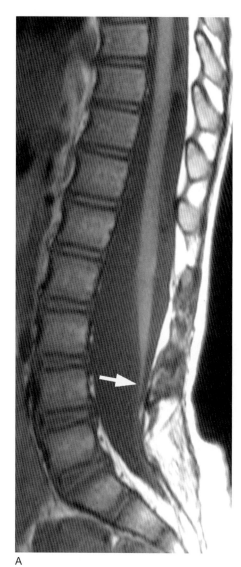

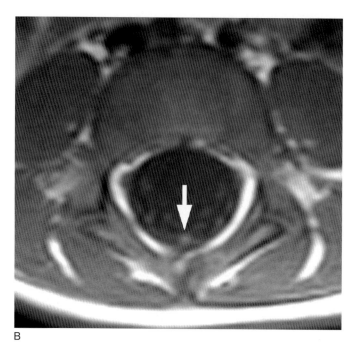

A

B

Figure 12.1.11 Tight filum terminale, 4-month-old girl with partial diastematomyelia (see Figure 12.1.20). (A) Sagittal T1-weighted image shows thickened filum terminale (arrow) with tethered, low conus medullaris. The spinal canal is abnormally large. (B) Axial T1-weighted image confirms thickening of the filum terminale (arrow).

DERMAL SINUS

The dermal sinus is an epithelium-lined fistula connecting the skin surface to the CNS and its meningeal coating. It is located more frequently in the lumbosacral region, although thoracic, cervical and occipital locations are also possible. On clinical examination, a midline dimple or pinpoint ostium is found, often in association with a hairy naevus, capillary haemangioma or hyperpigmented patches. While dermal sinuses are found above the intergluteal cleft and usually are directed superiorly, sacrococcygeal pits are found within the intergluteal cleft and extend either straight down or inferiorly; they are anatomically located below the termination of the thecal sac and do not require further imaging evaluation.

Complications of dermal sinuses include local infection, meningitis and abscesses that may result from bacteria invading the CNS along the tract.

Embryologically, dermal sinus tracts result from focal incomplete disjunction of the neuroectoderm from the cutaneous ectoderm. Dermal sinuses are easily recognized on midsagittal MR images as a thin hypointense stripe crossing the subcutaneous fat (Figure 12.1.12). Dermal sinuses are often associated with dermoids, which probably result from encystment of part of the dermal sinus tract (Figure 12.1.13). This association was found in 11.3% of cases in our series but may be higher. Dermoids are located at the level of the cauda equina or conus medullaris and show variable MRI features depending on their content. Infected

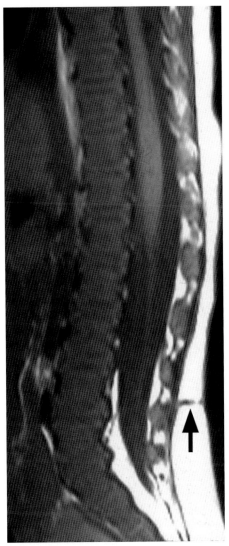

Figure 12.1.12 Dermal sinus, 1-month-old boy. Sagittal T1-weighted image shows dermal sinus coursing through the subcutaneous fat (arrow).

dermoids exhibit intense contrast enhancement, which may become ring-like with abscess formation.

PERSISTENT TERMINAL VENTRICLE

The 'fifth ventricle' of the historic scientific literature is a small ependyma-lined cavity within the conus medullaris that is always identifiable on postmortem examinations but must achieve a certain size to become visible on MRI (Figure 12.1.14). Embryologically, it is related to incomplete regression of the terminal ventricle during secondary neurulation. The persistent terminal ventricle is generally asymptomatic, although low-back pain, sciatica and bladder disorders have been reported. Enlargement of the terminal ventricle with cyst formation may be a developmental variant or may result from pathological changes leading to

obstruction of the terminal ventricle. Differentiation from hydromyelia is based on the location immediately above the filum terminale. Intramedullary tumours are ruled out by the lack of gadolinium enhancement. The size of the 'cyst' usually remains unchanged on follow-up.

FURTHER READING

Barkovich AJ, Edwards MSB, Cogen PH. MR evaluation of spinal dermal sinus tracts in children. American Journal of Neuroradiology 1991; 12:123–129.

Brown E, Matthes JC, Bazan C 3rd, Jinkins JR. Prevalence of incidental intraspinal lipoma of the lumbosacral spine as determined by MRI. Spine 1994; 19:833–836.

Coleman LT, Zimmerman RA, Rorke LB. Ventriculus terminalis of the conus medullaris: MR findings in children. American Journal of Neuroradiology 1995; 16:1421–1426.

Elton S, Oakes WJ. Dermal sinus tracts of the spine. Neurosurgery Focus (serial online). January 2001; 10:Article 4. Available at http://www.neurosurgery.org/focus/jan01/10-1-4.

Kernohan JW. The ventriculus terminalis: its growth and development. Journal of Comparative Neurology 1924; 38:10–125.

Raghavan N, Barkovich AJ, Edwards M, Norman D. MR imaging in the tethered spinal cord syndrome. American Journal of Neuroradiology 1989; 10:27–36.

Scotti G, Harwood-Nash DC. Congenital thoracic dermal sinus: diagnosis by computer assisted metrizamide myelography. Journal of Computer Assisted Tomography 1980; 4:675–677.

Sigal R, Denys A, Halimi P et al. Ventriculus terminalis of the conus medullaris: MR imaging in four patients with congenital dilatation. American Journal of Neuroradiology 1991; 12:733–737.

Tortori-Donati P, Cama A, Rosa ML, Andreussi L, Taccone A. Occult spinal dysraphism: neuroradiological study. Neuroradiology 1990; 31:512–522.

Tortori-Donati P, Rossi A, Biancheri R, Cama A. Magnetic resonance imaging of spinal dysraphism. Topics in Magnetic Resonance Imaging 2001; 12:375–409.

Tortori-Donati P, Rossi A, Cama A. Spinal dysraphism: a review of neuroradiological features with embryological correlations and proposal for a new classification. Neuroradiology 2000; 42:471–491.

Uchino A, Mori T, Ohno M. Thickened fatty filum terminale: MR imaging. Neuroradiology 1991; 33:331–333.

Warder DE. Tethered cord syndrome and occult spinal dysraphism. Neurosurgery Focus (serial online). January 2001; 10:Article 1. Available at http://www.neurosurgery.org/focus/jan01/10-1-1.

Weprin BE, Oakes WJ. Coccygeal pits. Pediatrics 2000; 105:E69.

Yundt KD, Park TS, Kaufman BA. Normal diameter of filum terminale in children: in vivo measurement. Pediatric Neurosurgery 1997; 27:257–259.

COMPLEX DYSRAPHIC STATES

Abnormal development of the notochord during gastrulation results in complex malformations, involving not only the spinal cord but also other organs deriving from or induced by the notochord. These malformations have been categorized into: (1) disorders of midline notochordal integration, which result in longitudinal notochordal splitting; and (2) disorders of notochordal formation, which result in the absence of a certain notochordal segment.

DISORDERS OF MIDLINE NOTOCHORDAL INTEGRATION

As mentioned above, during gastrulation notochordal cells derived from the Hensen's node stream in equal numbers from both sides

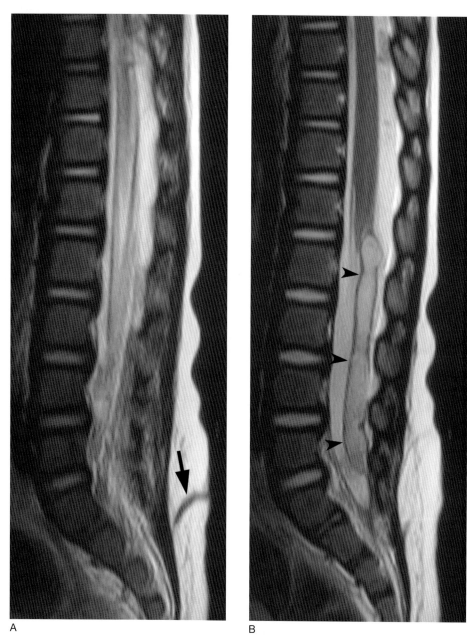

A   B

Figure 12.1.13 Dermal sinus with dermoid, 8-year-old girl. (A) Slightly parasagittal T2-weighted image shows sacral dermal sinus coursing obliquely downward in subcutaneous fat (arrow). (B) Midsagittal T2-weighted image shows huge dermoid in the thecal sac (arrowheads), extending upward to the tip of the conus medullaris. The mass gives slightly lower signal than cerebrospinal fluid and is outlined by a thin low-signal rim.

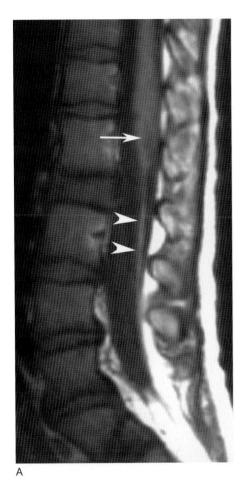

A

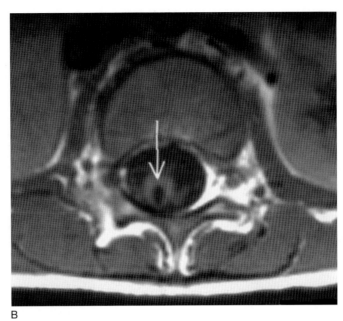

B

Figure 12.1.14 Persistent terminal ventricle. (A) Sagittal T1-weighted image shows faint hypointensity within the conus medullaris (arrow). There is concurrent filar lipoma (arrowheads). (B) Axial T1-weighted image confirms intramedullary cavity involving the conus medullaris (arrow) at the anatomical site of the terminal ventricle.

of the node to the interface between the ectoderm and the endoderm. Midline integration is the process by which notochordal cells integrate along the midline to form a single notochordal process. The cause of failed midline notochordal integration has stimulated much debate among authors. The eventual malformation basically depends on the severity of the insult and the efficiency of subsequent repair efforts. Several malformations belong to this wide group. Only the most important entities will be dealt with here.

Neurenteric cysts

The most severe, albeit the most rare, form of failed midline notochordal integration is dorsal enteric fistula, in which an abnormal canal connecting the skin surface with the bowel (neurenteric canal) crosses the intervening space between a duplicated spine. Neurenteric cysts are related to endodermal differentiation of primitive streak remnants that remain trapped between a split notochord; as such, they may be viewed as a localized form of dorsal enteric fistula. They are lined with a mucin-secreting, cuboidal or columnar epithelium that resembles the alimentary tract. Their content is variable and the chemical composition may be similar to CSF. The typical location is intradural in the cervicothoracic spine anterior to the cord (Figure 12.1.15), usually in close connection with vertebral abnormalities; however, neurenteric cysts

also may be found in the lumbar spine and even in the posterior fossa.

On MRI (Figure 12.1.15), neurenteric cysts usually are isointense to hyperintense relative to CSF on proton density and T2-weighted images. On T1-weighted images, they appear isointense or slightly hyperintense to CSF, consistent with a high protein content. Absence of contrast enhancement is the rule; however, we have seen one case of a neurenteric cyst that enhanced following intravenous gadolinium administration.

Diastematomyelia

Diastematomyelia refers to a variably elongated separation of the spinal cord into two usually symmetrical halves. Diastematomyelia may be best considered as a continuous spectrum of abnormality, ranging from partially cleft cord in a single dural tube to a completely duplicated cord within dual dural tubes with an intervening bony spur. The term 'split cord malformations' has been suggested to describe this continuum. We prefer the traditional denomination, which has the advantage of being widely recognized and accepted.

Embryologically, failed midline integration results in two paired notochordal processes separated by intervening primitive streak cells. Each heminotochord induces a separate neural plate. The resulting malformation depends on the developmental fate of the

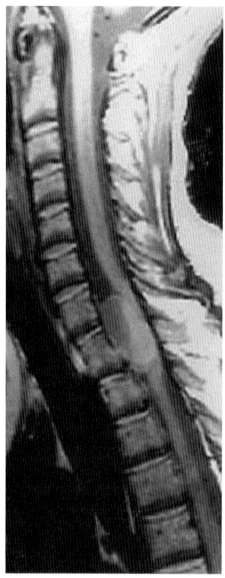

Figure 12.1.15 Neurenteric cyst. Sagittal PD-weighted image shows an intradural cyst ventral to the spinal cord at the C7-T2 level. (Reproduced with permission of American Medical Association from Martin AJ, Penney CC. Spinal neurenteric cyst. Archives of Neurology 2001; 58:126–127.)

diastematomyelia. Vertebral abnormalities are the rule and include bifid lamina, widened interpediculate distance, hemivertebrae, bifid vertebrae, fused vertebrae and narrowing of the intervertebral disc space. Scoliosis also is common and is seen in 30% to 60% of these individuals.

The radiological hallmark is the osteocartilaginous septum with resulting double dural tubes, each containing a hemicord. Although in most cases, the spur is osseous and connects the vertebral body to the neural arch along a midsagittal plane, 'atypical' spurs are not uncommon. The spur may course obliquely and be complete or incomplete (Figure 12.1.16). In most cases, the spur is located

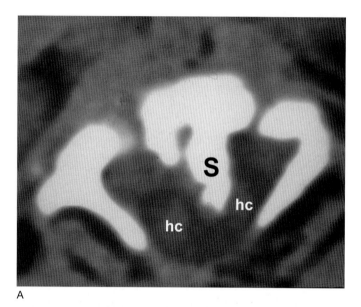

A

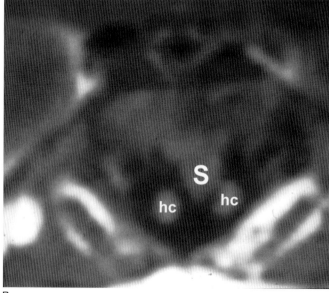

B

Figure 12.1.16 Diastematomyelia type I. (A) Axial CT scan shows bony spur (S) separating the spinal canal into two halves, each containing a hemicord (hc). This incomplete spur projects posteriorly from the vertebral body. Notice associated bony spina bifida. (B) Axial T1-weighted image shows the spur (S) and the dual dural tubes, each containing a hemicord (hc).

intervening primitive streak tissue. If it develops towards bone and cartilage, the two hemicords eventually will be contained into two individual dural sacs separated by an osteocartilaginous spur. Conversely, if the primitive streak tissue is reabsorbed or leaves a thin fibrous septum, the two hemicords will lie within a single dural tube. This represents the foundation of classification of diastematomyelia into two groups.

Diastematomyelia type I This consists of two hemicords contained within individual dural tubes, separated by a bony or osteocartilaginous septum that extends from the vertebral body to the neural arches. This rigid median septum is entirely extradural. Patients usually present with scoliosis and TCS. A hairy tuft located relatively cranial along the child's back is a reliable clinical marker of

at the thoracic or lumbar level and lies at the caudal end of the split cord. The two hemicords usually surround the spur tightly before fusing with each other to form a normal spinal cord below, whereas rostrally the splitting is much more elongated. Therefore, there is a craniocaudal sequence of partial clefting, complete diastematomyelia with single dural tube and diastematomyelia with dual dural tubes (Figure 12.1.17). Hydromyelia is commonly associated and may involve the normal cord both above and below the splitting, as well as one or both hemicords. Failure of neurulation of one hemicord produces a hemimyelo(meningo)cele.

Diastematomyelia type II This is characterized by a single dural tube housing both hemicords. Three variants exist: presence of an intervening fibrous septum, absence of a septum and partial cord splitting.

A midline, non-rigid, fibrous septum is sometimes detected at surgery, usually in patients presenting with TCS. These septa may be identified on high-resolution axial and coronal T2-weighted images as thin hypointense stripes interposed between the two hemicords (Figure 12.1.18). Absence of a septum is the most common occurrence in diastematomyelia type II (Figure 12.1.19). Although the diagnosis is relatively straightforward both on axial and coronal MR images, diastematomyelia may be difficult to appreciate on sagittal MR images, where the only tell-tale sign is an apparent thinning of the spinal cord that results from partial averaging with the intervening subarachnoid space between the two hemicords (Figures 12.1.18, 12.1.19). In rare instances, the cleft is partial and the splitting incomplete; these are the mildest forms in the diastematomyelia spectrum (Figure 12.1.20).

Hydromyelia may be present with the same features as in diastematomyelia type I. The conus medullaris is typically low and there is a strong association with tight filum terminale and filar lipomas. Associated vertebral anomalies are usually milder than in type I.

DISORDERS OF NOTOCHORDAL FORMATION

Programmed cell death, or apoptosis, is a process of cell elimination that occurs during normal development and represents a crucial phenomenon in the various steps of embryogenesis. If prospective notochordal cells are wrongly specified in terms of their rostrocaudal positional encoding, they will be eliminated by apoptosis. In such instances, fewer cells, or even no cells, will form the notochord at a given abnormal segmental level. The consequences of such a segmental notochordal paucity are manifold and affect the development of the spinal column and spinal cord as well as that of other organs that rely on the notochord as their inductor. If the prospective notochord is depleted, a wide array of vertebral malformations will result. Because of lack of neural induction, the neural tube will similarly be depleted. The resulting malformation essentially depends on the segmental level and the extent of the abnormality along the longitudinal embryonic axis, with subsequent interference on the processes of primary and/or secondary neurulation. In the vast majority of cases, the abnormality involves the caudal extremity of the embryo, resulting in the caudal agenesis constellation. Much more rarely, the abnormality involves an intermediate notochordal segment, thereby resulting in segmental spinal dysgenesis.

Caudal agenesis

Caudal agenesis (CA) comprises total or partial agenesis of the spinal column, anal imperforation, genital anomalies, bilateral renal dysplasia or aplasia, pulmonary hypoplasia and lower limb abnormalities. CA is also commonly, albeit inappropriately, called caudal regression syndrome; etymologically, the term 'caudal agenesis' should be preferred, as 'caudal regression' implies a concept of excessive regression of the embryonic tail that cannot be adequately applied in tail-less animals, such as humans (M. Catala, personal communication). CA may be part of syndromic complexes such as OEIS, VACTERL (<u>v</u>ertebral abnormality, <u>a</u>nal imperforation, <u>c</u>ardiac malformations, <u>t</u>racheo<u>e</u>sophageal fistula, <u>r</u>enal abnormalities, <u>l</u>imb deformities) and the Currarino triad (partial sacral agenesis, anorectal malformation and presacral mass: teratoma and/or meningocele). There is a definite association with maternal diabetes mellitus (1% of offspring of diabetic mothers). The congenital spectrum of vertebral abnormality in CA may range from agenesis of the coccyx to absence of the sacral, lumbar and lower thoracic vertebrae but the vast majority involve only the sacrum and coccyx. The sacrum may be totally or partially absent, with S1 through S4 present in individual cases.

Caudal agenesis has been categorized into two types depending on the location and shape of the conus medullaris: either high and abrupt (type I) or low and tethered (type II). Although these two types were once believed to be embryologically related to disordered primary or secondary neurulation, respectively, both are actually consistent with abnormality of gastrulation. In fact, segmental maldevelopment of the notochord secondarily interferes with either secondary neurulation alone, or both primary and secondary neurulation, depending on the longitudinal extent of the original notochordal damage. Therefore, the crucial embryological watershed between the two varieties is the interface between primary and secondary neurulation (i.e. the junction between the true notochord and the tail bud), corresponding to the caudal end of the future neural plate. This site has been the source of continuing debate among authors: recent results suggest that it corresponds to S3 through S5. As a consequence, the degree of spinal cord aplasia correlates with the severity of the spinal malformation, which is more severe in type I than in type II.

Type I CA (Figure 12.1.21) If not only the tail bud but also part of the true notochord fails to develop, both the processes of primary and secondary neurulation are affected. Depending on the severity of the original damage, the eventual degree of vertebral aplasia will range from absence of the coccyx and lower mid-sacrum to aplasia of all coccygeal, sacral, lumbar and lower thoracic vertebrae, although the last vertebra is L5 through S2 in the majority of patients. Owing to the same embryological mechanism, there is aplasia of the caudal metameres of the spinal cord, resulting in an abrupt spinal cord terminus that nearly always is club- or wedge-shaped (Figure 12.1.21). The spinal cord terminus is high (most often opposite T12) in most cases but it may lie opposite to L1 in a minority of cases. The thecal sac tapers below the cord terminus and ends at an unusually high level (Figure 12.1.21). Clinically, patients have a stable neurological defect due to their 'fixed' spinal cord dysplasia.

Type II CA (Figure 12.1.22) If the tail bud fails to develop but the true notochord is unaffected, primary neurulation occurs normally

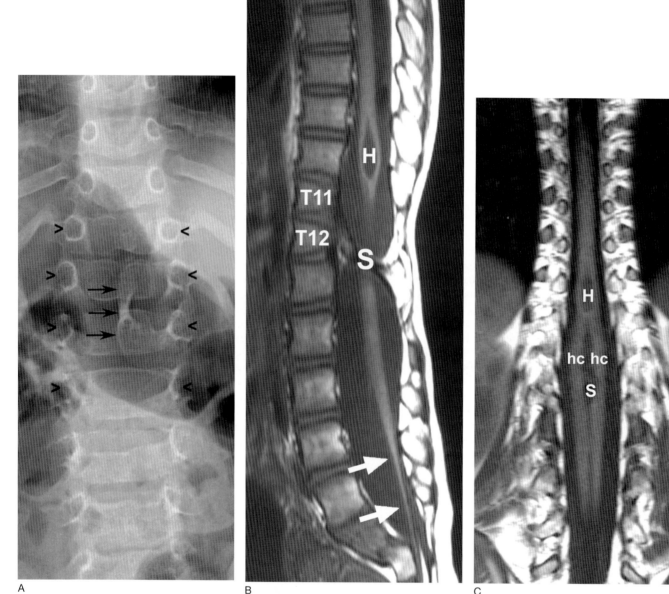

Figure 12.1.17 Diastematomyelia type I, 3-year-old girl. (A) Conventional x-rays, anteroposterior view, show increased interpeduncular distance (arrowheads) and a bony structure projecting into the spinal canal (arrows). (B) Sagittal and (C) coronal T1-weighted images show bony spur (S) projecting into the spinal canal. The spur is located at the T12-L1 level. The two hemicords are visible on the coronal plane (hc, C), whereas the intervening subarachnoid space between the two hemicords are seen above the spur on the midsagittal plane (B). There is a tight filum terminale that tethers the spinal cord inferiorly (arrows, B). There is also hydromyelia involving the spinal cord above the splitting (H). The T11 and T12 vertebral bodies are rudimentary (B). (D–F) Axial T2-weighted images show the malformation sequence from cephalad to caudad: (D) hydromyelia (H); (E) split spinal cord (hc) within single dural sac; and (F) split spinal cord (hc) with dual dural sacs and intervening bony spur (S) that connects the vertebral body to an abnormally thick neural arch. (G) Axial CT scan shows the sclerotic bony spur (S) connecting anteriorly with the vertebral body and posteriorly with a rudiment of the spinous process that is separated from the laminae by bony spina bifida (arrows). There are two dural sacs (asterisks) separated by the spur.

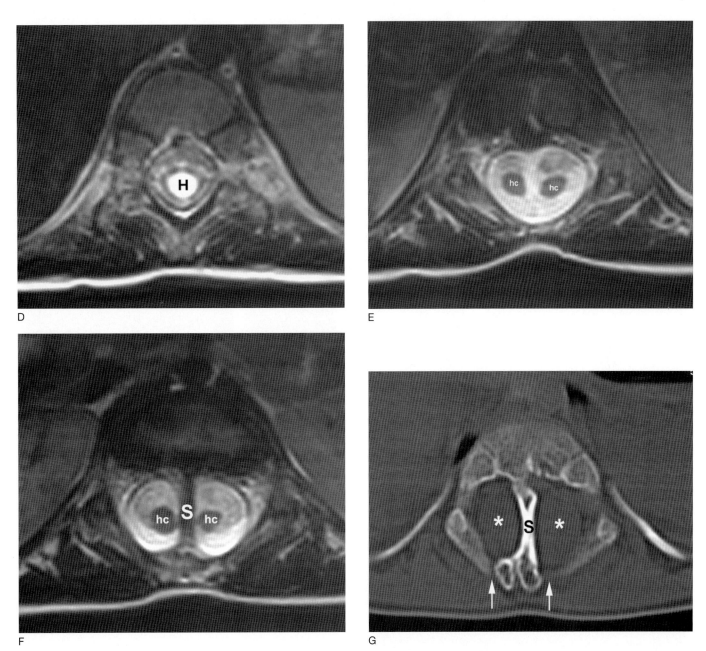

Figure 12.1.17 *Continued*

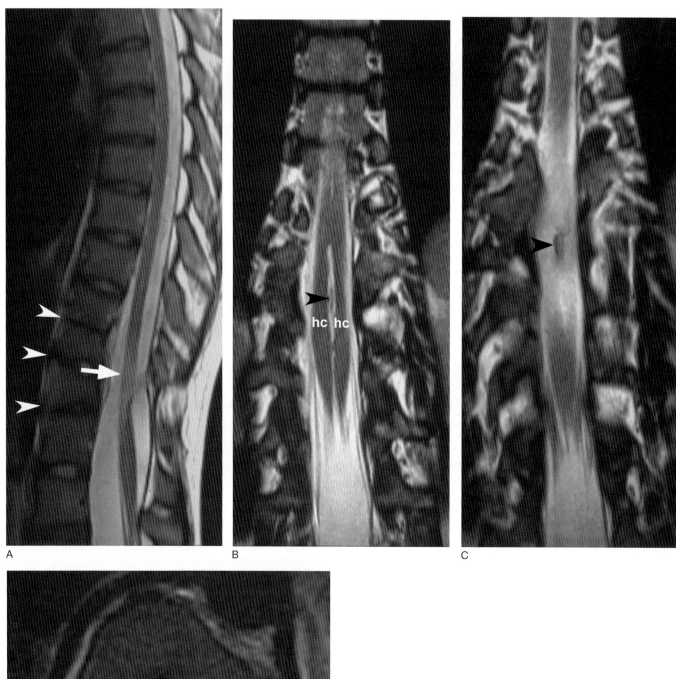

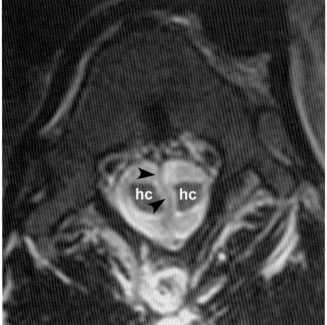

Figure 12.1.18 Diastematomyelia type II with fibrous septum, 11-year-old girl. (A) The only tell-tale sign of the abnormality on this sagittal T2-weighted image is an apparent thinning of the spinal cord (arrow), which actually results from the intervening subarachnoid space between the two hemicords. The spinal canal is enlarged. There are concurrent vertebral segmentation defects with rudimentary intervertebral discs (arrowheads). (B,C) Coronal and (D) axial T2-weighted images show the two hemicords (hc) are contained within a single dural sac, which is divided into two halves by an intervening hypointense band (arrowhead). A fibrous septum was found at surgery.

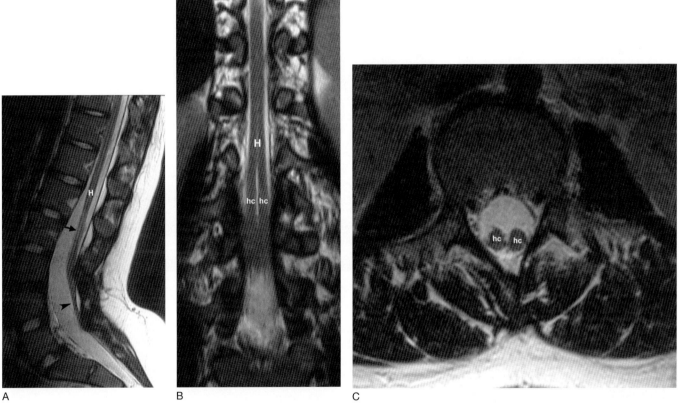

Figure 12.1.19 Diastematomyelia type II without septum, 13-year-old girl. (A) Sagittal T2-weighted image shows a low spinal cord with apparent focal thinning (arrow) resulting from partial averaging with the intervening subarachnoid space between the two hemicords. Hydromyelia (H) involves the cord above the splitting. There is associated tight filum terminale (arrowhead). (B) Coronal T2-weighted image shows split hemicords (hc) and cranial hydromyelia (H). (C) Axial T2-weighted image clearly shows the two hemicords (hc) contained in a single dural tube, with no intervening septum.

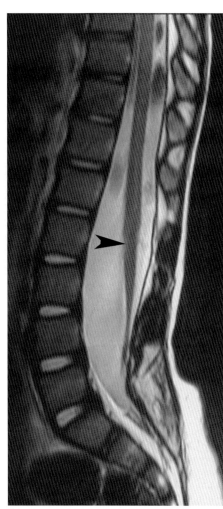

A

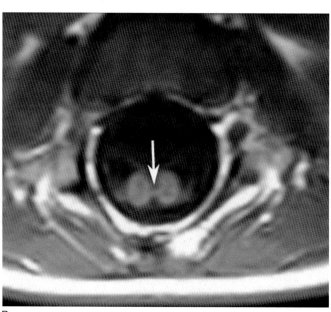

B

Figure 12.1.20 Diastematomyelia type II with partial splitting, 4-month-old girl. Same case as Figure 12.1.11. (A) Sagittal T2-weighted image shows faint thinning of the conus medullaris (arrowhead), which has a low position due to associated tight filum terminale. (B) Axial T2-weighted image shows incomplete cord splitting (arrow).

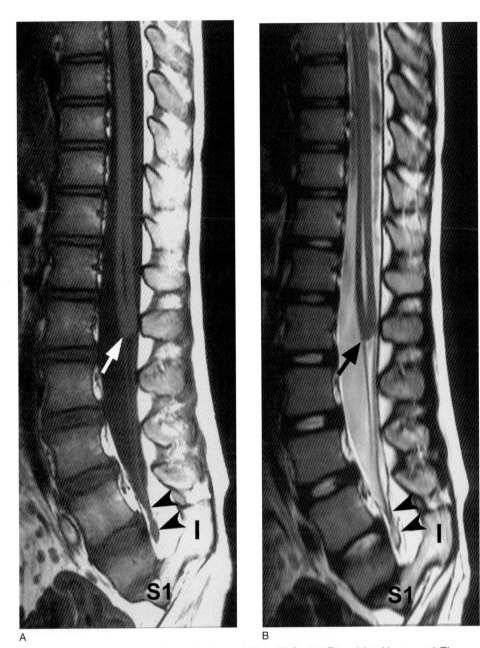

A   B

Figure 12.1.21 Caudal agenesis, type I, 8-year-old boy. (A) Sagittal T1-weighted image and (B) sagittal T2-weighted image show subtotal sacrococcygeal agenesis, with a rudiment of S2 as the last visible vertebra, articulating with medialized ileum (I). The cord terminus is blunt and lies opposite the lower half of L1 (arrow), a somewhat atypically 'low' position for type I CA. There is terminal hydromyelia and 'double bundle' arrangement of the nerve roots of the cauda equina. The dural sac tapers abruptly and ends abnormally high (arrowheads).

and there is interference only with the process of secondary neurulation. Therefore, vertebral dysgenesis is less severe than in type I, with up to S4 present as the last vertebra. Moreover, only the tip of the conus medullaris (corresponding to the metameres formed by secondary neurulation) is absent. In most cases, partial agenesis of the conus is difficult to recognize, because the conus itself is stretched caudally and tethered to a tight filum, lipoma (Figure 12.1.22), terminal myelocystocele, lipomyelomeningocele or anterior sacral meningocele. Unlike with CA type I, these patients will typically present with TCS.

Segmental spinal dysgenesis

The clinical-radiological definition of segmental spinal dysgenesis (SSD) includes: (1) segmental agenesis or dysgenesis of the lumbar or thoracolumbar spine; (2) segmental abnormality of the underlying spinal cord and nerve roots; (3) congenital paraplegia or paraparesis; and (4) congenital lower limb deformities. Segmental vertebral anomalies may involve the thoracolumbar,

lumbar or lumbosacral spine. Affected patients typically have a palpable gibbus of bony consistency along their back. As is the case with CA, the embryogenesis of SSD may be related to genetically induced notochordal derangement during gastrulation involving an intermediate, rather than the caudal-most, segment of the notochord (2,50).

In the most severe cases, the spinal cord at the level of the abnormality is thoroughly absent and the bony spine is focally aplastic. As a result, the spine and spinal cord are 'cut in two' (Figure 12.1.23), with resulting acute angle kyphosis. Between the two spinal segments, the spinal canal is extremely narrowed or even totally interrupted. The lower spinal cord segment is invariably bulky and low-lying. A horseshoe kidney is typically lodged in the concavity of the kyphosis. Newborns with severe SSD are paraplegic at birth and invariably show hypotrophic and deformed lower limbs with equinocavovarus feet.

In less severe cases, there is focal hypoplasia of the spinal cord, which will therefore appear narrower than normal on MRI studies (Figure 12.1.24). There is no disconnection of either the spinal cord or the spine, although bony stenosis of the spinal canal and minor vertebral abnormalities affect the pathological segment.

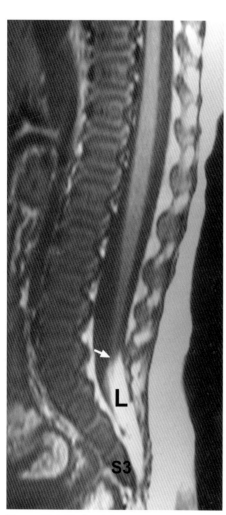

Figure 12.1.22 Caudal agenesis, type II, 3-month-old boy. Sagittal T1-weighted image shows the spinal cord is low and tethered (arrow) to an intradural lipoma (L). The vertebral anomaly is less severe than in type I, with S3 present in this case.

FURTHER READING

Barkovich AJ, Raghavan N, Chuang SH. MR of lumbosacral agenesis. American Journal of Neuroradiology 1989; 10:1223–1231.

Carey JC, Greenbaum B, Hall BD. The OEIS complex (omphalocele, exstrophy, imperforate anus, spinal defects). Birth Defects Original Article Series 1978; 14:253–263.

Currarino G, Coln D, Votteler T. Triad of anorectal, sacral, and presacral anomalies. American Journal of Roentgenology 1981; 137:395–398.

Dias MS, Azizkhan RG. A novel embryogenetic mechanism for Currarino's triad: inadequate dorsoventral separation of the caudal eminence from hindgut endoderm. Pediatric Neurosurgery 1998; 28:223–229.

Dias MS, Walker ML. The embryogenesis of complex dysraphic malformations: a disorder of gastrulation? Pediatric Neurosurgery 1992; 18:229–253.

Duhamel B. From the mermaid to anal imperforation: the syndrome of caudal regression. Archives of Disease in Childhood 1961; 36:152–155.

Faris JC, Crowe JE. The split notochord syndrome. Journal of Pediatric Surgery 1975; 10:467–472.

Gudinchet F, Maeder P, Laurent T, Meyrat B, Schnyder P. Magnetic resonance detection of myelodysplasia in children with Currarino triad. Pediatric Radiology 1997; 27:903–907.

Naidich TP, Blaser SI, Delman BN et al. Embryology of the spine and spinal cord. Proceedings of the American Society of Neuroradiology Congress 2002:3–13.

Naidich TP, Harwood-Nash DC. Diastematomyelia. Part I. Hemicords and meningeal sheaths. Single and double arachnoid and dural tubes. American Journal of Neuroradiology 1983; 4:633–636.

Nievelstein RAJ, Hartwig NG, Vermeji-Keers C, Valk J. Embryonic development of the mammalian caudal neural tube. Teratology 1993; 48:21–31.

Nievelstein RAJ, Valk J, Smit LME, Vermeji-Keers C. MR of the caudal regression syndrome: embryologic implications. American Journal of Neuroradiology 1994; 15:1021–1029.

Pang D. Sacral agenesis and caudal spinal cord malformations. Neurosurgery 1993; 32:755–779.

Pang D. Split cord malformation. Part II: clinical syndrome. Neurosurgery 1992; 31:481–500.

Pang D, Dias MS, Ahab-Barmada M. Split cord malformation. Part I: a unified theory of embryogenesis for double spinal cord malformations. Neurosurgery 1992; 31:451–480.

Prop N, Frensdorf EL. A postvertebral endodermal cyst associated with axial deformities: a case showing the 'endodermal-ectodermal adhesion syndrome'. Pediatrics 1967; 39:555–562.

Schlesinger AE, Naidich TP, Quencer RM. Concurrent hydromyelia and diastematomyelia. American Journal of Neuroradiology 1986; 7:473–477.

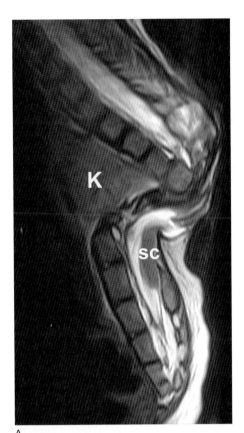

A

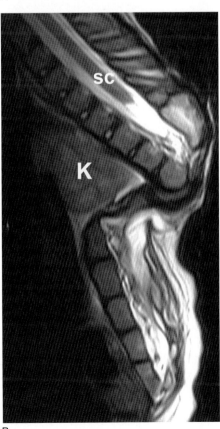

B

Figure 12.1.23 Segmental spinal dysgenesis, 2-year-old girl. (A,B) Sagittal T2-weighted images shows acute thoracolumbar kyphosis with complete interruption of the spinal column. There are two completely separated spinal cord segments (sc); the upper ends several vertebral levels above the gibbus (white arrowhead) and shows hydromyelia, whereas the lower is bulky and low (arrows). Notice horseshoe kidney (K) lodged into the kyphotic concavity, a typical arrangement in severe segmental spinal dysgenesis.

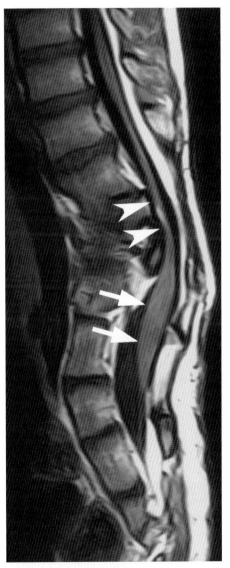

Figure 12.1.24 Segmental spinal dysgenesis, 8-year-old boy. Sagittal T1-weighted image shows indeterminate vertebrae at the upper lumbar level resulting in congenital kyphosis without complete disconnection of the spine. The spinal cord at the dysgenesis level is thin (arrowheads). The conus medullaris is bulky and low (arrows).

Smith NM, Chambers HM, Furness ME, Haan EA. The OEIS complex omphalocele-exstrophy-imperforate anus-spinal defects: recurrence in sibs. Journal of Medical Genetics 1992; 29:730–732.

Tortori-Donati P, Fondelli MP, Rossi A. Anomalie congenite del midollo spinale. In: Simonetti G, Del Maschio A, Bartolozzi C, Passariello R, eds. Trattato Italiano di risonanza magnetica. Naples: Idelson-Gnocchi; 1998:517–553.

Tortori-Donati P, Fondelli MP, Rossi A, Raybaud CA, Cama A, Capra V. Segmental spinal dysgenesis. Neuroradiologic findings with clinical and embryologic correlation. American Journal of Neuroradiology 1999; 20:445–456.

Tortori-Donati P, Rossi A, Biancheri R, Cama A. Magnetic resonance imaging of spinal dysraphism. Topics Magnetic Resonance Imaging 2001; 12:375–409.

Tortori-Donati P, Rossi A, Cama A. Spinal dysraphism: a review of neuroradiological features with embryological correlations and proposal for a new classification. Neuroradiology 2000; 42:471–491.

CONCLUSIONS

The MRI features of spinal dysraphisms may appear complicated and puzzling even to the experienced observer. However, a rational approach founded on a correlation of clinical, embryological and neuroimaging information greatly facilitates the diagnosis in the vast majority of cases. Neuroradiologists should pursue the maximum degree of collaboration with neurosurgeons and other specialists in order to improve their diagnoses and to increase the amount and accuracy of information that is made available to clinicians involved in the management of children with these disorders.

The Skull

*Nathalie Capon Degardin, Francis Brunelle,
Eric Arnaud, Elisabeth Lajeunie-Renier (deceased),
Dominique Renier*

The role of skull radiographs in the investigation of cranial disease has greatly diminished with the advent of cross-sectional imaging and though the skull x-ray may reflect intracranial pathology, it is so insensitive that it is no longer used; however, it still plays a role in the primary investigation of cranial lumps and bumps as many have a classical appearance. As described elsewhere in this chapter, skull x-rays are used in the primary assessment of abnormal skull shape. It is part of the routine skeletal survey in the work-up of suspected skeletal dysplasias and it may exhibit characteristic changes in generalized conditions such as the haemoglobinopathies, which may cause confusion.

A brief account of the more frequent conditions is given below.

SKULL SIZE

The relative proportion of face and skull vault changes throughout childhood, reaching almost adult proportions by about 10 years of age. Skull size is monitored by measuring it clinically and plotting the measurements on a growth chart. The anterior fontanelle closes by about 2 years of age. A persistently patent fontanelle is seen in many of the skeletal dysplasias.

Microcephaly (a small head) is associated with developmental delay, early anoxia from any cause, including intrauterine placental insufficiency and perinatal anoxia, congenital brain malformations and infections. Macrocephaly (a large head) may be familial but is also a feature of hydrocephalus, large extracerebral fluid spaces, sometimes referred to as benign macrocrania of infancy, chronic subdural effusions, intracranial fluid collections and hemimegalencephaly. In the latter two cases, the skull is often asymmetrical. In general, both large and small heads need investigation to establish the cause. This is best done by magnetic resonance imaging (MRI).

NORMAL VARIANTS AND ARTIFACTS

These may lead to an erroneous diagnosis of pathology.

PARIETAL FORAMINA

These are well corticated defects in the parietal bones which are of variable size but symmetrical. These defects gradually ossify and disappear with age (Figure 12.2.1).

OCCIPITAL THINNING

Congenital thinning of the occipital bones, which may create an appearance of radiolucency of the skull posteriorly, can be erroneously interpreted as a destructive lesion as it may cause a lucency over the diploic spaces (Figure 12.2.2).

ARTIFACTS

Hair styles, such as plaits, ponytails and the small tight plaits favoured by African-American children, cause density on x-ray. A similar artifact may be caused by a fold of loose skin of an infant (Figure 12.2.3).

SELLA TURCICA

Alterations in the size and shape of the sella are crude indicators of disease. An enlarged sella without erosion is found in children with chronic, often subclinical, hypothyroidism due to overstimulation. Craniopharyngiomas may expand and destroy the sella and are often accompanied by calcification. Erosion of clinoids is associated with raised intracranial pressure but is rarely seen in children because of the ease with which the sutures will separate in response to raised pressure. A J-shaped sella is associated with some of the skeletal dysplasias (Figure 12.2.4), in particular the mucopolysaccharidoses.

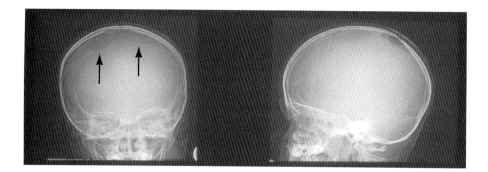

Figure 12.2.1 Frontal and lateral view of skull showing bilateral parietal defects.

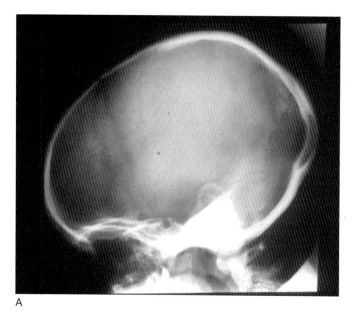

A

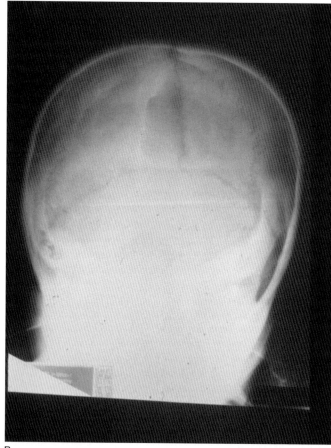

B

Figure 12.2.2 Lateral (A) and Towne's (B) skull radiographs showing typical appearances of occipital thinning.

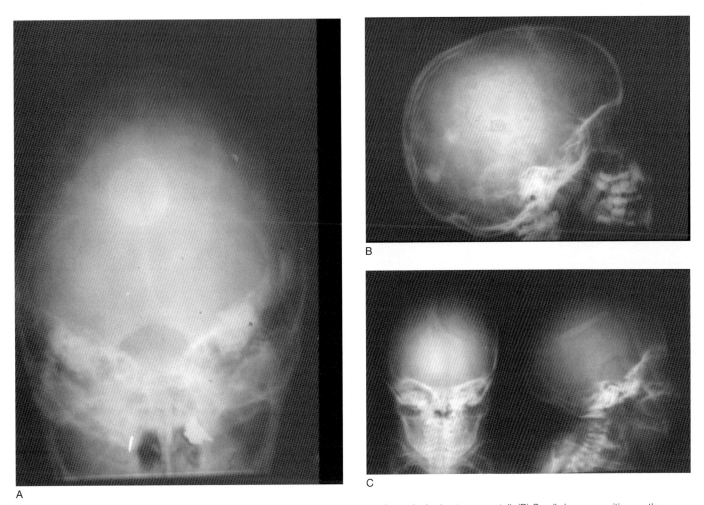

Figure 12.2.3 External artifact, which could simulate disease. (A) Round centre of opacity is due to a ponytail. (B) Small dense opacities on the lateral skull are due to the tiny hair plaits seen often on African-American children. (C) Two views of the skull showing typical skin fold artifact.

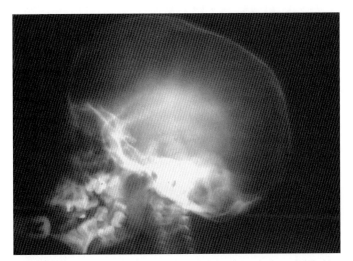

Figure 12.2.4 Lateral skull view showing J-shaped sella in a child with Morquio's disease.

WORMIAN BONES

These are sutural bones seen mostly in the posterior skull but may involve all sutures. They are a frequent normal variant especially in the lambdoid suture and in these circumstances are usually small and less than ten in number. Wormian bones are also a feature of many skeletal dysplasias. The most frequent are osteogenesis imperfecta (Figure 12.2.5), cleidocranial dysostosis, pyknodysostosis and hypophosphatasia.

OS INCA

This is an intraparietal bone situated posteriorly and lies between the lambdoid sutures laterally and the mendosal sutures inferiorly, which are joined by a transverse suture. It is a normal variant.

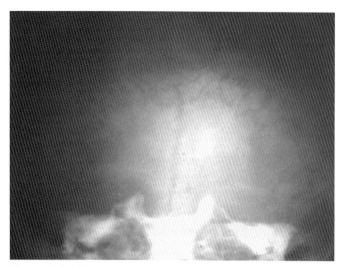

Figure 12.2.5 Towne's view of skull showing multiple wormian bones in a boy with osteogenesis imperfecta.

SKULL DENSITY

In the neonate, the vault is poorly ossified compared with the base and should not be mistaken for pathology. True poor ossification and hypomineralization of the skull vault occurs in osteogenesis imperfecta and hypophosphatasia and rickets.

Increased density is a feature of the skeletal dysplasias, which have a generalized increase in bone density. The reader is referred to the section on skeletal dysplasias in Chapter 2.7.

Increased density may also result from thickening of the diploic space such as occurs in fibrous dysplasia and the haemoglobinopathies. In fibrous dysplasia, there is marked activity on scintigraphy and the thickening of the diploic space shows as intermediate density on T1-weighted MRI (Figure 12.2.6). It may also result from metabolic conditions such as hypercalcaemia and hyperparathyroidism.

INCREASED THICKNESS OF THE SKULL VAULT

This occurs when there is increased marrow production such as occurs in sickle cell anaemia and thalassaemia (Figure 12.2.7). In both of these conditions, but especially in thalassaemia, the increased thickness is streaky and is described as 'hair standing on end appearance'. This generalized increase in marrow production may also cause thickening of the maxilla and obliteration of the sinuses.

Fibrous dysplasia in the skull affects mainly the sphenoid, the orbitofrontal regions and the base of skull, but the parietal and occipital bones are also sometimes involved. The underlying pathology is intraosseous proliferation of fibrous tissue. When the disease involves the skull base and the sphenoid bones there may

be encroachment on the cranial nerve foramina and complications include blindness and exophthalmos. Involvement of the maxilla gives a facial leonine appearance and is known as Leontiasis osseum.

BARE ORBIT

This describes the appearance of the orbit on the anteroposterior (AP) radiograph when there is erosion or elevation of the sphenoid wing so that it is not visualized. In children, this is most commonly associated with neurofibromatosis.

ASYMMETRY

This is most frequently seen with postural plagiocephaly. On correctly positioned skull radiographs, the borders of the cranial fossae should overlap as these are symmetrical structures. Displacement of one relative to the other implies that there is a long-standing space-occupying lesion in the cranial cavity. An example of this is an arachnoid cyst in the temporal lobe. Such cysts may also cause thinning of the skull vault.

CRANIOTABES

Congenital depression of the skull vault may arise by compression of the fetal head *in utero* by the infant hand or against the maternal sacrum (Figure 12.2.8). There is usually a history of oligohydramnios. These can be distinguished from birth 'ping pong' fractures by the absence of a history of instrumental delivery and absence of overlying scalp swelling.

INTRACRANIAL CALCIFICATION

Calcification may be detected on radiographs as an incidental finding but if it is important to identify calcification for diagnosis, a computed tomography (CT) scan should be performed as this is infinitely more sensitive than an x-ray both in detection and localization. Calcification may be detected on MRI as signal voids but microcalcification can appear as high signal. MRI is, however, more sensitive than CT in demonstrating any associated brain abnormalities, e.g. non-calcified tubers in tuberous sclerosis, so in many patients both techniques may be needed for full assessment.

The type of calcification and its location are aids to diagnosis. For example, basal calcification is seen with old TB meningitis. Periventricular calcification is seen in association with microcephaly in congenital toxoplasmosis or other congenital infections. A chronic calcified subdural haematoma lies peripherally. Vascular calcification is linear and seen in angiomatous malformations. Gyral calcification is seen in Sturge–Weber syndrome.

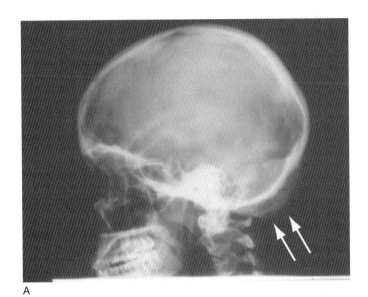

A

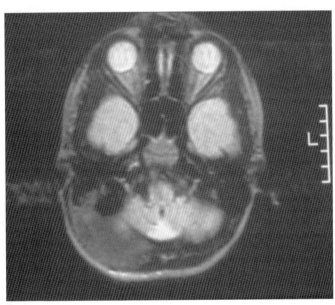

C

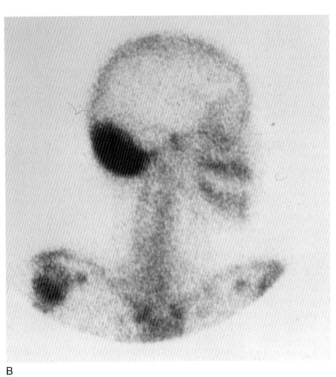

B

Figure 12.2.6 Fibrous dysplasia of the occipital bone on the right. (A) Radiograph. Note the thickened diploic space posteriorly. (B) Bone scintigraphy showing very hot activity in the lesion. (C) T1-W MR scan showing the thickening of the diploic space with intermediate density of the fibrous tissue in the diploic space.

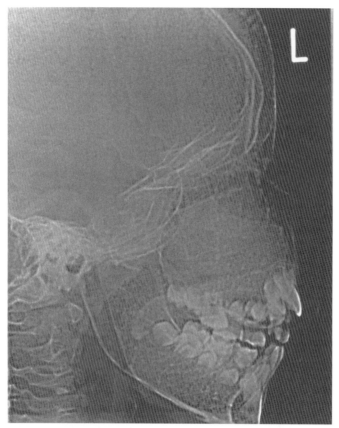

Figure 12.2.7 Lateral view of frontal part of the skull and facial bones in a girl with thalassaemia. Note the thickened diploic space in the frontal bone and the obliteration of the sinuses due to enlargement of the marrow cavity.

Calcification in tuberous sclerosis (Figure 12.2.9) is scattered through the brain in addition to being in the subependymal region. Causes of intracranial calcification are shown in Table 12.2.1. Many of these causes are very rare and also in many instances the precise cause is never found in spite of exhaustive investigation.

SKULL BONE TUMOURS

OSSIFYING FIBROMAS

These are dense fibrous tumours that tend to grow in the sinuses, especially the frontal sinuses, but may grow on the skull vault bones (Figure 12.2.10). They may block the ostia and cause sinusitis and even mucoceles. On radiographs they appear as dense opacities and are sometimes referred to as ivory osteomas. These may occur in isolation but are also found in association with Gardner's syndrome.

GORLIN'S SYNDROME

This is also known as the basal cell naevus syndrome. The main features of this are basal cell carcinomas and odontogenic cysts and mild prognathism. The carcinomas are rare in childhood but

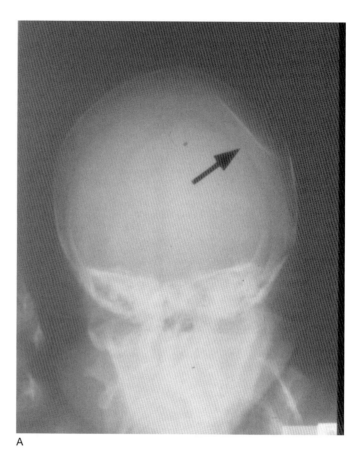

A

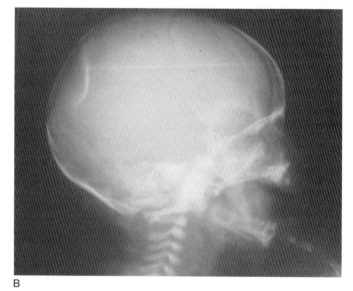

B

Figure 12.2.8 Frontal (A) and lateral (B) view of the skull showing the depression typical of craniotabes. This child had no history of instrumental delivery and was born with this defect.

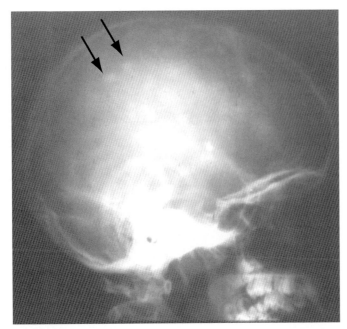

Figure 12.2.9 Lateral skull film showing multiple calcified opacities due to tuberous sclerosis.

Table 12.2.1 Causes of intracranial calcification in children (adapted from Nicer encyclopedia, Vol. 7: Paediatric imaging)

Physiological	Pineal gland
	Choroid plexus
Pathological tumours	Craniopharyngioma
	Lipoma of the corpus callosum
Meningeal	Chronic subdural haematoma
	Gorlin's syndrome
Gyrae	Sturge–Weber syndrome
Vascular	Vascular malformation
Infection	Toxoplasmosis
	Congenital rubella
	Cytomegalic virus
	Herpes simplex virus
	Cysticercosis
	AIDS
	TB (basal meninges)
	Measles
	Chickenpox
	Pertussis
	Coxsackie B virus
Congenital/ developmental	Familial idiopathic basal ganglion calcification
	Hastings–James syndrome
	Cockayne syndrome
	Neurofibromatosis
	Tuberous sclerosis
	Down's syndrome
	Lipid proteinosis
	Methaemoglobinopathy
	Oculocraniosomatic disease
Metabolic	Mitochondrial cytopathies
	Fahr's syndrome
	Hallervorden–Spatz disease
	Carbonic anhydrase deficiency type 11
Endocrine	Hypoparathyroidism
	Pseudohypothyroidism
	Pseudopseudohypothyroidism
	Hyperparathyroidism
	Hypothyroidism
Toxic	Hypoxia/anoxia
	Lead poisoning
	Radiation
	Methotrexate treatment
	Nephrotic syndrome

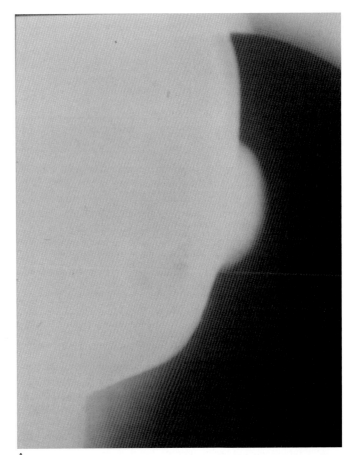

A

B

Figure 12.2.10 (A) Tangential soft tissue view of left parietal region and (B) CT scan showing an unusual location but a typical appearance of an osteoma.

the jaw lesions may present. Mental retardation and seizures are frequent. The typical feature in the skull is dense ossification of the dura, particularly in the falx and tentorium.

ANEURYSMAL BONE CYSTS

These may involve any skull bone but compared with the humerus and femur are rare with about 3% incidence in the skull. In the spine, they involve the neural arches. The histology is the same no matter where they occur in the body and are composed of fibrous and vascular tissue. They are vascular on angiography. They may become very large and cause expansion of the skull bones, which may compress the underlying brain. On CT and MRI the expansile nature is easily demonstrated and there may be fluid–fluid levels within the multilocular cysts.

DERMOIDS

These present as palpable masses and lie in the midline of the skull. On radiographs there is a well-demarcated lucency of the skull vault (Figure 12.2.11) as the lesions cause pressure erosion of the tables. They may involve both inner and outer tables, which can be seen in a tangential view but is much better assessed by thin-slice CT. Imaging is required before removal to ensure that there is no intracranial extension and to identify the relationship of the lesion to the underlying venous sinuses. This is best done with MRI.

Angular dermoids occur at the angle of the eye and are discussed in the section on the orbits.

EPIDERMOIDS

These are small masses that occur in young children but are not present at birth. They occur anywhere in the skull vault bones (Figure 12.2.12) and are often an incidental finding on radiographs done for trauma. They have a characteristic appearance with a central lucency and a fine though dense sclerotic margin. They do not erode the inner table. This can be confirmed by ultrasound (US).

LANGERHANS' CELL HISTIOCYTOSIS

This frequently involves the skull vault (Figure 12.2.13) and may present clinically with a palpable mass or may be discovered during the work-up of a patient. The lesions may be single or multiple. They are destructive lesions within the diploic spaces, but often involve both tables, are poorly defined and when large may coalesce. Localized extradural extension is frequent. The appearance is often described as a geographical appearance. With repair the edges become sclerotic. The mastoid is most frequently involved followed by the orbits, maxilla and mandible. Intracranial involvement of the pituitary gland causes diabetes insipidus. Symmetrical regions of abnormal signal may occur in the white matter of the cerebellar hemispheres, which may be interpreted as a demyelinating disease. These areas have low signal on T1-weighted (T1-W) and high signal on T2-weighted (T2-W) images.

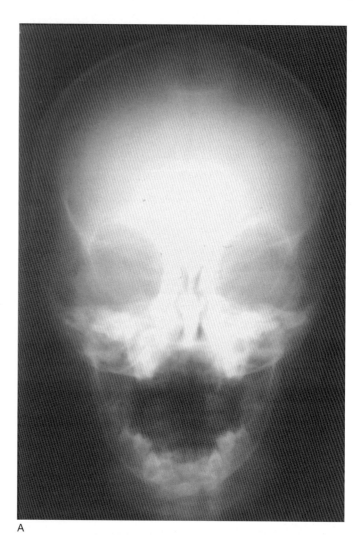

A

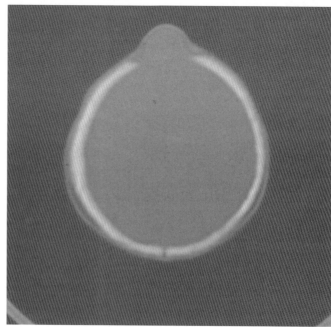

B

Figure 12.2.11 (A) Frontal radiograph and (B) axial CT scan of typical location and appearance of dermoid cyst. Note on the radiograph the central midline defect and associated soft tissue mass. The CT scan shows the dermoid cyst, which lies very close to the sagittal sinus.

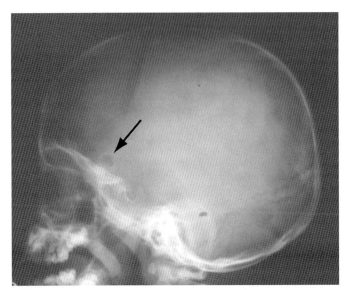

Figure 12.2.12 Lateral radiograph of the skull showing a radiolucent lesion with sclerotic margins above the sphenoidal wing typical of an epidermoid.

MALIGNANT PROCESSES AFFECTING THE SKULL

Malignant processes that affect the skull are leukaemia (Figure 12.2.14), neuroblastoma metastases, rhabdomyosarcoma, osteosarcoma, Ewing's sarcoma and, rarely, melanotic neuroectodermal tumour or progonoma. Other malignant tumours of the skull in children are excessively rare and are the subject of individual case reports or cancer registers and are not discussed here.

LEUKAEMIA AND NEUROBLASTOMA

These deposits have a predilection for the cranial sutures where they cause widening. These are easily differentiated from the suture widening of raised intracranial pressure by the associated clinical history and a degree of osteopenia. They may also cause destructive lesions anywhere in the skull.

LYMPHOMA OF BONE

This may rarely present in the skull vault. When it does the lesion tends to be sclerotic and there may be extension into the meninges. Primary meningeal involvement, if it extends superficially, is more likely to cause destructive lesions.

OSTEOSARCOMA AND EWING'S SARCOMA

These have similar appearances in the skull as elsewhere, that is mixed bone-forming and destructive lesions. They may have a

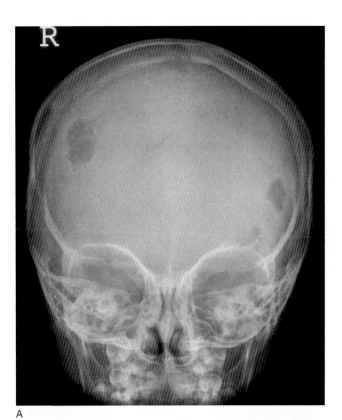

A

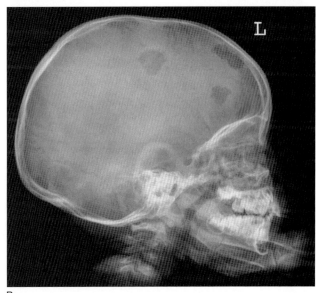

B

Figure 12.2.13 (A) AP and (B) Lateral radiographs of a child showing typical lytic lesions of histiocytosis.

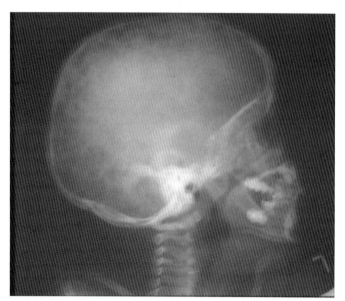

Figure 12.2.14 Lateral skull radiograph showing poorly defined destructive lesions typical of leukaemia or neuroblastoma. This child had leukaemia.

large extradural intracranial component. It is the location of the tumour in an unexpected location that causes confusion initially. Histology is required for tissue diagnosis but cross-sectional imaging suggests a primary bone tumour.

RHABDOMYOSARCOMA

This is the most frequent sarcoma in the skull. It may affect the facial bones, mastoid, orbit, the nasopharynx and the soft tissues. Clinical presentation is usually with a mass with or without associated pain depending on what adjacent structures it involves. Nasal or nasopharyngeal lesions may present with a blocked nose. It is mainly a soft tissue mass with secondary bone destruction. Any of the cell types may be present. The prognosis is poor compared to lesions elsewhere in the body. There is a high incidence of recurrence. The differential diagnosis is lymphoma and nasopharyngeal carcinoma, discussed in Chapter 14. Imaging is with CT and MRI. CT displays the extent of bone destruction and MRI the relationship to the meninges and brain. The mass is of intermediate signal on T1-W and high signal on T2-W images with moderate enhancement with gadolinium. Imaging must be performed in at least axial and coronal planes and should be performed in accordance with the tumour protocols.

MELANOTIC NEUROECTODERMAL TUMOUR

This is a rare tumour that typically arises from the maxilla in the first year of life but may arise from any part of the skull. It is a rapidly growing soft tissue mass with erosion of the skull and extradural intracranial extension. Because of the melanin content, the tumour may have high signal on T1-W and low signal on

T2-W images. Though locally invasive, the prognosis is good if there is complete excision.

CRANIOSYNOSTOSIS

Craniosynostosis is defined by a premature fusion of one or multiple cranial sutures. The frequency is 1 in 2100 births. In the vast majority of cases, this premature closure of the cranial sutures appears during the prenatal life, and the resulting craniofacial deformity is usually obvious at birth. Raised intracranial pressure is uncommon in single suture stenosis. This phenomenon depends on the type and number of sutures involved. Chronic increased intracranial pressure, resulting from a discrepancy between the brain growth and the restrained skull growth, has to be recognized as soon as possible in order to avoid intellectual or sensorial (visual) consequences.

Craniostenoses are usually isolated and sporadic, but familial forms are known. Syndromic forms are represented by the craniofaciosynostosis family, like Crouzon syndrome, Apert syndrome, Saethre–Chotzen syndrome and Pfeiffer syndrome. Recent work in the field of molecular genetics has provided some explanation for the origin of craniosynostosis. Numerous studies have demonstrated the involvement of fibroblast growth factor receptor (FGFR) and TWIST genes mutations in craniosynostoses, and not only in syndromic forms. However, the pathogenesis is only partly understood. The expressivity among subjects with the same mutations, within the same family, is not always the same: phenotypes can be numerous, ranging from a mild subnormal appearance to extremely abnormal craniofacial morphology. Furthermore, mutations within the same gene can result in several different craniofacial syndromes and, conversely, mutations in different genes can result in the same collection of clinical features and identical diagnoses (Table 12.2.2).

CLINICAL AND RADIOLOGICAL DIAGNOSIS

The clinical analysis of the deformity of the skull or the face is generally sufficient to recognize the pathology. Premature closure of a suture is responsible for an increased cranial diameter parallel to the pathological suture, and a decrease of the perpendicular diameter (Virchow statement). Thus, several morphological forms are known: scaphocephaly resulting in the premature fusion of the sagittal suture, trigonocephaly caused by metopic synostosis, brachycephaly involving both coronal sutures, plagiocephaly caused by unilateral coronal synostosis, and oxycephaly with fusion of both longitudinal and transversal suture.

Table 12.2.2 Gene mutations to craniosynostoses

Craniosynostosis	*Gene mutation*
Crouzon syndrome	*FGFR2*/(*FGFR3* + *Acanthosis nigrans*)
Pfeiffer syndrome	*FGFR1* (Pro252Arg)/*FRFG2*
Apert syndrome	*FGFR2* (Ser252Trp, Pro253Arg)
Saethre–Chotzen syndrome	*TWIST*
Coronal syndrome	*FGFR3* (Pro250Arg)

Table 12.2.3 Main brain malformations associated with craniosynostoses

Craniosynostosis type	Intracranial-associated malformations
Scaphocephaly	Non-specific
Bi-coronal synostosis	Non-specific
Uni-coronal synostosis	Non-specific
Trigonocephaly (metopic synostosis)	Corpus callosum agenesia
Lambdoid synostosis	Non-specific
Crouzon syndrome/Pfeiffer syndrome	Hydrocephalus (40%), Chiari-like malformation (70%)
Apert syndrome	Ventriculomegaly, corpus callosum agenesia, septum pellucidum cyst

The goals of the imaging investigation are multiple:

- to affirm or confirm the synostosis;
- to identify the cerebral consequences;
- to detect associated intracranial malformations (especially in syndromic forms) (Table 12.2.3); and
- to exclude other diseases such as secondary cranial deformity, hydrocephalus, microcephaly and postural deformity.

Postural deformity is frequent in neurologically impaired and premature infants and is a result of remaining in the same position for long periods of time.

IMAGING

Several imaging techniques can be used to study craniosynostosis:

- skull radiographs with AP and lateral (and Worms–Bretton) views;
- CT scan with bone and cerebral windows and 3D CT reconstruction;

- MRI and MR angiography; and
- Skeletal x-rays to exclude other malformation, and ultrasonography of the heart and kidney, as appropriate.

The indications for each of these investigations are summarized in a decision algorithm (Figure 12.2.15).

COMMON RADIOLOGICAL FEATURES

On x-rays, the diagnosis is based on the analysis of the cranial vault, of the sutures and of the cranial base.

A CT scan shows the extent of deformity of the pathological suture(s) and allows better assessment of the skull base deformity. A CT scan is necessary to assess any associated cerebral malformation (Table 12.2.3). MRI is sometimes needed to precisely determine cerebral problems. The CT scan may be performed using a low-dose technique.

The following radiological features may be found:

- Modifications of the pathological suture(s). On x-rays, the suture is absent on the whole of its length or is replaced by a thin, dense line. Sometimes, the diagnosis is not so obvious: the synostosed suture at the early fibrous stage can be radiolucent. Therefore, sutural inactivity signs can be sought, e.g. the linear appearance of the suture seems too narrow or there is sclerosis of the edges of the suture. A CT scan shows the thickening of the synostotic suture. Three-dimensional CT reconstructions can also demonstrate all these features but are not mandatory.
- Modifications of the patent sutures. The other sutures can also be modified by sutural hyperactivity: a widening and increased broken-line aspect of the suture may be seen.
- Associated signs of elevated intracranial pressure, such as bone erosions.
- 'Copper beating': increased skull markings, sometimes called a 'copper beaten' appearance, are frequent with craniosynostosis

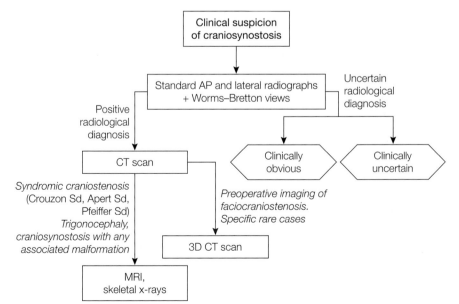

Figure 12.2.15 Algorithm for imaging investigations in craniostenosis.

and may, but do not necessarily, reflect raised intracranial pressure.

- Diminution of the posterior fossa volume may cause downward herniation of the cerebellar tonsils and brainstem, producing in some cases secondary hydrocephalus or syringomyelia.

SPECIFIC RADIOLOGICAL FEATURES

SCAPHOCEPHALY AND TRIGONOCEPHALY

Scaphocephaly or sagittal synostosis is the most frequent form of craniosynostosis, and is clinically diagnosed by identifying the transversally narrowed and longitudinally elongated skull. Radiographs show:

- on the lateral view, horizontalization of the skull base, lengthening of the anterior part (Figure 12.2.16) of the skull base

and digital impressions on parietal bones localized posteriorly; and

- on the frontal view, flattening of both parietal bones and a thick median sagittal crest.

A CT scan demonstrates the features of the skull shape. The brain usually conforms to the skull and is otherwise normal. Increased volume of anterior subarachnoid spaces is frequent.

Trigonocephaly or metopic synostosis is diagnosed clinically by a triangular forehead appearance (Figure 12.2.17) (obvious on axial views). Laterally, the forehead is flattened and medially, the metopic crest bulges. Hypotelorism is constant. On x-rays, the main sign is the upward/medial angled deformity of the orbits, producing a racoon-eye appearance (Figure 12.2.17B). Trigonocephaly is more frequently associated with chromosomal abnormality (chromosomes 7, 9, 11, 13) than the other craniosynostoses. It has been described in cases of prenatal valproic acid exposure.

In scaphocephaly and trigonocephaly, MRI should be routinely performed in order to detect brain malformations (Table 12.2.3).

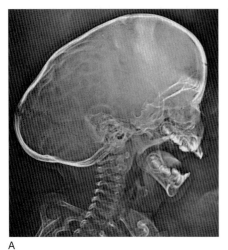

A

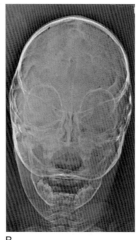

B

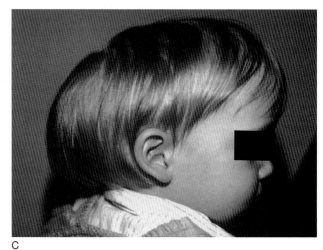

C

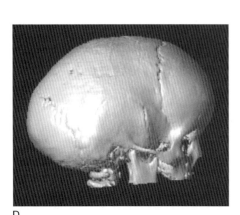

D

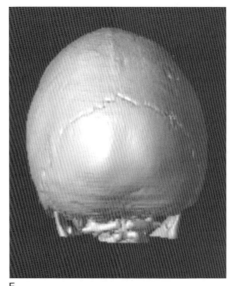

E

Figure 12.2.16 Lateral (A) and (B) frontal view of a child with scaphocephaly secondary to sagittal suture stenosis; (C) photograph of a child showing the typical shape of the head. (D) 3D reconstruction of another child with sagittal suture stenosis showing the typical cranial configuration. (E) 3D reconstruction shows patent lambdoid suture but fused sagittal suture, shown as a ridge centrally.

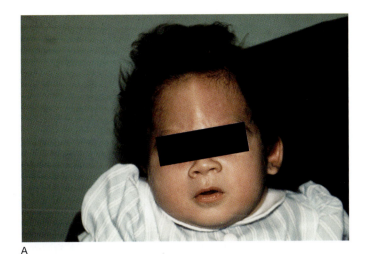

A

BRACHYCEPHALY

In brachycephaly or bilateral coronal synostosis, the sagittal diameter of the skull is diminished with a short, flat and sometimes concave forehead (Figure 12.2.18) and the transverse diameter is increased with bulging temporal bones. The superior development of the skull can give a turricephalic form. On the frontal views, upward displacement of the lesser wings of the sphenoid bone is significant and gives a 'mephistophelic' deformity of the orbits.

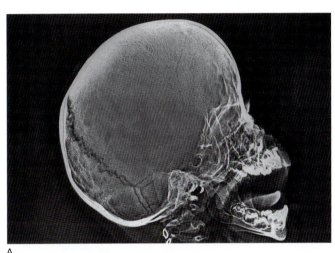

A

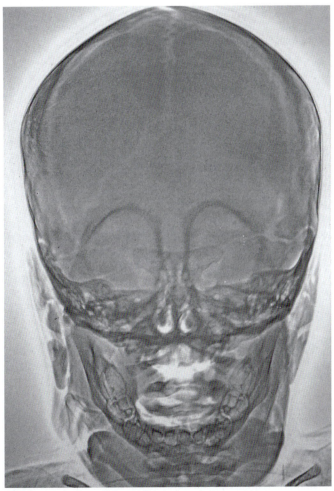

B

Figure 12.2.17 (A) Photograph and (B) frontal radiograph of a child with trigonocephaly. The photograph shows the bulging metopic crest with flattening of the forehead on either side. The radiograph shows the characteristic medial displacement of the orbits, which are closer together than normal due to hypotelorism. They also have adopted a vertical shape.

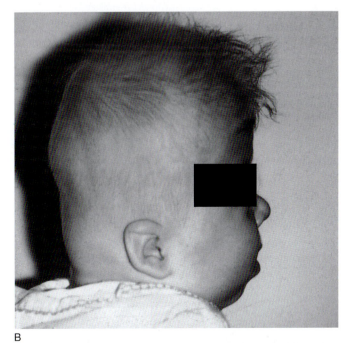

B

Figure 12.2.18 (A) Lateral radiograph and (B) lateral photograph of a child with bilateral coronal sutural stenosis. There is flattening of the forehead and elongation of the height of the skull. Note the absence of the sutures on the radiograph compared with the lambdoid sutures. The photograph shows the typical skull shape.

PLAGIOCEPHALY

Plagiocephaly or unilateral coronal synostosis confers an impressive asymmetrical aspect (Figure 12.2.19) to the face and skull: regression and flattening of the ipsilateral part of the forehead, deviation of the nose to the other side and facial scoliosis.

On imaging, there is elevation of the ipsilateral upper outer margin of the orbit (lesser wing of the sphenoid bone) and of the pterion, on the frontal views. The skull base is also involved with anterior displacement of the lesser wing of the sphenoid bone, temporal bulging and anterior displacement of the petrous bone.

LAMBDOID SYNOSTOSIS

Unilateral synostosis of the lambdoid suture (or posterior plagiocephaly) occurs rarely and must not be confused with postural or functional plagiocephaly (without any lambdoid sutural fusion, which is much more frequent). There is ipsilateral parieto-occipital flattening with compensatory temporal vaulting and, on the other side, occipital bulging. The diagnosis is made on standard skull radiographs, where the fusion of the suture can be easily seen (Figure 12.2.20).

Pachycephaly or bilateral lambdoid synostosis is also very infrequent. The main feature is the acute angle of the posterior skull – the term 'coup the serpe' (cut by a scythe) is used by the French to describe this acute angle (Figure 12.2.21). On x-rays, both lambdoid sutures have completely disappeared.

OXYCEPHALY OR SYNOSTOSIS OF BOTH CORONAL AND SAGITTAL SUTURES

The diagnosis for this condition is often made later than the other craniosynostoses, usually after the age of 1 year. This craniosynostosis is more common in the North African population. The forehead is flattened and oblique in a superior and posterior orientation. The skull is pointed with the bregma at the highest point of the skull. Proptosis is almost constant. Digital impressions ('copper beating') are very frequent and diffuse.

SYNDROMIC CRANIOSYNOSTOSES

These involve craniosynostosis and facial abnormalities and in some cases, there is malformation of the hands and feet.

CROUZON SYNDROME

This is an autosomal dominant syndrome of craniosynostosis and maxillary hypoplasia with reverse crossbite. Craniosynostosis is variable and often progressive. In most cases, both coronal sutures are involved (Figure 12.2.22). The facial abnormality is not always diagnosed at birth and is discovered later as the face grows. The ocular proptosis can be very impressive. Hypertelorism is almost constant. Hypodevelopment of the maxillary bone can be responsible for sleep apnoea. Hands and feet are normal. A chronic herniation of the cerebellar tonsils (Chiari-like malformation) and hydrocephalus must be systematically searched for on the MRI (Table 12.2.3).

APERT SYNDROME

This syndrome is described as an acrocephalosyndactyly, involving a bilateral coronal synostosis (brachycephaly), and osseous and membranous fingers and toes (syndactyly). Ocular proptosis, hypertelorism, strabismus, down-slanting lids, maxillary hypoplasia and mental retardation are other characteristics of this syndrome (Figure 12.2.23). Cleft palate, C5–C6 vertebral fusion, intracranial malformations, such as agenesis of the corpus callosum, cyst of the septum pellucidum and non-progressive ventriculomegaly are also described (Table 12.2.3).

CLOVER LEAF SKULL

Multiple stenosis of all sutures leads to ballooning of the thin bones between sutures giving a 'clover leaf' deformity (Figure 12.2.24).

PFEIFFER SYNDROME

This syndrome includes craniosynostosis involving variable sutures, and hands and feet anomalies, such as broad thumbs or medially deviated great toes (Table 12.2.3).

SAETHRE–CHOTZEN SYNDROME

This syndrome includes variable craniosynostosis (mostly bicoronal) with facial characteristics (eyelid ptosis, crux cymbae), membranous syndactylies and wide duplicated great toes.

IMAGING AND FOLLOW-UP

Most of the diagnosed craniosynostoses require surgical treatment. Imaging is required for the postsurgical follow-up, e.g. to assess the bone reconstitution, to verify absence of recurrence of the treated fused suture and to check for fusion of other sutures in children with clinically progressive craniosynostosis.

Sometimes, especially in some cases of mild scaphocephaly, simple observation of the child is the management. In such cases, clinical examination and regular radiographs may be performed to rule out evidence of developing increased intracranial pressure.

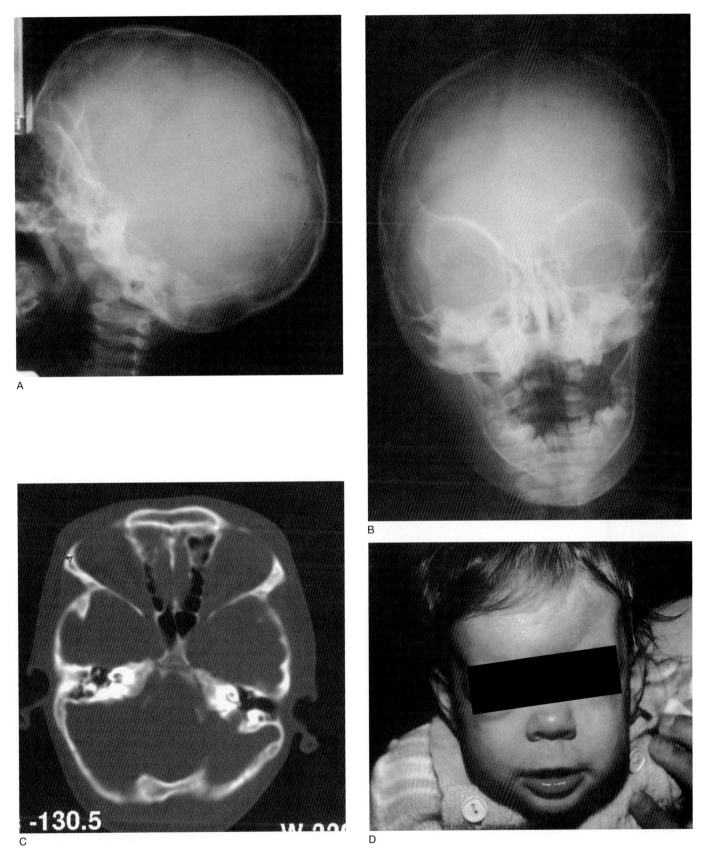

Figure 12.2.19 (A) Lateral radiograph (B) frontal radiograph of children with unilateral coronal suture stenosis. Note on the lateral radiograph the density of the stenosed suture and the asymmetry of the sphenoidal wings. On the frontal view, the elevation of the lateral aspect of the right orbit is typical. (C) Axial CT slice of the skull base showing the secondary asymmetry caused by the coronal suture stenosis. (D) Photograph of a child with the typical facial appearances.

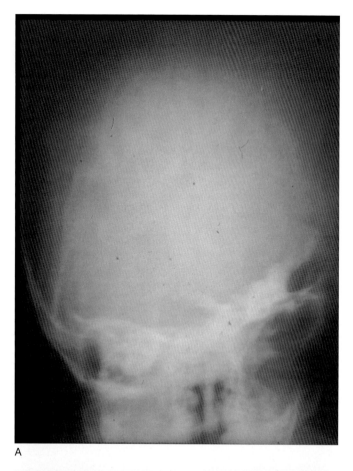

A

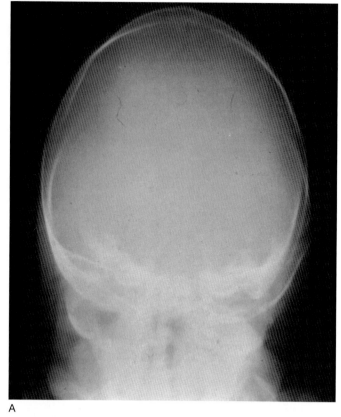

A

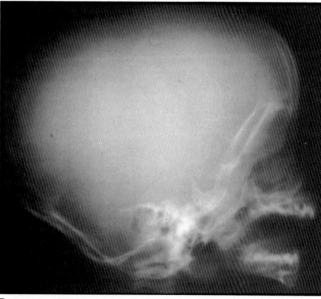

B

Figure 12.2.20 (A) Towne's view and (B) lateral view of a child with plagiocephaly due to unilateral lambdoid suture stenosis on the right. Note the asymmetry of the skull secondary to this.

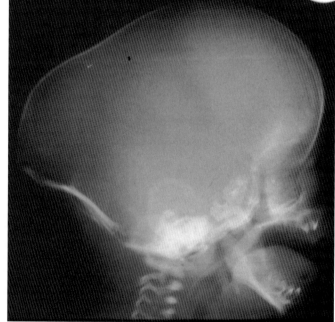

B

Figure 12.2.21 (A) Towne's and (B) lateral view of the typical configuration of bilateral lambdoid suture stenosis. Note the flattening of the occiput underneath the posterior fontanelle. This is typical of this condition.

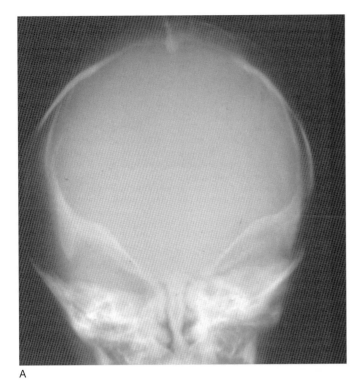

A

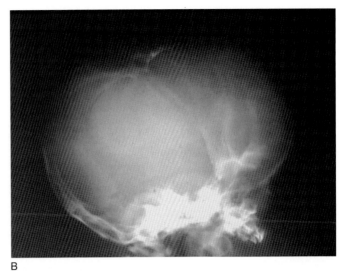

B

Figure 12.2.22 (A) Frontal and (B) lateral view of a child with Crouzon syndrome. There is stenosis of the sagittal and coronal sutures with some localized thinning of the skull. Note the density of the stenosed sutures near the skull vertex. The typical harlequin shape of the eyes is well seen.

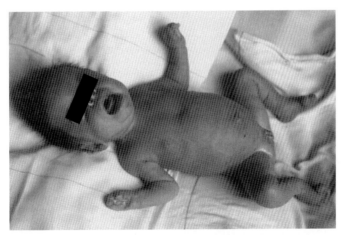

Figure 12.2.23 Photograph showing the typical changes of Apert syndrome. Note the syndactyly of the fingers and toes and the abnormal skull shape due to the coronal suture stenosis.

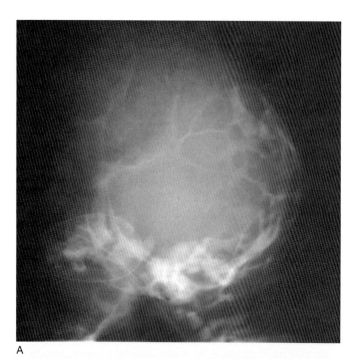

A

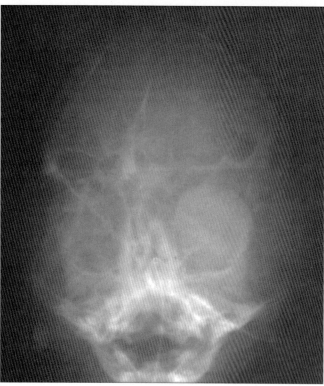

B

Figure 12.2.24 (A) Lateral and (B) frontal view of skull in a child with clover leaf skull due to multiple sutural stenosis. The opacity in the left orbit is due to gross proptosis. Note the ballooning of the membranous skull vault outwards between the stenosed sutures.

FURTHER READING

Anderson PF, Hall CM, Evans RD et al. The hands in Saethre-Chotzen syndrome. Journal of Craniofacial Genetic Developmental Biology 1996; 16:228–233.

Anderson PJ, Hall CM, Evans RD et al. The cervical spine in Saethre-Chotzen syndrome. Cleft Palate and Craniofacial Journal 1997; 34:79–82.

Anderson PJ, Hall CM, Evans RD et al. The feet in Pfeiffer's syndrome. Journal of Craniofacial Surgery 1998; 9:83–87.

Cinalli G, Sainte-Rose C, Kollar EM et al. Hydrocephalus and craniosynostosis. Journal of Neurosurgery 1998; 88:209–214.

Fernbach SK, Feinstein KA. Radiologic evaluation of the child with craniosynostosis. Neurosurgery Clinics of North America 1991; 2:569–585.

Huang MH et al. The differential diagnosis of abnormal head shapes: separating craniosynostosis from positional deformities and normal variants. Cleft Palate and Craniofacial Journal 1998; 35: 204–211.

Kreiborg S, Cohen MM Jr. Characteristics of the infant Apert skull and its subsequent development. Journal of Craniofacial Genetic Development Biology 1990; 10:399–410.

Lejeunie E, Barcik U, Thorne JA et al. Craniosynostosis and fetal exposure to sodium valproate. Journal of Neurosurgery 2001; 95:778–792.

Lajeunie E, Cameron R, El Ghouzzi V et al. Clinical variability in patients with Apert's syndrome. Journal of Neurosurgery 1999; 90:443–447.

Lajeunie E, Le Merrer M, Marchac D, Renier D. Syndromal and nonsyndromal primary trigonocephaly: analysis of a series of 237 patients. American Journal of Medical Genetics 1998; 75:211–215.

Lo JL, Marsh JL, Pilgrim TK, Vannier MW. Plagiocephaly: differential diagnosis based on endocranial morphology. Plastic and Reconstructive Surgery 1996; 97:282–291.

Marchac D, Renier D. Craniofacial Surgery for Craniosynostosis. Boston: Little, Brown & Co. 1982; p. 125.

Marchac D, Renier D. Faciocraniosynostosis: from infancy to adulthood. Childs Nervous System 1996; 12:669–677.

Muenke M et al. A unique point mutation in the fibroblast growth factor receptor 3 gene (FGFR3) defines a new craniosynostosis syndrome. American Journal of Human Genetics 1997; 60:555–564.

Persing JA, Jane JA, Shaffey M. Virchow and the pathogenesis of craniosynostosis: a translation of his original work. Plastic and Reconstructive Surgery 1989; 83:738–742.

Renier D, Lajeunie E, Arnaud E, Marchac D. Management of craniosynostoses. Childs Nervous System 2000; 16:645–658.

Swischuk LE. Imaging of the newborn, infant, and young child, 4th edn. Maryland: Williams & Wilkins; 1997.

Taybi H, Lachman R. Radiology of syndromes, metabolic disorders, and skeletal dysplasias. Year Book Medical Publishers Inc.; 1990.

Thompson DN, Harkness W, Jones BM et al. Aetiology of herniation of the hindbrain in craniosynostosis. An investigation incorporating intracranial pressure monitoring and magnetic resonance imaging. Pediatric Neurosurgery 1997; 26:288–295.

Thompson DN, Slaney SF, Hall CM et al. Congenital cervical spinal fusion: a study in Apert syndrome. Pediatric Neurosurgery 1995; 25:20–27.

Tokumary AM, Barkovich AJ, Ciricillo SF, Edwards MS. Skull base and calvarial deformities: association with intracranial changes in craniofacial syndromes. American Journal of Neuroradiology 1996; 17:619–630.

Vannier MW, Hildebolt CF, Marsh JL, Pilgrim TK et al. Craniosynostosis: diagnostic value of three-dimensional CT reconstruction. Radiology 1989; 173:669–673.

Imaging Brain Maturation

Nadine Girard

INTRODUCTION

Brain maturation is characterized by changes in brain morphology, which are illustrated by fetal brain imaging and by changes in brain composition; these are demonstrated by brain imaging in both the pre- and postnatal periods. Maturation of the brain begins in the second trimester and continues progressively to reach an adult-like pattern at approximately 2 years of age. Consequences of brain maturation are characterized by different windows of brain vulnerability and different diseases in infants and neonates compared to older children and adults. Although ultrasonography (US) and computer tomography (CT) can show the changes in brain morphology, these techniques are insensitive to myelination, which is one of the most important events occurring during brain maturation. Magnetic resonance imaging (MRI) is currently the method of choice to evaluate brain maturation.

FURTHER READING

Baierl P, Forster Ch, Fendel H, Naegele M, Fink U, Kenn W. Magnetic resonance imaging of normal and pathological white matter maturation. Pediatric Radiology 1988; 18:183–189.

Barkovich AJ, Kyos HC, Jackson DE, Norman D. Normal maturation of the neonatal and infant brains: MR imaging at 1.5 T. Radiology 1988; 166: 173–180.

Barkovich AJ. Pediatric neuroimaging, 3rd edn. Philadelphia: Lippincott Williams and Wilkins; 2000.

Boujraf S, Luypaert R, Shabana W et al. Study of pediatric brain development using magnetic resonance imaging of anisotropic diffusion. Magnetic Resonance Imaging 2002; 20:327–336.

Brody BA, Kinney HC, Kloman AS, Gilles FH. Sequence of central nervous system myelination in human infancy I : An autopsy study of myelination. Journal of Neuropathology and Experimental Neurology 1987; 46:283–301.

Girard N, Raybaud C, DuLac P. MRI study of brain myelination. Journal of Neuroradiology 1991; 18:291–307.

Kinney HC, Brody BA, Kloman AS, Gilles FH. Sequence of central nervous system myelination in human infancy. II. Patterns of myelination in autopsied infants. Journal of Neuropathology and Experimental Neurology 1988; 47:217–234.

Kinney HC, Armstrong DD. Perinatal neuropathology. In: Graham DI, Lantos PL (eds). Greenfield's neuropathology, 6th edn. London: Arnold; 1997:537–599.

Kinney HC, Karthigasan J, Borenshteyn NI, Flax JD, Kirschner DA. Myelination in the developing human brain: Biochemical correlates. Neurochemical Research 1994; 19:983–996.

Paus T, Collins DL, Evans AC et al. Maturation of white matter in the human brain: A review of magnetic resonance studies. Brain Research Bulletin 2001; 54:255–266.

Raybaud C, Girard N. Cerebral development and MRI. In: Garreau B (ed.) Neuroimaging in child neuropsychiatric disorders. Berlin: Springer-Verlag; 1998:59–88.

Van Der Knaap MS, Valk J. Magnetic resonance of myelin, myelination and myelin disorders, 2nd edn. Heidelberg: Springer-Verlag; 1995.

Volpe JJ. Neurology of the newborn, 3rd edn. Philadelphia: W.B. Saunders; 1995:675–729.

MRI TECHNIQUES

The most important factor in obtaining high-quality MR images is a still patient. This may require sedation or general anaesthesia, dependent on local hospital practice. In neonates, sedation is generally not necessary because immobility can be obtained by wrapping the baby in an air bag. Feeding can help by achieving sleep.

Parameters of the MR sequences have to be adapted to the brain composition of young infants especially for T2-weighted images (WI). Indeed the T1 values of brain structures are much higher than those seen in adults so that longer repetition time (TR) and echo time (TE) of T2-weighted images are necessary to evaluate adequately brain maturation compared to older children and adults. Heavily T2-weighted sequences are used in infants less than 12 months old. We routinely used a turbo spin echo sequence with a TR of 7500 ms and a TE of 163 ms. Fast spin echo techniques are known to provide similar information on myelination in a shorter time than the conventional spin echo sequences.

Fluid attenuated inversion recovery (FLAIR) sequences are considered highly efficient to look for regions of abnormal T2 prolongation. However, in young infants, FLAIR images are not very useful when looking for normal brain maturation probably because the standard sequence is not adapted to the infant brain composition. We do not use flair images in young infants because the time of inversion (TI) is unsustainable.

T1-weighted images can be obtained through spin echo (SE), turbo spin echo (TSE) and gradient echo (GE) sequences. We routinely use GE T1-weighted images because of excellent grey-white matter differentiation, especially in infants less than 6 months old. A three-dimensional GE T1-weighted sequence is also used in older infants allowing 1.2 mm contiguous slices, which can be reconstructed in any anatomical plane.

Inversion recovery (IR) sequences can also be used for T1-weighted images and give excellent images. We now routinely use this type of sequence in infants with the high resolution head coil (in which eight canals detect the signal).

High-resolution head coils are now available from some manufacturers and the parameters of each type of sequence we use are summarized in Table 12.3.1.

In neonates, T1 and T2 WI are obtained in three planes. In young infants, axial and coronal T2, sagittal and axial T1, coronal flair and IR images are routinely used. In older infants (beyond 6 months old), three-dimensional T1 WI are usually required.

Diffusion-weighted images are used mostly to look for pathology such as hypoxic-ischaemic changes. However, anisotropic changes can be seen in white matter tracts of the normal neonatal brain, tracts in which myelin is not detected with conventional T1 and T2 sequences.

Hydrogen MR spectroscopy can also be used to assess brain maturation. Spectroscopy is used mostly to look for pathology. A monovoxel technique with short and long TE is used with the high-resolution head coil. Parameters of the short echo sequence are characterized by a TR of 1500 ms, a TE of 30 ms and 128 acquisitions. Parameters of the long echo sequence are characterized by a TR of 1500 ms, a TE of 135 ms and 192 acquisitions. Peaks of N-acetylaspartate (NAA) and creatine increase along with brain maturation whereas choline and myoinositol peaks decrease. Peaks of glutamine and glutamate also decrease with brain maturation (Figure 12.3.1).

FURTHER READING

Girard N, Gambarelli D. Normal fetal brain. In: Brunelle F, Shaw D (eds). Magnetic resonance imaging. An atlas with anatomic correlations. Rickmansworth Brunelle & Shaw; 2001.

Girard N, Raybaud C, Gambarelli D. Pediatric neuroimaging : Fetal MR imaging. In: Demaerel PH (ed.). Recent advances in diagnostic neuroradiology. Berlin: Springer-Verlag; 2001:373–398.

Table 12.3.1 Parameters of the sequences used postnatally in the authors' experience

	TR (ms)	TE (ms)	TI (ms)	Flip angle	Matrix
T1 WI					
2D	345	4.98	–	90	512
3D	1520	4.48	920	15	512
T2 WI	7500	128	–	160	512
Neonate	7500	163	–	160	512
IR	7200	64	350	180	512
FLAIR	9000	115	2200	180	256
Diffusion	3200	94			128

TR, repetition time; TE, echo time; TI, time of inversion; WI, weighted images; IR, inversion recovery; FLAIR, fluid attenuated inversion recovery.

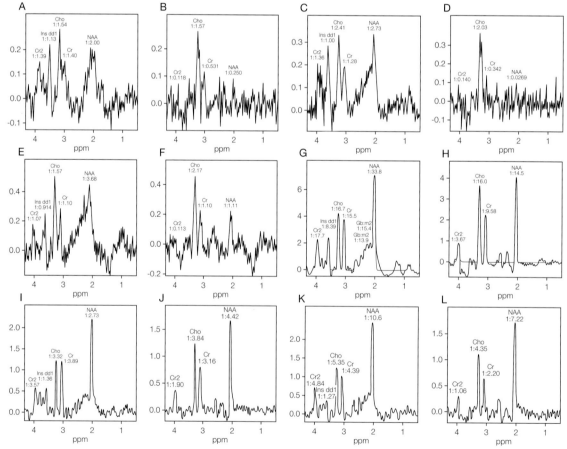

Figure 12.3.1 *In utero* spectra with short and long echo time obtained at 29 weeks (A,B), 33 weeks (C,D), 39 weeks (E,F). Postnatal spectra obtained at 7 months (G,H), 18 months (I,J) and 5 years (K,L). Short echo time (A,C,E,G,I,K) and long echo time (B,D,F,H,J,L).

Girard N, Raybaud C, Gambarelli D, Figarella-Branger D. Fetal brain MR imaging. Magnetic Resonance Imaging Clinics of North America 2001; 9:19–56.

Huppi SP, Posse S, Lazeyras F et al. Magnetic resonance in preterm and term newborns: 1H-spectroscopy in developing human brain. Pediatric Research 1991; 30:574–578.

Kato T, Nishina M, Matsushita K et al. Neuronal maturation and N-acetyl-L-aspartic acid development in human fetal and child brains. Brain Development 1997; 19:131–133.

Kreis R, Ernst T, Ross BD. Development of the human brain: In vivo quantification of metabolite and water content with proton magnetic resonance spectroscopy. Magnetic Resonance Medicine 1993; 30:424–437.

Le Bas JF, Esteve F, Grand S et al. Magnetic resonance spectroscopy and brain diseases: clinical applications. Journal of Neuroradiology 1998; 25:55–69.

Prayer D, Prayer L. Diffusion-weighted magnetic resonance imaging of cerebral white matter development. European Journal of Radiology 2003; 45:235–243.

Prenger EC, Beckett WB, Kollias SS, Ball WB. Comparison of T2-weighted spin-echo and fast spin-echo techniques in the evaluation of myelination. Journal of Magnetic Resonance Imaging 1994; 4:179–184.

Raybaud C, Girard N. Cerebral development and MRI. In: Garreau B (ed.). Neuroimaging in child neuropsychiatric disorders. Berlin: Springer-Verlag; 1998:59–88.

Vion-Dury J, Salvan AM, Confort-Gouny S, Cozzone PJ. Atlas of brain proton magnetic resonance spectra. Part I: General and methodological considerations. Journal of Neuroradiology 1998; 25:207–212.

IMAGING TECHNIQUES *IN UTERO*

Although ultrasonography is currently considered as the primary imaging method for routine examination of the fetal brain, MRI is highly accurate in illustrating the morphological changes of the developing brain as well as fetal brain abnormalities and thus constitutes a useful procedure when ultrasonography is inconclusive. Fetal MRI is widely used in both neuroradiology and paediatric radiology units. With the development in fast imaging, fetal MRI is useful in prenatal diagnosis. Experimental studies have shown no side effects for the embryo.

As MRI examinations are increasingly used in pregnancy, normal brain maturation of the developing fetal brain has to be understood so that brain abnormalities can be detected as early as possible during the pregnancy. Sedation of the mother in order to sedate the fetus and reduce movement is now not always necessary with the advent of T2-weighted sequences, which can be obtained in 30 s. T1-weighted images of good quality require longer sequences (from 1 to 3 min), so sedation of the mother is often necessary in order to obtain a complete evaluation of the brain including T1- and T2-weighted images as in the neonatal period. In breech presentation or in a transverse lie position, the fetal head moves with the mother's breathing. Fetal sedation is obtained by maternal premedication administered orally 15 min to 1 h before the MRI examination.

Image quality from *in utero* studies can be affected by a low signal-to-noise ratio related to the coil used, the fetal position and the fetal movement. In contrast to the neonatal period there is no coil devoted to the fetal brain itself. Images are obtained using a body coil alone or in combination with a surface coil. Consequently, high-resolution MRI (that is 3D T1-weighted acquisition of 1-mm-thick sections) is not possible *in utero* as it is in the neonatal period. On the other hand, 3D T2-weighted sequence (true fisp sequence) is possible *in utero* allowing 1.6-mm-thick contiguous sections, which are extremely helpful in evaluating the midline as well as the cortical sulcation.

Ultrasound is usually sufficient to ensure an accurate diagnosis of a structural brain abnormality before week 18–20 so *in vivo* MRI is usually performed during the second half of gestation (from 18 weeks on). Images are obtained routinely in sagittal, coronal and axial planes relative to the fetal head with both T1- and T2-weighted sequences. The coronal plane used is the plane following the axis of the brainstem. Axial images are obtained along the fronto-occipital axis of the cerebral hemispheres. The plane coursing from the anterior to the posterior commissures (that is the axial plane generally used postnatally) is difficult to obtain *in utero*.

For T1-weighted images, SE, TSE and GE images can be obtained. Gradient echo images (FLASH sequence, i.e. fast low angle shot) are used because of excellent differentiation between the cortical ribbon, the white matter and the ventricular walls compared with TSE images. Fetal head contrast can be improved on the 1.5 Tesla magnet by adding two bands of saturation that are positioned on the maternal subcutaneous fat of the abdominal wall and of the lower back, by using gradient echo images with fat saturation in order to suppress the signal from peritoneal fat.

Regarding T2 WI, TSE, HASTE images can be obtained. HASTE (half-Fourier single shot turbo spin echo) images are available only with a magnet of high-gradient strength and are acquired much more quickly than TSE images: about 2 s for each slice, i.e. 30 s for 15 slices. Images obtained from HASTE sequences are true T2-weighted images with low susceptibility weighting and sequential slice capability. This last advantage improves the management of fetal movement. The low susceptibility is in one way an advantage giving a very high contrast of the layering of the developing brain; in an other way, it is a disadvantage because of the difficulty in depicting old haemorrhage. Haste images with a matrix of 512 can currently be obtained: they give excellent identification of the parenchymal layering and have low chemical shift artifacts compared with haste images with a matrix of 256.

Other sequences can be used in special circumstances. Angiographic images are obtained at the Hopital Nord, Marseille by a sequential 2D FLASH sequence, which allows a good compromise between vascular and tissue contrast; inversion recovery images allow a very good delineation of the cortical ribbon, of the extra-cerebral spaces and, consequently, of lesions arising from the sub-arachnoid spaces.

Diffusion images (echo planar images) can also be performed as in the neonatal period to detect cytotoxic and/or vasogenic oedema. The acute response of the fetal brain to insult is not as common as the neonatal brain. On the other hand, the T2 diffusion images are extremely useful especially in detecting old haemorrhage. Diffusion images also have the capacity to show premyelinating tracts (Figure 12.3.2).

Techniques of parallel acquisitions are now available from some manufacturers and the parameters of the sequences *in utero* are summarized in Table 12.3.2.

Proton spectroscopy of the fetal brain can be performed *in utero*. Although the feasibility of spectroscopy has already been

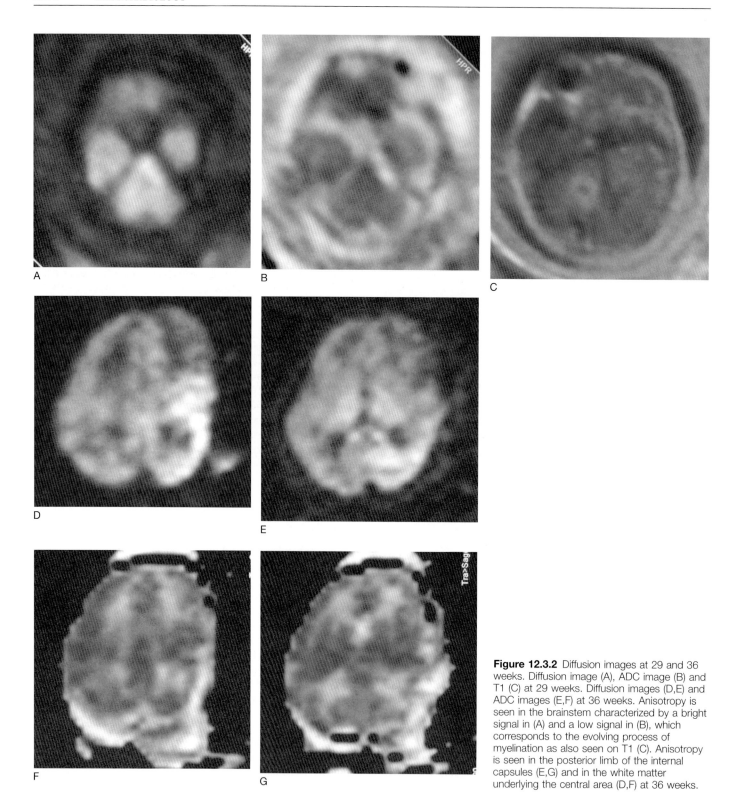

Figure 12.3.2 Diffusion images at 29 and 36 weeks. Diffusion image (A), ADC image (B) and T1 (C) at 29 weeks. Diffusion images (D,E) and ADC images (E,F) at 36 weeks. Anisotropy is seen in the brainstem characterized by a bright signal in (A) and a low signal in (B), which corresponds to the evolving process of myelination as also seen on T1 (C). Anisotropy is seen in the posterior limb of the internal capsules (E,G) and in the white matter underlying the central area (D,F) at 36 weeks.

demonstrated, metabolic mapping of the fetal brain at different gestational ages from 18 to 40 weeks is still needed. Proton spectroscopy may be highly effective in demonstrating white matter metabolic changes, such as in gliosis, not currently detectable on MR images. Technically, proton spectroscopy is more difficult to perform *in utero* compared with the postnatal period because head coils cannot be used. Body phased array coils are used in combination with spinal coils. The number of acquisitions is increased to get enough signal in the spectra. The acquisition time of 61/2 min is almost twice that in the postnatal period. Four spectra are

Table 12.3.2 Parameters of the sequences used *in utero* in the authors' experience

	TR (ms)	TE (ms)	TI (ms)	Flip angle	Matrix
T1 WI	570-600	11	–	90	256
T2 WI (HASTE)	1030	84	–	140	256
					512
IR	6730	61	350	180	256
3D T2 (true fisp)	4.3	2.15	–	68	256
Angio (2D TOF)	25	6.74	–	30	256
Diffusion	6000	99	–	–	128

HASTE, half-Fourier single shot turbo spin echo.

acquired: two are obtained from the body phased array coil and two from the spinal coils.

FURTHER READING

Brisse H, Fallet C, Sebag G et al. Supratentorial parenchyma in the developing fetal brain: in vitro MR study with histologic comparison. American Journal of Neuroradiology 1997; 18:1491–1497.

Bydder GM, Rutherford MA, Cowan FM. Diffusion-weighted imaging in neonates. Child's Nervous System 2001; 17:190–194

Bydder GM, Rutherford MA. Diffusion weighted imaging of the brain in neonates and infants. Magnetic Resonance Imaging Clinics of North America 2001; 9:83–98.

Chong BW, Babcook CJ, Salamat MS et al. A magnetic resonance template for normal neuronal migration in the fetus. Neurosurgery 1996; 39:110–116.

Girard N. Fetal MR imaging. European Radiology 2002; 12:1869–1871.

Girard N, Gambarelli D. Normal fetal brain. In: Brunelle F, Shaw D (eds). Magnetic resonance imaging. An atlas with anatomic correlations. Rickmansworth Brunelle & Shaw; 2001.

Girard NJ, Raybaud CA. In vivo MRI of fetal brain cellular migration. Journal of Computer Assisted Tomography 1992; 16:265–267.

Girard NJ, Raybaud CA. Ventriculomegaly and pericerebral CSF collection in the fetus: early stage of benign external hydrocephalus? Child's Nervous System 2001; 17:239 245.

Girard N, Raybaud C, D'Ercole C et al. In vivo MRI of the fetal brain. Neuroradiology 1993; 35:431–436.

Girard N, Raybaud C, Poncet M. In vivo MR study of brain maturation in normal fetuses. American Journal of Neuroradiology 1995; 16:407–413.

Girard N, Raybaud C, Poncet M. In vivo magnetic resonance imaging of the fetal brain. In: Guerrini R, Andermann F, Canapicchi R et al. (eds). Dysplasia of cerebral cortex and epilepsy. Philadelphia: Lippincot-Raven; 1996:101–103.

Girard N, Raybaud C, Gambarelli D. Pediatric neuroimaging: Fetal MR imaging. In: Demaerel PH (ed). Recent advances in diagnostic neuroradiology. Berlin: Springer-Verlag; 2001:373–398.

Girard N, Raybaud C, Gambarelli D, Figarella-Branger D. Fetal brain MR imaging. Magnetic Resonance Imaging Clinics of North America 2001; 9: 19–56.

Heerschap A, van den Berg PP. Proton magnetic resonance spectroscopy of human fetal brain. American Journal of Obstetrics and Gynecology 1994; 170:1150–1151.

Kok RD, van den Bergh AJ, Heerschap A, Nijland R, van den Berg PP. Metabolic information from the human fetal brain obtained with proton magnetic resonance spectroscopy. American Journal of Obstetrics and Gynecology 2001; 185:1011–1015.

Kok RD, van den Berg PP, van den Bergh AJ, Nijland R, Heerschap A. Maturation of the human fetal brain as observed by 1H MR spectroscopy. Magnetic Resonance Medicine 2002; 48:611–616 .

Liu AY, Zimmerman RA, Haselgrove JC, Bilaniuk LT, Hunter JV. Diffusion-weighted imaging in the evaluation of watershed hypoxic-ischemic brain injury in pediatric patients. Neuroradiology 2001; 43:918–926.

Stehling MK, Mansfield P, Ordidge RJ et al. Echo-planar imaging of the human fetus in utero. Magnetic Resonance Medicine 1990; 13:314–318.

Yamashita Y, Namimoto T, Abe Y et al. MR imaging of the fetus by a HASTE sequence. American Journal of Roentgenology 1997; 168:513–519.

MRI OF BRAIN MATURATION AND ORIGINS OF MR SIGNAL

Brain maturation is characterized by changes in brain morphology and composition.

BRAIN MORPHOLOGY

Changes in brain morphology include an increase in brain volume and weight, the changes in surface configuration that are due to the developing sulcation, the changes in ventricular shape and the decrease in volume of the subarachnoid spaces. These changes are mostly seen during the fetal period and are well illustrated by fetal brain MRI (Figures 12.3.3 to 12.3.8).

Brain weight increases rapidly during the fetal period. Brain weight is 12 gm at week 12, 20 gm at week 20, 350 gm at birth, 925 gm at 1 year, 1064 gm at 2 years, 1273 gm at 8 years and around 1400 gm in adults. Brain growth from midgestation through infancy is considered to reflect synaptogenesis, dendritic arborization and spine formation, axonal elongation and collateral formation, myelination, gliogenesis, neurotransmitter development, and vascular development.

The lateral cerebral ventricles are relatively large in young fetuses causing the so-called 'relative fetal hydrocephalus', especially at the level of the atrium, also known as 'colpocephaly'. The ventricular size is constant from 14 to 40 weeks. The normal ventricular size at the atria level on the axial plane is 7.6 ± 0.6 mm as shown from US studies. The upper limit of normal is generally agreed to be 10 mm. MRI data from the author's experience (Figure 12.3.9) show that the normal ventricular size at the atria level in the axial plane is below 9 mm except in young fetuses of 18–21 weeks in which the upper limit is 9.4 mm. The discrepancy between US and MRI data is probably related to anatomical factors: first, the germinal matrix, which is easily identified on MRI, is not included in the ventricular size; second, the axial plane used on MRI is that of the anteroposterior (AP) commissure and is not as oblique as the plane used on US studies.

The subarachnoid spaces are also prominent in young fetuses. A decrease in volume is seen from 30 weeks on. However, prominence of the subarachnoid spaces still persists in some fetuses at the parieto-occipital levels; it can be associated with mild uni- or bilateral ventriculomegaly and these aspects are thought to reflect the vacuolization of the primary meninges, which is known to occur from ventral to dorsal and posterior to anterior leading to posterior accumulation of cerebrospinal fluid (CSF).

Sulcation changes dramatically from 18 to 34 weeks, from an agyric brain to a convoluted pattern. The more significant sulcal markings appear as follows: the parieto-occipital fissure is well shaped and present at week 18; the calcarine fissure starts to fold at week 24 and shows its definite horizontal 'Y' shape at week 30; the central sulcus is seen at the surface of the brain at week 24 extending in depth to half of the cerebral hemisphere at week 28–29 and shows its classical orientation and depth at week 34–35; the callosomarginal fissure shows its definite shape at week 27–28; the pre- and postcentral sulci are identified at the surface of the

Text continued on p. 1720

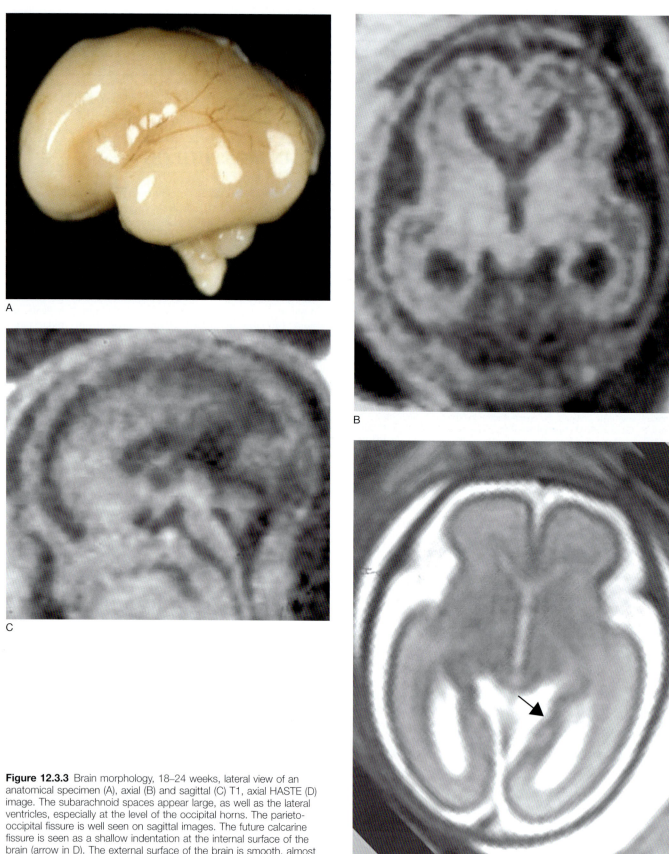

Figure 12.3.3 Brain morphology, 18–24 weeks, lateral view of an anatomical specimen (A), axial (B) and sagittal (C) T1, axial HASTE (D) image. The subarachnoid spaces appear large, as well as the lateral ventricles, especially at the level of the occipital horns. The parieto-occipital fissure is well seen on sagittal images. The future calcarine fissure is seen as a shallow indentation at the internal surface of the brain (arrow in D). The external surface of the brain is smooth, almost agyric, as seen on anatomical specimen. The sylvian fissures are widely opened.

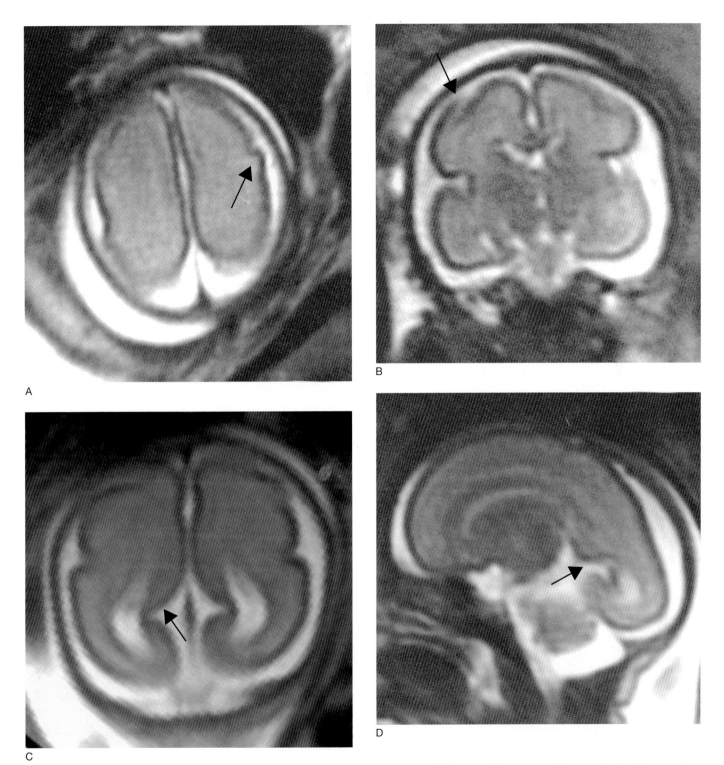

Figure 12.3.4 Brain morphology, 24–25 weeks, axial (A), coronal (B,C) and sagittal (D) HASTE images. The groove of the central sulcus is seen at the external surface of the brain (arrow in A and B); the calcarine fissure is better identified compared to the previous stage (arrow in C and D).

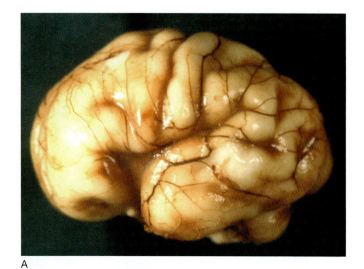

A

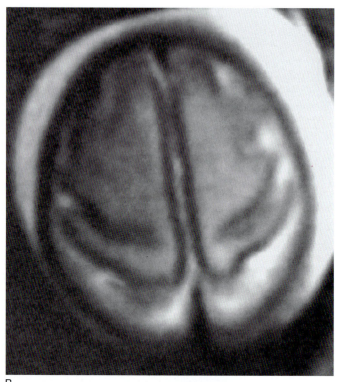

B

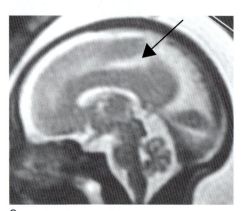

C

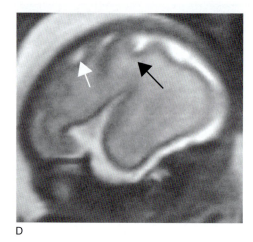

D

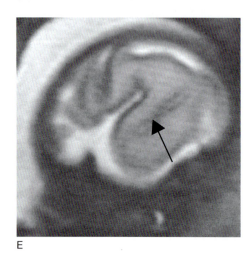

E

Figure 12.3.5 Brain morphology, 26–29 weeks; lateral view of an anatomical specimen (A), axial HASTE image (B) and sagittal HASTE images (C to E). The central sulcus has deepened. The callosomarginal sulcus (arrow in C) and the first temporal sulcus (arrow in E) are well seen. The pre- (white arrow in D) and postcentral (black arrow in D) are identified at the surface of the brain.

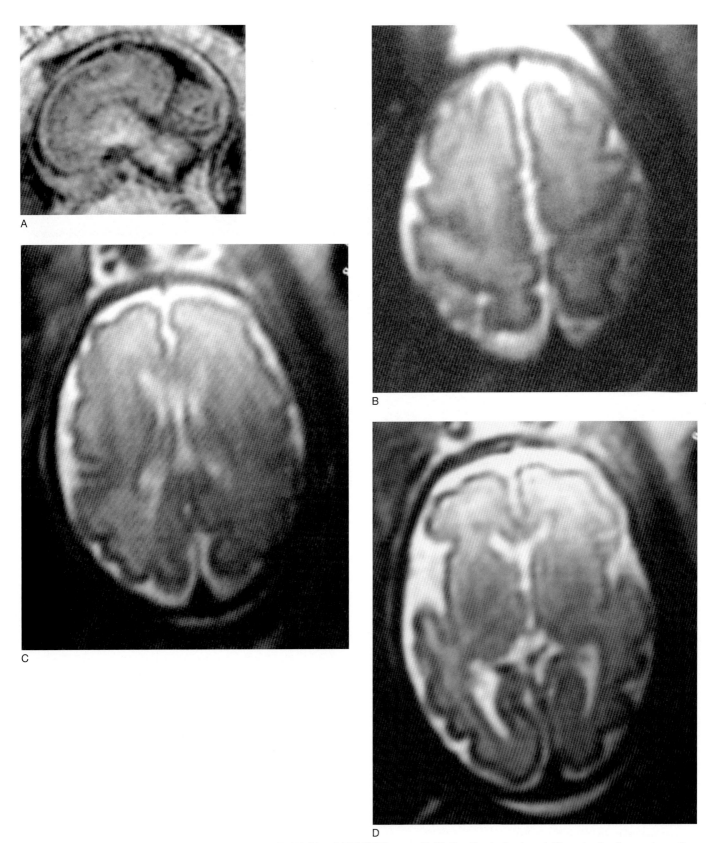

Figure 12.3.6 Brain morphology, 30–33 weeks, sagittal T1 WI (A), axial HASTE images (B–D). Gyration is developed. The calcarine fissure shows its definitive shape. The superior frontal sulcus is identified.

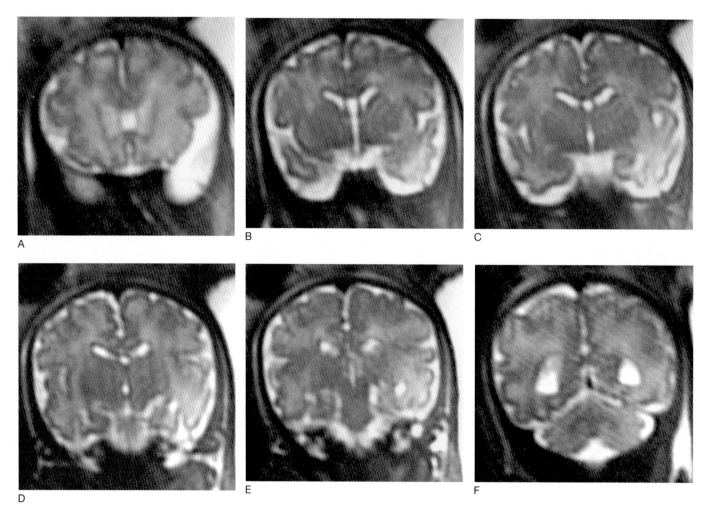

Figure 12.3.7 Brain morphology, 34–35 weeks, coronal HASTE images (A–F). Gyration has reached almost its definitive shape. Frontal, temporal and occipital sulci can be seen.

brain at week 27 and are deep at week 35–35; the first temporal sulcus is identified at week 28; the superior frontal sulcus is deep at week 32. Gyration almost has its definitive shape by week 35. The sylvian fissure is the last to be achieved and is dependent upon the development of the frontal and temporal operculum.

FURTHER READING

Brisse H, Fallet C, Sebag G, Nessmann C, Blot P, Hassan M. Supratentorial parenchyma in the developing fetal brain: in vitro MR study with histologic comparison. American Journal of Neuroradiology 1997; 18: 1491–1497.

Dooling EC, Chi JG, Gilles FH. Telencephalic development: Changing gyral patterns. In: Gilles FH, Leviton A, Dooling EC (eds). The developing human brain. Growth and epidemiologic neuropathology. Boston: John Wright PSG Inc.; 1983:94–104.

Girard N, Gambarelli D. Normal fetal brain. In: Brunelle F, Shaw D (eds). Magnetic resonance imaging. An atlas with anatomic correlations. Rickmansworth Brunelle & Shaw; 2001.

Girard NJ, Raybaud CA. In vivo MRI of fetal brain cellular migration. Journal of Computer Assisted Tomography 1992; 16:265–267.

Girard NJ, Raybaud CA. Ventriculomegaly and pericerebral CSF collection in the fetus: early stage of benign external hydrocephalus? Child's Nervous System 2001; 17:239–245.

Girard N, Raybaud C, Gambarelli D. Pediatric neuroimaging: Fetal MR imaging. In: Dmaerel PH (ed.). Recent advances in diagnostic neuroradiology. Berlin: Springer-Verlag; 2001: 373–398.

Girard N, Raybaud C, Gambarelli D, Figarella-Branger D. Fetal brain MR imaging. Magnetic Resonance Imaging Clinics of North America 2001; 9:19–56.

Holms GL. Morphological and physiological maturation of the brain in the neonate and young child. Journal of Clinical Neurophysiology 1986; 3:209–238.

Larroche JC. Developmental pathology of the neonate. Amsterdam: Elsevier/North-Holland Biomedical Press; 1977.

BRAIN COMPOSITION

Changes in brain composition are characterized by changes in cellularity, an increase in complex lipids content due to the evolving process of myelination, a decrease in water content (mostly in the white matter), a developing fibre network both in the white matter and the cortex, neurotransmitters and neurotransmitter–receptor interaction.

The effects on the MR signal are a shortening of T1 (bright signal on T1 WI) and a shortening of T2 (dark signal on T2 WI).

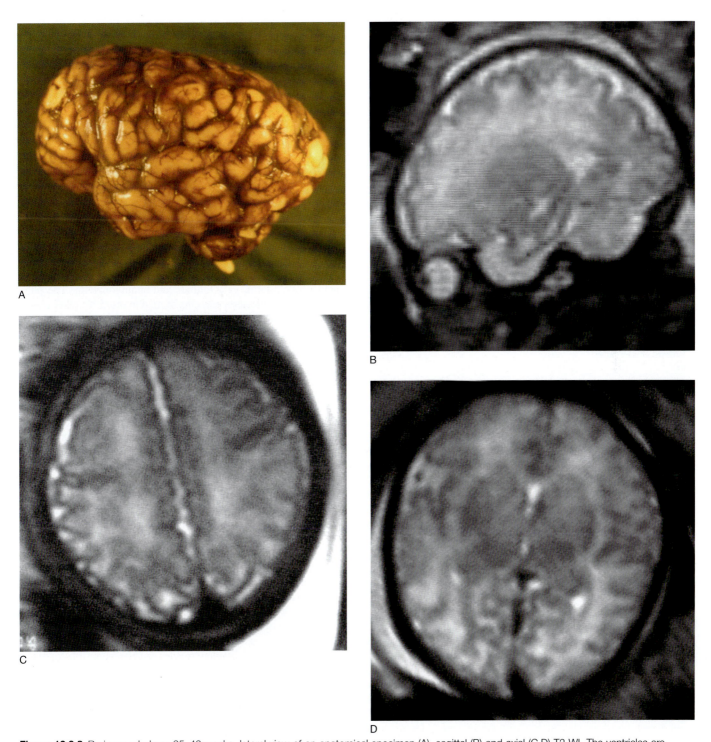

Figure 12.3.8 Brain morphology, 35–40 weeks, lateral view of an anatomical specimen (A), sagittal (B) and axial (C,D) T2 WI. The ventricles are small. The subarachnoid spaces have decreased in volume.

Primary mechanisms responsible for these effects are the water content, the cellular density and the MR properties of lipids. The most rapid changes in myelination occur between mid-gestation and the second postnatal year. Two partially overlapping stages can be identified: a period of oligodendrocyte proliferation and differentiation, and a period of rapid myelin synthesis and deposition.

The decrease in water content is mostly in the white matter of the maturing brain (Table 12.3.3).

The high cellular density and the cellular packing in the cortex, the basal ganglia and the germinal matrix are responsible for the multilayered pattern observed *in utero*. The intense proliferation of astrocytes to guide neuronal migration and of oligodendrocytes

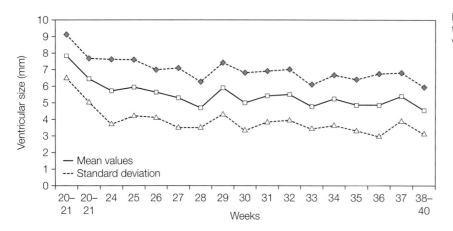

Figure 12.3.9 Ventricular size at the atria level in the axial plane. ◊, standard deviation +; □, mean values; △, standard deviation -.

Table 12.3.3 Changes in water, lipid and protein contents

	20–22 weeks	*Term*	*Mature*
Water			
Cerebral cortex	90%	90%	85%
Cerebral white matter	90%	90%	70%
Lipids			
Cerebral cortex	1.7%	2.7%	4.5%
Cerebral white matter	2.4%	2.7%	17%
Proteins			
Cerebral cortex	8.3%	7.6%	7.3%
Cerebral white matter	7.3%	10.5%	13%

before the onset of myelination (the so-called myelination gliosis) is seen as an intermediate layer within the white matter (Figure 12.3.10). This layer of migrating cells is transient and is seen up to 30 weeks. Premyelinating oligodendrocytes (preoligodendrocytes), which are present before axonal ensheathment begins, emit processes for identifying target axons. From 30 weeks on, some residual nests of cells can persist and appear as periventricular nodules predominantly in the frontal areas (Figure 12.3.11). Preoligodendrocytes coincide with the high-risk period for periventricular leukomalacia (PVL) in very premature neonates. Absence of this intermediate layer prior to 30 weeks on fetal MRI coincides with white matter damage whatever the cause of the damage. Signal changes in the basal ganglia are more conspicuous at week 29–30 compared to the previous stages. However, these conspicuous signal changes, especially on T1-weighted images, are transient. The germinal matrix (also named the ventricular zone, ependymal layer) is also highly cellular in young fetuses and appears as a thick layer on fetal MRI up to 29–30 weeks. Disruption or nodular appearance of the ventricular wall coincides with ependymal reactions to injury, especially ventricular dilatation, infection or inflammation.

Myelin is a highly organized multilamellar structure formed by the plasma membrane of oligodendrocytes. This membrane surrounds neuronal axons and facilitates the impulse conduction. Biochemically, myelin contains small numbers of specific proteins and lipids that are integrated into the membrane marked by a high degree of stability. Lipids constitute 70% of the dry weight of the myelin membrane. The major lipid components of CNS myelin

include cholesterol, galactolipids and sphingomyelin. The phospholipid and cholesterol contents of myelin resemble other plasma membranes; however, myelin differs in that it contains abundant quantities of galactolipids and plasmalogens, and a diverse group of glycerophospholipids. One-third of the myelin lipids consist of two galactolipids: the galactocerebrosides and sulphatides. Proteolipid-protein (PLP) is a specific protein that stabilizes the myelin membrane, although the mechanism remains unclear. PLP constitutes half of the protein in the mature myelin membrane. Myelin basic protein (MBP) is also a specific protein that interacts with the cytoplasmic faces of the sheath and facilitates the compaction of the myelin membrane. PLP and MBP are known as the major myelin proteins. Minor myelin proteins include the myelin-associated glycoprotein (MAG) and the 2'3'-cyclic-nucleotide 3'phosphohydrolase (CNPase). Galactocerebrosides and sulphatides occupy the extracellular face of the membrane and are known from animal models to transduce developmental signals, to facilitate the protein trafficking and stabilize the membrane, and to be responsible for axon–myelin interaction.

When wrapping around an axon, the oligodendrocytic extension undergoes a process of compaction. Loss of cytoplasm from the compaction is responsible for loss of mobile protons and, as a consequence, loss of MR signal, especially on T2 WI. A single oligodendrocyte can be responsible for the myelination of several axons simultaneously (up to 50 nerve fibres). Consequently, the destruction of a few oligodendrocytes can be responsible for extensive damage. On the other hand, oligodendrocytes are capable of proliferation, especially during maturation, which has implications in the reparative processes. Apart from the intense proliferation of oligodendrocytes before the onset of myelination, there is a period of greatly increased lipid synthesis in the oligodendrocytes. Lipids cause a decrease in T1 and T2, and an increase in the magnetization effect. Galactocerebroside is the major lipid responsible for the magnetization effect.

Other factors are also of importance such as the hydrophilic properties of some constituents of myelin. Cholesterol, glycolipids and portions of the myelin proteins are hydrophilic and bond strongly with water molecules leading to a decrease in the amount of free water and shortening of T1. Changes of MR signal from the myelination process are apparent first on T1 WI and then on T2 WI: this is probably due to the fact that T1 and T2 WI express different mechanisms. Signal changes from brain myelination are

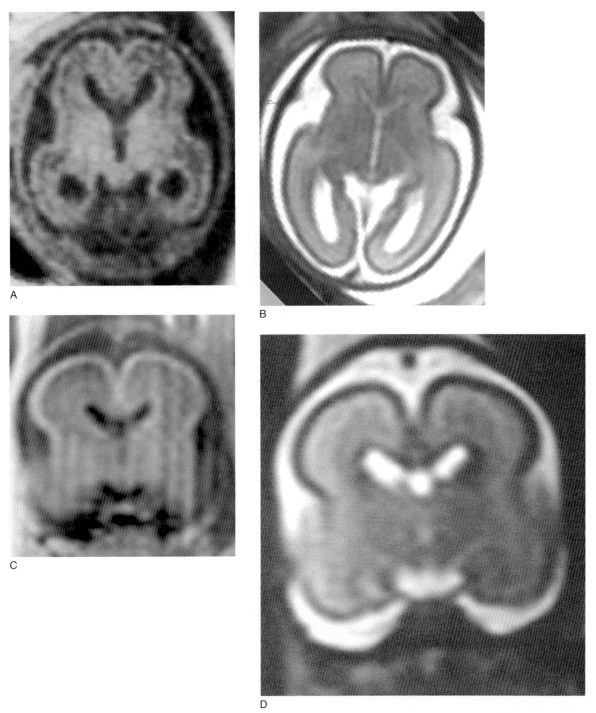

Figure 12.3.10 Effects of the high cellularity, coronal (A) and axial (B) T1 WI and HASTE (C,D) images at week 22–23. Typical multilayered pattern: the cortical ribbon, the intermediate layer and the germinal matrix are of high signal and low signal intensity, respectively, on T1 and T2 WI. Basal ganglia also show similar signal changes. The germinal matrix is thick at that gestational age.

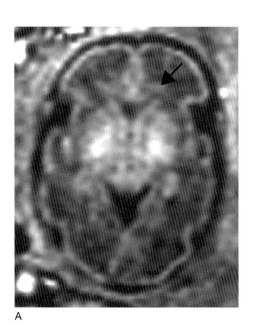

A

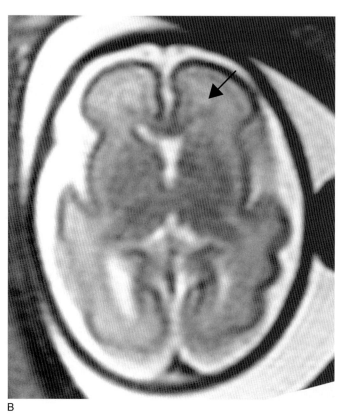

B

Figure 12.3.11 Effects of the high cellularity, axial T1 (A) and HASTE (B) images at week 29. Highly bright signal is seen on T1 WI within the basal ganglia. Also, note nodules in the frontal white matter corresponding to nests of residual cells (arrow in A and B). The intermediate layer of migrating cells is sparse. Note that the germinal matrix appears thinner than in the previous stage.

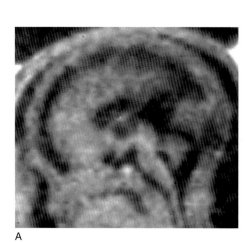

A

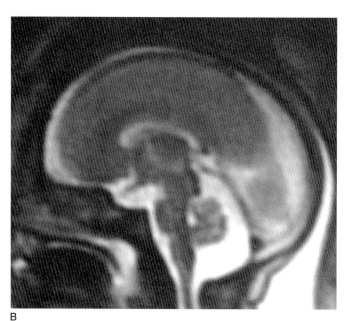

B

Figure 12.3.12 Signal changes from brain myelination, 22 weeks, sagittal T1 (A) and HASTE (B) images. Bright signal is seen in the posterior brainstem at the level of the medulla, pons and mesencephalum on T1 WI whereas low signal intensity is seen on T2 WI.

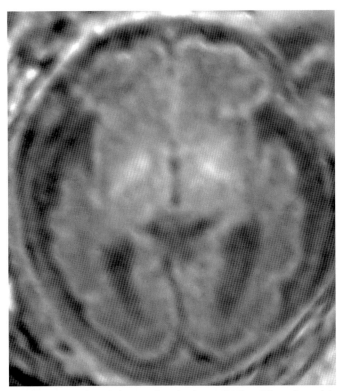

Figure 12.3.13 Signal changes from brain myelination, 33 weeks, axial T1 WI. Bright signal is seen within the posterior limb of the internal capsules.

seen in the posterior brainstem as early as 20 weeks (Figure 12.3.12), in the posterior limb of the internal capsule from 33 weeks on (Figure 12.3.13), in the optic tracts (Figure 12.3.14) and in the white matter underlying the central area from 35 weeks on (Figure 12.3.15).

Although oligodendrocytes are the cells responsible for myelination, astrocytes also play an important role especially for homeostasis of the neuronal extracellular milieu. Astrocytes are also functionally coupled with oligodendrocytes through the astrocytic processes in contact with oligodendrocytes. Astrocytes are also involved in the metabolism of the neurotransmitters glutamate and gamma-aminobutyric acid (GABA), in the detoxification of ammonia and in the glycogen pathway. Interactions between neurons and oligodendrocytes are also needed to achieve proper myelination. Indeed, spontaneous neuronal activity plays a major role in the initiation of myelination and induces the onset of the myelination process by oligodendrocytes.

The cellular and biochemical processes of brain maturation are complex and any failure in the synthesis of specific proteins or lipids will produce myelination disorders. Absence of the specific proteins will produce an unstable myelin. Absence of the PLP gene is currently known to produce Pelizaeus–Marzbacher disease (and its connate form, Seitelberger disease) with its absence of myelination. Absence of the specific MBP is part of the 18p- syndrome. Enzymatic defects in lipid synthesis, glycogen synthesis and others will produce the so-called leucodystrophies or metabolic diseases. Inability of astrocytes to realize their functions causes Alexander's disease and is due to a mutation in the glial fibrillary acidic protein (GFAP) gene, GFAP being a marker of astrocytes.

FURTHER READING

Aoki Y, Haginoya K, Munakata M et al. A novel mutation in glial fibrillary acidic protein gene in a patient with Alexander disease. Neuroscience Letters 2001; 312:71–74.

Back SA. Recent advances in human perinatal white matter injury. Progress in Brain Research 2001; 132:131–147.

Barkovich AJ, Kyos HC, Jackson DE, Norman D. Normal maturation of the neonatal and infant brains: MR imaging at 1.5 T. Radiology 1988; 166:173–180.

Barkovich AJ. Pediatric neuroimaging, 3rd edn. Philadelphia: Lippincott Williams and Wilkins; 2000.

Baumann N, Pham-Dinh D. Biology of oligodendrocyte and myelin in the mammalian central nervous system. Physiological Reviews 2001; 81:871–927.

Berry M, Butt AM. Structure and function of glia in the central nervous system. In: Graham DI, Lantos PL (eds). Greenfield's neuropathology, 6th edn. London: Arnold; 1997:63–83.

Bosio A, Bussow H, Adam J, Stoffel W. Galactosphingolipids and axono-glial interaction in myelin of the central nervous system. Cell and Tissue Research 1998; 292:199–210.

Coetzee T, Suzuki K, Nave K-A, Popko B. Myelination in the absence of galactolipids and proteolipids proteins. Molecular and Cellular Neuroscience 1999; 14:41–51.

Coetze T, Suzuki K, Popko B. New perspectives on the function of myelin galactolipids. Trends in Neuroscience 1998; 21:126–130.

Compston A, Zajicek J, Sussman J et al. Glial lineages and myelination in the central nervous system. Journal of Anatomy 1997; 190:161–200.

Demerens C, Stankoff B, Logak M et al. Induction of myelination in the central nervous system by electrical activity. Proceedings of the National Academy of Sciences, USA 1996; 93:9887–9892.

Deng W, Poretz RD. Oligodendroglia in developmental neurotoxicity. Neuro Toxicology 2003; 24:161–178.

Dupree JL, Coetzee T, Blight A, Suzuki K, Popko B. Myelin galactolipids are essential for proper node of Ranvier formation in the CNS. Journal of Neuroscience 1998; 18:1642–1649.

Fralix TA, Ceckler TL, Wolff SD, Simon SA, Balaban RS. Lipid bilayer and water proton magnetization transfer: Effect of cholesterol. Magnetic Resonance Medicine 1991; 18:214–223.

Gilles FH, Shankle W, Dooling EC. Myelinated tracts: Growth patterns. In: Gilles FH, Leviton A, Dooling EC (eds). The developing human brain. Growth and epidemiologic neuropathology. Boston: John Wright PSG Inc.; 1983:117–183.

Girard N, Raybaud C, DuLac P. MRI study of brain myelination. Journal of Neuroradiology 1991; 18:291–307.

Greer JM, Lees MB. Molecules in focus. Myelin proteolipid protein – the first 50 years. International Journal of Biochemistry and Cell Biology 2002; 34:211–215.

Haran M, Chowdhury A, Manohar C, Bellare J. Myelin growth and coiling. Colloids and Surfaces A: Physicochemical and Engineering Aspects 2002; 205:21–30.

Hardy RJ, Friedrich VL. Progressive remodeling of the oligodendrocyte process arbor during myelinogenesis. Developmental Neuroscience 1996; 18:243–254.

Kaye EM. Update on genetic disorders affecting white matter. Pediatric Neurology 2001; 24:11–24.

Knapp PE. Proteolipid protein: Is it more than just a structural component of myelin? Developmental Neuroscience 1996; 18:297–308.

Koenig SH. Cholesterol of myelin is the determinant of gray-white contrast in MRI of brain. Magnetic Resonance Medicine 1991; 20:285–291.

Koenig SH, Brown III RD, Spiller M, Lundbom N. Relaxometry of brain: Why white matter appears bright in MRI. Magnetic Resonance Medicine 1990; 14:482–495.

Kucharczyk W, MacDonald PM, Staniz GH, Henkelman RM. Relaxivity and magnetization transfer of white matter lipids at MR imaging : Importance of cerebrosides and pH. Radiology 1994; 192:521–529.

Kursula P. The current status of structural studies on proteins of the myelin sheath (Review). International Journal of Molecular Medicine 2001; 8:475–479.

Larroche JC, Amakawa H. Glia of myelination and fat deposit during early myelogenesis. Biology of the Neonate 1973; 12:421–435.

Marcus J, Popko B. Galactolipids are molecular determinants of myelin development and axo-glial organization. Biochimica et Biophysica Acta 2002; 1573:406–413.

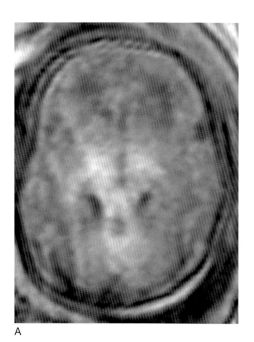
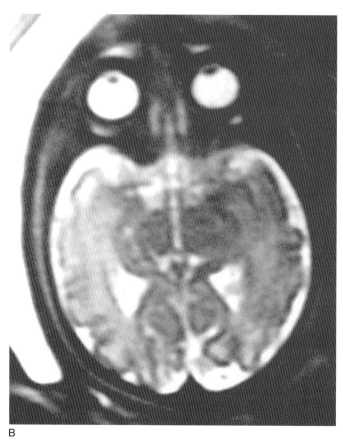

A   B

Figure 12.3.14 Signal changes from brain myelination, 35 weeks, axial T1 (A) and T2 (B). Bright signal is seen in the optic tracts on T1 whereas a low signal is detected on T2.

Pribyl TM, Campagnoni CW, Kampf K et al. Expression of the myelin basic protein gene locus in neurons and oligodendrocytes in the human fetal central nervous system. Journal of Comparative Neurology 1996; 374:342–353.

Rogister B, Ben-Hur T, Dubois-Dalcq M. From neural stem cells to myelinating oligodendrocytes. Molecular and Cell Neuroscience 1999; 14:287–300.

Sarnat HB. Ependymal reactions to injury. A review. Journal of Neuropathology and Experimental Neurology 1995; 54:1–15.

Vyas AA, Schnaar RL. Brain gangliosides: Functional ligands for myelin stability and the control of nerve regeneration. Biochimie 2001; 83:677–682.

Wolff SD, Balaban RS. Magnetization transfer contrast (MTC) and tissue water proton relaxation in vivo. Magnetic Resonance in Medicine 1989; 10:135–144.

Woodward K, Malcolm S. Proteolipid protein gene. Pelizaeus–Merzbacher disease in humans and neurodegeneration in mice. Trends in Genetics 1999; 15:125–128.

Yakovlev PI, Lecours AR. The myelogenetic cycles of regional maturation of the brain. In: Minkowski A (ed.). Regional development of the brain in early life. Oxford: Blackwell Scientific Publications; 1967:3–70

GENERAL SEQUENCES OF CENTRAL NERVOUS SYSTEM MYELINATION

The general rules of brain myelination are well known from histological studies. CNS myelination progresses in predictable sequences from caudal (spinal cord and brainstem) to rostral (telencephalon). It begins at 12–13 weeks in the spinal cord and continues well after birth (at least into the third decade) in the intracortical fibres of the cerebral cortex. In the cortex, myelination progresses in a concentric fashion whereas in the subcortical white matter myelination follows functionally defined bundles. Sensory pathways myelinate before the motor pathways. Associative areas are the last to be myelinated. In a given cortical-subcortical functional unit the cortex is generally myelinated first. Myelination of different parts of the brain develops at different times, at different speeds and at a variable speed for a given structure: indeed, the rate of myelination in a particular pathway may change across time, such that the onset of myelination prior or at birth is not necessarily associated with early myelination. As an example, a bright signal is seen in the posterior limb of the internal capsule as early as 33 weeks whereas the low signal on T2 WI will be seen at 2 months postnatally. On the other hand, the optic tracts show signal changes on both T1 and T2 WI by week 35. In telencephalic sites, myelination progresses from the central sulcus outward towards all poles; the occipital pole myelinates before the frontal pole, which in turn myelinates before the temporal pole. At birth, large areas of the cortex are already myelinated whereas the subcortical white matter is not. Primary areas of the cortex (central area, calcarine area, auditive area of the medial temporal lobe) show low signal intensity on T2 WI. Cortical and subcortical myelination are not necessarily interrelated.

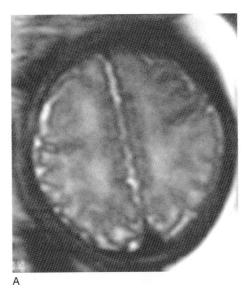
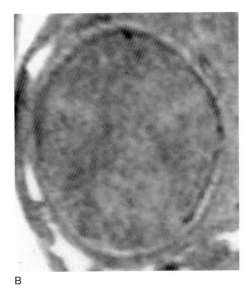

A   B

Figure 12.3.15 Signal changes from brain myelination, 36 weeks, axial T2 (A) and T1 (B). Bright signal is seen in the white matter underlying the central sulcus on T1 whereas a low signal is detected on T2, corresponding to myelination in projection fibres. Also, note the similar marked signal changes of the central sulcus compared to the remaining cortex.

Biochemical sequences closely follow the anatomical sequences. Sphingomyelin is followed simultaneously by cerebrosides, MBP, PLP and non-hydroxy sulphatide, followed by hydroxy sulphatide. Biochemical sequences are identical in the different sites of myelination but occur at different times. This probably contributes to the regional variability of many inborn disorders of CNS white matter.

FURTHER READING

Gilles FH, Shankle W, Dooling EC. Myelinated tracts: Growth patterns. In: Gilles FH, Leviton A, Dooling EC (eds). The developing human brain. Growth and epidemiologic neuropathology. Boston: John Wright PSG Inc.; 1983:117–183.

Holms GL. Morphological and physiological maturation of the brain in the neonate and young child. Journal of Clinical Neurophysiology 1986; 3:209–238.

Kinney HC, Armstrong DD. Perinatal neuropathology. In: Graham DI, Lantos PL (eds). Greenfield's neuropathology, 6th edn. London: Arnold; 1997:537–599.

Kinney HC, Brody BA, Kloman AS, Gilles FH. Sequence of central nervous system myelination in human infancy. II. Patterns of myelination in autopsied infants. Journal of Neuropathology and Experimental Neurology 1988; 47:217–234

Kinney HC, Karthigasan J, Borenshteyn NI, Flax JD, Kirschner DA. Myelination in the developing human brain: Biochemical correlates. Neurochemical Research 1994; 19:983–996.

Larroche JC. Developmental pathology of the neonate. Amsterdam: Elsevier/North-Holland Biomedical Press; 1977.

Yakovlev PI, Lecours AR. The myelogenetic cycles of regional maturation of the brain. In: Minkowski A (ed.). Regional development of the brain in early life. Oxford: Blackwell Scientific Publications; 1967:3–70

POSTNATAL MRI TIMETABLES

MRI will illustrate identical anatomical sequences as histology but with a time delay compared to histological studies. However, the postnatal timetables as seen by MRI can be summarized as follows: at birth (Figure 12.3.16) the medulla and the mesencephalon display a bright signal on T1 and a low signal on T2, whereas the anterior part of the pons is not yet myelinated completely. The white matter underlying the central area also shows a bright signal on T1 and a low signal on T2. Cortical ribbon at the level of the rolandic, calcarine and hippocampal areas is brighter on T1 and of low signal on T2 compared to the cortex of other cerebral regions. Optic tracts are also seen to be myelinated. The posterior limb of the internal capsule displays a bright signal on T1 but is not yet myelinated on T2. At 2 months of age (Figure 12.3.17) the posterior limb of the internal capsules appears of low signal intensity on T2. The beginning of myelination is seen on T2 within the optic radiations but is subtle. The cerebellum and the brainstem are now of low signal intensity compared to the previous stage. At 4 months of age (Figure 12.3.18) the entire internal capsule (anterior and posterior limbs) is now of low signal intensity on T2 as are the periventricular optic radiations. Myelination of the white matter within the centrum semi ovale has reached the pre- and postcentral areas. The splenium of the corpus callosum also shows low signal intensity on T2 whereas the anterior part is not yet myelinated. At 7–8 months of age (Figure 12.3.19) the entire corpus callosum appears of low signal on T2 because myeli-

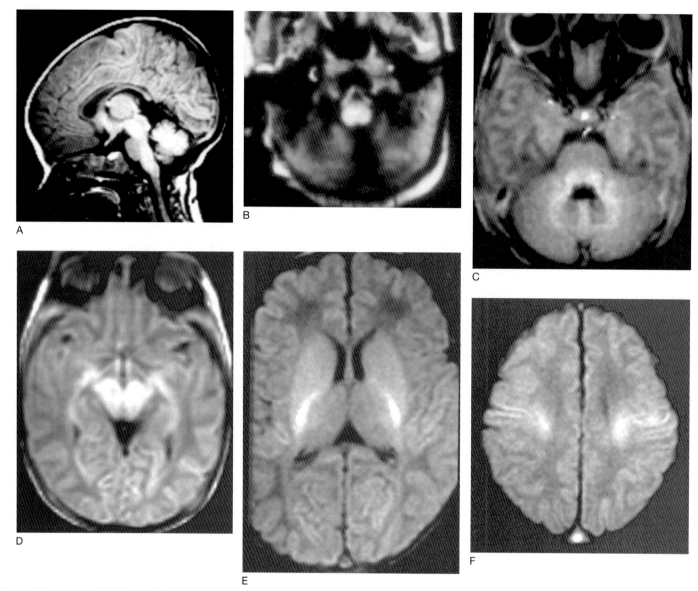

Figure 12.3.16 Neonate, T1 (A–F), T2 (G–L). The posterior part of the pons, the mesencephalon and the medulla show a myelinated pattern of bright signal on T1 and low signal on T2 as well as the white matter underlying the central area. Posterior limb of the internal capsules are bright on T1. Remaining white matter of the cerebral hemispheres is of dark signal on T1 and of bright signal on T2. Note that the central sulci and the cortex of the occipital lobes appear brighter on T1 and of lower signal on T2 compared to the other cerebral regions.

nation has reached the genu. Although the white matter of the cerebral hemispheres shows a bright signal on T1, it is not myelinated on T2. At 18–24 months (Figure 12.3.20) a mature pattern of the white matter is seen and the subcortical 'U' fibres also show a low signal intensity on T2 WI.

Although the mature pattern is reached at 18–24 months, the myelination of the brain is known to go on far beyond that age, at least until 20 years.

CONCLUDING REMARKS

MRI gives normal milestones of brain maturation especially of brain myelination. MRI detects simple anatomical structures, which appear at determined periods, thereby providing an easy and reliable approach to the morphological evaluation of the brain

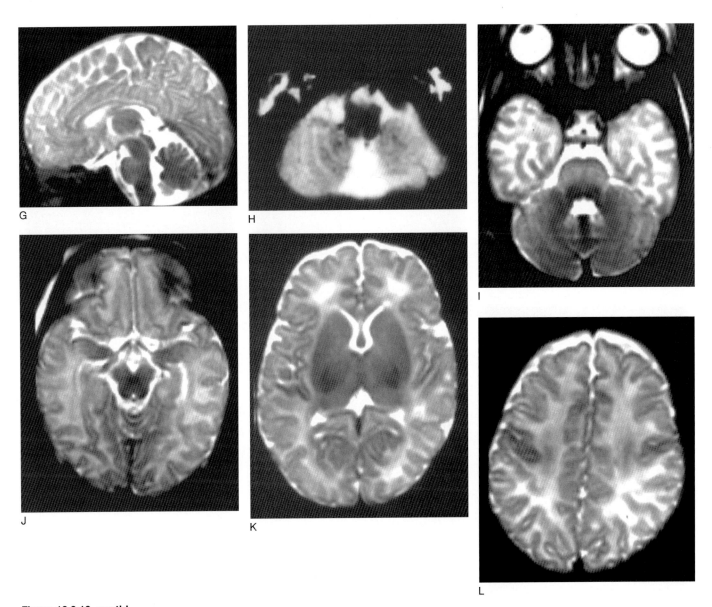

Figure 12.3.16, cont'd.

development and maturation. Hence, the potential benefits of prenatal MRI are to recognize disorders of brain development as early as possible. MRI is also used as a follow-up imaging tool in the prediction of outcome, especially in birth asphyxia or in neonates at risk of brain damage (i.e. neonates of very low birth weight and very premature). MRI also provides the illustration of the windows of vulnerability of both the grey and white matter. In addition to

the anatomical and biochemical sequences of brain myelination, brain maturation also includes the maturation of neurotransmitters. Glutamate is one of the neurotransmitters known to be responsible for the selective vulnerability of the neurons (of the basal ganglia and deep layers of the cortex) to hypoxia beyond 34 weeks and for the selective vulnerability of the white matter before 32 weeks.

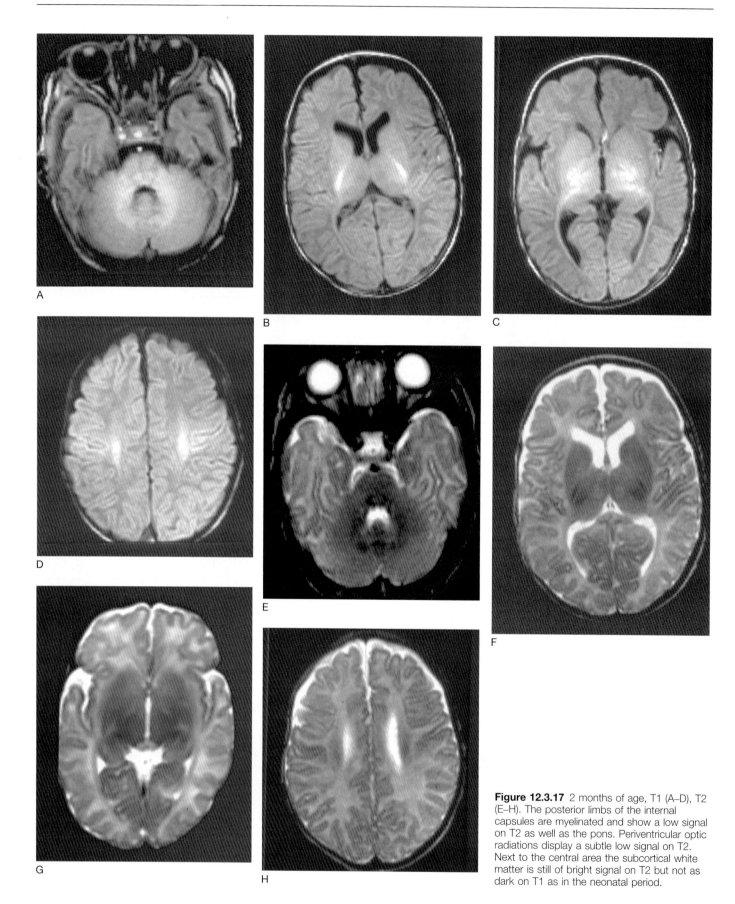

Figure 12.3.17 2 months of age, T1 (A–D), T2 (E–H). The posterior limbs of the internal capsules are myelinated and show a low signal on T2 as well as the pons. Periventricular optic radiations display a subtle low signal on T2. Next to the central area the subcortical white matter is still of bright signal on T2 but not as dark on T1 as in the neonatal period.

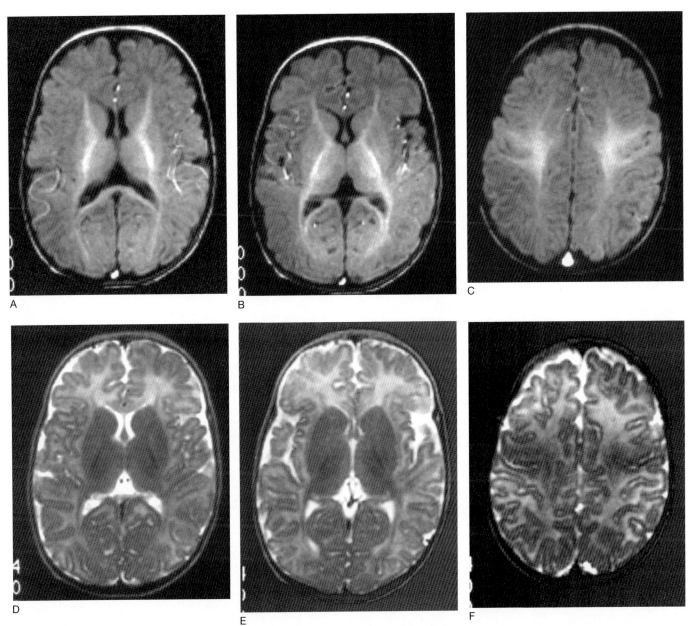

Figure 12.3.18 4 months of age, T1 (A–C), T2 (D–F). Entire internal capsules and the periventricular optic radiations are well identified and show a low signal intensity on T2. Myelination of the white matter of the centrum semi ovale has reached the pre- and postcentral areas. Splenium of the corpus callosum also shows a low signal on T2 whereas the anterior part of the corpus callosum is not yet myelinated.

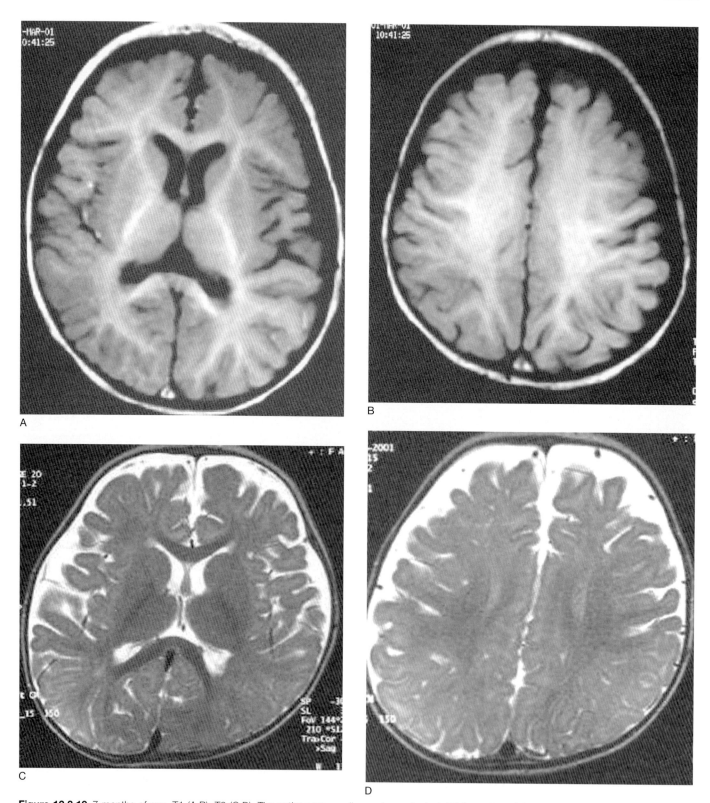

Figure 12.3.19 7 months of age, T1 (A,B), T2 (C,D). The entire corpus callosum is myelinated. White matter of the cerebral hemispheres display a bright signal as in the mature pattern but is not yet myelinated on T2.

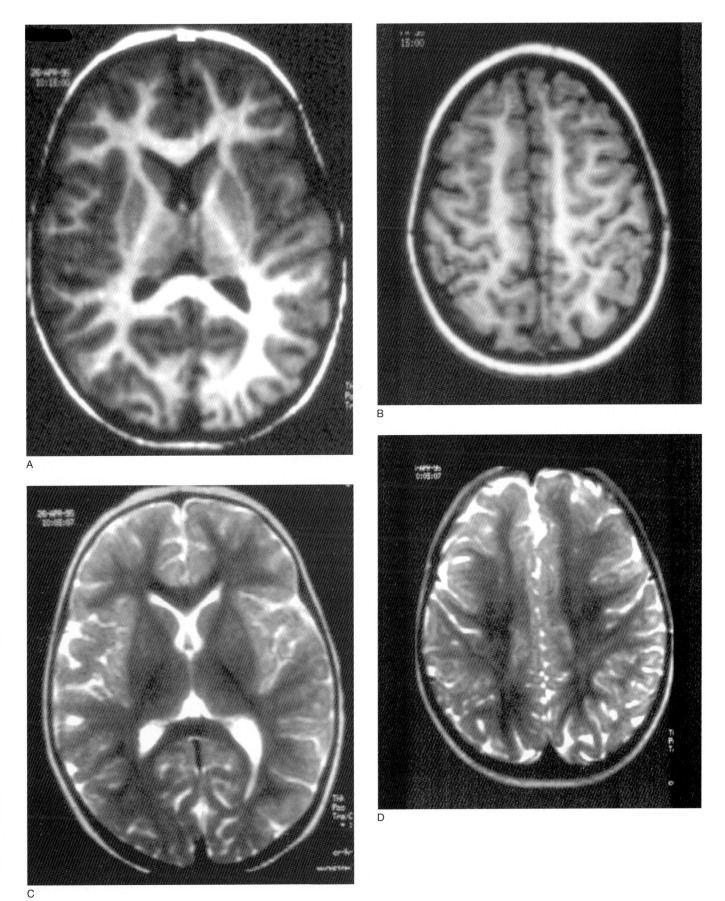

Figure 12.3.20 18 months of age, T1 (A,B), T2 (C,D). A mature pattern is seen. White matter appears of low signal on T2 and of bright signal on T1.

Congenital Cerebral Malformations

Philippe Demaerel, Francis, Brunelle, Valérie Chigot, Hussein Aref

INTRODUCTION

There has been considerable advance in our knowledge of the congenital cerebral malformations. The progress in genetics and the improvements in image resolution are the main reasons for this advance. A good and flexible classification for the cortical developmental malformations is now available, which allows the inclusion of new observations.

Following a brief review of the embryology, a review will be given of the more common congenital abnormalities of cleavage and sulcation. It is important to realize that most malformations can display mild, moderate or extensive changes and that different malformations often occur simultaneously.

EMBRYOLOGY

A brief review of the embryology of the brain is necessary to understand the malformations that tend to occur regularly.

The neural plate can be recognized at approximately 17 days. The neural plate will develop and end in the formation of a neural tube. The closure of this structure begins in the most rostral part and will reach the posterior end within a few days.

The anterior part of the neural tube will form the prosencephalon, mesencephalon and rhombencephalon around 30 days of gestation. At this time, the corpus callosum will develop from the commissural plate at the rostral end. The so-called meninx primitiva develops in the groove of the commissural plate and is necessary for the correct progression in guiding of axons that cross the midline. The genu of the corpus callosum is formed before the truncus and the splenium, followed by a more anterior part of the genu and the rostrum. This sequence of formation is important when analyzing partial agenesis of the corpus callosum. It is thought that remnants of the meninx primitiva give rise to interhemispheric lipomas. The prosencephalon will divide into the diencephalon and telencephalon. The diencephalon is the precursor of the deep cerebral structures while the telencephalon consists of the putamen, the caudate nucleus and the hemispheres. In holoprosencephaly, there is a failure of cleavage into hemispheres and sometimes even a failure of separation of the telencephalon from the diencephalon. The rhombencephalon will divide into the metencephalon and the myelencephalon.

The formation of the cerebral cortex begins during the 7th week of gestation. First, the germinal layers become visible in the walls of the telencephalon. This is the period of neuronal and glial proliferation. The second period consists of a migration of the neurons from the germinal zone along the so-called guiding radial glial fibres. This process takes place between the 8th and 24th week of gestation. There is now sufficient genetic evidence that the cytoskeleton plays an important role in the neuronal migration. The cells of layer 1 arrive first at their final superficial destination in the cortex. Then, the layers 6, 5, 4, 3 and 2 follow in this order. The six-layered cortex can be recognized in the 16th fetal week. The thickness does not exceed 4.5 mm.

The period of migration is followed by the cortical organization, leading to the complex three-dimensional structure of the mature cortex.

Up to the 18th week, the hemispheric surface is smooth. At this time, the callosal and parieto-occipital sulci and the calcarine fissure are visible. From 20 weeks onwards, early operculization of the posterior part of the insula can be seen and most major sulci and gyri are present by the 25th week of gestation. In the following 3 weeks, there is a significant increase in the number of sulci and gyri and between the 32nd and 34th week all sulci and gyri can be outlined. It is known that there is a delay of approximately 13 days between the fetal magnetic resonance imaging (MRI) observations versus neuroanatomy.

PATHOLOGY

CEPHALOCELES (MENINGOCELES AND ENCEPHALOCELES) AND RELATED MALFORMATIONS

The term encephalocele describes a defect in the skull vault through which there is herniation of the intracranial content extracranially. The cause of the malformation is not fully understood. Theories include failure of neural tube closure, failure of cranial bone development, focal dysgenesis of the dura, and in the case of basal encephaloceles, failure of union of the basal ossification centres. Some authors suggest that cephaloceles may occur after neural tube closure. At many of the sites of dermoid sinuses, as in the frontonasal region at the fonticulus nasofrontalis and in the occipital or, less commonly, vertex regions, diverticulation of the meninges is a normal feature present for a limited period at some stage of development. At these sites a sac containing cerebrospinal fluid (CSF), or brain or both may persist and form cephaloceles. Four types of cephaloceles are described. (1) A meningocele is a sac containing CSF and meninges but no brain tissue. (2) An encephalocele is a sac containing in addition to meninges and CSF, brain tissue. These are also known as meningoencephaloceles. (3) Atretic meningocele is the term used to describe a form fruste of a meningocele. There is a meningofibrous cord extending through a skull defect. These occur most frequently in the parietal and occipital areas. In addition, a nest of hamartomatous neural tissue forming a gliomatous mass may occur at any of these sites. (4) Gliocoeles describe a cyst, lined with glial tissue and containing CSF. The location of the cephalocele in relation to the bone in which the defect occurs is used to name the cephalocele, e.g. an occipital cephalocele protrudes through a defect posteriorly in the occipital bone or in the midline between them. External lesions are easy to diagnose but some cephaloceles may protrude centrally as occurs with a frontoethmoidal cephalocele and only become clinically apparent by associated facial deformity or because of symptoms such as a blocked nose or feeding problems due to obstruction by the cephalocele. Similarly, occult cephaloceles may occur in the orbit or in the temporal bone.

Cephaloceles occur in 1/4000 to 1/5000 live births. They are of unknown aetiology and may occur in isolation or in association with other malformations or as part of a syndrome complex such as HARD +/− E (hydrocephalus agyria retinal dysplasia and encephalocele) or Walker–Warburg syndrome.

Cephaloceles vary markedly in size from tiny bulges to masses larger than the head. They may form a simple rounded swelling or a more complex lobulated structure and may be cystic and translucent or appear solid. When the cephalocele is large the head is often microcephalic due to loss of the volume of herniated brain substance. When there is hydrocephalus the head may be large. The cephalocele is distended and tender. It may reduce in size or disappear after surgical shunting of the ventricles.

The skin over the cephalocele may appear normal but stretching may result in marked thinning with ulceration and secondary infection.

The contents of the cephalocele vary from:

1. CSF alone in continuity with the subarachnoid space (meningocele);
2. recognizable brain tissue, but often deformed or damaged usually by ischaemic or haemorrhagic events, in continuity with intracranial components and sometimes with parts of the ventricular system (meningoencephalocele); and
3. disorganized neural/glial tissues ('glioma').

Antenatal diagnosis is now frequent since the advent of routine ultrasound (US). MRI is required to precisely define the exact content of the sac and to identify associated abnormalities such as corpus callosum agenesis.

The purpose of imaging is to determine:

1. The anatomy of the bone defect. This is often evident on standard X-ray but is well defined by high-resolution computed tomography (CT) (Figure 12.4.1). In practice, CT is only required for internal lesions to enable planning of repair and any subsequent reconstructive surgery.
2. MRI is used to determine:
   (a) The contents of the cephalocele. Herniations of neural tissue and/or meninges containing CSF reflect the appropriate signal; gliosis may result in higher T2-weighted (T2-W) signal from damaged tissue. Hamartomatous lesions also reflect signal similar to normal neural tissue.
   (b) The normality or otherwise of the remainder of the intracranial and/or spinal contents, and in particular the presence or absence of: (i) hydrocephalus, which may need treatment prior to repair of a cephalocele; and (ii) additional malformations such as Dandy–Walker or Chiari malformations;
   (c) The vascular anatomy of the venous sinuses as these and other vessels may be present in the sac.

T1- and T2-weighted sequences in axial, sagittal and coronal planes are required.
Cephaloceles are classified by location (Figure 12.4.2).

OCCIPITAL AND OCCIPITOCERVICAL CEPHALOCELES

These are the most frequent types seen in the Western hemisphere and represent 80% of lesions in this population. The bone defect may involve:

1. the occipital bone plus adjacent cervical posterior arches (Figure 12.4.3);
2. the occipital bone alone below the external occipital protuberance (Figure 12.4.4);
3. the occipital bone above the protuberance and tentorial insertion (Figure 12.4.5); and
4. the combined supraprotuberal and infraprotuberal defect.

The cephaloceles may contain the occipital lobes and/or cerebellum (Figure 12.4.5): the insertion of the tentorium may be low and then both infratentorial and supratentorial structures, unilaterally or bilaterally, may enter the cephalocele. The brainstem may be pulled posteriorly, particularly when a Chiari type III malformation is associated. The Chiari III malformation is defined by the association of an occipital or upper cervical meningoencephalocele and herniation of the tonsils (Figure 12.4.3). The major veins and sinuses may be in normal position. The lateral sinuses are usually above the superior margins of the defect. The straight sinus torcula may be absent or fenestrated and the superior sagittal sinus may be duplicated round the margins of a high skull defect (Figure 12.4.6). Microcephaly is frequently associated (10% to 25%); hydrocephalus occurs with 20% of meningoceles and 65% of encephaloceles.

Rarely, an occipital cephalocele may contain:

1. A cystic extension of the fourth ventricle arising from the roof or a lateral recess. Hydrocephalus is usual and dysgenesis of the corpus callosum may be present.
2. A deformed bifid cerebellum with absent vermis, each part containing a dilated segment of the fourth ventricle attached to a forked tectum.

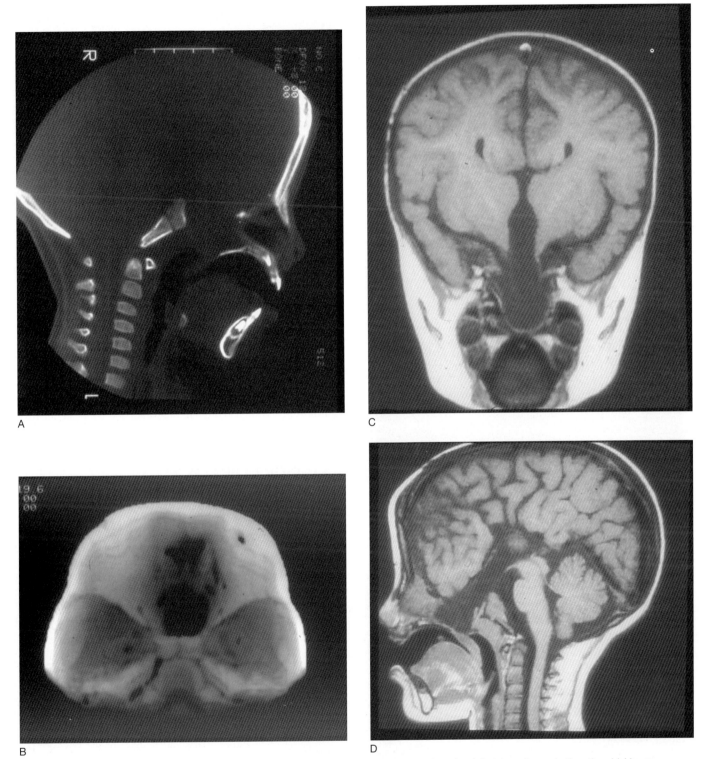

A

B

C

D

Figure 12.4.1 (A) Sagittal reconstruction of an ethmoidal encephalocele. (B) 3D reconstruction, the defect is well seen in the ethmoidal bone. (C,D) coronal and sagittal T1-W MRI. The defect is seen as well as its content. The third ventricle and the pituitary gland are seen in the encephalocele. Absent corpus callosum.

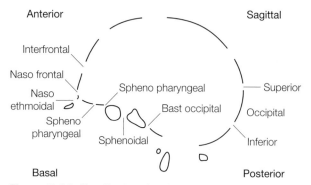

Figure 12.4.2 Classification of cephaloceles by location.

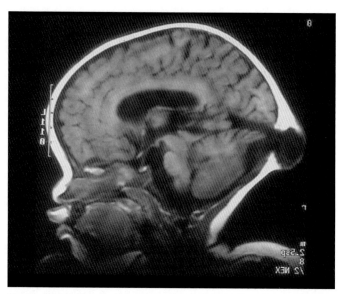

Figure 12.4.5 The meningocele is seen below the torcular, part of the vermis is seen in the sac.

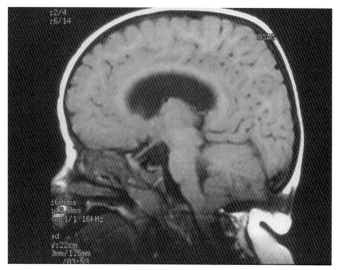

Figure 12.4.3 Occipital cephalocele associated with Chiari malformation. This represents the Chiari III malformation.

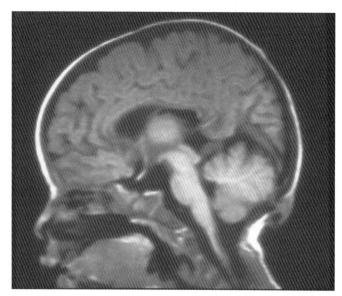

Figure 12.4.4 Occipital cephalocele situated between the external protuberance and the cervical spine.

Other posterior fossa malformations associated with occipital cephaloceles include the Chiari III and the Dandy–Walker and the Walker–Warburg syndromes (Figure 12.4.7).

MRI will clearly define the abnormal anatomy including relationships of the spinal cord and brainstem and the posterior fossa vessels as well as any of the associated malformations.

ANTERIOR CEPHALOCELES

Anterior cephaloceles occur in about 1/35 000 live births but are more common in Asia. They are often associated with facial clefts, callosal dysgenesis or lipoma and other cerebral malformations, and sometimes pituitary insufficiency. Many cases present with a clinically evident mass or deformity such as hypertelorism, which is present in all patients, but in some cases this is not a prominent feature and other presentations include chiasmatic syndromes, airway obstruction, CSF rhinorrhoea and meningitis. CSF rhinorrhoea is usually secondary to inadvertent biopsy of a choanal obstructing mass.

MRI is necessary to distinguish simple meningoceles from encephaloceles and to define structures contained within the latter.

Anterior cephaloceles are subdivided by location into:

1. Syncipital cephaloceles: these form masses above the nose passing through a bone defect, which may be intrafrontal, frontonasal (Figure 12.4.8), frontoethmoidal, or nasoethmoidal. Hypertelorism and/or a mass at the base of the nose are presenting features. These may also be associated with craniofacial abnormalities.
2. Nasopharyngeal or nasal encephaloceles include transsphenoidal cephaloceles, which pass through the body of the sphenoid bone, leaving the dorsum sellae intact, into the nasopharynx (Figure 12.4.9). Contents may include parts of the optic pathway, anterior third ventricle and anterior cerebral arteries. It is important that the pituitary gland is identified and localized by MRI prior to surgery, to ensure that it is not

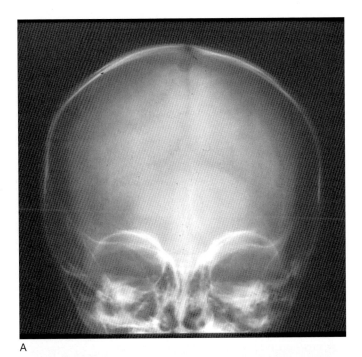

A

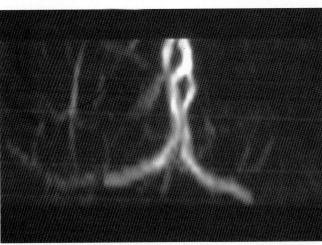

B

Figure 12.4.6 (A) Interparietal meningocele. The bony defect is seen on the anteroposterior (AP) view of the skull. (B) Magnetic resonance arteriography (MRA), the sagittal sinus is duplicated at the level of the bony defect.

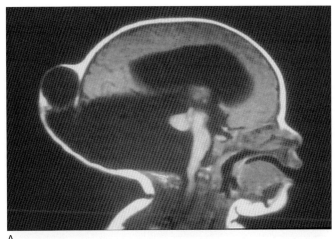

A

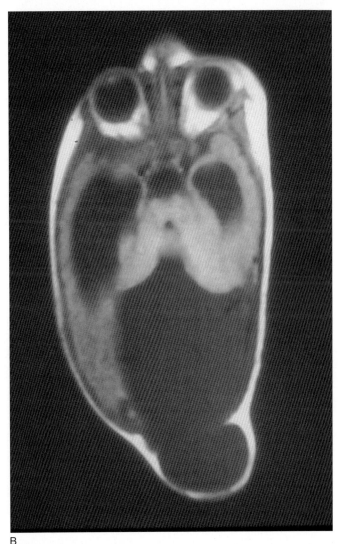

B

Figure 12.4.7 (A,B) Sagittal and axial MRI T1-W images; the meningocele is associated with a Dandy–Walker malformation.

inadvertently injured. Sphenoethmoidal cephaloceles passing through the lamina cribrosa and transethmoidal encephaloceles are other variants of nasopharyngeal cephaloceles. All may present as intranasal masses causing choanal obstruction and respiratory distress in the newborn. They may also descend into the nasopharynx and cause feeding difficulties.

3. Cephaloceles involving the orbit. Spheno-orbital cephaloceles (Figure 12.4.8) extend laterally through the superior orbital fissure or an adjacent osseous defect into the orbit. Spheno-maxillary cephaloceles extend into the pterygopalatine fossa through the inferior orbital and ocular and optic pathway abnormalities.

4. Parietal cephaloceles pass through a midline defect between the bregma and lambda. They vary in size. Meningoceles and

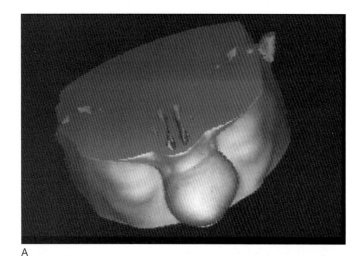

A

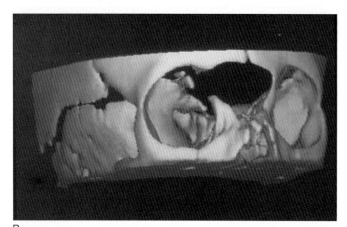

B

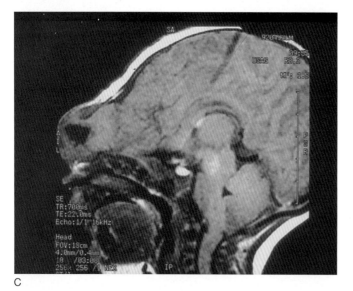

C

Figure 12.4.8 (A,B) 3D reconstruction, soft tissues and bone window. The soft tissue mass is seen in between the two orbits. The sphenoorbital defect is evident. (C) the content of the mass is made of cerebral tissue.

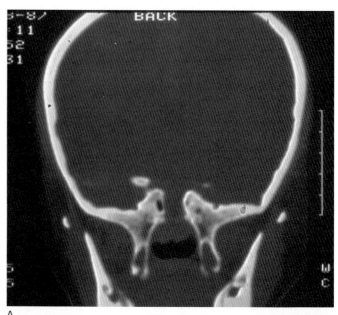

A

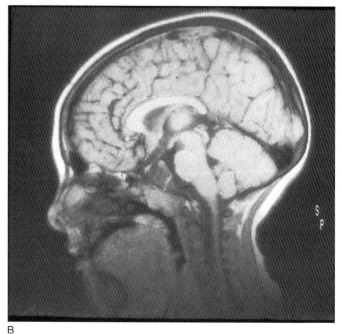

B

Figure 12.4.9 (A) Coronal CT scan shows the defect at the level of the sella turcica. (B) Sagittal MRI shows that the content of the sac is made of the third ventricle and pituitary gland.

encephaloceles are equal in frequency. The prognosis is related to be presence of brain in the cephalocele and associated malformations: it is generally poor, mental retardation being usual, though meningocele patients may develop normally. Almost 50% of cases develop hydrocephalus *in utero*, and a further 25% after birth. Midline malformations of the brain are usually present including callosal dysgenesis usually with a dorsal interhemispheric cyst, Dandy–Walker malformation, Chiari II malformation holoprosencephaly and defects of neuronal migration. The superior sagittal sinus is generally fenestrated around the lesion; this should be recognized because it may be a source of bleeding at surgery. The leaves of the falx may fail to fuse with widening of the interhemispheric fissure and the tentorium also may be fenestrated.

5. Lateral cephaloceles are rare. They may occur along the coronal or lambdoid sutures or pass through the greater wing of the sphenoid into the pterygoid fossa. The latter contain temporal lobe and may present with seizures.

6. Temporal cephaloceles: herniation of brain substance through the tegmen antri or tegmen tympani is usually due to previous surgery, infection or trauma and is uncommonly a congenital anomaly. The herniated brain, which is mature with microglial reaction, is not usually covered by dura and clinical presentation is with CSF leak or meningitis or occasionally with epilepsy.

ANTENATAL DIAGNOSIS

With the advent of routine ultrasound, the diagnosis is often suspected in the fetus. MRI confirms the diagnosis and shows encephaloceles as hyperintense fluid-filled masses in the occipital region (Figure 12.4.10). Large encephaloceles are not compatible with life (Figure 12.4.11).

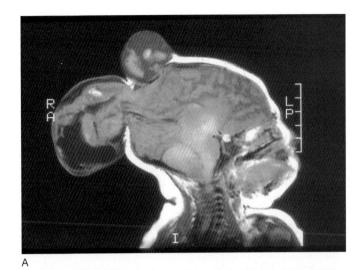

A

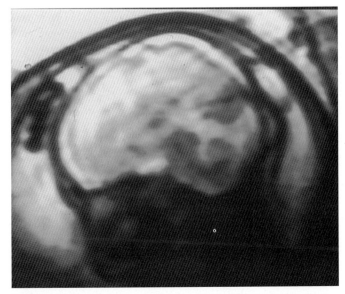

Figure 12.4.10 Sagittal antenatal, T2-weighted MRI of a fetus with an occipital encephalocele.

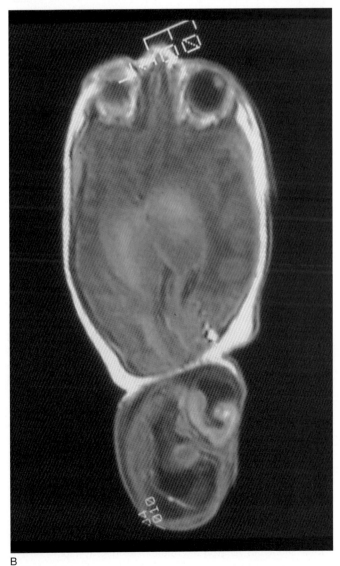

B

Figure 12.4.11 (A,B) Sagittal and axial T1-weighted MRI; a large interparietal defect containing brain tissue is demonstrated.

EXENCEPHALY AND ANENCEPHALY

Related severe malformations include exencephaly and anencephaly, in which the membranous bones of the vault are absent. These lesions are diagnosed *in utero*, where antenatal ultrasound screening is available. Termination of pregnancy is performed as the conditions are incompatible with life. Imaging is therefore rarely, if ever, indicated in these conditions. In exencephaly, the neural tissue protrusion is covered by connective tissue and presents as a mass with adherent vascular dura and skin. The neural tissue is either an undifferentiated mass or composed of disarranged neurones, glial tissue and its precursors. Some cases of exencephaly may be caused by amniotic bands and/or adhesions. Characteristic features of these bands include constrictions, amputations of peripheral digits or limbs and deep linear defects.

Anencephaly occurs in 1/500 live births. It is more common in females (3:1) and in diabetic pregnancies. The baby dies within days of birth. It is probably secondary to early ischaemic damage of the brain. Antenatal ultrasound is diagnostic and leads to interruption of pregnancy.

Absence of the cranial vault is associated with malformation of the base. The orbits are shallow with exophthalmos and the optic nerves do not reach the foramina. The cribiform plate is imperforate. The sella turcica is small and the posterior pituitary is often absent. There is an amorphous mass of vascular neuroglial tissue termed the area cerebrovasculosa adjacent to the base and there is no evidence of a cerebellum, tentorium or falx.

APLASIA CUTIS CONGENITA

Aplasia cutis congenita (congenital scalp defect, congenital ulcer of the newborn) is focal absence of the scalp usually in the midline overlying the superior sagittal sinus near the vertex, but may be occipital, postauricular or in about 25% of cases multiple. The lesions are usually less than 2.5 cm diameter but may be as large as 8 cm. About 25% of cases are familial and the majority of these (80%) are inherited as autosomal dominants. Limb abnormalities may be associated. In about 30%, the bone underlying the scalp defect is absent and then any secondary infection with ulceration may cause haemorrhage from the sinus, which can be fatal, or meningoencephalitis. Distinction from cephalocele is clinically simple but meningocele, lipomeningocele and midline malformations of the brain have been associated but the brain is usually normal.

MRI is the modality of choice to show the depth of the defect, involvement of bone and the relationship of the adjacent venous sinus. Treatment is directed towards covering the defect with full thickness skin grafts.

CT scanning with 3D reconstruction shows the extent of the bony defect. This resolves progressively with age.

OTHER MIDLINE DYSRAPHISMS

Minor anomalies seen on the midline are true dysraphisms. The atretic meningoceles in the occipital region are such (Figure 12.4.12). They present as small soft tissue masses in the occipital region. The skin may be abnormal. The implantation, colour or length of the hair is abnormal as seen in diastematomyelia. An angioma can be seen.

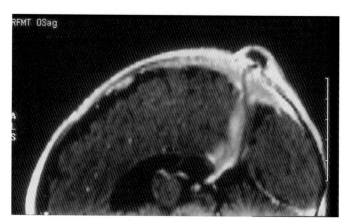

Figure 12.4.12 Atretic interparietal meningocele. Gadolinium injection shows the presence of an hypervascular stalk.

MRI should be done to assess the venous anatomy. The longitudinal sinus may enter the anomaly. It is often duplicated. The fibrous stalk may be attached to the tentorium. The resection of the lesion should be complete as it may recur.

Pathological examination reveals meningeal and fibrous tissues and the mass may contain choroid plexus as well as dermoid or neural tissues.

ANTERIOR ATRETIC MENINGOCELE

An atretic meningocele can be seen at the roof of the nasal bridge. It is clinically seen as a small mass associated with an enlargement of the nasal bridge (Figure 12.4.13) or a fistula that discharges small drops of CSF.

MRI should be done:

1. to confirm the diagnosis by showing the extension and nature of the mass; and
2. to check the intracranial extension of a possible cyst or meningocele.

If the lesion is purely nasal, excision surgery can be performed (Figure 12.4.14). On the other hand, if a meningocele is present a combined neurosurgical and nasal approach should be done to completely resect the lesions and to close the meningeal and dural opening.

Pathological examination will reveal lipomas, dermoid or neural tissues.

The term 'nasal glioma' is technically incorrect and refers to this type of lesion containing neural tissue.

PERSISTENT DERMAL SINUS REMNANTS

Dermal sinuses are developmental epithelial-lined tracts that extend from the skin surface towards the central nervous system. They may terminate within superficial tissues, extend through a bony channel to the epidural region, pass through the dura into the subarachnoid space or further into neural tissue. The normal event of separation of cutaneous from neural ectoderm occurs almost simultaneously with the closure of the neural tube, which explains why a sinus may be included between the dorsal columns and terminate in or near the central canal of the spinal cord. Tethering of

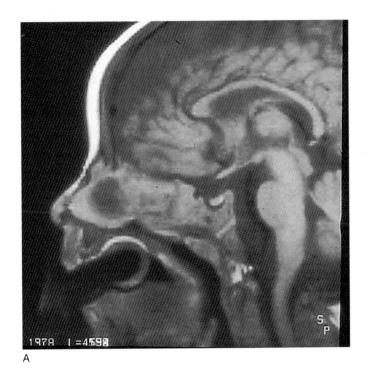

A

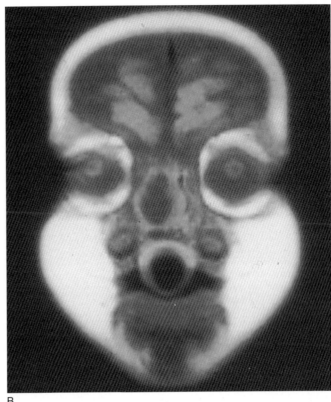

B

Figure 12.4.13 (A,B) Sagittal and coronal T1-weighted MRI shows the presence of an hypointense mass in the right nostril. Biopsy, if performed, would lead to a CSF leak.

the cord is commonly associated. Dermal sinuses may occur anywhere in the neural system in the midline, including frontally.

A dermal sinus may be patent and present with CSF leakage, or more usually with ascending infection, which may result in meningitis, often recurrent, or epidural, intradural or parenchymal abscess or granuloma formation. Irregular or ring enhancement, which could indicate abscess or granuloma formation in the lower spine, foramen magnum/vermis region or midline subfrontal region should suggest the possibility of an underlying dermal sinus: a bone defect should be sought (Figure 12.4.12).

The sinus may be closed but remnants of the dermal structure may be manifest as epidermoid or dermoid masses anywhere along the course of the track (Figure 12.4.15).

These congenital anomalies and their complications are best imaged by MRI.

The dermal sinuses have the characteristics of fibrous tissue and reflect low signal relative to subcutaneous tissue. A defect in the bone through which the sinuses pass is best shown by wide window CT, though any vessels around its margin are best shown by MRI.

DERMOID OR EPIDERMOID TUMOURS

These are sometimes associated with dermal sinuses but more commonly are isolated lesions. They account for between 0.2% and 1% of all intracranial tumours and are benign and slow

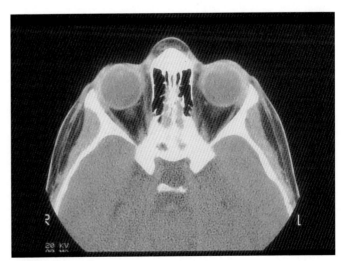

Figure 12.4.14 Axial scan shows a nasal atretic meningocele with content is purely fat. Nasal lipoma is diagnosed.

growing, so that conservative management is often appropriate once the diagnosis is established. They may develop at any depth within the closing neural groove and overlying ectoderm and hence may be located superficially or within the spinal or intracranial subarachnoid space. Intracranial lesions are usually found in the basal cisterns and most frequently in a cerebellopontine angle.

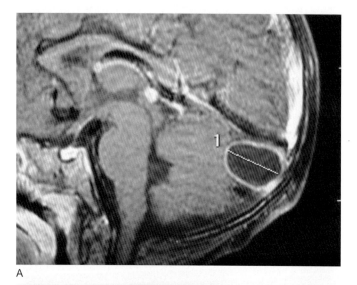

A

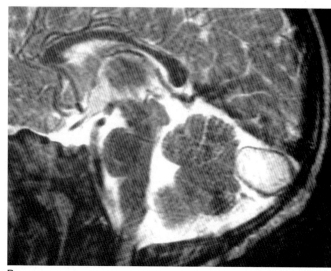

B

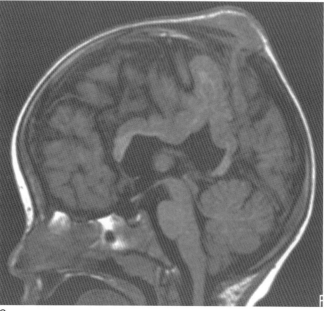

C

Figure 12.4.15 (A) Sagittal T1-W MRI with gadolinium injection. A dermoid cyst the walls of which are enhancing is seen. (B) On T2-W images, the content of the cyst is hyperintense. (C) Sagittal T1-weighted image of a different child with a midline vertex dermoid cyst connected by a sinus track to the level of the vein of Galen.

Less commonly, they occur within cord or brain substance or within the ventricular system.

Epidermoids are composed of stratified squamous epithelium and form cysts containing keratin and cholesterol. Occasionally, haemosiderin may be present in the cyst fluid.

Dermoids may be composed of any or all of the dermal structures. The cyst fluid often contains fat. If rupture occurs, the fat may be recognized on both CT and MRI in the ventricles and/or subarachnoid space.

Typically, both tumours are well-defined encapsulated and usually lobulated masses of low density on CT, and dermoids often have fatty components; occasionally calcification is present in the capsule.

On MRI, dermoids may have regions with very short T1-W and T2-W relaxation due to the presence of fat (Figure 12.4.16).

Epidermoids (Figure 2.4.17) have longer T1-W and T2-W relaxation relative to neural tissue, commonly reflecting signal on T1-

W sequences similar to CSF. On long T2-W sequences, the signal returned is usually hyperintense and often inhomogeneous; occasionally, the presence of haemosiderin may result in regions of low signal return from parts of the cyst contents. Enhancement is usually absent but may occur in the capsules and in the presence of infection.

In the subarachnoid space, epidermoids may not be clearly defined on MRI, especially in the spinal canal.

The intracranial masses may present with local pressure symptoms, seizures or, uncommonly, with meningitic reaction due to leakage of irritant contents into the CSF.

Dermoid/epidermoids also occur in the midline in the subgaleal or subperiosteal space, separate from the skin. In the occipital region, they are often associated with a midline occipital bone defect, duplicated longitudinal sinus and a communicating mass involving the vermis. Near the vertex the tumours cause pressure erosion on the bone but are almost never associated with deep exten-

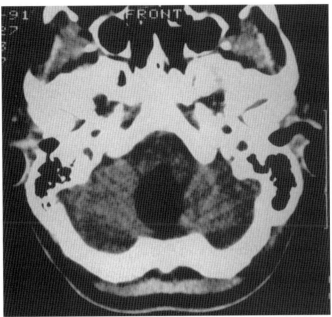

A

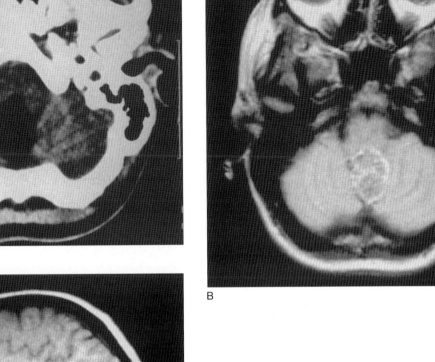

B

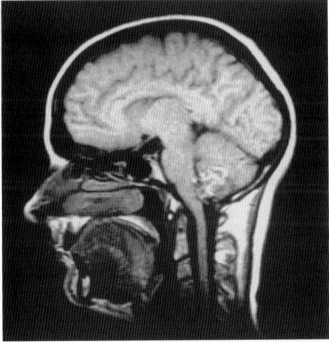

C

Figure 12.4.16 Posterior fossa dermoid. (A) Cranial CT scan shows a low density mass compressing the brainstem and separating the cerebellar hemispheres. (B) Axial and (C) sagittal T1-weighted MRI. There is a heterogeneous mass in the same location. The bright areas are due to fat. The dark strands were proven to be due to hair at surgery.

sion. More laterally situated tumours are often confined within the diploe: they form a lobulated lucency with sclerotic edges expanding the bone. A common site is the outer angle of the orbit, where they may encroach on the orbital fat and displace the globe.

An intraorbital dermoid/epidermoid presents as a well-defined extraconal mass compressing the adjacent structures and causing corticated erosion of bone in the superolateral or superomedial angles of the orbit.

FURTHER READING

Bolger WE, Reger C. Temporal lobe encephalocele appearing as a lytic lesion of the skull base and pterygoid process. Ear Nose and Throat Journal 2003; 82:269–272.

Formica F, Iannelli A, Paludetti G, Di Rocco C. Transphenoidal meningoencephalocele. Childs Nervous System 2002; 18:295–298.

Fraioli B, Conti C, Lunardi P et al. Intrasphenoidal encephalocele associated with cerebrospinal fluid fistula and subdural hematomas: technical case report. Neurosurgery 2003; 52:1487–1490.

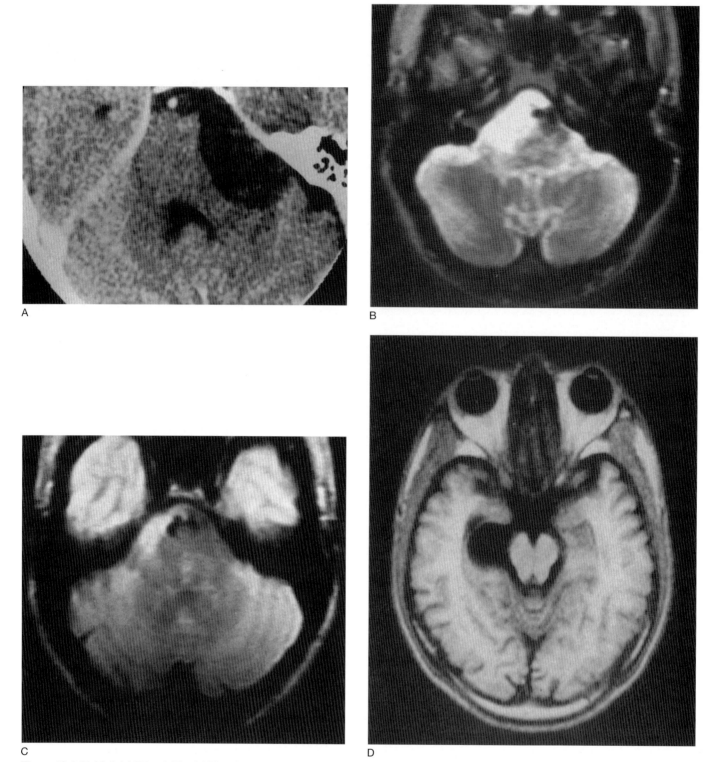

A

B

C

D

Figure 12.4.17 (A) Axial CT and (B) axial T2-weighted MRI. (C) T1-weighted MRI and (D) T1-weighted MRI of a different patient. The epidermoid cyst in (A), (B) and (C) shows as a low attenuation lesion on CT and on MRI as a mixed, slightly lobulated lesion in the cerebello pontine angle displacing the brainstem. In (D) there is a low-density mass on the right in the choroidal fissure with a similar signal to CSF.

Mahapatra AK, Suri A. Anterior encephaloceles: a study of 92 cases. Pediatric Neurosurgery 2002; 36:113–118.

Posnick JC, Costello BJ. Dermoid cysts, gliomas, and encephaloceles: evaluation and treatment. Atlas of Oral Maxillofacial Surgery Clinics of North America 2002; 10:85–99.

Tubbs RS, Wellons JC 3rd, Oakes WJ. Occipital encephalocele, lipomeningomyelocele, and Chiari I malformation: case report and review of the literature. Childs Nervous System 2003; 19:50–53.

CORPUS CALLOSUM ABNORMALITIES

As stated above, the corpus callosum forms from the commissural plate at the 7th week of gestation. The genu is formed before the truncus and the splenium. By the 20th week of gestation, the anterior part of the splenium and the rostrum are formed (Figure 12.4.18).

The terms hypogenesis or complete agenesis are the preferred terms for partial or complete absence of the corpus callosum. In hypogenesis, the anterior part of the corpus callosum is usually present (Figure 12.4.18). The term dysgenesis of the corpus callosum is reserved for truly abnormal formation of the corpus callosum in patients with holoprosencephaly (see holoprosencephaly).

The imaging findings of agenesis are quite specific. A radial pattern can be seen on sagittal images (Figure 12.4.19). This is due to the eversion of the cingulate gyri and radial orientation of the medial hemispheric sulci from the region of the roof of the third ventricle. The longitudinal bundles of Probst can be seen on the

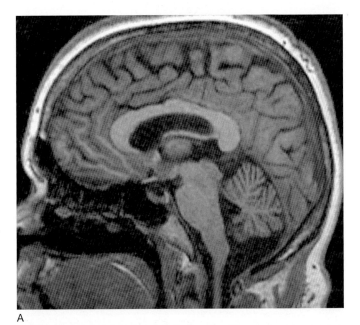

A

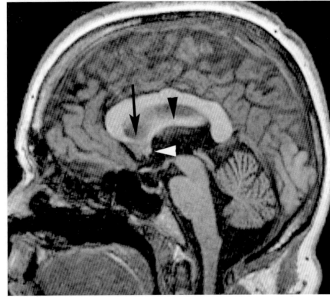

B

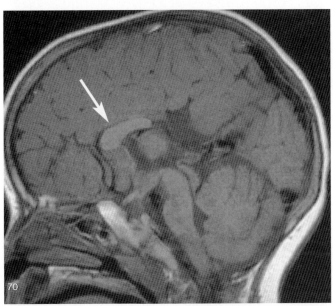

C

Figure 12.4.18 Normal corpus callosum and hypogenesis. Sagittal T1-weighted images (A–C). Note the presence of the rostrum (B, arrow). The anterior commissure (B, white arrowhead) and the fornix (B, black arrowhead). In a child with hypogenesis, only part of the genu and truncus are formed (C, arrow).

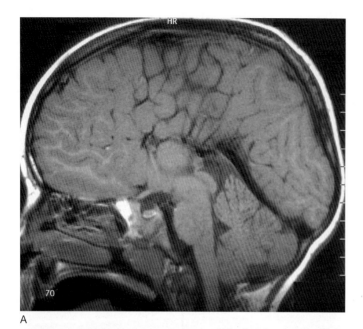

A

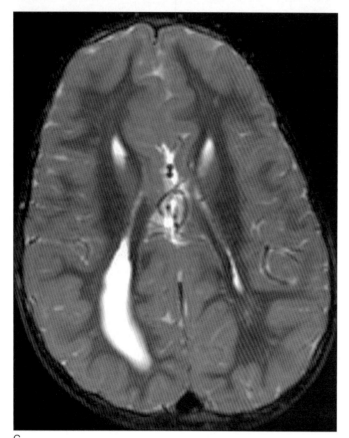

C

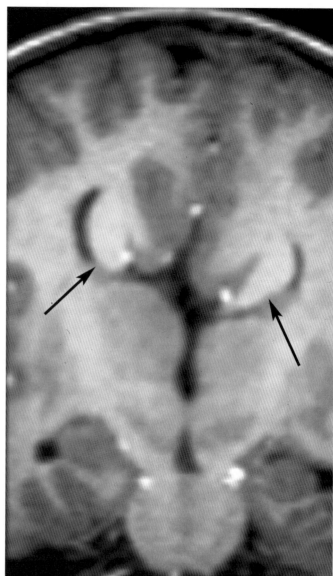

B

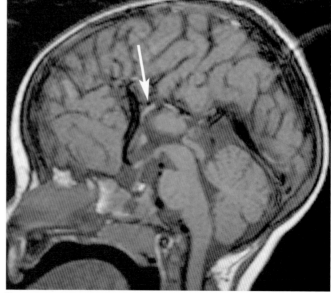

D

Figure 12.4.19 Agenesis of the corpus callosum. Sagittal T1-weighted (A,D), coronal T1-weighted (B) and axial T2-weighted (C) images. The typical radial pattern on a mid-sagittal image is due to the radial orientation of the medial hemispheric sulci (A). The longitudinal bundles of Probst cause an impression on the lateral ventricles (B, arrows). The dilatation of the posterior horns of the lateral ventricles is best seen on an axial image (C). The enlarged hippocampal commissure mimicks the truncus of the corpus callosum (D, arrow).

coronal images (Figure 12.4.19). These bundles represent the callosal fibres that, instead of crossing the midline, impress into the medial walls of the lateral ventricles. The temporal horns are enlarged inferolaterally due to hypoplasia of the tapetum. Colpocephaly, corresponding to the dilatation of the trigones and posterior horns of the lateral ventricles, is typically seen on axial images (Figure 12.4.19). The dilatation is due to the absence of the splenium, which normally defines the ventricular borders. For the same reason, the third ventricle is widened and extends superiorly. The anterior commissure is usually present. The hippocampal commissure is usually absent but may be large and mimic hypogenesis of the corpus callosum (Figure 12.4.19).

Interhemispheric cysts can be associated with corpus callosal developmental abnormalities and different subtypes have been recognized. In type 1, there is communication with the ventricular system. In type 2, there are associated cortical developmental abnormalities (Figure 12.4.20). The interhemispheric cysts in type 3 do not communicate with the ventricles.

Interhemispheric lipomas have frequently been described in association with partial or complete absence of the corpus callosum. A curvilinear type of lipoma often appears to be an incidental finding, while the tubulonodular lipoma is usually associated with a more severe abnormality of the corpus callosum and tends to be symptomatic (Figure 12.4.21). Calcification can be observed and the tubulonodular lipoma often extends bilaterally through the choroidal fissure into the choroid plexus of the lateral ventricle.

Callosal abnormalities are frequently associated with other congenital malformations and can be observed in many syndromes. Intracranial lipomas can be found in different locations, usually in the midline (Figure 12.4.21).

HOLOPROSENCEPHALY

The underlying cause for the complete or partial failure of cleavage of the hemispheres remains uncertain but may be the result of a defective cranial mesenchyme.

Alobar, semilobar and lobar holoprosencephaly have been distinguished but significant overlap exists between the different types. The septum pellucidum and the olfactory bulb are always absent in the three subtypes. The alobar form is the most severe and the child rarely survives. Facial dysmorphism and microcephaly are frequent. The falx, interhemispheric fissure and corpus callosum are absent. There is a horseshoe-shaped monoventricle, which often communicates with a dorsal cyst. In the semilobar form, the midline structures are somewhat better developed. There is a rudimentary third ventricle with attempted division of the monoventricle. The interhemispheric structures are partially formed posteriorly (Figure 12.4.22). Dysgenesis of the corpus callosum is seen and has been attributed to abnormalities of the rostral floor plate. This results in a defect of the rostral lamina terminalis

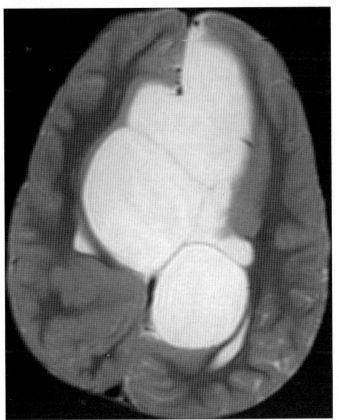

A

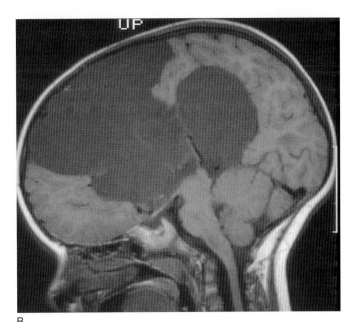

B

Figure 12.4.20 Agenesis of the corpus callosum and interhemispheric cyst. Axial T2-weighted (A) and sagittal T1-weighted (B) images. Note the presence of heterotopic grey matter (A).

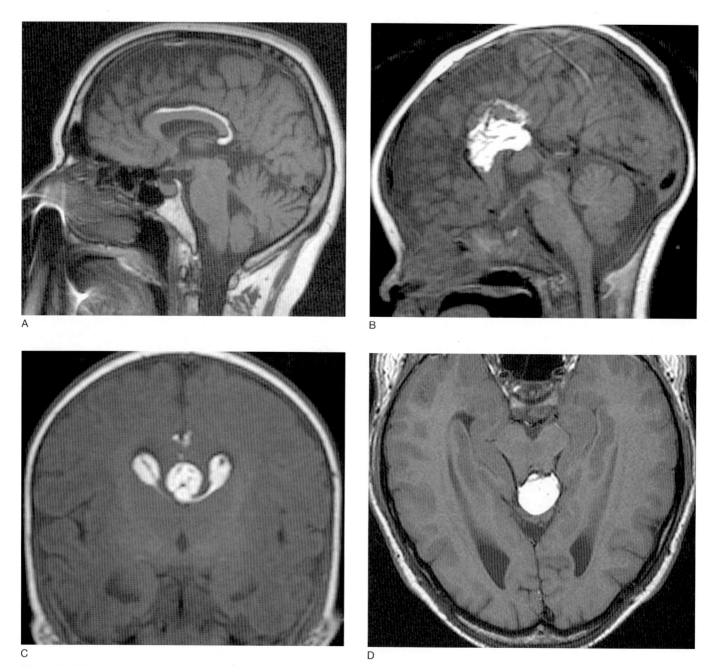

A

B

C

D

Figure 12.4.21 Hypogenesis of the corpus callosum and interhemispheric lipoma. Sagittal T1-weighted (A,B), coronal T1-weighted (C) and axial T1-weighted (D) images. The curvilinear lipoma is usually associated with a mild degree of hypogenesis of the corpus callosum (A). The tubulonodular lipoma is often associated with agenesis (B). The tubulonodular lipoma often extends into the choroid plexus of the lateral ventricle (C). Intracranial lipomas can be found in different locations where remnants of the meninx primitiva can be found (D).

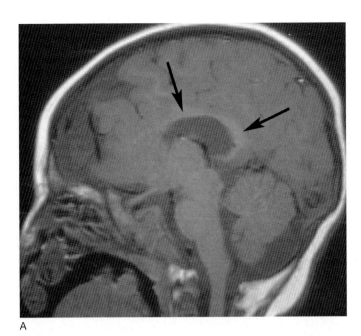

A

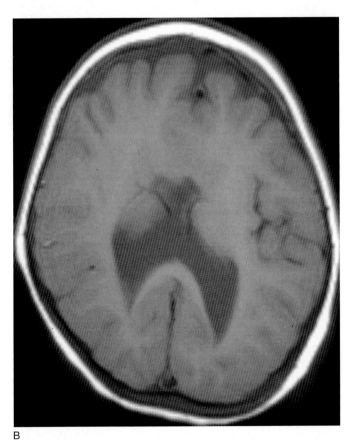

B

Figure 12.4.22 Semilobar holoprosencephaly. Sagittal (A) and axial (B) T1-weighted images. There is dysgenesis of the corpus callosum (A, arrows). The interhemispheric fissure is partially formed in its posterior segment (B).

and no secretion of netrins (which guide axons to the midline) leading to absence of the anterior part of the corpus callosum. Syntelencephaly is a peculiar form of the semilobar holoprosencephaly where the midline structures are present in the frontal and occipital region but remain fused in the middle part of the brain (Figure 12.4.23). Clinically, endocrine dysfunction and choreoathetosis are absent in this variant of holoprosencephaly.

The lobar form is the least severe from the clinical point of view and the abnormalities can sometimes be very subtle. Usually, the frontal horns appear hypoplastic related to the absence of the septum pellucidum. This latter form is also closely related to septo-optic dysplasia (Figure 12.4.24).

SEPTO-OPTIC DYSPLASIA

Also known as de Morsier's syndrome, consists of hypoplasia of the optic nerves and chiasm with absence of the septum pellucidum. Normally, the septum pellucidum is a thin membrane extending from the inferior border of the corpus callosum to the fornix. MR imaging has been used to further classify patients with optic nerve hypoplasia. In one review, in 25% of the patients, no associated abnormalities were demonstrated. The septum pellucidum was absent in 20% of the children. An ectopic neurohypophysis was observed in 15% of the patients (Figure 12.4.24). An associated cortical developmental abnormality was found in 15% of the patients with optic nerve hypoplasia (Figure 12.4.24). There was evidence of antenatal or prenatal brain injury in the remaining 25% of the children.

CORTICAL DEVELOPMENTAL MALFORMATIONS

Compared to the mid eighties, there has been a tremendous advance in our knowledge of the cerebral cortical developmental malformations. MR imaging played a key role in this progress. There has been confusion about the terminology, e.g. cortical dysplasia has been used to cover several other malformations such as polymicrogyria and schizencephaly while nowadays the term is preferably used for a well-described entity called the focal cortical dysplasia of Taylor.

The classification of Barkovich – based on imaging, genetic and pathological observations – consists of a flexible framework that includes all known malformations. It is clear that the classification may undergo alterations and additions in the future as our knowledge in genetics improves.

Three groups of malformations are distinguished: (1) abnormalities of neuronal and glial proliferation; (2) abnormalities of neuronal migration; and (3) abnormalities of cortical organization.

These malformations can result from several environmental factors including maternal exposure to ethanol and radiation, ischaemia or *in utero* infection but an increasing number of genetic causes are being identified. It is important to know that antenatal tissue destruction may not be easy to prove in lesions occurring before 26 weeks, because of the difficult

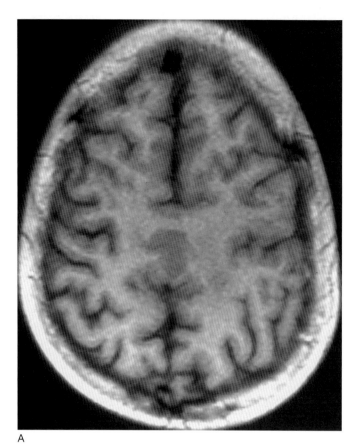

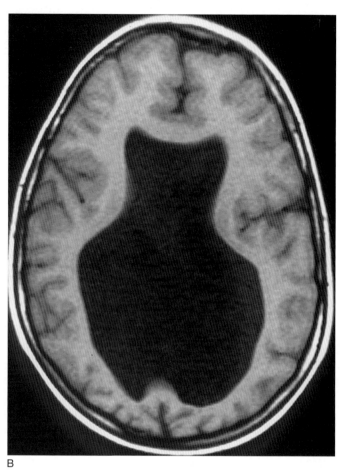

A
B

Figure 12.4.23 Syntelencephaly. Axial T1-weighted images (A,B). There is a fusion of the middle part of the brain (A). The septum pellucidum is absent (B).

differentiation from developmental malformation. The main reason for this is the absence of scar or gliosis formation in the first part of gestation.

These malformations are an important cause of developmental disabilities and epilepsy.

ABNORMALITIES OF NEURONAL PROLIFERATION

These malformations occur in the early days of the cortical development and they often return a high signal on T2-weighted images. We will only discuss the abnormalities that tend to be seen on a regular basis. Some tumours (e.g. dysembryoplastic neuroepithelial tumour, ganglioglioma, gangliocytoma) and the tuberous sclerosis complex are included in this group but will be discussed elsewhere in this section.

FOCAL CORTICAL DYSPLASIA

This entity, first described by Taylor, consists of a focal disorganized cortex with abnormally large neurons, called balloon cells because of their histopathological appearance. Apart from the abnormal cortex, there is also an abnormal focal myelination.

On imaging, the cortex may appear normal or thinner than normal, usually with blurring of the grey–white matter interface, a useful sign to differentiate focal cortical dysplasia from polymicrogyria. The high signal on T2-weighted images may be due to gliosis and/or the presence of balloon cells (Figure 12.4.25). Gadolinium enhancement has occasionally been reported.

Mesial temporal sclerosis has been observed together with focal cortical dysplasia.

It is now accepted that there is an overlap between focal cortical dysplasia and the cortical tubers, which can be observed in tuberous sclerosis. Imaging of infants younger than 3 months has demonstrated cortical malformations with low signal on T2-W and high signal on T1-W images, relative to immature white matter (Figure 12.4.26).

Focal transmantle dysplasia is histopathologically similar to focal cortical dysplasia but extends from the wall of the ventricle to the cortex. This imaging finding has been called the 'transmantle sign' (Figure 12.4.27).

HEMIMEGALENCEPHALY

This malformation may involve part of one hemisphere or the whole hemisphere and hemicranium. The affected area appears significantly enlarged and returns heterogeneous signals reflecting

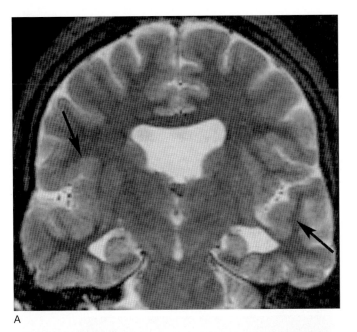

A

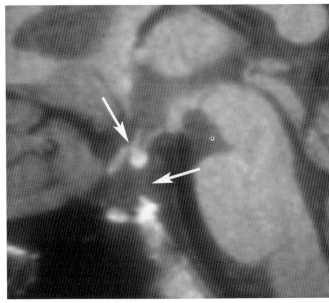

C

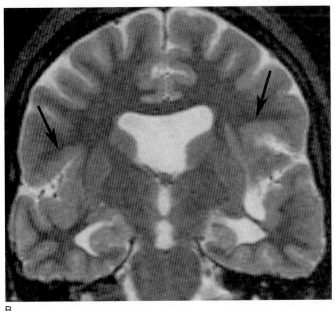

B

Figure 12.4.24 Septo-optic dysplasia. Coronal T2-weighted (A,B) and sagittal T1-weighted (C) images. Bilateral polymicrogyria can be seen in the region of the insular cortex (A,B, arrows). The septum pellucidum is absent. Note the ectopic neurohypophysis (C, arrow) and the absence of the pituitary stalk in another child. The bony sella turcica and the adenohypophysis are hypoplastic (C).

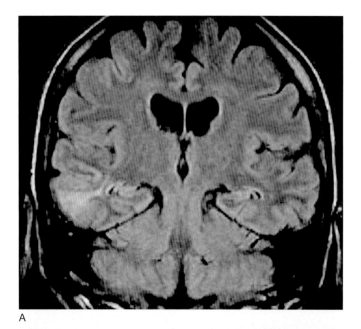

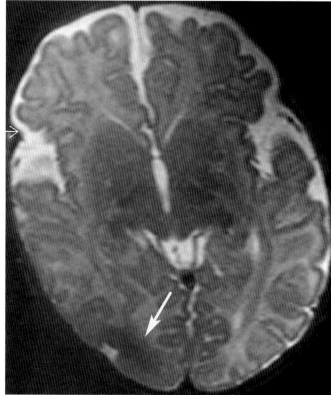

A

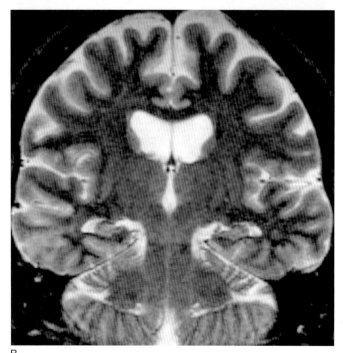

B

Figure 12.4.25 Focal cortical dysplasia of Taylor. Coronal fluid-attenuated inversion recovery (A) and T2-weighted (B) images. The abnormalities in the cortex and in the subcortical white matter of the right temporal lobe are shown.

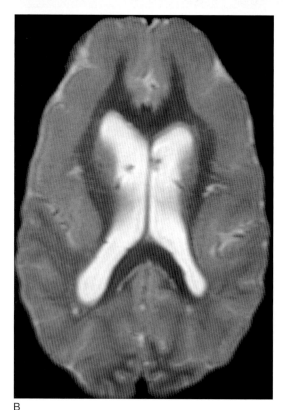

B

Figure 12.4.26 Cortical tuber. Axial T2-weighted (A) and T1-weighted (B) images. In infants younger than 3 months, the tubers may return a low T2-W signal and a high T1-W signal relative to the immature white matter (arrows).

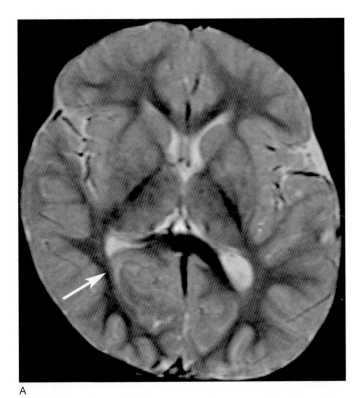

A

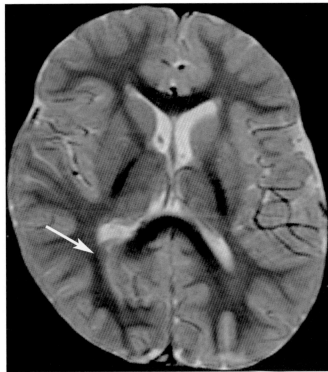

B

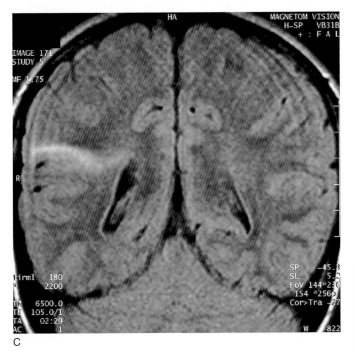

C

Figure 12.4.27 Focal transmantle dysplasia. Axial T2-weighted (A,B) and coronal fluid-attenuated inversion recovery (C) images. An abnormal signal is seen on the axial images in the right occipital lobe (A, arrow). Note the extension towards the ventricle (B, arrow) and the so-called transmantle sign (C). (Reproduced with permission from Ph. Demaerel. Cortical developmental malformations. Recent Advances in Diagnostic Neuroradiology 2001:325–345.)

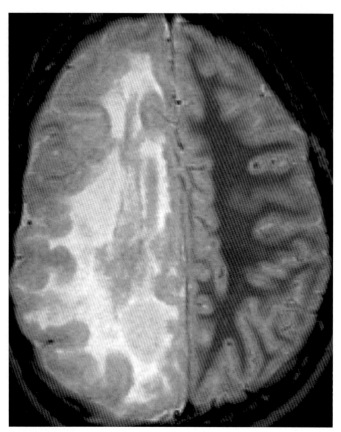

Figure 12.4.28 Hemimegalencephaly. Axial T2-weighted image. The right hemisphere appears enlarged and abnormalities can be seen both in the grey and in the white matter.

dysmyelination and abnormalities of proliferation, migration and cortical organization (Figure 12.4.28). It is important to evaluate the contralateral hemisphere to exclude abnormalities, which would render any treatment unsuccessful. The abnormalities may undergo changes over time.

ABNORMALITIES OF NEURONAL MIGRATION

These malformations occur during the migration of the neurons from the germinal matrix to their final destination, the cortex. They typically return a signal similar to that of grey matter.

LISSENCEPHALY

This entity is also referred to as agyria-pachygyria complex. The classical (type I) lissencephaly can be differentiated from the cobblestone (type II) lissencephaly (Figure 12.4.29). Some patients have been shown to have chromosomal mutations, the best known clinical entity being the autosomal dominant form of the Miller–Dieker syndrome. The locus (LIS-1) has been mapped to chromo-

some 17p13.3 and the genes identified. A variable involvement of the cortex can be observed, usually correlating with the severity of the symptoms. Relative sparing of the frontal lobes (LIS-1 mutations) and of the occipital lobes (XLIS mutations) have been reported. In agyria, imaging usually demonstrates the thin outer cortex (corresponding to a molecular and a disarranged outer cellular layer) and a thick 'inner' cortex (corresponding to the arrested neurons) with a cell-sparse band of white matter in between. The thicker the heterotopic band the higher the chances of finding a pachygyric cortex. In agyria, the cortex is smooth with only the shallow sylvian fissures. The infants present with seizures and hypotonia.

In pachygyria, the cortex is thickened and the sulci are incompletely formed. The junction between grey and white matter is regular as opposed to the junction in polymicrogyria (Figure 12.4.30).

The cobblestone lissencephalies represent what has been called the type II lissencephalies. The cortex is thickened and lacks a layered structure, consisting of a disorganized outer layer and an inner layer representing remnants of the cortical plate. It has been typically described in Fukuyama congenital muscular dystrophy, muscle-eye-brain disease and Walker–Warburg syndrome. Recently, it has been suggested these abnormalities be considered as part of the 'cobblestone complex' rather than lissencephaly type II. Patients with band heterotopia are nowadays classified as an X-linked form of lissencephaly (see grey matter heterotopia).

Another type of lissencephaly, caused by a mutation of reelin, has recently been described. A hypoplastic cerebellum without lobulation is typically associated. Histologically and on MR imaging, the cell sparse zone, which is typically seen in DCX and LIS1 mutations, cannot be recognized in the reelin mutant cortex.

GREY MATTER HETEROTOPIA

Heterotopic grey matter can be located in the subependymal region, in the subcortical region or in between at any point along the route of migration from the subependymal region to the subcortex (Figure 12.4.31). Heterotopia refers to normal structures in an abnormal site.

Bilateral periventricular nodular heterotopia (BPNH) has been linked to mutations in filamin-1 (FLN1), a molecule that plays a role in the communication between the cell surface and the cytoskeleton (Figure 12.4.32). The X-linked BPNH is more frequent in females with prenatal lethality in males and 50% recurrence risk in the female siblings of women with BPNH. Heterozygous females show epilepsy and coagulopathy.

Laminar or band heterotopia or the so-called 'double cortex' has been seen in association with mutations in the DCX gene, which was found to encode a protein doublecortin (Figure 12.4.33). The entity is also classified as an X-linked form of lissencephaly (X-LIS). The abnormality consists of a band of grey matter, usually in both hemispheres, within the white matter. Pachygyria is typically more severe in the frontal lobes. The main clinical manifestations are developmental delay and epilepsy. In some families with epilepsy, some men with classical lissencephaly had mothers or sisters with band heterotopia. The more severe the pachygyria and the thicker the band heterotopia, the higher the chances of

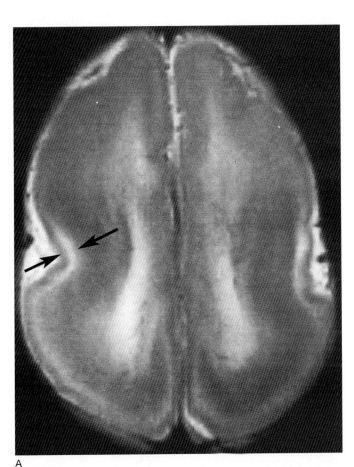

A

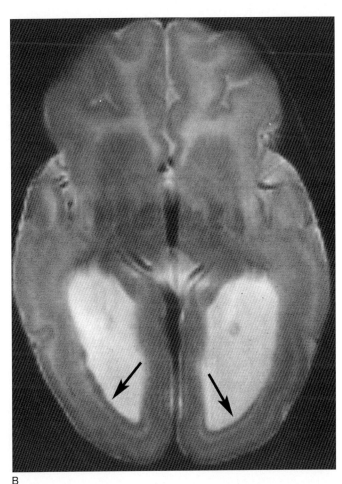

B

Figure 12.4.29 Lissencephaly type I. Axial T2-weighted images (A,B). Between the thin outer cortex and the band of arrested neurons, the cell-sparse band of white matter is clearly seen (A, arrows). Note the presence of subependymal heterotopic grey matter at the level of the temporal and occipital lobes (B, arrows).

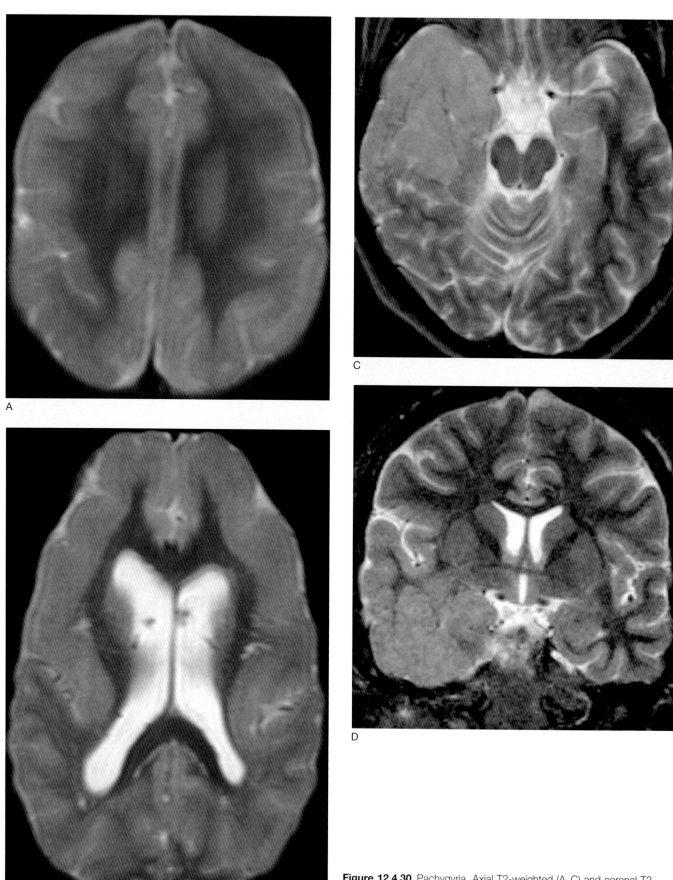

Figure 12.4.30 Pachygyria. Axial T2-weighted (A–C) and coronal T2-weighted (D) images. Diffuse pachygyria (A) and pachygyria with symmetrical predominantly frontal and temporal involvement are shown (B). Focal extensive pachygyria in the right temporal lobe is demonstrated (C,D).

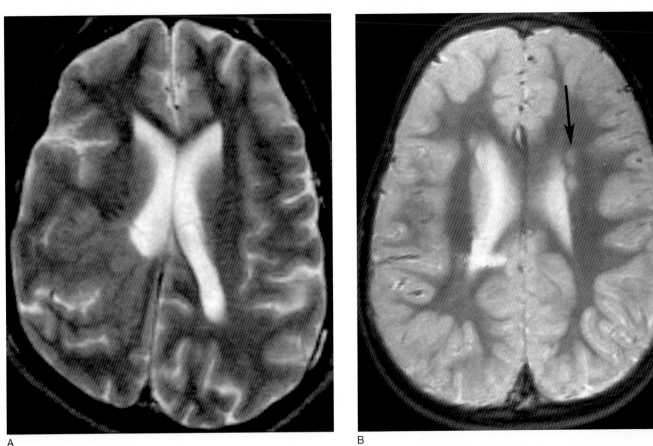

A

B

Figure 12.4.31 Subcortical heterotopia. Axial T2-weighted images (A,B). Extensive right parietal subcortical heterotopia is shown in the presence of a smaller right hemisphere. Note the abnormal appearance of the cortex of the right frontal lobe. Small heterotopic grey matter nodules are seen at some distance from the ventricles in the left frontal white matter (B, arrow).

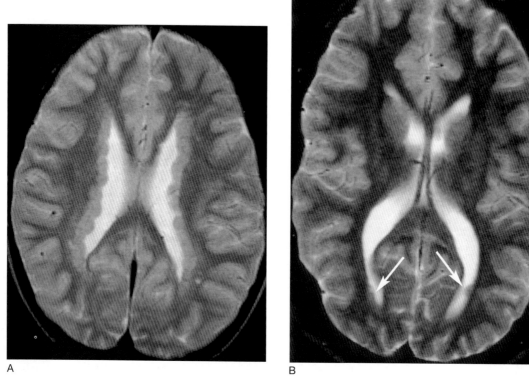

Figure 12.4.32 Bilateral periventricular nodular heterotopia. Axial T2-weighted images (A,B). Diffuse (A) involvement and limited occipital (B, arrows) involvement are illustrated.

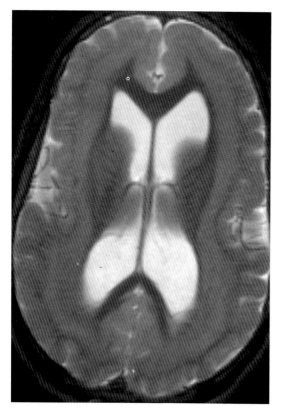

Figure 12.4.33 Band heterotopia. Axial T2-weighted image. A band of grey matter is seen within the white matter of both hemispheres.

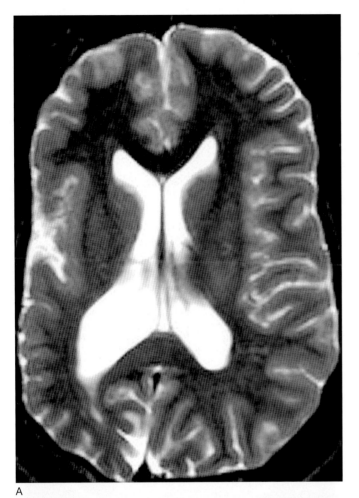

A

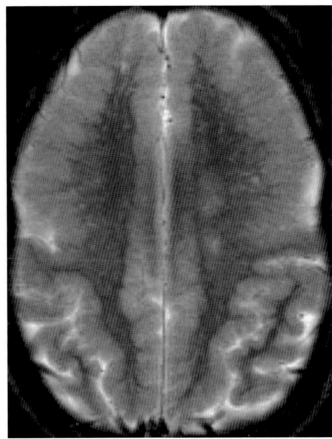

B

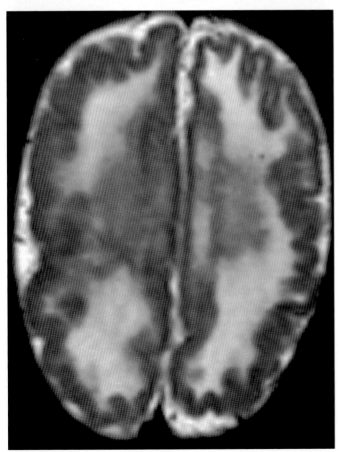

C

Figure 12.4.34 Polymicrogyria. Axial T2-weighted images (A–C). Three different degrees of involvement are shown: focal right insular and parietal polymicrogyria (A), symmetrical predominantly frontal polymicrogyria (B) and diffuse polymicrogyria following cytomegalovirus infection (C).

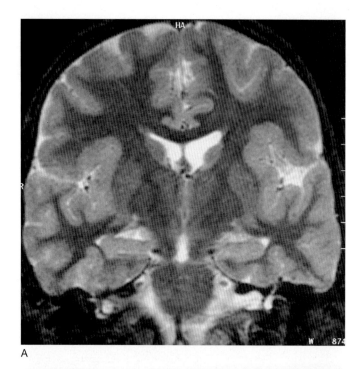

A

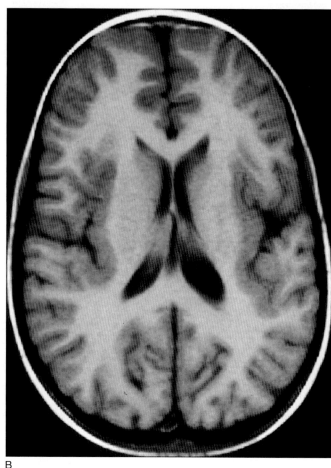

B

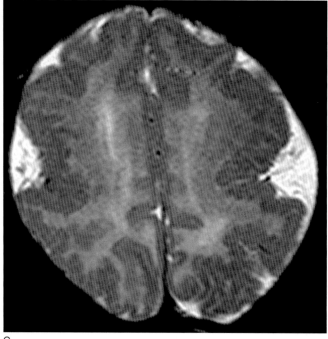

C

Figure 12.4.35 Bilateral perisylvian polymicrogyria. Coronal T2-weighted (A), axial T1-weighted (B) and axial T2-weighted (C) images. Note the bilateral perisylvian cortical involvement (A,B). The symmetrical peri-Rolandic abnormalities represent abnormal cortical infolding (C).

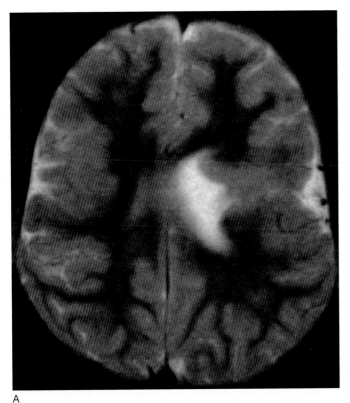

A

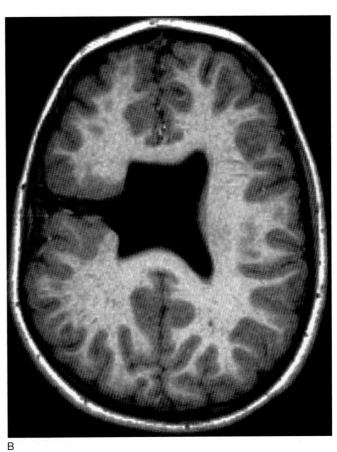

B

Figure 12.4.36 Schizencephaly. Axial T2-weighted (A) and axial T1-weighted (B) images. Unilateral left closed-lip schizencephaly is shown (A). Note the abnormal frontal cortex on the right side (A). An example of right open-lip schizencephaly is shown (B). The septum pellucidum is absent. Note the polymicrogyria that lines the cleft in both children.

developing Lennox–Gastaut syndrome or some other generalized epilepsy.

ABNORMALITIES OF CORTICAL ORGANIZATION

After the migration, a complex organization of the neurons will lead to the normal six-layered cortex. The more common malformations that may occur will be discussed below.

BILATERAL PERISYLVIAN POLYMICROGYRIA

Polymicrogyria refers to an abnormal gyration consisting of an increased number of gyri. The cortical maldevelopment is due to a process affecting mainly the deep cortical layers, reducing the vascularization and arresting growth (Figure 12.4.34). The excessive proliferation of the outer layers results in the increased number of gyri. Whereas in the past it was debatable whether polymicrogyria could be diagnosed on MR imaging or only histopathologically, it is now accepted that the diagnosis can be given on imaging. Microscopically, two types have been recognized. Both the unlayered and the four-layered polymicrogyria may be seen together in the same patient, indicating that they may represent one entity with a variable expression. The inner border is sharp but irregular, which allows the differential diagnosis with pachygyria, where the inner border is sharp but smooth. The abnormal arterial supply is often associated with anomalous venous drainage. In some cases, polymicrogyria may be due to a gene mutation but it is likely that a vascular insult in layer 5 of the cortex may cause the abnormality between the 20th and 24th week of gestation. Polymicrogyria has been described following cytomegalovirus infection (Figure 12.4.34). The cerebral and cerebellar cortex can be affected.

Bilateral perisylvian polymicrogyria is a well-recognized entity (Figure 12.4.35). Clinical presentation includes congenital hemiplegia, facial-lingual diplegia with seizures, pseudobulbar palsy and mental retardation. Usually, the opercular and perisylvian cortex are involved. Several families have been reported, indicating genetic heterogeneity.

SCHIZENCEPHALY

The term schizencephaly merely refers to an abnormal cleft, which is the reason why 'agenetic porencephaly' has been suggested. The cleft is lined by a polymicrogyric cortex and extends from the subependymal region to the pia. Bilateral and unilateral schizencephaly can be observed, most often in the perisylvian area. The terms open- and closed-lip schizencephaly refer to the separated and adjacent walls of the cleft (Figure 12.4.36). Patients with bilateral clefts usually have microcephaly, developmental delay and spastic quadriparesis. Open-lip schizencephaly results in more severe impairment. Heterozygous mutations in the EMX2 gene have been reported.

Schizencephaly is associated with septo-optic dysplasia in about one-third of the cases. Recently, a correlation was found between the location of the clefts and the absence of the septum pellucidum. The patients with absent septum pellucidum had their clefts in the frontal lobe, confirming the hypothesis that the septum pellucidum forms from the 'medial medullary velum' of the frontal lobe. These observations suggest a developmental disorder rather than a destructive insult. The ventricles are usually dilated and a diverticulum can be identified where the pia and ependyma join to form the pia-ependymal seam.

ACKNOWLEDGEMENTS

We gratefully thank Paul Casaer, MD, PhD, Lieven Lagae MD, PhD and Gunnar Buyse MD, PhD from the Department of Paediatrics, for referring their patients.
We acknowledge Wolfgang Desmedt for his photographic assistance.

FURTHER READING

Aida N. Fukuyama congenital muscular dystrophy: a neuroradiologic review. Journal of Magnetic Resonance Imaging 1998; 8:317–326.

Barkovich AJ. Congenital malformations of the brain and skull. In: Barkovich AJ, ed. Pediatric neuroimaging, 2nd edn. Philadelphia: Lippincott-Raven Publishers; 1996:177–276.

Barkovich AJ. Magnetic resonance imaging: role in the understanding of cerebral malformations. Brain and Development 2002; 24:2–12.

Barkovich AJ. Neuroimaging manifestations and classification of congenital muscular dystrophies. American Journal of Neuroradiology 1998; 19:1389–1396.

Barkovich AJ, Kuzniecky RI, Bollen AW et al. Focal transmantle dysplasia: a specific malformation of cortical development. Neurology 1997; 49: 1148–1152.

Barkovich AJ, Kuzniecky RI, Dobyns WB et al. A classification scheme for malformations of cortical development. Neuropediatrics 1996; 27:59–63.

Barkovich AJ, Simon EM, Clegg NJ et al. Analysis of the cerebral cortex in holoprosencephaly with attention to the sylvian fissures. American Journal of Neuroradiology 2002; 23:143–150.

Barkovich AJ, Simon EM, Walsh CA. Callosal agenesis with cyst: a better understanding and new classification. Neurology 2001; 56:220–227.

Baron Y, Barkovich AJ. MR imaging of tuberous sclerosis in neonates and young infants. American Journal of Neuroradiology 1999; 20:907–916.

Blaser SI, Jay V. Disorders of cortical formation: radiologic-pathologic correlation. Neurosurgery Clinics of North America 2002; 13:41–62.

Bronen RA, Vives KP, Kim JH et al. Focal cortical dysplasia of Taylor, balloon cell subtype: MR differentiation from low-grade tumor. American Journal of Neuroradiology 1997; 18:1141–1151.

Chan S, Chin SS, Goodman RR et al. Prospective magnetic resonance imaging identification of focal cortical dysplasia including the non-balloon cell subtype. Annals of Neurology 1998; 44:749–757.

Chen C-Y, Zimmerman RA, Faro S et al. MR of the operculum: abnormal opercular formation in infants and children. American Journal of Neuroradiology 1996; 17:1303–1311.

Demaerel Ph, Vandegaer Ph, Wilms G et al. Interhemispheric lipoma with variable callosal dysgenesis: relationship between embryology, morphology, and symptomatology. European Radiology 1996; 6:904–909.

Golden JA. Cell migration and cerebral cortical development. Neuropathology and Applied Neurobiology 2001; 27:22–28.

Grant PE, Barkovich AJ, Wald LL et al. High-resolution surface-coil MR of cortical lesions in medically refractory epilepsy: a prospective study. American Journal of Neuroradiology 1997; 18:291–301.

Gropman AL, Barkovich AJ, Vezina LG et al. Pediatric congenital bilateral perisylvian syndrome: clinical and MRI features in 12 patients. Neuropediatrics 1997; 28:198–203.

Guerrini R, Carrozzo R. Epilepsy and genetic malformations of the cerebral cortex. American Journal of Medical Genetics 2001; 106:160–173.

Hahn JS, Pinter JD. Holoprosencephaly: genetic, neuroradiological, and clinical advances. Seminars in Pediatric Neurology 2002; 9:309–319.

Hanefeld F, Kruse B, Holzbach U et al. Hemimegalencephaly: localized proton magnetic resonance spectroscopy in vivo. Epilepsia 1995; 36:1215–1224.

Hayashi N, Tsutsumi Y, Barkovich AJ. Polymicrogyria without porencephaly/schizencephaly. MRI analysis of the spectrum and the prevalence of macroscopic findings in the clinical population. Neuroradiology 2002; 44:647–655.

Iannetti P, Spalice A, Atzei G et al. Neuronal migrational disorders in children with epilepsy: MRI, interictal SPECT and EEG comparisons. Brain and Development 1996; 18:269–279.

Ickowitz V, Eurin D, Rypens F et al. Prenatal diagnosis and postnatal follow-up of pericallosal lipoma: report of seven new cases. American Journal of Neuroradiology 2001; 22:767–772.

Landrieu P, Husson B, Pariente D et al. MRI-neuropathological correlations in type 1 lissencephaly. Neuroradiology 1998; 40:173–176.

Leventer RJ, Phelan EM, Coleman LT et al. Clinical and imaging features of cortical malformations in childhood. Neurology 1999; 53:715–722.

Lewis AJ, Simon EM, Barkovich AJ et al. Middle interhemispheric variant of holoprosencephaly: a distinct cliniconeuroradiologic subtype. Neurology 2002; 59:1860–1865.

Li LM, Cendes F, Cunha Bastos A et al. Neuronal metabolic dysfunction in patients with cortical developmental malformations. A proton magnetic resonance spectroscopic imaging study. Neurology 1998; 50:755–759.

Mitchell TN, Stevens JM, Free SL et al. Anterior commissure absence without callosal agenesis: a new brain malformation. Neurology 2002; 58: 1297–1299.

Montenegro MA, Guerreiro MM, Lopes-Cendes I et al. Interrelationship of genetics and prenatal injury in the genesis of malformations of cortical development. Archives of Neurology 2002; 59:1147–1153.

Rakic P. Principles of neural cell migration. Experientia 1990; 46:882–891.

Raybaud C, Girard N, Levrier O et al. Schizencephaly: correlation between the lobar topography of the cleft(s) and absence of the septum pellucidum. Childs Nervous System 2001; 17:217–222.

Raymond AA, Fish DR, Sisodiya SM et al. Abnormalities of gyration, heterotopias, tuberous sclerosis, focal cortical dysplasia, microdysgenesis, dysembryoplastic neuroepithelial tumour and dysgenesis of the archicortex in epilepsy. Brain 1995; 118:629–660.

Rolland Y, Adamsbaum C, Sellier N et al. Opercular malformations: clinical and MRI features in 11 children. Pediatric Radiology 1995; 25: S2–S8.

Ruoss K, Lovblad K, Schroth G et al. Brain development (sulci and gyri) as assessed by early postnatal MR imaging in preterm and term newborn infants. Neuropediatrics 2001; 32:69–74.

Sato N, Hatakeyama S, Shimizu N et al. MR evaluation of the hippocampus in patients with congenital malformations of the brain. American Journal of Neuroradiology 2001; 22:389–393.

Sidman RL, Rakic P. Development of the human central nervous system. In: Haymaker W, Adams RD, eds. Histology and histopathology of the central nervous system. Springfield: Thomas; 1982:3–145.

Sisodiya SM, Free SL, Stevens JM et al. Widespread cerebral structural changes in patients with cortical dysgenesis and epilepsy. Brain 1995; 118:1039–1050.

Spreafico AC, Battaglia G, Arcelli P et al. Cortical dysplasia. An immunocy-tochemical study of three patients. Neurology 1998; 50:27–36.

Van Bogaert P, David P, Gillain CA et al. Perisylvian dysgenesis: clinical, EEG, MRI and glucose metabolism features in 10 patients. Brain 1998; 121:2229–2238.

Woo CL, Chuang SH, Becker LE et al. Radiologic-pathologic correlation in focal cortical dysplasia and hemimegalencephaly in 18 children. Pediatric Neurology 2001; 25:295–303.

Yagishita A, Arai N, Maehara T et al. Focal cortical dysplasia: appearance on MR images. Radiology 1998; 203:553–559.

Congenital Cerebellar Malformations

Philippe Demaerel

INTRODUCTION

The increasing number of reports on cerebellar malformations is the best proof of the renewed interest in the cerebellum. A reference classification is certainly not yet available but interesting proposals have been put forward on the basis of anatomy and embryology. Our understanding of the role played by genes in the genesis of the cerebellum is steadily improving. Our insight into cerebellar malformations, although far from complete, is more advanced. In this chapter, an outline classification of cerebellar malformations based on our own experience and on the recent reports in the literature will be described.

CEREBELLAR ANATOMY AND EMBRYOLOGY

Our understanding of cerebellar embryology is still limited and incompletely understood. Fetal magnetic resonance imaging (MRI) has been used to study the development of the cerebellum and is capable of visualizing the cerebellar primordium from the 10th week of gestation. However, due to the limited resolution, the imaging findings were 5–6 weeks behind the known histological observations. Recent advances in the field of neurogenetics have improved our insight into cerebellar development. Several genes, proteins and molecules are involved in the various stages of cerebellar development. It is thought that the so-called midbrain-hindbrain organizer or isthmus regulates the development of the cerebellum. This region is a source of hormonal factors and signalling molecules that regulate the proliferation of ventricular cells and is controlled by several genes, e.g. *Gbx 2* homeobox gene and *Otx 2*.

At approximately 3 weeks, the neural tube is divided into the prosencephalon, mesencephalon and rhombencephalon. When the neural tube closes, during the 4th week, the rhombencephalon divides into the metencephalon (pons and cerebellum) and the myelencephalon (medulla oblongata). Following the proliferation of cells in the alar plate, the rhombic lip is formed at around 6 weeks of gestation. In a recent report it was suggested that the traditional view of the rhombic lip as a paired structure should be questioned. Sidman and Rakic proposed the cerebellar primordium as an unpaired structure. It has been suggested that the cerebellar primordium develops in the roof of the metencephalon, which will become divided into a median vermis and a pair of hemispheres, due to rotational forces directed outwards with eversion of the cerebellum and resulting in a so-called fissure fracture between the vermis and the hemispheres. The hemispheres, which develop from the lateral parts (rhombic lips) of the cerebellar primordium, grow more rapidly and the cerebellum will rotate around its transverse axis in the caudal direction.

The cavity of the rhombencephalon, the rhombencephalic vesicle, expands considerably to become the fourth ventricle. The roof is divided into two membranous areas by the plica choroidea: (1) an anterior membranous area, which disappears upon formation of the choroid plexus; and (2) a posterior membranous area, which will communicate with the subarachnoid space of the cisterna magna at the foramen of Magendie, occurring between the 11th and 16th week of gestation according to the literature. The Blake's pouch is a temporary structure that arises from the posterior membranous area and is considered the precursor of the foramen of Magendie. The foramina of Luschka open after the 16th week of gestation.

Between the 9th and 13th week of gestation, the Purkinje cells and the neurons of the deep cerebellar nuclei migrate radially outward from the germinal matrix. This process depends on the expression of several genes. The generation of granular cells and their tangential migration will result in a transient external granular cell layer. This secondary germinal matrix persists until approximately the age of 18 months. Cells in this secondary matrix will proliferate and migrate inward, forming the internal granular cell layer.

At about the 12th week of gestation, cerebellar fissures begin to form. The posterolateral fissure, which separates the flocculonodular lobe from the rest of the cerebellum, is the first to be formed. The flocculonodular lobe develops first and is therefore often referred to as archicerebellum. By 13 weeks, the anterior lobe is separated from the posterior lobe by the primary fissure and consists of the three lobules in the vermis: lingula, central lobule and culmen. The second and third lobules have hemispheric extensions. The terms paleocerebellum and neocerebellum refer respectively to the vermis plus flocculi and the hemispheres except the flocculi.

The vermis is formed by approximately 16 weeks of gestation, 4–8 weeks before the formation of the cerebellar hemispheres. It is clear that the formation of the vermis and the hemispheres are closely related. The vermian and hemispheric parts of the anterior lobe and of the posterior part of the posterior lobe develop together. The processes of foliation and fissuration occur at least partly simultaneously. The onset of the foliation is triggered by the migration and the local increase of cells. The migration and maintenance of the Purkinje cells and the generation and migration of granular cells are under genetic control and play a critical role in these processes, as has been recently demonstrated in animal experiments. Meningeal cells also play a role in the foliation. Fetal MR imaging showed the foliation after the 16th week of gestation.

The vermis is divided into an anterior lobe, a posterior lobe and the nodulus. The nine lobules are separated from each other by fissures. Each lobule can be subdivided into sublobules, which contain a variable number of folia.

Axial and coronal T2-weighted images are particularly important in the demonstration of abnormalities of foliation and fissuration. The normal aspect of the cerebellum is shown here as a reference for comparison with illustration of the pathology (Figure 12.5.1).

It is important to realize that not all changes should be considered as being of pathological significance. The significance of the megacisterna magna remains controversial although most authors consider this abnormality as a normal variant rather than a mal-

formation (see Dandy–Walker malformation). The Dandy–Walker malformation is considered to be the result of persistence of the anterior membranous area, while the megacisterna magna and the persisting Blake's pouch are considered to be the result of a deficient posterior membranous area.

Developmental venous anomalies can also occur in the cerebellum and should not be considered as a pathological finding (Figure 12.5.2).

Dilated perivascular spaces of Virchow–Robin can also be observed at the level of the dentate nuclei but usually have no pathological significance (Figure 12.5.2).

CLASSIFICATION

In the past, the cerebellum attracted less attention from radiologists who had an interest in congenital malformations. This was mainly due to the relatively small volume of the cerebellum com-

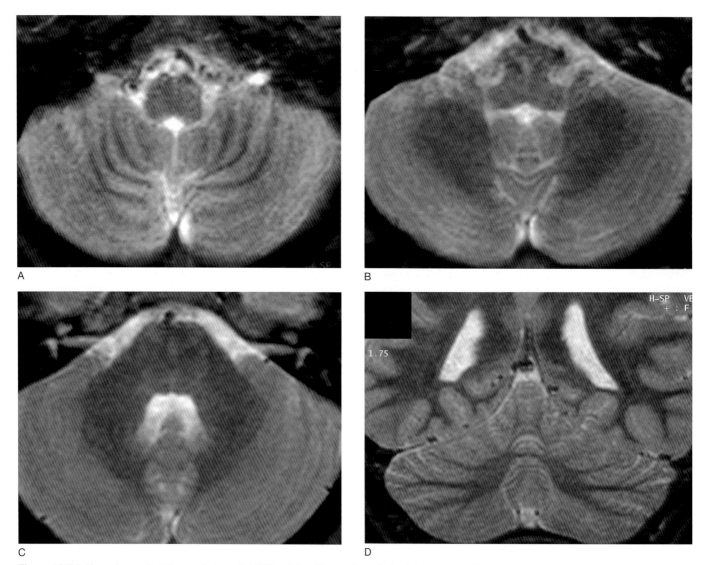

Figure 12.5.1 Normal aspect of the cerebellum. Axial T2-weighted image through the inferior vermis (A,B) and through the fourth ventricle (C). Coronal T2-weighted image shows the normal orientation of the vermian fissures and the normal arborization of the white matter (D).

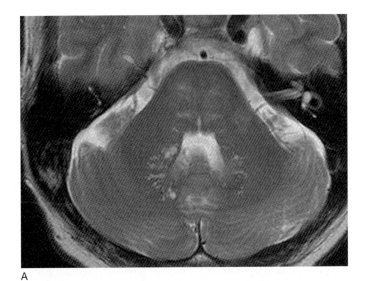

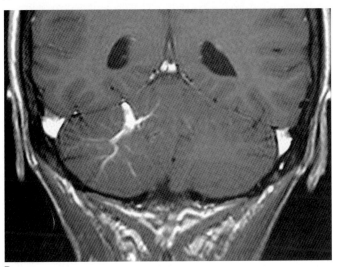

Figure 12.5.2 Perivascular spaces of Virchow–Robin in the dentate nuclei. Axial T2-weighted image shows several cyst-like structures (A). (Courtesy of Dr A. Broeders, Department of Radiology, Damiaan Hospital, Ostend, Belgium.) Coronal gadolinium-enhanced T1-weighted image demonstrates the contributing veins and the large draining vein of a developmental venous anomaly in the right cerebellar hemisphere (B).

pared to the cerebrum. Small lesions were easily missed or were not visible on routine 5–6-mm images. With the recent improvements in coil design, it is now possible to obtain a much better image quality than a few years ago.

At present, there is no widely accepted classification for cerebellar abnormalities. The genetic control of the cerebellar development is emerging but it would be premature to attempt to classify cerebellar abnormalities on this basis. The cerebellar anatomy and embryology and the known histopathological observations can be used as the framework for a classification.

An interesting classification was based on the presence of ataxia. Pure non-progressive congenital ataxia included a hereditary subtype with/without cerebellar hypoplasia and a non-hereditary subtype, including the Dandy–Walker malformation, Chiari malformation and posterior fossa cyst. The other group, the ataxic syndromes, included the molar tooth malformations.

The recent proposal of Patel and Barkovich to classify cerebellar abnormalities as either hypoplasia or dysplasia is an interesting way to create a frame. The authors based their classification on a retrospective analysis of 70 patients. Nineteen patients with a Dandy–Walker malformation and six patients with focal hypoplasia were classified in the group of patients with 'hypoplasia'. Twelve patients with a molar tooth malformation, eight with rhombencephalosynapsis, ten with congenital muscular dystrophy and six with CMV infection were classified in the group of patients with 'dysplasia'.

In this chapter, we will discuss the Chiari malformations separately, followed by the hypoplasia of the cerebellum. The latter includes the different forms of focal hypoplasia and the Dandy–Walker malformation. We will include a brief description of tectocerebellar dysraphia and persistent dermal sinus remnants in this group although we realize that it is not completely straightforward to classify these malformations in this group. Both entities reflect a dysraphism while the infratentorial abnormalities in tectocerebellar dysraphism are partly similar to what can be observed in the Dandy–Walker malformation. The posterior fossa arachnoid cyst will also be discussed together with the Dandy–Walker malformation, although it is not associated with hypoplasia.

Finally, we will review those cerebellar malformations that are associated with cerebellar dysgenesis. We classified these malformations according to the involvement of the vermis and/or the hemispheres.

At the present time, it seems inevitable that there will be overlap between hypoplasia and dysgenesis. Cerebellar hypoplasia can be associated with abnormal foliation and it can sometimes be extremely difficult to differentiate vermian dysgenesis from vermian hypoplasia.

CEREBELLAR PATHOLOGY

CHIARI MALFORMATIONS

Chiari originally described three malformations: Chiari I, II and III. The extremely rare Chiari III malformation consists of an associated cephalocele. The term Chiari IV is no longer used.

The Chiari I malformation, to be clinically significant, is defined as a caudal displacement of the cerebellar tonsils over a distance of at least 5 mm through the foramen magnum. MR imaging is far superior to computed tomography (CT) for assessing the herniation of the cerebellar tonsils. In a series of 22 591 patients, 0.77% fitted the criteria of Chiari I malformation. Fourteen per cent of these patients were asymptomatic and MR imaging was not found to be useful in differentiating these patients from symptomatic patients. The Chiari 1 malformation represents a congenital anomaly in most cases and syringomyelia is associated in approximately 20% (Figure 12.5.3). The posterior fossa is small and the clivus shortened. The diameter of the foramen magnum in the axial plane is important. The typical symptom is headache when coughing but often the presentation is more ambiguous leading to misdiagnoses such as multiple sclerosis, fibromyalgia or even psychiatric disorders. There is an association with congenital anomalies of the skull and/or skull base, which predispose to tonsillar displacement.

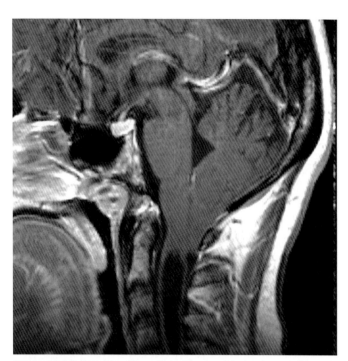

Figure 12.5.3 Chiari I malformation with associated syringomyelia. Sagittal T1-weighted image shows the descent of the cerebellar tonsils through the foramen magnum.

Chiari I malformation can also be acquired. Several aetiologies have been described, for example, children who develop tonsilar herniation following shunting for hydrocephalus or following lumboperitoneal shunting. The adult type of Chiari I malformation is likely to be the result of an underdeveloped occipital bone inducing overcrowding of the posterior fossa and its contents. Posterior fossa decompression is indicated when there are neurological signs. It is worth mentioning that syringomyelia may develop following the surgical intervention.

The Chiari II malformation is a complex malformation that is associated with a myelomeningocele in more than 85% of cases. The underlying problem is thought to be the lack of expression of surface molecules that cause a persisting aperture of the posterior neuropore. As a result of a failure of ventricular expansion the posterior fossa remains too small to harbour the developing cerebellum. There is a large foramen magnum and the tentorium is in a low position. The cerebellum, which is small and underdeveloped, becomes squeezed and extends downward through the foramen magnum and upward through the tentoral hiatus (Figure 12.5.4). The pons becomes stretched, the hemispheres extend anterolaterally around the brainstem and the clivus gets a concave outlining as a result of the pressure. Tectal beaking and medullary kinking can be observed. Occasionally, the fourth ventricle can herniate behind the medulla and caudal to the vermis leading to an entrapment of the ventricle.

Persistent cerebellar herniation may cause degeneration in the cerebellar tissue in the long term, probably due to mechanically induced ischaemia. This phenomenon is called the 'vanishing cerebellum' (Figure 12.5.5). The cognitive consequences of this finding are being studied.

HYPOPLASIA

VERMIAN AND/OR HEMISPHERIC HYPOPLASIA

A variable degree of hypoplasia can be seen with involvement of the vermis and/or the hemispheres (Figure 12.5.6). It should be realized that it may be extremely difficult, if not impossible, to differentiate vermian hypoplasia from vermian dysgenesis. The posterior fossa has a normal size and the straight sinus is in a normal position. In pontoneocerebellar hypoplasia, there is marked brain stem hypoplasia, flattening of the cerebellum and the vermis. These patients present with severe neurological signs in the neonatal period. All lobules are present and this allows the differential diagnosis with partial cerebellar agenesis. On a clinical basis, pontoneocerebellar hypoplasia has been divided into: type 1 with spinal horn degeneration and a poor prognosis (abnormal pattern of foliation has been observed); and type 2 (progressive macrocephaly and chorea/dystonia) with a slightly better prognosis according to Barth.

Cerebellar hypoplasia with enlarged flocculi is a feature of trisomy 21. A small inferior vermis with increase in the volume of the fourth ventricle has been noted in fragile X syndrome. Brain stem hypoplasia is commonly associated in many diffuse cerebellar anomalies.

Partial or complete absence of the cerebellum may also be due to destruction, possibly following infarction or inflammation *in utero* or early in life. Genetic defects can also result in a more or less severe hypoplasia of the cerebellum.

DANDY–WALKER MALFORMATION

In the 1980s, it was suggested that the Dandy–Walker complex covered a continuum ranging from the megacisterna magna, through the Dandy–Walker variant to the Dandy–Walker malformation. But there has always been controversy and confusion with regard to definition of the different entities. More recently, the terms mild or severe Dandy–Walker malformation have been proposed. It appears increasingly likely that a genetic mutation is involved in this anomaly.

The abnormalities consist: of (1) a partial or complete agenesis of the vermis; (2) a cystic dilatation of the fourth ventricle; and (3) an enlarged posterior fossa with upward displacement of the tentorium. The superior medullary velum and the remaining superior vermis is rotated anterosuperiorly (Figure 12.5.7). The cerebellar hemispheres are hypoplastic and appear 'winged outward' due to the presence of the cyst on the midline. The cyst wall is sometimes visible and consists of three layers: the ependyma, the squeezed neuroglial tissue and the pia. The cyst never extends anterior to the lateral edge of the cerebellum (Figure 12.5.7). Hydrocephalus is almost always present and requires shunting. Agenesis of the corpus callosum and occipital meningocele are frequently associated abnormalities.

It is thought that an aberrant development of the roof of the fourth ventricle, between the 4th and 7th week of gestation, causes the abnormalities. In normal circumstances, the roof is divided into an anterior and a posterior membranous area by the developing choroid plexus. The anterior membranous area is incorporated into

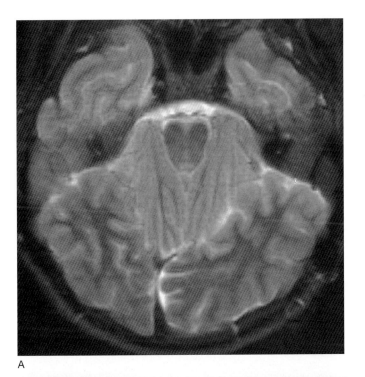

A

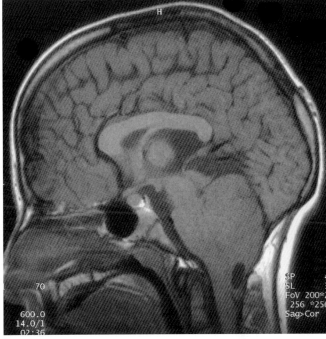

B

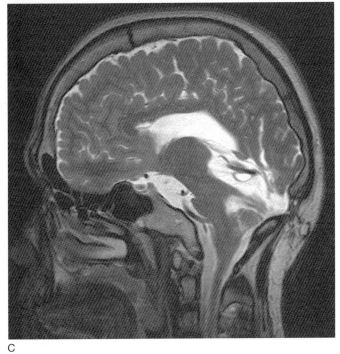

C

Figure 12.5.4 Chiari II (A,B) and Chiari III malformation (C). The abnormal orientation of the folia with their extension on both sides of the brainstem is shown on an axial T2-weighted image. Tectal beaking and descent of cerebellar tissue through the foramen magnum, with a cyst-like structure, is seen on the sagittal T1-weighted image (B). A Chiari II malformation with an associated occipital cephalocele is shown (C). Note the attraction of the cerebellum towards the occipital bone defect.

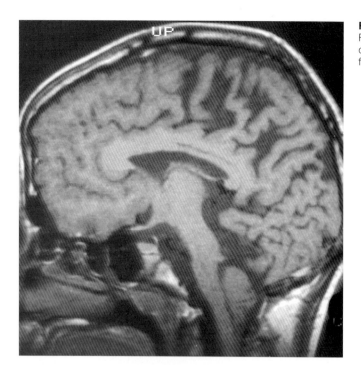

Figure 12.5.5 Chiari II malformation. Sagittal T1-weighted image. Follow-up examination in a 10-year-old boy demonstrates the degeneration of the cerebellar tissue. Note the absence of the pontine flexure.

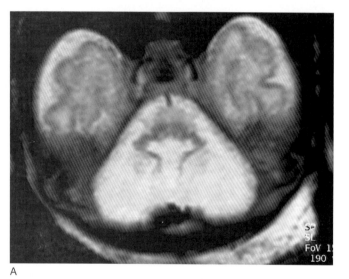

A

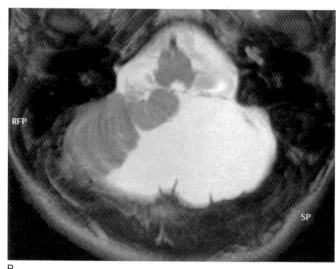

B

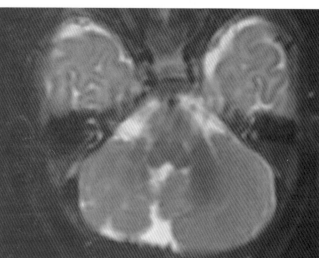

C

Figure 12.5.6 Cerebellar hypoplasia. Three different degrees of hypoplasia are shown on axial T2-weighted images: vermian and hemispheric aplasia (A), unilateral aplasia (B) and right-sided hemispheric hypoplasia with normal vermis (C).

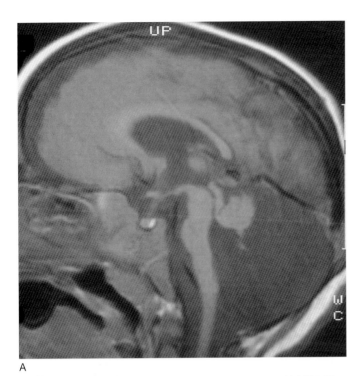

A

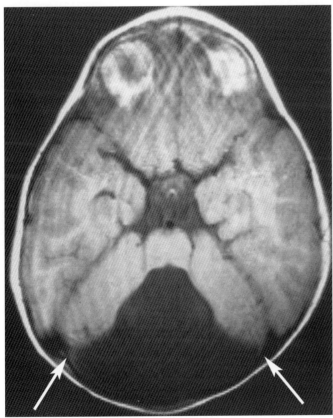

B

Figure 12.5.7 Dandy–Walker malformation. Sagittal (A) and axial (B) T1-weighted images. Note the enlarged posterior fossa with absence of the inferior vermis and part of the superior vermis. The superior medullary velum and the remaining superior vermis are rotated anterosuperiorly (A). On the axial image, the typical 'winged-outward' appearance of the hypoplastic cerebellar hemispheres is seen. Note that the 'posterior fossa cyst' does not extend beyond the cerebellar hemispheres (B, arrows).

the choroid plexus while the posterior area forms the foramen of Magendie. If these processes do not occur, the roof of the fourth ventricle balloons posteriorly and a cyst is formed. Others have argued that the Dandy–Walker malformation may be the result of a vermian maldevelopment.

Treatment is necessary when hydrocephalus or compression of the posterior fossa cyst occurs. A ventriculoperitoneal shunt is the easiest option but is associated with more shunt obstruction or overshunting. A cystoperitoneal shunt is preferable but is technically more difficult to position and secure. Both shunting procedures may be necessary in the same patient.

The Dandy–Walker malformation can be part of several intracranial malformations and has been reported in numerous syndromes. The PHACE syndrome is a recently described entity, consisting of extracranial cutaneous capillary haemangiomas with associated intracranial meningeal lesions, posterior fossa malformations (including Dandy–Walker malformation), arterial anomalies, eye abnormalities and coarctation of the aorta.

The megacisterna magna results from an insult in the posterior membranous area, perhaps due to a late opening of the foramen of Magendie, which can remain widened on imaging. The abnormalities may extend in any direction and, in 25% of cases, even into the supratentorial space (Figure 12.5.8). There are no clinical signs and hydrocephalus is always absent. The posterior fossa is usually slightly enlarged with scalloping of the occipital bone and sometimes even mild vermian compression. The megacisterna magna can mimic an arachnoid cyst. An arachnoid cyst can be differentiated by the clinical signs (ataxia and/or headache) and by mass-effect on the cerebellum (Figure 12.5.9). Arachnoid cysts are enclosed within the layers of the arachnoidea. It should be stressed that not all arachnoid cysts are symptomatic. It can be very difficult to differentiate an arachnoid cyst from a choroid plexus cyst.

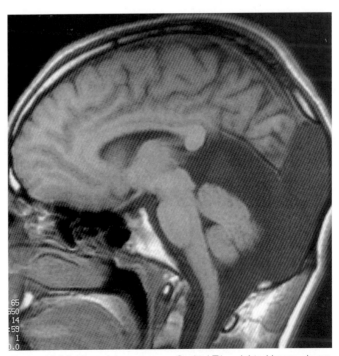

Figure 12.5.8 Megacisterna magna. Sagittal T1-weighted image shows a huge megacisterna magna extending into the supratentorial space. There is no evidence of cerebellar compression.

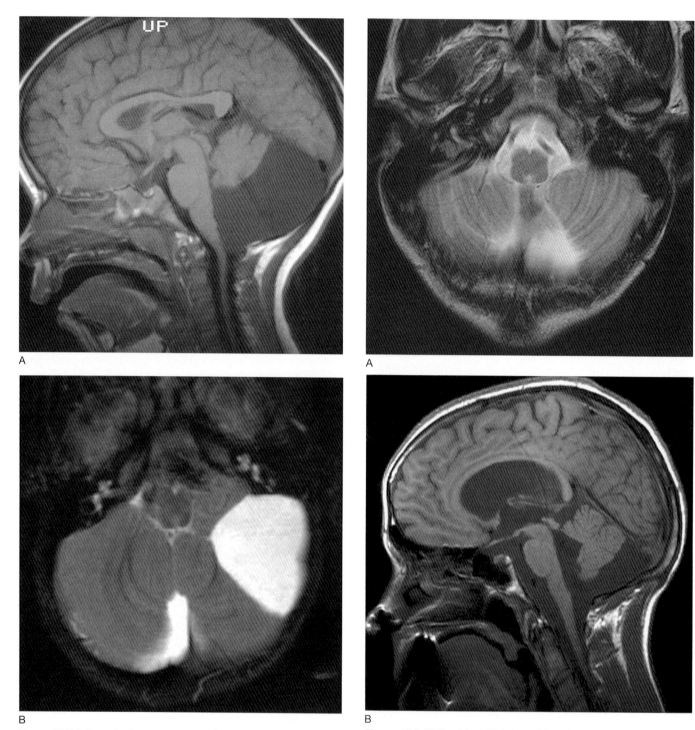

Figure 12.5.9 Posterior fossa arachnoid cyst. Sagittal T1-weighted (A) and axial T2-weighted (B) images. On the sagittal image, the arachnoid cyst is seen, compressing the cerebellum (A). Another example is shown of an arachnoid cyst on the left lateral side of the cerebellum, a common location of infratentorial arachnoid cysts (B).

Figure 12.5.10 Persistent Blake's pouch. Axial T2-weighted (A) and sagittal T1-weighted (B) images. Note the displacement of the hemispheres on the axial image with evidence of a cerebrospinal fluid flow artifact (A). Note the continuity with the fourth ventricle and the supratentorial hydrocephalus (B).

The extension of the cyst anterior to the cerebellar hemispheres differentiates this from the Dandy–Walker cyst.

The persisting Blake's pouch occurs secondary to a non-perforation of the foramen of Magendie and probably associated anomalies of the foramina of Luschka resulting in severe obstruction. The imaging findings resemble those of megacisterna magna but hydrocephalus is invariably present (Figure 12.5.10).

TECTOCEREBELLAR DYSRAPHISM

The posterior fossa abnormalities in tectocerebellar dysraphism or inverse cerebellum with occipital encephalocele are similar to some extent to those observed in Dandy–Walker malformation. In addition, there is an occipital cephalocele with traction of the brainstem towards the bone defect. An intracranial dermoid or lipoma can also be seen (Fig. 12.5.11). Occipital cephaloceles may contain cerebellum, brainstem, occipital lobes, vascular structures or cerebrospinal fluid and glial remnants only. The bone defect can be found above or below the torcular (Figure 12.5.11). Tecto-cerebellar dysraphism shows similarities with Walker–Warburg syndrome, an autosomal recessive disorder with agyria, hydrocephalus and retinal dysplasia.

PERSISTENT DERMAL SINUS REMNANTS

Dermal sinuses are developmental epithelia-lined tracts that extend from the skin surface towards the central nervous system. A dermal sinus may be patent and present with cerebrospinal fluid (CSF) leakage or, more commonly, with ascending infection, which may result in meningitis. The dermal sinuses have the characteristics of fibrous tissue and reflect low signal relative to subcutaneous tissue. Dermoid or epidermoid tumours are sometimes associated with dermal sinuses (Figure 12.5.12). In the occipital region, dermoids are often associated with a midline occipital bone defect, duplicated longitudinal sinus and a communicating mass involving the vermis.

DYSGENESIS

VERMIAN DYSGENESIS

MOLAR TOOTH MALFORMATIONS

This term is now preferred to classify malformations where the typical imaging finding is the 'molar tooth' appearance of the midbrain on axial images (Figure 12.5.13). It is now well known that patients with the Joubert syndrome only represent some of these patients. Clinically, the Joubert syndrome consists of episodic hyperpnoea/apnoea, severe hypotonia, ataxia, mental retardation and abnormal eye movements. The syndrome is inherited as an autosomal recessive trait.

Histopathologically, the lack of decussation of the superior cerebellar peduncles, pontine tracts and corticospinal tracts have been demonstrated. This causes the horizontal course of the superior cerebellar peduncles and the narrow pontomesencephalic junction, which is best seen on sagittal images. Partial (usually involving the posterior lobe) or complete vermian agenesis is seen with the presence of a midline cleft and a particular shape of the fourth ventricle. The upper part of the ventricle has a bat-wing or umbrella shape and the midportion a triangular shape (Figure 12.5.13).

In a series of children with congenital ocular motor apraxia, inferior vermian hypoplasia/dysgenesis was the most common abnormality. Associated renal and liver problems have been described.

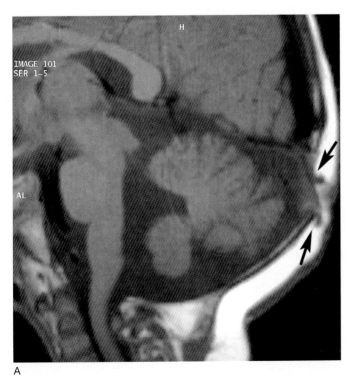

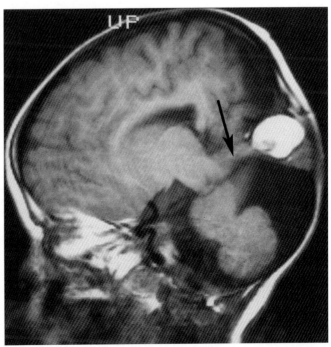

A   B

Figure 12.5.11 Occipital cephalocele and tectocerebellar dysraphia. Sagittal T1-weighted images. Note the abnormal shape of the fourth ventricle and the displacement of the cerebellum towards the cephalocele (A, arrows). The intracranial lipoma and the displacement of the cerebellum towards the cephalocele is seen (B, arrow).

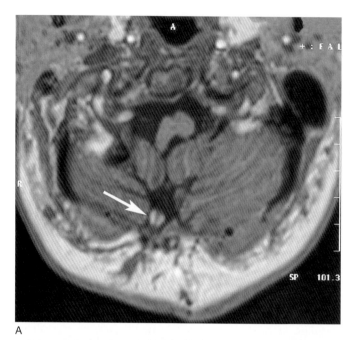

A

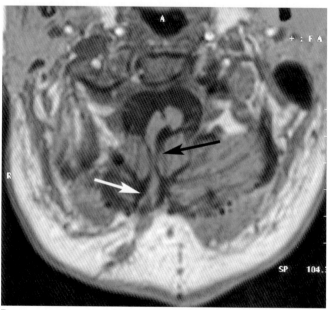

B

Figure 12.5.12 Dorsal dermal sinus with associated dermoid cyst. Axial T1-weighted images show the epithelial-lined sinus tract from the skin to the medulla (B, arrows). The small dermoid cyst can be identified (A, arrow). (Reproduced with permission from Buyse GG, Caekebeke J, Demaerel P, Plets C. Primary brain stem tethering: a rare cause of geniculate neuralgia. Journal of Laryngology and Otology 1999; 113: 945–947.)

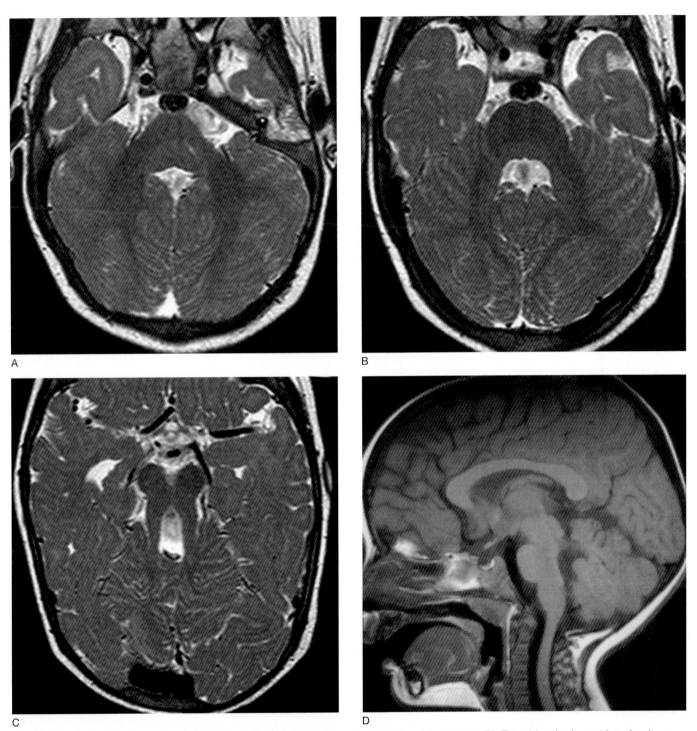

Figure 12.5.13 Molar tooth syndrome. Axial T2-weighted images (A–C) and sagittal T1-weighted image (D). The midportion has a triangular shape (A) while the upper part has an umbrella shape (B). The typical 'molar tooth' aspect of the midbrain due to the horizontal course of the superior cerebellar peduncles is shown (C). Partial vermian agenesis is seen with the presence of a midline cleft and a particular shape of the fourth ventricle (A,D). Note the high position of the fourth ventricle (D).

RHOMBENCEPHALOSYNAPSIS

Rhombencephalosynapsis is a rare disorder consisting typically of vermian agenesis or severe hypogenesis, fusion of the hypoplastic cerebellar hemispheres (with typical transverse orientation of the folia) and apposition or fusion of the dentate nuclei (Figure 12.5.14). The fourth ventricle often has a keyhole shape on axial images. Over 40 cases have been reported since Obersteiners' report in 1914 and recently a review of the literature has been published. Supratentorial abnormalities can be encountered. Ventriculomegaly, fusion of the thalami and absence of the septum pellucidum are commonly associated.

It has recently been suggested that the embryological defect affects the 'isthmic organizer' at the mesencephalic–metencephalic border. Molecular analysis of dorsalizing genes, such as *Lmx1a*, which regulate early developmental events at the pontomesencephalic junction, may reveal a mutation or mutations unique to rhombencephalosynapsis. The abnormality is likely to be the result of an insult between the 4th and 6th week of gestation. Therefore, the term metencephalosynapsis might be preferred because the rhombencephalon has divided into the metencephalon and the myelencephalon during the 4th week.

In the traditional view, rhombencephalosynapsis was considered to be an abnormal development of the vermis with subsequent fusion of the hemispheres. In the more recent view, rhombencephalosynapsis is considered to be a failure of vermian differentiation with undivided development of the hemispheres.

An association with septo-optic dysplasia has been observed. A wrong expression of genes involved in the early patterning centres of the brain has been suggested. The FGF8 gene is active both in the region of the septum pellucidum and that of the cerebellar primordium.

VERMIAN AND/OR HEMISPHERIC DYSGENESIS

ABNORMALITIES OF FOLIATION AND FISSURATION TYPE 1A AND 1B

Patients with malorientation of the fissures in the anterior lobe of the vermis are encountered on a regular basis. This abnormality is particularly well seen on coronal images and may represent an incidental finding (Figure 12.5.15). Symptoms are not related to the cerebellar lesions. Extension of the abnormal fissuration into the hemispheres is only rarely observed in our experience. We have called this group of abnormalities the type 1a anomalies.

In some patients, there is an associated abnormal foliation of the anterior lobe of the vermis and of part of the posterior lobe (Figure 12.5.15). In this group, extension of the abnormalities into the

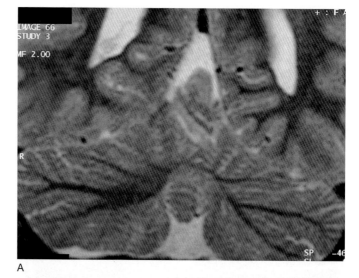

A

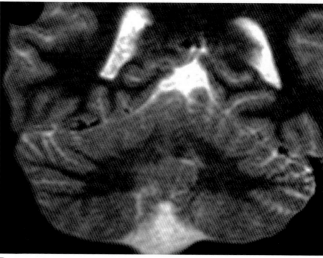

B

Figure 12.5.15 Abnormality of foliation and fissuration type 1. Coronal T2-weighted images. In the type 1a, there is only an abnormal orientation of the fissures (A). In the type 1b, there is an associated abnormal foliation of the anterior lobe of the vermis with some extension into the right hemisphere (B).

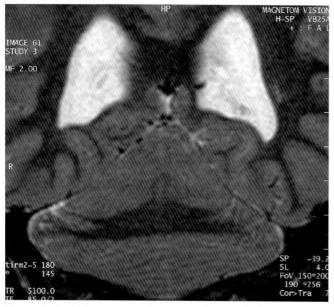

Figure 12.5.14 Rhombencephalosynapsis. Coronal T2-weighted image. The fusion of the grey and white matter of both hemispheres is seen in the absence of a vermis.

hemispheres is more frequently seen. This group of abnormalities is called type 1b. Clinical cerebellar signs are frequently seen.

ABNORMALITIES OF FOLIATION AND FISSURATION TYPE 2

It is important to realise that minor alterations were found in the cerebellar cortex of 85% of 147 newborns without any other structural abnormality. We classified our 17 patients with cerebellar hemispheric abnormalities of foliation and fissuration together in the type 2 group. None of our patients had Fukuyama congenital muscular dystrophy or Walker–Warburg syndrome but similar findings have been described in these syndromes. It is interesting to note that more than 60% of these patients also had type 1b anomalies.

The hemispheric changes included cortical dysgenesis and/or cortical hypertrophy and/or aberrant orientation of the folia (Figure 12.5.16). It is important not to consider the hypertrophy of the cortex as Lhermitte–Duclos disease, because the MRI appearances are completely different (see Lhermitte–Duclos disease). The hypertrophy may resemble the Spiegel malformation, which consists of a diffuse hemihypertrophy. This malformation is also different from another entity called macrocerebellum. In these patients, the cerebellum appears abnormally large without architectural abnormalities. Clinically, global developmental delay, tone abnormalities, delayed maturation of the visual system and delayed myelination of the cerebrum are found. The pathogenesis is not yet clear but it seems likely that this finding represents a marker for disturbed cerebral development.

More than 50% of the patients with type 2 abnormalities had cerebral abnormalities.

The term cortical dysgenesis has no histopathological connotation and is preferred over the term cortical dysplasia. On imaging, a bumpy grey–white matter interface is seen. Small cyst-like structures of uncertain origin can sometimes be seen. They may represent engulfed loculations of the subarachnoid space and they have been frequently described in patients with Fukuyama congenital muscular dystrophy. Cystic cerebellar lesions have also been described following infection.

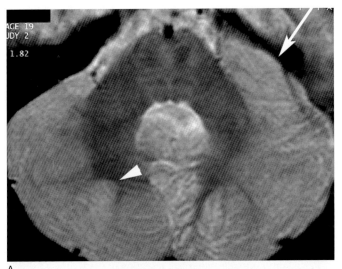

A

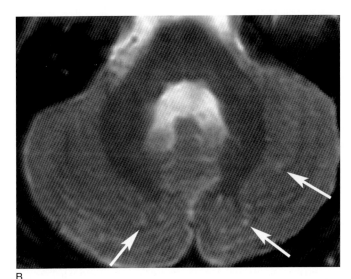

B

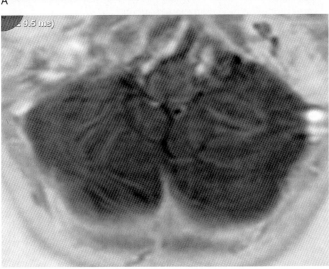

C

Figure 12.5.16 Abnormalities of foliation and fissuration type 2. Axial T2-weighted (A,B) and T1-weighted images. Three entities can be encountered: cortical dysgenesis (A, arrowhead), cortical hypertrophy (A, arrow) and abnormal pattern of foliation (C). Note the presence of cyst-like cortical lesions in a child with cortical dysgenesis.

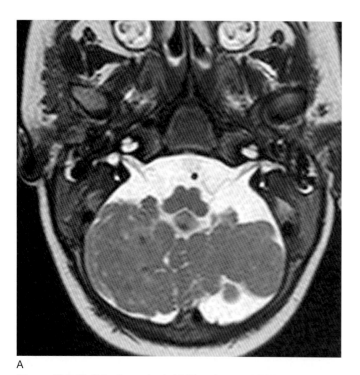

A

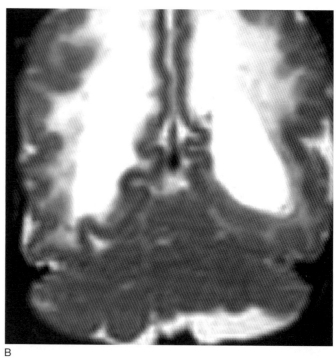

B

Figure 12.5.17 Polymicrogyria. Axial (A) and coronal (B) T2-weighted images. The abnormal cerebellar cortex and the abnormal pattern of foliation can be seen (A and B). Note the associated supratentorial polymicrogyria and extensive white matter disease (B).

In patients with congenital cytomegalovirus, the cerebellar cortex may appear similar to the polymicrogyric cerebral cortex (Figure 12.5.17). The clinical features include developmental delay, neurocognitive defects, eye movement disorders, hypotonia, vestibulo-ocular apraxia and language retardation.

LHERMITTE–DUCLOS–COWDEN SYNDROME

Lhermitte and Duclos reported the first patient with this syndrome in 1920. Despite the recent insights into its pathogenesis, this fascinating entity remains a mystery, particularly as to whether this represents a neoplastic or a malformation lesion. According to the World Health Organization (WHO), the lesion is classified as a dysplastic gangliocytoma. An association with Cowden disease is now accepted. Cowden disease or 'multiple hamartoma syndrome' is an autosomal dominant phakomatosis with an increased frequency of malignancies.

The abnormality may be discovered incidentally or the patient may present with unsteadiness of gait, cranial nerve palsies or neurological deterioration due to hydrocephalus. The MR imaging appearances typically consist of a mass-like lesion with a non-enhancing striated pattern of the enlarged folia. The abnormality returns a high signal on T2-weighted imaging (Figure 12.5.18). It

should be mentioned that pial enhancement has been reported in a few cases. Usually only the hemispheres are involved but vermian extension has been described. Occasionally, the differential diagnosis can be difficult with cerebellitis, where the interface with the normal structures appears smoother (Figure 12.5.19).

Histopathologically, there is a widening of the molecular layer and a hypertrophy of the granule cell layer. The Purkinje cells are absent and the ganglion cells are abnormal but there is no evidence to indicate a neoplastic nature. An underlying genetic cause is likely, because mutations in the PTEN gene have been detected in some patients with Lhermitte–Duclos–Cowden syndrome.

Partial or, if possible, complete resection of the lesion is the procedure of choice in symptomatic patients.

ACKNOWLEDGEMENTS

We gratefully thank Paul Casaer, MD, PhD, Lieven Lagae MD, PhD and Gunnar Buyse MD, PhD from the Department of Paediatrics, University Hospitals K.U. Leuven, for referring their patients. We acknowledge Wolfgang Desmedt for his photographic assistance.

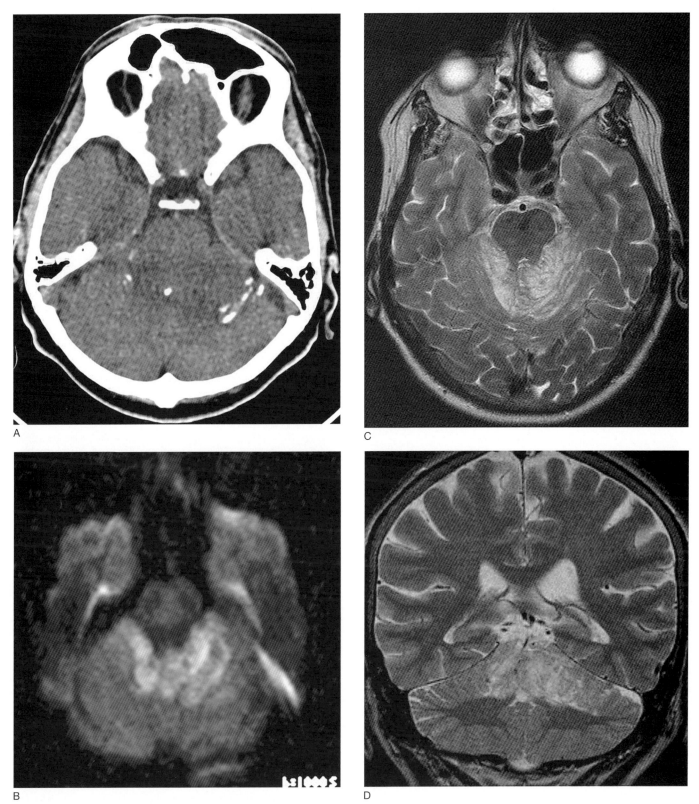

Figure 12.5.18 Lhermitte–Duclos–Cowden disease. Axial CT (A), axial diffusion-weighted (B), axial (C) and coronal T2-weighted (D) images. Calcification is best seen on CT (A). The lesion returns a typical high signal on a diffusion-weighted image (B). On T2-weighted images, the abnormality returns a high signal with some preservation of the cerebellar folia.

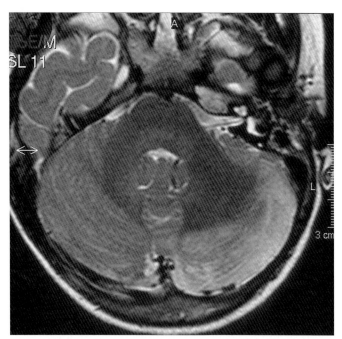

Figure 12.5.19 Acute cerebellitis. Axial T2-weighted image. The high signal in the left cerebellar cortex appears much more homogeneous with a smoother interface than in a patient with Lhermitte–Duclos–Cowden syndrome.

FURTHER READING

Aida N, Yagishita A, Takada K et al. Cerebellar MR in Fukuyama congenital muscular dystrophy: polymicrogyria with cystic lesions. American Journal of Neuroradiology 1994; 15:1755–1759.

Altman NR, Naidich TP, Braffman BH. Posterior fossa malformations. American Journal of Neuroradiology 1992; 13:690–724.

Barkovich AJ, Kjos BO, Norman D et al. Revised classification of posterior fossa cysts and cystlike malformations based on the results of multiplanar MR imaging. American Journal of Neuroradiology 1989; 11:188–191.

Bodensteiner JB, Schaefer GB, Keller GM et al. Macrocerebellum: neuroimaging and clinical features of a newly recognized condition. Journal of Child Neurology 1997; 12:365–368.

Boltshauser E, Schneider J, Kollias S et al. Vanishing cerebellum in myelomeningocele. European Journal of Pediatric Neurology 2002; 6:109–113.

Buyse GG, Caekebeke J, Demaerel P et al. Primary brain stem tethering: a rare cause of geniculate neuralgia. Journal of Laryngology and Otology 1999; 113:945–947.

Calabro F, Arcuri T, Jinkins JR. Blake's pouch cyst: an entity within the Dandy-Walker continuum. Neuroradiology 2000; 42:290–295.

Chiari H. Uber Veränderungen des Kleinhirns infolge von Hydrocephalie des Grosshirns. Deutsch Med Wochenschr 1891; 17:1172–1175.

Chong BW, Babcook CJ, Pang D et al. A magnetic resonance template for normal cerebellar development in the human fetus. Neurosurgery 1997; 41:924–929.

Dandy WE. The diagnosis and treatment of hydrocephalus due to occlusion of the foramina of Magendie and Luschka. Surgical Gynecology and Obstetrics 1921; 32:112–124.

Demaerel P. Abnormalities of cerebellar foliation and fissuration: classification, neurogenetics and clinicoradiological correlations. Neuroradiology 2002; 44:639–646.

Demaerel P, Lagae L, Baert AL. MR of cerebellar cortical dysplasia. American Journal of Neuroradiology 1998; 19:984–986.

Demaerel P, Wilms G, Marchal G. Rostral vermian cortical dysplasia: MRI. Neuroradiology 1999; 41:190–194.

Domingo Z, Peter J. Midline developmental abnormalities of the posterior fossa: correlation of classification with outcome. Pediatric Neurosurgery 1996; 24:111–118.

Friede RL. Uncommon syndromes of cerebellar vermis aplasia: II. Tecto-cerebellar dysraphia with occipital encephalocele. Developmental Medicine and Child Neurology 1978; 20:764–772.

Gil Z, Rao S, Constantini S. Expansion of Chiari I-associated syringomyelia after posterior fossa decompression. Childs Nervous System 2000; 16:555–558.

Inamdar SD. Concept of the development of the mammalian cerebellum based on physical rotation forces. Medical Hypotheses 1982; 38:88–91.

Jeffery N. Differential regional brain growth and rotation of the prenatal human tentorium cerebelli. Journal of Anatomy 2002; 200:135–144.

Joubert M, Eisenring JJ, Robb JP et al. Familial agenesis of the cerebellar vermis: a syndrome of episodic hyperpnea, abnormal eye movements, ataxia, and retardation. Neurology 1969; 19:813–825.

Larsell O. The development of the cerebellum in man in relation to its comparative anatomy. Journal of Comparative Neurology 1947; 87:85–129.

Lhermitte J, Duclos P. Sur un ganglioneurome diffus du cortex du cervelet. Byull Assoc Fr Etude Cancer 1920; 9:99–107.

Meadows J, Kraut M, Guarnieri M et al. Asymptomatic Chiari type I malformations identified on magnetic resonance imaging. Journal of Neurosurgery 2000; 92:920–926.

Neumann PE, Garretson JD, Skabardonis GP et al. Genetic analysis of cerebellar folial pattern in crosses of C57BL/6 and DBA/2J inbred mice. Brain Research 1993; 619:81–88.

Nishikawa M, Sakamoto H, Hakuba A et al. Pathogenesis of Chiari malformation: a morphometric study of the posterior cranial fossa. Journal of Neurosurgery 1997; 86:40–47.

Oberdick J, Baader S, Schilling K. From zebra stripes to postal zones: deciphering patterns of gene expression in the cerebellum. Trends in Neuroscience 198; 21:383–390.

Obersteiner H. Ein Kleinhirn ohne Wurm. Arbeiten dus den Neurologischen Institut an der Wienen Universität (Wien) 1914; 21:124–136.

Padberg GW, Schot DL, Vielvoye GJ et al. Lhermitte-Duclos disease and Cowden disease: a single phakomatosis. Annals of Neurology 1991; 29:517–523.

Patel S, Barkovich AJ. Analysis and classification of cerebellar malformations. American Journal of Neuroradiology 2002; 23:1074–1087.

Quisling R, Barkovich A, Maria B. Magnetic resonance imaging: features and classification of central nervous system malformations in Joubert syndrome. Journal of Child Neurology 1999; 14:628–635.

Sargent MA, Poskitt KJ, Jan JE. Congenital ocular motor apraxia: imaging findings. American Journal of Neuroradiology 1997; 18:1915–1922.

Sidman RL, Rakic P. Development of the human central nervous system. In: Haymaker W, Adams RD, eds. Histology and histopathology of the nervous system. Springfield, Ill: Thomas; 1982:3–145.

Soto-Ares G, Delmaire C, Deries B et al. Cerebellar cortical dysplasia: MR findings in a complex entity. American Journal of Neuroradiology 2000; 21:1511–1519.

Soto-Ares G, Devisme L, Jorriot S et al. Neuropathologic and MR imaging correlation in a neonatal case of cerebellar cortical dysplasia. American Journal of Neuroradiology 2002; 23:1101–1104.

Steinlin M. Non-progressive congenital ataxias. Brain and Development 1998; 20:199–208.

Sutphen R, Diamond TM, Minton SE et al. Severe Lhermitte-Duclos disease with unique germline mutation of PTEN. American Journal of Medical Genetics 2000; 82:290–293.

Takanashi J, Sugita K, Barkovich AJ et al. Partial midline fusion of the cerebellar hemispheres with vertical folia: a new cerebellar malformation. American Journal of Neuroradiology 1999; 20:1151–1153.

Toelle SP, Yalcinkaya C, Kocer N et al. Rhombencephalosynapsis: clinical findings and neuroimaging in 9 children. Neuropediatrics 2002; 33:209–214.

Tortori-Donati P, Fondelli M, Rossi A et al. Cystic malformations of the posterior cranial fossa originating from a defect of the posterior membranous area: mega cisterna magna and persisting Blake's pouch: two separate entities. Childs Nervous System 1996; 12:303–308.

Tortori-Donati P, Fondelli MP, Rossi A et al. Intracranial contrast-enhancing masses in infants with capillary haemangioma of the head and neck: intracranial capillary haemangioma? Neuroradiology 1999; 41:369–375.

Truwit CL, Barkovich AJ, Shanahan R et al. MR imaging of rhomben-cephalosynapsis: report of three cases and review of the literature. American Journal of Neuroradiology 1991; 12:547–549.

Utsunomiya H, Takano K, Ogasawara T et al. Rhombencephalosynapsis: cerebellar embryogenesis. American Journal of Neuroradiology 1998; 19:547–549.

Wassef M, Joyner AL. Early mesencephalon/metencephalon patterning and development of the cerebellum. Perspectives in Developmental Neurobiology 1997; 5:3–16.

Yachnis AT. Rhombencephalosynapsis with massive hydrocephalus: case report and pathogenetic considerations. Acta Neuropathologica 2002; 103:301–304.

Yachnis A, Rorke L. Neuropathology of Joubert syndrome. Journal of Child Neurology 1999; 14:655–659.

Neurocutaneous Syndromes

In-One Kim

Neurocutaneous syndromes (phakomatoses) are a heterogeneous group of disorders that share the common features of an abnormal proliferation of ectodermal, mesenchymal and neuroectodermal tissues. These disorders generally manifest as prominent neurological abnormality and skin lesions. Frequently, hamartomatous tumours develop within the central nervous system, the skin and genitourinary tracts. The commonly encountered disorders of childhood included in the neurocutaneous syndromes are neurofibromatosis, tuberous sclerosis, Sturge–Weber syndrome, ataxia telangiectasia and von Hippel–Lindau disease, which are listed together with other less common conditions in Table 12.6.1.

NEUROFIBROMATOSIS

Neurofibromatosis is a group of heterogeneous diseases with several variants, but two distinct types have the greatest clinical impact: neurofibromatosis type 1 (NF-1, von Recklinghausen disease or peripheral neurofibromatosis) and neurofibromatosis type 2 (NF-2, bilateral acoustic schwannoma or central neurofibromatosis).

NEUROFIBROMATOSIS TYPE 1

Neurofibromatosis type 1 is the most common of all the neurocutaneous syndromes and accounts for more than 90% of all neurofibromatosis cases. NF-1 is the most frequent form arising in childhood and the incidence ranges from 1 per 2000 to 3000 live births. The responsible gene is on the long arm of chromosome 17 in about 50% of cases and inheritance is autosomal dominant with high penetrance. Diagnosis is based on the presence of two or more of the following criteria:

1. At least six café-au-lait macules over 5 mm.
2. One plexiform neurofibroma or two or more neurofibromas.
3. Two or more iris Lisch nodules (pigmented hamartomas).
4. Axillary or inguinal freckles.
5. Optic nerve glioma.
6. Presence of a characteristic bone lesion such as sphenoid wing dysplasia, lambdoid bony defect or pseudoarthrosis of the tibia.
7. First-degree relative with NF-1.

Central nervous system (CNS) manifestations occur in about 15%–20% of cases of NF-1 including neoplasms such as gliomas or plexiform neurofibroma and non-neoplastic hamartomatous lesions in the basal ganglia or white matter. Skull or meningeal dysplasia and spine, cord or nerve root lesions can be present. Other manifestations of mesodermal dysplasia include skeletal abnormalities such as kyphoscoliosis or limb deformity, genitourinary involvement of neurofibromas or neurofibrosarcomas and vascular abnormalities.

NON-NEOPLASTIC HAMARTOMATOUS LESIONS

The characteristic magnetic resonance imaging (MRI) findings of CNS involvement in NF-1 consists of high signal intensity lesions on T2-weighted images (T2-WI) involving the globus pallidus, posterior thalamus, optic radiation, brainstem and cerebellar white matter. The lesions in the globus pallidus can be seen as high signal intensity on T1-weighted images (T1-WI). These abnormal signal intensity lesions are frequently well demarcated and nodular in shape and uncommonly they can show mass effect or contrast enhancement (Figure 12.6.1). These so-called hamartomatous lesions are present in nearly 80% of the patients and children generally remain asymptomatic. Pathologically, these lesions are considered as malformed dysplastic glial proliferation or abnormal myelination. They typically diminish with age but can increase in size or number in early childhood. These lesions do not represent a neoplastic condition and they do not need intervention or biopsy.

NEOPLASMS

Glial neoplasms of the brain are characteristic of NF-1. The commonest intracranial tumour in NF-1 is an optic pathway glioma that is usually a low-grade astrocytoma (Figure 12.6.2). Optic

Table 12.6.1 Neurocutaneous syndromes of childhood

Neurofibromatosis
   NF type 1 (von Recklinghausen disease)
   NF type 2 (bilateral acoustic neuroma)
Tuberous sclerosis
Sturge–Weber syndrome
Von Hippel–Lindau disease
Ataxia-telangiectasia
Other neurocutaneous syndromes
   Incontinentia pigmenti
   Epidermal naevus syndrome
   Neurocutaneous melanosis
   Hereditary haemorrhagic telangiectasia (Osler–Rendu–Weber disease)
   Klippel–Trenaunay–Weber syndrome
   Basal cell naevus syndrome
   Hypomelanosis of Ito

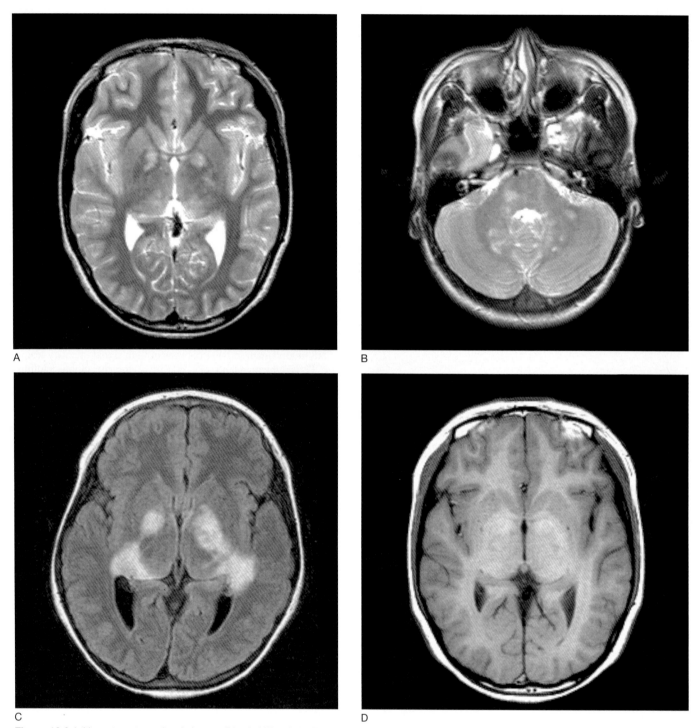

Figure 12.6.1 Hamartomatous signal abnormalities in NF-1. Axial T2 image shows high signal lesions in the globus pallidus and posterior thalamus (A), and the pons and cerebellar white matter (B). Flair image shows nodular high signal lesions along the optic tracts (C). T1 image shows subtle linear high signals in the both globus pallidus (D).

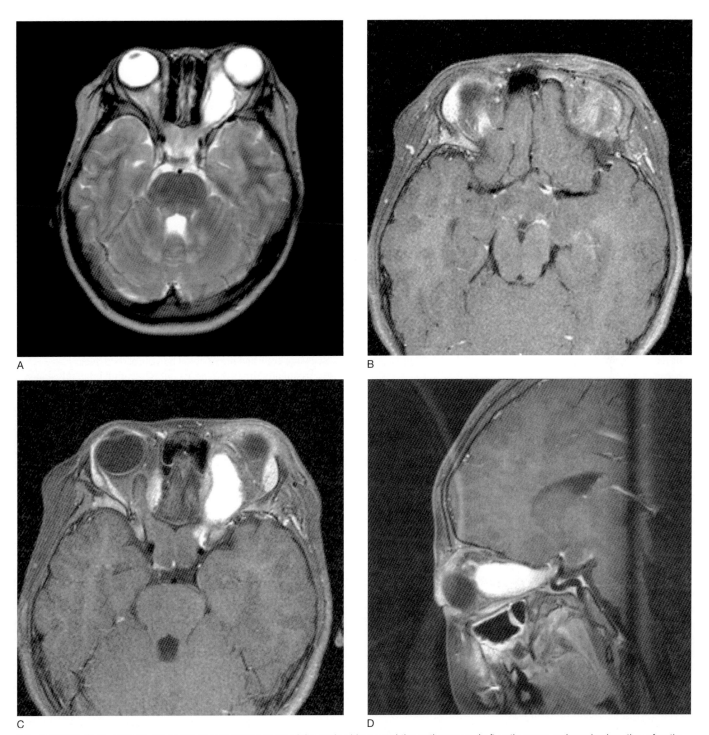

A

B

C

D

Figure 12.6.2 Optic gliomas. T2 image shows enlargement of the optic chiasm and the optic nerves. Left optic nerve and proximal portion of optic chiasm show abnormal high signal intensity. Dural ectasia of the optic nerve is seen as linear high signals along the optic nerves (A). Enlargement of the optic chiasm and enhancement of the left optic nerve is seen on the postcontrast fat-saturated T1 images (B–D).

nerve gliomas can involve one or both optic nerves and commonly extend into the chiasm. Posterior involvement of the optic tracts, lateral geniculate body and optic radiations can occur. These tumours grow slowly over a prolonged period of time. Optic pathway gliomas are typically isointense and homogeneous on T1-WI and hyperintense on T2-WI. Enhancement is usually absent or minimal but can be striking when extension along the posterior pathway is present. Occasionally, asymptomatic optic nerve thickening is present. Other glial neoplasms include hypothalamic gliomas, cerebellar and brainstem gliomas, and gliomas of the cerebral hemisphere, thalamus or basal ganglia (Figures 12.6.3 and 12.6.4). Fourth ventricle gliomas, ependymomas and glioblastomas can occur but are rare.

Plexiform neurofibromas are the primary tumour of NF-1, which are found in about one-third of patients. They are seen as multiple, tortuous, cord-like masses infiltrating along the involved nerve. The plexiform neurofibromas are isointense on T1-WI, hyperintense on T2-WI and show strong enhancement (Figure 12.6.5). Craniofacial plexiform neurofibromas commonly occur along the trigeminal nerve forming periorbital and intraorbital mass and may extend to the cavernous sinus. Sphenoid dysplasia and pulsating exophthalmos are often associated with periorbital plexiform neurofibromas. Sarcomatous degeneration of peripheral soft tissue neurofibromas can occur in 5%–15% of NF-1 cases.

SKULL, MENINGEAL AND OSSEOUS LESIONS

Macrocrania, calvarial defects (lambdoid defect), dural ectasia and hypoplasia of the greater wing of sphenoid with orbital herniation of the temporal lobe associated with plexiform neurofibromas are common in NF-1. Enlargement of the internal auditory canal or diffuse optic nerve enlargement can be secondary to dysplastic dural ectasia. Tibial bowing, pseudoarthrosis, twisted-ribbon ribs or overgrowth of a digit or a limb are distinctive features of osseous lesions in NF-1.

SPINE, SPINAL CORD AND NERVE ROOTS

Spinal anomalies are primarily the result of mesenchymal dysplasia involving bone and dura primarily associated with NF-1. The characteristic bony deformities include kyphoscoliosis, vertebral scalloping and hypoplasia of the pedicles or processes. Cervical kyphosis associated with vertebral scalloping and wedging is highly suspicious for neurofibromatosis. Enlargement of one or multiple neural foramina is most often associated with neurofibromas along the nerve root but it can be caused by dural ectasia or diverticulum (lateral meningocele) or arachnoid cysts. Spinal neurofibromas typically present as intradural extramedullary masses and the neurofibromas on the exiting spinal nerves form dumb-bell tumours. Posterior vertebral scalloping is secondary to dysplastic dural ectasia. The occurrence of malignant schwannoma is one of the complications of neurofibromatosis. Low-grade astrocytoma can occur as an intramedullary tumour in NF-1.

VASCULAR ABNORMALITIES

Most of the reported vascular abnormalities are segmental or diffuse stenosis. Basal telangiectatic collaterals with narrowing of the internal carotid artery can be present as a moyamoya syndrome (Figure 12.6.6). Aneurysms or non-aneurysmal vascular ectasia can occur in association with NF-1.

NEUROFIBROMATOSIS TYPE 2

Neurofibromatosis type 2 is a distinct form of the disease that is different clinically and radiologically. It is much less common than NF-1 and is more common in young adults than in children. NF-2 has been identified with defects of chromosome 22 and the transmission mode is autosomal dominant inheritance. Bilateral masses of the eighth nerves are diagnostic for NF-2. Other CNS tumours such as glioma, meningioma and schwannoma can be present. Cutaneous manifestations are less common than NF-1 and cutaneous neurofibromas or iris Lisch nodules are not features of NF-2.

NEOPLASMS

Neoplasms of NF-2 are associated with tumours of coverings such as Schwann cells and meninges. The vestibulocochlear nerve is the most frequently involved nerve in NF-2 and bilateral acoustic schwannomas are the hallmark of NF-2. Acoustic tumours typically arise from the vestibular nerve and displace or engulf the cochlear and facial nerves. The next most frequently involved nerve is the trigeminal nerve and other nerves such as the oculomotor, trochlear or abducens nerve can be involved. Multiple cranial nerve schwannomas should be suspected for the diagnosis of NF-2 (Figure 12.6.7). On MRI, schwannomas appear as well-demarcated round masses that are iso- to hyperintense on T2-WI with strong heterogeneous enhancement. Intracranial meningiomas are also common in NF-2 and they are often multiple.

SPINAL CORD AND NERVE ROOT

Multiple intradural, extramedullary soft tissue masses are common and they are meningiomas or schwannomas (Figure 12.6.8). Multiple masses along the spinal nerve roots can also be present in NF-2 and they are usually schwannomas. Ependymomas, occurring as intramedullary tumours, are also common in NF-2.

TUBEROUS SCLEROSIS

Tuberous sclerosis (TS, Bourneville disease) is an autosomal dominant disease with multisystem involvement including neurological, cutaneous, ocular, renal, cardiac, pulmonary and other organs. The incidence of the disorder is estimated to be between 1 per 10 000 to 100 000 live births but sporadic cases are probably much more common. Specific deletions in chromosome 9 and perhaps chromosome 11 have been identified. The classical clinical triads are seizures, mental retardation and adenoma sebaceum, all of which are found in less than half the patients. The diagnosis of TS is made on the finding of one of the following: adenoma sebaceum, ungual or subungual fibromas, cortical or subependymal hamartomas or giant cell tumours. A presumptive

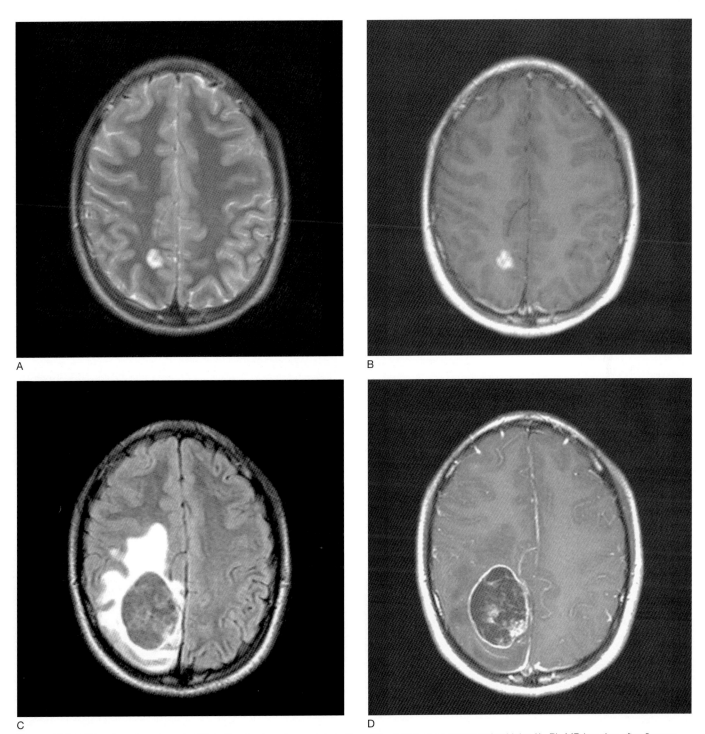

A

B

C

D

Figure 12.6.3 Pilocytic astrocytoma in NF-1. Focal enhancing nodule in the white matter of posterior parietal lobe (A, B). MR imaging after 3 years reveals enlargement of the nodule with peritumoural oedema. The mass shows discrete peripheral enhancement and speckled internal enhancement (C, D).

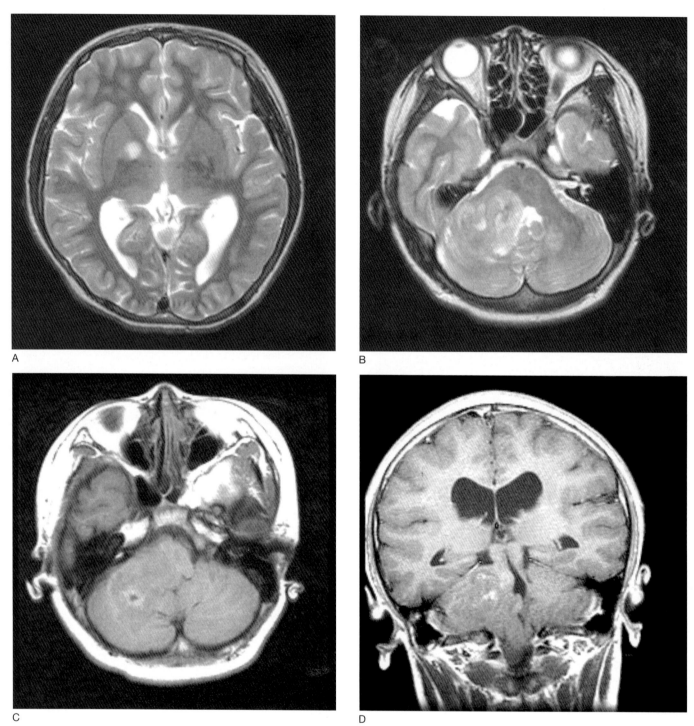

Figure 12.6.4 Cerebellar astrocytoma in NF-1.

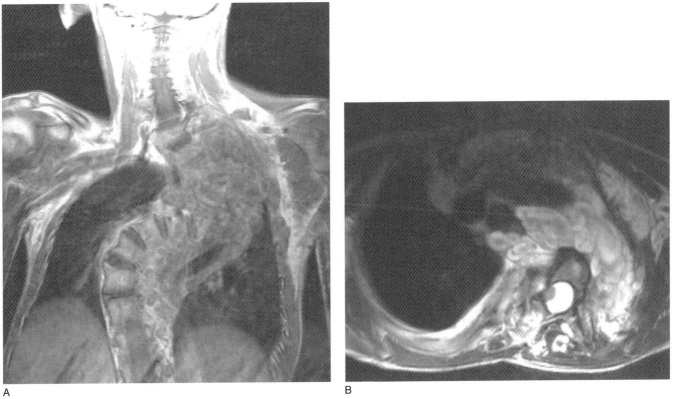

Figure 12.6.5 Plexiform neurofibroma. Coronal image shows kyphoscoliotic curvature of the cervicothoracic spine with paraspinal soft tissue masses (A). T2 image shows nodular masses arranged in a tortuous cord-like fashion surrounding the spine. The individual mass reveals as a target-like high signal nodule containing central low signal. Dilated dural sac causes posterior scalloping of the vertebra (B).

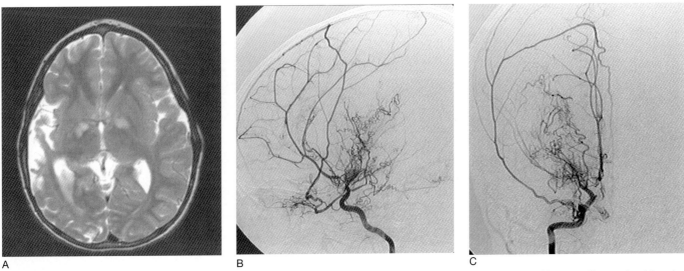

Figure 12.6.6 Moyamoya syndrome in NF-1. Internal carotid arteriography shows severe narrowing of the internal carotid artery with prominent basal collateral vessels.

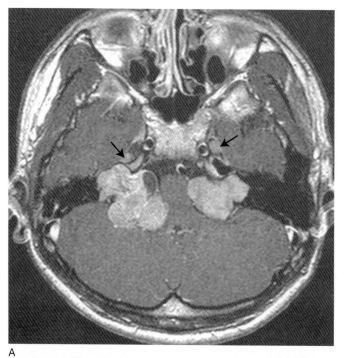

A

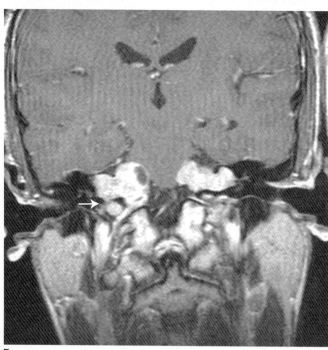

B

Figure 12.6.7 Bilateral acoustic neuromas in NF-2. Postcontrast T1 axial image shows bilateral acoustic neuromas and enhancing nodules (arrows) within the cavernous sinus (A). Coronal image shows enhancing nodule (arrow) below the acoustic neuroma (B).

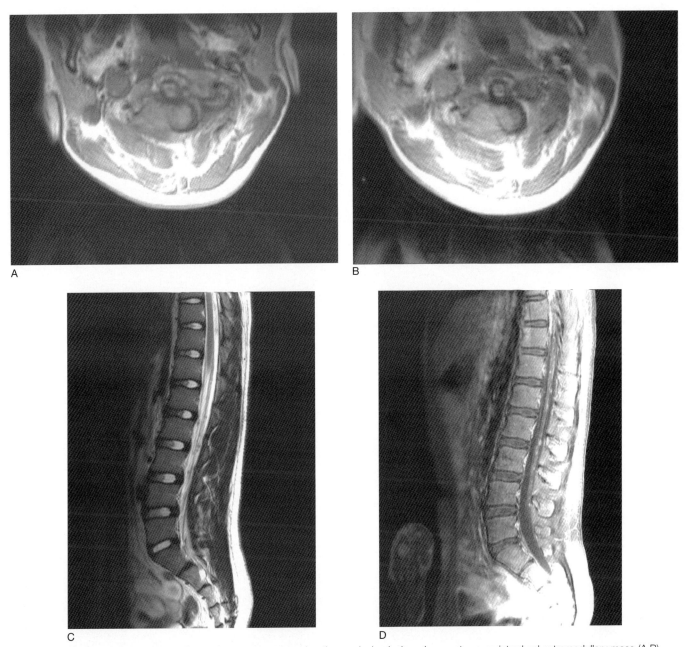

Figure 12.6.8 Meningiomas in NF-2. Enhancing mass compressing the cervical spinal cord presents as an intradural extramedullary mass (A,B). Multiple enhancing nodules along the nerve roots are also present (C,D).

diagnosis can be made with any of two of the following: hypopigmented macule, shagreen patches, infantile spasm, retinal hamartomas, renal hamartomas or cysts, cardiac rhabdomyomas, or first-degree relative with TS. Over 90% of patients with TS have skin lesions and brain hamartomas. Many patients have seizure onset before the age of 2 years and some degree of mental retardation. Hydrocephalus can occur due to a large periventricular hamartoma or giant cell tumour. Renal angiomyolipomas and cysts are usually asymptomatic in children and cardiac rhabdomyomas may be asymptomatic or result in arrhythmia or blood flow obstruction (Figure 12.6.9). Cardiac rhabdomyomas usually regress spontaneously. Pulmonary cysts or lymphangioleiomy-

omatosis may develop in adults but is rare in children. Progressive vascular degenerative changes can cause aneurysms of the thoracic and abdominal aorta.

The principal manifestations of the CNS are cortical tubers (Figure 12.6.10), white matter abnormalities (Figure 12.6.11), subependymal nodules and subependymal giant cell astrocytoma. These CNS lesions are thought to be caused by a migration abnormality of the dysgenetic neurons, which have giant cell clusters on microscopic examinations. Other CNS manifestations include retinal hamartomas and mild non-obstructive ventricular enlargement. Moyamoya syndrome with TS can be caused by progressive occlusion of the craniocervical arteries.

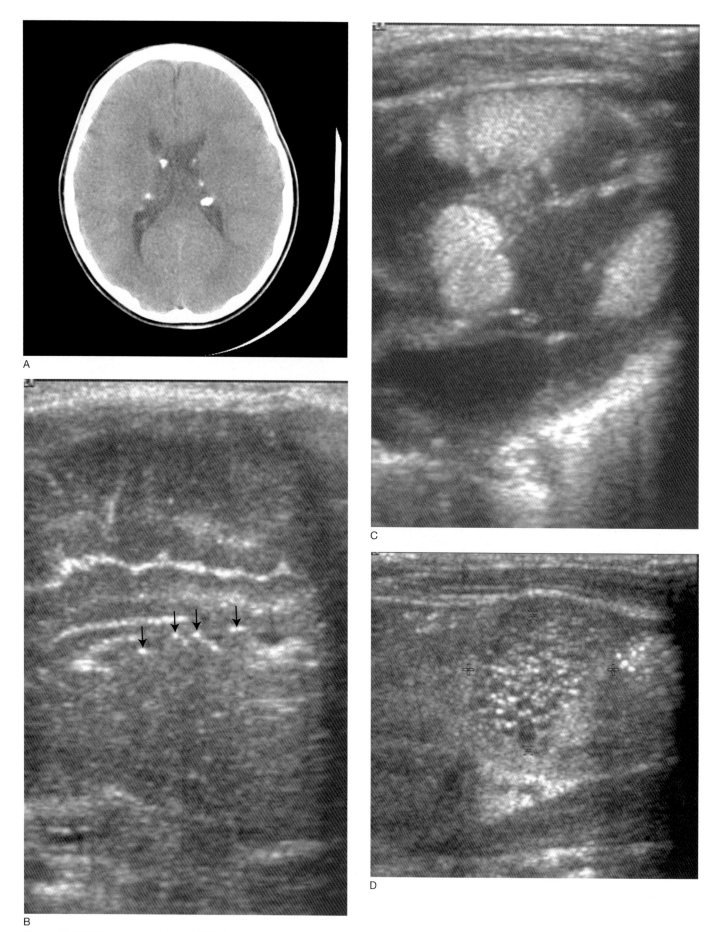

Figure 12.6.9 Tuberous sclerosis. Axial CT shows calcified subependymal nodules (A). Sonography of the newborn with tuberous sclerosis (B,C,D). Sagittal sonography of the brain shows multiple subependymal nodules (arrows) along the striatothalamic groove (B). Cardiac sonography shows rhabdomyomas as multiple echogenic masses (C). Sonography of the kidney shows conglomerated cystic mass (D).

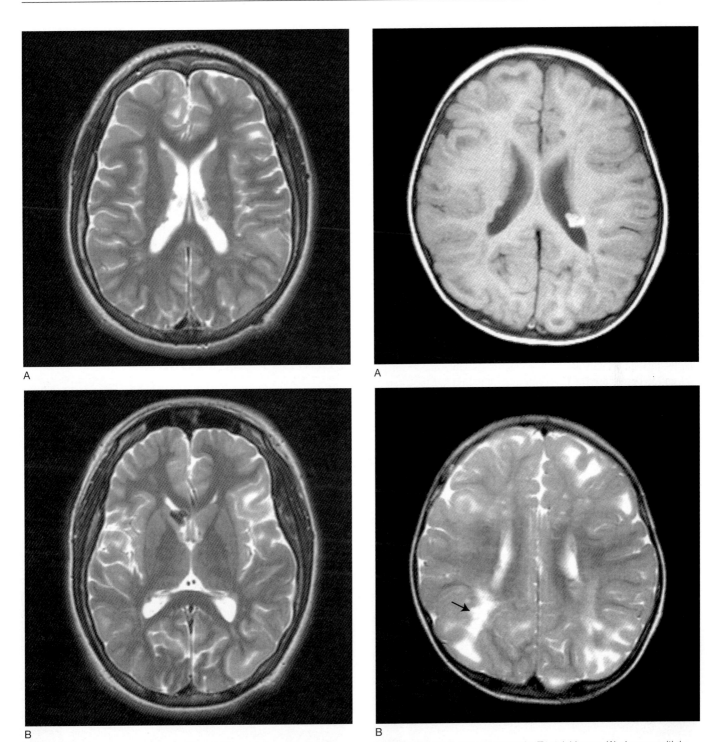

Figure 12.6.10 Tuberous sclerosis. T2 axial images show multiple low signal nodules along the lateral wall of the ventricles. A very low signal lesion in the right frontal horn represents a calcified nodule. Cortical tubers are seen as multiple subcortical low signal lesions with flattened overlying gyri in both cerebral hemispheres.

Figure 12.6.11 Tuberous sclerosis. T1 axial image (A) shows multiple cortical tubers and subependymal nodules. The tubers are seen as flat, expanded gyri with low signal of the subcortical white matter. The subependymal nodules along the lateral ventricles are isointense with the white matter. T2 axial images (B) show high signal of the subcortical tubers and white matter lesions (arrow).

CORTICAL TUBERS

Cortical tubers are the most characteristic lesions of TS. The tubers are seen as sclerotic plaques within an expanded and thickened cortex more often frontally and infrequently in the cerebellum. MR appearances of the cortical tubers are usually hypointense on (T1-WI) and hyperintense on T2-WI but they can be seen as hyperintense on T1-WI and hypointense on T2-WI in neonates and young children (Figure 12.6.12). Enhancement of the tubers after contrast administration can be seen infrequently. CT demonstrates the cortical tubers as low-density lesions and calcification of the tubers increases with age.

WHITE MATTER LESIONS

The white matter lesions can be a continuous lesion with the cortical tuber or primary deep white matter abnormality. They can be seen as straight or curvilinear bands extending from the ventricle toward the cortex or wedge-shaped focal lesion or non-specific conglomerate foci within the white matter. Like the cortical tubers, the lesions are seen as iso- to hypointense to white matter on T1-WI and hyperintense on T2-WI in older children but they can be seen as hyperintense on T1-WI and hypointense on T2-WI in infants. Pathologically, these are hamartomatous lesions containing various areas of focal migration abnormalities, astrogliosis, dysmyelination or even low-grade neoplastic changes.

SUBEPENDYMAL NODULES

Subependymal nodules (tubers) are the most familiar lesions composed of giant cells with neural or glial features. They can be located anywhere along the ventricular margin, most commonly near the caudate nucleus along the striothalamic groove of the lateral ventricles just behind the foramen of Monro. The third and fourth ventricles are infrequent sites. On MRI, the nodules are seen as variable sized nodules projecting towards the ventricle. The signal is isointense with the white matter but frequently hypointense on T2-WI because of calcification. Calcification of the nodule is common with age. Subependymal nodules can enhance after contrast administration but enhancement does not represent neoplastic transformation. Giant cell astrocytomas usually occur from the subependymal nodules near the foramen of Monro and the most important feature of the neoplastic transformation is increment of the size of nodules.

SUBEPENDYMAL GIANT CELL ASTROCYTOMAS

Subependymal giant cell astrocytomas occur in about 8%–12% of patients with TS. The tumours are closely related to the subependymal tuber near the foramen of Monro. They are very slow-growing tumours and frequent causes of obstructive hydrocephalus. The

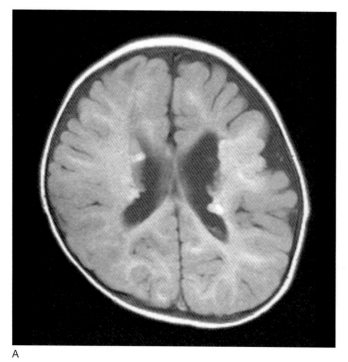
A

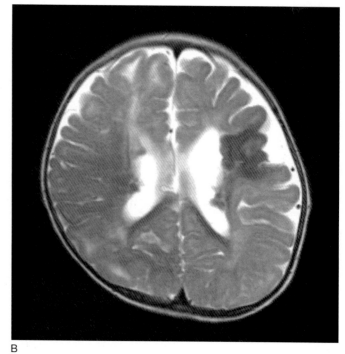
B

Figure 12.6.12 Tuberous sclerosis in an infant. T1 image (A) shows high signal subependymal nodules and a cortical tuber of the left frontal lobe that is hyperintense compared to the normal parenchyma and extends from the cortex to the ventricle. T2 image (B) shows low signal intensity of the cortical tuber. Cortical tubers of the right frontal lobe show high signal intensity.

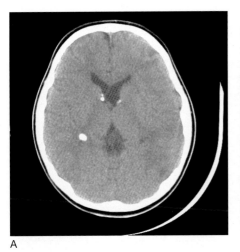 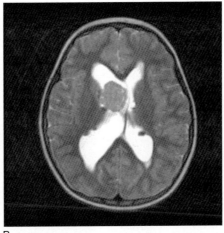 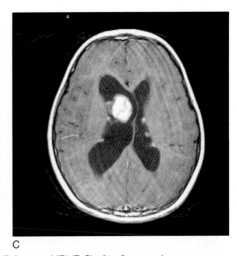

A   B   C

Figure 12.6.13 Giant cell astrocytoma. Non-contrast CT (A) shows calcified subependymal nodules. Follow-up MRI (B,C) after 3 years shows a mass within the right frontal horn near the foramen of Monro and dilatation of the right lateral ventricle. The mass shows homogeneous high signal after contrast enhancement.

tumours are frequently heterogeneous on CT or MRI due to cystic components or calcifications and show strong but somewhat heterogeneous enhancement after contrast administration. The diagnosis of giant cell tumour is based on the demonstration of slow growth over time, which indicates the need for periodic follow-up scans of the enhancing lesions near the foramen of Monro (Figure 12.6.13).

STURGE–WEBER SYNDROME

Sturge–Weber syndrome (encephalotrigeminal angiomatosis) is characterized by a facial port-wine naevus in the first division of the trigeminal nerve and ipsilateral leptomeningeal angiomatosis. Unilateral involvement is far more common than bilateral involvement. Angiomas are typically distributed in the parieto-occipital region but hemispheric, temporal and frontal regions can be involved. Common clinical manifestations are seizure, mental retardation, hemiplegia, hemianopsia, buphthalmos and glaucoma. The leptomeningeal malformation consists of abnormal venous structures between the arachnoid and pial membranes, which is probably due to faulty development of cortical venous drainage (Figure 12.6.14). Chronic venous stasis and congestion leads to hypoxia of the affected brain and results in slow progressive cortical atrophy and dystrophic calcification of the cortical grey matter. Angiomas may also involve the choroid plexus of the lateral ventricles and ocular choroidal or scleral angioma is frequent. The patients with angiomas of the choroid and sclera may present with ocular pain from glaucoma. Sturge–Weber syndrome can be found in association with angiomas of the viscera and extremities, such as the Klippel–Trenaunay–Weber syndrome.

IMAGING

Gyral calcifications and cortical atrophy are the common radiological findings usually beginning in late infancy and progressing with age. The calcification of the cortex shows a classical gyral pattern often described as tram-track in appearance, which is often better demonstrated by CT than by MRI. The calcifications eventually become dense enough to be seen on plain skull radiographs. These are most prominent in the occipital or parieto-occipital lobes ipsilateral to the facial angioma. The calcifications are sometimes difficult to see on T1-weighted MR imaging studies but are readily identified with T2-weighted images as tram-like low signal intensity along the gyri. The cortical and subcortical enhancement is another important feature of Sturge–Weber syndrome, which can be seen in early infancy and before the appearance of calcification. The enhancement usually represents pial angioma but gyral enhancement can be due to cortical ischaemia (Figure 12.6.15). Due to the chronic venous stasis, prominent collateral venous drainage may be seen such as angiomatous enhancement of the ipsilateral choroid plexus or prominent medullary or subependymal veins. Contrast-enhanced MR is the most accurate imaging method to show the enhancement and to indicate the extent of the pial angioma, which is important for the planning of surgery for seizure control. MR venography can demonstrate the venous anomalies including engorgement of the deep veins and the absence of the superficial cortical veins in the involved region. In the infant with Sturge–Weber syndrome, the white matter of the involved region shows a hypointense signal on T2-weighted images compared with the remainder of the brain. It might represent the result of increased deoxyhaemoglobin in capillaries and veins due to the impaired superficial venous drainage, although accelerated myelination was postulated as another aetiological hypothesis. The involved hemisphere becomes atrophic in most patients and the affected cortex shows slight hyperintensity on T2-weighted images representing gliosis in the ischaemic brain. The ipsilateral calvarial vault is thickened and paranasal sinuses are enlarged due to the impaired brain growth of the affected site (Figure 12.6.16).

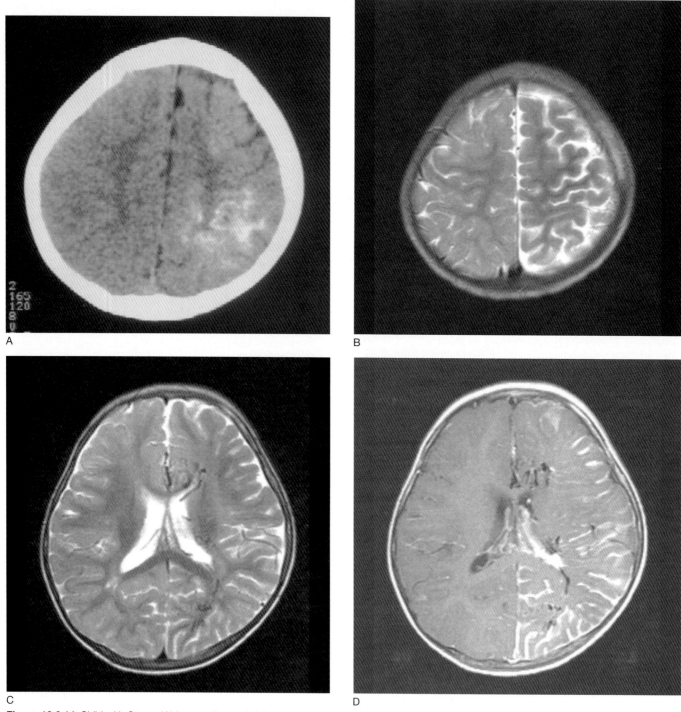

Figure 12.6.14 Child with Sturge–Weber syndrome. Axial non-contrast CT shows curvilinear calcifications involving the left frontal and parietal lobe with mild atrophy of the left hemisphere (A). Axial T2 image shows prominent low signal intensity of the white matter and gyral atrophy of the left hemisphere (B). Axial T2 image through the lateral ventricle shows dilated deep veins adjacent to the left lateral ventricle (C). Postcontrast axial image shows prominent leptomeningeal enhancement over the entire left hemisphere with enlargement of the left choroid plexus (D). Postcontrast coronal image shows leptomeningeal enhancement over the left hemisphere and enlarged left choroid plexus. Prominent fine nodular enhancement (arrow) over the surface of the brain beneath the left calvarium is also seen (E). MR venography shows absence of superficial venous drainage and prominent deep veins in the left cerebral hemisphere (F).

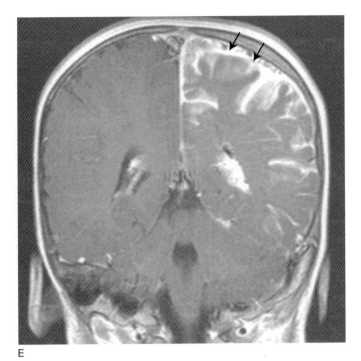

E

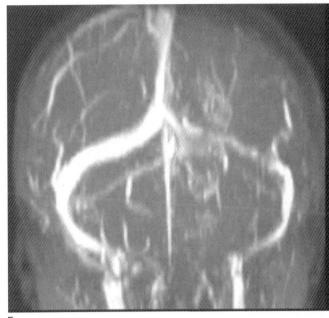

F

Figure 12.6.14 (Continued)

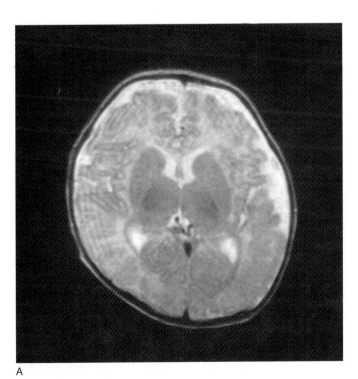

A

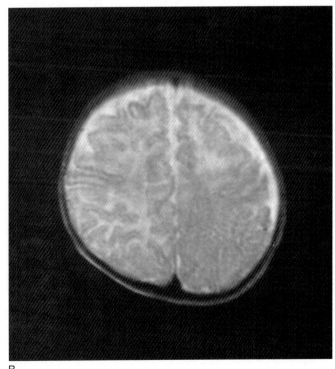

B

Figure 12.6.15 Progressive atrophy in an infant with Sturge–Weber syndrome. T2 image shows relative low signal intensity of the left parieto-occipital lobe. Parenchymal atrophy is not seen (A,B). Follow-up MRI shows gyral atrophy of the left parieto-occipital lobe (C,D). Postcontrast image shows leptomeningeal enhancement of the left parieto-occipital lobe (E).

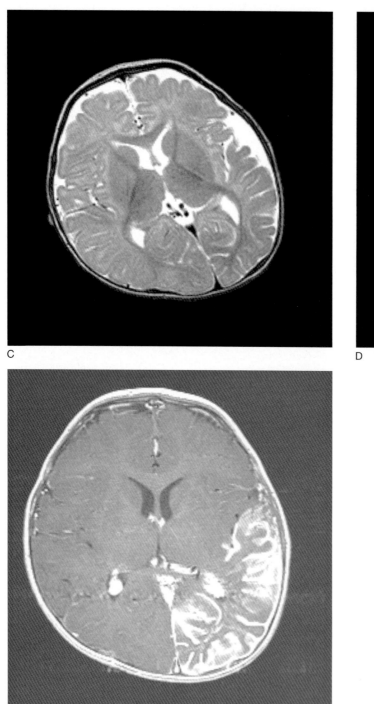

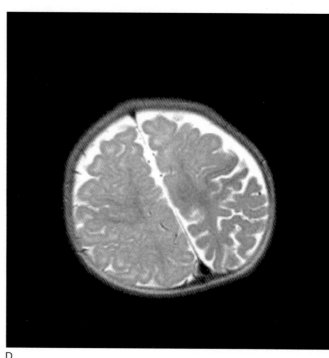

C

D

E

Figure 12.6.15 (*Continued*)

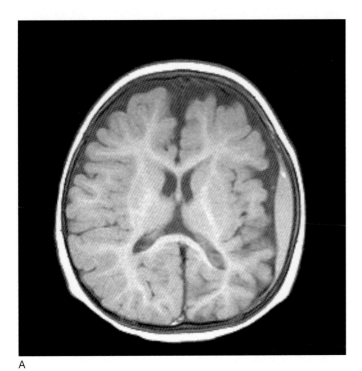

A

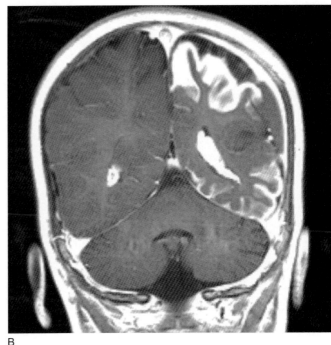

B

Figure 12.6.16 Sturge–Weber syndrome with subdural hygroma. T1 axial image shows gyral atrophy of the left temporoparietal lobe with old subdural haemorrhage (A). Postcontrast coronal image shows prominent enhancement of the atrophic gyral surface and enlargement of the left choroid plexus (B).

VON HIPPEL–LINDAU DISEASE

Von Hippel–Lindau disease is an autosomal dominant disorder with a variable penetrance. Principal manifestations include retinal angioma, cerebellar and spinal cord haemangioblastomas and multiorgan neoplasm of the abdominal viscera. The diagnosis can be made with more than one haemagioblastoma of the CNS, one CNS haemangioblastoma plus visceral involvement. Visceral lesions include renal cell carcinoma, pheochromocytoma, cyst of the kidney, liver, pancreas or epididymis. Retinal angioma (haemangioblastoma) occur in over half of the patients and may be multiple and bilateral. Cerebellar haemangioblastomas occur in more than half of the patients and may be multiple. Less commonly involved sites are the brainstem or spinal cord, particularly the cervical or thoracic cord (Figure 12.6.17). Supratentorial haemangioblastomas are very rare. Neurological abnormalities include increased pressure, cerebellar dysfunction, haemorrhage or myelopathy. Although retinal angioma may appear in childhood, the patients usually become symptomatic after 20 s. The peak incidence for haemangioblastoma is in the fourth or fifth decade of life.

IMAGING

Cerebellar haemangioblastomas occur as a cystic mass with a small, non-calcified vascular mural nodule in about 80% and as a solid tumour in about 20% of cases. In contrast, the tumours of the spinal cord are predominantly solid or partially cystic. On MRI, the cyst shows somewhat higher signal than CSF and the cyst wall does not show contrast enhancement. The mural nodule or solid tumour shows isointensity on T1-weighted images and slight hyperintensity on T2-WI, and shows strong homogeneous enhancement after contrast administration. Occasionally, flow voids of the feeding artery and draining vein of the tumour can be identified. On cerebral angiography, the haemangioblastomas show a characteristic intense vascular nodule in the early arterial phase with a dense, prolonged vascular staining.

ATAXIA-TELANGIECTASIA

Ataxia-telangiectasia is an autosomal recessive disorder that consists of oculocutaneous telangiectasia and cerebellar ataxia. The patients also have severe immune deficiencies and predisposition to malignant tumours (Figure 12.6.18). The gene abnormality is located on chromosome 11, which results in derangement of the detection of DNA damage or cellular repair. Ataxia and mucocutaneous telangiectasia appears in early childhood and recurrent bacterial and viral sinopulmonary infection occurs leading to pulmonary insufficiency. Malignant tumours such as lymphomas and leukaemia develop in more than 10% of younger patients, whereas epithelial malignancies can occur in adults.

Major radiological abnormalities are cerebellar cortical atrophy, which is more marked in the vermis, showing prominent cerebellar folia and a dilated fourth ventricle. Haemorrhage can occur from the rupture of parenchymal telangiectasia. Cerebellar atrophy and progressive neurological deterioration should raise the question of ataxia-telangiectasia.

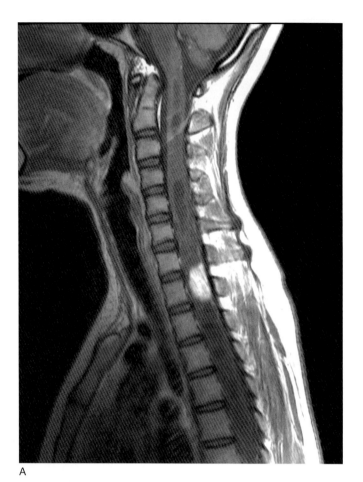

A

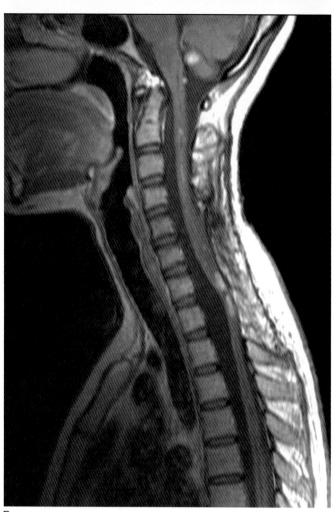

B

Figure 12.6.17 Recurrent haemangioblastoma in a child with von Hippel–Lindau disease. Postcontrast sagittal image of the spine shows a homogeneous strong enhancing mass with cyst-like low signal of the distal spinal cord. Heterogeneous low signal intensities of the spinal cord are seen proximal to the enhancing mass (A). Follow-up imaging after the removal of the haemangioblastoma in the lower cervical cord revealed a round enhancing nodule in the cerebellar tonsil (B).

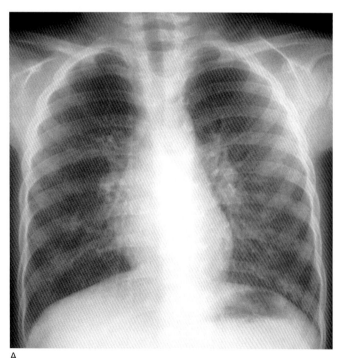

A

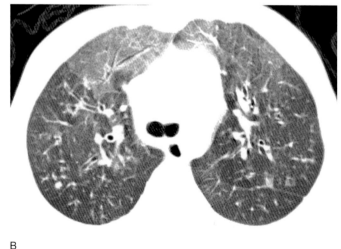

B

Figure 12.6.18 Recurrent respiratory infection in a child with ataxia-telangiectasia. Plain chest radiography and high resolution CT of the lung shows ground glass opacity with focal sparing suggesting bronchopneumonia (A,B). Follow-up chest radiograph shows progressive bronchopneumonia over the entire lung field (C). T2 axial image shows prominent folia in the entire cerebellum (D). The patient had a telangiectatic skin lesion that was proved as lymphoma histologically. T2 axial image shows mild expansile high signal lesion involving the right temporal lobe with focal low signal (E). The right temporal lesion shows oedematous low signal intensity with mild leptomeningeal enhancement (F). The lesion was removed and diagnosed as a lymphoma.

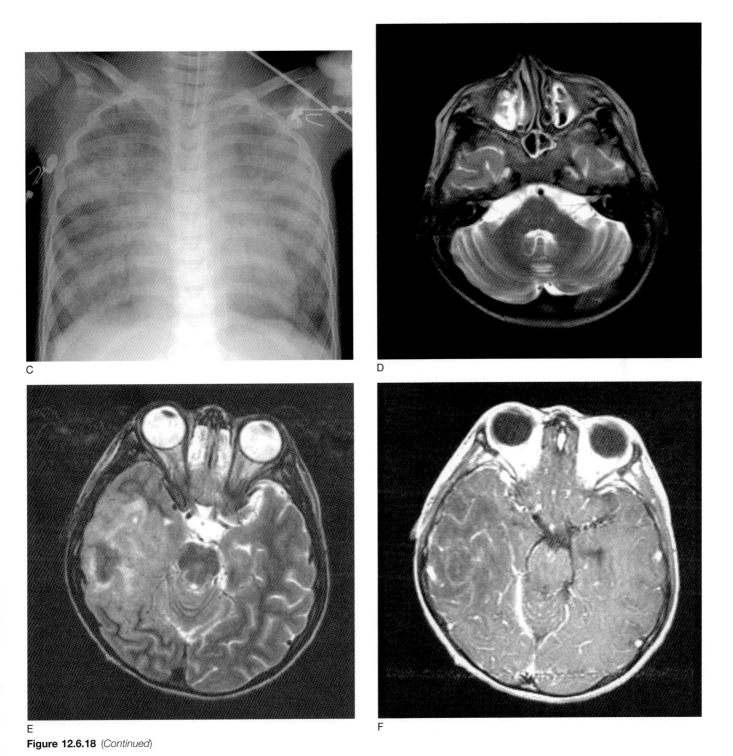

Figure 12.6.18 (*Continued*)

INCONTINENTIA PIGMENTI

Incontinentia pigmenti is an uncommon X-linked disorder with characteristic skin lesions, dental and skeletal dysplasia, ocular abnormalities and non-progressive CNS involvement. The erythematous skin lesions appear early in infancy and become verrucous and hyperpigmented. Seizures, quadriplegia, ataxia and mental retardation are frequent. Neuroimaging abnormalities include ischaemic brain lesions involving the cortex and underlying white matter in watershed zones. Periventricular white matter can be involved resulting in a feature suggesting periventricular leucomalacia. The ocular globes may show findings of persistent hyperplastic primary vitreous (Figure 12.6.19).

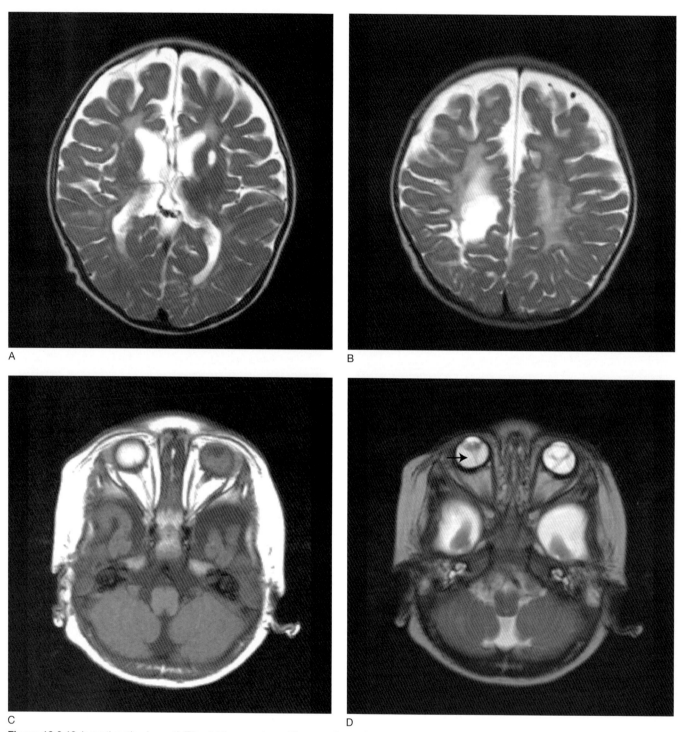

Figure 12.6.19 Incontinentia pigmenti. T2 axial images show diffuse gyral atrophy most prominent in the frontal region. The lateral ventricles show mild dilatation and slight undulation in the convexity level. The periventricular white matter show high signal intensity and focal leucomalacia is seen in the posterolateral portion. Focal tissue loss is also seen in the left basal ganglia (A,B). Axial images through the orbit show bilateral microphthalmia and abnormal signals of the vitreous suggesting retinal detachment. Linear structures (arrow) within the vitreous represent a persistent hyaloid vessel suggesting persistent hyperplastic primary vitreous (C,D).

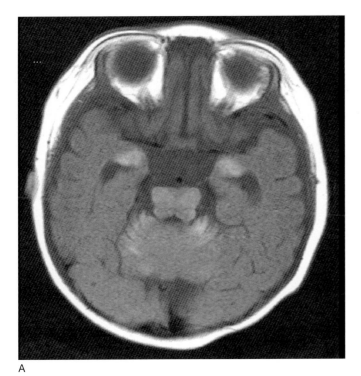
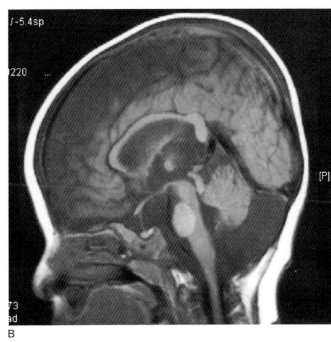

A   B

Figure 12.6.20 Neurocutaneous melanosis in an infant with seizure. T1 images show bilateral symmetrical focal high signal intensity in the anterior temporal lobes, cerebellar folia (A) and diffuse high signal of the pons (B). Retrocerebellar fluid collection suggests Dandy–Walker variant. (Courtesy of Dr Ji-Hye Kim.)

EPIDERMAL NAEVUS SYNDROME

Epidermal naevus syndrome is a sporadic disorder characterized by a linear epidermal naevus, and skeletal and CNS abnormalities. Clinical presentations can be mental retardation, seizure and hemihypertrophy. Ocular abnormalities such as ptosis, coloboma, and Coat's disease can occur. CNS involvement may include hemimegalencephaly, focal cortical malformation, heterotopia and cerebellar vermian hypoplasia. CNS vascular abnormalities such as infarcts, porencephaly, vascular dysplasia or arteriovenous malformations can be seen.

NEUROCUTANEOUS MELANOSIS

Neurocutaneous melanosis is a syndrome composed of giant congenital melanocytic naevi on the head and neck or dorsal spine area. Clinical manifestations include seizures, increased intracranial pressure and chronic meningitis. CNS symptoms typically develop at less than 2 years of age. Symptomatic neurocutaneous melanosis has poor prognosis and the patients have increased risk of cutaneous and CNS melanoma. This disorder is thought to represent an error of migration and differentiation of embryonal neu-

roectoderm. Pathologically, abnormal meningeal pigmentation and thickening due to melanocytic proliferation can be seen at the meninges and the brain especially involving the cerebellum, brainstem and basal ganglia. MRI shows foci of T1 shortening due to the presence of free radicals in melanin, most commonly in the anterior temporal lobe, cerebellar nuclei, cerebellar white matter and brainstem (Figure 12.6.20). Hydrocephalus, Dandy–Walker malformation and arachnoid cysts can be present.

FURTHER READING

Adamsbaum C, Pinton F, Rolland Y et al. Accelerated myelination in early Sturge–Weber syndrome; MRI-SPECT correlations. Pediatric Radiology 1996; 26:759–762.

Aoki S, Barkovich AJ, Nishimura K et al. Neurofibromatosis type 1 and 2: cranial MR findings. Radiology 1989; 172:527–534.

Barkovich AJ. The phakomatoses. In: Barkovich AJ (ed) Pediatric neuroimaging, 3rd edn. Philadelphia: Lippincott Williams & Wilkins; 2000:383–441.

Ciemins JJ, Horowitz AL. Abnormal white matter signal in ataxia telangiectasia. American Journal of Neuroradiology 2000; 21:1483–1485.

Conway JE, Chou D, Clatterbuck RE et al. Hemangioblastomas of the central nervous system in von Hippel–Lindau syndrome and sporadic disease. Neurosurgery 2001; 48:55–62; discussion 62–63.

Cure JK, Holden KR, Van Tassel P. Progressive venous occlusion in a neonate with Sturge–Weber syndrome: demonstration with MR venography. American Journal of Neuroradiology 1995; 16:1539–1542.

Demirci A, Kawamura Y, Sze G, Duncan C. MR of parenchymal neurocutaneous melanosis. American Journal of Neuroradiology 1995; 16: 603–606.

DiPaolo DP, Zimmermann RA, Rorke LB et al. Neurofibromatosis type 1: pathologic substrate of high signal intensity foci in the brain. Radiology 1995; 195:721–724.

Farina L, Uggetti C, Ottolini A et al. Ataxia-telangiectasia: MR and CT findings. Journal of Computer Assisted Tomography 1994; 18:724–727.

Griffiths PD, Martland TR. Tuberous sclerosis complex: the role of neuroradiology. Neuropediatrics 1997; 28:244–252.

Herron J, Darrah R, Quaghebeur G. Intra-cranial manifestations of the neurocutaneous syndromes. Clinical Radiology 2000; 55:82–98.

Hyman MH, Whittemore VH. National Institutes of Health consensus conference: tuberous sclerosis complex. Archives of Neurology 2000; 57:662–665.

Inoue Y, Nemoto Y, Murata R et al. CT and MR imaging of cerebral tuberous sclerosis. Brain Development 1998; 20:209–221.

Mukonoweshuro W, Griffiths PD, Blaser S. Neurofibromatosis type 1: the role of neuroradiology. Neuropediatrics 1999; 30:111–119.

Pascual-Castroviejo I, Roche MC, Martinez Fernandez V et al. Incontinentia pigmenti: MR demonstration of brain changes. American Journal of Neuroradiology 1994; 15:1521–1527.

Portilla P, Husson B, Lasjaunias P, Landrieu P. Sturge–Weber disease with repercussion on the prenatal development of the cerebral hemisphere. American Journal of Neuroradiology 2002; 23:490–492.

Smirniotopoulos JG, Murphy FM. The phakomatoses. American Journal of Neuroradiology 1992; 13:725–746.

Hypoxic and Ischaemic Brain Insults in Newborns and Infants

Robert A Zimmerman, Alex Mun-Ching Wong, Larissa T Bilaniuk

INTRODUCTION

Injury to the brain of the fetus, or to that of the newborn in the perinatal period, whether premature or term, has the potential risk of producing cerebral palsy and mental retardation. The deficits associated with these insults remain for the rest of the life of the patient. The consequences of such insults can range from death, vegetative stage, motor and cognitive impairment, to minimal or no clinical evidence of injury. The more severely injured patients represent a tremendous burden to the family, both emotionally and financially, and a cost to the community and to the society that helps to care for them. This chapter reviews the more common patterns of injury found in premature and term infants that are sustained *in utero*, perinatally or during the immediate postnatal period.

In the United States, of the four million live births per year, the incidence of cerebral palsy has been estimated to be between 2–3 per thousand live births. It is thought that approximately 12% of infants with cerebral palsy are the result of asphyxia, a deprivation of oxygen. Thus, of the 8000–12 000 patients with cerebral palsy born per year in the US, between 960 and 1440 would be as a result of asphyxia. Often the injury is not simply due to asphyxia, a reduction in oxygen, but also to ischaemia, because reduction in oxygenation in the fetus or infant can affect the heart, causing bradycardia. Thus, both a decrease in oxygen and a decrease in blood flow are important risk factors in the production of brain injury. The term for this type of injury to the brain is hypoxic ischaemic encephalopathy (HIE), reflecting both the decrease in the oxygen and the decrease in the blood flow to the brain. In the study of the pathophysiology of HIE, the important factors are the oxygen, CO_2 and glucose content of the blood and the cerebral blood flow in millilitres per minute per hundred grams of tissue, as well as the length and severity of the single insult or multiple insults. The type and severity of injury also depends on the degree of maturity or lack thereof of the cerebral tissues. The concept of selective vulnerability of tissues (e.g. neurons) is seen in the metabolically active thalamus and putamen in the term infant, when there is a sudden decrease in oxygenation and blood flow. Much of the rest of the grey matter/neuronal tissue, with the exception of the pre- and postcentral gyri, are not as mature at term and therefore have lower metabolic rates. Thus, insults associated with a profound asphyxia, such as a period of fetal bradycardia for 15–30 min, tend to more commonly produce neuronal necrosis in the putamen, thalamus and rolandic cortex. Provided there is relatively rapid return of oxygenation and flow, such as happens with Caesarean section, delivery and resuscitation, the vast areas of neuronally immature cortex appear unaffected.

Similar selective vulnerability is seen in the premature infant, where the fragile germinal matrix containing venules with single cell layer walls is injured, resulting in rupture and germinal matrix haemorrhage (GMH).

FURTHER READING

Barkovich AJ, Truwit CL. MR of perinatal asphyxia: correlation of gestational age with pattern of damage. American Journal of Neuroradiology 1990; 11:1087–1096.

Chugani HT, Phelps ME, Mazziotta JC. Positron emission tomography study of human brain functional development. Annals of Neurology 1987; 22:487–497.

Hagberg B, Hagberg G, Zetterstrom R. Decreasing perinatal mortality – increase in cerebral palsy morbidity. Acta Paediatrica Scandanavica 1989; 78:664–670.

Kuban KCK, Leviton A. The epidemiology of cerebral palsy. New England Journal of Medicine 1994; 330:188–195.

Nelson KB. What proportion of cerebral palsy is related to birth asphyxia? [editorial] Journal of Pediatrics 1988; 112:572–574.

Nelson KB, Ellenberg JH. Antecedents of cerebral palsy: multivariate analysis of risk. New England Journal of Medicine 1986; 315:81–86.

Pasternak JF, Predey TA, Mikhael MA. Neonatal asphyxia: vulnerability of basal ganglia, thalamus, and brainstem. Pediatric Neurology 1991; 7:147–149.

Rorke LB, Zimmerman RA. Prematurity, postmaturity and destructive lesions in utero. American Journal of Neuroradiology 1992; 13:517–536.

Taylor DL, Edwards AD, Mehmet H. Oxidative metabolism, apoptosis and perinatal brain injury. Brain Pathology 1999; 9:93–117.

Torfs CP, van den Berg B, Oechsli FW, Cummins S. Prenatal and perinatal factors in the aetiology of cerebral palsy. Journal of Pediatrics 1990; 116:615–619.

GREY MATTER INJURY

Among the classifications of neuronal injury that have been utilized in HIE, one consists of: (1) diffuse neuronal injury; (2) cerebral cortical and deep nuclear neuronal injury; (3) deep nuclear and brainstem injury; and (4) pontosubicular injury.

Diffuse neuronal injury is seen primarily with markedly prolonged partial asphyxia. Because of the diffuse involvement of the cortex beyond the typical watershed, there is a decreased level of consciousness and the presence of seizures. Sucking, swallowing and tongue motion may be abnormal because of involvement of brainstem cranial nerve nuclei. Long-term effects in this group of patients is decreased intellect, spasticity, seizures in 10–30% and loss of vision. Abnormalities of sucking and swallowing frequently persist, requiring a feeding tube.

Cortical and deep nuclear neuronal injury causes increased tone, dystonia with extrapyramidal involvement. There are long-term feeding difficulties requiring a feeding tube and, in half of these patients, cognition is abnormal. Chorioathetotic problems with dystonia are found with bilateral basal ganglia involvement and intact pyramidal tracts. The onset of these extrapyramidal abnormalities may be late, often not apparent between 6 and 12 months but developing later. The symptoms of chorioathetotic cerebral palsy can present between 1 and 4 years of age and, in some cases, as late as 7–14 years of age. The intellect in patients with chorioathetotic cerebral palsy is often intact.

Deep nuclear and brainstem neuronal injury typically involves the basal ganglia and thalami and has abnormalities as described in the preceding paragraph. Third nerve palsies, ventilatory disturbances and impaired suck and swallowing are not uncommon.

Selective neuronal injury involving the neurons of the basis pontis and the subiculum of the hippocampus is the least common form of neuronal injury. It occurs in the premature infant but can be seen at term. There is an association with periventricular leukomalacia (PVL).

FURTHER READING

Colamaria V, Curatolo P, Cusmai R, Dalla Bernardina B. Symmetrical bithalamic hyperdensities in asphyxiated full-term newborns: an early indicator of status marmoratus. Brain Development 1988; 10:57–59.

Goodwin TM, Belai I, Hernandez P. Asphyxial complications in the term newborn with severe umbilical acidemia. American Journal of Obstetrics and Gynecology 1992; 167:1506–1512.

Maller AI, Hankins LL, Yeakley JW, Butler IJ. Rolandic type cerebral palsy in children as a pattern of hypoxic-ischaemic injury in the full-term neonate. Journal of Child Neurology 1998; 13:313–321.

Pasternak JF, Gorey MT. The syndrome of acute near-total intrauterine asphyxia in the term infant. Pediatric Neurology 1998; 18:391–398.

Roland EH, Jan JE, Hill A, Wong PK. Cortical visual impairment following birth asphyxia. Pediatric Neurology 1986; 2:133–137.

Roland EH, Poskitt K, Rodriguez E. Perinatal hypoxic-ischaemic thalamic injury: clinical features and neuroimaging. Annals of Neurology 1998; 44:161–166.

Rosenbloom L. Dyskinetic cerebral palsy and birth asphyxia. Developmental Medicine and Child Neurology 1994; 36:285–289.

Winkler P, Zimmerman RA. Perinatal brain injury. In: Zimmerman RA, Gibby WA, Carmody RF, eds. Neuroimaging: clinical and physical principles. New York: Springer; 2000:531–538.

WHITE MATTER INJURY

In the term infant, white matter injury can occur not only relatively close to the ventricle, so-called periventricular leukomalacia (PVL), but also much further from the ventricle, in the subcortical region. Much of this subcortical leukomalacia appears to be that related to partial prolonged asphyxia, without gross cortical infarction. It reflects the shift of the watershed zone between vascular territories to the more peripheral aspects of the brain. In the premature infant, the relatively less well developed and poorly vascularized periventricular white matter, with a passive pressure-dependent blood flow, is more vulnerable to injury and, thus, PVL results. That this happens within the white matter, from the ependyma of the lateral ventricles to the subcortical region, can be seen with the distribution of PVL lesions as the fetus or infant matures from 26 weeks of gestation to term. The area most vulnerable to white matter damage, when the damage is relatively limited, will tend to migrate away from the ependymal surface of the ventricle and present more peripherally in the white matter with increase in gestational age.

Frequently, when there has been damage to the white matter and to the oligodendroglia, myelination in the surviving white matter is either delayed or will not take place. This can be best recognized on a combination of T1- and T2-weighted images. Short tau inversion recovery (STIR) images give a very heavily T1-weighted image that can be quite useful for recognizing absence of myelination. Myelination on a T1-weighted image is generally complete by age 8 months. Myelination on a T2-weighted image is mostly complete between 18 and 24 months, and is complete even in the subcortical U-fibres by 3 years of age. Blood products at the site of haemorrhagic leukomalacia are best demonstrated by conventional spin echo T2-weighted images or gradient echo 2D FLASH (fast low angle shot) susceptibility sequences.

FURTHER READING

Childs AM, Ramenghi LA, Evans DJ et al. MR features of developing periventricular white matter in preterm infants: evidence of glial cell migration. American Journal of Neuroradiology 1998; 19:971–976.

Greisen G, Borch K. White matter injury in the preterm neonate: the role of perfusion. Developmental Neuroscience 2001; 23:209–212.

Miyawaki T, Matsui K, Takashima S. Developmental characteristics of vessel density in the human fetal and infant brains. Early Human Development 1998; 53:65–72.

Rezaie P, Dean A. Periventricular leukomalacia, inflammation and white matter lesions within the developing nervous system. Neuropathology 2002; 22:106–132.

Rutherford MA, Pennock JM, Counsell SJ et al. Abnormal magnetic resonance signal in the internal capsule predicts poor neurodevelopmental outcome in infants with hypoxic-ischaemic encephalopathy. Pediatrics 1998; 102:323–328.

ADDITIONAL CAUSES OF BRAIN INJURY

Not every newborn patient, whether premature or term, who suffers a brain injury does so from hypoxic ischaemic injury due to asphyxia. Acute vascular occlusions resulting in infarction, often in the middle cerebral artery territory, occur for a variety of reasons, including emboli from distal sources, thrombi from hypercoagulable states, etc. Birth trauma, related to the use of forceps or vacuum, particularly in cases of cephalopelvic disproportion, can result in scalp, calvarial and underlying brain injury. Traumatic lesions may occur with or without the presence of asphyxia. Trauma is not limited to the brain and its coverings alone but can also occur in the cervical and thoracic spinal cord region, as a consequence of forces associated with delivery. Hypoglycaemia can also produce brain injury but is recognized more often as a postnatal complication in the infant who is several days of age when oral intake is extremely poor. Infections, such as encephalitides due to herpes simplex virus (HSV) and/or cytomegalovirus (CMV) and meningitides, can be transplacentally transmitted to the fetus but some infections can also occur during the passage through the birth canal. Some inborn errors of metabolism, such as neonatal Leigh's disease, can present as acute brain injury in the immediate postpartum period. It is also important to recognize that the birth process may be complicated by a pre-existing *in utero* injury that makes the fetus more vulnerable to HIE at the time of delivery, producing an infant with low Apgar scores and signs of distress. Each case needs to be evaluated as fully as possible with the radiological imaging performed promptly, properly and completely, to document the location and nature of the disease process. Initial studies combined with follow-up examinations to monitor evolution and resolution of the disease process can document the extent and nature of the disease process in a specific patient, and can increase our overall understanding of the nature of the various lesions that can occur in newborns.

In evaluating the neuroimaging studies obtained after the birth in cases where hypoxic ischaemic injury is alleged to have occurred, one must consider factors that could point to a prenatal, an intrapartum or a postnatal time of the event (Table 12.7.1). One must try to figure out whether the events were single or multiple, and whether they were prolonged or sudden and catastrophic. What the mother reports and what the obstetrician observes do not always add up to what actually happened. An attempt should be made to correlate the results of the neuroimaging studies with the medical history and clinical findings. In most instances, when there is infant distress at the time of birth, the clinical, radiographic and

Table 12.7.1 Factors that may adversely affect the fetal brain (adapted with permission from Perinatal brain injury. In: Winkler P, Zimmerman RA, eds. Neuroimaging: clinical and physical principles. Heidelberg: Springer-Verlag; 2000)

Maternal risk factors
Placental failure, abruption or haemorrhage
Vascular or coagulation disorder affecting the placenta
Prolonged rupture of membranes
Complications of labour and delivery
Chorioamnionitis
Cardiovascular disease, failure or acute events, including marked hypotensive episodes and shock, such as in sepsis, eclampsia, haemorrhage and severe anaphylaxis
Diabetes
Drug abuse (alcohol, narcotic, cocaine) and smoking
Intoxication (i.e. with carbon monoxide)
Infection, septicaemia
Adverse effects of anaesthesia

Fetal risk factors
Infectious disease
Iatrogenic (intrauterine invasive diagnosis or treatment)
Twin pregnancy (monozygotic twins)
Umbilical cord abnormality or malposition
Increased blood viscosity and hypercoagulation
Genetic/chromosomal abnormalities, including metabolic disorders
Hypoglycaemia

laboratory observations are made at that point in time. However, there are patients in whom clinical manifestations do not become apparent until the infant reaches or fails to reach certain developmental milestones, such as those associated with sitting, standing, verbalizing, etc. Rigidity of a hand may be the initial manifestation of a middle cerebral artery infarction in the contralateral hemisphere, while spasticity of the lower extremities may be indicative of periventricular leukomalacia. These findings are often not apparent in the first months of life but when they become evident, require further investigation both clinically and with neuroimaging.

RADIOGRAPHIC EVALUATION

ULTRASOUND

Currently, the initial imaging of the central nervous system (CNS) of the fetus is performed by ultrasound (US). Often this is done at 18–20 weeks of gestation and, if abnormal, leads to further clinical (amniocentesis) or radiographic (fetal magnetic resonance imaging) evaluation. In the past 5 years, ultrafast magnetic resonance imaging (MRI) techniques have enabled successful examination of the fetus between 18 and 40 weeks of gestation, with the recognition of such conditions as hydrocephalus, hypoxic ischaemic brain injury, congenital malformations and *in utero* neoplasms.

Ultrasound is limited to the neonatal and infant age group because of the need for an acoustic window, e.g. the anterior fontanel. Once the fontanel closes, the window is gone. The advantages of US are its portability to the crib-side of sick infants, its lack of need for sedation and its relatively quick study time. Ventricular enlargement or compression, the presence of central brain bleeds, the shift of the midline structures and the presence of gross areas of brain oedema can be demonstrated with US. The disadvantages are that large areas of the brain are usually not visualized and therefore not examined, such as portions of the frontal lobes and the posterior parietal and occipital lobes. The posterior fossa is rarely studied successfully unless additional acoustic windows are utilized. The differentiation of haemorrhage within the white matter from ischaemic infarction is not accurate and the recognition of small areas of PVL or even large symmetrical areas of PVL is not necessarily easy. The use of US in infants is operator dependent and, therefore, it is the skill of the technician or doctor who performs the examination that either maximizes or minimizes the obtainable information.

In the premature infant, following delivery, the initial study of choice, when the patient is unstable, is the cranial ultrasound examination (Figure 12.7.1). This is done to ascertain whether or not there is intracranial haemorrhage either in the ventricles or within the brain tissue. The size and morphology of the ventricles is shown, whether they are dilated as in hydrocephalus, or compressed by brain oedema. The echogenicity of the brain parenchyma can give evidence of calcifications as in cases of *in utero* infections (such as CMV) as well as show changes due to haemorrhages and/or brain oedema. The two most prevalent lesions that affect the premature brain are germinal matrix haemorrhage occurring in the low birth weight infant and

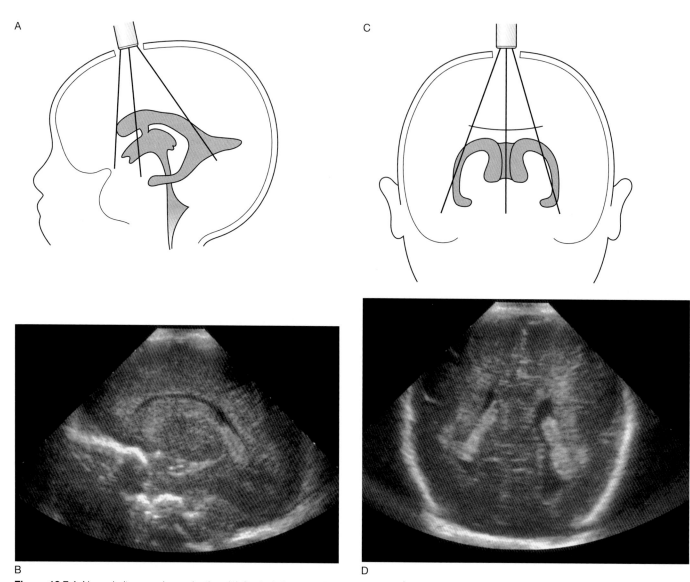

Figure 12.7.1 Normal ultrasound examination. (A) Sagittal diagram of ventricular system shows probe in anterior fontanelle position with lines indicating coronal planes of imaging. (B) Normal 26-week-old infant, coronal US through level of the atria of the lateral ventricle. (C) Coronal diagram of the lateral ventricles shows probe in anterior fontanelle with lines indicating sagittal planes for US imaging. (D) Sagittal US through the lateral ventricle in a normal 26-week-old infant.

periventricular leukomalacia seen in many premature infants (Figures 12.7.2 and 12.7.3).

In the term infant (37–42 weeks), depending upon the stability of the infant, the initial study also may be an US examination to determine the size of the ventricles and to check for the presence of abnormal echogenicity, as manifestations of brain swelling and/or haemorrhage or hydrocephalus. In the term infant, routine US through the anterior fontanelle misses peripheral portions of the frontal lobes and the parietal-occipital lobes, the site of the parasagittal watershed infarctions that accompany partial prolonged asphyxia with reduced oxygenation and/or hypotension. Ultrasound is limited in its evaluation of the structures of the posterior fossa when performed through the anterior fontanelle. The anatomy of the posterior fossa can be displayed when the probe is centred over the mastoid sutures.

Transcranial Doppler (TCD) US is another US technique that requires skilled acquisition of data. TCD is used to measure the velocity of flow in centimetres per second in the major vessels at the circle of Willis. Knowledge of the vascular anatomy is critical if reproducible results are to be obtained. With good data, TCD can be used to demonstrate both reduced and increased velocity of flow in the internal carotid artery and middle cerebral arteries, which reflects change in calibre of a vessel, e.g. stenosis or absence of flow in cases of occlusion.

FURTHER READING

Chow PP, Horgan JC, Taylor KJ. Neonatal periventricular leukomalacia: real-time sonographic diagnosis with CT correlation. American Journal of Roentgenology 1985; 145:155–160.

Cohen HL, Blitman NM, Sanchez J. Neurosonography of the infant: the normal examination. In: Timor-Tritsch IE, Monteagudo A, Cohen HL, eds. Ultrasonography of the prenatal and neonatal brain, 2nd edn. New York: McGraw-Hill; 2001:403–422.

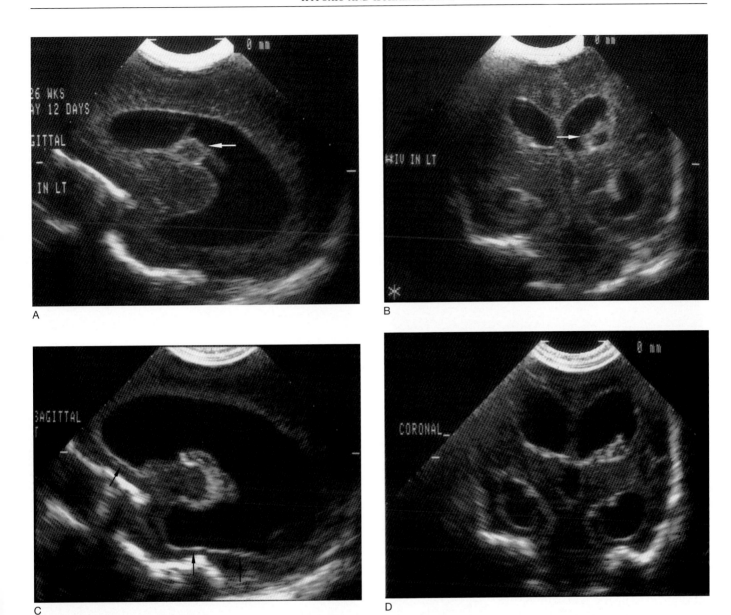

Figure 12.7.2 Germinal matrix haemorrhage, ultrasound examination. (A) 26-week-old premature infant. 12 days post delivery, shows a caudothalamic area of increased echogenicity consistent with haemorrhage on the sagittal (A) and coronal (B) US images (arrows). The lateral ventricles are enlarged. Follow-up US examination 9 days later shows, on sagittal (C) and coronal (D) images, further ventricular enlargement due to hydrocephalus. Note increased echogenicity of the walls of the ventricles (arrows) indicating siderosis. The haemorrhage in the germinal matrix appears smaller.

de Vries LS, Eken P, Kubowitz LM. The spectrum of leukomalacia using cranial ultrasound. Behavioral Brain Research 1992; 49:1–6.

de Vries LS, Wigglesworth JS, Regev R, Dubowitz LM. Evolution of periventricular leukomalacia during the neonatal period and infancy: correlation of imaging and postmortem findings. Early Human Development 1988; 17:205–219.

Ment LR, Bada HS, Barnes P et al. Practice parameter: neuroimaging of the neonate. Report of the Quality Standards Subcommittee of the American Academy of Neurology and the Practice Committee of the Child Neurology Society. Neurology 2002; 58:1726–1738.

Nwaesei CG, Allen AC, Vincer MJ. Effect of timing of cerebral ultrasonography on the prediction of later neurodevelopmental outcome in high-risk preterm infants. Journal of Pediatrics 1988; 112:970–975.

Skranes J, Vike T, Nilsen G. Can cerebral MRI at age 1 year predict motor and intellectual outcomes in very-low-birthweight children? Developmental Medicine and Child Neurology 1998; 40:256–262.

Weisglas-Kuperus N, Baerts W, Fetter W, Sauer P. Neonatal cerebral ultrasound, neonatal neurology and perinatal conditions as predictors of neurodevelopmental outcome in very low birthweight infants. Early Human Development 1992; 31:131–148.

COMPUTED TOMOGRAPHY

Computed tomography (CT) in both the premature and term infant gives a more comprehensive evaluation of the whole head/brain than does US, including the tissues of the scalp, the bones of the calvarium, the brain parenchyma and the CSF spaces, both within and outside of the brain tissue.

Computed tomography is often the initial imaging test in stable neonates presenting with acute HIE, whether it is suspected to be due to ischaemic infarction or to a haemorrhagic bleed within the

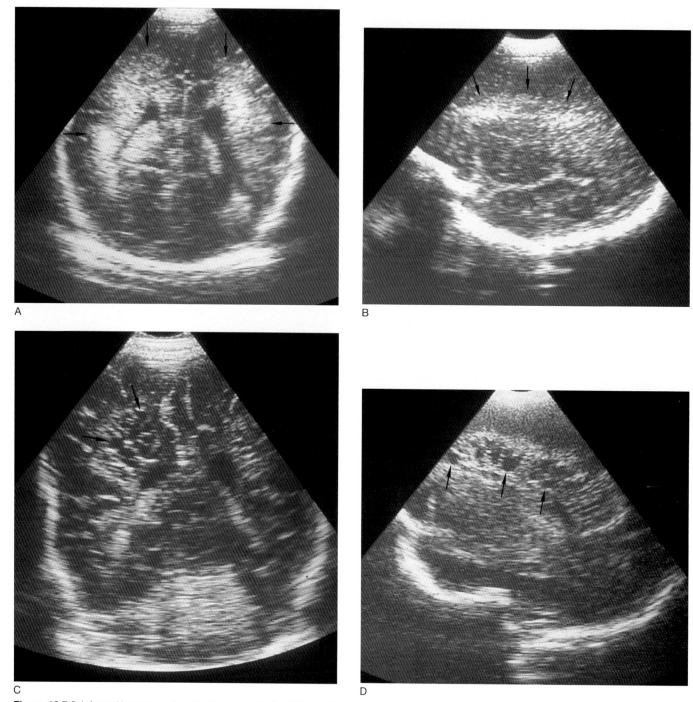

A

B

C

D

Figure 12.7.3 Infant with acute periventricular leukomalacia (PVL) evolving into cystic PVL. Coronal (A) and sagittal (B) US on day 3 of life shows hyperechoic changes in the periventricular white matter consistent with acute PVL (arrows). Follow-up examination at 21 days of life shows cystic changes (arrows) on the coronal (C) and sagittal (D) US examination.

brain. Unless an arteriovenous malformation, infection or a tumour is suspected, CT is done without contrast enhancement. Single-slice helical or spiral scanning takes only minutes to perform a whole brain study. Multiple-slice CT (4–16 slice) takes on the order of 10–20 s. These rapid scan times have decreased the need for sedation. Strokes are shown as loss of grey–white matter differentiation and as hypodensity of the involved area of the brain with mass effect depending on the size and age of the infarction (Figure 12.7.4). Mass effect in larger hypoxic ischaemic injuries is seen by 24 h postictus and progresses for several days and then resolves (Figure 12.7.5). Contrast enhancement occurs at the site of infarction, once the blood–brain barrier (BBB) becomes open with the ingrowth of new vessels. Generally, some enhancement can be seen as early as 3–5 days postinjury and it can last for 3–5 weeks. Reabsorption of infarcted tissue produces encephalomalacia. In the basal ganglia, thalamus and brainstem, chronic cystic changes are referred to as lacunar infarctions. Atrophy in the form of ventricular dilatation and sulcal prominence accompanies the chronic stages of larger cerebral infarctions.

Demonstration of acute haemorrhage is a particularly important aspect of CT. The globulin molecule of haemoglobin is dense (shows increased attenuation), absorbing more of the x-ray beam than the adjacent brain. Hounsfield units (HU) for acute blood clots are in the 50–100 range, denser than brain, less dense than calcification. Localization of the site of blood, whether parenchymal,

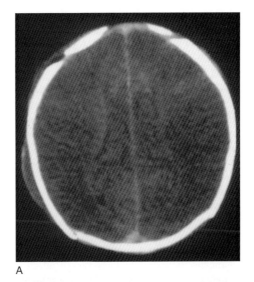

A

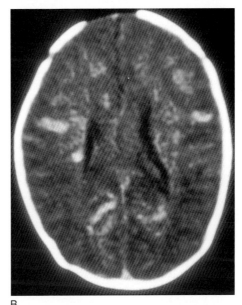

B

Figure 12.7.5 Global hypoxic ischaemic brain injury demonstrated acutely and subacutely by CT examination. (A) Axial non-contrast enhanced CT at 41 h post delivery shows marked hypodensity involving both grey and white matter with compression of the lateral ventricles. (B) Follow-up CT examination 9 days later shows scattered foci of abnormal increased density involving areas of the cortex and periventricular white matter, consistent with necrosis. The ventricles have returned to normal size.

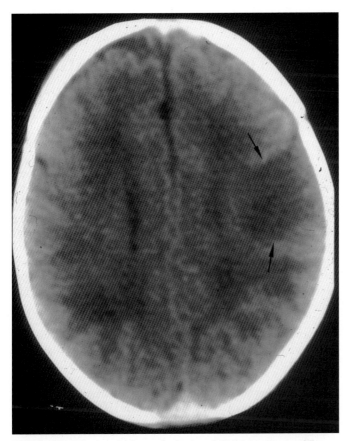

Figure 12.7.4 Acute middle cerebral artery (MCA) infarction on CT. Axial CT without contrast material shows a focal hypodensity (arrows) involving cortex and subcortical white matter in the posterior left frontal region.

ventricular, subarachnoid (SAH), subdural or epidural is relatively accurate with CT (Figure 12.7.6). SAH is best seen on CT, with fluid attenuated inversion recovery (FLAIR) MRI sequence as a second option. Blood within the brain takes approximately 3 h to undergo clot retraction, during which time serum exudes and the haematoma becomes more dense. The extruded serum may be helpful in outlining the haematoma. Surrounding vasogenic oedema within the adjacent brain is also not uncommon, a manifestation of adjacent cerebral injury secondary to the process producing the bleeding as well as the bleeding itself. With time, the globulin molecule breaks down and the density of the clot is lost. For example, it takes about 24 days for a 2.5 cm clot to become isodense to the brain and still later, to become hypodense. Ultimately, all but a slit-like collection of haemosiderin will remain along with adjacent changes due to the damage caused by the bleed. When the haematoma is chronic and no longer dense it may be misdiagnosed on contrast-enhanced CT for an abscess or tumour, because it will enhance peripherally. In such case, absence of mass effect and oedema should indicate old haematoma but MRI can directly detect the old blood products.

Computed tomography has limitations in that the white matter of the newborn, whether preterm or term, is watery and unmyelinated, and may not show the presence of acute white matter injury successfully because both the white matter and the lesion are of low density (decreased attenuation). Ultrasound may be better at showing this and MRI using diffusion and/or spectroscopy is more sensitive for lesions in the acute stage of the injury process. The main issue in obtaining CT or MRI is that the patient has to be transported to the site of the scanners and needs monitoring and support during the scanning process. Ultrasound has the distinct advantage of being portable to the Neonatal Intensive Care Unit, with the study being performed with minimal manipulation or risk to the patient.

FURTHER READING

Adsett DB, Fitz CR, Hill A. Hypoxic-ischaemic cerebral injury in the term newborn: correlation of CT findings with neurological outcome. Developmental Medicine and Child Neurology 1985; 27:155–160.

Fitzhardinge PM, Flodmark O, Ashby S. The prognostic value of computed tomography of the brain in asphyxiated premature infants. Journal of Pediatrics 1982; 199:476–481.

Flodmark O, Roland EH, Hill A, Whitfield MF. Periventricular leukomalacia: radiologic diagnosis. Radiology 1987; 162:119–124.

Ishida A, Nakajima W, Arai H. Cranial computed tomography scans of premature babies predict their eventual learning disabilities. Pediatric Neurology 1997; 16:319–322.

Lipp-Zwahlen AE, Deonna T, Chrzanowski R. Temporal evolution of hypoxic-ischaemic brain lesions in asphyxiated full-term newborns as assessed by computerized tomography. Neuroradiology 1985; 27:138–144.

Ment LR, Bada HS, Barnes P et al. Practice parameter: neuroimaging of the neonate. Report of the Quality Standards Subcommittee of the American Academy of Neurology and the Practice Committee of the Child Neurology Society. Neurology 2002; 58:1726–1738.

Yokochi K, Horie M, Inukai K. Computed tomographic findings in children with spastic diplegia: correlation with the severity of their motor abnormality. Brain Development 1989; 11:236–240.

MAGNETIC RESONANCE IMAGING

Magnetic resonance imaging provides the best morphological and physiological information about the newborn infant brain, whether premature or full term.

On the T2-weighted images and FLAIR, there is a lack of contrast between areas of periventricular leukomalacia and unmyelinated white matter because the brain is both watery and relatively unmyelinated in the premature and term infant (Figure 12.7.7). However, haemorrhagic and calcific lesions can be detected on T1-weighted and gradient echo or susceptibility scans and most acute infarcts can be demonstrated on diffusion scans. In older infants and children, once myelination of the brain is complete, standard T1- and T2-weighted pulse sequences can demonstrate acute, subacute and chronic infarcts, blood products and vascular flow voids in a manner sufficient to diagnose many vascular problems. In the child, FLAIR imaging (fluid attenuated inversion recovery) demonstrates water within tissue to a much greater degree and more exquisitely than T2 turbo spin echo imaging. With FLAIR, the water within the ventricles and sulci is black but the water within the injured, infarcted or gliotic brain generates a very bright signal intensity (Figure 12.7.8). Gadolinium enhancement with T1-weighted images is used to demonstrate BBB disturbances in subacute infarction. Enhancement may be seen 3 days after infarction and can last for a variable period of time ranging from many weeks to months.

Haemorrhage can be detected and its evolution characterized by MRI and it shows different intensity depending on its stage and on the MR sequence. T1-weighted images show oxyhaemoglobin as

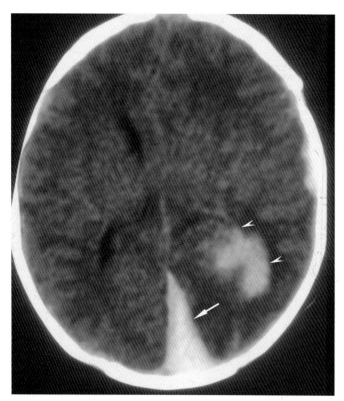

Figure 12.7.6 Traumatic brain injury at time of birth, CT. Axial non-contrast enhanced CT performed on a 1-day-old male shows a large posterior left parafalcine subdural haematoma (arrow) and an intraparenchymal periatrial bleed (arrowheads). Note that there is mass effect with shift of the right lateral ventricle to the right. Subdural haemorrhage can be seen along the inner table of the skull on the left.

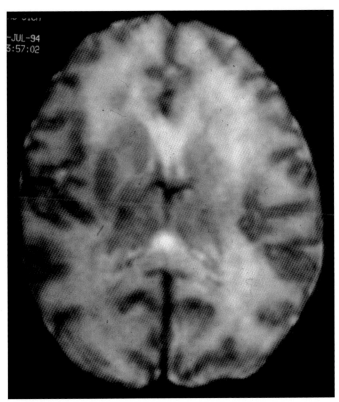

Figure 12.7.7 Newborn infant with acute PVL, MRI. Axial T2-weighted image shows hyperintense white matter, which could be normal or abnormal. Proton spectroscopy showed elevated lactate in the periventricular white matter and follow-up examination showed cystic PVL.

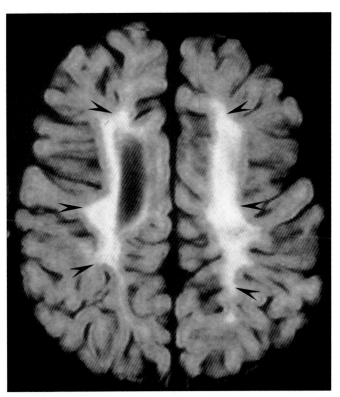

Figure 12.7.8 Gliosis from PVL shown on FLAIR sequence of MRI. Hyperintense signal in the periventricular white matter (arrowheads) is shown in the brain of a 20-month-old female with PVL.

isointense, deoxyhaemoglobin as slightly hypointense, methaemoglobin as hyperintense and haemosiderin as dark signal intensity (Figure 12.7.9). T2-weighted image oxyhaemoglobin is hyperintense (bright), deoxyhaemoglobin is hypointense (dark), intracellular methaemoglobin is hypointense (dark), extracellular methaemoglobin is hyperintense (bright) and haemosiderin is hypointense (dark) (Figure 12.7.10).

Gradient echo 2D FLASH T2-weighted imaging (susceptibility scan) is a valuable adjunct to routine MRI sequences. It demonstrates with great sensitivity blood products within cerebral tissue by a loss of signal (blackness) at the affected sites (Figure 12.7.11). The black foci of no signal are produced by dephasing of the protons that occur secondary to the paramagnetic effects of iron in the components and by-products of blood.

FURTHER READING

Aida N, Nishimura G, Hachiya Y et al. MR imaging of perinatal brain damage: comparison of clinical outcome with initial and follow-up MR findings. American Journal of Neuroradiology 1998; 19:1909–1921.

Cowan F, Rutherford M, Goenendaal F et al. Origin and timing of brain lesions in term infants with neonatal encephalopathy. Lancet 2003; 361:736–742.

Fedrizzi E, Inverno M, Bruzzone MG. MRI features of cerebral lesions and cognitive functions in preterm spastic diplegic children. Pediatric Neurology 1996; 15:207–212.

Inder TE, Huppi PS, Warfield S. Periventricular white matter injury in the premature infant is associated with a reduction in cerebral cortical gray matter volume at term. Annals of Neurology 1999; 46:755–760.

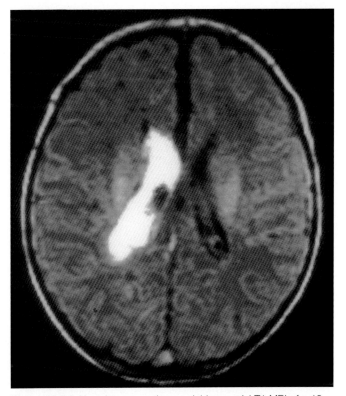

Figure 12.7.9 Hyperintense methaemoglobin on axial T1 MRI of a 12-day-old female post germinal matrix haemorrhage. High signal intensity methaemoglobin is present in the right lateral ventricle.

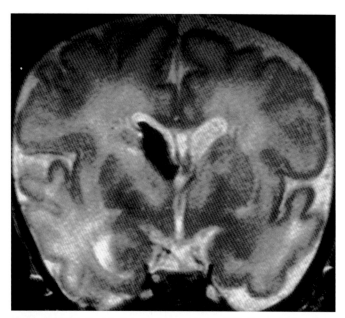

Figure 12.7.10 Germinal matrix haemorrhage, MRI. Coronal T2-weighted image shows a subependymal bleed at the site of the right caudothalamic groove.

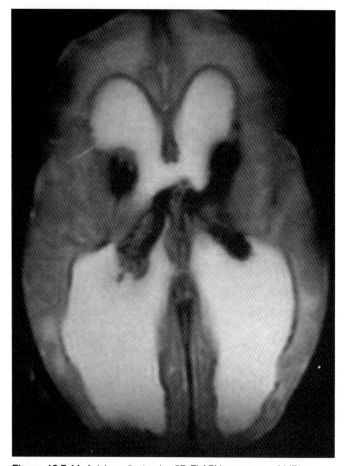

Figure 12.7.11 Axial gradient echo 2D FLASH sequence of MRI performed on a 34-week-old gestational premature infant, 2 weeks post delivery, shows great sensitivity in detection of blood products. Note hydrocephalus with enlargement of the lateral ventricles. The choroid plexi are coated by blood products and the ependyma of both lateral ventricles is lined by hypointense haemosiderin.

Johnson AJ, Lee BC, Lin WL. Echoplanar diffusion-weighted imaging in neonates and infants with suspected hypoxic-ischaemic injury: correlation with patient outcome. American Journal of Roentgenology 1999; 172:219–226.

Ment LR, Bada HS, Barnes P et al. Practice parameter: neuroimaging of the neonate. Report of the Quality Standards Subcommittee of the American Academy of Neurology and the Practice Committee of the Child Neurology Society. Neurology 2002; 58:1726–1738.

Mercuri E, Rutherford M, Cowan F. Early prognostic indicators of outcome in infants with neonatal cerebral infarction; a clinical, electroencephalogram, and magnetic resonance imaging study. Pediatrics 1999; 103:103–139.

Rollins NK, Morriss MC, Evans D, Perlman JM. The role of early MR in the evaluation of the term infant with seizures. American Journal of Neuroradiology 1994; 15:239–248.

Rutherford MA, Pennock JM, Counsell SJ. Abnormal magnetic resonance signal in the internal capsule predicts poor neurodevelopmental outcome in infants with hypoxic-ischaemic encephalopathy. Pediatrics 1998; 102:323–328.

Rutherford MA, Pennock JM, Dubowitz L. Cranial ultrasound and magnetic resonance imaging in hypoxic-ischaemic encephalopathy: a comparison with outcome. Developmental Medicine and Child Neurology 1994; 36:813–825.

Rutherford MA, Pennock JM, Schwieso J. Hypoxic-ischaemic encephalopathy: early and late magnetic resonance imaging findings in relation to outcome. Archives of Diseases in Children 1996; 75:F145–F151.

MAGNETIC RESONANCE ARTERIOGRAPHY (MRA) AND VENOGRAPHY (MRV)

Today, MRA and MRV are performed to demonstrate arteries and veins and to help characterize the nature of vascular abnormalities (Figure 12.7.12). This can be done with 3D time-of-flight, 2D time-of-flight, 3D phase and 2D phase contrast MRA. When there is haemorrhage present at the site of vessels being investigated,

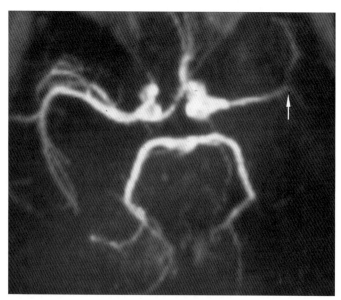

Figure 12.7.12 Magnetic resonance arteriography of a left middle cerebral artery (MCA) infarct. The patient suffered an infarct in and around the time of birth. The MRA was performed at age 8 months. There is occlusion of the horizontal portion of the MCA at the bifurcation (arrow).

phase contrast MRA is utilized to avoid incorporation of the high signal intensity of the methaemoglobin of the haematoma into the image of vascular flow. Three-dimensional time-of-flight and 2D time-of-flight are used respectively for arteries and veins. A saturation pulse is applied at the top of the head when venous flow needs to be removed from the image. A saturation pulse is applied at the bottom of the brain when arteries need to be removed, such as when an MRV is performed.

FURTHER READING

Edelman RR, Mattle HP, Atkinson DJ, Hoogewoud HM. MR angiography. American Journal of Roentgenology 1990; 154:937–946.

Ruggieri PM, Laub GA, Masaryk TJ, Modic MT. Intracranial circulation: pulse-sequence considerations in three-dimensional (volume) MR angiography. Radiology 1989; 171:785–791.

MAGNETIC RESONANCE DIFFUSION WEIGHTED IMAGING

Random motion of water molecules arises predominantly from diffusion but also the flow of blood from the capillary bed contributes to this effect. Although these effects can be separated, the techniques for doing this are difficult, so that usually the combined effect is measured and is called the apparent diffusion coefficient (ADC). The apparent diffusion can be measured in any desired direction (x-, y- or z-axis) by acquiring images in the presence of very large field gradients applied in that direction. Acquisition of a series of images with different gradients allows the ADC to be accurately quantitated. The effect of the motion of water molecules decreases the signal intensity from that expected as a result of the usual contrast mechanisms (T1, T2, T2*); regions of tissue with higher ADC will be less intense on the images.

FURTHER READING

Sorenson AG, Buonanno FS, Gonzales RG. Hyperacute stroke: evaluation with combined multi-section diffusion-weighted and haemodynamically weighted echo-planar MRI. Radiology 1996; 199:391–401.

Wolf RL, Zimmerman RA, Clancy R, Haselgrove JC. Quantitative ADC measurements in term neonates for early detection of hypoxic-ischaemic brain injury: initial experience. Radiology 2001; 218:825–833.

TRACE

The 'trace' is the average of the ADC in three perpendicular directions. This value is relatively easy to measure and, like the anisotropy, is indicative of the physiological state of the tissue. In normal adult brain, the ADC values fall broadly into three different ranges that are characteristic of the three categories of material in the brain.

FURTHER READING

Brunberg JA, Chenevett TL, McKever PE. In vivo MR determination of water diffusion coefficients and diffusion anisotropy: correlation with structural alteration in gliomas of the cerebral hemispheres. American Journal of Neuroradiology 1995; 16:361–371.

CSF AND FLUID SPACES

The ADC values are those expected from unrestricted diffusion. The trace ADC values of CSF are about 3.0×10^{-3} mm^2/s and are the same in all directions (anisotropy).

GREY MATTER

Tissue restricts the diffusion of water, so that the trace ADC values for grey matter are lower than that for CSF, lying in the range of $0.8–1.2 \times 10^{-3}$ mm^2/s. However, the restriction is the same in all directions, so there is no isotropy.

FURTHER READING

Le Bihan D, Turner R, Douek P. Diffusion MR imaging: clinical applications. American Journal of Roentgenology 1992; 159:591–599.

WHITE MATTER

The axon sheath acts as a significant barrier to the diffusion in a direction perpendicular to the fibre axis and, thus, the ADC of white matter in the brain is isotropic, varying with the direction of measurement of the diffusion. The trace value is somewhat less than that of grey matter and falls in the range $0.4–0.6 \times 10^{-3}$ mm^2/s.

Following birth, the ADC changes in a fashion commensurate with the expected postnatal myelination. The ADC of white matter decreases and becomes more isotropic during the first 6 months.

While there are many factors that affect the ADC, it is possible to explain the main features of the changes that occur in oedema in terms of the redistribution of water between two compartments. In the intracellular compartment, the diffusion of water is highly restricted so that the ADC is low, and in the extracellular compartment, the diffusion of water is less than that in free water (or CSF) but nonetheless, is significantly higher than in the intracellular compartment. The measured ADC is essentially an average of these two values, weighted according to the relative volumes of water in the two compartments. When cytotoxic oedema occurs the extracellular water moves into the cell and increases the fraction of water in the compartment with the lower ADC, so that ADC value falls. In cases of vasogenic and interstitial oedema, the water is predominantly extracellular and so the component with the larger ADC dominates and the ADC is larger than normal.

Brain oedema secondary to ischaemia has been the focus of many studies using diffusion-weighted imaging. Within the first hours, when acute cytotoxic oedema develops, the ADC decreases and the lesion appears brighter on diffusion-weighted images (DWI) (Figure 12.7.13). Changes are visible on DWI before any change can be appreciated on conventional CT or T1- and T2-weighted images. With time, as the vasogenic oedema develops, the lesion darkens on DWI because the ADC increases. The regions of abnormal brain indicated on DWI and on the T2-weighted images are similar but not identical. The region in which the diffusion is changed is in general greater than the region in which the T2 is altered.

Diffusion imaging has revolutionized our ability to see abnormalities in tissue due to change in the movement of water molecules due to acute infarctions secondary to hypoxic ischaemic brain injury.

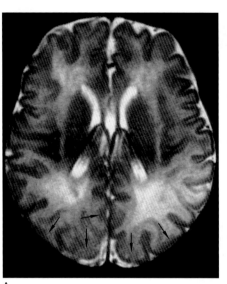 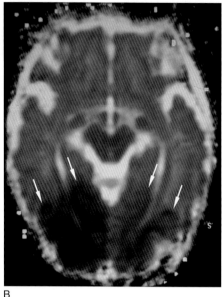 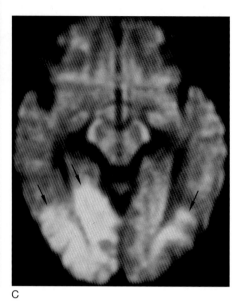

A B C

Figure 12.7.13 Diffusion-weighted imaging of bilateral temporal occipital watershed infarctions due to partial prolonged asphyxia in a 7-day-old male. Axial T2-weighted image (A) shows loss of cortical grey matter signal intensity (arrows) in the bilateral temporal occipital regions (arrows). There is increased signal intensity in the underlying white matter. The ADC map (B) shows low signal at the site of infarctions, whereas on the diffusion-weighted image (C) the signal is high (arrows).

FURTHER READING

Barkovich AJ. MR and CT evaluation of profound neonatal and infantile asphyxia. American Journal of Neuroradiology 1992; 13:959–972.

Cambray-Deakin M, Foster A, Burgoyne R. The expression of excitatory amino acid binding sites during neuritogenesis in the developing rat cerebellum. Developmental Brain Research 1990; 54:265–271.

Matsumoto K, Lo EH, Pierce AR. Role of vasogenic edema and tissue cavitation in ischaemic evolution on diffusion-weighted imaging: comparison with multiparameter MR and immunohistochemistry. American Journal of Neuroradiology 1995; 16:1107–1115.

Ment LR, Bada HS, Barnes P et al. Practice parameter: neuroimaging of the neonate: report of the Quality Standards Subcommittee of the American Academy of Neurology and the Practice Committee of the Child Neurology Society. Neurology 2002; 58:1726–1738.

Phillips MD, Zimmerman RA. Diffusion imaging in pediatric hypoxic ischaemic injury. Neuroimaging Clinics of North America 1999; 9:41–52.

Roelants-van Rijn AM, Nikkels PG, Groenendaal F et al. Neonatal diffusion-weighted MR imaging: relation with histopathology or follow-up MR examination. Neuropediatrics 2001; 32:286–292.

Schneider H, Ballowitz L, Schachinger H, Hanefeld F, Droszus J-U. Anoxic encephalopathy with predominant involvement of basal ganglia, brain stem, and spinal cord in the perinatal period: report on seven newborns. Acta Neuropathologica 1975; 32:287–298.

Wimberger DM, Roberts TP, Barkovich AJ. Identification of 'premyelination' by diffusion-weighted MRI. Journal of Computer Assisted Tomography 1995; 19:28–33.

Wolf RL, Zimmerman RA, Clancy R, Haselgrove JC. Quantitative ADC measurements in term neonates for early detection of hypoxic-ischaemic brain injury: initial experience. Radiology 2001; 218:825–833.

MAGNETIC RESONANCE PERFUSION

There are two techniques for looking at vascular perfusion in the brain. These are the tracer techniques, one involving a bolus gadolinium injection with T1-weighted imaging and the other, arterial spin labelling (ASL), without gadolinium injection, in which the incoming blood is altered by an RF pulse placed over the carotid artery in the neck and then is imaged in the brain. Quantification of blood flow by either technique is difficult, but relative perfusion can be determined. With bolus techniques, measurement of time to peak enhancement and production of maps of the relative cerebral blood volumes throughout the brain have proven useful. With ASL, quantification of blood flow in ml/100 g of tissue has recently been achieved.

FURTHER READING

Edelmann RR, Siewert B, Darby DG. Qualitative mapping of cerebral blood flow and functional localization with echo-planar MR imaging and signal targeting with alternating radio frequency. Radiology 1994; 192:513–520.

Jezzard P. Advances in perfusion MR imaging. Radiology 1998; 208:296–299.

MAGNETIC RESONANCE SPECTROSCOPY (MRS)

Acute infarction in the brain alters the measurable levels of cerebral metabolites seen with MRS. *N*-acetylaspartate (NAA) decreases as neurons are destroyed while lactate, a by-product of anaerobic metabolism not normally seen, becomes elevated (Figure 12.7.14). With total tissue necrosis, the MRS shows complete absence of cerebral metabolites. MRS can be obtained as a single voxel, set of voxels at one level (2D CSI) or as multiple sets of levels with multiple voxels (3D CSI). The time to echo (TE) is important. With a TE of 135–144 ms, lactate is inverted because of J-coupling, allowing separation of lactate and lipids, which, with studies performed at short echo times (e.g. TE 10–30 ms), is not possible and then the lactate and lipid peaks overlap.

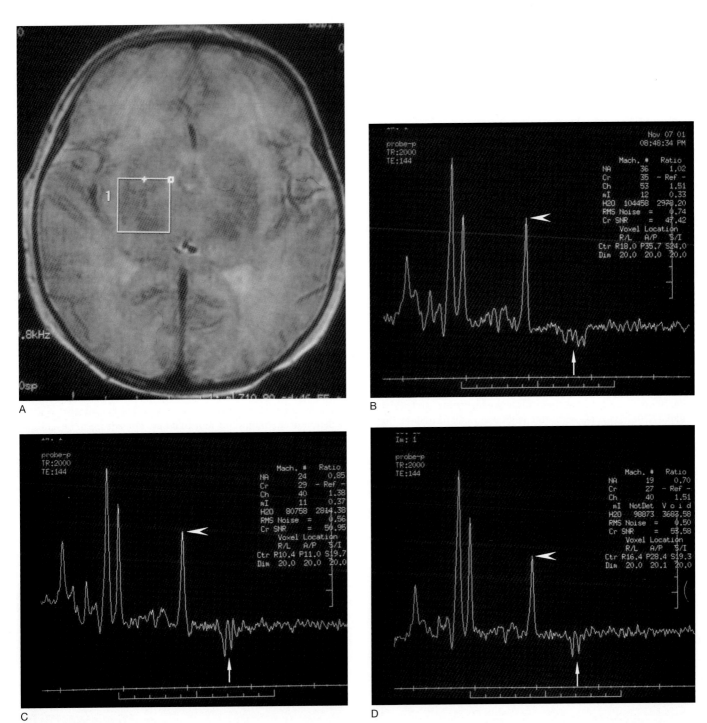

Figure 12.7.14 Newborn infant examined on day 2 of life, after profound asphyxic injury. (A) Localization of the TE 144 ms proton spectroscopy in the right basal ganglia is shown by the white square. (B) Proton spectrum at day 2 shows lactate as an inverted doublet at 1.3 ppm (arrow) with relatively normal NAA (arrowhead). (C) Follow-up proton spectroscopy from the same site at day 3 shows a decrease in NAA (arrowhead) and an increase in lactate (arrow). (D) Follow-up at day 12 of life from the right basal ganglia shows a further decrease in NAA (arrowhead) and less lactate (arrow) than on the prior examination.

FURTHER READING

Ashwal S, Holshouser BA, Tomasi LG. 1H-magnetic resonance spectroscopy determined cerebral lactate and poor neurological outcomes in children with central nervous system disease. Annals of Neurology 1997; 41:470–481.

Barkovich AJ, Baranski K, Vigneron D. Proton MR spectroscopy for the evaluation of brain injury in asphyxiated, term neonates. American Journal of Neuroradiology 1999; 20:1399–1405.

Groenendaal F, van der Grond J, Witkamp TD, de Vries LS. Proton magnetic resonance spectroscopic imaging in neonatal stroke. Neuropediatrics 1995; 26:243–248.

Robertson NJ, Cox IJ, Cowan FM. Cerebral intracellular lactic alkalosis persisting months after neonatal encephalopathy measured by magnetic resonance spectroscopy. Pediatric Research 1999; 46:287–296.

Vigneron DB, Barkovich AJ, Noworolski SM et al. Three-dimensional proton MR spectroscopic imaging of premature and term neonates. American Journal of Neuroradiology 2001; 22:1424–1433.

FETAL BRAIN IMAGING

As imaging of the *in utero* fetus has improved over the past decade, both with US and fetal MRI, greater detection of *in utero* fetal brain injury has occurred. Fetal MRI is not a screening technique and is only performed after a fetal US has raised an issue of an abnormality. Destruction of the wall of the lateral ventricle (in association with hydrocephalus), germinal matrix haemorrhage, infarctions of the cortex and subadjacent white matter and periventricular leukomalacia, with and without cystic formation, have been shown by improved imaging techniques (Figure 12.7.15). Fetal MRI is performed with a combination of ultrafast imaging, the HASTE sequence, in which each individual slice is a separate acquisition, so that movement during one portion of the study does not affect the rest of the study. Image acquisition times are on the order of 0.5 s, with a set of images in one plane taking approximately 20 s. Overall study time is on the order of 20–30 min. In addition to the T2-weighted HASTE, gradient echo T1-weighted images are obtained, as well as echo planar T2-weighted images. T2-weighted images show a pattern of parenchymal intensity as well as the gross sulcal and gyral morphology and ventricular size, enabling the diagnosis of most abnormalities. T1-weighted gradient echo images are utilized for showing myelination in the brain as well as hyperintense blood products. EPI T2-weighted images are used to show blood products, such as germinal matrix haemorrhage or intraparenchymal bleeding, as well as to show the osseous structures of the calvarium and spine. Acute middle cerebral infarctions have been demonstrated in fetuses *in utero* by diffusion imaging.

The studies are performed in the axial, coronal and sagittal planes. As the fetus moves, it is important to adjust the imaging planes rapidly, in order to have anatomical orthogonal planes and not oblique planes of section, which may be impossible to interpret and could lead to misdiagnosis. Comparison of one side of the brain to the other is an important way of establishing what is and is not normal. The images also supply information about the blood vessels within the brain, arteries and veins, which may be seen as flow voids, and enlarged in the case of a vein of Galen malformation (Figure 12.7.16). The rest of the fetus and the amniotic fluid and placenta and umbilical cord are also seen and evaluated. Anomalies of the spinal canal such as myelomeningoceles and anomalies of the chest and abdomen, such as diaphragmatic hernias or omphaloceles, are well demonstrated. These MRI studies are performed from 18 weeks gestation onwards, without sedation of the mother or fetus, and are considered to be safe.

FURTHER READING

Bilaniuk LT. Magnetic resonance imaging of the fetal brain. Seminars in Roentgenology 1999; 34:48–61.

Girard N, Raybaud C, Gambarelli D, Figarella-Branger D. Fetal brain MR imaging. Magnetic Resonance Imaging Clinics of North America 2001; 9:19–56.

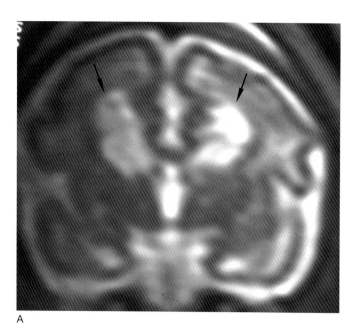

A

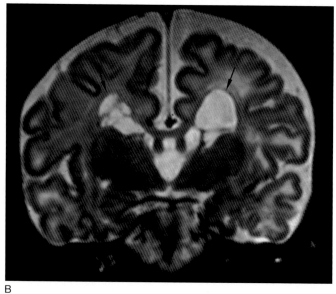

B

Figure 12.7.15 *In utero* PVL demonstrated with fetal MRI. (A) Coronal T2-W imaging performed *in utero* at 32 weeks of gestation shows cystic PVL in the periventricular region (arrows). (B) Coronal T2-W imaging at 2 months of age shows the same cystic PVL (arrows).

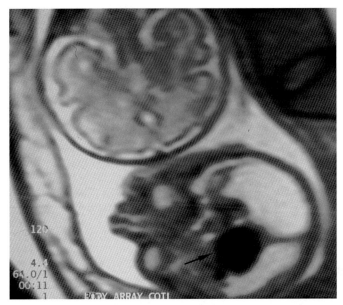

Figure 12.7.16 Fetal MRI utilizing an ultrafast T2-W imaging sequence (HASTE) shows twins at 32 weeks' gestation, one normal and the other with vein of Galen malformation and severe brain atrophy. Note the large flow void due to the dilated vein of Galen (arrow) and the absence of brain tissue surrounding markedly dilated lateral ventricles representing ex vacuo enlargement.

Righini A, Bianchini E, Parazzini C et al. Apparent diffusion coefficient determination in normal fetal brain: a prenatal MR imaging study. American Journal of Neuroradiology 2003; 24:799–804.

IMAGING OF PREMATURE INFANT BRAIN

This section looks at injuries occurring to the brain of infants born between 24 weeks (time of viability) and 37 weeks of gestation. The period from 37 weeks to 42 weeks will be considered term. Beyond 42 weeks is post-term. Premature infants have different responses to hypoxia and ischaemia from term infants, depending upon their gestational age. Very premature infants (between 24 and 26 weeks) have a poor astrocytic response to injury, so that scar tissue (gliosis) does not occur at the site of injury. When injury to the periventricular white matter occurs at this time, the tissue is reabsorbed and focal loss of tissue is found (Figure 12.7.17). Insults occurring between 26 and 28 weeks can cause injury with early gliotic response, with scar tissue starting to form. Beyond 28 weeks, gliosis is expected (Figure 12.7.18). In the premature infant, the vulnerability of tissue also appears to be related to both the weight of the infant and the gestational age. The germinal matrix, the site at which the neurons are produced prior to 22 weeks of gestation, and which subsequently functions to produce glial tissue, involutes by 32 weeks and is gone by 36 weeks. The two major types of injury seen in the premature infant are germinal matrix haemorrhage, which affects primarily the low birth weight, early gestational infants, and periventricular leukomalacia, which affects both the youngest as well as the oldest of the premature infants, as well as term infants.

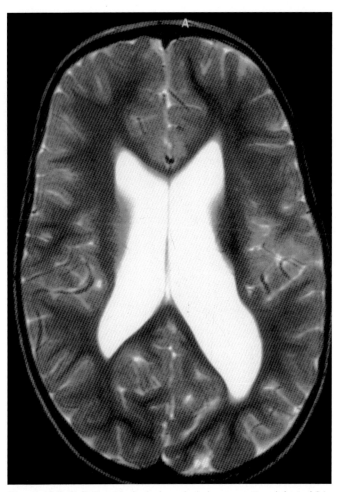

Figure 12.7.17 Periventricular leukomalacia in a premature infant of 24 weeks' gestation. MRI, T2-W imaging, performed at age 2. There is atrophic enlargement of the lateral ventricles with loss of surrounding white matter without evidence of gliosis.

GERMINAL MATRIX HAEMORRHAGE

In the United States, there are approximately 55 000 infants born each year with a birth weight of under 1500 g. This represents an incidence of approximately 1.25% of live births. This incidence has stayed relatively unchanged in the last few decades. Because of the current ability of the neonatologists to care for these neonates, 85% of them survive. The overall incidence of germinal matrix haemorrhage (GMH) in infants under 1500 g is given as 15%.

Germinal matrix haemorrhage is graded according to: whether or not the bleed extends from the germinal matrix into the ventricle; what happens to the size of the ventricle as a result of the bleeding; and whether or not the bleed extends into the surrounding brain tissue. A Grade I germinal matrix haemorrhage is a subependymal bleed without intraventricular or intraparenchymal extension (Figure 12.7.10). The haemorrhages can be bilateral or unilateral. The most common site for GMH to occur is the

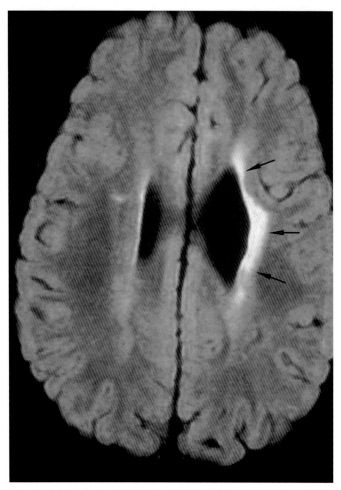

Figure 12.7.18 Periventricular gliosis, MRI. FLAIR image performed at age 3 years for right-sided weakness shows enlargement of the left lateral ventricle with abnormal increased signal intensity in the periventricular white matter (arrows).

caudathalamic groove, where between 28 and 32 weeks the germinal matrix is the thickest. It should be noted that the germinal matrix extends all the way around both lateral, 3rd and 4th ventricles, and that bleeding can occur in any portion of the germinal matrix not only that located at the caudathalamic groove. Grade II germinal matrix haemorrhage is associated with some intraventricular extension. Grade III is sufficient extension of haemorrhage into the ventricle to produce ventricular enlargement (Figure 12.7.19). Grade IV is germinal matrix haemorrhage that has extended into the surrounding brain tissue, producing an intracerebral haematoma (Figure 12.7.19). Grade IV haemorrhage has also been attributed to periventricular haemorrhagic venous infarctions (Figure 12.7.19). Grade IV haemorrhages can also have intraventricular haemorrhage. Approximately 15% of germinal matrix haemorrhages have a Grade IV parenchymal haematoma, the incidence being higher in the lower birth weight neonates. GMH may be associated with some degree of periventricular leukomalacia. Seventy-five per cent of infants who die with GMH have some degree of periventricular leukomalacia.

The pathogenesis of the germinal matrix haemorrhage is thought to be related to prematurity, cerebral blood flow, cerebral blood pressure and cerebral blood volume. It is also related to the platelet capillary function as regards blood clotting. Fluctuations in blood pressure and cerebral blood flow such as occur secondary to rapid volume expansion, seizures, hypoxia, and hypotension followed by hypertension, are thought to be causes of germinal matrix bleeding. It is possible that positive pressure breathing, by raising the venous pressure, may lead to GMH. Relative thrombocytopenia occurring in low birth weight infants is thought to be a factor that increases the incidence of GMH. Because they consist of a single cell layer wall, the venules within the germinal matrix are fragile and vulnerable to injury as the tissue surrounding them is destroyed. With injury to the germinal matrix tissue, rupture of the venules occurs, producing haemorrhage. If that haemorrhage is able to extend, as may occur in thrombocytopenic infants, then intraventricular and/or intraparenchymal bleeding can ensue.

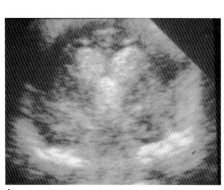

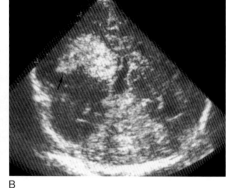

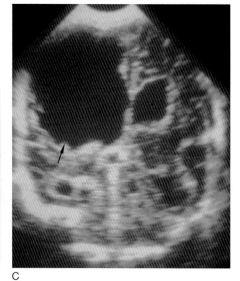

A   B   C

Figure 12.7.19 Germinal matrix haemorrhages (GMH) diagnosed by US in coronal plane. (A) Grade III germinal matrix haemorrhage with blood distending both lateral and third ventricles. (B) Grade IV germinal matrix haemorrhage, 32-week gestation newborn, hyperechoic bleed extends from the right caudothalamic groove into the brain tissue (arrow). (C) Follow-up US of a patient who had a Grade IV GMH and now has an ex vacuo porencephaly of the right lateral ventricle (arrow).

It should be noted that in 50% of infants with intraventricular haemorrhage, there are no clinical signs. Patients with germinal matrix haemorrhage have been divided into three clinical syndromes: (1) catastrophic with rapid onset of coma, seizures, decreasing haematocrit and bulging fontanelle; (2) slow deterioration with subtle alteration of consciousness and hypotonia; (3) silent (50%). It is thought that at least half of the germinal matrix haemorrhages occur within a day of birth, that a quarter occur by the second day and the other quarter between the third and fourth days. Seventy-five per cent of the germinal matrix haemorrhages fall into the Grade I and II categories, Grade III incidence is 25% and Grade IV is 15%. Severe forms of germinal matrix haemorrhage when accompanied by significant PVL have an incidence of recognizable neurological sequelae of between 35% and 90%.

FURTHER READING

Golden JA, Gilles FH, Rudewlli R. Frequency of neuropathological abnormalities in very low birth weight infants. Journal of Neuropathology and Experimental Neurology 1997; 56:472–478.

Guyer B, Hoyert DL, Martin JA. Annual summary of vital statistics: 1998. Pediatrics 1999; 104:1229–1246.

Horbar JD, Badger GJ, Lewit EM. Hospital and patient characteristics associated with variation in 28-day mortality rates for very low birth weight infants. Pediatrics 1997; 99:149–156.

Kiely JL, Susser M. Preterm birth, intrauterine growth retardation, and perinatal mortality. American Journal of Public Health 1992; 82:343–344.

Papile LA, Brustein J, Burstein R, Koffer H. Incidence and evolution of subependymal and intraventricular haemorrhage: a study of infants with birth weights less than 1500 gm. Journal of Pediatrics 1978; 92:529–534.

Perlman JM, Volpe JJ. Intraventricular haemorrhage in extremely small premature infants. American Journal of Diseases of Children 1986; 140:1122–1124.

Takashima S, Mito T, Ando Y. Pathogenesis of periventricular white matter haemorrhages in preterm infants. Brain Development 1986; 8:25–30.

Wilcox AJ, Skjoerven R. Birth weight and perinatal mortality: the effect of gestational age. American Journal of Public Health 1992; 82:378–382.

IMAGING OF GERMINAL MATRIX HAEMORRHAGE

ULTRASOUND

Ultrasound, because it is portable to the infant in the Neonatal Intensive Care Unit, does not require sedation and is sensitive for detection of both germinal matrix and intraventricular bleeding, is the initial procedure of choice, and is a relatively routine procedure for follow-up of these patients during the neonatal period, up until the anterior fontanelle closes. The acute bleed, once clotting has occurred, appears hyperechoic and is characterized by its location and extension (Figure 12.7.20). Blood extending into the ventricular system can be seen coating the choroid plexus and pooling in the occipital horn, often as a blood–CSF level (Figure 12.7.19). Blood extending from the germinal matrix into the brain tissue, a Grade IV haemorrhage, is also identifiable by its size and extent (Figure 12.7.19). Large enough haemorrhages lead to mass effect, with displacement of the adjacent ventricular structures. The clot will break down over a number of weeks, the central portion of the clot becoming progressively less echoic than the more peripheral portions (Figures 12.7.2 and 12.7.19).

In follow-up of the germinal matrix haemorrhage by US, attention is paid to the size of the ventricles, as hydrocephalus can be

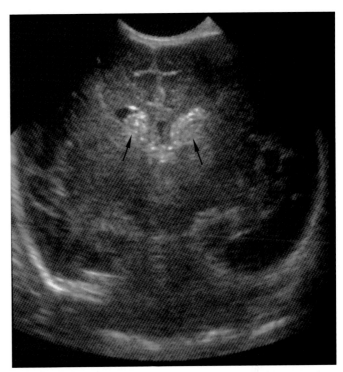

Figure 12.7.20 Bilateral acute Grade I GMH in a newborn infant, US. Coronal US shows bilateral hyperechoic bleeds at the site of the caudothalamic grooves (arrows).

a significant complication (Figures 12.7.2 and 12.7.19). Blood within the foramen of Monro, aqueduct of Sylvius and 4th ventricle, can lead to obstruction of these relatively narrow spaces, producing one or more sites of occlusion. The most common site of obstruction is the aqueduct of Sylvius, followed by the outlets of the 4th ventricle. Multiple levels of obstruction, both in the aqueduct and outlets of the 4th ventricle, are not uncommon and can lead to trapping of the 4th ventricle, the 'isolated' 4th ventricle. In the latter situation, shunting of the lateral ventricle will decompress the lateral ventricles if they communicate through the foramen of Monro and the 3rd ventricle, which they usually do, but if the 4th ventricle is trapped, then separate shunting of the 4th ventricle may be necessary. In the GMH patient, the US examination is not only performed to detect the presence of blood but also PVL. PVL is seen acutely and subacutely as hyperechoic changes around the margins of the ventricles, most commonly along the bodies of the lateral ventricles in the frontoparietal region. When symmetrical, recognition may be more difficult than when asymmetrical. Initial sites of PVL are hyperechoic but with time they become progressively less echoic and finally hypoechoic with the development of cystic changes. As the cysts develop, the ventricles become larger in an atrophic fashion. Small areas of periventricular leukomalacia are difficult to recognize by US.

FURTHER READING

Adcock LM, Moore PJ, Schlesinger AE. Correlation of ultrasound with postmortem neuropathologic studies in neonates. Pediatric Neurology 1998; 19:263–271.

Dolfin T, Skidmore MB, Fong KW. Incidence, severity, and timing of subependymal and intraventricular haemorrhages in preterm infants born in a perinatal unit as detected by serial real-time ultrasound. Pediatrics 1983; 71:541–546.

Kuban K, Sanocka U, Leviton A. White matter disorders of prematurity: association with intraventricular haemorrhage and ventriculomegaly. Journal of Pediatrics 1999; 134:539–546.

Leviton A, Pagano M, Kuban KC. The epidemiology of germinal matrix haemorrhage during the first half-day of life. Developmental Medicine and Child Neurology 1991; 33:138–145.

Maalouf EF, Duggan PF, Counsell SJ et al. Comparison of findings on cranial ultrasound and magnetic resonance imaging in preterm infants. Pediatrics 2001; 107:719–727.

Partridge JC, Babcock DS, Steichen JJ. Optimal timing for diagnostic cranial ultrasound in low-birth-weight infants: detection of intracranial haemorrhage and ventricular dilation. Journal of Pediatrics 1983; 102:281–287.

Schellinger D, Grant EG, Manz HJ. Intraparenchymal haemorrhage in preterm neonates: a broadening spectrum. American Journal of Roentgenology 1988; 150:1109–1115.

Shackelford GD, Volpe JJ. Cranial ultrasonography in the evaluation of neonatal intracranial haemorrhage and its complications. Journal of Perinatal Medicine 1985; 13:293–304.

COMPUTED TOMOGRAPHY

Computed tomography is performed in the axial plane with sections of between 3 and 5 mm in thickness, without the injection of contrast material. Contrast is indicated when the differential diagnosis includes intracranial infection or brain tumour. CT has proven to be outstanding in the demonstration of acute bleeding both within and outside of the brain tissue. Acute and subacute haemorrhage into the germinal matrix is clearly identified as an area of increased density, increased attenuation and the intraventricular extent and the size of the ventricles are also demonstrated. The presence of blood in the 3rd and 4th ventricles and cisterna magna can be clearly shown (Figure 12.7.21). Demonstration of blood in the 4th ventricle and cisterna magna can be difficult by US. CT is poor at showing changes consistent with PVL because of the high water content and lack of myelination of the premature infant's brain. CT is of value in the follow-up of the GMH patient. It will demonstrate the size of the ventricles, cisterns and subarachnoid space. Enlargement of the ventricles may be due both to developing hydrocephalus, as well as to loss of white matter from PVL (Figure 12.7.11). The density of the blood products in the brain tissue will decrease with time as the globulin molecule is broken down. Typically, the haematoma may become isodense in a period of several weeks to 1 month. It depends on the size of the clot. The larger the clot, the longer the time to isodensity. Increased density seen even later at the site of the GMH may reflect calcification. Unclotted subarachnoid blood loses its density in approximately 1 week. In older premature infants, coexisting choroid plexus bleeding along with GMH can be seen. Closer to term, haemorrhage into the ventricle arises most commonly as a result of rupture of vessels within the choroid plexus. This is most often within the glomus of the choroid plexus in the atria of the lateral ventricles.

FURTHER READING

Krishnamoorthy KS, Fernandez RA, Momose KJ. Evaluation of neonatal intracranial haemorrhage by computerized tomography. Pediatrics 1977; 59:165–172.

Pevsner PH, Garcia-Bunuel R, Leeds N. Subependymal and intraventricular haemorrhage in neonates: early diagnosis by computed tomography. Radiology 1976; 119:111–114.

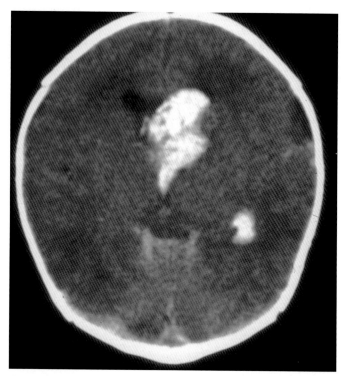

Figure 12.7.21 Germinal matrix haemorrhage, CT. Left caudothalamic GMH projecting into the left lateral ventricle. Blood is present in the 3rd and lateral ventricles.

Rumack CM, McDonald MM, O'Meara OP. CT detection and course of intracranial haemorrhage in premature infants. American Journal of Roentgenology 1978; 131:493–497.

Scott WR, New PF, Davis KR. Computerized axial tomography of intracerebral and intraventricular haemorrhage. Radiology 1974; 112:73–80.

Siegel MJ, Patel J, Gado MH. Cranial computed tomography and real-time sonography in full-term neonates and infants. Radiology 1983; 149: 111–116.

MAGNETIC RESONANCE IMAGING

Usually MRI requires significant time for each acquisition (minutes) during which it is necessary that the patient remain still. In a sick neonate, this can be a problem and, in addition, such patients require support and monitoring of vital signs during the scanning. However, MRI provides the best definition of brain anatomy and pathology. T1-weighted imaging (T1-WI), T2-weighted imaging (T2-WI), susceptibility gradient imaging, diffusion imaging and perfusion imaging offer the most complete information about the nature and extent of brain injury in neonates, and thus influence management, therapy and prognostication. Diffusion tensor imaging (DTI) has a significant potential future role in understanding how tracts are affected by various insults. It should be noted that postgadolinium T1-weighted imaging is not included in this initial evaluation. The reason for this is that, in general, the imaging is done to ascertain the site of bleeding and to evaluate the patency of CSF pathways and ventricular size. Contrast material is used primarily to demonstrate abnormalities of the blood–brain barrier, such as can occur subacutely in an infarcted area, to demonstrate abnormal enhancement in an intracranial infection, and to help to demonstrate the vascular bed, when a vascular malformation (e.g. venous malformation) is present.

MRI provides information about blood products in the brain and in the ventricular system, which varies depending on the chemical nature of the blood at the time of the imaging. Hyperacute haemorrhage consists mostly of oxyhaemoglobin, which is isointense on T1-WI and hyperintense on T2-WI. As clotting occurs the oxyhaemoglobin becomes deoxyhaemoglobin and the signal on T1-WI is slightly hypointense, while the signal on T2-WI becomes markedly hypointense (Figure 12.7.10). Over several days, deoxyhaemoglobin becomes methaemoglobin. Methaemoglobin, while intracellular, is bright on T1-WI and dark on T2-WI (Figure 12.7.9). Following rupture of the red blood cells, the extracellular methaemoglobin becomes bright on both T1-WI and T2-WI. With reabsorption of the globulin molecule by macrophages, haemosiderin is left in the tissue, usually within the macrophages. Haemosiderin is dark on both T1-WI and T2-WI. Blood within the subarachnoid space and within the ventricles, if not clotted, will increase the protein content of CSF, and will appear bright on FLAIR imaging. It is possible for subarachnoid and intraventricular blood to clot, and undergo changes similar to that described for intraparenchymal haemorrhage. Susceptibility scanning (gradient echo imaging), most often done as a 2D FLASH sequence, lacks the 180 degree pulse of the spin echo sequence. This brings out the inhomogeneity in the field, which can be caused by the presence of blood products and is shown as a loss of signal – an area of blackness (Figure 12.7.22). Such a pulse sequence should be used whenever blood products are thought to be present and there is a need for them to be demonstrated.

Diffusion imaging can be used to show acute cytotoxic oedema in the germinal matrix at the site of injury (Figure 12.7.22). Diffusion can also show acute periventricular leukomalacia, accompanying the germinal matrix injury. Proton spectroscopy during the acute stage of PVL can demonstrate elevation of lactate. Blood products will affect the voxels, at the site of bleeding, causing a loss of information.

MRI has been particularly successful in the follow-up of GMH by being able to demonstrate blood products that have caused occlusion of the aqueduct of Sylvius and outlets of the 4th ventricle and have led to obstructive hydrocephalus (Figure 12.7.23). Siderosis of the ependymal lining of the ventricles, due to deposition of blood products, can be seen both on T2-WI and on susceptibility scanning as focal loss of signal along the ependyma (Figure 12.7.24).

FURTHER READING

Barkovich AJ. Pediatric neuroimaging, 2nd edn. New York: Raven Press; 1995.
Blankenberg FG, Norbash AM, Lane B et al. Neonatal intracranial ischaemia and haemorrhage: diagnosis with US, CT, and MR imaging. Radiology 1996; 199:253–259.

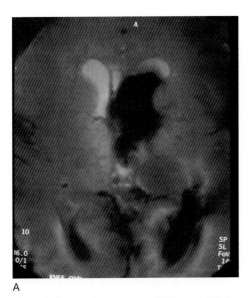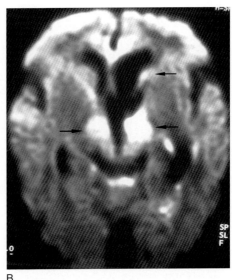

Figure 12.7.22 Germinal matrix haemorrhage, susceptibility and diffusion scanning, MRI. (A) Axial 2D FLASH susceptibility scan shows loss of signal at the site of blood in the left GMH with intraventricular extension. (B) Axial diffusion-weighted imaging (B1000) shows abnormal restricted diffusion at the site of the germinal matrix infarcts (arrows).

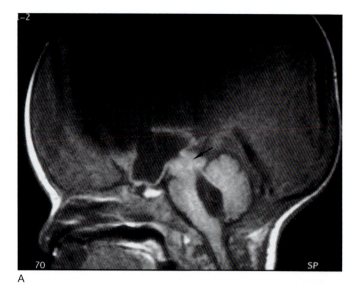

A

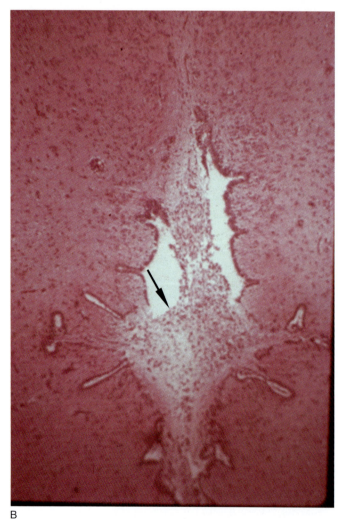

B

Figure 12.7.23 Germinal matrix haemorrhage with hydrocephalus due to aqueductal occlusion by blood. (A) Sagittal T1-WI shows marked hydrocephalus of the lateral and third ventricles. Aqueduct of Sylvius is occluded by blood products (arrow). (B) Pathological specimen of aqueduct of Sylvius from another patient shows obstructing clot within the aqueduct (arrow).

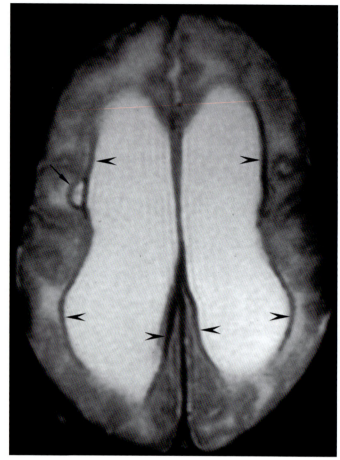

Figure 12.7.24 Siderosis of the lateral ventricles with obstructive hydrocephalus from germinal matrix haemorrhage. Axial 2D FLASH susceptibility scan shows siderosis of the ependyma (arrowheads) of the markedly enlarged lateral ventricles. Note on the right a small area of cavitation (arrow) from prior haemorrhage.

Bozzao A, Di Paolo A, Mazzoleni C et al. Diffusion-weighted MR imaging in the early diagnosis of periventricular leukomalacia. European Radiology 2003; 13:1571–1576.

Counsell SJ, Maalouf EF, Rutherford MA. Periventricular haemorrhagic infarct in a preterm neonate. European Journal of Paediatric Neurology 1999; 3:25–28.

Felderhoff-Mueser U, Rutherford MA, Squier WV et al. Relationship between MR imaging and histopathologic findings of the brain in extremely sick preterm infants. American Journal of Neuroradiology 1999; 20: 1349–1357.

Maalouf EF, Duggan PF, Counsell SJ et al. Comparison of findings on cranial ultrasound and magnetic resonance imaging in preterm infants. Pediatrics 2001; 107:719–727.

Mahle WT, Tavani F, Zimmerman RA et al. An MRI study of neurological injury before and after congenital heart surgery. Circulation 2002; 106(12 Suppl 1):I109–114.

McArdle CB, Richardson CJ, Hayden CK. Abnormalities of the neonatal brain: MR imaging. I. Intracranial haemorrhage. Radiology 1987; 163: 387–394.

Roelants-van Rijn AM, Nikkels PG, Groenendaal F et al. Neonatal diffusion-weighted MR imaging: relation with histopathology or follow-up MR examination. Neuropediatrics 2001; 32:286–294.

PERIVENTRICULAR LEUKOMALACIA

In the premature infant, the vulnerability of specific sites to hypoxic ischaemic injury relate to the relative lack of development of the brain (prematurity) and vascularity, as well as absence of autoregulation of cerebral blood flow, which is passive pressure dependent. The deep white matter, compared to the subcortical white matter, is relatively poorly vascularized at the end of the second trimester and the cerebral blood flow is passive, pressure dependent, so that with either a decrease in cerebral blood flow (ischaemia) and/or a decrease in oxygenation (hypoxia), injury to the white matter can occur. There is resultant periventricular coagulative necrosis, with possible subsequent cystic necrosis followed by reabsorption of damaged tissue and/or the formation of scar tissue.

The current overall incidence of PVL in infants less than 1500 g, as determined by US, is estimated to be between 5% and 10%. This is much less than that found at autopsy. This represents, to some degree, the lack of sensitivity of US and the fact that the patients who died and underwent autopsy were sicker to begin with than those who survived. At autopsy, in those infants weighing less than 1500 g, the incidence of PVL is 45%. Approximately 20% of PVL is without intraventricular haemorrhage and from 53% to 75% is associated with intraventricular haemorrhage. As gestational age increases, the incidence of PVL found at autopsy decreases. With gestational age around or less than 33/34 weeks, the incidence is between 26% and 38%, and with gestational age less than 38 weeks, 24%.

In the pathogenesis of PVL, lesions in the white matter should be considered as infarctions in the border zone, one that in the premature infant is between the penetrating arterial vessels coming in from the cortex and those arising deep along the margins of the ventricle and extending out. The oligodendroglia (cells that form myelin) are vulnerable to the effects of ischaemia, which leads to the release of free radicals, cytokines, glutamate and other noxious agents. These substances injure the oligodendroglia, impairing or preventing myelination at sites of injury. Cytokines are also released by infectious/inflammatory stimuli, such as occurs with chorioamniitis, and have been shown in prematures to have a direct effect on the white matter, producing PVL.

Following injury, coagulation necrosis occurs over the course of the first day, producing a bland area of infarction (Figure 12.7.25).

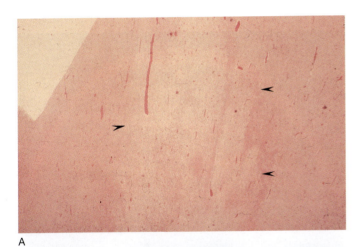

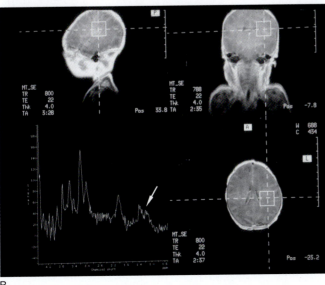

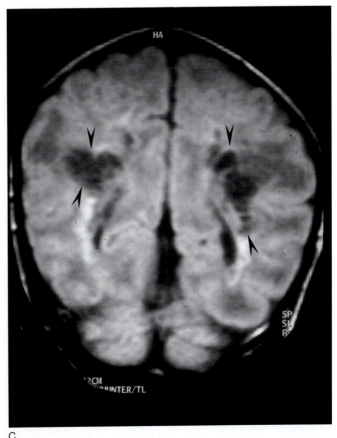

Figure 12.7.25 Acute periventricular leukomalacia. (A) Pathological section through an area of acute PVL shows bland infarction (arrowheads). (B) Proton spectroscopy, using a 270 ms TE, through the periventricular white matter on the left shows elevated lactate peak at 1.3 ppm (arrow). (C) Follow-up coronal proton density image at 3 weeks of age in the same patient as shown in B, shows cystic PVL (arrowheads) bilaterally.

Subacutely, macrophages migrate into the area and vessels on the periphery dilate, a reaction to the injury. Microscopic calcifications develop, which while not seen on CT, are often demonstrated by MRI as T1-hyperintense lesions, because of their paramagnetic effects (Figure 12.7.26). Tissue dissolution at the site of injury occurs producing areas of microcystic formation, first recognizable by US from 2 to 3 weeks postinjury, in a few lasting for the rest of the patient's life but in most disappearing completely. Depending on the age at injury, gliosis either will or will not be present. Prior to 26 weeks of gestation, the damaged tissue is reabsorbed and scar tissue is not seen (Figure 12.7.27A). After 26 weeks of gestation, there is an increasing likelihood that scar tissue will form and will be demonstrated on images. Scar tissue (gliosis) produces an increase in water content and is best shown on MRI with proton density or FLAIR sequence (Figure 12.7.27B). Haemorrhagic changes at sites of PVL are relatively uncommon, with a top estimate of incidence being up to 25%. MRI with conventional spin echo T2-WI or with susceptibility scanning is the most sensitive technique for the detection of haemorrhagic PVL (Figure 12.7.28).

Initial clinical manifestations of the injury process will depend to some extent upon the process producing the PVL and may or may not be apparent. Early deficits, if recognized, can include weakness of the lower extremity and problems with visual-evoked potentials. Much of the brain at risk for injury by PVL in the newborn, premature or term infant, at the time of injury, is not at a functional level. Therefore, much of the sequelae of PVL only become apparent with time. Spastic diplegia is the most common manifestation, developing over the course of the first 1–2 years of life. This usually involves the lower extremities but when the upper extremities are involved, there is often more extensive disease and a likelihood of intellectual deficits developing. Visual deficits are not uncommon when PVL involves the periatrial white matter, in the region of the occipital optic radiations. While PVL is thought of as an injury related to prematurity, it is also seen in term infants and post-term infants. The location of injury in the term infant is usually not adjacent to the ependymal surface of the ventricle but at a distance from the ependyma. PVL is not an infrequent injury seen postsurgical repair of congenital heart disease, where hypothermia and total cardiac bypass are utilized. For PVL

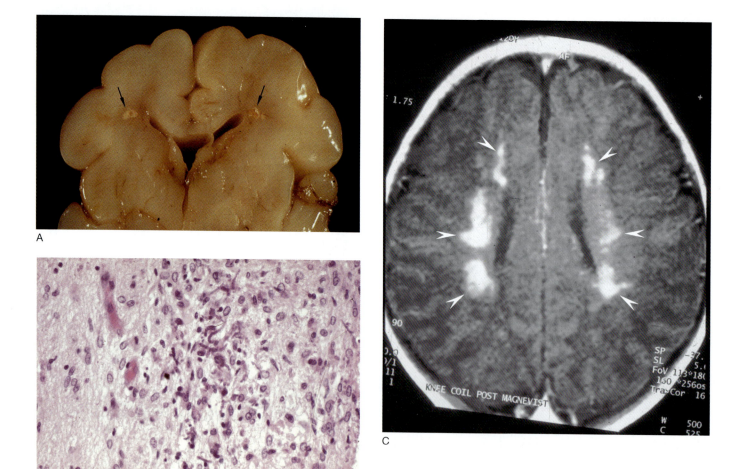

Figure 12.7.26 Subacute periventricular leukomalacia. (A) Pathological specimen, coronal view, shows bilateral plaques of PVL (arrows). (B) Subacute histological reaction with calcification at the site of PVL. (C) Axial MRI T1-WI shows hyperintense paramagnetic effect of calcification in the periventricular white matter (arrowheads).

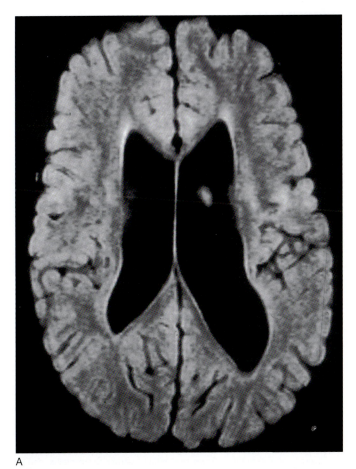
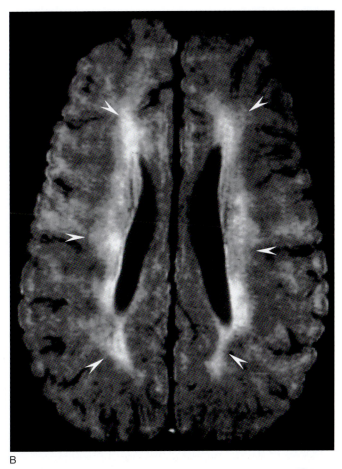

A

B

Figure 12.7.27 Periventricular leukomalacia, 24 weeks vs 29 weeks on MRI with FLAIR imaging. (A) Axial FLAIR in a 24-week gestation infant with PVL seen as volume loss at age 2 years. (B) Axial FLAIR in a 29-week gestation child with PVL, examined at age 15 months. Gliosis (arrowheads) is present in the periventricular white matter.

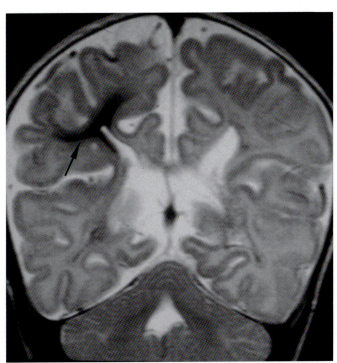
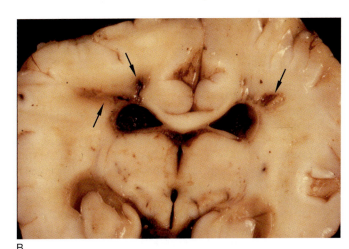

A

B

Figure 12.7.28 Haemorrhagic periventricular leukomalacia, MRI. (A) Coronal T2-WI shows hypointense blood products in the right periventricular region (arrow) with loss of white matter volume. (B) Coronal pathological specimen from a different patient shows bilateral haemorrhagic PVL (arrows).

in association with GMH see 'Germinal matrix haemorrhage' above.

FURTHER READING

Banker BQ, Larroche JC. Periventricular leukomalacia of infancy. Archives of Neurology 1962; 7:386–410.

DeVries LS, Wigglesworth JS, Regev R, Dubowitz LM. Evolution of periventricular leukomalacia during the neonatal period and infancy: correlation of imaging and postmortem findings. Early Human Development 1988; 17:205–219.

Gressens P, Richelme C, Kadhim HJ, Gadisseux J-F, Evrard P. The germinative zone produces the most cortical astrocytes after neuronal migration in the developing mammalian brain. Biology of the Neonate 1992; 61: 4–24.

Hagberg H, Wennerholm UB, Savman K. Sequelae of chorioamnionitis. Current Opinions in Infectious Disease 2002; 15:301–316.

Iida K, Takashima S, Ueda K. Immunohistochemical study of myelination and oligodendrocyte in infants with periventricular leukomalacia. Pediatric Neurology 1995; 13:296–304.

Kuban KCK, Allred EN, Dammann O et al. Topography of cerebral white-matter disease of prematurity studied prospectively in 1607 very-low-birth-weight infants. Journal of Child Neurology 2001; 16:401–408.

Leviton A, Gilles F. Ventriculomegaly, delayed myelination, white matter hypoplasia, and "periventricular" leukomalacia: how are they related? Pediatric Neurology 1996; 15:127–136.

Nelson MD Jr, Gonzalez-Gomez I, Gilles FH. The search for human telencephalic ventriculofugal arteries. American Journal of Neuroradiology 1991; 12:215–222.

Rezaie P, Dean A. Periventricular leukomalacia, inflammation and white matter lesions within the developing nervous system. Neuropathology 2002; 22:106–132.

Shuman RM, Selednik LF. Periventricular leukomalacia: a one-year autopsy study. Archives of Neurology 1980; 37:231–235.

Takashima S, Iida K, Deguchi K. Periventricular leukomalacia, glial development and myelination. Early Human Development 1995; 43: 177–184.

Zupan V, Gonzalez P, Lacaze-Masmonteil T. Periventricular leukomalacia: risk factors revisited. Developmental Medicine and Child Neurology 1996; 38:1061–1067.

ULTRASOUND

Because PVL is most common in premature infants and because premature infants have a variety of problems due to immaturity, such as those associated with ventilation of the immature lungs as well as apnoeic episodes associated with prematurity, imaging is most often done at the bedside in the Neonatal Intensive Care Unit by US via the anterior fontanelle. Ultrasound is relatively insensitive in detection of PVL, especially small areas of PVL and those that are bilaterally symmetrical. There is also a normal reflectivity of the periventricular white matter that can, but should not, be confused with PVL. During the acute stage of PVL when there is coagulation necrosis (a form of infarction) and oedema in the white matter, hyperechoic changes are seen on US (Figure 12.7.3). Over the course of the subsequent 1–2 weeks these areas become less hyperechoic, and between 14 and 21 days and beyond, if there was extensive injury, hyperechoic cysts can be found at the site of injury (Figure 12.7.3). These cysts usually disappear as the ventricles enlarge and the damaged tissue is reabsorbed. Haemorrhagic PVL is also hyperechoic and may be difficult to differentiate by US from non-haemorrhagic PVL.

FURTHER READING

Baarsma R, Laurini RN, Baerts W, Okken A. Reliability of sonography in non-hemorrhagic periventricular leucomalacia. Pediatric Radiology 1987; 17: 189–191.

Carson SC, Hertzberg BS, Bowie JD, Burger PC. Value of sonography in the diagnosis of intracranial haemorrhage and periventricular leukomalacia: a postmortem study of 35 cases. American Journal of Neuroradiology 1990; 155:595–601.

Dammann O, Leviton A. Duration of transient hyperechoic images of white matter in very-low-birthweight infants: a proposed classification. Developmental Medicine and Child Neurology 1997; 39:2–5.

De Vries LS, Wigglesworth JS, Regev R, Dubowitz LM. Evolution of periventricular leukomalacia during the neonatal period and infancy: correlation of imaging and postmortem findings. Early Human Development 1988; 17:205–219.

Dipietro MA, Brody BA, Teele RL. Periventricular echogenic "blush" on cranial sonography; pathologic correlates. American Journal of Neuroradiology 1986; 7:305–310.

Holling EE, Leviton A. Characteristics of cranial ultrasound white matter echolucencies that predict disability – a review. Developmental Medicine and Child Neurology 1998; 41:136–139.

Hope PL, Gould SJ, Howard S. Precision of ultrasound diagnosis of pathologically verified lesions in the brains of very preterm infants. Developmental Medicine and Child Neurology 1988; 30:457–471.

Maalouf EF, Duggan PJ, Counsell SJ et al. Comparison of findings on cranial ultrasound and magnetic resonance imaging in preterm infants. Pediatrics 2001; 107:719–727.

Paneth N, Rudelli R, Monte W, Rodriguez E. White matter necrosis in very low birth weight infants: neuropathologic and ultrasonographic findings in infants surviving six days or longer. Journal of Pediatrics 1990; 116:975–984.

Sie LT, van der Knapp MS, van Wezel-Meijler G et al. Early MR features of hypoxic-ischaemic brain injury in neonates with periventricular densities on sonograms. American Journal of Neuroradiology 2000; 21:852–861.

van Wezel-Meijler G, van der Knaap MS, Sie LT et al. Magnetic resonance imaging of the brain in premature infants during the neonatal period. Normal phenomena and reflection of mild ultrasound abnormalities. Neuropediatrics 1998; 29:89–96.

COMPUTED TOMOGRAPHY (CT)

Computed tomography is not the procedure of choice in the diagnosis of acute PVL. CT is more often done when there is an issue of haemorrhage. Because the unmyelinated brain is already watery and of low density, the addition of more water due to infarction often results in an insufficient further reduction in density for the acute damage to be recognized as a density difference. In very extensive injuries to the supratentorial white matter, there may be bilateral oedema with decreased density of the white matter, with sufficient mass effect to produce ventricular compression. This can be difficult to recognize on CT when each hemisphere is symmetrically involved. Here, comparison of the involved supratentorial white matter to the uninvolved infratentorial cerebellar white matter can prove useful. Haemorrhagic PVL is a relatively unusual finding on CT, unless the bleeds are large enough to be recognized (Figure 12.7.29).

In the follow-up of the infant with PVL, CT can be useful. Cysts are rarely shown but loss of volume along the margins of the lateral ventricles, with dilatation of the ventricular system and with the cortical grey matter extending deeper towards the ventricular walls, can be recognized. Irregularity of the margins of the ventricles is another sign, although not a specific sign, of PVL (Figure

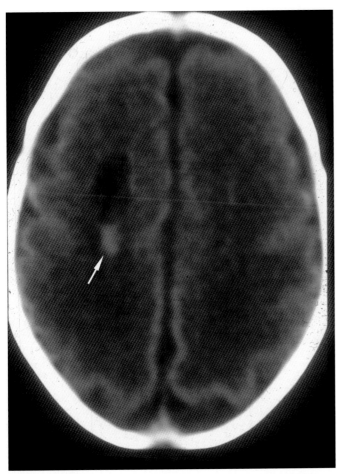

Figure 12.7.29 Acute haemorrhagic PVL, CT appearance. Axial CT shows an area of increased density (arrow) in the periventricular white matter on the right, consistent with haemorrhagic PVL.

MAGNETIC RESONANCE IMAGING

During the acute injury stage of PVL, both T1- and T2-weighted MR sequences do not demonstrate the injury (Figure 12.7.7). This is because there is not enough contrast between the normal unmyelinated, watery brain of the premature and term infant, and the oedematous area due to infarction. However, diffusion weighted imaging (DWI) can demonstrate acute infarcts due to restriction of motion of water in the periventricular white matter, seen as bright signal on diffusion images and as dark areas on ADC maps (Figure 12.7.31). In the very young patients, the changes in the white matter evolve very rapidly, losing their diffusion positivity within a week. Proton spectroscopy performed either as single or multivoxel study of the damaged white matter can show elevation of lactate at the site of injury (Figure 12.7.25B). Follow-up scanning over the ensuing 1–2 weeks can show a subacute phase during which there is evidence of contrast enhancement at the site of PVL (Figure 12.7.32). Subacutely, calcific changes occur transiently in the white matter at the sites of injury, and produce focal T1 hyperintensities at the sites of injury (Figure 12.7.26C). This appears to represent a paramagnetic effect due to the small size of the calcifications. With follow-up, over the ensuing weeks, cystic changes occasionally may be shown on T1-WI or T2-WI and these rarely persist throughout the patient's life (Figure 12.7.33). Most often, cysts are not visible. In patients who are old enough to form scar tissue at the time of injury, hyperintense gliottic changes at the sites of PVL can be seen once myelination has occurred. These are best seen on T2-W, proton density and FLAIR images (Figure 12.7.27B). There is associated thinning of the white matter volume and of the corpus callosum, related to a decreased number of crossing axons (Figure 12.7.34). When the injury has occurred, before the second trimester, there is merely a loss of white matter without evidence of gliottic change (Figure 12.7.27A).

12.7.30); however, gross undulation of the ventricular walls is fairly typical of PVL. Irregularity of the ventricular margin can be seen as a result of ventriculitis, intraventricular bleeding or with tumour dissemination. With significant loss of periventricular white matter, the developing brain becomes narrower and the head may have an elongated appearance. This may be another clue to PVL, although an elongated head is also seen in sagittal suture craniosynostosis.

FURTHER READING

Di Chiro G, Arimitsu T, Pellock JM, Landes RD. Periventricular leukomalacia related to neonatal anoxia: recognition by computed tomography. Journal of Computer Assisted Tomography 1978; 2:352–355.

Flodmark O, Becker LE, Harwood-Nash DC. Correlation between computed tomography and autopsy in premature and full-term neonates that have suffered perinatal asphyxia. Radiology 1980; 137:93–103.

Flodmark O, Roland EH, Hill A, Whitfield MF. Periventricular leukomalacia: radiologic diagnosis. Radiology 1987; 162:119–124.

Schellinger D, Grant EG, Richardson JD. Cystic periventricular leukomalacia: sonographic and CT findings. American Journal of Neuroradiology 1984; 5:439–445.

FURTHER READING

Aida N, Nishimura G, Hachiya Y. MR imaging of perinatal brain damage: comparison of clinical outcome with initial and follow-up MR findings. American Journal of Neuroradiology 1998; 19:1909–1921.

Bozzao A, Di Paolo A, Mazzoleni C et al. Diffusion-weighted MR imaging in the early diagnosis of periventricular leukomalacia. European Radiology 2003; 13:1571–1576.

Cioni G, Bertuccelli B, Boldrini A et al. Correlation between visual function, neurodevelopmental outcome, and magnetic resonance imaging findings in infants with periventricular leucomalacia. Archives of Disease in Childhood and Fetal Neonatal Education 2000; 82:F134–F140.

Felderhoff-Mueser U, Rutherford MA, Squier WV et al. Relationship between MR imaging and histopathologic findings of the brain in extremely sick preterm infants. American Journal of Neuroradiology 1999; 20: 1349–1357.

Feldman HM, Scher MS, Kemp SS. Neurodevelopmental outcome of children with evidence of periventricular leukomalacia on late MRI. Pediatric Neurology 1990; 6:296–302.

Flodmark O, Lupton B, Li D. MR imaging of periventricular leukomalacia in childhood. American Journal of Neuroradiology 1989; 10:111–118.

Groenendaal F, van der Grond J, Eken P et al. Early cerebral proton MRS and neurodevelopmental outcome in infants with cystic leukomalacia. Developmental Medicine and Child Neurology 1997; 39:373–379.

Hoon AH, Lawrie WT, Melhem ER et al. Diffusion tensor imaging of periventricular leukomalacia shows affected sensory cortex white matter pathways. Neurology 2002; 59:752–756.

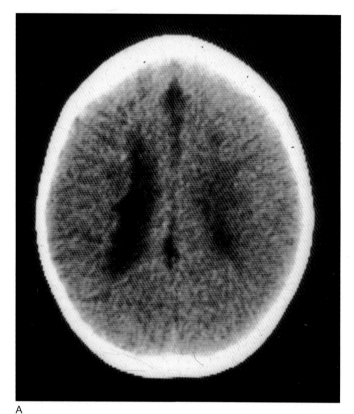

A

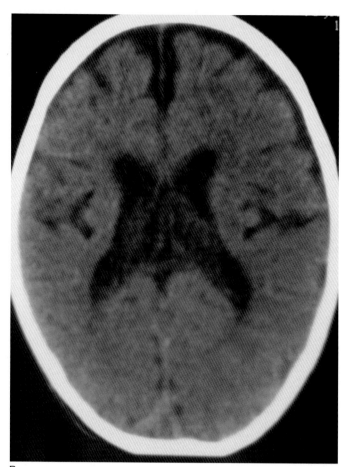

B

Figure 12.7.30 PVL, chronic; CT appearance. (A) Axial non-contrast enhanced CT shows dilatation of the bodies of the lateral ventricles, with irregular margins to the ventricles due to loss of subependymal and periventricular tissue. (B) Axial non-contrast enhanced CT shows dilated ventricles with decreased white matter volume.

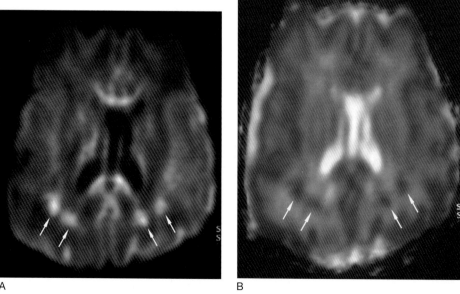

A   B

Figure 12.7.31 MRI of acute PVL, diffusion imaging. There is restricted motion of water (arrowheads) on the B1000 (A) and on the ADC map (B) in the brain of a 1500-g triplet.

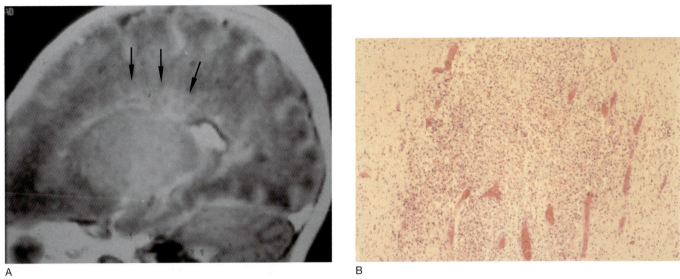

Figure 12.7.32 Subacute PVL, MRI. (A) Sagittal T1 post contrast enhancement shows striated pattern of enhancement of the periventricular white matter (arrows). (B) Pathological specimen in another patient with subacute PVL showing dilated blood vessels and macrophage infiltration at the site of damage.

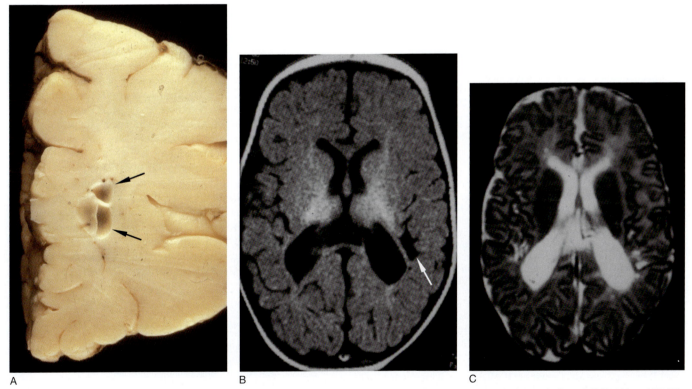

Figure 12.7.33 Cystic PVL, MRI. (A) Pathological specimen shows periventricular cysts representing cystic PVL (arrows). (B and C) T1-WI and T2-WI show dilated atria of the lateral ventricles with reduced white matter; cyst on T1 in the left periatrial region (arrow) and bilateral high signal gliosis on T2.

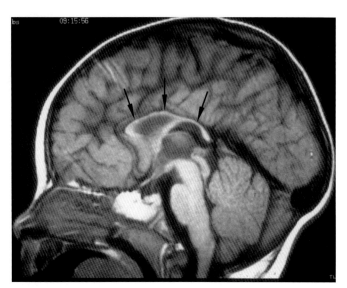

Figure 12.7.34 Chronic PVL with corpus callosal thinning, MRI. Sagittal T1-WI in a 10-month-old female shows marked thinning of the entire corpus callosum (arrows).

Huppi PS, Murphy B, Maier SE et al. Microstructural brain development after perinatal cerebral white matter injury assessed by diffusion tensor magnetic resonance imaging. Pediatrics 2001; 107:455–460.

Inder T, Huppi PS, Zientara GP et al. Early detection of periventricular leukomalacia by diffusion-weighted magnetic resonance imaging techniques. Journal of Pediatrics 1999; 134:631–634.

Inder TE, Huppi PS, Warfield S et al. Periventricular white matter injury in the premature infant is followed by reduced cerebral cortical gray matter volume at term. Annals of Neurology 1999; 46:755–760.

Maalouf EF, Duggan PJ, Counsell SJ et al. Comparison of findings on cranial ultrasound and magnetic resonance imaging in preterm infants. Pediatrics 2001; 107:719–727.

Maalouf EF, Duggan PJ, Rutherford MA. Magnetic resonance imaging of the brain in a cohort of extremely preterm infants. Journal of Pediatrics 1999; 135:351–357.

Mahle WT, Tavani F, Zimmerman RA et al. An MRI study of neurological injury before and after congenital heart surgery. Circulation 2002; 106(12 Suppl 1):I109–114.

Melhem ER, Hoon AH Jr, Ferrucci JT Jr et al. Periventricular leukomalacia: relationship between lateral ventricular volume on brain MR images and severity of cognitive and motor impairment. Radiology 2000; 1:199–204.

Miller SP, Vigneron DB, Henry RG et al. Serial quantitative diffusion tensor MRI of the premature brain: development in newborns with and without injury. Journal of Magnetic Resonance Imaging 2002; 16:621–632.

Olsen P, Paakko E, Vainionpaa L, Pyhtinen J, Jarvelin MR. Magnetic resonance imaging of periventricular leukomalacia and its clinical correlation in children. Annals of Neurology 1997; 41:754–761.

Roelants-van Rijn AM, Nikkels PG, Groenendaal F et al. Neonatal diffusion-weighted MR imaging: relation with histopathology or follow-up MR examination. Neuropediatrics 2001; 32:286–294.

Shouman-Clays E, Henry-Feugeas M-C, Roset F. Periventricular leukomalacia: correlation between MR imaging and autopsy findings during the first 2 months of life. Radiology 1993; 189:59–64.

Sie LT, van der Knaap MS, Oosting J et al. MR patterns of hypoxic-ischaemic brain damage after prenatal, perinatal or postnatal asphyxia. Neuropediatrics 2000; 31:128–136.

Sie LT, van der Knapp MS, van Wezel-Meijler G et al. Early MR features of hypoxic-ischaemic brain injury in neonates with periventricular densities on sonograms. American Journal of Neuroradiology 2000; 21:852–861.

Truwit CL, Barkovich AJ, Koch TK, Ferriero DM. Cerebral palsy: MR findings in 40 patients. American Journal of Neuroradiology 1992; 13:67–78.

van Wezel-Meijler G, van der Knaap MS, Sie LT et al. Magnetic resonance imaging of the brain in premature infants during the neonatal period. Normal phenomena and reflection of mild ultrasound abnormalities. Neuropediatrics 1998; 29:89–96.

TERM INFANT

INTRAVENTRICULAR BLEEDING IN THE TERM INFANT

In the premature infant, the germinal matrix is the primary source of intraventricular bleeding. However, the germinal matrix involutes and disappears by 36 weeks of gestation. Even in the premature infant, haemorrhage from the germinal matrix may be associated with choroid plexus haemorrhage. In the term infant (post 37 weeks), the most common source of intraventricular haemorrhage is the choroid plexus. Infants with congenital heart disease and normal vaginal delivery that have been studied by MRI have been found to have a 33% incidence of intrachoroidal haemorrhage, most without rupture into the ventricle (Figure 12.7.35A–C). With stress, such as that produced by congenital heart disease surgery, including total cardiac bypass, the incidence of intrachoroidal bleeding increases significantly. Stress on the choroid plexus can lead to rupture of intrachoroidal haemorrhage producing intraventricular bleeding (Figure 12.7.35C). The presence of blood within the ventricle where it is not accompanied by hypoxic ischaemic brain injury has little significance other than the risk that the blood can produce irritation and adhesions at the site of CSF pathway narrowings; such as the aqueduct or outlets of the 4th ventricle, leading to obstructive hydrocephalus and/or a trapped 4th ventricle. When this happens, the situation is similar to that of the patient with germinal matrix haemorrhage, in that the decision has to be made as to the necessity of shunting the ventricles. More extensive bleeding from the choroid plexus can produce acute obstruction of the ventricle and compression of the surrounding brain, which can result in permanent parenchymal brain injury. Bleeding rarely extends into the surrounding brain parenchyma, producing brain injury.

Intraventricular haemorrhage in term infants can have a variety of other aetiologies. Haemorrhage can be associated with reperfusion of infarction, such as that occurring in a watershed distribution and, if large enough, intraventricular extension of the bleed is possible. Haemorrhage with intraventricular extension can arise from large traumatic contusions, rupture of aneurysms and arteriovenous malformations, or from haematomas associated with cortical vein thrombosis with haemorrhagic infarction.

FURTHER READING

Tavani F, Zimmerman RA, Clancy RR, Licht DJ, Mahle WT. Incidental intracranial haemorrhage after uncomplicated birth: MRI before and after neonatal heart surgery. Neuroradiology 2003; 45:253–258.

PARTIAL PROLONGED ASPHYXIA

With development of the brain during gestation, as the fetus approaches term, there is a shift in the vascular watershed of the brain from the periventricular white matter out towards the cortex, between the territories of the anterior and middle cerebral arteries

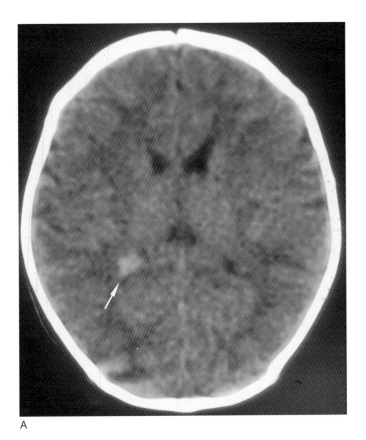

A

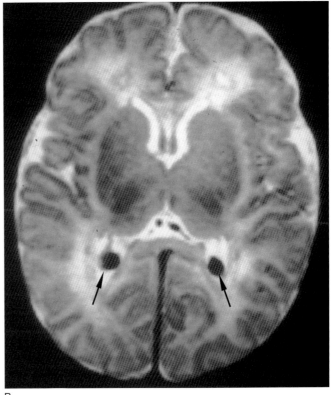

B

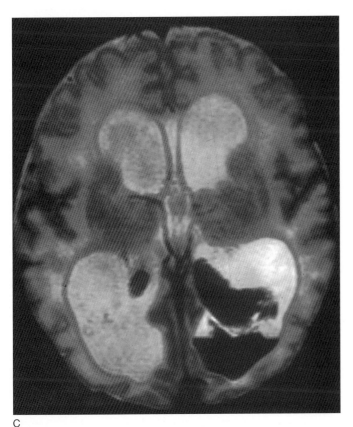

C

Figure 12.7.35 Term infant, intrachoroidal glomus haemorrhage. (A) Axial non-contrast enhanced CT in newborn shows increased density in the choroid plexus on the right (arrows). (B) T2-weighted axial image shows bilateral intrachoroidal glomus haemorrhages as hypointensities (arrows). (C) Axial T2-WI demonstrates bilateral choroid plexus haemorrhages; the one on the left has extended into the lateral ventricle. There is accompanying hydrocephalus with siderosis of the ependyma.

anteriorly and between the middle and posterior arteries posteriorly. These vascular watersheds involve the cortex and subadjacent white matter (Figure 12.7.36). Injury to these watersheds is associated with relatively long periods of time (hours to portions of the day), during which there is suboptimal oxygenation and/or perfusion to the brain. The watershed infarcts can also be seen with a hypotensive episode, occurring before, during and after delivery. Examples of situations in which this type of injury occurs are the presence of a nuchal cord with intermittent tightening, chorioamniotis with intermittent cord spasm, episodes of moderate fetal bradycardia, postdelivery respiratory distress and postdelivery septic shock. Problems in resuscitation of the newborn infant can also result in this type of injury. Similar injury can occur in the postnatal period especially when there is difficulty with feeding, which results in dehydration, leading to hypotension, apnoea and respiratory arrest. In the symptomatic neonate with parasagittal watershed infarction, weakness of the proximal limbs (upper greater than lower extremities) may be found as an early neurological finding, along with all of the potential consequences such as neonatal seizures and depressed level of consciousness. Long-term sequelae vary and in more severe cases, there is abnormality of the motor function and cognition, such as spasticity, and language and visual problems.

FURTHER READING

Adams JH, Brierley JB, Connor RC, Treip CS. The effects of systemic hypotension upon the human brain: clinical and neuropathological observations in 11 cases. Brain 1966; 89:235–268.

Pryds O, Greisen G, Lou H, Friis-Hansen B. Vasoparalysis associated with brain damage in asphyxiated term infants. Journal of Pediatrics 1990; 117:119–125.

Takashima S, Armstrong DL, Becker LE. Subcortical leukomalacia: relationship to development of the cerebral sulcus and its vascular supply. Archives of Neurology 1978; 35:470–472.

Volpe JJ, Pasternak JF. Parasagittal cerebral injury in neonatal hypoxic-ischaemic encephalopathy: clinical and neuroradiologic features. Journal of Pediatrics 1977; 91:472–476.

ULTRASOUND

Ultrasound when performed through the anterior fontanelle can miss significant changes in the brain of the patient suffering from a partial prolonged asphyxic event. The parasagittal involvement between the vascular territories tends to involve the anterior and posterior poles of the brain. These are the areas that are not seen at all or only very poorly on US performed through the anterior fontanelle. If the area immediately under the ultrasound is involved, then changes can be detected (Figure 12.7.37). If the event produces sufficient oedema and mass effect, there can be decrease in the size of lateral ventricles as oedema develops and compresses adjacent ventricles and structures. It is possible, with reperfusion of the infarcted tissue, to have haemorrhages develop within the areas of watershed infarction. During an acute stage when demonstrated by US, the infarction, oedema and haemorrhage all appear as hyperechoic areas, and may not be differentiated. In this type of injury, most often the basal ganglia and thalami are not involved, unless there has been a mixed picture of both partial prolonged and profound asphyxia.

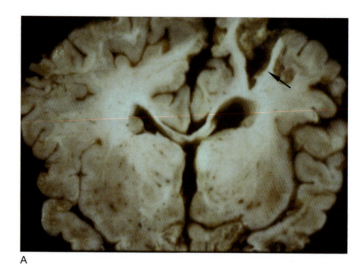

A

B

Figure 12.7.36 Watershed injury. (A) Coronal pathological specimen shows watershed infarction (arrow) between the left anterior and middle cerebral artery vascular territory, involving both cortex and subadjacent white matter, with underlying enlargement of the left lateral ventricle. (B) Artist's illustration of bilateral extensive frontal and posterior watershed infarctions (grey colour) between middle and anterior cerebral artery territories anteriorly and between middle and posterior cerebral artery territories posteriorly.

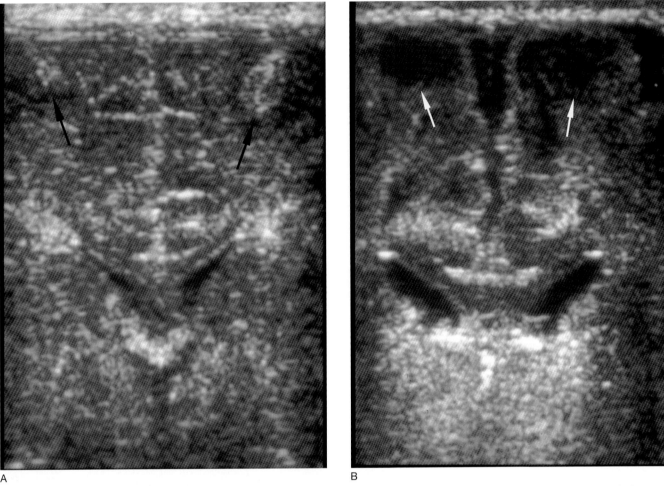

Figure 12.7.37 Partial prolonged asphyxia with watershed parasagittal infarction. US examination. (A) US acutely shows areas of hyperechoic change, bilaterally in the parasagittal watershed territories (arrows). The interhemispheric fissure is narrow. (B) Follow-up US 6 days later shows enlargement of the interhemispheric fissure and hypoechoic necrotic areas bilaterally in the parasagittal watershed infarcts (arrows). The lateral ventricles are larger than on the prior examination.

FURTHER READING

Rutherford M, Pennock JM, Dubowitz L. Cranial ultrasound and magnetic resonance imaging in hypoxic-ischaemic encephalopathy: a comparison with outcome. Developmental Medicine and Child Neurology 1994; 36:813–825.

COMPUTED TOMOGRAPHY

During the acute stage of injury secondary to partial prolonged asphyxia, CT reveals oedema with decreased density and loss of grey–white matter definition in the anterior and/or posterior watershed areas (Figure 12.7.38). There is frequently associated mass effect with obliteration of overlying sulci and if the area of involvement is extensive enough, there is also compression of the lateral ventricles. Very prolonged partial prolonged asphyxia can lead to an acute injury that extends well beyond the usual watershed territory, involving a much greater extent of the supratentorial cortex. The oedema in the brain is cytotoxic oedema. In cytotoxic oedema, the cells swell and the extracellular space becomes restricted.

During the evolution of the injury, the opening of the blood–brain barrier (BBB) contributes a component of vasogenic, interstitial oedema to the picture. After injury, the identification of cortical oedema by CT takes time. The neonatal brain is already relatively watery and unmyelinated. Therefore, the time that it takes to increase the water content of the damaged brain sufficiently so that it stands out from the adjacent normal brain and can be detected, differs from that of the adult/adolescent or child's brain.

The earliest oedematous changes, with obliteration of grey–white matter junctions, can be seen in some by 18 h, but in most only by 24 h. The oedema increases progressively from 24 to 72 h, becoming maximal at this point in time. Relatively severe swelling with hypodensity and ventricular obliteration can be seen between 48 and 96 h. Following that, the oedema regresses, although the brain injury remains. The ventricular system begins to reappear, often looking relatively normal in size, by the 6th to 7th day postinjury. The injured grey/white matter junction near the cerebral cortex can also reappear, looking almost normal on a non-contrast enhanced CT. This can be seen around the 8th day postinjury and will persist until atrophy starts to occur. This so-called

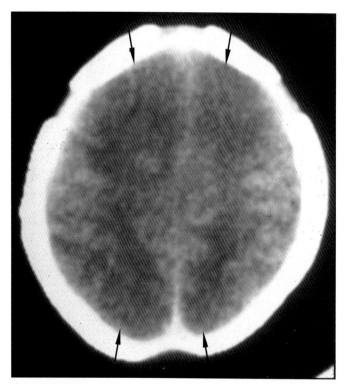

Figure 12.7.38 Partial prolonged asphyxia with bilateral watershed infarctions. Non-contrast enhanced CT shows hypodensities involving the right and left parasagittal watershed distribution (arrows). Cortex density is abnormally decreased and the lesions extend into the subadjacent white matter bilaterally.

'reversal of brain injury' is not actually a return to normal. It is the early development of cortical laminar necrosis at the site of injury. The cortex can become even more dense, reflecting 'calcification' in the cortex, which may be transiently present, when neurons are mummified. Iodinated contrast can show disturbances in the blood–brain barrier at sites of cortical injury but this takes 3–5 days to occur (Figure 12.7.39). With time, necrosis of tissue will produce atrophy. Necrosis will typically affect the cortex that has been injured, leading to a diminution in the size of the gyri and an increase in the CSF spaces of the adjacent sulci. Ulgyria describes a mushroom-shaped gyrus where the damage is greatest at the depth of the sulcus, based on the vascular anatomy. The ulgyric changes are not infrequent in the parasagittal watershed injury.

Depending on the extent of involvement, the underlying ventricular system can enlarge to some degree, in an atrophic fashion. Early atrophy can be identified at approximately 12 days postinjury but this depends on the severity of the insult and with time the atrophy becomes more severe, being progressive over the course of up to several months.

When haemorrhage has occurred, because of reperfusion, high-density blood products may be found in association with the infarcted tissue. It is important to realize that the areas of haemorrhage may be asymmetrical and that they can occur at less common watershed areas, such as the inferior temporal lobe, between middle and posterior cerebral arteries. However, when this is the only finding, a phase contrast MRA and follow-up studies are indicated in order to exclude an underlying vascular anomaly and/or cortical vein occlusion as the aetiology of the bleed.

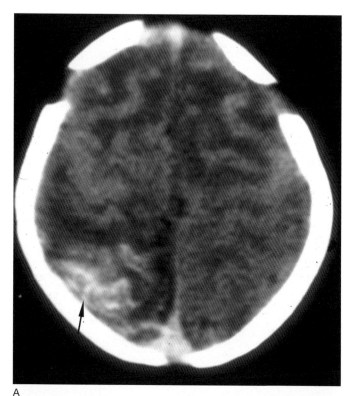

A

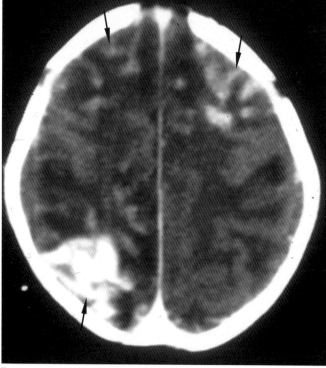

B

Figure 12.7.39 Subacute watershed infarctions, CT. The mass effect has resolved; there is hypodensity at the site of the bilateral injuries. (A) The right posterior parietal region shows increased density indicative of calcification or bleeding (arrow). (B) Following contrast material injection there is enhancement at the sites of watershed infarction in both frontal lobes and at the site of the increased density seen precontrast in the right parietal lobe (arrows).

Partial prolonged asphyxic injuries that are not clinically recognized and studied initially can present later in infancy or childhood. The imaging pattern of injury is often characteristic. The reason for the injury is not necessarily deducible from the image and requires clinical correlation, if such exists. The pattern of injury to the brain in partial prolonged asphyxic injuries is not limited to the term infant. This occurs well beyond infancy.

FURTHER READING

Pasternak JF. Parasagittal infarction in neonatal asphyxia. Annals of Neurology 1987; 21:202–204.

MAGNETIC RESONANCE IMAGING

The advent of diffusion weighted imaging with ADC maps has revolutionized the ability of MRI to demonstrate the watershed injury of partial prolonged asphyxia (Figure 12.7.40). With acute cytotoxic oedema, the motion of water is restricted. On the B1000 diffusion image, restricted motion of water appears high in signal intensity (bright). The anatomical distribution of this change can be easily demonstrated. Diffusion imaging can be obtained both axially and coronally. Diffusion imaging is routinely performed in the axial plane while coronal is often done for purposes of better anatomical localization. The ADC map that is generated from the x-, y-, and z-gradient direction B1000 images shows the area of restricted motion of water due to infarction as a black or hypointense area. Measurement of the degree of restriction can be made on the MRI console. This can be correlated to normal areas of the brain and to data on normalcy from the literature. In the acute injury phase, diffusion is often positive within hours to several days of the insult. However, the T2-weighted images, which will show the injury to the cortex as a loss of normal low-signal intensity, with an increase in signal at this site is a phenomenon that takes closer to 24 h to become evident. T1-weighted images and FLAIR images are usually not useful during the acute period. Susceptibility scans are useful in demonstrating the presence of blood products secondary to reperfusion and haemorrhage at the site of infarction, a less frequent phenomenon (Figure 12.7.41).

Given the choice of three techniques, US, CT and MRI, the first choice is MRI. With MRI, diffusion and T2-weighted axial and coronal images provide the most information. Additional valuable information can be obtained from the performance of proton spectroscopy. By putting the voxel at the site of the watershed region, lactate elevation can be demonstrated in the first 24 h, followed by both a decrease in lactate and NAA with time.

The follow-up of the watershed injury due to partial prolonged asphyxia, shows a loss of cortex and subcortical white matter at the site of injury. Not infrequently, there is subcortical cystic encephalomalacia, ulgyria or gliosis at the site of injury (Figure 12.7.42). All of these are associated with a resultant atrophy, enlargement of the sulci and often enlargement of the lateral ventricles. These changes are irreversible. In the follow-up of these patients, there may be times when there are T1-weighted hyperintensities seen at the sites of injury, the aetiology of which may be calcification of the neurons or evidence of bleeding at the site of injury.

FURTHER READING

Barkovich AJ, Hallam D. Neuroimaging in perinatal hypoxic-ischaemic injury. MRDD Research Review 1997; 3:1–14.

Barkovich AJ, Baranski K, Vigneron D et al. Proton MR spectroscopy for the evaluation of brain injury in asphyxiated, term neonates. American Journal of Neuroradiology 1999; 20:1399–1405.

Chateil JF, Quesson B, Brun M et al. Localised proton magnetic resonance spectroscopy of the brain after perinatal hypoxia: a preliminary report. Pediatric Radiology 1999; 29:199–205.

Cowan FM, Pennock JM, Hanrahan JD, Manji KP, Edwards AD. Early detection of cerebral infarction and hypoxic ischaemic encephalopathy in neonates using diffusion-weighted magnetic resonance imaging. Neuropediatrics 1994; 25:172–175.

Groenendaal F, van der Grond J, Eken P et al. Early cerebral proton MRS and neurodevelopmental outcome in infants with cystic leukomalacia. Developmental Medicine and Child Neurology 1997; 39:373–379.

Kuenzle C, Baenziger O, Martin E. Prognostic value of early MR imaging in term infants with severe perinatal asphyxia. Neuropediatrics 1994; 25:191–200.

Mahle WT, Tavani F, Zimmerman RA et al. An MRI study of neurological injury before and after congenital heart surgery. Circulation 2002; 106(12 Suppl 1):I109–114.

Martin E, Barkovich AJ. Magnetic resonance imaging in perinatal asphyxia. Archives of Disease in Childhood 1995; 72:F62–F70.

McKinstry RC, Miller JH, Snyder AZ et al. A prospective, longitudinal diffusion tensor imaging study of brain injury in newborns. Neurology 2002; 59:824–833.

Phillips MD, Zimmerman RA. Diffusion imaging in pediatric hypoxic ischaemic injury. Neuroimaging Clinics of North America 1999; 9:41–52.

Robertson RL, Ben-Sira L, Barnes PD et al. MR line-scan diffusion-weighted imaging of term neonates with perinatal brain ischaemia. American Journal of Neuroradiology 1999; 20:1658–1670.

Rollins NK, Morriss MC, Evans D, Perlman JM. The role of early MR in the evaluation of the term infant with seizures. American Journal of Neuroradiology 1994; 15:239–248.

Rutherford M, Pennock JM, Dubowitz L. Cranial ultrasound and magnetic resonance imaging in hypoxic-ischaemic encephalopathy: a comparison with outcome. Developmental Medicine and Child Neurology 1994; 36:813–825.

Rutherford M, Pennock J, Schwieso J. Hypoxic-ischaemic encephalopathy: early and late magnetic resonance imaging findings in relation to outcome. Archives of Disease in Childhood 1996; 75:F145–F151.

Rutherford MA, Pennock JM, Schwieso JE. Hypoxic ischaemic encephalopathy: early magnetic resonance imaging findings and their evolution. Neuropediatrics 1995; 26:183–191.

Sie LT, van der Knaap MS, Oosting J et al. MR patterns of hypoxic-ischaemic brain damage after prenatal, perinatal or postnatal asphyxia. Neuropediatrics 2000; 31:128–136.

Wolf RL, Zimmerman RA, Clancy R, Haselgrove JH. Quantitative apparent diffusion coefficient measurements in term neonates for early detection of hypoxic-ischaemic brain injury: initial experience. Radiology 2001; 218:825–833.

Yokochi K. Clinical profiles of subjects with subcortical leukomalacia and border-one infarction revealed by MR. Acta Paediatrica 1998; 87:879–883.

Yokochi K, Fujimoto S. Magnetic resonance imaging in children with neonatal asphyxia: correlation with developmental sequelae. Acta Paediatrica 1996; 85:88–95.

PROFOUND ASPHYXIA

Profound asphyxia occurs when there is a sudden, marked or catastrophic decrease in cerebral blood flow and/or in oxygenation to the brain of the fetus or newborn infant. One such example would be the fetus, just prior to emergency Caesarean section, with a fetal heart rate of 60–80 beats per min (normal = 120–140) lasting 15–30 min. The usual clinical scenarios during which this occurs

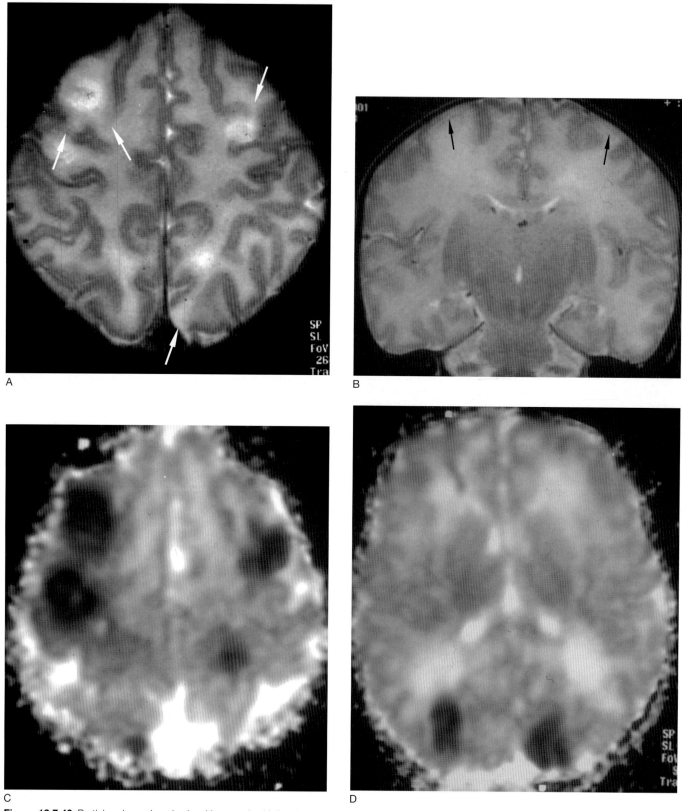

Figure 12.7.40 Partial prolonged asphyxia with watershed infarctions, MRI. (A) Axial T2-WI shows bilateral loss of normal cortical signal intensity (arrows) with increased signal in the white matter in the watershed distribution between middle and anterior cerebral arteries. (B) Coronal T2-WI shows loss of normal cortical signal intensity (arrows) in the watershed distribution bilaterally. (C and D) Axial ADC maps show restricted motion of water in the bilateral infarcted areas superiorly (C) and inferiorly (D).

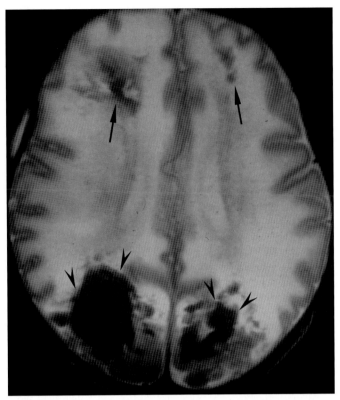

Figure 12.7.41 Haemorrhagic watershed infarct in partial prolonged asphyxia, MRI. Axial T2-WI shows hypointense haemorrhage, bilaterally in both anterior (arrows) and posterior (arrowheads) sites of watershed infarction.

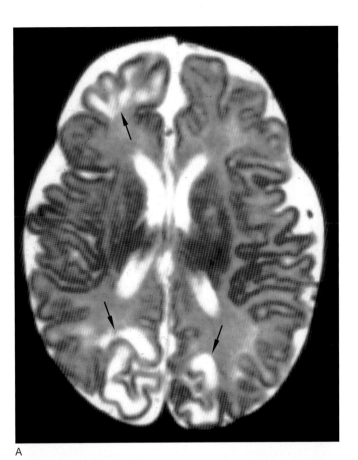

A

are ruptured uterus during vaginal delivery (a finding that may be associated with prior section), placental abruption or cord prolapse occurring during the course of delivery. With a sudden decrease in oxygen and blood flow, there is little time for the cerebral circulation to shift its flow to the more vulnerable, metabolically active structures, such as the central grey matter portions of thalami and putamina, which are neuronally mature at the time of term. In the majority of profound asphyxic injuries at term, these two structures are injured (the ventral lateral nucleus of the thalami and the posterior putamina). Increasing severity leads to greater injury, and the next most common site is the pre- and postcentral gyri, the rolandic cortex region that lies along the central sulcus. Not only is the rolandic cortex vulnerable but also the subrolandic white matter. The subrolandic white matter represents an area of active myelination at term. It is thought that the maturity of the neurons in the cortex and the active myelination are the reasons why this region is vulnerable. More severe injuries involve the hippocampi, typically bilaterally, and can also involve the midbrain. When the injury is much more severe, a diffuse cortical injury occurs involving most of the cerebral hemispheres, supratentorially.

FURTHER READING

Hill A. Current concepts of hypoxic-ischaemic cerebral injury in the term newborn. Pediatric Neurology 1991; 7:317–325.

Pasternak JF, Gorey MT. The syndrome of acute near-total intrauterine asphyxia in the term infant. Pediatric Neurology 1998; 18:391–398.

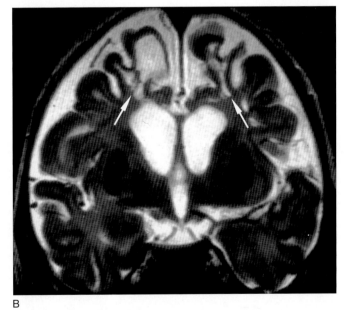

B

Figure 12.7.42 Chronic cystic subcortical encephalomalacia at sites of watershed infarction, MRI. (A) Six-week-old male, axial T2-WI shows right frontal and bilateral temporo-occipital cystic encephalomalacia (arrows). (B) Three-month-old female, coronal T2-WI, shows parasagittal watershed subcortical and cortical cystic encephalomalacia (arrows). The lateral ventricles are enlarged.

Roland EH, Poskitt K, Rodriguez E. Perinatal hypoxic-ischaemic thalamic injury: clinical features and neuroimaging. Annals of Neurology 1998; 44: 161–166.

Rosenbloom L. Dyskinetic cerebral palsy and birth asphyxia. Developmental Medicine and Child Neurology 1994; 36:285–289.

Kreusser KL, Schmidt RE, Shackelford GD, Volpe JJ. Value of ultrasound for identification of acute haemorrhagic necrosis of thalamus and basal ganglia in an asphyxiated term infant. Annals of Neurology 1984; 16:361–363.

Shen EY, Huang CC, Chyou SC. Sonographic finding of the bright thalamus. Archives of Disease in Childhood 1986; 61:1096–1099.

ULTRASOUND

Ultrasound examination may demonstrate the injury process once oedema develops in the central grey matter, approximately 24 h from the time of injury, as a hyperechoic change in the thalamus and putaminal region (Figure 12.7.43). Calcifications develop as a result of neuronal injury and may also come to contribute to the hyperechoic changes seen towards the end of the first week postinjury and even later. If the central grey matter injury is sufficiently swollen, then there may be compression of the 3rd ventricle by oedema at the time of the initial hyperechoic changes shown on US. If there is additional, wider injury, either from associated partial prolonged asphyxia or from more extensive injury to the pre- and postcentral gyri, it is possible to have brain swelling that produces lateral ventricular compression (Figure 12.7.43C). It is also possible for the US to be insensitive to small areas of injury, such as can be seen when just the ventral lateral nucleus of the thalamus and posterior putamen are involved. Thus, US may not demonstrate the injury process. This is especially true when the US is performed early, following the injury, before oedema has had a chance to develop. Timing of insults often requires serial studies, including those done by other imaging modalities such as CT and MRI.

FURTHER READING

Cabanas F, Pellicer A, Perez-Higueras A. Ultrasonographic findings in thalamus and basal ganglia in term asphyxiated infants. Pediatric Neurology 1991; 7:211–215.

Connolly B, Kelehan P, O'Brien N. The echogenic thalamus in hypoxic ischaemic encephalopathy. Pediatric Radiology 1994; 24:268–271.

Donn SM, Bowerman RA, DiPietro MA, Gebarski SS. Sonographic appearance of neonatal thalamic-striatal haemorrhage. Journal of Ultrasound in Medicine 1984; 3:231–233.

COMPUTED TOMOGRAPHY

The most significant and common CT finding in the profound asphyxic injury is a decrease in density of the central grey matter structures of the thalamus and posterior putamen region (Figure 12.7.44B). CT resolution is often not sufficient to separate the posterior putamen from the lateral thalamic region. As with US, development of sufficient oedema in the central grey matter is necessary so that it can be seen as a low density, which takes about 24 h or possibly 18 h for appearance of an early blurring of definition of structures. The hypodensity often involves more than the area that is subsequently demonstrated as injured on follow-up MRI. This relates to the fact that some neurons are more vulnerable to insults than others, and the oedema that develops is both cytotoxic and vasogenic and does not reflect just the sites of cell death. If the involvement of the central grey matter is of sufficient size, the oedema will result in compression of the 3rd ventricle. With more extensive injury, especially with an associated partial prolonged asphyxia leading to a profound asphyxia, a more generalized brain swelling with compression of the lateral ventricles will be present along with hypodensity involving cortex and subcortical areas (Figure 12.7.44C). Subacutely, the central swelling will resolve over the first week, and grey–white matter definition in the central structures of the brain will transiently appear falsely more normal. With time, over the ensuing weeks, the thalamus may shrink in size, the 3rd ventricle enlarge and focal areas of increased density may appear within the thalami, representing sclerosis (calcifications) (Figure 12.7.44D). It is possible to develop focal cavitary necrosis in either/or both the thalamus and putamen (Figure 12.7.44E). Haemorrhagic change can also be seen as increased density at the site of injury and can be difficult to differentiate from the calcifications by CT, but not by MRI. Shrinkage of cortex in the vicinity of the pre- and postrolandic gyri occurs and may be

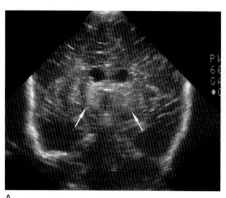 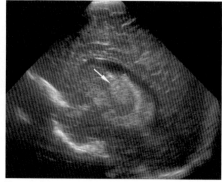 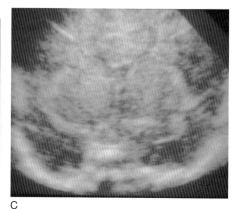

A   B   C

Figure 12.7.43 Profound asphyxia. (A and B) Coronal and sagittal US through the thalamic basal ganglionic region demonstrates hyperechoic changes at site of acute damage (arrows). (C) Coronal image shows hyperechoic changes involving the thalami basal ganglia, along with more diffuse white matter and grey matter swelling producing marked compression of the lateral and third ventricles.

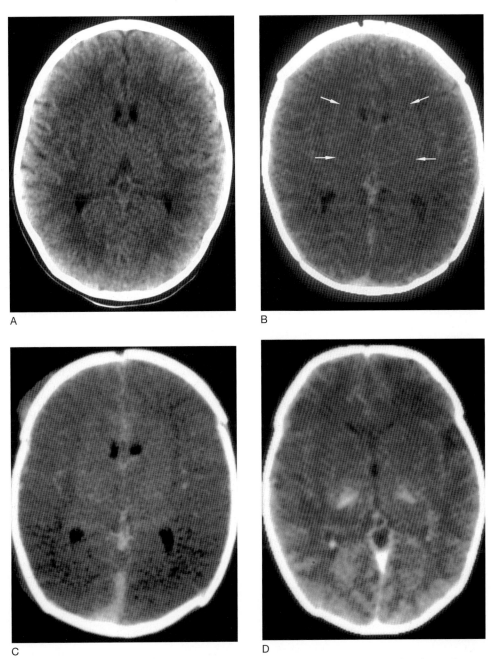

Figure 12.7.44 Profound asphyxia, CT findings. (A) Normal CT in newborn infant demonstrates normal density of central grey matter involving the basal ganglia and thalamus. (B) Axial CT of acute profound asphyxia shows hypodensity involving central grey matter (arrows). (C) Axial CT of profound asphyxia shows early changes of acute injury, with brain swelling, not only involving central grey matter but cortex peripherally. (D) Subacute profound asphyxia, hyperdensities in bilateral thalami consistent with either blood or calcification. Note increased density in the right choroid plexus consistent with blood.

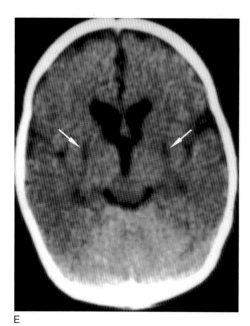

E

Figure 12.7.44 *continued* (E) Chronic injury shown on CT. The ventricles have enlarged and there is local decreased density in the bilateral putamina (arrows) consistent with cystic infarction.

recognized on CT. If the subcortical white matter underlying the pre- and postcentral gyri is injured, then there may not be loss of cortex and enlargement of sulci at this site. Damage to the hippocampi, if severe enough, can result in temporal horn enlargement, which can be seen on CT. Midbrain injury can occasionally be seen on CT, acutely as hypodensity, and subsequently as an atrophic damaged area.

FURTHER READING

Colamaria V, Curatolo P, Cusmai R, Dalla Bernardina B. Symmetrical bithalamic hyperdensities in asphyxiated full-term newborns: an early indicator of status marmoratus. Brain Development 1988; 10:57–59.

Kotagal S, Toce SS, Kotagal P, Archer CR. Symmetric bithalamic and striatal haemorrhage following perinatal hypoxia in a term infant. Journal of Computer Assisted Tomography 1983; 7:353–355.

Phillips MD, Zimmerman RA. Diffusion imaging in pediatric hypoxic ischaemic injury. Neuroimaging Clinics of North America 1999; 9:41–52.

Shewmon DA, Fine M, Masdeu JC, Palacios E. Postischaemic hypervascularity of infancy: a stage in the evolution of ischaemic brain damage with characteristic CT scan. Annals of Neurology 1981; 9:358–365.

MAGNETIC RESONANCE IMAGING

While CT is frequently the most successful early study in identifying injury consistent with profound asphyxia, MRI has become the most definitive. Diffusion-weighted imaging in the first days after injury can demonstrate restricted motion of water in the central grey matter of the thalami and putamen. This is seen as high signal intensity on the B1000 image and as low signal on the ADC map (Figure 12.7.45). Similarly, when the injury is more extensive, involving the rolandic cortex and subcortical white matter, the hippocampi and the brainstem, it can be demonstrated as well (Figure 12.7.45). The timing of the diffusion-weighted imaging is not clearcut. It is spectroscopy, in some instances, that may be more sensitive to the early injury, with increased lactate and subsequently decreased NAA, whereas diffusion abnormalities may evolve more or less slowly compared to the more rapidly appearing changes on the proton spectroscopy (Figure 12.7.14).

On T2-weighted images, the signal intensity of the acutely injured grey matter is increased due to the presence of increased water (Figure 12.7.46). Marked hypointensity can occasionally be seen and most often represents blood products at the site of injury. Loss of the normal low signal intensity of the myelinated posterior portion of the posterior limb of the internal capsule can be another sign of oedema on T2-WI in a term infant with central grey matter injury. Beyond 5 or 6 days, the diffusion abnormalities are often normalized in the central grey matter, as neuronal necrosis leads to calcification. In follow-up of subacute injury, the T1-WI shows hyperintense signal in the damaged neurons of the thalamus and posterior putamen. This is a paramagnetic effect of the microscopic calcifications of the mummified necrotic neurons, producing T1 shortening (Figure 12.7.47A). This is anatomically different from the normal term infant's high T1 signal representing myelination in the posterior limb of the internal capsule. Similarly, T1 hyperintensity can be seen at the site of damaged neurons of the pre- and postcentral gyri, the hippocampus and the midbrain. Further evolution of the injury occurs with time and becomes more evident as the child's brain becomes more myelinated (18 months and beyond), showing the sites of damage on T2-WI as areas of high signal intensity due to the presence of gliosis (scar tissue) (Figure 12.7.47B). Focal atrophy of the brain, the dilatation of sulci around the affected gyri, the enlargement of the 3rd ventricle, the temporal horns and the lateral ventricles often occur with more severe injuries. In general, contrast enhancement has not proven to be useful in demonstrating this type of injury.

FURTHER READING

Barkovich AJ. MR and CT evaluation of profound neonatal and infantile asphyxia. American Journal of Neuroradiology 1992; 13:959–972.

Barkovich AJ, Baranski K, Vigneron D et al. Proton MR spectroscopy for the evaluation of brain injury in asphyxiated, term neonates. American Journal of Neuroradiology 1999; 20:1399–1405.

Barkovich AJ, Westmark KD, Bedi HS et al. Proton spectroscopy and diffusion imaging on the first day of life after perinatal asphyxia: preliminary report. American Journal of Neuroradiology 2001; 22:1786–1794.

Chateil JF, Quesson B, Brun M et al. Localized proton magnetic resonance spectroscopy of the brain after perinatal hypoxia: a preliminary report. Pediatric Radiology 1999; 29:199–205.

Hanrahan JD, Cox IJ, Azzopardi D et al. Relation between proton magnetic resonance spectroscopy within 18 hours of birth asphyxia and neurodevelopment at 1 year of age. Developmental Medicine and Child Neurology 1999; 41:76–82.

Kuenzle C, Baenziger O, Martin E. Prognostic value of early MR imaging in term infants with severe perinatal asphyxia. Neuropediatrics 1994; 25:191–200.

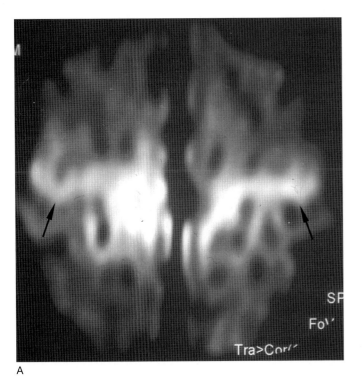

A

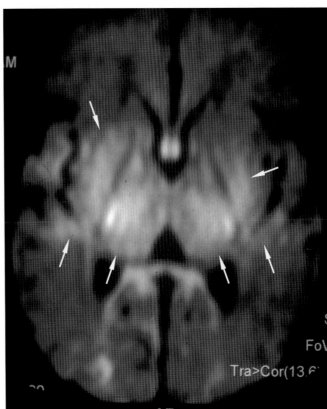

B

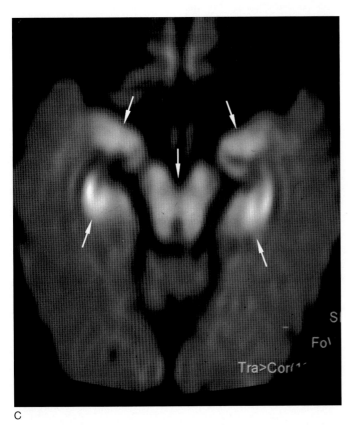

C

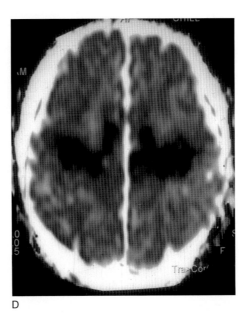

D

Figure 12.7.45 Profound asphyxia, MR diffusion imaging and ADC maps. Three-day-old female, post 15 min cardiac arrest at time of delivery. (A–C) Diffusion images at B1000: (A) abnormal high signal in bilateral rolandic regions (arrows); (B) abnormal high signal involves thalami, putamina and portions of insular cortex (arrows); and (C) abnormal high signal involving the hippocampi and amygdala regions as well as the midbrain (arrows). (D–F) ADC maps of the same regions as seen on the diffusion where motion of water is seen as hypointense signal: (D) rolandic region;

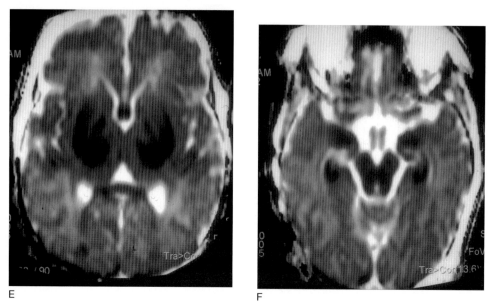

E F

Figure 12.7.45 *continued* (E) basal ganglia, putamina and insular region; and (F) hippocampi, amygdala and midbrain region.

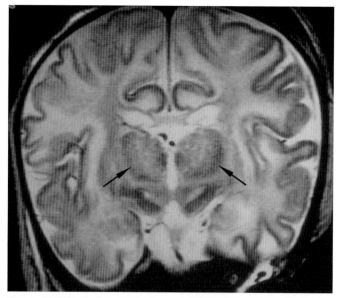

Figure 12.7.46 Profound asphyxia in subacute stage, MRI. T2-WI coronal image shows hyperintense signal (arrows) in the thalami and posterior putamina.

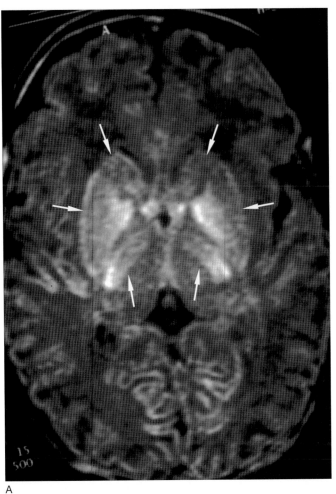

A

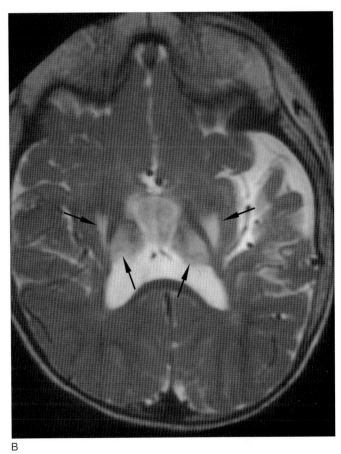

B

Figure 12.7.47 Subacute and chronic changes following profound asphyxia, MRI. (A) Axial T1-WI at 5 days of age. Abnormal increased T1 signal intensity involves the thalami, lenticular nuclei and caudate nuclei (arrows). (B) Follow-up T2-weighted MRI at age 3 years shows hyperintense signal consistent with gliosis in the posterior putamina and thalami bilaterally (arrows). Thalami are reduced in size.

McKinstry RC, Miller JH, Snyder AZ et al. A prospective, longitudinal diffusion tensor imaging study of brain injury in newborns. Neurology 2002; 59:824–833.

Menkes J, Curran JG. Clinical and magnetic resonance imaging correlates in children with extrapyramidal cerebral palsy. American Journal of Neuroradiology 1994; 15:451–457.

Pasternak JF, Gorey MT. The syndrome of acute near total intrauterine asphyxia in the term infant. Pediatric Neurology 1998; 18:391–398.

Robertson RL, Ben-Sira L, Barnes PD et al. MR line-scan diffusion-weighted imaging of term neonates with perinatal brain ischaemia. American Journal of Neuroradiology 1999; 20:1658–1670.

Roland EH, Poskitt K, Rodriguez E, Lupton BA, Hill A. Perinatal hypoxic-ischaemic thalamic injury: clinical features and neuroimaging. Annals of Neurology 1998; 44:161–166.

Rutherford M, Pennock JM, Dubowitz L. Cranial ultrasound and magnetic resonance imaging in hypoxic-ischaemic encephalopathy: a comparison with outcome. Developmental Medicine and Child Neurology 1994; 36:813–825.

Sie LT, van der Knaap MS, Oosting J et al. MR patterns of hypoxic-ischaemic brain damage after prenatal, perinatal or postnatal asphyxia. Neuropediatrics 2000; 31:128–136.

Wolf RL, Zimmerman RA, Clancy R, Haselgrove JH. Quantitative apparent diffusion coefficient measurements in term neonates for early detection of hypoxic-ischaemic brain injury: initial experience. Radiology 2001; 218:825–833.

DESTRUCTIVE CYSTIC BRAIN INJURY

There are three cystic destructive brain lesions, which are mentioned separately here as they may cause confusion on imaging and are often discussed as separate entities. Both porencephaly and multicystic encephalomalacia have been mentioned above. Hydranencephaly is an extreme form of infarction of the brain.

PORENCEPHALY

Porencephalic cavities are a consequence of germinal matrix haemorrhage that has expanded in the cerebral parenchyma but they may occur from any cause of cerebral destruction. On imaging they appear as smooth-walled cysts, which contain fluid that is isointense to CSF on all sequences and imaging techniques (Figure 12.7.48). The brain around these cavities is normal. The cavities

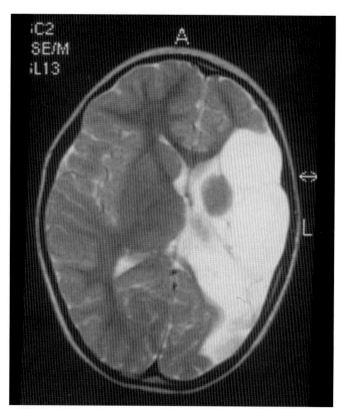

Figure 12.7.48 Porencephaly. T2-weighted image. Note the large porencephalic cyst on the left, which is in communication with the ventricle. This lesion has occurred in the middle cerebral artery territory and probably reflects an arterial thrombosis.

may merge with the ipsilateral ventricle to cause apparent ventricular enlargement. They may lie adjacent to the ventricle and depending on the size, compress it or depending on the location and the extent of destruction, parts of the ventricle may be relatively normal in size and shape and the rest may be in communication with one of these porencephalic cavities. Porencephalic cysts may develop in a cerebral hemisphere and remain extraventricular. When large they may cause enlargement of the hemicranium, which may be visible on a skull x-ray. There is minimal or no glial reaction detectable by imaging around these smooth-walled cavities.

The timing of the destructive insult determines the pathological description of these lesions. Those that occur before the 26th week of gestation may be lined with dysplastic grey matter and are similar to schizencephaly and are sometimes described as agenetic porencephaly. Those that occur later in the second trimester are termed encephaloclastic porencephaly. They are regarded as a destructive brain lesion and result from a severe ischaemic injury to the brain of vascular origin, which may be precipitated by a variety of insults. The insult causes liquefaction and brain necrosis, which results in these cavities.

FURTHER READING

Debus O, Koch HG, Kurlemann G et al. Factor V Leiden and genetic defects of thrombophilia in childhood porencephaly. Archives of Disease in Childhood. Fetal and Neonatal Edition 1998; 78:121–124.

Ho SS, Kuzniecky RI, Gilliam F et al. Congenital porencephaly: MR features and relationship to hippocampal sclerosis. American Journal of Neuroradiology 1998; 19:135–141.

HYDRANENCEPHALY

In this situation, there is replacement of both cerebral hemispheres by large dilated CSF-filled cysts (Figure 12.7.49). There is no cortical mantle but there is usually preservation of the basal regions of the temporal lobes and the inferomedial aspects of the frontal lobes, and sometimes remnants in the parafalcine regions. The thalami and brainstem appear normal or small. The cerebellum is usually normal. The skull size may be normal, small or enlarged. The underlying pathology is not fully understood but is likely to be vascular in origin in many cases but infection and genetic causes have been implicated. Children with hydranencephaly are severely handicapped. Distinguishing hydranencephaly from severe hydrocephalus can be difficult. In hydrocephalus, it is usually still possible to distinguish a rim of cortex around the dilated ventricles on MRI but it may be impossible on CT. Distinguishing the two is important as relieving the hydrocephalus may result in improved cognitive and motor function.

FURTHER READING

Castro-Gago M, Alonso A, Pintos-Martinez E et al. Congenital hydranencephalic-hydrocephalic syndrome associated with mitochondrial dysfunction. Journal of Child Neurology 1999; 14:131–135.

Greco F, Finocchiaro M, Pavone P, Trifilette RR, Parano E. Hemihydranencephaly: case report and literature review. Journal of Child Neurology 2001; 16:218–221.

MULTICYSTIC ENCEPHALOMALACIA

Both porencephaly and hydranencephaly must be distinguished from severe destructive multicystic encephalomalacia. Pathologically, this is characterized by destructive cavities that have glial septae within the destroyed areas of the brain, because there is an astrocytic response (Figure 12.7.50). This is seen on MR imaging as prolongation of the T1 and T2 relaxation times. Multicystic encephalomalacia results from diffuse and severe hypoxic ischaemic insult to the brain of whatever underlying aetiology, late in the third trimester, during birth, perinatally or after birth. The cavities that form are variable in size. Those associated with major vessel injury will be in the distribution of that vessel, e.g. the middle cerebral artery. Other insults, such as partial prolonged asphyxia can produce lesions in the watershed regions of the cortex and subcortical white matter. Very severe ischaemia may result in destruction of much of the brain including the basal ganglia. This type of lesion can superficially resemble hydranencephaly on CT but with MRI it is usually easy to distinguish the glial septae that characterize severe multicystic encephalomalacia.

FURTHER READING

Okumura A, Hayakawa F, Kato T, Kuno K, Watanabe K. MRI findings in patients with spastic cerebral palsy. I: Correlation with gestational age at birth. Developmental Medicine and Child Neurology 1997; 39:363–368.

Weidenheim KM, Bodhireddy SR, Nuovo GJ, Nelson SJ, Dickson DW. Multicystic encephalopathy: review of eight cases with etiologic considerations. Journal of Neuropathology and Experimental Neurology 1995; 54:268–275.

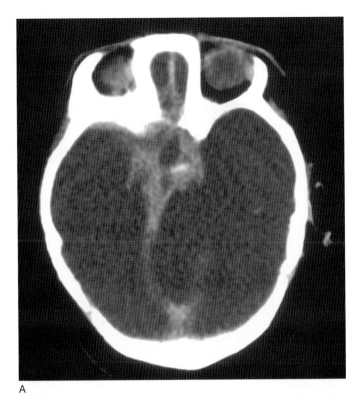

A

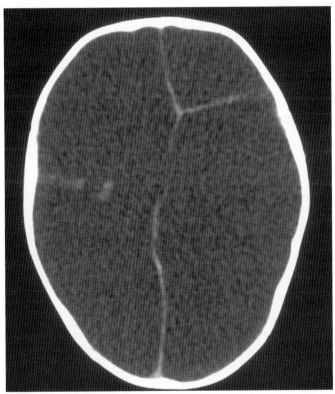

B

Figure 12.7.49 Hydranencephaly. (A and B) Two slices of a CT series showing very severe hydranencephaly with virtually no preservation of brain tissue.

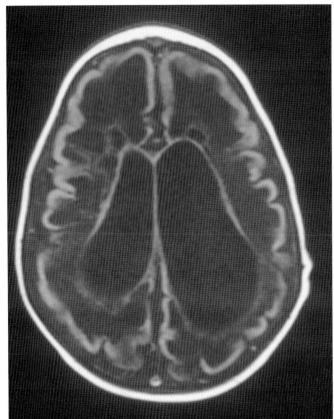

A

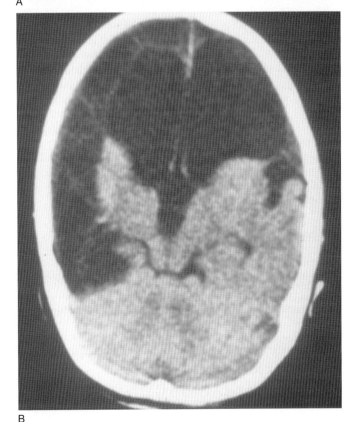

B

Figure 12.7.50 Multicystic encephalomalacia. (A) T1-weighted sequence of a child who had severe birth asphyxia. Note the microcephaly, ex vacuo dilatation of the ventricles and replacement of the cortical mantle by a cystic cavity, which on the right has some discrete cysts. (B) In this child the appearances superficially resemble hydranencephaly but note the preservation of the dilated ventricles and the glial septae within the encephalomalacic brain.

TRAUMATIC BIRTH INJURY

Injury due to trauma sustained during the birth process can involve the extracranial soft tissues, the calvarium, the intracranial space surrounding the brain or the brain tissue itself. In addition, injuries to the spinal cord and cervical vertebrae can occur and produce neurological dysfunction. All of these injuries are associated with some type of force, which may be associated with the use of instruments such as forceps or vacuum extractors, or related to disproportion between the head and the pelvis.

Extracranial haematomas are of three types: caput seccedaneum, a haemorrhagic oedema of the soft tissues; subgaleal haematoma, located beneath the aponeurosis covering the scalp; and cephalohaematoma, a subperiosteal collection of blood. Caput seccedaneum is seen in ordinary vaginal deliveries but is more frequent with vacuum deliveries. Moulding of the skull and scalp oedema that crosses sutures commonly occur when there is vertex presentation. This can be seen on both CT and MRI as scalp swelling. If not very haemorrhagic, CT shows scalp oedema as an enlargement of the scalp of decreased density and MRI as high signal on T2-weighted images. Subgaleal haematoma lies beneath the aponeurosis covering the scalp and connecting the frontal and occipital portions of the occipito frontalis muscle. This type of haematoma can spread into and dissect the soft tissues of the neck. Vacuum extraction can be associated with this type of injury and results in a firm, fluctuant mass, increasing in size after birth. The presence of haemorrhage within the scalp can lead to a decrease in the haematocrit of the neonate and to an elevated bilirubin because of the breakdown of the blood products. Cephalohaematoma is a haematoma confined by the cranial sutures, lying under the periosteum of the outer table of the skull (Figure 12.7.51). It has a 1–2% incidence in live births and is more common in males than females. It is more common in the first born than in subsequent siblings. It is more frequent in babies delivered with the aid of forceps. Fractures are associated with 10–25% of cephalohaematomas. The appearance is that of a firm tense mass and it may be bilateral. Resolution takes weeks to months, some haematomas undergoing calcification and even ossification, resulting occasionally in a calvarial deformity.

FURTHER READING

Govaert P, Vanhaesebrouck P, Depraeter C. Vacuum extraction, bone injury and neonatal subgaleal bleeding. European Journal of Pediatrics 1992; 151:532–535.

Sutton LN, Wang Z, Duhaime AC et al. Tissue lactate in pediatric head trauma: a clinical study using 1H NMR spectroscopy. Pediatric Neurosurgery 1995; 22:81–87.

SKULL FRACTURES AND INTRACRANIAL HAEMATOMAS

Most skull fractures associated with misapplication of forceps are linear and non-displaced. Depressed fractures are possible and are most often of the ping-pong variety, found in the parietal bone (Figure 12.7.52). Separation of the sutures on a traumatic basis can also be seen, with haemorrhage at the site of the separated suture.

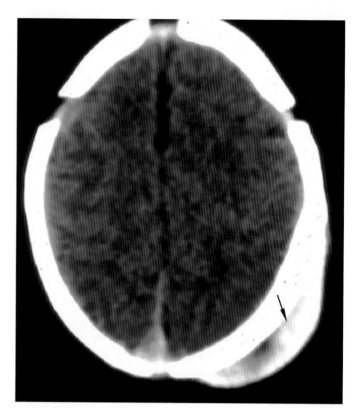

Figure 12.7.51 Cephalohaematoma. Axial CT without contrast material shows a left parietal high density cephalohaematoma (arrow).

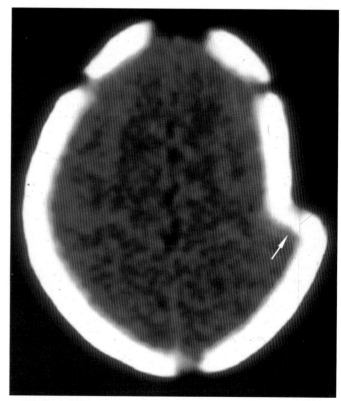

Figure 12.7.52 Depressed skull fracture. Axial CT shows a depressed fracture of the left parietal bone (arrow).

With fractures or traumatic sutural diastasis, it is necessary to look for bleeding both outside the brain and also within the skull, either in the subdural or epidural space. Epidural haemorrhage (Figure 12.7.53) is relatively uncommon, occurring in only 2% of all cases of neonatal haemorrhage observed at autopsy in whom there was increased intracranial pressure. Subdural intracranial haemorrhage, involving primarily the posterior falx and the tentorium,

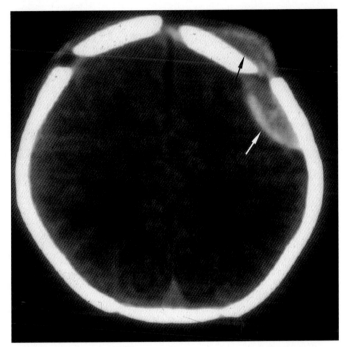

Figure 12.7.53 Acute epidural haematoma and cephalohaematoma in a 2-day-old male. Axial CT shows increased density bleeds both intra- and extracranially (arrows).

is the most common type of bleeding when there is excessive moulding and vertical elongation of the head in the passage through the birth canal, such as with vaginal vertex deliveries (Figure 12.7.54). Even in normal deliveries, MRI has been able to demonstrate an incidence in the 50% range for small amounts of bleeding along the tentorium and posterior falx. This type of bleeding is usually not associated with parenchymal injury. With more marked elongation of the head, the haemorrhages may become more extensive causing compression of adjacent brain. Pronounced elongation and distortion of the head could cause disruption of veins that drain the cerebellum into the straight sinus and vein of Galen and this could result in a significant haematoma, which could compress the 3rd ventricle and cerebral aqueduct, giving rise to obstructive hydrocephalus. Impedance of venous drainage could lead to intraparenchymal haemorrhage, such as within the cerebellar hemisphere, resulting in a parenchymal brain injury (Figure 12.7.55).

Subdural haematoma can occur in association with forceps delivery, vacuum extraction and cephalopelvic disproportion. Intracerebral haematomas are relatively uncommon. They can occur in association with a bleeding contusion due to focal blunt trauma. Their presentation is associated with seizures and focal motor deficits, depending on their location. The dropping of an infant in the delivery or recovery room, or in the neonatal nursery can result in traumatic injury with fracture and intracerebral contusion/haematoma.

Fetal distress may be the reason for rapid extraction of the infant and in such circumstances, there may be hypoxic ischaemic injury in addition to traumatic lesions (Figure 12.7.56).

FURTHER READING

Harwood-Nash DD, Hendrick EB, Hudson AR. The significance of skull fracture in children: a study of 1,187 patients. Radiology 1971; 101:151.

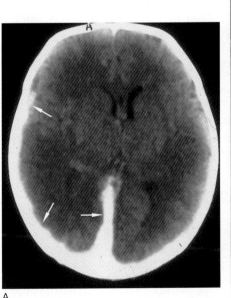
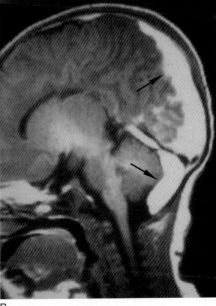
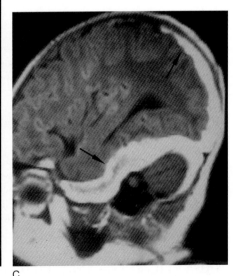

A   B   C

Figure 12.7.54 Acute subdural haemorrhage secondary to traumatic delivery. (A) Axial CT without contrast material shows a right-sided falx based subdural haematoma (arrow) extending laterally (arrows) with mass effect on the right hemisphere. (B and C) Sagittal T1 MRI images show hyperintense subdural haematomas both infra- and supratentorially (arrows).

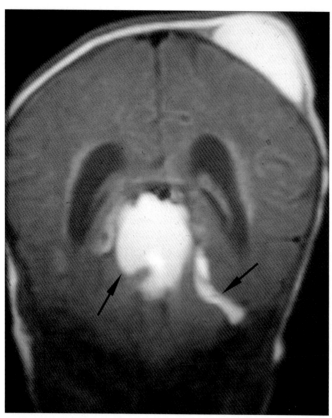

Figure 12.7.55 Cephalohaematoma, cerebellar haematoma and subtentorial subdural haematoma. Coronal T1-WI shows high signal intensity methaemoglobin in a left parietal cephalohaematoma in a subdural haemorrhage along the left tentorium and in a large haematoma that extends into the superior vermis (arrows).

Lindenberg R, Freytag E. Morphology of brain lesions from blunt trauma in early infancy. Archives of Pathology 1969; 87:298.

Takagi T, Nagai R, Wakabayashi S. Extradural haemorrhage in the newborn as a result of birth trauma. Childs Brain 1978; 4:306.

ULTRASOUND

US can show mass effect on the ventricular system from an intraparenchymal haematoma and can show oedema in the brain from hypoxic ischaemic brain injury, depending on the timing of the US examination.

COMPUTED TOMOGRAPHY

CT is the gold standard for the evaluation of the traumatized newborn. CT will show and characterize the extracranial soft tissue injury as well as fractures of the calvarium, the extra-axial haematomas and intraparenchymal brain swelling with ventricular compression, depending on the timing of the examination from the time of the injury (Figures 12.7.51 to 12.7.54A).

MAGNETIC RESONANCE IMAGING

MRI is as valuable as CT – not in detecting a fracture or subarachnoid haemorrhage, which CT does much better, but by

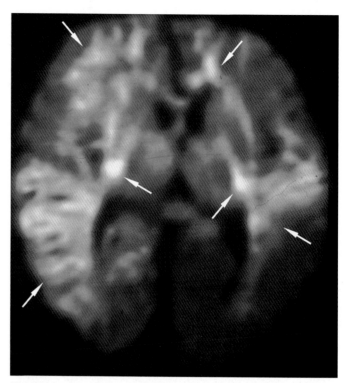

Figure 12.7.56 Hypoxic ischaemic brain injury in a patient who sustained trauma at birth, MRI. Axial diffusion-weighted imaging shows extensive right- and left-sided cortical, subcortical and basal ganglionic restricted diffusion (arrows).

showing the condition of the extracranial soft tissues and showing whether there is haemorrhage or not. MRI is ideal for showing blood products in the subdural space, in demonstrating the intactness or lack thereof of the dural venous sinuses, as well as delineating intracerebral bleeding and characterizing parenchymal injury from hypoxic ischaemia (Figures 12.7.54B to 12.7.56). The combination of T1-WI, T2-WI, diffusion imaging, susceptibility scanning and MRV can provide invaluable information that can lead to prompt and correct management.

FURTHER READING

Govaert P, Vanhaesebrouck P, Depraeter C. Vacuum extraction, bone injury and neonatal subgaleal bleeding. European Journal of Pediatrics 1992; 151:532–535.

Hankins GDV, Leicht T, Van Hook J, Uckan EM. The role of forceps rotation in maternal and neonatal injury. American Journal of Obstetrics and Gynecology 1999; 180:231–234.

SPINAL CORD INJURY

The overall incidence of injury to the spinal cord at the time of birth is unknown. With breech presentations, injury occurs to the lower cervical and upper thoracic spinal cord, while with vertex presentations, the upper to mid cervical spinal cord is most frequently injured. Pathologically, there are haemorrhages and lacerations within the cord, and haemorrhage is present in the epidural and intraspinal space. The mechanism of injury is stretching causing laceration and tears. Vertebral lesions are less frequent and subluxation is possible but are not often shown unless there has been a major distraction. With pulling, the dura may rupture, leading to an audible snap heard in the delivery room. Depending on the location of the spinal cord injury, the resultant changes may be death from lack of respiration (upper cervical cord to brainstem injury), progressive respiratory depression with high cervical cord injury, and hypotonia or flacidity of the lower extremities resulting from lower cervical to upper thoracic cord injury. Accompanying asphyxia with spinal cord injury can either be present as a result of the cord injury with depressed respirations or may be present when an asphyxiated infant has been urgently and traumatically delivered.

FURTHER READING

Grabb PA, Pang D. Magnetic resonance imaging in the evaluation of spinal cord injury without radiographic abnormality in children. Neurosurgery 1994; 35:406–414.

MacKinnon JA, Perlman M, Kirpalani H. Spinal cord injury at birth: diagnostic and prognostic data in twenty-two patients. Journal of Pediatrics 1993; 122:431–437.

Menticoglou SM, Perlman M, Manning FA. High cervical spinal cord injury in neonates delivered with forceps: report of 15 cases. Obstetrics and Gynecology 1995; 86:589–594.

Rossitch E, Oakes WJ. Perinatal spinal cord injury: clinical, radiographic and pathologic features. Pediatric Neurosurgery 1992; 18:149–152.

PLAIN RADIOGRAPHS

Plain radiographs are used to identify distraction or subluxation of one vertebra relative to another (Figure 12.7.57). Because of the ligamentous laxity in infants of this age, significant cord injury can exist, with normal spinal radiographs. Of the x-rays performed, a well-centred and exposed lateral is the most critical.

COMPUTED TOMOGRAPHY

CT is used to look for fractures, subluxations and distractions of the cervical spine. With good-quality CT, it may be possible to demonstrate blood within the spinal canal, an indication of traumatic bleeding. Adequate visualization of the spinal cord is usually not possible with CT, without the use of intrathecal contrast.

MAGNETIC RESONANCE IMAGING

MRI is the best modality for evaluation of the spine when a traumatic lesion is suspected. It will provide information as to the intactness of the cervical cord, the presence of ligamentous injury and whether there is abnormal alignment of vertebral bodies due to distraction or subluxation. Sagittal and axial T1-WI and T2-WI are used. Susceptibility scanning can be useful with sagittal imaging in showing blood products within the cord (Figure 12.7.58B). Acutely, cord swelling is demonstrated on the T2-WI as high signal intensity (Figure 12.7.58A). Blood products are most often seen acutely as low signal intensity on T2-WI. With passage of time, over the ensuing weeks, the cord at the site of

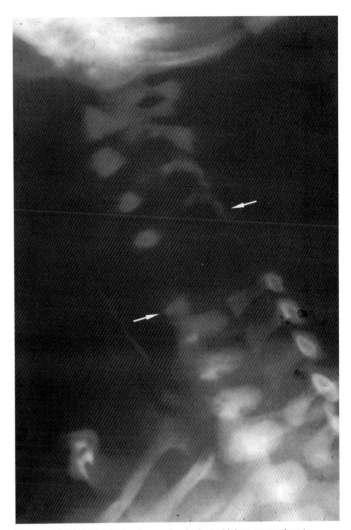

Figure 12.7.57 Cervical spine and spinal cord injury secondary to traumatic delivery, plain films. Oblique lateral cervical spine radiograph shows marked distraction of C4 from C5 vertebra (arrows).

injury shrinks and becomes focally atrophic (Figure 12.7.58C–D). There may be only small areas of hypointensity on T1-WI and increased signal on T2-WI but they may be sufficient to indicate sites of prior injury. Complete trans-section of the cord is unusual.

BRACHIAL PLEXUS INJURY

Brachial plexus injuries are more common than spinal cord injuries by a factor of 10 or more. The incidence is estimated to be about 0.5 per thousand live births, occurring primarily in term infants. The injuries involve nerve roots that supply the brachial plexus, rather than the brachial plexus itself. Erb's palsy is the most common form, typically involving C5 and C6 nerve roots with deficit in the proximal upper extremity. C5 and C6 nerve roots unite to form the upper trunk of the brachial plexus. Klumpke's palsy usually involves the C8 and T1 nerve roots, which form the lower trunk of the brachial plexus. Only 10% of the brachial plexus palsies are of the Klumpke's type. The aetiology of the injury appears to be traction with stretching of the roots anchored at the

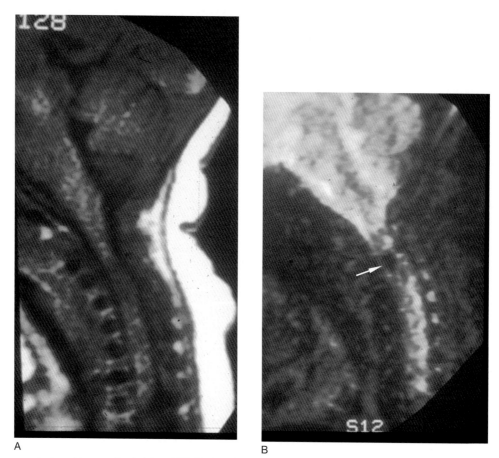

Figure 12.7.58 Upper cervical cord haemorrhagic injury, MRI. Sagittal (A) T1 image and (B) susceptibility scan 1 day following birth show upper cervical cord swelling with a focal area of haemorrhage demonstrated on the susceptibility scan (arrow).

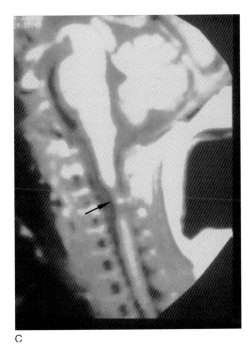 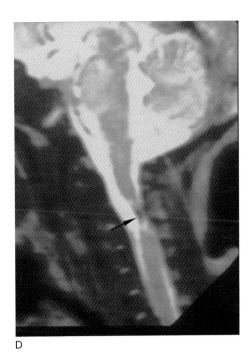

C   D

Figure 12.7.58 *continued* (C and D) Follow-up examination 6 weeks later shows cord atrophy with residual hypointensity indicating the site of blood products (arrow) shown on the T2 image (D).

cervical spine and spinal cord. Traction is usually applied to the head or shoulder and occurs in both vertex and breech presentations. Large fetal size and abnormal presentation are factors, as is shoulder dystocia.

Radiographic evaluation with plain films and CT is usually normal. MRI has the best sensitivity, demonstrating the presence of pseudomeningoceles at the site of the avulsed nerve roots, with fluid-filled pouches seen on T2-weighted coronal, sagittal and axial images (Figure 12.7.59).

FURTHER READING

Gudinchet F, Maeder P, Oberson JC, Schnyder P. Magnetic resonance imaging of the shoulder in children with brachial plexus birth palsy. Pediatric Radiology 1995; 25 (Suppl 1):S125–128.

Miller SF, Glasier CM, Griebel ML, Boop FA. Brachial plexopathy in infants after traumatic delivery: evaluation with MR imaging. Radiology 1993; 189:481–484.

Molnar GE. Brachial plexus injury in the newborn infant. Pediatric Review 1984; 6:110–115.

Nocon JJ, McKenzie KD, Thomas LF, Hansell RS. Shoulder dystocia: an analysis of risks and obstetric maneuvers. American Journal of Obstetrics and Gynecology 1993; 168:1732–1739.

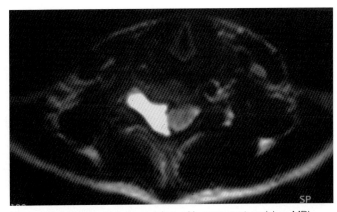

Figure 12.7.59 Brachial plexus injury with nerve root avulsion, MRI. Axial T2-WI shows a fluid collection in the right C7–T1 neural foramen at the site of the nerve root avulsion.

HYPOGLYCAEMIA

In the newborn infant, hypoglycaemic blood level is defined as one below 30 mg/dl blood glucose level and in the preterm infant as a level below 20 mg/dl. Whether or not these represent the threshold for injury to the brain in the newborn is unknown. While hypoglycaemia can be a factor in an asphyxiated infant, it is often less clearcut as to its role in an ensuing brain injury. Hypoglycaemic brain injury that is more clearcut occurs in the postnatal period, when the infant feeds poorly, and because of decreased oral intake, develops severe hypoglycaemia. Postnatal hypoglycaemic events occur in newborn infants, in the days subsequent to birth, who have hyperinsulinaemia and hypoglycaemia. Prolonged decreased glucose blood levels can lead to injury by affecting neurons and glia. The injury occurs primarily in the cortex and subcortical white matter, and presents as a posterior temporal, parietal occipital injury.

ULTRASOUND

Through the anterior fontanelle, the area of interest, the posterior, temporal, parietal and occipital lobes are not well visualized. Ultrasound tends to miss the injury associated with hypoglycaemia.

COMPUTED TOMOGRAPHY

The manifestation of hypoglycaemic brain injury on CT is decreased density in the cortex and subadjacent white matter of the posterior supratentorial brain, in the posterior temporal and parietal occipital regions. There is focal brain swelling with mass effect acutely, seen 24 h or more after the onset of injury, resulting eventually in atrophy of the involved structures with loss of cortex and white matter. The occipital horns may become enlarged with atrophy.

MAGNETIC RESONANCE IMAGING

Magnetic resonance imaging, with diffusion, can show restricted motion of water at the site of injury relatively early during the acute stage of insult (Figure 12.7.60). On T2-weighted images, the cortex is too bright and the differentiation between white and grey matter is lost (Figure 12.7.60). Focal posterior brain swelling is seen. In addition to the injury to the posterior portion of the brain, in a lesser number of cases, damage to the globus pallidus has been seen.

FURTHER READING

Anderson JM, Milner RDG, Strich SJ. Effects of neonatal hypoglycaemia on the nervous system: a pathological study. Journal of Neurology, Neurosurgery and Psychiatry 1967; 30:295.

Barkovich AJ, Ali FA, Rowley HA. Imaging patterns of neonatal hypoglycaemia. American Journal of Neuroradiology 1998; 19:523–528.

Cornblath M, Hawdon JM, Williams AF. Controversies regarding definition of neonatal hypoglycaemia: suggested operational thresholds. Pediatrics 2000; 105:1141–1145.

Cornblath M, Schwartz R, Aynsley-Green A. Hypoglycaemia in infancy: the need for a rational definition. Pediatrics 1990; 85:834–837.

Kinnala A, Rikalainen H, Lapinleimu H. Cerebral magnetic resonance imaging and ultrasonography findings after neonatal hypoglycaemia. Pediatrics 1999; 103:724–729.

Spar JA, Lewine JD, Orrison WW. Neonatal hypoglycaemia: CT and MR findings. American Journal of Neuroradiology 1994; 15:1477–1478.

Traill Z, Squier M, Anslow P. Brain imaging in neonatal hypoglycaemia. Archives of Disease in Childhood and Fetal Neonatal Education 1998; 79:F145–F147.

KERNICTERUS

Elevation of unconjugated bilirubin, as a result of a haemolytic process, such as can occur with Rh incompatibility or due to the breakdown of a collection of blood in the scalp or intracranially can lead to the risk of neurotoxicity from the unconjugated biliru-

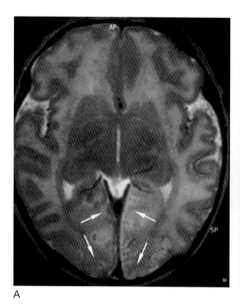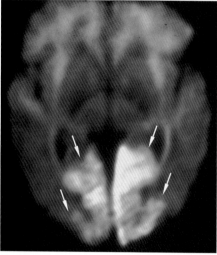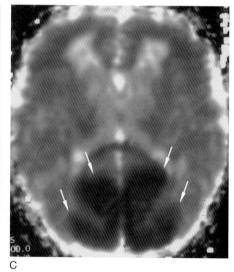

Figure 12.7.60 Hypoglycaemic brain injury, 3 days postbirth, MRI. (A) Axial T2-WI shows bilateral loss of normal cortical signal intensity in the temporo-occipital regions (arrows). (B) Axial diffusion images show high signal at the site of injury (arrows). (C) Axial ADC map shows decreased signal at site of restriction of motion of water molecules (arrows).

bin. This was a more significant problem in the past when Rh incompatibility was a problem. However, in recent years, with very rapid discharge of the newborn from the hospital, the kernicterus has reappeared as a problem.

The normal physiological breakdown of blood, which results in elevation of bilirubin levels, can be seen in term infants in the first 5 days up to a level of 6 mg/dl. In premature infants, this may go as high as 10–12 mg/dl. The elevated bilirubin can persist in the premature infant for a longer period of time, up to 3–4 weeks. The danger of marked elevation of unconjugated bilirubin is its toxicity to the neurons, which produces permanent damage. This appears to be due to the selective susceptibility of specific neurons to this type of toxicity. The neurons that are affected are primarily those in the globus pallidus, subthalamic nucleus and hippocampus. Damage can occur to cranial nerve nuclei that involve cranial nerve 3, the vestibular and cochlear nerves, the facial nerve, the reticular system within the pons, the inferior olivary nuclei and the dentate nucleus in the cerebellum. The anterior horn cells in the spinal cord can also be involved. Early on there is neuronal swelling, followed by dissolution at the end of the first week, with later mineralization and astroglial proliferation. The treatment is phototherapy in the early stage before the bilirubin level is too elevated. Once it has reached the range of 20–25 mg/dl, then treatment is by exchange transfusion.

MAGNETIC RESONANCE IMAGING

On MRI, T1-weighted images can show abnormal early increased signal intensity at the site of injury within the globus pallidus in comparison to age-matched normal patients. Follow-up studies, conducted weeks to months later, will show eventual atrophy of the globus pallidus, with persistent abnormal increased signal intensity on T2-weighted images (Figure 12.7.61). So far, there are no reports of series of patients with kernicterus that have been studied by diffusion imaging. Ultrasound and CT are unrewarding.

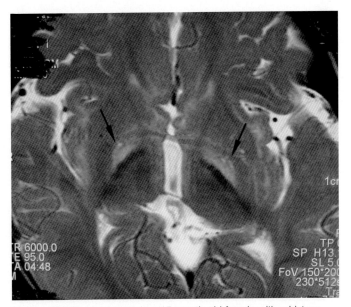

Figure 12.7.61 Kernicterus in a 15-month-old female with a history of perinatal hyperbilirubinaemia, MRI. Axial T2-WI shows abnormal increased signal intensity in the globus pallidi bilaterally (arrows).

FURTHER READING

Bratlid D. How bilirubin gets into the brain. Clinical Perinatology 1990; 17:449–465.

Harris MC, Bernbaum JC, Polin JR. Developmental follow-up of breast-fed term infants with bilirubin brain injury: resolution of clinical signs. Pediatric Research 1998; 43:217A.

Martich-Kriss V, Kollias SS, Ball WS Jr. MR findings in kernicterus. American Journal of Neuroradiology 1995; 16 (Suppl 4):819–821.

Penn AA, Enzmann DR, Hahn JS. Kernicterus in a full-term infant. Pediatrics 1994; 93:1003–1006.

Wiley CC, Lai N, Hill C. Nursery practices and detection of jaundice after newborn discharge. Archives of Pediatric and Adolescent Medicine 1998; 152:972–975.

Yokochi K. Magnetic resonance imaging in children with kernicterus. Acta Paediatrica 1995; 84:937–939.

FOCAL INFARCTION IN AN ARTERIAL VASCULAR TERRITORY

The imaging demonstration of an acute infarction in the middle cerebral artery (MCA) territory during the postpartum period is not a very rare event. Nor is the discovery of a previously clinically unrecognized old infarct in a vascular territory a rare event in the infant during the first year of life. Infarctions do occur in neonates and infants and may be evidenced acutely by the presence of seizures, or may remain asymptomatic until, with further development, signs such as fisting of the hand or paresis of an extremity become evident. Autopsy data from infants reveal a 5.4% incidence of arterial occlusions that result in strokes. The incidence of infarcts increases from prematurity to term. Of the acute infarctions in a vascular territory diagnosed by imaging, 90% are unilateral, while 10% are bilateral. The vast majority are unilateral middle cerebral artery (MCA) infarcts, 75% occurring in the left MCA. Multiple possible aetiologies exist for these infarcts. Infarctions can be caused by emboli or thrombus from placental fragments associated with placental infarction. Clots related to involution of placental vessels or formed in the umbilical vein can be sources of emboli that pass from the venous circulation through the foramen ovale of the fetal heart to the brachiocephalic vessels and into the brain. The direction of flow appears to be into the left common carotid artery. The exact reason for this is uncertain.

A second aetiology for occlusion of the MCA is abnormality of blood volume and coagulability. With polycythaemia there is a possibility of sludging of blood flow and thrombosis. Genetic coagulation abnormalities, such as protein C and S deficiencies, antiphospholipid antibodies, and factor 5 Leiden mutation, all may come to play a role in producing thrombosis, either in the umbilical venous circulation, which can act as a source of emboli, or in the internal carotid/middle cerebral artery circulation. The abnormalities of coagulation may not be those inherent to the fetus but those that develop in the mother who is under the stress of the pregnancy, and who then transmits the abnormality through the placenta to the fetus. Other aetiologies of vascular occlusion include vasospasm, such as can occur with the use of cocaine by the mother during the time of fetal development. Vasospasm may also accompany marked subarachnoid haemorrhage that results from trauma at the time of birth. Vascular distortion, such as can occur with extremes of rotation or extension during the delivery process, may be another source of vascular injury and occlusion. However, despite the multiple aetiologies outlined above, in some cases the cause is not found and they remain idiopathic. In general, infarctions within arterial vascular territories do not correlate to more global deprivation of oxygen with hypoxia or deprivation of flow with ischaemia from hypotension. While both hypoxic ischaemic insult and embolism or thrombosis might occur in the same patient, producing both types of injury, that occurrence appears to be infrequent. It should be noted that with the emergence of fetal MRI and fetal diffusion imaging, acute infarctions in the middle cerebral artery vascular territory have been diagnosed *in utero*, thus proving that these infarctions can occur before birth.

ULTRASOUND

On US, acute infarctions present as hyperechoic zones within the vascular territory (Figure 12.7.62). If large enough, they may have mass effect on the ventricles, producing a shift. Some infarcts are haemorrhagic but US may not detect the blood. With US it is difficult to differentiate a bland from a haemorrhagic infarct. Transcranial Doppler offers the possibility of demonstrating the vascular occlusion at the site of the MCA or ICA. A small percentage of infarcts are in the distribution of the posterior cerebral artery and may not be readily apparent on US, as this area can be missed on US.

COMPUTED TOMOGRAPHY

Computed tomography is the most common technique used to diagnose focal vascular infarctions of the newborn. The infarcts are recognized 24 h or more after their onset. They are seen as a loss in density of the cortex, and as hypodensity involving both grey and white matter within the vascular distribution (Figure 12.7.4). Occasionally, high density can be seen in the proximal

MCA or internal carotid artery at the site of the thrombus or placental embolus. Placental emboli may contain calcifications. The infarcts behave in a fashion similar to the changes seen in a hypoxic ischaemic brain, except that they are at the site of the tissue distal to the vascular occlusion. Swelling with mass effect will occur in infarcts that are large enough, the swelling peaking at about 72 h after the onset. Resolution of the mass effect takes approximately 6–7 days. Following oedema, calcification at the site of infarction is not an unusual phenomena in the neonate. This may be mistaken for haemorrhage because of the high density within the cortex. MRI is the way to distinguish between the calcification and haemorrhage: by using a 2D FLASH susceptibility scan, the haemorrhage will 'blossom', becoming markedly hypointense, whereas the calcification may be relatively invisible. There may be more than one site of infarction/ischaemia with multiple emboli. If the area is ischaemic, follow-up studies may show resolution of the changes seen initially after insult. Contrast enhancement of the infarcted tissue starts 3–5 days after the insult and lasts for a period of up to a number of weeks. Eventually, the infarcted tissue is reabsorbed, resulting in multicystic encephalomalacia. Many of the late presenting cases, towards the end of the first year of life, are found on imaging to have such areas of cystic encephalomalacia (Figure 12.7.63). There is often not a clear history as to when the infarct occurred.

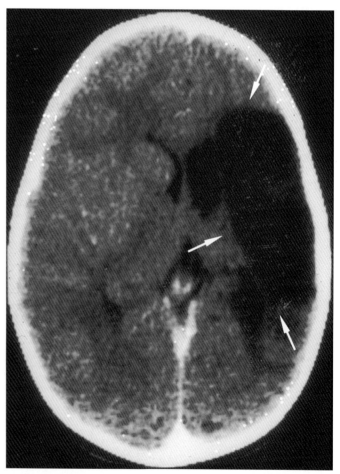

Figure 12.7.63 Chronic infarction of the left middle cerebral artery, CT. Axial CT shows hypodensity (arrows) involving the left MCA territory with enlargement of the frontal horn of the left lateral ventricle and reduction in size of the left cerebral hemisphere.

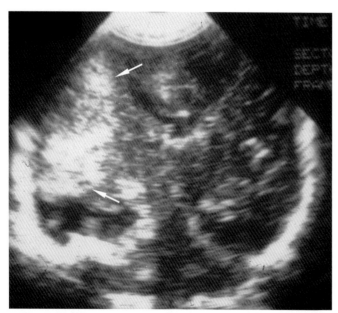

Figure 12.7.62 Acute middle cerebral artery infarction, US examination. Coronal image shows hyperechoic changes (arrows) in the territory of the right middle cerebral artery.

MAGNETIC RESONANCE IMAGING/ MR ANGIOGRAPHY

Magnetic resonance imaging is the procedure of choice for the evaluation of the acute, subacute and chronic arterial vascular territory infarction. With the watery infant brain, recognition of the loss of definition of the cortical grey matter's hypointensity is initially difficult and takes time following the onset of infarction (Figure 12.7.64A). Whether or not it is 24 hours, remains to be resolved. The difficulty in recognition and the time of detection is different from that seen in the older child, adolescent and adult when myelination has occurred and the brain is less watery. Diffusion imaging, demonstrating acute cytotoxic oedema, is the most sensitive sequence and shows the earliest manifestation, even before the T2-weighted images become positive. Restriction of the motion of water at B1000 produces hyperintense signal on the diffusion image, which is present in the x-, y- and z-gradient direction, and on the ADC map the area is markedly hypointense, with measurement revealing low values for diffusion coefficient (Figure 12.7.64B). Comparison of the ADC values from one side of the brain to the other side is usually sufficient, as there is often unilateral involvement. However, when bilateral diffuse disease is present, the cerebellum of the posterior fossa can be utilized and normative values can be used.

The presence of blood products, either in the thrombosed MCA or in the brain tissue, associated with reperfusion after breakup of an embolus, can be demonstrated by the use of various pulse sequences including T1-WI, T2-WI and gradient echo 2D FLASH susceptibility scanning (Figure 12.7.65). Also, the B0 EPI diffusion image can be used for its susceptibility to show blood products. Mass effect on the adjacent sulci and ventricular system is well demonstrated on coronal and axial T2-weighted MRI. Contrast enhancement occurs at the site of infarction, 3–5 days after onset, and lasts for a number of weeks. MR angiography may be utilized during the acute phase, for demonstration of occlusion or stenosis or decreased flow within the affected MCA and/or internal carotid artery (Figure 12.7.12). With recanalization of the vessel later on, there may be no evidence of an embolus on follow-up months to years afterwards. During the second week postinfarction, the diffusion-weighted imaging will become less positive, normalizing, and then showing increased motion of water molecules as encephalomalacia and cystic changes develop at the site of infarction (Figure 12.7.66). MRI with T2-WI and diffusion sequence is the best method of demonstrating whether there is more than one area of infarction, and in demonstrating whether or not there is also the presence of HIE.

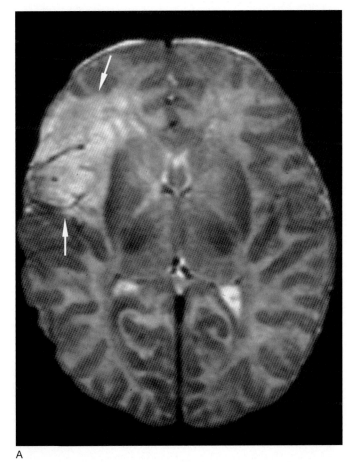

A

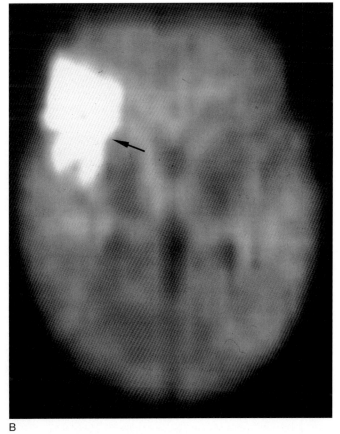

B

Figure 12.7.64 Acute infarction of the anterior division of the right middle cerebral artery in a 4-day-old female, MRI. (A) Axial T2-WI shows loss of cortical signal and increased signal intensity at the site of the infarction (arrows). (B) Axial diffusion image shows hyperintense signal at the site of restricted motion of water (arrow).

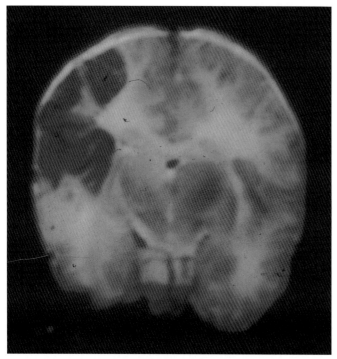

Figure 12.7.65 Haemorrhagic middle cerebral artery infarction, MRI. Coronal T2-WI shows hypointense blood products at the site of right MCA embolic infarction with reperfusion.

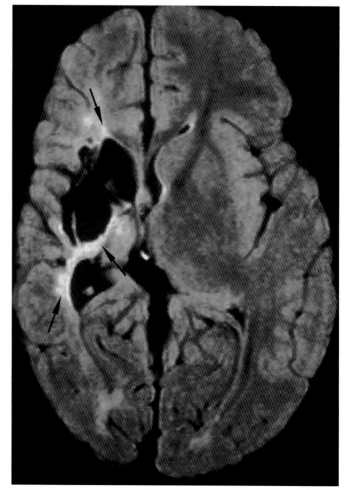

Figure 12.7.66 Cystic encephalomalacia at the site of a chronic old right MCA infarct, MRI. Axial FLAIR image shows hypointensity within the fluid-filled cystic encephalomalacic spaces, which are surrounded by hyperintense gliotic tissue (arrows).

FURTHER READING

Amato M, Huppi P, Herschkowitz N, Huber P. Prenatal stroke suggested by intrauterine ultrasound and confirmed by magnetic resonance imaging. Neuropediatrics 1991; 22:100–102.

Baram TZ, Butler IJ, Nelson MD Jr, McArdle CB. Transverse sinus thrombosis in newborns: clinical and magnetic resonance imaging findings. Annals of Neurology 1988; 24:792–794.

Barmada MA, Moossy J, Shuman RM. Cerebral infarcts with arterial occlusion in neonates. Annals of Neurology 1979; 6:495–502.

Bode H, Strassburg HM, Pringsheim W, Kunzer W. Cerebral infarction in term neonates: diagnosis by cerebral ultrasound. Childs Nervous System 1986; 2:195–199.

Cowan FM, Pennock JM, Hanrahan JD, Manji KP, Edwards AD. Early detection of cerebral infarction and hypoxic ischaemic encephalopathy in neonates using diffusion-weighted magnetic resonance imaging. Neuropediatrics 1994; 25:172–175.

deVeber G, Monagle P, Chan A. Prothrombotic disorders in infants and children with cerebral thromboembolism. Archives of Neurology 1998; 55:1539–1543.

de Vries LS, Groenendaal F, Eken P. Infarcts in the vascular distribution of the middle cerebral artery in preterm and fullterm infants. Neuropediatrics 1997; 28:88–96.

Fujimoto S, Yokochi K, Togari H. Neonatal cerebral infarction: symptoms, CT findings and prognosis. Brain Development 1992; 14:48–52.

Gould RJ, Black K, Pavlakis SG. Neonatal cerebral arterial thrombosis: protein C deficiency. Journal of Child Neurology 1996; 11:250–251.

Hernanz-Schulman M, Cohen W, Genieser NB. Sonography of cerebral infarction in infancy. American Journal of Roentgenology 1988; 150:897–902.

Krishnamoorthy KS, Soman TB, Takeoka M, Schaefer PW. Diffusion-weighted imaging in neonatal cerebral infarction: clinical utility and follow-up. Journal of Child Neurology 2000; 15:592–602.

Mercuri E, Rutherford M, Cowan F. Early prognostic indicators of outcome in infants with neonatal cerebral infarction; a clinical, electroencephalogram, and magnetic resonance imaging study. Pediatrics 1999; 103:103–139.

Pegelow CH, Ledford M, Young JN, Zilleruelo G. Severe protein S deficiency in a newborn. Pediatrics 1992; 89:674–676.

Pellicer A, Cabanas F, Garciaalix A. Stroke in neonates with cardiac right-to-left shunt. Brain Development 1992; 14:381–385.

Rorke LB. Anatomical features of the developing brain implicated in pathogenesis of hypoxic-ischaemic injury. Brain Pathology 1992; 2:211–221.

Smith CD, Baumann RJ. Clinical features and magnetic resonance imaging in congenital and childhood stroke. Journal of Child Neurology 1991; 6:263–272.

Thorarensen O, Ryan S, Hunter J, Younkin DP. Factor V Leiden mutation: an unrecognized cause of hemiplegic cerebral palsy, neonatal stroke, and placental thrombosis. Annals of Neurology 1997; 42:372–375.

Varelas PN, Sleight BJ, Rinder HM. Stroke in a neonate heterozygous for factor V Leiden. Pediatric Neurology 1998; 18:262–264.

Wong VK, LeMesurier J, Franceschini R. Cerebral venous thrombosis as a cause of neonatal seizures. Pediatric Neurology 1987; 3:235–237.

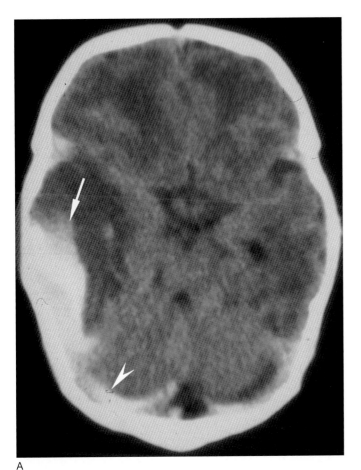

A

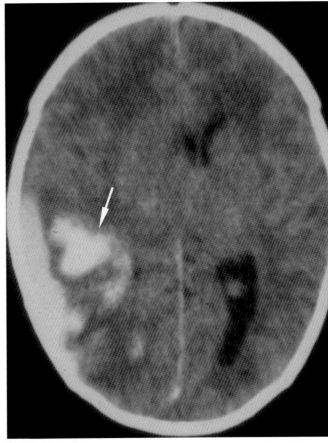

B

Figure 12.7.67 Acute haemorrhagic infarction secondary to venous thrombosis, CT. (A and B) Axial non-contrast enhanced CTs show acute haemorrhage in the right temporal lobe (arrow). Thrombus is present in the right transverse venous sinus (arrowhead) and straight sinus. Significant mass effect is being exerted on the right lateral ventricle and there is a shift of the midline of the brain to the left side.

VENOUS INFARCTION

Occlusion of the dural venous sinuses and/or deep cerebral veins is unusual at the time of birth and does not typically present as a pattern of infarction that could be mistaken for an arterial vascular distribution such as the MCA. Demonstration of clot as high signal intensity on T1-WI and/or T2-WI within the affected veins, and the absence of flow on MRV performed with phase contrast or 2D T2 time of flight (when there is no increased signal on T1-WI due to methaemoglobin), are usually sufficient for diagnosis of venous occlusive disease. Most cases of venous occlusive disease in neonates occur during the weeks after birth, when dehydration can develop secondary to hyperosmotic load when infant formula milk is incorrectly mixed, or due to loss of fluids with diarrhoea or lack of oral intake of fluids. Venous occlusion can also occur in conjunction with coagulation disorders and coagulation problems associated with sepsis. Infarcts due to venous occlusion differ from the arterial territorial infarcts and depend on whether there is a cortical vein thrombosis or a generalized occlusion of the superficial and/or deep venous territorial drainage. There is a tendency for venous infarcts to be haemorrhagic (Figure 12.7.67). With obstruc-

tion of the major dural venous sinuses, problems with significant swelling of the brain due to lack of venous drainage can occur. With deep venous thrombosis of the internal cerebral veins, vein of Galen and straight sinus oedema and/or infarction in the thalami is not uncommon.

FURTHER READING

Baram TZ, Butler IJ, Nelson MD Jr, McArdle CB. Transverse sinus thrombosis in newborns: clinical and magnetic resonance imaging findings. Annals of Neurology 1988; 24:792–794.

Govaert P, Achten E, Vanhaesebrouck P, De Praeter C, Van Damme J. Deep cerebral venous thrombosis in thalamo-ventricular haemorrhage of the term newborn. Pediatric Radiology 1992; 22:123–127.

Hanigan WC, Tracy PT, Tadros WS, Wright RM. Neonatal cerebral venous thrombosis. Pediatric Neuroscience 1988; 14:177–183.

Konishi Y, Kuriyama M, Sudo M. Superior sagittal sinus thrombosis in neonates. Pediatric Neurology 1987; 3:222–225.

Rivkin MJ, Anderson ML, Kaye EM. Neonatal idiopathic cerebral venous thrombosis: An unrecognized cause of transient seizures or lethargy. Annals of Neurology 1992; 32:51–56.

Shevell MI, Silver K, O'Gorman AM. Neonatal dural sinus thrombosis. Pediatric Neurology 1989; 5:161–165.

Wong VK, LeMesurier J, Franceschini R. Cerebral venous thrombosis as a cause of neonatal seizures. Pediatric Neurology 1987; 3:235–237.

Cranial and Spinal Ultrasound of the Newborn Infant

Gillian Cattell, Josephine M McHugo

INTRODUCTION

The introduction of cranial ultrasound in 1978 was an important step forward in the monitoring and understanding of the pathogenesis of the lesions associated with prematurity that lead to mortality and neurodevelopmental morbidity. Since the early reports there have been huge improvements in equipment that have given better insights into the lesions. Cranial ultrasound is now routine and has become an established and integral part of the monitoring and care of preterm babies and term babies who are at risk for intracerebral complications or who exhibit clinical symptoms. Most infant cranial ultrasound is concerned with the pathology associated with prematurity and hypoxic ischaemic encephalopathy but cranial malformations may be initially identified by ultrasound either pre- or postnatally. Ultrasound is also the technique used to monitor the progress of posthaemorrhagic hydrocephalus in these infants, being supplemented by computed tomography (CT) or magnetic resonance imaging (MRI) as clinically indicated.

The identification of structural deficits is important for the immediate and future care of the child, facilitates critical clinical management decisions and enables parents to be given important information about prognosis. Cranial ultrasound has therefore become an established and integral part of neonatal care and in the main is performed in sick infants in the incubator but can safely be carried out in stable children in the ultrasound department.

The anterior fontanelle provides an acoustic window to the infant brain and is easily accessible in the smallest and sickest infants who are most at risk of haemorrhagic and ischaemic injury (Figure 12.8.1). Access can also be obtained through patent sutures and the posterior fontanelle, but with a more limited field of view. Although there are no proven deleterious effects associated with ultrasound the ALARA (*as low as reasonably achievable*) principle should be adhered to as best practice. This is particularly applicable in cranial ultrasound where there is a persistent tissue/bone interface with the increased risk of heating. As with all ultrasound examinations however the highest risks are those associated with the competency of the operator to perform the exam, and to record and interpret the results accurately and in a timely fashion.

EQUIPMENT AND TRAINING

Optimal diagnostic images require high resolution equipment with a small footprint phased array or sector probe suitable to access the smallest fontanelle. Most modern ultrasound machines now have multifocus probes (5–12 mHz) but the minimum requirements are 5 mHz for the term infant and 7 mHz for the more premature. A small footprint linear probe is also useful for assessing the pericortical areas and the dural sinuses. It is important that the operator is familiar with their equipment and uses standard settings where possible to enable comparison of subtle echotexture changes to be observed. Most imaging diagnosis is made using real-time 2D imaging but advanced imaging techniques include both pulsed and colour flow Doppler.

Multiple focal zones with an adequate frame rate and colour/pulsed wave Doppler are also essential tools for these imaging techniques. The potential of 3D ultrasonography in neonatal neurosonography is more recently described and may further improve the demonstration of the vasculature and the anatomy.

Competency is paramount and appropriate supervised training is essential for safe practice. It is inappropriate to attempt a diagnosis without these skills.

ARCHIVING AND DOCUMENTATION

Serial imaging requires a good archiving system for diagnostic purposes, audit, teaching and training. Modern equipment enables digital images to be taken and is the preferred method for long-term storage. Thermal images are useful for inclusion in the patient notes but have a short shelf life and poor resolution for diagnostic purposes. Increasingly, real-time video images are also appropriate allowing retrospective viewing when unexpected pathology is diagnosed weeks or months after birth.

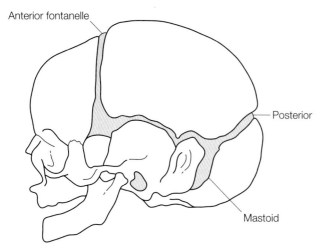

Figure 12.8.1 Sutures. Diagram of the skull demonstrating the position of the anterior fontanelle, the posterior fontanelle and the mastoid suture.

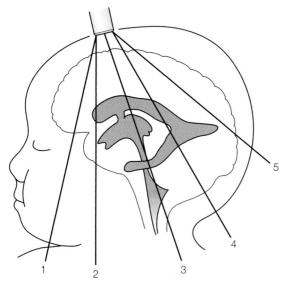

Figure 12.8.2 Diagram of coronal sections: (1) anterior to frontal horns; (2) through anterior horns at level of sylvian fissure; (3) at level of intraventricular foramen and 3rd ventricle; (4) through posterior horns to include choroid plexus; and (5) superior to the lateral ventricles through the parenchyma.

TECHNICAL STANDARDS

Standard hygiene procedures for handling infants should be applied. These include handwashing and cleaning of the probe with an alcohol-based wipe before and after each exam. A probe cover is appropriate for infected babies. Liaison with neonatal nurses will ensure optimal timing of scans to fit with nursing care and their advice must be taken if the infant develops complications during the procedure. Attention must be given to the pressure applied to the fontanelle as intracranial pressure can be easily raised in the smallest and sickest infants and may result in bradycardias. Immobilization of the infant's head will aid the operator to achieve a

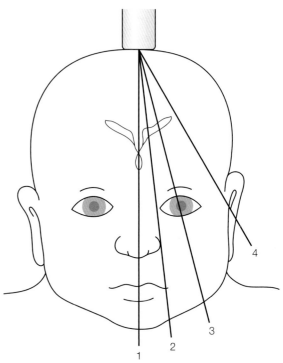

Figure 12.8.3 Diagram of sagittal sections: (1) midline through 3rd ventricle, cavum and 4th ventricle; (2) medial to each ventricle to include caudothalamic groove; (3) through each lateral ventricle to include frontal, occipital and temporal horns; and (4) lateral to each ventricle to include frontal and parietal parenchyma.

good examination. Care should be taken of ventilator/CPAP tubing and hats, which may limit access.

ORIENTATION AND TECHNIQUE

A consistent approach to image production is required to facilitate serial comparisons. Views should be taken in a minimum of two planes with orientation standardized to comply with similar views taken at MRI or CT exams with the right of the head on the left of the screen for coronal images and the nose to the left of the image for sagittal views. Care should be taken in probe frequency selection as there is a trade-off between resolution and penetration, but should be the highest that is clinically appropriate. Representative views can then be imaged by appropriate angulation of the probe through the anterior fontanelle. Standard sagittal and coronal views should be taken at every examination with supplemental views as required to image abnormal areas (Figures 12.8.2 and 12.8.3; Tables 12.8.1 and 12.8.2).

Normal appearances at the varying section levels are demonstrated in Figure 12.8.4.

VENTRICULAR INDEX

It is necessary to have a means of assessing progressive ventricular enlargement and the best recognized of these is the ventricular index (Figure 12.8.5).

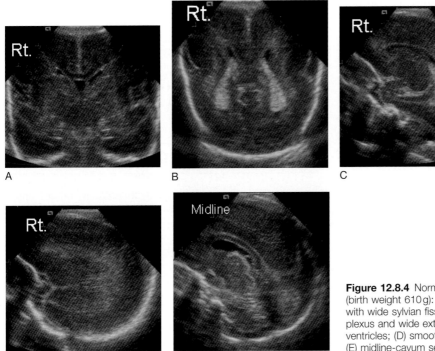

A   B   C

D   E

Figure 12.8.4 Normal appearances at 23+ weeks' gestation at age 7 h (birth weight 610 g): (A) coronal – narrow frontal horns and 3rd ventricle with wide sylvian fissure; (B) narrow posterior horns filled by choroid plexus and wide extracortical space; (C) parasagittal – narrow lateral ventricles; (D) smooth parenchyma with no sulci/gyri seen; (E) midline-cavum septum pellucidum is seen inferior to the corpus callosum and superior to the 3rd ventricle.

Table 12.8.1 Coronal

1. Anterior to the frontal horns of the lateral ventricles
2. At the level of the anterior horns and the sylvian fissure
3. At the level of the 3rd ventricle and intraventricular foramen to include the thalami
4. At the posterior horns to include the choroid plexi
5. Posterior/superior to the lateral ventricles (parenchyma)

Table 12.8.2 Sagittal

1. Midline through the 3rd ventricle, cavum septum pellucidum and cerebellum to include the 4th ventricle and foramen magnum
2. Medial to each ventricle to include the caudo-thalamic groove
3. Through each lateral ventricle to include frontal, occipital and temporal horns
4. Lateral to each ventricle to include frontal and parietal white matter

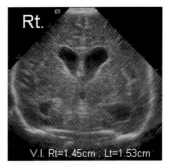

Figure 12.8.5 Ventricular index – 35 weeks, birth weight 2200 g. On day 18 the ventricles were found to be unchanged in size since transfer from another hospital on day 9. No evidence seen of IVH. Ventriculomegaly of unknown cause. In coronal section at the level of intraventricular foramen, the frontal horns and 3rd ventricle. Two measurements taken from each lateral ventricular wall to the midline.

The measurement is a linear measurement from the falx to the outer limit of the lateral ventricle on the coronal view at the level of the third ventricle. The validity of the measurement is based on an original cohort of 273 preterm infants and is recognized as the best measurement for the purpose. It has the disadvantage that it can only be used if there is no midline shift, as such a change makes any sequential measurements meaningless. Ventriculomegaly has been defined by some as 4 mm above the 97th centile for the patient age.

CHALLENGES

The size of the acoustic window is the limiting factor to the quality of achievable images with angulation of the probe being restricted by overriding sutures and a small very anteriorly placed fontanelle. The use of supplemental views using the posterior fontanelle and the mastoid approach may aid diagnosis in technically difficult examinations. Access through any of the sutures is possible but difficult to interpret without constant practice. Oblique views may also help in the diagnosis of more peripheral pathology suspected on standard views. The use of colour flow and pulsed wave Doppler may give additional information in cases of suspected ischaemia and vascular malformations.

DOPPLER ULTRASOUND

Imaging the vascular physiology in real time using colour Doppler aids the diagnosis and prognosis of many disease processes in the infant brain. As a research tool it has revolutionized the understanding of both normal and abnormal haemodynamics of the developing fetal and infant brain.

Perfusion of the infant brain is very dynamic and using colour Doppler it is possible to assess this in real time in the neonatal intensive care unit. However, the exact role of cerebral Doppler ultrasound in clinical practice has yet to be fully established. It is now widely used in routine practice in Europe but is less commonly used in the UK.

Using colour Doppler cranial ultrasound it has been established that the immature infant is unable to autoregulate arterial flow resulting in marked hyperperfusion following a period of hypotension or hypoxia. It is this hyperperfusion that results in some of the severe intracerebral damage seen in the neonate with long-term sequelae.

TECHNIQUE

Using the anterior fontanelle it is possible to image the anterior and middle cerebral arteries and their larger branches as well as the venous drainage. A trans temporal approach allows visualization of the vein of Galen and the terminal veins if these are not visualized via the anterior fontanelle. A posterior approach using the posterior fontanelle will enable visualization of the posterior cerebral arteries and branches and the distal basilar and internal carotid arteries. Whatever the approach, the image should be electronically magnified to the area of interest to enhance the colour sensitivity with the colour gain set to maximize the flow signal and minimize the background noise. Low flow should be assessed by setting the band pass filter to the lowest possible setting. The goal of colour imaging is to show not only the major arteries and veins but more importantly to colour map the smaller branch vessels.

Once the vessels have been identified then Doppler interrogation of the waveform is performed. Spectral analysis should include both blood velocities and resistive index. There is a progressive increase in both the peak systolic and end diastolic flow from 30 weeks gestational age to 8 months post term (Table 12.8.3).

Assessment of blood velocities is preferred to resistive indices (RI) as RI in the first month of life can be misleading as low flow, which is abnormal, may result in a RI that is in the normal range.

Table 12.8.3 Arterial velocities (cm/s)

		32 weeks	40 weeks	6 months
Anterior cerebral artery	PSV	43.1	52.9	91.2
	EDV	9.6	13.2	34.2
	TAV	21.9	28.7	59.7
Basilar artery	PSV	37.6	54.2	84.3
	EDV	8.2	13.0	31.3
	TAV	19.6	28.9	52.5
Internal carotid artery	PSV	43.3	60.0	92.1
	EDV	9.7	13.7	31.6
	TAV	22.2	31.9	59.2

PSV, peak systolic velocities; EDV, end diastolic velocities; TAV, time averaged velocities.
Reproduced from Couture A, Veyrac C, Baud C, Saguintaah M, Ferran J L. Advanced cranial ultrasound transfontanellar Doppler imaging in neonates. European Radiology 2001; 11:2399–2410.

VENOUS FLOW

Two patterns of normal venous flow are seen:

- sinusoidal (low amplitude flow) is seen in larger vessels, e.g. sagittal sinus and the vein of Galen; and
- monophasic (continuous flow) is seen in the smaller vessels.

ROLE OF DOPPLER IN INFANTS

There is increasing evidence of a potential role of colour Doppler in the following clinical situations, both in identifying those at risk as well as in established disease:

1. intraventricular haemorrhage;
2. hydrocephalus;
3. anoxic – ischaemic damage;
4. venous thrombosis; and
5. congenital malformations.

It must, however, be remembered that Doppler velocities in individual vessels represent the haemodynamic situation only at the time of scanning. Abnormal results have predictive or prognostic value. The pathophysiology of cerebral circulation is very dynamic being affected not only by brain pathology but also by non-intracranial factors such as transducer pressure, cardiac output, cardiac rhythm and the presence of arterial shunts, e.g. patent ductus arteriosus.

Venous thrombosis most commonly occurs in the sagittal sinus and vein of Galen, both of which can be directly visualized in the neonate. In agenesis of the corpus callosum, either complete or partial, the position of the pericallosal artery is diagnostic, whereas complex venous flow in cystic spaces posterior to the third ventricle is diagnostic of a vein of Galen aneurysm.

Therefore, using colour mapping to define the position of the vessels and measurements of velocities for haemodynamic assessment in addition to 2D ultrasound it is possible to further define normal and abnormal in the sick neonate.

TIMING OF EXAMINATIONS

The timing and frequency of examinations is dependent on locally available resources. However, many clinically silent problems can be missed without appropriate protocols for routine examination. Little published data is available but the following protocols are suggested as a minimum standard. Preterm infants, especially those with a birth weight of less then 1000 g, are accepted as being at high risk for both germinal matrix and intraventricular haemorrhage (IVH), which commonly occurs within 72 h of birth. Therefore, all infants born before 33 completed weeks' gestation should have a routine scan before day 7. Regardless of normality on the initial scan, further examination during the second week of life and again at 28 days and/or prior to discharge will facilitate the diagnosis of most significant pathology. Indeed, in one observational study, approximately 30% of infants had a previously unsuspected abnormal predischarge examination and 12% of these were severe

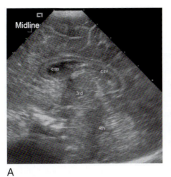 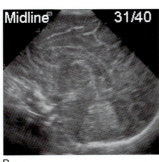 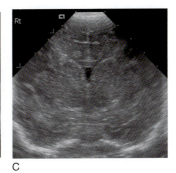

A   B   C

Figure 12.8.6 Cavum septum pellucidum and vergae. Midline fluid-filled space seen in all premature infants. Variable size and rate of closure through the gestations. Closure occurs posteroanteriorly with the vergae closing early in many cases. Twins born at 31 weeks' gestation, imaged on days 35 and 37. (A) Closure of vergae. (B) Almost complete closure of cavum septum pellucidum. (C) Image of a term child who has diffuse, widespread increased parenchymal echogenicity with loss of gyral/sulcal delineation. The ventricles are compressed. The persistent cavum septum pellucidum is seen in the midline on this coronal image.

abnormalities. If there is any suspicion of IVH or increased parenchymal echogenicity, appropriate follow-up is useful with timing governed by the clinical course as many cases of PVL will present late. Routine postnatal scans should also be considered for infants of all gestational ages born as a result of high-risk pregnancies, e.g. monochorionic twinning. Antenatal scans even in the hands of experienced fetal medicine teams may miss significant pathology, usually because of limitations of suitable access to the fetal head *in utero*. High-risk pregnancies include mothers with significant coagulopathy and prolonged rupture of membranes.

NORMAL APPEARANCES

An understanding of normal brain development is crucial to the accurate diagnosis of common pathology. What is normal at the limits of viability is abnormal at term, with many variables in between.

At 24 weeks' gestation the brain is smooth in appearance with only major sulci present. The longitudinal fissure, insula and extra-cortical spaces are markedly widened between 24 and 27 weeks but become increasingly less so with advancing gestational age. Gyral formation is again variable but starts from about 28 weeks and is easily demonstrated in sagittal views. From 32 to 35 weeks medial and lateral gyri become increasingly more prominent with the typical "cobblestone" appearance at term.

The cavum septum pellucidum is a fluid-filled space in the midline inferior to the corpus callosum and is present in all structurally normal preterm infants but varies considerably in size and appearance. Closure of the cavum occurs from the posterior aspect (vergae) at a variable rate towards term, with the body narrowing before the vergae closes completely. This may result in the appearance of apparent thickened septations and should not be confused with the finer septations associated with infective processes. Absence/closure of the cavum in the very preterm is always associated with structural abnormalities but is normal in most term infants (Figure 12.8.6). The cavum septum pellucidum has disappeared by 2 months of age in 85% of all infants.

The lateral ventricles are comma shaped, with walls that are smooth in outline and lie anteriorly close to the midline but more

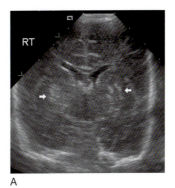 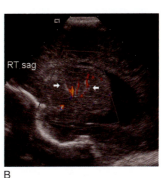

A   B

Figure 12.8.7 Lenticular striate echodensities. Linear echodensities that follow the path of the striate arteries and are of no known clinical significance. These commonly become apparent with increasing gestational age in the preterm infant. (A) Coronal: linear echodensities lateral to the thalami. (B) Parasagittal: echodensities following the pathway of the striate arteries demonstrated with colour Doppler.

posteriorly are angled towards the cortex due to the impingement of the parieto-occipital sulcus. Ventricular size can vary considerably within the normal spectrum but in general preterm infants have fuller ventricles than at term when they are usually slit-like anteriorly. Asymmetry of the ventricles can also be within the normal spectrum but care should be taken to note head position on serial scans to confirm gravity-dependent normality.

NORMAL VARIANTS

The choroid plexus extends from the temporal horn anteriorly to the foramen of Monro where it extends caudally into the 3rd and 4th ventricles. The caudate thalamic groove marks the anterior extension of the choroid plexus in the lateral ventricles. Any high signal anterior to this represents haemorrhage. Normal appearances vary with gestational age and the size of the ventricles. Irregularities in echogenicity and outline can be within the normal spectrum in the older infant but in the preterm may be indicative of adherent blood clot and may be a marker for early IVH. In the

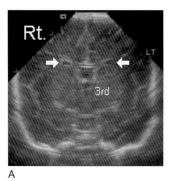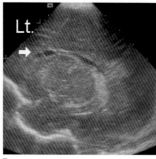

A   B

Figure 12.8.8 Frontal horn thin-walled cysts. One of di-chorionic twins of different sexes born at 30 weeks' gestation both having similar appearances – no known clinical significance. Septated fluid-filled structures lying inferior and lateral to the narrow frontal horns. Seen bilaterally on first routine scan and persisted on scan prior to discharge. (A) Coronal: fluid-filled pear-shaped structures seen bilaterally inferior to the frontal horns. (B) Parasagittal: septated elongated fluid-filled structure lying immediately lateral to the frontal horn and difficult to demonstrate as separate to it in all cases.

preterm infant, thin echogenic lines radiating out along the arterial pathways of the striate arteries anterior to the thalamus are often seen and are a clinically benign finding (Figure 12.8.7). Also said to be benign are thin-walled frontal horn cysts lying immediately adjacent to the anterior horn of the lateral ventricles and must not be confused with periventricular leucomalacia (Figure 12.8.8).

CHOROID PLEXUS CYSTS

Choroid plexus cysts are recognized in about 1% of pregnancies and have been seen in up to 3% of newborns. Whilst some of the antenatally diagnosed cases are associated with chromosome anomalies (most notably trisomy 18) the postnatally persistent ones are often unchanged and are of no clinical importance.

Cysts have been described as causing ventricular dilatation by obstructing the foramen of Munro. Large cysts (>2 cm) are sometimes associated with symptoms.

Subependymal cysts have sometimes been confused with choroid plexus cysts but can usually be identified by their specific situation at the junction of the ventricle and the choroids, whereas the choroid plexus cysts can lie anywhere within the choroid plexa.

ABNORMALITIES

The developing fetal and neonatal brain responds differently to hypoxia depending on the gestational age of the insult and the resulting injuries show very different ultrasound appearances. The aetiology of the injuries are thought to be on the basis of localized or generalized ischaemia. Autoregulation is easily compromised in the premature neonate and relative hypoperfusion of the brain is common. Haemorrhagic lesions may arise from the vascular bed of the germinal matrix and extend into the ventricular system but may also occur into ischaemic areas of cerebral white matter. Historically, haemorrhage was graded 1–4 to reflect the clinical implications of the diagnosis, however this is no longer thought to be

useful by many as it excludes certain types of haemorrhage and is seen not to fit the pathophysiology of both haemorrhagic and ischaemic lesions. Classification should therefore be by common easily described ultrasound appearances.

Ventriculomegaly is defined as an increase in the dimension of the ventricular system above the normal range. Where there is a subjective suspicion of dilatation the ventricular index should be recorded (Figure 12.8.5). It is vital to differentiate obstructive and progressive hydrocephalus that is appropriate for ventricular shunting to relieve the raised pressure from non-obstructive hydrocephalus that will not respond to surgical intervention. In order to differentiate these two conditions, serial scans are essential to differentiate obstructive from non-obstructive hydrocephalus. In obstructive hydrocephalus, there will be progressive increase in the ventricular dilatation associated with an increase in the head circumference and fullness and tension in the anterior fontanelle in response to the increased intracranial pressure. Ventriculomegaly can also occur secondary to cerebral atrophy (ex vaccuo) and neural tissue loss with normal intracranial pressures.

Injuries in the immature brain are to the periventricular area with sparing of the subcortical white matter and cerebral cortex. After 34–36 weeks of gestation the pattern of ischaemic injury changes and the areas at most risk are in the subcortical white matter and cerebral cortex at the watershed regions of arterial supply. Not only is the maturity of the brain important in the injury following a hypotensive episode but also the duration of that injury – severe anoxia of longer than 10–15 min results in damage that is limited initially to the thalami, hippocampus and adjacent regions. Prolonged insult results in damage to the superior vermis optic radiations and calcarine cortex. If the anoxia is further prolonged then all the grey matter is damaged; this type of injury typically occurs after 25–30 min.

BRAIN INJURY IN THE PRETERM INFANT

Hypoperfusion in the immature infant is followed by a period of hyperperfusion as the vascular autoregulatory mechanisms are underdeveloped in the immature brain. This hyperperfusion, particularly in the presence of increased venous pressure, results in rupture of the capillaries and parenchymal haemorrhage. Haemorrhage in the preterm infant is most common in the germinal matrix. The germinal zones are most active from 8 to 28 weeks of gestation and after this the activity and therefore the vascularity decreases. Germinal matrix haemorrhage is uncommon after 34 weeks. Choroid plexus bleeds are also common at this gestation and are often seen in association with germinal matrix haemorrhage (Figures 12.8.9 to 12.8.11).

Periventricular leucomalacia is the ischaemic parenchymal lesion typically seen in the deep white matter adjacent to the lateral ventricles. These lesions typically show evolution over time and this differentiates them from echodensities that show no progression and subsequent resolution. These transient periventricular echodensities probably represent transient oedema. PVL lesions show evolution over time with ultimately cavitation and cystic formation once liquefaction of the necrotic white matter has occurred (Figures 12.8.12 and 12.8.13). Cavitation occurs 2–6 weeks after

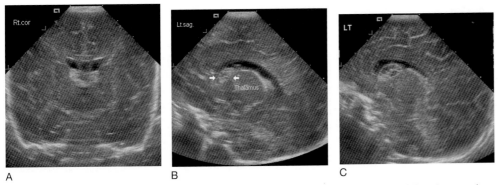

Figure 12.8.9 Germinal matrix haemorrhage in an infant born at 30 weeks' gestation. (A) Day 4: coronal section demonstrating bilateral germinal matrix echo densities inferior to the ventricle and anterior to the intraventricular foramen and superior to the 3rd ventricle. (B) Day 17: sagittal section demonstrating the caudothalamic groove. Subtle cystic components. (C) Day 45: multiple cystic components – haemorrhage resolving.

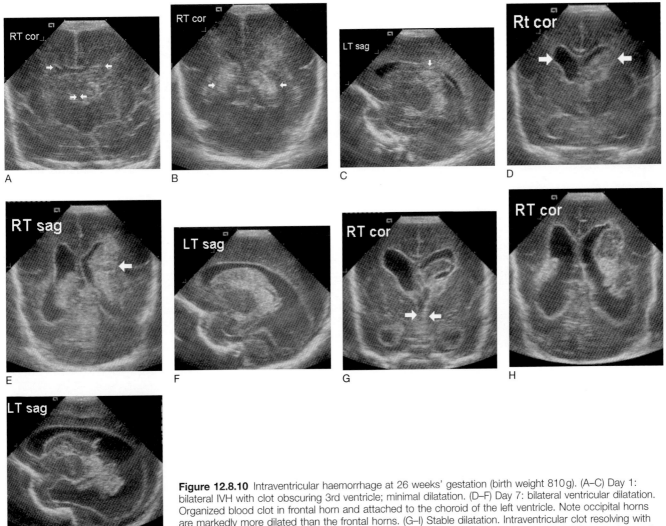

Figure 12.8.10 Intraventricular haemorrhage at 26 weeks' gestation (birth weight 810 g). (A–C) Day 1: bilateral IVH with clot obscuring 3rd ventricle; minimal dilatation. (D–F) Day 7: bilateral ventricular dilatation. Organized blood clot in frontal horn and attached to the choroid of the left ventricle. Note occipital horns are markedly more dilated than the frontal horns. (G–I) Stable dilatation. Intraventricular clot resolving with no further dilatation. Note hyperechogenicity of the ventricular walls. At discharge, ventricles were increasing in size along the centiles.

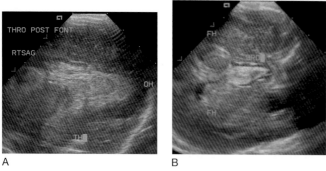

Figure 12.8.11 Alternative views: 28 weeks' gestation (birth weight 1225 g). Day 1: small bilateral IVH (no dilatation). Day 2: clinical suspicion of further bleed. It was difficult to demonstrate the extent of the haemorrhage through the small anterior fontanelle. Further views demonstrated extensive clot throughout the ventricular system. (A) Sagittal view through the posterior fontanelle (B) Axial view through the mastoid suture. OH, occipital horn; TH, temporal horn; FH, frontal horn; 3ʳᵈ, third ventricle.

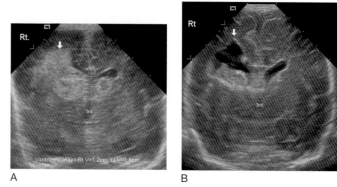

Figure 12.8.12 Porencephalic cyst. First of twins born at 28 weeks' gestation with a birth weight of 1300 g. (A) Day 3: coronal – bilateral intraventricular haemorrhage with adjacent right frontal white matter haemorrhage. Cavum septum pellucidum compressed and not seen due to raised intraventricular pressure. Day 31: resolving haemorrhage. Day 62: small communication with ventricle seen. (B) Out-patient follow-up at 6 months showed a large porencephalic cyst.

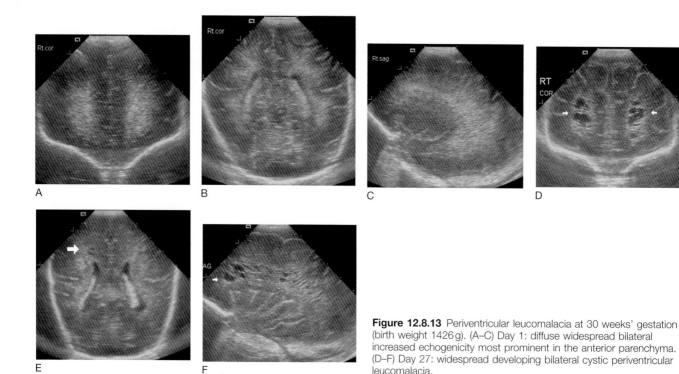

Figure 12.8.13 Periventricular leucomalacia at 30 weeks' gestation (birth weight 1426 g). (A–C) Day 1: diffuse widespread bilateral increased echogenicity most prominent in the anterior parenchyma. (D–F) Day 27: widespread developing bilateral cystic periventricular leucomalacia.

the injury (typically < 3 weeks) and this is an important issue in the timing of the ischaemic insult. Cavitation may communicate with the ventricle and cause an irregular outline.

SEVERE ISCHAEMIC LESIONS IN THE PRETERM INFANT

Severe and prolonged hypotension or cardiac arrest show a different pattern of cerebral injury in the immature neonate. In this situation, there is injury to the deep grey matter nuclei and the brainstem. These are the areas that are most developed and there-

fore have the highest metabolic rate making them most susceptible to ischaemic injury. Initially, the ultrasound finding will be normal followed by increased echodensities in the basal ganglia and thalami, by day 2–3.

Ischaemic lesions are most common in the very preterm in the periventricular white matter. The most vulnerable areas are the zones at the end of the arteries, which are most prone to hypoperfusion and ischaemia. The resultant ultrasound appearances are typically 'fan-shaped' areas of increased echogenicity and occur typically lateral to the anterior horns of the ventricles whilst increased echogenicity in the more posterior periventricular region is often described as a 'flare'. It is the persistence of this echogenicity over time that is the predictor of outcome. Transient flares are

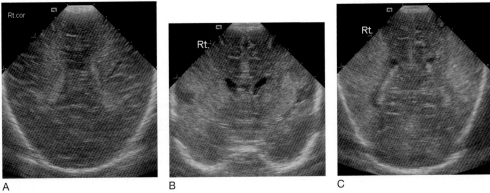

Figure 12.8.14 Hypoxic ischaemic encephalopathy (HIE). Term infant with a history of seizures. (A) Day 1: diffuse widespread minimally increased parenchymal echogenicity with some loss of gyral/sulcal delineation. Narrow lateral ventricles. Note persistent cavum septum pellucidum. (B,C) Day 12: widespread increased echogenicity of the parenchymal white matter with sparing of the sylvian fissures and medial structures. Lateral ventricles are demonstrated better.

difficult to interpret clinically without consistent serial scans to monitor the ultrasound changes, but those that do persist are markers for periventricular leucomalacia, with the cystic changes usually evident from 10 days after the ischaemic event. On serial scans the ultrasound appearances are progressive and initially appear as areas of irregular echogenicity that become more homogeneous over time before discrete echopenic areas develop. However, as some 'flares' are transient this stage can be missed in between scans and in the absence of serial scans a predischarge examination should be performed for all infants born before 33 weeks of completed gestation. Ischaemic lesions can also occur in the subcortical regions and can be difficult to diagnose on routine views. Oblique or angled coronal views are helpful here to interpret findings. Less commonly, the thalami and basal ganglia can be involved.

POSTHAEMORRHAGIC HYDROCEPHALUS

This is a complication of ischaemic injury of the newborn and is in part due to arachnoiditis but also may result from fibrosis in areas of brain destruction. On ultrasound, multiple fibrous strands are seen in the ventricles, often making the ventricle multilocular. These are easier to appreciate with ultrasound than CT. Choroid plexus may become wrapped around an intraventricular catheter and lead to shunt malfunction. This too is easily appreciated with ultrasound.

INJURY TO THE TERM INFANT

Diffuse cerebral oedema is manifested by generalized loss of grey–white matter interfaces, a small ventricular system and loss of the normal appearances of the sulci relating to generalized cerebral oedema (Figure 12.8.14). It is vital that all the technical factors are correctly set while performing the ultrasound in order that the generalized increase in echodensities can be appreciated. However,

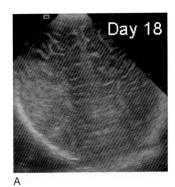
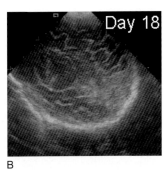

Figure 12.8.15 MCA infarct in a term infant requiring ventilation. Days 2 and 5: US appearances within normal spectrum. Day 9: diffuse echogenicity. Day 18: well-delineated irregular echogenicity. Day 23: decreased echogenicity. Normal appearances at out-patient follow-up. (A) Day 18: coronal. (B) Day 18: sagittal.

outcome cannot be predicted on the basis of ultrasound alone. Hypoxic-ischaemic injury to the infant after 32–34 weeks' gestation results in a different pattern of injury. At this gestation the brain is most susceptible to injury at the boundaries between the anterior and middle cerebral arteries and the middle and posterior cerebral arteries. The ultrasound findings are increased echogenicity by day 2–3 followed in the more severe cases by discrete cystic changes that correspond to the arterial boundaries (Figure 12.8.15).

The origins and timing of neonatal encephalopathy in term infants remain obscure in many cases, but most infants present in the first 1–3 days of life with abnormal neurological signs and/or seizures, subsequent to perinatal asphyxia, with late onset seizures suggestive of meningitis or hypocalcaemia. Hypoxic ischaemic encephalopathy stages 2 and 3 that persist for more than 7 days is associated with neurological impairment and death. There is associated ex vacuo dilatation of the adjacent lateral ventricles.

CONGENITAL ABNORMALITIES

The rapid increase in the use of antenatal ultrasound both as a screening and diagnostic tool means that a considerable number of structural intracranial abnormalities can now be identified antenatally.

The full extent of the abnormality is often unknown prior to delivery. This is particularly true of abnormalities of the cerebral cortex that are difficult to image in the late third trimester due to the fetal head position being low in the pelvis or the increasing ossification of the cranial vault bones. Transvaginal scanning can improve the definition but significant abnormalities, particularly of migration disorders, are usually not apparent prenatally or in the neonatal period. Following delivery ultrasound forms an important part of the initial investigation of these infants. However, MRI is more accurate and often a complete diagnosis is not possible until an age at which myelination should have been completed.

Agenesis of the corpus callosum is amenable to antenatal diagnosis and the postnatal ultrasound findings are classical of this abnormality (Figure 12.8.16). Associated migration disorders, however, require MRI also to define.

In Dandy–Walker syndrome there is hypoplasia or agenesis of the vermis of the cerebellum associated with a posterior fossa cyst that communicates directly with the 4th ventricle. There may be associated dilatation of the third and lateral ventricle (Figure 12.8.17). Imaging the posterior fossa in the term infant is difficult and the transparietal or posterior fontanelle approach may be helpful. Again, the complete anatomical abnormalities will require additional imaging.

SPINAL ULTRASOUND

Ultrasound of the spinal cord is feasible before the spinal arches ossify as the cord in the neonate and infant is a relatively superficial structure. It is a useful screening tool but if abnormalities are detected, most infants will require MRI for delineation of the full extent of the lesion.

TECHNIQUE

The incompletely ossified neural arches provide an acoustic window. The infant is placed prone with a folded nappy or small pillow under the abdomen to induce slight kyphosis, which separates the spinous processes and enhances the access. The probe is placed initially over the midline and then parallel to it but slightly lateral to determine the best view. A linear array high frequency probe gives the best images in neonates. Scans are obtained in the longitudinal and transverse planes carefully annotating the level of the scan in relation to the vertebral body. The whole cord from the cervical region distally may be thus examined.

NORMAL APPEARANCES

The spinal cord is seen as a hypoechoic central tubular structure with parallel echogenic walls (Figure 12.8.18). It tapers distally as

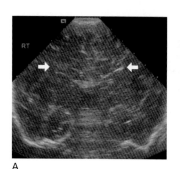
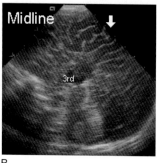

A   B

Figure 12.8.16 Postnatal follow-up of term infant with antenatally diagnosed agenesis of the corpus callosum. (A) Coronal: widely spaced frontal horns with absence of the normal characteristic = superior to the 3rd ventricle. Colpocephaly of posterior horns (not shown). (B) Sagittal: corpus callosum not seen. Note abnormal gyral figuration (Probst bundles) seen radiating from the normal anatomical position of the corpus callosum superior and posterior to the 3rd ventricle.

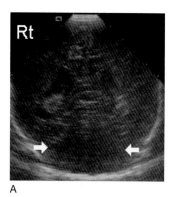
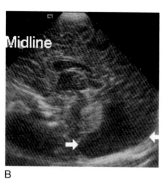

A   B

Figure 12.8.17 Posterior fossa. Term infant with no antenatal care requiring ventilation from birth. Routine scan on day 1. Subsequent chromosomal analysis diagnosed trisomy 18. (A) Coronal: poorly demonstrated fluid-filled posterior fossa. (B) Sagittal midline: normally placed corpus callosum, cavum and 3rd ventricle with large posterior fossa and small cerebellum.

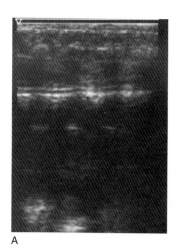
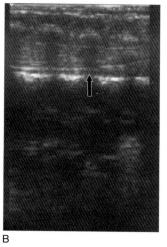

A   B

Figure 12.8.18 Ultrasound images in the sagittal plane of the spinal cord (A) at the lower thoracic level and (B) at L2 extending towards the sacrum. Note the typical appearances of the normal cord, the hypoechoic central tubular structure within parallel echogenic walls. In (B) the tapering of the cord distally is shown. The arrow marks the normal dura.

it becomes the conus at the level between the lower border of T12 and the lower border of L1. The conus is continuous with the echogenic filum, which can be traced into the sacral canal. The filum is echogenic as it is fibrous. It is surrounded by the echogenic nerve roots. Pulsation is seen in the normal cord, which is vascular. The cord also moves in a longitudinal plane with flexion of the neck. The dura is an echogenic linear structure that lies parallel to the cord. Between this and the cord is the hypoechoic arachnoid fluid. The ventriculus terminalis, which is a normal cystic dilatation of the lower cord, may sometimes be seen and should not be confused with a syrinx. The epidural veins can be seen with Doppler ultrasound.

INDICATIONS FOR NEONATAL SPINAL ULTRASOUND

Spinal cord ultrasound is usually performed in infants who have a neurocutaneous marker that is associated with a tethered cord and sometimes occult dysraphism. It is an inexpensive, non-invasive method of determining the normal location of the conus and excluding a tethered cord, cord malformation such as a syrinx, diastematomyelia (Figure 12.8.19) or diplomyelia.

Though it is possible to examine overt dysraphic lesions with ultrasound, full demonstration of these will require MRI (see Chapter 12.1 for a full description). Neurocutaneous markers for underlying cord pathology include, sacral tufts and dimples, lipomas, haemangiomas over the spinal canal and dorsal dermal sinuses. The latter, which are epithelialized fistulous tracks, also require MRI to demonstrate the extent of the connection between the skin surface and the spinal canal. A patent connection renders the child at risk for meningitis. Both haemangiomas and dorsal dermal sinuses may weep intermittently.

Dorsal dermal sinus tracks appear as hypoechoic connections extending from the skin surface to the canal. They are associated with an intraspinal lipoma, epidermoid or dermoid. The cord is often tethered to these. Lipomas are hyperechoic. The dermoid and epidermoid lesions also have increased signal. MRI is required to demonstrate the full extent of the lesion before surgery.

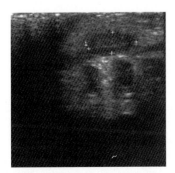

Figure 12.8.19 Transverse section of the cord at the level of diastematomyelia. Note the splitting of the cord. Superficially, there is a small echogenic collection, which represented a haemangioma at the level of the lesion that was in the midthoracic region in this child.

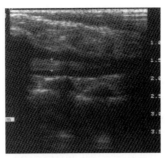

Figure 12.8.20 Tethered cord. Sagittal section at the level of L5. Note the thickened filum secondary to the tethering.

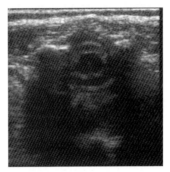

Figure 12.8.21 Sagittal section across the cord at midthoracic level showing a large central cavity due to a syrinx.

TETHERED CORD

Tethering of the cord is a feature of spinal dysraphism (Figure 12.8.20). The cord is tethered to a neural placode within the canal. In covered dysraphism, the cord is also tethered to a placode. In the absence of dysraphism, other lesions associated with cord tethering are a fibrolipoma of the filum or a thickening of the filum terminale, known as a tight filum syndrome. The normal filum is 2 mm or less in diameter. In a tight filum syndrome, the conus is low and the filum thickened. Once suspected, MR should be performed to assess fully. Fibrolipomas of the filum are, as the name implies, fibrofatty aggregations within the filum. They are of variable size and consistency. On sonography they appear as echogenic masses with the filum tethered to them. When the cord is tethered, no matter what the cause is, there is dampening of cord motion.

SYRINX

A syrinx appears as a hypoechoic expansile lesion within the cord (Figure 12.8.21). It may be at any level and, rarely, the whole cord may be involved. It has a high association with Chiari malformations. Both brain and full spinal cord MR imaging will be required in any infant in whom a syrinx is detected on sonography.

FURTHER READING

American College of Radiology. ACR Standard for the performance of the Pediatric Neurosonology examination. Paediatric Neurosonology 1999; 571–573.

Anderson NG, Hay R, Hutchings M, Whitehead M, Darlow B. Posterior fontanelle cranial ultrasound: anatomic and sonographic correlation. Early Human Development 1995; 42:141–152.

British Society of Paediatric Radiologists. Technical Standard for Cranial Ultrasound. Guidelines section BSPR website http://www.bspr.org.uk 2003.

Carteaux P, Cohen H, Check J et al. Evaluation and development of potentially better practices for the prevention of brain hemorrhage and ischemic injury in very low birth weight infants. Pediatrics 2003; 111:489–496.

Clinical Safety Statement for Diagnostic Ultrasound. European Federation of Societies for Ultrasound in Medicine and Biology 2002.

Coley BD, Siegel MJ. Spinal ultrasonography. In: Pediatric sonography, 3rd edn. Philadelphia: Lippincott, Williams & Wilkins; 2002:673–699.

Couture A, Veyrac C, Baud C, Sagiuintaah M, Ferran JL. Advanced cranial ultrasound: transfontanellar Doppler imaging in neonates. European Radiology 2001; 11:2399-2410.

Cowan F, Rutherford M, Groenendaal F et al. Origin and timing of brain lesions in term infants with neonatal encephalopathy. Lancet 2003; 361:713–714.

de Vries LS, Eken P, Groenendaal F et al. Antenatal onset of haemorrhagic and/or ischaemic lesions in preterm infants. prevalence and associated obstetric variables. Archives of Diseases in Childhood 1998; 78:F51–F56.

di Salvo D. A new view of the neonatal brain: Clinical utility of supplemental neurologic US imaging windows. Radiographics 2001; 21:943–955.

Fetus and Newborn Committee, Canadian Paediatric Society. Routine screening cranial ultrasound examinations for the prediction of long term neurodevelopmental outcomes in preterm infants. Pediatrics and Child Health 2001; 6:39–43.

Goetz MC, Gretebeck RJ, Oh KS, Hermansen MC. Incidence, timing and follow-up of periventricular leukomalacia. American Journal Perinatology. 1995; 12:325–327.

Higham J, Crawford S. In: Carty H, Greenwich, eds. Paediatric ultrasound. London: Medical Media; 2001.

Levene M. Measurement of the growth of the lateral ventricles in preterm infants with real-time ultrasound. Archives of Diseases in Childhood 1981; 56:900–904.

Luna JA, Goldstein RB. Sonographic visualization of neonatal posterior fossa abnormalities through the posterolateral fontanelle. American Journal of Roentgenology 2000; 174:561–567.

Makhoul IR, Eisenstein I, Sujov P et al. Neonatal lenticulostriate vasculopathy: further characterisation. Archives of Diseases in Childhood 2003; 88:F140–F414.

Pal BR, Preston PR, Morgan MEI, Rushton DI, Durbin GM. Frontal horn thin walled cysts in preterm neonates are benign. Archives of Diseases in Childhood 2001; 85:F187–F193.

Papile L, Burstein J, Burstein R, Koffler H. Incidence and evolution of subependymal and intraventricular haemorrhage: a study of infants with birthweights less than 1500 g. Journal of Pediatrics 1978; 92:529–534.

Perlman JM, Rollins N. Surveillance protocol for the detection of intracranial abnormalities in premature neonates. Archives of Pediatrics and Adolescent Medicine 2000; 154:822–826.

Pierrat V, Duquennoy C, van Haastert IC et al. Ultrasound diagnosis and neurodevelopmental outcome of localised and extensive cystic periventricular leucolmalacia. Archives of Diseases in Childhood 2001; 84:F151–F156.

Rennie JM. Neonatal seizures. European Journal of Paediatrics 1997; 156:83–87.

Reynolds PR, Dale RC, Cowan FM. Neonatal cranial ultrasound interpretation: a clinical audit. Archives of Diseases in Childhood 2001; 84:F92–F95.

Riccabona M, Nelson T, Weitzer C, Resch B, Pretorius D. Potential of three-dimensional ultrasound in neonatal and paediatric neurosonography. European Radiology 2003; 13:2082–2093.

Riebel T, Nasir R, Weber K. Choroid plexus cysts: a normal finding on ultrasound. Pediatric Radiology 1992; 22:410–412.

Shaw CM, Alvord EC Jr. Cava septi pellucidi et vergae: their normal and pathological states. Brain 1969; 92:213–214.

Hydrocephalus and Arachnoid Cysts

Dan Greitz, Olof Flodmark

THE PHYSIOLOGY OF CEREBROSPINAL FLUID AND HYDROCEPHALUS

INTRODUCTION

The conventional view on the cerebrospinal fluid (CSF) circulation is that of a bulk flow, from the site of production at the choroid plexus to the site of absorption at the pacchionian granulations (Figure 12.9.1). The driving force of bulk flow is the CSF pressure at the production site being slightly in excess of the pressure at the absorption site (Figure 12.9.2). The CSF bulk flow theory explains hydrocephalus as an imbalance between CSF formation and absorption. An obstruction to the CSF flow, inside or outside the ventricular system, causes obstructive and communicating hydrocephalus, respectively. The intracranial pressure is thought to be dependent on the balance between production and absorption of CSF. This indicates that patients with hydrocephalus should have increased intracranial pressure. The bulk flow theory makes pathophysiology of hydrocephalus both easy to understand and possible to briefly summarize. However, the theory has proven incorrect, mainly because the pacchionian granulations do not exist in small infants and hence it is unlikely that the granulations absorb CSF, when developing at 18 months of age.

The application of the bulk flow theory on hydrocephalus originates from Dandy, who made the first experimental studies on hydrocephalus in 1914. He plugged the aqueduct in dogs and found that the ventricles dilated proximal to the obstruction. This was the first evidence that CSF is produced in the ventricles and that the intraventricular absorption of CSF is less than this production. Although Dandy proved that an intraventricular CSF obstruction causes obstructive hydrocephalus, he recognized that decreased bulk flow across the pacchionian granulations could not cause communicating hydrocephalus. He questioned that the pacchionian granulations absorb CSF and stated that the ventricles should not dilate if there is a CSF blockage at the pacchionian granulations. Such an obstruction cannot cause a higher pressure in the ventricle than in the subarachnoid space but would instead dilate the subarachnoid space (Figure 12.9.2D). By estimating the absorption of an intrathecally injected colour tracer, Dandy pro-

vided compelling evidence that the CSF absorption is a diffuse process occurring everywhere in the capillaries of the subarachnoid space. Since the CSF absorption capacity of the cranial subarachnoid space exceeds the CSF production, he excluded idiopathic communicating hydrocephalus from the bulk flow theory and left this condition unexplained.

Later, O'Connel and Hakim described patients with the clinical syndrome of idiopathic normal pressure hydrocephalus (NPH), i.e. communicating hydrocephalus with normal ventricular pressure. NPH, a condition occurring in the elderly and less commonly in children, is also incompatible with the bulk flow theory. The ventricles should not dilate without an increase of the CSF pressure and the CSF pressure, in turn, should increase at CSF outflow obstructions. Greitz, using flow-sensitive magnetic resonance imaging (MRI) and radionuclide cisternography, rediscovered that the brain capillaries absorb CSF (Figure 12.9.1B,C). Other researchers, using different CSF tracers, have recently verified this. This revised view on the CSF circulation prompts a new explanation for the development of communicating hydrocephalus. Even in 1942, O'Connel correctly postulated that increased CSF pulse pressure in the ventricles, without increase of mean CSF pressure, could cause communicating hydrocephalus. Consequently, modern theories emphasize the importance of vascular pulsations and vascular absorption of CSF for the pathophysiology of communicating hydrocephalus.

DEFINITIONS AND TERMINOLOGY

The word hydrocephalus means abnormal accumulation of fluid in the brain or cranial vault and the term is thus applicable to such disparate conditions as cerebral atrophy and obstruction to flow of cerebrospinal fluid (CSF) due to a blockage of the interventricular foramen of Monro. Hence, any discussion using the term hydrocephalus must include a definition clearly stating the context in which the term is used.

In this chapter, 'hydrocephalus' is used to describe the situation resulting from obstruction to CSF flow within the ventricular system causing accumulation of CSF upstream to the obstruction. Hydrocephalus is also used to describe the condition caused by a disturbance in the hydrodynamic balance within the intracranial cavity, usually known as communicating hydrocephalus.

A

B

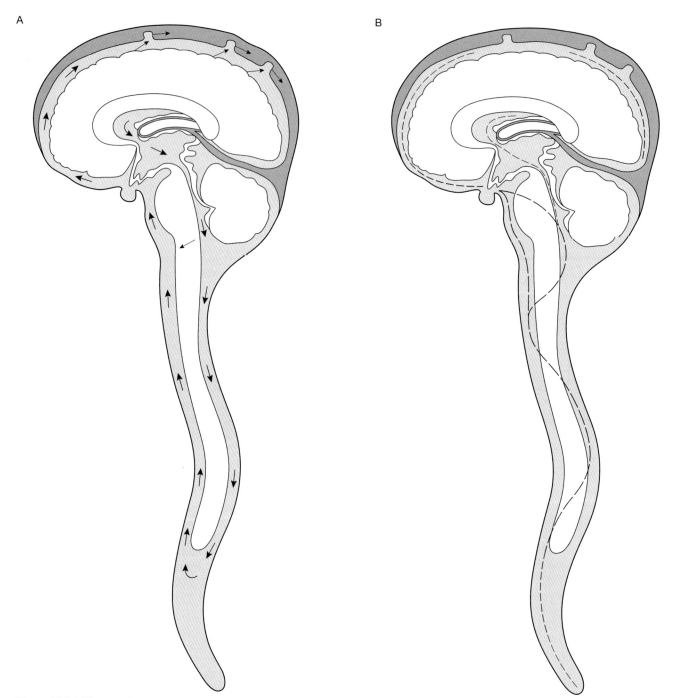

Figure 12.9.1 Diagram showing the bulk flow model (A) and the two types of cerebrospinal fluid circulation related to the revised concept of circulation (B,C). (A) Cerebrospinal fluid is produced in the choroid plexus and is transported by bulk flow to the arachnoid granulations at the venous sinuses where it is absorbed by a valvular mechanism. (B) There is a dominant pulsatile CSF flow, which is responsible for the transport of CSF. The transport of CSF occurs by mixing caused by intracranial arterial pulsations. The length of the segments of the dashed line indicates the magnitude of CSF velocity. There is a fast CSF velocity and transport compartment in the brainstem–cord area and slow CSF velocity and transport compartments in the upper and lower ends of the subarachnoid space. The caudal systolic and the cranial diastolic CSF flows in the spinal canal follow one main channel along the spinal convexities. (C) The minute CSF bulk flows are exaggerated for more clear illustration. The thickness of the arrows is related to the magnitude of bulk flow, which decreases in both directions from the foramen magnum. The cerebrospinal fluid is absorbed everywhere in the central nervous system by the circulating blood. (Reproduced with permission from AJNR 1996; 17:431–438.)

C

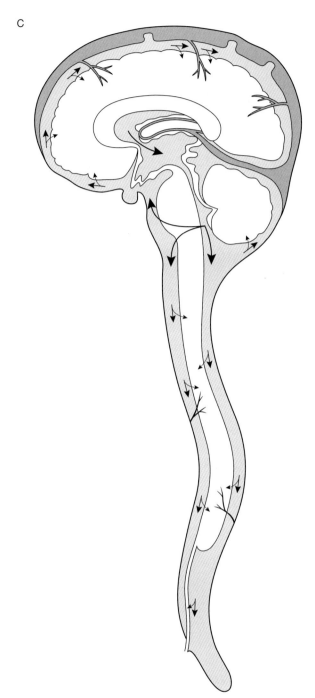

Figure 12.9.1 *Continued.*

NORMAL CSF PHYSIOLOGY AND BRAIN WATER

CSF is produced everywhere in the central nervous system. The main production occurs in the choroid plexus and absorption of CSF occurs in the capillaries of the central nervous system (Figure 12.9.1C). Transport of CSF occurs by vascular pulsations in the subarachnoid space causing rapid mixing of CSF (Figure 12.9.1B). Mixing is a diffuse, random process and the transport of CSF tracers occurs in all directions, down the concentration gradient of the tracer. Although there are intraventricular pulsations causing mixing of CSF, the unidirectional bulk flow from the ventricles to the subarachnoid space dominates the flow of CSF in the ventricles. The main purpose of the CSF is to protect the brain from mechanical damage and serve as a cushion for the brain. The immersion of the brain into a liquid reduces its weight substantially (97%) and CSF dampens the effects of intra- and extracranial forces. CSF also serves as transport vehicle for different neurotransmitters and other metabolites produced in the brain.

The choroid plexus produces 500 ml of CSF per 24 h but the total CSF volume in an adult is 120–150 ml; therefore, CSF is recycled over three times per day. The brain capillaries also produce a significant amount of fluid. The interstitial fluid (ISF) originating from the brain capillary adequately substitutes the CSF in the subarachnoid space, at intraventricular CSF obstructions. The total volume of the interstitial fluid is twice that of the CSF and the chemical composition of the fluids is similar. There is a rapid diffusion and mixing of CSF and interstitial fluid, aided by arterial pulsations, across the outer surface of the brain. This makes it impossible to separate the fluids despite their different origins. Thus, fluid outside the brain defines CSF and fluid within the interstitial space of the brain defines interstitial fluid. Although there are minor variations of the chemical CSF composition in different regions of the subarachnoid space, the CSF and interstitial fluid cannot be separated by differences in composition. The most characteristic feature of unbound brain water (CSF and interstitial fluid) is its low protein concentration amounting to 0.4% of the protein concentration in plasma.

The intimate relationship between the formation of CSF and interstitial fluid is also important for the absorption of CSF. Since there is net production of CSF in the choroid plexus, there is also net flow of CSF from the subarachnoid space into the brain and spinal cord (Figure 12.9.3). The absorption of CSF by the brain capillaries occurs in the same way as capillaries in the other parts of the body absorb interstitial fluid. The brain capillary actively absorbs the macromolecules and plasma proteins in the CSF. One of the pivotal properties of the arteriole and brain capillary is to regulate and maintain fluid homeostasis at a normal intracranial pressure (Figure 12.9.3B).

Atrophy will be used to describe loss of brain tissue rather than the somewhat confusing term 'hydrocephalus ex vacuu'. 'Ventriculomegaly' is a purely descriptive term implying larger than normal ventricular system without any reference to the cause of such dilatation. 'Colpocephaly' is sometimes used to describe a condition in which the occipital horns of the lateral ventricles are dilated out of proportion compared to other parts of the ventricular system.

DEFINITION OF HYDROCEPHALUS AND TRANSMANTLE PULSATILE STRESS

The definition of hydrocephalus is enlarged ventricles at the expense of a narrowed subarachnoid space. This indicates the

Figure 12.9.2 (A,B) Schematic drawing of a river with interconnected lakes and outflow through a dam. There is a pressure drop from the source to the dam. When the dam is closed, there is an enlargement of the fluid space just upstream to the obstruction (B). (C,D) The bulk flow concept. The driving force of the cerebrospinal fluid circulation is a pressure drop from the choroid plexus to the arachnoid granulation. As is the case in the river, the subarachnoid space, not the ventricular system, would dilate when the outflow through the arachnoid granulation is closed (D).

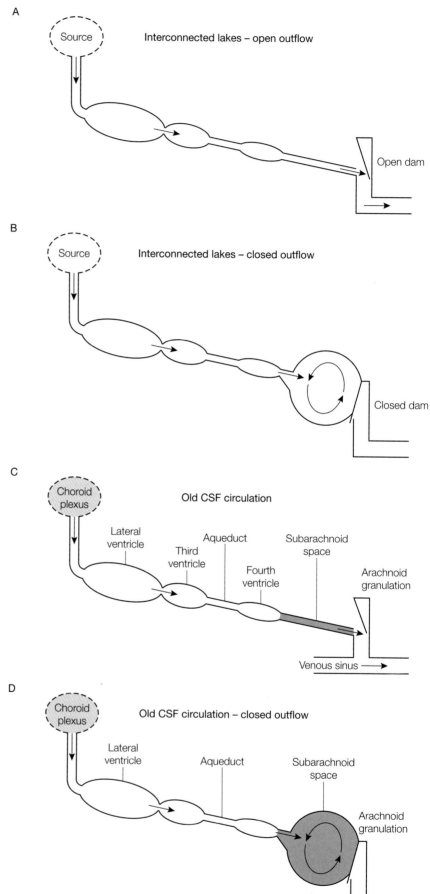

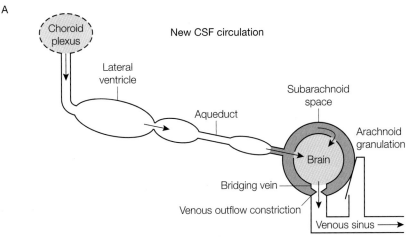

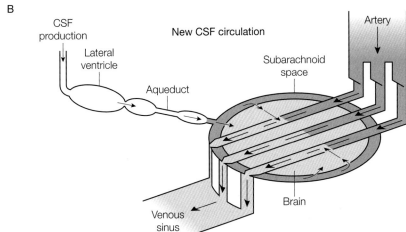

Figure 12.9.3 Revised CSF circulation and its relation to cerebral blood circulation. (A) The brain capillaries absorb the CSF. (B) The absorption of CSF means a minimal addition to the major diffusion of water through the brain caused by the circulation of blood. The intracranial pressure is regulated by filtration and absorption of fluid in the capillaries. The arterioles and capillaries regulate the intracranial pressure at a slightly positive level. This positive CSF pressure causes slight obstruction of the venous outlets, which explains the prompt pressure drop from the bridging veins to the venous sinus (A,B). The venous outflow resistance facilitates blood flow by distending the upstream-located cerebral veins and capillaries.

presence of an increased regional force directed from the ventricles towards the subarachnoid space, i.e. an increased transmantle pressure gradient. Hydrocephalus differs from processes lacking a transmantle gradient such as cerebral atrophy, where both the ventricles and subarachnoid space enlarge. The transmantle pressure gradient is very small. Studies using direct intraventricular and subarachnoid pressure monitoring have reported gradients ranging from 0 to 5 cm of water in hydrocephalus. However, in some studies a transmantle gradient was not discernible. The transmantle pressure gradient exists as a dynamic phenomenon acting over time. Owing to the law of Pascal, it can only exist transiently in a fluid-filled cavity and requires repeated pulse waves to persist. Since direct pressure measurements have been equivocal, the transmantle pressure gradient should be renamed 'transmantle pulsatile stress' to stress its dynamic nature and its dependence on the pulse wave.

Most biological tissues are characterized by plasticity and therefore respond to local forces by local displacement, deformation and remoulding. Small pressure gradients may deform the brain, since it has a high plasticity. Deformation of the brain and the CSF spaces defines hydrocephalus. The brain is displaced towards the skull and the cortical gyri are often compressed or flattened. The transmantle pressure gradient is the only possible force that could be responsible for such deformation. The normalization of the CSF spaces following shunting indicates that the transmantle pressure gradient can be narrowed or reversed, which is further support that it really exists.

According to modern theories, the cumulative effect of many pulse waves slowly remoulding the brain is the cause of the ventricular enlargement in chronic hydrocephalus. As mentioned above, the deformation of the brain and CSF spaces indicates the presence of local pressure differences. Computed tomography (CT) and MRI are excellent tools to demonstrate anatomy. By analyzing the anatomy in hydrocephalus, it is thus possible to demonstrate the accumulated effect of local pressure differences, which are undetectable at direct pressure measurement. Later, we will return to this simple concept of analyzing pressure gradients by using CT and MR imaging, because it may increase the understanding of communicating hydrocephalus, and may give new insights into the hydrocephalic process.

NORMAL INTRACRANIAL HYDRODYNAMICS

OVERVIEW

The Monro–Kellie doctrine states that the total volume of the four main intracranial components, i.e. the brain, the CSF, the arterial and the venous blood, is constant and that any volume increase in one component causes a matching decrease in the other components. The doctrine is a consequence of fluids being incompressible. The systolic expansion of the intracranial arteries is thus balanced by a matching expulsion of CSF through the foramen magnum and expulsion of blood from the veins into the dural venous sinuses (Figure 12.9.4). The systolic expansion of the arteries compresses the venous outlets of the bridging vein and causes a systolic flow in the venous sinuses. The compression occurs at the venous outlets because the dural sinuses are, from a functional point of view, located outside the cranial cavity and the pressure drop is maximal at this site. The pulsating intracranial arteries cause the CSF to flow back and forth in the spinal canal.

When the pulse wave enters the cranium there is an immediate increase in the CSF pressure that, according to Pascal's law, will be evenly distributed in the whole intracranial space. Consequently, intracranial pressure differences equilibrate rapidly. However, temporary pressure gradients arise during the cardiac cycle because flow effects cause shifts in the intracranial fluids. The flows and gradients are largest at the openings of the cranial cavity, i.e. at the foramen magnum and at the venous outlets into the venous sinuses.

The speed of the pulse pressure is inversely proportional to compliance. In a non-compliant cavity, the transmission of pulse pressure occurs with the speed of sound (1540 m/s in water). Because the intracranial veins and the spinal thecal sac are compliant, the speed of the intracranial pulse pressure is decreased to 5 m/s, i.e. much slower than in a non-compliant cavity. The time for the intracranial pulse wave to pass from the arteries to the bridging veins is about 30 ms. Therefore, it is possible to monitor the effects and the timing of the pulse wave by flow-sensitive MRI, since its time resolution is about 15 ms.

Figure 12.9.4 Normal intracranial hydrodynamics. The relative thickness of the arrows in the artery indicates the magnitude of pressure. The relative thickness of the arrows in the venous system and subarachnoid space indicates the magnitude of flow. (A) Presystole. No pressure gradients are present in the brain. CSF is flowing upward into the cranial cavity from the compliant spinal canal. The normal venous outflow obstruction is not shown for clearer demonstration of the changes occurring during systole. (B) Early systole. The systolic pulse wave causes a large expansion of the arteries with a concomitant and significant dampening of the arterial pulse pressure. The pressure is immediately transmitted to the entire subarachnoid space. The expansion of the arteries causes a large volume conduction of CSF that compresses the outlets of the cortical veins and increases the systolic blood flow in the venous sinus. Simultaneously, the arterial expansion causes a large systolic expulsion of CSF into the compliant spinal canal. (C) Mid systole. After some delay (60 ms), the small and dampened pulse wave in the artery (thin arrows) is transmitted into the brain capillaries. This causes a slight brain expansion and a transmantle stress of normal magnitude. (Modified from International Journal of Neuroradiology 1997; 3:367–375.)

A

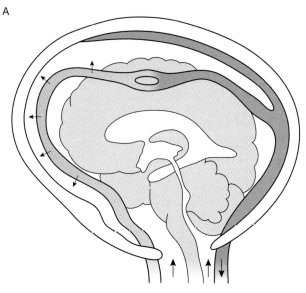

Normal – presystole

B

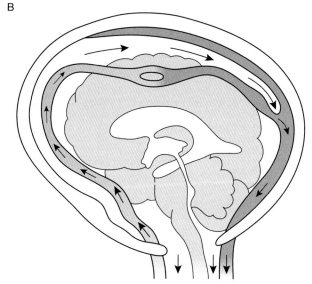

Normal – early systole

C

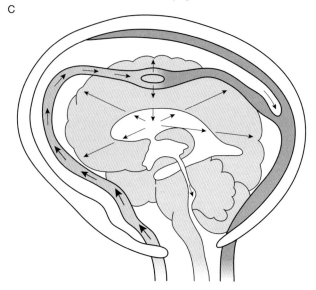

Normal – mid systole

Intracranial hydrodynamics is dependent on the compliance of the thecal sac and the compressible bridging veins. Compliance is the capacity of a buffer system to accommodate a volume change and is defined as volume change divided by pressure change. It is a dynamic phenomenon and cannot be measured directly since the system must be subjected to a volume change or a pressure change. Flow-sensitive MRI and intracranial pressure monitoring can measure volume and pressure changes induced by the arterial pulsations. Intracranial compliance can be determined by combining the two methods.

DYNAMICS IN HEALTHY INDIVIDUALS

Flow-sensitive MRI studies gives precise information of intracranial dynamics in all dimensions, both spatially and temporally. For the first time it is possible to differentiate the arterial expansion from the brain (capillary) expansion. The arterial expansion differs significantly from the brain expansion both in timing and in magnitude. The volume increase of the intracranial arteries is 1.5 ml and equals the sum of the systolic stroke volumes at the foramen magnum and in the venous sinuses (Figure 12.9.4B). The volume increase of the brain is about 0.03 ml. The brain expansion is thus only 2% of the arterial expansion. The minute brain expansion occurs inwards towards the ventricular system and thus equals the systolic flow in the aqueduct (stroke volume = 0.03 ml/beat). The brain expansion, in turn, is caused by the systolic expansion of the brain capillaries (Figure 12.9.4C). The arterial expansion has a fixed duration of about 300 ms. The brain expansion starts 60 ms later than the arterial one and occupies half of the cardiac cycle, i.e. 400 to 500 ms.

Of upmost importance to intracranial dynamics is the direct volume conduction of the pulse wave from the expanding arteries, via the CSF, to the veins and spinal canal, thereby bypassing the brain and its capillaries (Figure 12.9.4B). Arteries are compliant and act as an elastic reservoir. The expanding arterial wall absorbs part of the hydraulic energy in the pulse wave, which is released in diastole to maintain constant capillary flow. This is known as the 'windkessel' mechanism. It transforms the pulsating arterial flow into a continuous and almost non-pulsating capillary flow. The windkessel effect of the arteries may be compared to a bagpipe where the elastic capacitance of the bag (artery) transforms the pulsatile inflow of air into a continuous non-pulsatile outflow through the pipe (capillary). The presence of intracranial compliance, which allows the arteries to expand, is a mandatory prerequisite for the windkessel mechanism. The intracranial windkessel mechanism demonstrates large arterial expansion and almost absent capillary expansion, as described above.

ABNORMAL INTRACRANIAL HYDRODYNAMICS

OVERVIEW

As realized by Dandy, communicating hydrocephalus cannot be caused by an obstructed bulk flow of CSF at the pacchionian granulations (Figure 12.9.2D and 12.9.7A). Communicating hydrocephalus is instead caused by decreased intracranial compliance. Virtually all available hydrocephalus tests demonstrate decreased

intracranial compliance or the consequences of decreased compliance, especially when followed over longer periods. Most invasive tests interfere with intracranial compliance to some extent, since CSF infusion decreases compliance and CSF diversion increases compliance. The clinical improvement following CSF diversion using the lumbar CSF tap test or shunt placement is due to a forced compensatory dilation of the compressed intracranial veins. The forced dilation of the veins is a consequence of the Monro–Kellie doctrine since successful shunting is based on a slight overdrainage of CSF, which must be compensated by a matching increase in venous and capillary blood volume. The dilated vessels increase intracranial venous compliance and cerebral blood flow. Shunting is thus not only a treatment but may also be regarded as a test of restored venous compliance and cerebral blood flow. Some clinicians define hydrocephalus depending on whether the patients improve after shunting or not. Intrathecal bolus and infusion tests demonstrate decreased intracranial compliance as well as increased outflow resistance of CSF through the compressed capillaries. As explained earlier, the outflow of the injected mock CSF occurs through the compressed cerebral capillaries and veins, not through the pacchionian granulations.

The expression of decreased compliance in communicating hydrocephalus is increased intracranial pulse pressure and decreased intracranial stroke volume. Thus, intracranial pressure monitoring demonstrates increased CSF pulse pressure as well as increased incidence of intermittent high-pressure waves of vascular origin, the so-called A and B waves. The elevation of the pulsatility index (PI) on transcranial Doppler ultrasound indicates increased pulsatility in the major intracranial arteries. The increased pulsatility is a consequence of decreased intracranial compliance and breakdown of the windkessel mechanism, decreasing the diastolic flow in the arteries. Decreased intracranial compliance also increases the vascular impedance, i.e. resistance to pulsating flow, causing a decreased mean blood flow. Decreased intracranial compliance has hitherto been a little known cause of reduced cerebral blood flow. The compressed capillaries and veins also increase the vascular resistance to the convective blood flow. Studies using flow-sensitive MRI report significantly decreased systolic stroke volumes of CSF and blood into the cervical spinal canal and venous sinuses, i.e. decreased intracranial stroke volume.

The consequences of decreased compliance in hydrocephalus has until now not been fully appreciated. One reason for this may be that communicating hydrocephalus represents an unfamiliar condition where decreased compliance occurs at normal or near-normal intracranial pressure. Since the decreased intracranial compliance interferes with cerebral blood flow, it is conceivable that it may be responsible for the salient features of communicating hydrocephalus. In fact, the clinical signs and symptoms as well as ventricular dilation, reduced cerebral blood flow, malabsorption of CSF, intracranial pressure waves, increase of mean CSF pressure, increased CSF pulse pressure, increased pulsatility index and decreased intracranial stroke volumes may all be explained by decreased intracranial compliance.

DYNAMICS IN COMMUNICATING HYDROCEPHALUS

Flow-sensitive MRI in communicating hydrocephalus has shown that the stroke volume is decreased by 50% at the craniocervical junction and by one-third in the venous sinuses. This indicates that the total intracranial stroke volume in communicating hydrocephalus is about half that in normal individuals. Intracranial pressure monitoring reports a six-fold increase of the CSF pulse pressure as compared to normal individuals. Intracranial compliance is thus decreased by one order of magnitude in communicating hydrocephalus, since compliance is the ratio between volume change and pressure change. This explains why the impact of the pulse wave may have such importance for the pathophysiology of communicating hydrocephalus.

Decreased intracranial compliance restricts the expansion of the arteries, causing breakdown of the windkessel mechanism with increased pulsations in the brain capillaries (Figure 12.9.5). Since the artery cannot expand, there is decreased attenuation of pulse wave in the artery. The direct volume conduction from the artery to the bridging vein, which bypasses the brain capillaries, is decreased (Figure 12.9.5B). Due to conservation of momentum, there must be a forced pressure and volume transmission of the pulse wave, from the artery into the capillary and brain tissue (Figure 12.9.5C). The hydraulic energy of the pulse wave is absorbed in the capillary and the brain, instead of the artery. This results in a diminished pressure difference between the vascular system and brain tissue.

The systolic pressure transmission from capillary to brain tissue increases cerebral venous pressure, diminishes perfusion pressure and decreases cerebral blood flow. It also diminishes the transcapillary pressure difference between blood and tissue, which decreases the fluid exchange across the capillary wall. Decreased intracranial compliance also increases the pressure transmission in the opposite direction, from the CSF to the vascular system. The pressures in the CSF and blood are closely coupled and equilibrate more rapidly at decreased intracranial compliance. Thus, an increase in CSF pressure does not sufficiently increase the pressure difference between CSF and blood, which is needed to absorb CSF. Since brain capillaries absorb the CSF, this is probably an important factor behind the malabsorption of CSF and behind the increased outflow resistance at CSF infusion tests. Other important mechanisms for CSF malabsorption are decreased cerebral blood flow and increased vascular resistance in the compressed brain capillaries.

Figure 12.9.5 Hydrodynamics of communicating hydrocephalus. Labels as in Figure 12.9.4. (A) Presystole. The intracranial capacitance vessels are narrow and intracranial compliance is decreased. (B) Early systole. The decreased intracranial compliance restricts the arterial expansion, so little or no damping of the pulse pressure occurs in the artery. The artery behaves as if it were a rigid tube. Due to decreased volume conduction of CSF, the systolic flows in the dural sinus and in the subarachnoid space at the foramen magnum are decreased. The decreased arterial expansion causes a decreased volume conduction of CSF and decreased compression of the bridging veins at their outlets into the dural sinus. As a result, the venous outflow resistance is decreased and cannot dilate the upstream-located cerebral veins and capillaries any longer. The capacitance vessels are instead prone to collapse. The total vascular resistance is increased. (C) Mid systole. The high pulse pressure in the artery (thick arrows) is transmitted undamped into the brain capillaries, giving rise to a large capillary expansion, an increased CSF pulse pressure, a large systolic flow in the aqueduct, an increased transmantle stress and ventricular dilatation. The increased transmantle stress compresses the intracranial veins in their entire length, which in turn decreases intracranial compliance, increases vascular resistance and decreases cerebral blood flow. (Modified from International Journal of Neuroradiology 1997; 3:367–375.)

A

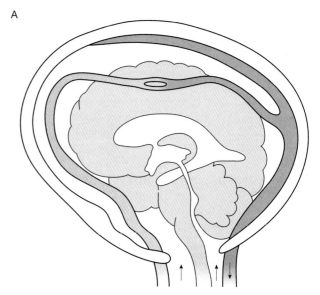

Hydrocephalus – presystole

B

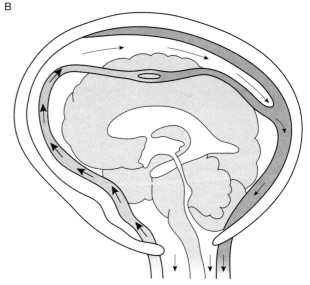

Hydrocephalus – early systole

C

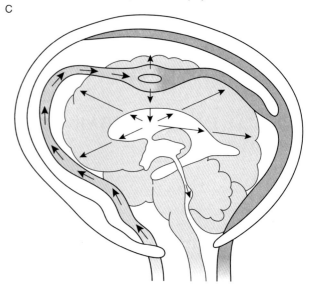

Hydrocephalus – mid systole

The increased brain expansion, directed inwards towards the ventricles, increases intraventricular pulse pressure and causes a hyperdynamic CSF flow in the aqueduct. The increased intraventricular pulse pressure, in turn, dilates the ventricular system and compresses the brain (Figure 12.9.5C). This dynamic rebound phenomenon is not obvious and may seem counterintuitive as discussed in the section of the transmantle pulsatile stress. The transmantle pulsatile stress may be explained by 'self-compression of the brain against the ventricular system during a systole', since ventricular fluid is incompressible and brain plasticity is high. Because of Pascal's law, the counterforce from the ventricles equals the force from the expanding brain.

The transmantle pulsatile stress compresses the capacitance vessels, i.e. the cerebral capillaries, cerebral veins and cortical veins. This increases vascular resistance and decreases cerebral blood flow (Figure 12.9.6). The increased vascular resistance also causes an increase in mean CSF pressure. The compressed capacitance vessels further decrease intracranial compliance and a vicious circle is formed. The mismatch between intracranial compliance and the blood circulation disturbs the autoregulation of cerebral blood flow and increases the incidence of intermittent high-pressure waves. The regulation of the arterioles is grossly maintained but arteriolar dilation causes increased pressure instead of increased cerebral blood flow. This explains the occurrence of the A and B high-pressure waves of vascular origin.

It is often necessary to combine clinical data with intracranial pressure monitoring or radiological follow-up studies to decide whether the hydrocephalic process is in an active or non-active state. Progressive ventricular enlargement is a sign of decreased compliance and enhanced transmantle pulsatile stress. It is not a sign of increased CSF pressure since the pressure usually is near normal but the pressure can also be significantly increased. In fact, the volume of the ventricles is inversely dependent on the CSF pressure, statistically. It is impossible to predict the CSF pressure based on the ventricular volume in an individual case. Due to proximity to the compliant spinal sac, infratentorial compliance is usually less decreased than supratentorial compliance. This explains why the supratentorial ventricles may enlarge out of proportion to the fourth ventricle, which often is of normal or even small size (Figure 12.9.7A). Consequently, obstructions to the pulsatile CSF flow in the prepontine cistern or in the cervical spinal canal are common when all four ventricles are enlarged. The decreased compliance in the posterior fossa increases the 'transcerebellar pulsatile stress' and dilates the fourth ventricle.

To sum up, communicating hydrocephalus is a disorder of intracranial pulsations, caused by decreased compliance. Decreased compliance restricts the arterial expansion and causes a breakdown of the windkessel mechanism. Therefore, communicating hydrocephalus has also been termed 'restricted arterial pulsation hydrocephalus'. Of upmost importance is the abnormal pressure and volume transmission into the brain capillaries, which increases ventricular pulse pressure, increases the pulsatile CSF flow in the aqueduct and dilates the ventricles.

DYNAMICS IN OBSTRUCTIVE HYDROCEPHALUS – ACUTE PHASE

Any process that restricts the intraventricular bulk flow of CSF, e.g. an intraventricular block by mass lesion or adhesions, may

A

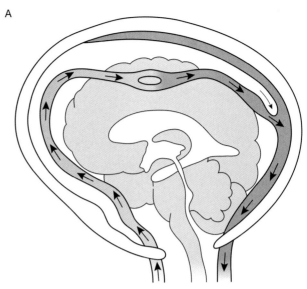

Normal – blood flow

B

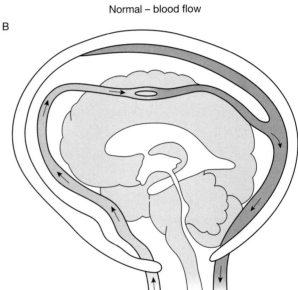

Hydrocephalus – blood flow

Figure 12.9.6 Cerebral blood flow in healthy individuals (A) and in communicating hydrocephalus (B). (A) The arterial windkessel mechanism, the wide intracranial vessels with small vascular resistance and the small venous outflow resistance that keep the cerebral veins distended maintain the high normal blood flow. The small venous outflow resistance is caused by a small positive intracranial pressure and is increased during systole. The venous outflow resistance is a mandatory prerequisite for the pressure drop occurring from the cortical veins to the venous sinus (c.f. Figure 12.9.3). (B) In communicating hydrocephalus, the increased transmantle pulsatile stress and the ventricular dilation compresses the cerebral veins and capillaries in their entire length. This significantly increases the vascular resistance and decreases the blood flow. The venous outflow resistance is reduced and the normal pressure drop from the subarachnoid space to the venous sinus (c.f. Figure 12.9.3) disappears. (This phenomenon cannot be explained by the bulk flow concept, since a pressure drop caused by a CSF obstruction at the arachnoid granulations would increase the pressure drop from the subarachnoid space to the sinus, not decrease it.) The reduced venous outflow resistance facilitates collapse of the compressed capacitance vessels, which further decreases cerebral blood flow.

A

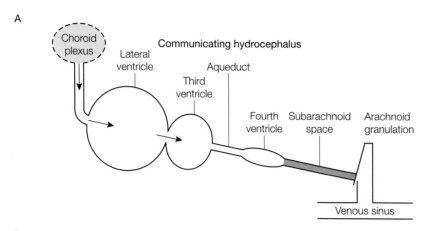

B

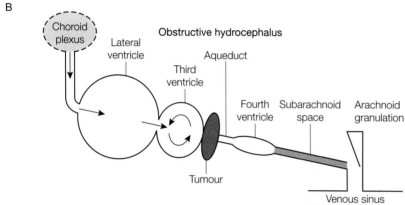

Figure 12.9.7 (A) Communicating hydrocephalus is characterized by enlargement of the ventricles, mainly the lateral and third ventricle, and a narrow subarachnoid space. This anatomy cannot be explained by an obstruction to the bulk flow at the arachnoid granulations. It is obvious that we have to search for other explanations (c.f. Figure 12.9.5) than obstructed bulk flow of CSF as the cause of ventricular enlargement in communicating hydrocephalus. (B) Obstructive hydrocephalus is easy to understand since the ventricles dilate proximal to an intraventricular obstruction to the bulk flow of CSF. An obstruction of the intraventricular foramen of Monro causes enlargement of the corresponding lateral ventricle and so on. This schematic drawing shows a tumour in the aqueduct that dilates the third and lateral ventricles.

cause obstructive hydrocephalus (Figure 12.9.7B). The intraventricular block prevents the CSF from reaching its main absorption site at the outer surface of the brain. The ventricles increase in volume because the periventricular capillaries can only absorb part of the CSF produced in the choroid plexus. The pressure in the ventricles and brain becomes elevated. The ventricular dilation displaces the surface of the brain towards the skull and compresses the cortical veins, mainly at their outlets close to the venous sinuses. This leads to venous congestion with increased blood volume and increased intracranial pressure. Hence, acute obstructive hydrocephalus is also termed 'venous congestion hydrocephalus'. The venous congestion and ensuing brain swelling counteracts the ventricular dilation, otherwise the ventricular dilatation would be fatal. At some point, a new equilibrium is achieved at higher pressure than normal. An important feature of acute hydrocephalus is the compression of the venous outlets, which is the main reason for the increased intracranial pressure. The venous outflow obstruction dilates the cerebral veins and capillaries upstream to the obstruction, which decreases the vascular resistance. This explains why the cerebral blood flow usually is only slightly decreased in the acute phase of obstructive hydrocephalus.

The arteriolar and capillary regulation of fluid absorption in the periventricular brain capillaries eventually balances the excess production of CSF from the trapped ventricle. The CSF pressure decreases and a new equilibrium is established at near-normal pressure in the chronic phase of obstructive hydrocephalus.

DYNAMICS IN OBSTRUCTIVE HYDROCEPHALUS – CHRONIC PHASE

As described above, the CSF pressure decreases in the chronic phase of obstructive hydrocephalus. The CSF production and CSF absorption is balanced in the trapped ventricles. The venous outflow compression and venous congestion disappears. Consequently, there is no force to counteract the ventricular dilation any longer and the capacitance vessels become compressed. This decreases intracranial compliance. This condition mimics the disorder of intracranial pulsations occurring in communicating hydrocephalus (Figure 12.9.5). The decreased intracranial compliance causes a breakdown of the arterial windkessel mechanism with increased capillary expansion, increased CSF pulsations and hyperdynamic CSF flow in the trapped ventricle. The increased intraventricular pulse pressure increases the transmantle pulsatile stress, which continues to dilate the ventricles even if the mean CSF pressure is normal. MRI may disclose the hyperdynamic intraventricular pulsations by increased 'flow void' in the foramina of Monro or in the aqueduct, within the trapped ventricles. Intracranial pressure monitoring demonstrates significantly increased CSF pulse pressure with normal or only a slight increase of the mean CSF pressure.

INTRACRANIAL DYNAMICS FOLLOWING TREATMENT (BY THIRD VENTRICULOSTOMY, SHUNTING OR POSTERIOR FOSSA DECOMPRESSION) OF CHRONIC HYDROCEPHALUS AND ACUTE HYDROCEPHALUS

CHRONIC HYDROCEPHALUS

Since communicating hydrocephalus and chronic obstructive hydrocephalus share the same clinical symptoms, the same pathophysiology and can be treated by the same methods, it is logical to group these conditions under the heading of 'chronic hydrocephalus'. Shunting, third ventriculostomy and, in some cases, posterior fossa decompression are established methods to treat obstructive hydrocephalus. Shunting has hitherto been the only available method to treat communicating hydrocephalus but recently there have been several preliminary reports of successful treatment by third ventriculostomy for this condition. This is not surprising when considering the dynamics of communicating hydrocephalus as explained above. The primary aim of performing ventriculostomy or inserting a shunt in chronic hydrocephalus is not to increase the CSF absorption but rather to increase intracranial compliance. Third ventriculostomy increases the systolic outflow from the ventricles, decreases the intraventricular pulse pressure and decreases the width of the ventricles. This would dilate the compressed capacitance vessels and increase intracranial compliance. Similarly, shunting restores venous compliance because the CSF diversion causes a forced dilatation of the compressed capacitance vessels.

ACUTE HYDROCEPHALUS

In acute obstructive hydrocephalus, a third ventriculostomy decreases the size of the ventricles and reduces the intracranial pressure by bypassing the intraventricular obstruction and re-establishing the bulk flow of CSF from the ventricles to the subarachnoid space. Similarly, shunting reduces the intracranial pressure by diverting fluid from the trapped ventricles.

POSTERIOR FOSSA DECOMPRESSION

Chiari malformations and other mass lesions at the craniocervical junction, which are thought to obstruct the CSF flow from the fourth ventricle, can be successfully treated by posterior fossa decompression. However, the hydrocephalus caused by Chiari I and II malformations is often of the communicating type. Achondroplasia also causes communicating hydrocephalus. All these conditions with communicating hydrocephalus can be treated by posterior fossa decompression. The underlying mechanism is that the posterior fossa decompression increases the intracranial compliance by recreating a communication with the compliant spinal thecal sac.

To sum up, acute hydrocephalus is characterized by venous outflow compression with dilated capacitance vessels. Chronic hydrocephalus is characterized by compressed capacitance vessels and decreased compliance. Thus, from a clinical and physiological point of view, hydrocephalus could be divided into acute hydrocephalus and chronic hydrocephalus where the former is of obstructive type and the latter may be either of communicating type or of obstructive type. It is interesting to note that it is possible to treat acute as well as chronic hydrocephalus by shunting, third ventriculostomy or posterior fossa decompression. In the acute phase, it is important to reduce the intracranial pressure by draining fluid from the obstructed ventricles. In the chronic phase, it is important to increase intracranial compliance by dilating the capacitance vessels or by restoring communication with the compliant spinal canal.

CLINICAL SYMPTOMS OF HYDROCEPHALUS

The clinical symptoms of hydrocephalus are a consequence of raised intracranial pressure, decreased intracranial compliance and the expansion of intracranial CSF-filled spaces, particularly the ventricular system. The raised intracranial pressure in communicating hydrocephalus is a consequence of decreased intracranial compliance compressing the capacitance vessels and increasing the vascular resistance. The clinical expression of these pathologies depends on the age of the child. In small babies, a rapidly increasing head size is the most important clinical marker of hydrocephalus. The cranial sutures widen allowing for an increased volume of the intracranial cavity, thus accommodating the dilating ventricular system. The soft skull allows the absolute value of the intracranial pressure to be only slightly elevated or just at the upper limits of normal. In premature babies, the extra-cerebral CSF-containing spaces are wide and will compress first before an increasing head circumference becomes obvious. Hence, ventriculomegaly, which may be due to hydrocephalus, can initially be clinically silent.

The classical symptoms of raised intracranial pressure include headaches, nausea, vomiting and visual disturbances. All depend on a rigid skull for their expression. These symptoms are therefore present in older children and adults in whom the sutures do not readily widen or split when the intracranial pressure increases. Children up to an age of 4–6 years can still accommodate a gradual increase in intracranial pressure by splitting of sutures. Other frequently described findings are a prominent forehead and 'sun-set' phenomena in the eyes.

Except in small babies, in whom the open fontanelle can be palpated, a non-invasive method to measure the intracranial pressure is not available. Evaluation of the fundi for possible papilloedema is difficult for the inexperienced and is of no use in the smaller children and babies who do not develop a high enough intracranial pressure to cause papilloedema. The most important information is often available from the head circumference charts in which the head growth is followed by serial measurements. Most children's heads grow at a normal pace and are known to follow their own growth 'channel'. Babies with large heads will often maintain a large head through infancy and may follow the normal growth pattern in the 97% percentile or even higher. This is not a pattern suggesting the presence of hydrocephalus. Much more suspicious is a growth chart illustrating crossing of percentiles, particularly at a steep angle, even though the absolute head size may be within normal limits for age. It is not uncommon for this to be the only clinical sign indicating a hydrocephalus under development. Thus, it is not the absolute measurement of head size that is most interesting but indeed the pattern of growth over time. Frequent use of a tape measure is a far more efficient tool in the diagnosis of hydrocephalus than a single or even repeated neuroradiological investigations. Thus, macrocephaly is a common but not obligatory finding in hydrocephalic children. By the same logistics, hydrocephalus is an uncommon association with microcephaly but the combination is not impossible.

RADIOLOGICAL INVESTIGATION OF SUSPECTED HYDROCEPHALUS

The neuroradiological work-up of infants and children with suspected hydrocephalus should focus on two issues that may require different strategies or may be solved concurrently. First, the clinical suspicion of hydrocephalus must be confirmed or disproved. This task may indeed be the most challenging requiring sophisticated investigations. Once the diagnosis is established, further investigations must concentrate on finding the cause for hydrocephalus.

Infants suspected of suffering from hydrocephalus are often first investigated using cranial ultrasound. This imaging method is eminently well suited to demonstrate the size and shape of the third and lateral ventricles. Thus, cranial ultrasound can be used to confirm the presence of hydrocephalus when associated with dilatation of the third and lateral ventricles. It may also show the cause of hydrocephalus if an intraventricular haemorrhage or tumour is visualized and is therefore useful in infants in whom the cause of hydrocephalus is known, such as intraventricular haemorrhage in premature neonates. However, examination of the posterior fossa is quite difficult and the structures located there are at best incompletely studied. Cranial ultrasound is further limited to those infants with a persisting and sizable anterior fontanelle. The use of alternate acoustic windows, such as the posterior fontanelle and the occipitotemporal sutures, has been advocated and is sometimes useful. However, this is only useful on occasion and then only in the hands of very skilled sonologists well experienced in paediatric neuroradiology. Cranial ultrasound is not sufficient if the cause of raised intracranial pressure is questionable or if the clinical suspicion of hydrocephalus is high and the ventricular size equivocal.

Complete evaluation of a child suspected of having hydrocephalus may be achieved with CT scanning but may require further evaluation using MRI. Both techniques allow direct visualization of the brain and all CSF-filled spaces within the skull. Although MRI has many advantages over CT, absence of ionizing radiation being most important in a paediatric population, CT is readily available and fast imaging on modern equipment often makes the use of sedation or anaesthesia unnecessary, a major advantage as repeated examinations are often necessary in the follow-up in the treatment of hydrocephalus. Whatever the imaging modality used, enhancement with intravenous contrast injection is necessary if the aetiology of hydrocephalus is unknown during initial work-up.

Increased size and a change in shape of the lateral ventricles is the most common finding in hydrocephalus. The frontal but also the occipital horns may acquire a more rounded shape while the temporal horns are often considered the parts of the lateral ventricles to be dilated first and thus the parts most sensitive to an obstruction in the ventricular system or decreased intracranial compliance. Symmetrical dilatation of both lateral ventricles is the rule. When asymmetrical dilatation is present, this can be due to a unilateral CSF obstruction in the lateral ventricle but more frequently this is caused by a concurrent loss of brain tissue that may or may not be associated with the aetiology of hydrocephalus. Dilatation of the occipital horns that is excessive in comparison with the dilatation elsewhere is common in neonates and infants. This is sometimes called colpocephaly. However, this is purely a descriptive term and is non-specific in relation to aetiology or severity of hydrocephalus. The reason for this observation is unknown. Excessive dilatation of the occipital horns is also thought to be the cause of a diverticulum forming in the medial wall of the occipital horn. This diverticulum may extend through the tentorial notch and down into the posterior fossa and appear there as a cystic mass lesion.

An observation often regarded as a reliable sign of hydrocephalus is enlargement of the anterior and posterior recesses of the third ventricle as seen in sagittal MR images. Periventricular high content of water is common in the acute phase of obstructive hydrocephalus. This image is likely explained by water leaking from the ventricles through the ependyma into brain tissue, thus increasing the interstitial water. The concentration around the frontal and occipital horns is due to marked CSF pulsations in the ventricles causing leakage where the ependyma is subjected to the strongest pulsating forces. This finding is highly suggestive of raised intraventricular pressure but is not an obligatory finding. It is most often seen in the early stages of an acute obstructive hydrocephalus. However, the absence of such periventricular high signal on MRI, or low attenuation on CT, does not exclude elevated intraventricular pressure. Absence of periventricular oedema, despite sometimes very high pressures, is common in children who have been shunted and are experiencing shunt failure.

The aqueduct of Sylvius is often prominent in hydrocephalus. In patients with an obstruction of the aqueduct, the proximal part often dilates massively and narrows rapidly down to a tapering end at the obstruction.

CSF FLOW-SENSITIVE MR IMAGING

It is very important to differentiate communicating hydrocephalus from obstructive hydrocephalus. MRI should be performed when CT or sonography are equivocal. MRI evaluates the anatomy in the posterior fossa better than CT and ultrasound. Once the cause of hydrocephalus has been established, however, CT and ultrasound are excellent for following the size of the ventricles. As opposed to CT, MRI can detect and estimate the CSF flow in the narrow parts of the ventricles, i.e. the foramen Monro, the aqueduct and the outflows of the fourth ventricle. On routine T2-weighted MR scans, CSF flow can be detected by signal loss or 'flow void' in areas of rapid or turbulent flow. In the majority of cases, it is sufficient to use sagittal T2-weighted standard spin echo sequences with 3 mm thickness and a 0.5 mm gap. Since the 180-degree refocusing pulses in fast spin echo sequences are flow compensating, we prefer using the old-fashioned dual echo sequence without flow compensation to detect CSF flow (Figure 12.9.8D,E). To decrease the scan time, a short TR of 1.5 s, $^3/_4$ NEX and reduced spatial resolution can be used. This dual echo sequence without flow compensation reliably demonstrates 'flow void' in the region of the aqueduct or the third ventriculostomy secondary to pulsatile flow. Fischbein et al. found that sagittal 3- to 4-mm fast spin echo sequences were as sensitive as phase contrast MR imaging to examine the patency or occlusion of a third ventriculostomy. Phase contrast studies are thus not needed in the routine evaluation of obstructions in the CSF pathways. Phase contrast MR imaging is a special technique that uses the relative phase angle of moving spins to quantify intracranial CSF flows. Sagittal phase contrast studies of CSF flow may be used as an adjunct diagnostic tool. We use phase contrast studies in a plane perpendicular to the CSF flow for complimentary radiological evaluation of CSF obstructions,

and as a research tool for quantification of the stroke volume of CSF.

Prior to a third ventriculostomy, sagittal high-resolution T2-weighted fast spin echo or high-contrast sagittal 3D CISS (constructive interference in steady-state) sequences can be used to detect thin subarachnoid membranes in the ventricles and in the prepontine cistern. It is important to surgically penetrate adhesions and membranes such as Liljequist's membrane in the upper prepontine cistern to establish a free CSF communication to the compliant spinal CSF spaces. Liljequist's membrane is an arachnoid condensation extending from the upper border of dorsum sellae to the anterior edge of the mammillary bodies.

SPECIAL INVESTIGATIONS

Even though MR imaging, using flow sensitive or other advanced dynamic sequences, is capable of providing most of the information necessary to understand the mechanisms behind obstructive hydrocephalus, there are situations in which cisternography using positive intrathecal contrast material is necessary for full understanding of the pathophysiology. This is particularly important in situations when a balance has been achieved and study of CSF flow

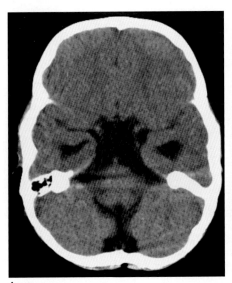

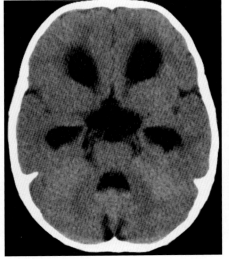

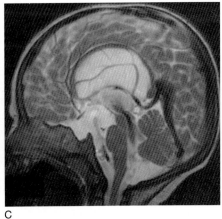

A   B   C

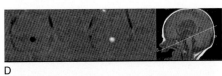

D

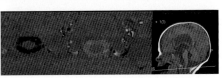

E

Figure 12.9.8 This girl of 9 months of age presented with abnormally increasing head circumference. She is found to have an arachnoid cyst of the suprasellar cistern. (A,B) CT scan shows marked dilatation of the lateral ventricles. The third ventricle is difficult to delineate as a large arachnoid cyst replaces it. The most anterior part of the third ventricle is seen anterior to the cyst in (B). (C) Mid sagittal T2-weighted image. Note the large cyst occupying the suprasellar cisterns. The cyst lifts the floor of third ventricle, pushes the mesencephalon posteriorly away from the clivus, herniates into the sella and lifts the chiasm up and anteriorly. Note also the hyperdynamic flow in the aqueduct causing flow artifacts in the third and fourth ventricles. Hydrocephalus is obvious and due to the cyst occupying the cistern and decreasing compliance in the basal cisterns. (D,E) Flow sequences over the aqueduct and foramen magnum showing hyperdynamic flow in these two locations. Hence, the cyst is not causing any obstruction to CSF flow out of the ventricular system but does not allow the basal cisterns to vary in size with vascular pulsations. Hydrocephalus in this case is of the communicating type.

does not detect any appreciable flow or exchange of fluid. This situation is often the case where arachnoid or ependymal cysts cause obstruction to CSF flow within or outside the ventricular system or where postinflammatory membranes form more or less complete barriers to normal CSF flow.

Nowadays, cisternography using positive contrast material is done using CT following a lumbar injection of isotonic and non-ionic contrast. The contrast is transferred to the basal cisterns by lowering the patient's head. Pulsations in the region of the foramen magnum usually provide an excellent mixing of contrast with CSF. However, asking the patient to rotate on the table usually ensures good mixing. Imaging is performed within minutes and should, with modern equipment, be aimed at providing imaging data of such quality that good reformatted images can be obtained in any desired plane. If, when using this technique, contrast does not readily enter the ventricular system or spread evenly throughout the basal cisterns, delayed imaging following a couple of hours rest in horizontal position may prove extremely helpful in understanding the dynamics of CSF in fluid-filled spaces with varying degree of communication with the subarachnoid space or ventricles.

Cisternography using a radionuclide as tracer has been used extensively in the past to investigate CSF flow, particularly in cases of suspected communicating hydrocephalus. However, new understanding of the pathophysiology behind this condition has rendered this investigation obsolete on this indication.

CAUSES OF ACUTE OBSTRUCTIVE HYDROCEPHALUS

The most straightforward and easiest to understand type of hydrocephalus is that caused by a blockage or obstruction to the flow of CSF within or out from the ventricular system. Two types of condition may cause this: a mass lesion compressing the normal conduit for CSF and a membrane or adhesions obstructing the passage of CSF (Figure 12.9.9).

In certain types of mass lesions, hydrocephalus is the typical presentation of the disease. Here, hydrocephalus with increased intraventricular pressure causes clinical symptoms long before the mass lesion itself causes symptoms. Mass lesions in critical locations, such as the interventricular foramen of Monro or adjacent to the aqueduct of Sylvius, can cause obstruction despite the limited size of the mass lesion itself. A foramen of Monro cyst, which is often a small cyst containing a colloid, can obstruct one or both of the foramina, thus causing a life-threatening situation with the potential for very high intracranial pressure and subsequent transtentorial herniation. The content of the colloid cyst is most commonly of high attenuation on CT but may be isodense with surrounding brain or even hypodense. The cyst may be easier to see on MRI but even here the pattern of signal in the cyst is highly variable.

A mass lesion only obstructing one of the two interventricular foramina can cause unilateral hydrocephalus. This is not an uncommon complication to tuberous sclerosis as a mostly benign giant cell astrocytoma with a predilection for this particular location is a common association in this disease.

Mass lesions in the region of the aqueduct of Sylvius can deform and obstruct the aqueduct. Small periaqueductal gliomas can

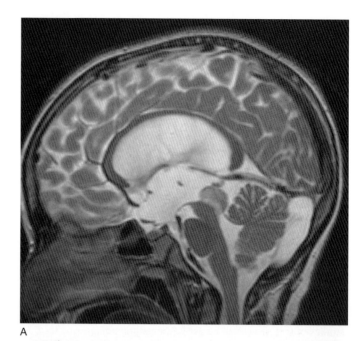

A

B

Figure 12.9.9 Girl of 8 years with obstructive hydrocephalus due to astrocytoma grade 2 in the quadrigeminal plate. (A) Mid sagittal T2-weighted image. Note the expansion of the third ventricle and the stretched corpus callosum caused by ventricular dilatation in an obstructive hydrocephalus. Hydrocephalus is caused by a mass in the quadrigeminal plate narrowing the aqueduct and causing obstruction to CSF flow out of the ventricular system. The 4th ventricle is of normal size. (B) Mid sagittal T2-weighted image. Two years later, the girl has been treated with a ventriculocisternostomy through the floor of the third ventricle creating a communication thus bypassing the obstructed aqueduct. Note the obvious flow artifact caused by CSF pulsating back and forth through the stoma.

obstruct the narrow aqueduct while tumours in the quadrigeminal cistern do not have to be very large before causing obstruction. Periaqueductal tumours tend to be low-grade gliomas with very slow or no growth. Long-term follow-up of children thought to have a primary obstruction of the aqueduct of Sylvius have been found, when imaged by MRI rather than CT, to have such mass lesions causing hydrocephalus rather than primary aqueductal stenosis. Inadvertent long-term follow-up, without specific therapy directed to the tumour, shows that these tumours often have a very low potential for malignancy. A tumour located ventral to the aqueduct, such as a brainstem glioma, rarely causes hydrocephalus until the tumour is very large, while a tumour located posterior to the aqueduct tends to cause kinking of the aqueduct and hydrocephalus is an early feature in this case. Thus, symptoms of raised intracranial pressure is a common presentation of primitive neuroectodermal tumours of the posterior fossa, often originating in the vermis, while hydrocephalus is a late and often terminal sign in patients with brainstem gliomas.

Periventricular oedema indicates obstructive hydrocephalus and reflects the high intraventricular pressure (Figure 12.9.10).

An important cause of obstructive hydrocephalus is arachnoid cysts that may show mass effect and obstruct CSF flow. Most difficult to identify as a cause of hydrocephalus is a cyst originating in the suprasellar region. Such a cyst may expand upwards and invaginate into the third ventricle by pushing the thin floor of the ventricle ahead of the expanding cyst. This invagination may expand and fill the entire third ventricle with subsequent obstruction of the lateral ventricles. This condition may mimic an aqueductal stenosis on CT and MRI and may be very difficult to differentiate from this condition, but it requires very different therapy. Failure to correctly identify the arachnoid cyst may lead to uncontrollable expansion of the cyst when the ventricular system is decompressed. This expansion may seriously damage suprasellar structures like the basal ganglia and the optic chiasm and cause visual impairment.

A less common cause of obstruction giving a similar appearance to an invaginating suprasellar arachnoid cyst is a true ependymal cyst in the third ventricle. Such a structure can have interesting properties as it may vary in size over time and may be pedunculated. Both these properties can cause intermittent obstruction over time or depending on position of the head as the pedunculated cyst may move and position itself differently in the third ventricle depending on the position of the head.

The most typical and best known expression of membranous obstruction to CSF flow is stenosis of the aqueduct of Sylvius. Knowledge from numerous air studies revealed that this obstruction was caused by adhesions obstructing the canal and sometimes splitting the aqueduct into two or more tiny channels. The cranial part of the aqueduct becomes grossly enlarged and narrows rapidly down to a funnel-like ending at the membrane. The condition caused symmetrical enlargement of both lateral ventricles and the third ventricle while the fourth ventricle remained normal in size or was even small. This is a very obvious pattern well known from pneumoencephalography studies that may also be recognized using CT or MRI; however, in general, caution is advised in drawing too great a conclusion from the relative size of the different CSF-containing compartments on CT or MRI. Thus, it is sometimes difficult to distinguish obstructive from communicating hydrocephalus on anatomical imaging alone. The cause of the obstruction may in some cases be a known infection but this condition is in many cases of unknown origin and not uncommonly present at birth.

Infections, in particular neonatal cerebral infections, have a tendency to cause ventriculitis with associated formation of septations, adhesions and membranes. Thus, the ventricular system can

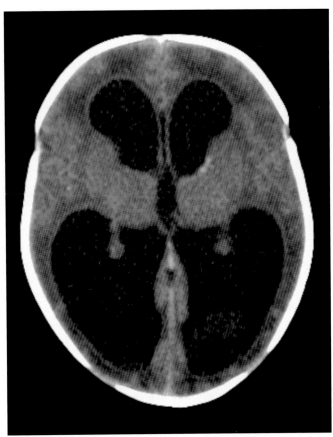

Figure 12.9.10 This 1-day-old boy suffered an intraventricular haemorrhage *in utero* and was born with a larger than normal head. Note the marked ventricular dilatation and periventricular low attenuation particularly marked anteriorly indicating periventricular oedema.

be divided into many compartments with poor intercommunication. This is an extremely difficult situation to deal with as successful treatment may require multiple shunts and shunt systems. Each compartment may require its own drainage as marsupialization of the membranes by endoscopic surgery usually has rather limited success. A special form of this condition is known as isolated or trapped fourth ventricle (Figure 12.9.11). Here, the fourth ventricle has lost its communication both in retrograde direction, to the third ventricle, and in antegrade direction, to the basal cisterns. It is important to recognize this condition as the expanding fourth ventricle may case symptoms of a posterior fossa mass lesion rather than poorly decompressed hydrocephalus. A trapped fourth ventricle only occurs following multiple shunt revisions, presumably with infections, and should be considered a complication of shunting.

CAUSES OF COMMUNICATING HYDROCEPHALUS

Communicating hydrocephalus in childhood can be caused by a variety of conditions with decreased intracranial compliance, some of which are also seen in adults (Figure 12.9.8). Obliteration of the

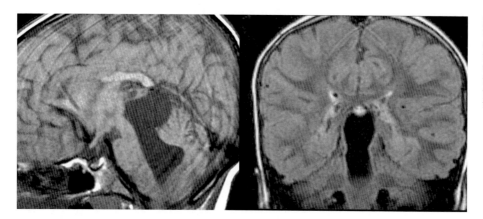

Figure 12.9.11 This 7-year-old boy has over the years had many shunt revisions. On the current MR investigation all ventricles except the fourth ventricle are small. The fourth ventricle is dilated and herniates up through the tentorial notch. A dilated and isolated fourth ventricle acts as a mass in the posterior fossa.

subarachnoid space is seen in a number of conditions such as subarachnoid haemorrhage, meningitis and other infections, trauma and following surgical interventions. More specific paediatric causes relate to hydrocephalus following intraventricular haemorrhage of the newborn, achondroplasia, Chiari II malformation with myelomeningocele and tumours of the spinal canal, all of which cause decreased intracranial compliance.

Posthaemorrhagic hydrocephalus following intraventricular haemorrhage of the newborn generated significant interest when reliable diagnostic opportunities arose with sonographic detection of intraventricular haemorrhage in premature neonates. It became clear that most preterm neonates with intraventricular haemorrhage developed ventriculomegaly, usually within days. Much effort was spent on early, active and aggressive treatment with repeated ventricular taps and early shunting, even before hydrocephalus was obvious with an enlarging head. However, the rate of complication turned out to be very high and most neonates suffered significant brain damage despite aggressive treatment. It is now recognized that most premature children develop ventriculomegaly as a temporary reaction to the haemorrhage and only develop hydrocephalus in need of permanent shunting in about 10% of all cases with haemorrhage. It is also now recognized that some of the ventriculomegaly is due to periventricular brain tissue damage, such as periventricular leucomalacia, and the dilatation is therefore caused by loss of brain tissue rather than elevated intraventricular pressure. A conservative approach is now exercised and shunting only performed when hydrocephalus is obvious and the infant's head is expanding out of control.

An interesting observation is that although premature neonates appear to manage their intraventricular haemorrhage very well with conservative care, intraventricular haemorrhage in the term neonate most often results in hydrocephalus in need of permanent shunting. The reason for this discrepancy is not known.

Children with a skeletal dysplasia such as achondroplasia have been known for a long time to have larger and more rapidly growing heads than a normal population. Neuroradiological investigations confirm that not only the ventricular system but also the subarachnoid spaces are larger than normal, a constellation of findings suggestive of communicating hydrocephalus. The skeletal abnormality in achondroplasia includes smaller than normal foramina in the base of the skull (Figure 12.9.12). Thus, not only the jugular foramen is smaller but, in particular, the foramen magnum is also smaller than usual and has commonly a keyhole shape. Previous studies have showed a venous pressure gradient over the jugular foramen suggesting that higher venous pressure may play a role in the pathophysiology of hydrocephalus. However, new research suggests that the narrow foramen magnum is more important as it impairs the flow of CSF to and from the spinal canal, thus creating a situation in which there will be a restriction of the arterial pulsations in the subarachnoid space, the now well established pathophysiology behind communicating hydrocephalus.

Obstruction of the foramen magnum is also seen in children with Chiari II malformations in whom a low-lying cerebellum is responsible for impaired flow of CSF over the foramen magnum. The same mechanism is implied as an explanation for hydrocephalus found in some cases of spinal cord tumours in which case a tumour mass obstructs the rapid to-and-fro flow of CSF between the cranial cavity and the compliant spinal canal, thus decreasing intracranial compliance.

A childhood tumour with a strong association with hydrocephalus is choroid plexus papilloma. In textbooks, this tumour is often mentioned as an example of overproduction of CSF causing hydrocephalus. Although excessive production of CSF has been shown to occur in this tumour, the capacity of re-absorption of CSF into the cerebral circulation, as discussed above, is of such magnitude that it appears extremely unlikely that an overproduction of CSF could cause hydrocephalus. Choroid plexus papilloma is an intraventricular tumour and is prone to bleed and increases CSF protein levels thus interfering with CSF physiology in the subarachnoid space, resulting in communicating hydrocephalus.

HYDROCEPHALUS AND CONGENITAL MALFORMATIONS

Hydrocephalus may be an integral part of some congenital malformations of the brain. The hydrocephalus can be of the communicating type, as described above in Chiari II malformation in which the obstruction at the level of foramen magnum causes impairment of the pulsatile flow of CSF between the cranial cavity and the compliant spinal canal.

Hydrocephalus is also associated with other malformations, the most common being arachnoid cysts. Such cysts may be of such a size and in a such location that normal flow of CSF out from the ventricular system is impaired. The most important of these cysts to recognize is the suprasellar cyst, discussed above in 'Causes of

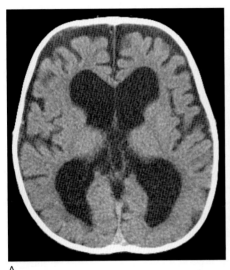
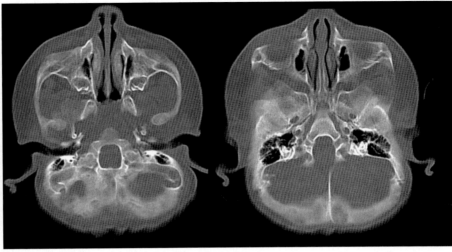

A   B

Figure 12.9.12 This 1-year-old boy with achondroplasia has a very large head that is accelerating in growth: + 7 SD (standard deviations) from normal on the usual normogram but + 2 SD on the normogram for achondroplasts. He has marked and distended cutaneous veins around both orbitae. (A) This CT scan shows the typical appearance with dilated ventricles and generous subarachnoid spaces over both cerebral hemispheres. Hydrocephalus is of the communicating type and is due to a combination of obstruction to venous return through small jugular foramina and reduced CSF flow across a small foramen magnum. (B) From the same CT scan, images of the skull base show a small foramen magnum as well as all other foramina in the skull base. Foramen magnum typically has a more pronounced keyhole shape than in this patient. Achondroplasia has abnormal formation of cartilaginous bone. The skull base is formed from cartilage while the calvarial bones are of membranous origin and hence normal in patients with achondroplasia.

Acute Obstructive Hydrocephalus'. Arachnoid cysts may also be located in the posterior fossa and by acting as a posterior fossa mass cause obstruction in the same manner as any other mass.

Children with callosal agenesis may have an associated cyst or cysts in the interhemispheric fissure. Some of these cysts communicate with the third ventricle and one or both lateral ventricles. The cyst is located on either side of the falx and may, despite communication with the ventricular system, have mass effect on the medial aspects of the cerebral hemisphere. In more complicated cases, the cysts may be multiloculated and without communication with the ventricular system. Such cysts can be very large and compress parts of the ventricular system, which is then difficult to identify. It may indeed be difficult to identify the cysts as cystic structures separate from the ventricular system. Callosal agenesis in its most pure form, without an associated interhemispheric cyst, is characterized by dilatation of the occipital horns, a feature sometimes referred to as colpocephaly.

A cystic structure also plays a role in creating the conditions for hydrocephalus in Dandy–Walker syndrome. Here, outlets of the fourth ventricle are initially atretic and the ventricle itself dilates early forming a large cyst expanding the posterior fossa. Hydrocephalus usually develops within the first months of life and is present in most children at the time of diagnosis. Shunting of the fourth ventricle is sometimes an effective treatment of hydrocephalus but more complex malformations exist in which full control over the hydrocephalus is not reached until an additional supratentorial shunt is inserted.

FETAL VENTRICULOMEGALY

Since prognosis in hydrocephalus is thought to be dependent on successful treatment of the condition rather than the degree of ven-

tricular dilatation at diagnosis, early diagnosis and treatment is felt to be important. However, the aetiology behind hydrocephalus has proved even more important for long-term prognosis than early treatment and the degree of ventricular dilatation at diagnosis. This has proved to be the difficulty associated with fetal diagnosis of hydrocephalus and *in utero* treatment.

Early attempts to diagnose ventriculomegaly using ultrasound and subsequent *in utero* intervention proved not to be very encouraging, as the results were poor. The reason for this is the difficulty in establishing the cause of hydrocephalus by using ultrasonography alone. Many unborn children with large ventricles not due to hydrocephalus were shunted *in utero* with disastrous results.

Prenatal MR imaging is providing new ways for detailed imaging of the fetal brain. The challenge now is not to identify ventriculomegaly but to identify the cause of this condition and hence define those cases in which treatment of hydrocephalus is felt to be associated with a good prognosis. Whether or not such optimal treatment must be undertaken during pregnancy or following early termination of the pregnancy is a different matter.

TREATMENT OPTIONS IN HYDROCEPHALUS

The optimal treatment for a child with hydrocephalus is to remove the cause of hydrocephalus and restore normal flow of CSF or normal haemodynamic conditions in the central nervous system. Treatment aimed at removing the cause of hydrocephalus will often concentrate on the removal of tumours or other masses like arachnoid cysts. Such action is dependent on precise and detailed information of the condition causing hydrocephalus. This option is extremely important to explore as the alternative (diversion of CSF using a shunt system) will condemn the child to lifelong dependence on advanced neurosurgical care as maintaining the proper function of the shunt is a prerequisite for normal life style and life expectancy.

In searching for the cause of hydrocephalus, it is of particular interest to study the dynamics of CSF as well as the communication between various CSF-containing spaces. MR imaging sequences sensitive to CSF flow as well as contrast injection into various spaces form the foundation for this diagnosis.

There are two main options for treatment when the cause of the hydrocephalus is not accessible for treatment. If the obstruction to CSF flow is found within the ventricular system or at the outflows from the fourth ventricle, a third ventriculostomy may successfully treat an obstructive hydrocephalus. The procedure is usually carried out using an endoscopic technique by which the thin floor of the third ventricle is opened thus creating a communication between the third ventricle and the suprasellar cisterns. The patency of such a third ventriculostomy can be checked using MR imaging as the pulsatile flow at the stoma can be seen on flow-sensitive sequences.

The most common treatment of hydrocephalus, irrespective of aetiology, is insertion of a permanent CSF diversion by means of a shunt system. There are many different kinds of shunt systems but they all have the same principal parts. The intraventricular tubing is usually located in one of the two lateral ventricles. The tip of the tube may have several holes over a short distance of the tubing. Thus, the shunt may be well functioning even if the tip of the shunt appears to be embedded in brain tissue. The ventricular catheter exits the cranial cavity through a burr hole and is then connected by means of a nipple to a shunt mechanism. The mechanism has two main functions: to provide a resistance of counter-pressure to CSF flow and to prevent back flow in the shunt system. The shunts often contain metal causing artifacts on MR imaging.

Some shunt systems allow adjustment of the resistance by the use of externally applied magnets. This is important for the radiologist to know, as this setting may be influenced and changed by the magnetic field in the MR scanner. The setting of the counter-pressure of the shunt mechanism is usually checked by means of a simple x-ray of the system. Many shunt mechanisms also include, proximal to the valve, a reservoir that can be punctured through the scalp.

The shunt system may in some cases be amended by adding an anti-siphon device to the system. This device prevents siphoning of CSF from the ventricular system to the abdominal cavity in an upright body position. The shunt mechanism is then connected through a nipple to the distal tubing, usually placed with its tip in the abdominal cavity. The shunt mechanism is usually cast in one piece that rarely disintegrates while disconnections are common at the nipples between the shunt mechanism and the distal tubing and less commonly between the ventricular tube and the shunt mechanism. X-ray examination of the shunt system to check patency must include images of the entire system in at least two projections. Too short a tube may lead to the lower end being projected over the liver on the anteroposterior (AP) view, only to be shown to lie subcutaneously on the lateral view. Calcification may develop around the subcutaneous tubing in the neck and chest and cause an irregular appearance of the tubing. Puncture of the reservoir in the shunt and injection of a radioisotope is an effective way of showing patency of the distal part of the shunt system.

Complications of an intraperitoneal shunt tip include migration through the hiatus into the pleural cavities causing a pleural effusion, perforation of the colon or bladder and, rarely, presentation in the vagina or rectum. Ultrasound of the abdomen with a normally functioning intraperitoneal tube tip will show some free fluid. Infection may lead to the formation of a large encysted CSF collection around the intraperitoneal tip. Even though it is infected, this infection is not usually gross and the fluid is sonolucent.

The primary aim of the treatment in acute obstructive hydrocephalus is to decrease the size of the ventricles and restore a normal intraventricular pressure. Inserting a CSF shunt, performing a third ventriculostomy or in some cases a posterior fossa decompression divert the excess volume of CSF produced within the trapped ventricles, restoring anatomy and CSF pressure. The reduction of the intracranial pressure also causes a secondary increase of intracranial compliance.

The primary aim of treatment of chronic obstructive hydrocephalus or communicating hydrocephalus is to restore intracranial compliance. The diversion of CSF following shunting causes a forced dilation of the compressed cortical veins. This increases venous compliance, decreases vascular resistance and increases cerebral blood flow. An alternative treatment would be a third ventriculostomy. This surgically created opening into the subarachnoid space ultimately reduces the intraventricular pulse pressure, due to increased expulsion of ventricular CSF during systole. This in turn will reduce the transmantle pulsatile stress, reduce ventricular size and expand the subarachnoid spaces including the compressed cortical veins, thus again restoring intracranial compliance and cerebral blood flow. In posterior fossa decompression, intracranial compliance is restored simply by recreating communication with the compliant spinal canal. Consequently, shunting, third ventriculostomy and posterior fossa decompression all increase intracranial compliance and decrease the transmantle pulsatile stress, which is causing the ventricular dilatation in chronic hydrocephalus.

Thus, the dynamic view of hydrocephalus presented here offers a logical explanation for the successful treatment of communicating hydrocephalus by third ventriculostomy and posterior fossa decompression. It cannot be explained by the CSF bulk flow theory, because a third ventriculostomy or a posterior fossa decompression cannot influence a 'decreased absorption of CSF at the pacchionian granulations'. This supports the view that communicating hydrocephalus is not caused by decreased absorption of CSF but rather by decreased intracranial compliance. The indications for treating communicating hydrocephalus at Chiari I malformations by posterior fossa decompression is well established and is now the preferred method. The indications for treatment of communicating hydrocephalus by third ventriculostomy have not yet been fully tested and remain to be determined. It seems that the clinical success rate for treatment by third ventriculostomy is somewhat lower in young children below the age of 1 year. Third ventriculostomy offers an alternative treatment to shunting and vice versa. It may also be used to replace the shunt when the child is older. This strategy has been successful in shunted premature children with posthaemorrhagic hydrocephalus. In this way, many children may become shunt independent. In this context, it should be pointed out that once a child has been treated by shunting or third ventriculostomy, they should be closely followed clinically until adulthood. The reason for this is that chronic hydrocephalus is a dynamic disease and there are reports of sudden death after minor head trauma as well as following a late closure of the shunt or stoma.

RADIOLOGY OF SHUNT FAILURE

Shunt failure may be due to many things, outgrowth of the shunt system, blockage and infections being the most common causes. In order to properly evaluate possible shunt dysfunction it is useful to have access to a previous examination as a baseline. For reasons explained above, such a baseline examination must be delayed until some time after the shunting and when the child is thought to have a well-functioning shunt system. Routine follow-up of shunt function is not advised as intervention should not be prompted by imaging alone but should depend on clinical symptoms and possible imaging evidence of shunt failure. Further, a normal follow-up does not protect from shunt failure the next day.

Clinical symptoms of shunt failure may include general symptoms of raised intracranial pressure. However, these symptoms are usually quite individual and the same child often expresses the same symptoms each time the shunt is not functioning properly. Hence, it is usually the parents who first suspect that the shunt may not be working properly and much emphasis should be placed on their evaluation of the situation rather than objective symptoms of raised intracranial pressure or decreased intracranial compliance.

With clinical symptoms of shunt failure imaging of the entire brain is necessary. The most subtle finding of shunt failure is the absence of the usual discrepancy of ventricular size seen when the shunt is working properly. Increased ventricular size is the more common finding when the shunt is not working properly.

Many children submitted to a shunt procedure will show very small ventricular size when clinically the shunt is felt to be functioning properly. This collapse of the ventricles may appear not to be desirable but is common and should not be taken as evidence of overdrainage and thus requiring adjustment of the shunt.

Excessive drainage of the ventricular system may occur and will cause specific symptoms in which the symptoms of headaches and nausea are relieved in horizontal position and provoked in upright position. This is a situation where an anti-siphon device may be useful. Following successful shunting, the reduction in ventricular size is usually readily apparent. However, the optimal ventricular size is not easily determined. If a child with marked hydrocephalus and a large head were shunted, the optimal course would be a gradual reduction in ventricular size as the head size adjusts to the size of the brain. If the intraventricular pressure is too low, the transmantle pressure gradient is reduced to zero and may be reversed. As a result, fluid will accumulate outside the brain rather than in the ventricular system and subdural haemorrhage or hygroma may appear without any other cause than the shunt. This is not considered to be a desirable consequence of shunting and the counterpressure of the shunt will have to be increased or an anti-siphon device added. Gradual adjustment of ventricular size and the delayed achievement of optimal ventricular size is the desired result following shunting.

SLIT VENTRICLE SYNDROME

Slit ventricle syndrome is a difficult concept. The typical imaging finding is narrow ventricles with no or quite subtle change in ventricular size. It mimics the condition in children who are shunted and when shunt failure occurs rapidly become very sick with symptoms of very high intracranial pressure and often very fast deterioration. According to Di Rocco, the diagnosis of slit ventricle syndrome should be limited to those shunted children with slit-like ventricles and patent CSF shunt devices who suffer from episodic headaches, vomiting and impaired consciousness secondary to decreased intracranial compliance. It is generally agreed that slit ventricle syndrome is caused by chronic overdrainage or siphoning following shunting. One explanation for this is that the shunting procedure is not as physiological as, for example, third ventriculostomy. It is difficult to regulate the CSF diversion in the shunting system, which may lead to chronic overdrainage of CSF. The condition is often described as the skull being one size to small. The skull cannot accommodate the normal volume of the brain plus the normal physiological volume changes in the vascular system, i.e. the intracranial compliance is significantly decreased. The mismatch between intracranial compliance and the blood circulation is more pronounced than in communicating hydrocephalus and intracranial high-pressure waves are more common.

The treatment of slit ventricle syndrome is difficult since the old shunt is functioning and no decrease in ventricular volume can be achieved by reshunting. Some surgeons advocate removal of the shunt to increase the size of the ventricles, followed by third ventriculostomy if the condition of the child deteriorates within the next few days. Some of the children may recover after shunt removal alone while others may recover after shunt removal combined with third ventriculostomy, regardless of the aetiology of hydrocephalus. This is another example of communicating hydrocephalus treated by third ventriculostomy and that third ventriculostomy can make children shunt independent. Lumboperitoneal shunting has also been used. Subtemporal decompression or cranial expansion, a more extensive operation, is used to increase the intracranial volume by making the skull larger.

VENTRICULOMEGALY DUE TO HIGH VENOUS PRESSURE – VEIN OF GALEN

In a skull with closed sutures, venous hypertension causes pseudotumour cerebri, not hydrocephalus. Venous hypertension or venous congestion levels out the transmantle pressure gradient and counteracts ventricular enlargement. Therefore, venous congestion is the main limiting factor for the ventricular enlargement in acute hydrocephalus. Before the closure of the fontanelles, there are special conditions in small infants since increased intracranial pressure may cause the skull to grow. In small infants, venous congestion may therefore cause ventriculomegaly. This is a special type of communicating hydrocephalus with mixed features resembling pseudotumour and acute obstructive hydrocephalus. The venous congestion often enlarges the subarachnoid space, since the transmantle pressure gradient is small or even reversed. In malformations of the vein of Galen, there is an arteriovenous fistula, which increases the pressure in the central veins. This increases the pressure and decreases the capillary fluid absorption in the central part of the brain. In combination with skull growth, this often leads to ventriculomegaly. It is important not to shunt the patients in this condition since the loss of intracranial counter-pressure following shunting may lead to a fatal disturbance of the intracranial blood circulation and subsequent brain damage.

Another cause of increased intracranial pressure is sinus thrombosis, which usually presents with narrow ventricles. Sinus thrombosis is a well known cause of pseudotumour. The vascular adaptation, with development of venous collaterals, usually decreases intracranial pressure in the chronic phase of thrombosis. Exceptionally, this may lead to communicating hydrocephalus in the chronic phase. The reason for the development of hydrocephalus is not decreased CSF absorption in the pacchionian granulations, but rather decreased venous compliance in the thrombosed cortical veins and venous sinuses. Communicating hydrocephalus in achondroplasia, which is caused by decreased intracranial compliance due to narrow foramen magnum and narrow jugular foramina, often demonstrates slightly increased subarachnoid spaces. This could be due to a component of slight venous stasis although the mean CSF pressure usually is not increased in this condition.

FURTHER READING

Aleman J, Jokura H, Higano S, Akabane A, Shirane R, Yoshimoto T. Value of constructive interference in steady-state, three-dimensional, Fourier transformation (CISS) magnetic resonance imaging for the neuroendoscopic treatment of hydrocephalus and intracranial cysts. Neurosurgery 2001; 48:1291–1295.

Barkovich AJ, Edwards MSB. Applications of neuroimaging in hydrocephalus. Pediatric Neurosurgery 1992; 18:65–83.

Barkovich AJ. Hydrocephalus. In: Barkovich AJ, ed. Pediatric neuroimaging, 3rd edn. Philadelphia: Lippincott Williams & Williams. 2000:581–620.

Baskin JJ, Manwaring KH, Rekate HL. Ventricular shunt removal: the ultimate treatment of the slit ventricle syndrome. Journal of Neurosurgery 1998; 88:478–484.

Borgesen SE, Gjerris F. Relationships between intracranial pressure, ventricular size, and resistance to CSF outflow. Journal of Neurosurgery 1987; 67:535–539.

Bradley WG Jr, Scalzo D, Queralt J et al. Normal-pressure hydrocephalus: evaluation with cerebrospinal fluid flow measurements at MR imaging. Radiology 1996; 198:523–529.

Bradley WG, Whittemore AR, Kortman KE et al. Marked cerebrospinal fluid void: Indicator of successful shunt in patients with suspected normal-pressure hydrocephalus. Radiology 1991; 178:459–466.

Casey AT, Kimmings EJ, Kleinlugtebeld AD et al. The long-term outlook for hydrocephalus in childhood. Pediatric Neurosurgery 1997; 27:63–70.

Conner EC, Foley L, Black PM. Experimental normal-pressure hydrocephalus is accompanied by increased transmantle pressure. Journal of Neurosurgery 1984; 61:322–327.

Dandy WE, Blackfan KD. Internal hydrocephalus. An experimental, clinical and pathological study. American Journal of Disease in Childhood 1914; 8:406–481.

Di Rocco C. Is the slit ventricle syndrome always a slit ventricle syndrome? Childs Nervous System 1994; 10:49–50.

Di Rocco C, McLone DG, Shimoji T, Raimondi AJ. Continuous intraventricular cerebrospinal fluid pressure recording in hydrocephalic children during wakefulness and sleep. Journal of Neurosurgery 1975; 42:683–689.

Di Rocco C, Pettorossi VE, Caldarelli M, Mancinelli R, Velardi F. Communicating hydrocephalus induced by mechanically increased amplitude of the intraventricular cerebrospinal fluid pressure: Experimental studies. Experimental Neurology 1978; 59:40–52.

Egnor M, Rosiello A, Zheng L. A model of intracranial pulsations. Pediatric Neurosurgery 2001; 35:284–298.

Egnor M, Zheng L, Rosiello A, Gutman F, Davis R. A model of pulsations in communicating hydrocephalus. Pediatric Neurosurgery 2002; 36:281–303.

Enzmann DR, Pelc NJ. Normal flow patterns of intracranial and spinal cerebrospinal fluid defined with phase-contrast cine MR imaging. Radiology 1991; 178:467–474.

Fischbein NJ, Ciricillo SF, Barr RM et al. Endoscopic third ventriculocisternostomy: MR assessment of patency with 2-D cine phase-contrast versus T2-weighted fast spin echo technique. Pediatric Neurosurgery 1998; 28:70–78.

Fukuhara T, Luciano MG, Kowalski RJ. Clinical features of third ventriculostomy failures classified by fenestration patency. Surgical Neurology 2002; 58:102–110.

Gideon P, Thomsen C, Gjerris F, Sorensen, Henriksen O. Increased self-diffusion of brain water in hydrocephalus measured by MR imaging. Acta Radiologica 1994; 6:514–519.

Gosalakkal JA. Intracranial arachnoid cysts in children: a review of pathogenesis, clinical features, and management. Pediatric Neurology 2002; 26:93–98.

Greitz D. Cerebrospinal fluid circulation and associated intracranial dynamics. A radiologic investigation using MR imaging and radionuclide cisternography. Acta Radiologica 1993; 34 (Suppl 386):1–23.

Greitz D, Franck A, Nordell B. On the pulsatile nature of the intracranial and spinal CSF-circulation demonstrated by MR imaging. Acta Radiologica 1993; 34:321–328.

Greitz D, Greitz T, Hindmarsh T. A new view on the CSF-circulation with the potential for pharmacological treatment of childhood hydrocephalus. Acta Paediatrica 1997; 86:125–132.

Greitz D, Greitz T. The pathogenesis and hemodynamics of hydrocephalus. A proposal for a new understanding. International Journal of Neuroradiology 1997; 3:367–375.

Greitz T, Grepe A, Kalmer M, Lopez J. Pre- and postoperative evaluation of cerebral blood flow in low-pressure hydrocephalus. Journal of Neurosurgery 1969; 31:644–651.

Greitz D, Hannerz J, Bellander B-M, Hindmarsh T. Restricted arterial expansion as a universal causative factor in communicating hydrocephalus. Neuroradiology (Suppl) 1995; 37:14–18.

Greitz D, Hannerz J. Rähn T, Bolander H, Ericsson A. MR imaging of cerebrospinal fluid dynamics in health and disease. On the vascular pathogenesis of communicating hydrocephalus and benign intracranial hypertension. Acta Radiologica 1994; 35:204–211.

Greitz D, Jan Hannerz J. A proposed model of cerebrospinal fluid circulation: Observations with radionuclide cisternography. American Journal of Neuroradiology 1996; 17:431–438.

Greitz D, Wirestam R, Franck A et al. Pulsatile brain movement and associated hydrodynamics studied by magnetic resonance phase imaging. The Monro-Kellie doctrine revisited. Neuroradiology 1992; 34:370–380.

Hakim S, Adams R. The special clinical problems of symptomatic hydrocephalus with normal cerebrospinal fluid pressure. Journal of Neurological Science 1965; 2:307–327.

Hirabuki N, Watanabe Y, Mano T et al. Quantitation of flow in the superior sagittal sinus performed with cine phase-contrast MR imaging of healthy and achondroplastic children. American Journal of Neuroradiology 2000; 21:1497–1501.

Hoffmann KT, Hosten N, Meyer BU et al. CSF flow studies of intracranial cysts and cyst-like lesions achieved using reversed fast imaging with steady-state precession (FISP) MR sequences. American Journal of Neuroradiology 2000; 21:493–502.

Hill A, Volpe JJ. Normal pressure hydrocephalus in the newborn. Pediatrics 1981; 68:623–629.

Jindal A, Mahapatra AK. Correlation of ventricular size and transcranial Doppler findings before and after ventricular peritoneal shunt in patients with hydrocephalus. Journal of Neurology, Neurosurgery and Psychiatry 1998; 65:269–271.

Kim DS, Choi JU, Huh R, Yun PH, Kim DI. Quantitative assessment of cerebrospinal fluid hydrodynamics using a phase-contrast cine MR image in hydrocephalus. Childs Nervous System 1999; 15:461–467.

McComb JG. Recent research into the nature of the cerebrospinal fluid formation and absorption. Journal of Neurosurgery 1983; 59:369–383.

McComb JG. Cerebrospinal fluid physiology of the developing fetus. American Journal of Neuroradiology 1992; 13:595–599.

Mitchell P, Mathew B. Third ventriculostomy in normal pressure hydrocephalus. British Journal of Neurosurgery 1999; 13:382–385.

Mohanty A, Vasudev MK, Sampath S, Radhesh S, Sastry Kolluri VR. Failed endoscopic third ventriculostomy in children: management options. Pediatric Neurosurgery 2002; 37:304–309.

Murphy BP, Inder TE, Rooks V et al. Posthaemorrhagic ventricular dilatation in the premature infant: natural history and predictors of outcome. Archives of Disease in Childhood. Fetal and Neonatal Edition 2002; 87:F37–F41.

O'Connel JEA. The vascular factor in intracranial pressure and the maintenance of the CSF circulation. Brain 1943; 66:204–228.

Parkkola RK, Komu ME, Aarimaa TM, Alanen MS, Thomsen C. Cerebrospinal fluid flow in children with normal and dilated ventricles studied by MR imaging. Acta Radiologica 2001; 42:33–38.

Quencer RM, Post MJD, Hinks RS. Cine MR in the evaluation of normal and abnormal CSF flow: intracranial and intraspinal studies. Neuroradiology 1990; 32:371–391.

Rekate HL. Classification of slit-ventricle syndrome using intracranial pressure monitoring. Pediatric Neurosurgery 1993; 19:15–20.

Sainte-Rose C, LaCombe J, Pierre-Khan A, Reiner D, Hirsch JF. Intracranial venous sinus hypertension: Cause or consequence of hydrocephalus in infants? Journal of Neurosurgery 1984; 60:727–736.

Schroeder HWS, Niendorf WR, Gaab MR. Complications of endoscopic third ventriculostomy. Journal of Neurosurgery 2002; 96:1032–1040.

Sgouros S, Malluci C, Walsh AR, Hockley AD. Long-term complications of hydrocephalus. Pediatric Neurosurgery 1995; 23:127–132.

Steinbock P, Hall J, Flodmark O. Hydrocephalus in achondroplasia. The possible role of intracranial venous hypertension. Journal of Neurosurgery 1989; 71:41–48.

Stephensen H, Tisell M, Wikkelso C. There is no transmantle pressure gradient in communicating or noncommunicating hydrocephalus. Neurosurgery 2002; 50:763–771.

Taylor AG, Peter JC. Advantages of delayed VP shunting in post-haemorrhagic hydrocephalus seen in low-birth-weight infants. Childs Nervous System 2001; 17:328–333.

Taylor GA, Madsen JR. Neonatal hydrocephalus: hemodynamic response to fontanelle compression – correlation with intracranial pressure and need for shunt placement. Radiology 1996; 210:685–689.

White DN, Wilson KC, Curry GR, Stevenson RJ. The limitation of pulsatile flow through the aqueduct of Sylvius as a cause of hydrocephalus. Journal of Neurological Science 1979; 42:11–51.

ARACHNOID CYSTS

An arachnoid cyst is a congenital malformation of the arachnoid. The walls of the arachnoid cyst consist of arachnoid cells secreting CSF into the cyst. Thus, accumulation of CSF in the cyst is an active process that, for yet unknown reasons, may in some cases cause a very large cyst with increased pressure and in other more common situations cause cysts without high pressure but still capable of displacing brain and eroding bone.

A true arachnoid cyst must be differentiated from a leptomeningeal cyst, i.e. a collection of CSF usually caused by a traumatic tear in the dura with arachnoid herniating through the tear and causing a collection of CSF surrounded by arachnoid scarring. These leptomeningeal cysts, commonly associated with 'growing skull fractures', often cause mass effect and corrective surgery should in most cases be considered.

Some locations for arachnoid cysts are more common than others. It is thought that half of all arachnoid cysts are found close to the Sylvian fissures (Figure 12.9.13). About 1 in 10 cysts are found in the suprasellar region, quadrigeminal cistern, cerebellopontine angle cistern and posterior infratentorial midline cistern. The remaining cysts are found over the hemispheres or in the interhemispheric fissure. Although these numbers are well accepted, they are developed from earlier studies of large series of patients found to have arachnoid cysts. With higher anatomical definition using new imaging methods, the incidental finding of arachnoid cysts, particularly in the middle cranial fossa, is now so common

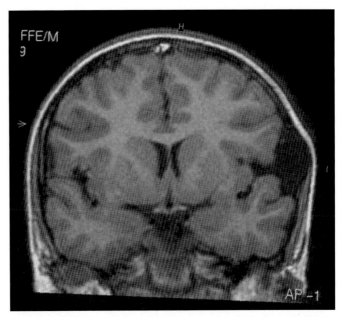

Figure 12.9.13 Coronal T1-weighted image of a child with an incidental finding of an arachnoid cyst associated with the left Sylvian fissures. Note the bulging of the skull vault over the lesion.

that our previous knowledge regarding frequencies must be questioned (Figures 12.9.14 and 12.9.15).

CLINICAL SYMPTOMS

Clinical symptoms of arachnoid cysts relate to location, size and age of the patient. Small cysts are almost always found incidentally and their relationship to non-specific symptoms such as headaches must be viewed with extreme care. Hydrocephalus may be caused by suprasellar cysts affecting the influence the cyst may have on the hydrodynamics of CSF (Figure 12.9.8). Suprasellar arachnoid cysts usually cause communicating hydrocephalus while large posterior fossa or quadrigeminal cistern cysts may distort the anatomy and cause aqueductal stenosis and thus obstructive hydrocephalus. Although an important association, hydrocephalus is associated with arachnoid cysts in only 1 in 10 cases. Suprasellar arachnoid cysts may also cause other symptoms relating to focal effects on surrounding structures, visual loss and hypothalamic dysfunction being the most important. Thus, an arachnoid cyst in the suprasellar cistern may cause precocious puberty.

Large arachnoid cysts in the middle cranial fossa may be found in patients imaged for occasional non-specific symptoms such as headaches, seizures, developmental delay or focal neurological signs. It is always difficult to assess the possible connection between the arachnoid cyst and such symptoms. A controversial issue is what effect the cyst may have had on the brain. When a cyst occupies the middle cranial fossa, the temporal lobe does not have a normal appearance and major parts may appear to be missing. It is tempting to assume that particularly early drainage of cyst will allow the brain to re-expand into the space previously occupied by the cyst, although this may not always be the case. Large cysts in small children may cause abnormally rapid head

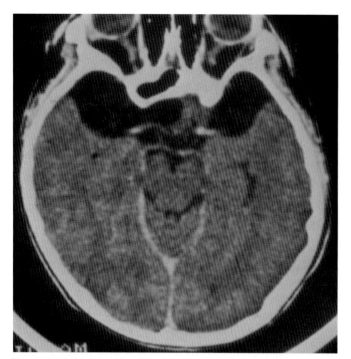

Figure 12.9.14 Axial T1-weighted image of a child with bilateral arachnoid cysts in the middle temporal fossa discovered during an investigation for epilepsy.

growth or abnormal shape to the head, even if hydrocephalus is not present.

Rarely, acute symptoms or deterioration may be due to haemorrhage in an arachnoid cyst. Such haemorrhages may occur spontaneously or following trauma and are due to damage to cortical veins close to the cyst. Large middle cranial fossa haemorrhages in small children are rare but may have occurred in a pre-existing arachnoid cyst.

RADIOLOGY

Arachnoid cysts appear on imaging as well demarcated unilocular cysts, usually with local mass effect. The space-occupying character of large cysts is obvious while even smaller cysts appear to have a focal mass effect. If the cysts are superficial, focal erosion of the skull is common. The signal and attenuation characteristics are those of CSF on MRI and CT, respectively.

Arachnoid cysts in the middle cranial fossa represent probably the most common location and are thought to have no clinical significance. Small cysts may be very common and occupy the most anterior portion of the middle cranial fossa without any deformation of bone and just minor displacement of the anterior tip of the temporal lobe. CT easily misses these cysts while they are clearly seen using MRI. Larger cysts in the middle cranial fossa typically

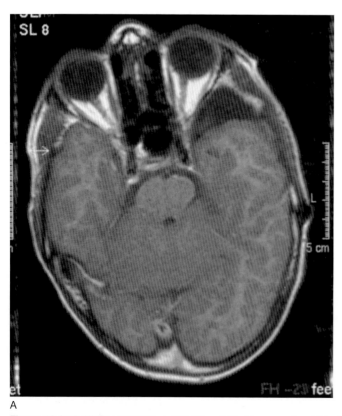

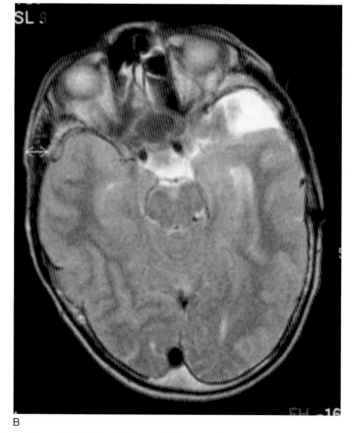

A   B

Figure 12.9.15 (A) T1-weighted and (B) T2-weighted images of a child with a unilateral, left-sided middle cranial fossa arachnoid cyst, discovered incidentally during investigation of headaches. Note the forward bowing of the sphenoidal bone by the cyst.

expand the bony walls of the middle cranial fossa with ballooning of the wing of sphenoid anteriorly. Very large cysts in this location are clearly expanding and may cause macrocephaly and displace the midline structures of the brain, particularly when found in neonates. Some large cysts in this location may declare themselves clinically with a spontaneous haemorrhage or may bleed following minor trauma. With blood filling the cyst, the underlying diagnosis of an arachnoid cyst may be difficult. However, recognition of the expanded bony middle cranial fossa gives the diagnosis away. Haemorrhage into these cysts is known to rupture into the subdural space causing subdural haemorrhage.

Clinically, the most important location of arachnoid cysts is in the suprasellar region. Here the cyst may be difficult to recognize unless very large. Smaller cysts may only occupy the suprasellar cistern and herniate into the third ventricle by pushing the floor of the ventricle in a cranial direction; thus, a diagnosis should be made only if the radiologist is aware of this potential diagnostic trap. When expanding, these cysts will expand in all directions: inferiorly into the pituitary fossa, laterally into the middle cranial fossae and anteriorly pushing on the chiasm and optic nerves. The most important expansion is posteriorly up into the third ventricle into which it may entirely invaginate and occupy. By doing this the cyst may occlude both foramen of Monro and even posteriorly kink and compress the aqueduct. This extension may explain an obstructive hydrocephalus while the most common mechanism behind hydrocephalus associated with these cysts may be occupying the basal cisterns, thereby reducing their compliance and thus causing communicating hydrocephalus. The cyst may compress the hypothalamus and even disrupt the pituitary stock, thus causing endocrine symptoms such as precocious puberty.

Arachnoid cysts in the basal cisterns must be distinguished from epidermoid tumours. This is best done using diffusion-weighted MR imaging since the two entities may be impossible to distinguish from each other on standard spin echo sequences. Intrathecal contrast injection followed by CT scanning may be an alternative way to identify the arachnoid cysts. However, some of these cysts are not completely separated from the subarachnoid space and may indeed only be ballooned membranes, much like a windsock, with contrast entering the incomplete cyst being only slightly delayed.

Posterior fossa arachnoid cysts in the posterior midline are diagnostically important since they may mimic a Dandy–Walker malformation. It then becomes important to identify the arachnoid cyst as being separate from the fourth ventricle. This is usually possible using sagittal MR imaging with special attention paid to flow-sensitive sequences. Cysts in the cerebellopontine angle may be quite large and must be distinguished from epidermoid tumours, a quite possible look-alike lesion.

TREATMENT

Indications for treatment are sometimes very difficult to establish. It may be impossible to predict if the cysts will totally or partially collapse when treated. Treatment decisions are particularly difficult in older children and adults since complications are common and the outcome difficult to evaluate. Causation between the presence of a cyst and clinical symptoms is not clear in this group of patients. Best results, from an imaging point of view, are usually achieved when cysts are treated in small children and neonates. Two principally different surgical techniques are used, fenestration of shunting using a low-pressure system to the peritoneal cavity. Imaging following surgery is particularly important in children with hydrocephalus, as it may be difficult at surgery to establish sufficient decompression of the usually suprasellar cysts. If the hydrocephalus alone is treated with a shunt but not the cyst, the suprasellar cyst may expand rapidly as counterpressure from the ventricles no longer exists. Such an expanding cyst may rapidly damage the optic chiasm and nerves, resulting in blindness.

FURTHER READING

Barkovich AJ, Simon EM, Walsh CA. Callosal agenesis with cyst: a better understanding and new classification. Neurology 2001; 56:220–227.

Daneyemez M, Gezen F, Akboru M, Sirin S, Ocal E. Presentation and management of supratentorial and infratentorial arachnoid cysts. Review of 25 cases. Journal of Neurosurgical Science 1999; 43:115–121.

Galarza M, Pomata HB, Pueyrredon F et al. Symptomatic supratentorial arachnoid cysts in children. Pediatric Neurology 2002; 27:180–185.

Gelabert-Gonzalez M, Fernandez-Villa J, Cutrin-Prieto J, Garcia-Allut A, Martinez-Rumbo R. Arachnoid cyst rupture with subdural hygroma: report of three cases and literature review. Childs Nervous System 2002; 18:609–613.

Gosalakkal JA. Intracranial arachnoid cysts in children: a review of pathogenesis, clinical features, and management. Pediatric Neurology 2002; 26:93–98.

Hoffmann KT, Hosten N, Meyer BU et al. CSF flow studies of intracranial cysts and cyst-like lesions achieved using reversed fast imaging with steady-state precession MR sequences. American Journal of Neuroradiology 2000; 21:493–502.

Kirollos RW, Javadpour M, May P, Mallucci C. Endoscopic treatment of suprasellar and third ventricle-related arachnoid cysts. Childs Nervous System 2001; 17:713–718.

Mohn A, Schoof E, Fahlbusch R, Wenzel D, Dorr HG. The endocrine spectrum of arachnoid cysts in childhood. Pediatric Neurosurgery 1999; 31:316–321.

Sgouros S, Chapman S. Congenital middle fossa arachnoid cysts may cause global brain ischaemia: a study with 99Tc-hexamethylpropyleneamineoxime single photon emission computerized tomography scans. Pediatric Neurosurgery 2001; 35:188–194.

Yalcin AD, Oncel C, Haymaz A, Kuloglu N, Forta H. Evidence against association between arachnoid cysts and epilepsy. Epilepsy Research 2002; 49:255–260.

CHAPTER

Metabolic Disorders

Zoltán Patay

12.10

INTRODUCTION

Metabolic diseases are generally considered to be rare. It is certainly true that the individual disease entities are not frequently encountered in the practice of the general radiologist. Nevertheless, the group of metabolic disorders, as a whole, represents a significant proportion of the pathologies involving the central nervous system in the paediatric population. Metabolic diseases often show specific ethnic or geographical preponderance but many of them are panethnic and may occur sporadically anywhere. Awareness of the different entities and their clinical and imaging manifestations is mandatory in order to raise or reach the diagnosis of these often under-recognized diseases.

GENERAL CONSIDERATIONS

CLASSIFICATION OF METABOLIC DISORDERS

Metabolic disorders are classically divided into inborn errors of metabolism and acquired metabolic diseases. Acquired metabolic diseases usually occur in specific or suggestive clinical settings, such as kernicterus in neonatal hyperbilirubinaemia, hypovitaminoses in malnutrition or neonatal hypoglycaemia in premature infants. Toxic encephalopathies are special, exogenous forms of acquired metabolic diseases.

Inborn errors of metabolism represent a vast and complex group of pathologies. Many classifications exist, all of them with the aim of facilitating the systematic approach to these diseases. Unfortunately, none of the currently available classifications is fully appropriate to guide the imaging evaluation. They are however useful, since each of them points to one of the many essential aspects of these pathologies.

CLASSIFICATION ACCORDING TO ORGAN SYSTEM INVOLVEMENT

This is mainly a clinically oriented classification, which takes into account the pattern of organ system involvement.

DISEASES WITHOUT INVOLVEMENT OF THE CENTRAL NERVOUS SYSTEM

The best known of the diseases in this group are the so-called glycogen storage disorders.

DISEASES WITH SYSTEMIC AND CENTRAL NERVOUS SYSTEM INVOLVEMENT

These diseases often present with visceral involvement (cardiac, musculoskeletal, hepatic abnormalities in mucopolysaccharidoses) and/or systemic metabolic derangements (lactic acidosis) in conjunction with central nervous system involvement.

DISEASES WITH INVOLVEMENT OF THE CENTRAL NERVOUS SYSTEM ONLY

In this group, the metabolic abnormality manifests exclusively with signs and symptoms of central nervous system involvement. This group of pathologies is often referred to as neurometabolic disorders, in the strict sense of the term. The best known of these pathologies are L-2-hydroxyglutaric aciduria, type 1 glutaric aciduria, 4-hydroxybutyric aciduria, alfa-ketoglutaric aciduria and *N*-acetyl aspartic aciduria (Canavan disease).

CLASSIFICATION ACCORDING TO CELLULAR ORGANELLE DYSFUNCTION

The cellular organelles have distinctly different functions in the metabolism; the mitochondria are involved mainly in energy metabolism, lysosomes in the degradation of macromolecules (lipids, lipoproteins, mucopolysaccharides) and peroxisomes in both anabolic and catabolic functions.

MITOCHONDRIAL DISORDERS

This term is somewhat confusing. Actually, many metabolic disorders are due to enzyme deficiencies within the mitochondria (some of the urea cycle defects, organic acidurias, such as type 1 glutaric aciduria, etc.), therefore could be referred to as mitochondrial disorders. In fact, true mitochondrial disorders comprise abnormalities of the mitochondrial energy metabolism, notably oxidative phosphorylation, fatty acid oxidation, ketogenesis and ketolysis.

LYSOSOMAL DISORDERS

Lysosomes are cellular organelles, the primary role of which is breakdown of macromolecules, mainly lipids and lipoproteins. This group comprises disorders of sphingolipids (Krabbe disease, metachromatic leucodystrophy, GM1 and GM2 gangliosidosis, Niemann–Pick disease, Gaucher disease, Fabry disease, Farber disease), mucopolysaccharides (Hunter disease, Scheie disease, Hunter–Scheie disease, Hurler disease, Sanfilippo disease, Morquio, Maroteaux–Lamy disease, Sly disease) and cystine (cystinosis) metabolism.

PEROXISOMAL DISORDERS

Peroxisomes are cellular organelles that are involved in both anabolic and catabolic processes. On the one hand, one of their primary roles is synthesis of phospholipids, which are essential components of myelin, but on the other, very long chain fatty acids and phytanic acids are degraded within the peroxisomes too.

A whole spectrum of quite different diseases falls into this category, the clinical manifestations of which are heavily dependent on the age of onset. Neonatal onset diseases include Zellweger syndrome and its variants, neonatal adrenoleucodystrophy, pseudoneonatal adrenoleucodystrophy, multifunctional enzyme deficiency, pipecolic aciduria, mevalonic aciduria and rhizomelic chondrodysplasia punctata. Early infantile onset diseases include infantile Refsum disease, pseudoinfantile Refsum disease as well as milder forms of Zellweger syndrome and neonatal adrenoleucodystrophy, and mevalonic and pipecolic acidurias. Childhood and juvenile onset diseases include X-linked adrenoleucodystrophy and classical Refsum disease, whereas adrenomyeloneuropathy is typically of adult onset.

GOLGI COMPLEX DISORDERS

These are rare disorders, characterized by the defect of glycosylation.

CLASSIFICATION ACCORDING TO THE BIOCHEMICAL/LABORATORY ABNORMALITY

This classification provides some help for the radiologist, since disease groups such as organic acidurias or aminoacidaemias have common, sometimes suggestive clinical and imaging features. There is however some overlap between these two groups of diseases too, e.g. aminoacidaemias are frequently associated with organic acidurias.

Disorders of the metal transport represent a peculiar group of pathologies, which is quite difficult to fit into any classification scheme.

ORGANIC ACIDOPATHIES

The best-known organic acidopathies are: primary lactic acidosis, propionic, methylmalonic and isovaleric acidaemias, 3-methylglutaconic, 4-hydroxybutyric, L-2-hydroxyglutaric acidurias and HMG-coenzyme A lyase deficiency.

AMINO ACIDOPATHIES

The most frequently encountered amino acidopathies are phenylketonuria, tyrosinaemia, alkaptonuria, homocystinuria, maple syrup urine disease, non-ketotic hyperglycinaemia and the so-called urea cycle defects.

DISORDERS OF METAL METABOLISM

The best known of these diseases are those related to copper transport (Menkes disease and Wilson disease). Other metals, which may be involved in inherited metabolic diseases, are iron, magnesium, selenium, zinc, manganese and molybdenum.

CLASSIFICATION ACCORDING TO BRAIN SUBSTANCE INVOLVEMENT

This classification is the one that serves best the purposes of the radiologist. This classification takes into account the dominance of substance involvement (grey matter, white matter or both) within the brain, usually best shown by magnetic resonance imaging (MRI).

LEUCODYSTROPHIES

Diseases that present with white matter abnormalities are referred to as leucodystrophies. The underlying metabolic abnormalities, however, span over a very wide range and include peroxisomal disorders (X-linked adrenoleucodystrophy) or lysosomal storage disorders (metachromatic leucodystrophy, Krabbe disease). In many other so-called classical leucodystrophies, the underlying metabolic abnormality is not known (Alexander disease, vanishing white matter disease, Van der Knaap disease, Aicardi–Goutiere syndrome) and there are others that have never been referred to as leucodystrophies but, from the imaging point of view, appear to be predominantly white matter diseases (GM2 gangliosidosis, L-2-hydroxyglutaric aciduria, many amino acidopathies, some forms of congenital muscular dystrophy).

In leucodystrophies or leucodystrophy-like conditions, the underlying pathological process may be quite different, notably delayed myelination, dysmyelination or demyelination or a combination of both. The differentiation between these categories is often difficult or impossible by imaging, nevertheless the concept is important. Myelination is a very energy and nutrient-dependent process and any systemic (cardiac, respiratory, etc.) or central nervous system disease (meningoencephalitis, neurometabolic disease, etc.) during the most active period of myelination (from birth to the age of 18 months) may lead to delay in the normal myelination process. In these cases, however, the constitution of the myelin is normal. Conversely, in dysmyelinating processes the chemical structure of the myelin is abnormal, leading to fragile myelin that is prone to early or abnormal breakdown, resulting in partial or complete loss of the myelin. The term demyelination refers to the loss of primarily normal myelin, the possible causes of which represent a wide range of pathologies, including inflammatory, toxic, metabolic and many other causes, as well as dysmyelination.

POLIODYSTROPHIES

This group comprises diseases that present with predominantly grey matter abnormalities. Some degree of white matter involvement, however, is often present. Classical disease categories are respiratory chain disorders (so-called 'mitochondrial diseases') and organic acidopathies.

PANDYSTROPHIES

In fact, the majority of the metabolic disorders fall into this category, since exclusive involvement of the grey or white matter structures is quite exceptional. It is nevertheless sometimes impossible to determine whether the often-present white matter abnormalities in 'poliodystrophies' are primary or secondary to neuronal degeneration and, conversely, whether the quite frequent signal changes within the basal ganglia in classical 'leucodystrophies' represent just myelin breakdown or genuine neuronal damage.

FURTHER READING

Hoffmann GF, Gibson KM, Trefz FK et al. Neurological manifestations of organic acid disorders. European Journal of Pediatrics 1994; 153 (Suppl 1):94–100.

THE CONCEPT OF SELECTIVE VULNERABILITY

Some of the metabolic disorders present with rather unremarkable, 'generic' features from the imaging point of view, such as atrophy and hypo- or delayed myelination. Nevertheless, one of the most striking imaging and pathological characteristics of many metabolic disorders is the often peculiarly selective involvement of the different brain structures. Depending on the disease entity, some brain structures may be severely damaged whereas others are completely normal. This is called selective vulnerability. The involved structures and the non-involved areas together often describe a pattern (often referred to as 'gestalt'), which may be quite consistent in the given disease entity.

The underlying pathomechanisms explaining the phenomena of selective vulnerability in most cases are rather poorly understood; nevertheless, a few hypotheses have been proposed.

DIRECT TOXIC EFFECT

In some diseases, a direct toxic effect of an abnormal metabolite has been identified. In urea cycle defects, for example, hyper-

ammonaemia is the cause of brain oedema. Increased blood concentration of homocystine in homocystinuria is known to be destructive to fibrillin in connective tissues, the result of which may be blood vessel wall damage or lens subluxation.

INDIRECT TOXIC EFFECT

Indirect mechanisms are also known. They include enzyme inhibition by an abnormal metabolite and activation of alternative metabolic pathways for an excess metabolite, resulting in the synthesis of another toxic metabolite.

ENZYME INHIBITION

Propionyl and methylmalonyl coenzyme A in propionic and methylmalonic acidurias is known to inhibit pyruvate carboxylase, which results in hypoglycaemia and ketosis. At the same time the glycine cleavage system may also be impaired, leading to hyperglycinaemia (explaining why propionic acidaemia is also referred to as ketotic hyperglycinaemia).

ACTIVATION OF ALTERNATIVE METABOLIC PATHWAYS

Hyperammonaemia in urea cycle defects leads to increased synthesis of glutamate, which is known to be an excitotoxic metabolite to the brain parenchyma. Excess tryptophan may be degraded through an alternate catabolic pathway towards quinolinic acid, which is also believed to be toxic to the basal ganglia, providing one of the possible explanations to basal ganglia disease in type 1 glutaric aciduria.

FURTHER READING

Johnston MV, Hoon AH Jr. Possible mechanism in infants for selective basal ganglia damage from asphyxia, kernicterus, or mitochondrial encephalopathies. Journal of Child Neurology 2000; 15:588–591.
Lipton SA, Rosenberg PA. Excitatory amino acids as a final common pathway for neurologic disorder. New England Journal of Medicine 1994; 330:613–622.

PRINCIPLES OF IMAGING IN METABOLIC DISORDERS

Imaging strategies in inborn errors of metabolism rely heavily on the concepts of selective vulnerability and pattern recognition. The imaging work-up of the patients with suspected metabolic disorders is designed to obtain the best possible visualization and characterization of the lesions within the central nervous system, which is obviously the most important prerequisite of the application of the concept of pattern recognition in the process of image analysis. The individual lesions represent the imaging substrates of the selective vulnerability and the sum of the lesions with the resultant lesion patterns correspond to the imaging phenotypes of the various disease entities.

IMAGING MODALITIES

CONVENTIONAL X-RAY

Conventional x-ray studies have a very limited role in the diagnostic imaging work-up of metabolic disorders. They may be used to demonstrate involvement of the skeletal system. Skull x-ray studies show deformities of the sella or abnormalities of the bony elements of the craniocervical junction, and skeletal x-rays are used to diagnose changes in mucopolysaccharidosis.

ULTRASOUND (US)

Transfontanel ultrasound is helpful in macrocephalic neurometabolic disorders to rule out hydrocephalus. In type 1 glutaric aciduria, the characteristic bilateral Sylvian fissure abnormalities may also be identified.

COMPUTED TOMOGRAPHY (CT)

Computed tomography is usually performed after an MRI examination in order to demonstrate calcifications, for example. In acute metabolic crisis, stroke or stroke-like presentations it may also be used to rule out vascular aetiologies or complications (ischaemia or intracerebral bleeding) as an emergency imaging modality.

MAGNETIC RESONANCE IMAGING (MRI)

Magnetic resonance imaging has an inherently high sensitivity in demonstrating normal or abnormal myelination, differentiating white and grey matter, and detecting structural and signal changes within the brain. The typical criticism of MRI is its low specificity, since most abnormalities present with increase of T1 and T2 relaxation (hyposignal with T1- and hypersignal on T2-weighted imaging). This shortcoming of MRI, however, may be significantly reduced by the systematic use of the concept of pattern recognition, through which disease-specific patterns may be identified.

IMAGING STRATEGIES

The protocol in magnetic resonance imaging of the brain should be adapted to the specific needs of image evaluation. The most important prerequisites for lesion detection are the selection of the optimal imaging planes, high spatial resolution and high-contrast resolution.

OPTIMAL IMAGING PLANE

Accurate assessment of the different anatomical structures of the brain requires appropriate imaging plane selection. For example, the dentate and subthalamic nuclei are best visualized in the coronal plane. The basal ganglia in general are well appreciated in the axial plane; nevertheless, involvement of the body of the caudate nucleus may require coronal cuts. The cerebellar vermis and the corpus callosum are the most adequately delineated in sagittal images.

OPTIMAL SPATIAL RESOLUTION

Some of the brain structures are quite well visualized in low resolution (256 matrix) images, because of their considerable volume (basal ganglia, thalami, centrum semiovale). Some other structures, such as the cerebral and cerebellar cortex, the claustra, the brainstem structures, the subcortical U-fibres, etc. are smaller; therefore, the use of high resolution (512 matrix) is indispensable in their accurate evaluation. Ultra-high resolution matrix (1024) may have potential in the future but is not currently used.

OPTIMAL CONTRAST RESOLUTION

T1-weighted imaging is essential in the evaluation of the normal or abnormal myelination process in infants under the age of 12 months. In older children, T1-weighted imaging may also be useful in the assessment of the pattern of a demyelinating process (sparing of perivascular white matter in metachromatic leucodystrophy or of the subcortical U-fibres in some other white matter diseases). The T1 contrast can be enhanced by the use of the real inversion recovery (rIR) technique.

T2-weighted imaging is useful in the assessment of both the grey and the white matter at any age. It is usually more sensitive than the T1-weighted imaging in lesion detection. Fluid-attenuated inversion recovery (FLAIR) imaging is less frequently used in children than in adults. Its sensitivity is inferior to conventional T2-weighted imaging, especially in brainstem lesions. Conversely, modular inversion recovery (mIR) technique sometimes allows very accurate delineation of small lesions within the brainstem and the deep grey matter nuclei.

EVALUATION OF THE MR IMAGES

The evaluation of the MR images in metabolic disorders is based on the application of the concept of pattern recognition. Pattern recognition means the recognition of the imaging manifestations of the selective tissue or structure vulnerability within the central nervous system. Some of the abnormalities are easy to recognize, others may be subtler, requiring sophisticated imaging techniques and meticulous evaluation. In order to obtain the most complete data set for pattern recognition, a systematic and extensive evaluation of the brain structures is mandatory. The most relevant white or grey matter structures of the brain are listed in Table 12.10.1.

WHITE MATTER STRUCTURES

The cerebral white matter is assessed globally but also separately in the different (frontal, parietal, occipital and temporal) lobes, since their involvement may be different or similar in the various diseases. Depending on the magnitude of involvement in the different lobes, anteroposterior or posteroanterior gradients may be identified. Similarly, central and peripheral white matter structures may show different degrees of damage, therefore centripetal or

Table 12.10.1 The most important white and grey matter structures of the brain to be analyzed in metabolic disorders

White matter structures	Grey matter structures
Cerebral (lobar) white matter	Cerebral cortex
Subcortical U-fibres	Claustrum
Extreme capsule	Caudate nucleus
External capsule	Putamen
Internal capsule	Globus pallidus
Lamina medullaris	Thalamus
Corpus callosum	Subthalamic nucleus
Anterior commissure	Red nucleus
Mamillary bodies	Dentate nucleus
Posterior tegmental brainstem tract	Cerebellar cortex
Cortical-spinal tract	
Cerebellar white matter	

centrifugal progression patterns may be found. Special attention should be paid to the subcortical U-fibres, the sparing or involvement of which may be characteristic to specific disease entities (metachromatic leucodystrophy versus Canavan disease). It is also important to analyze the deep white matter layers. The internal capsule may be entirely or partially affected, therefore the anterior limb, the genu and the posterior limb have to be evaluated separately. The external and extreme capsules may be normal or abnormal too. The medial and lateral laminae medullares separate the pars medialis of the globus pallidus from the pars lateralis and the pars lateralis of the globus pallidus from the putamen, respectively. The corpus callosum usually reflects the magnitude and possible gradient of involvement of the hemispheric white matter. Signal abnormalities and volume changes (swelling or atrophy) may be found.

To date no data is available about the possible involvement of the anterior commissure in demyelinating processes but it is probably because little or no attention has been paid to this potentially important structure so far. The mamillary bodies are also prone to damage; the best-known example is Wernicke encephalopathy. The central tegmental structures of the pons are frequent sites of lesions in metabolic and neurodegenerative processes. The pyramidal spinal tracts should be carefully analyzed from the precentral gyrus all the way down to the decussation at the level of the medulla oblongata, including their course through the posterior limbs of the internal capsule and the cerebral peduncles. The cerebellar hemispheric white matter is perhaps less frequently involved than the cerebral white matter in metabolic diseases, but the presence of signal abnormalities can be a useful element in pattern recognition.

GREY MATTER STRUCTURES

The cerebral cortex is quite difficult to assess for atrophic changes, nevertheless in some diseases (GM2 gangliosidosis, Van der Knaap disease, Canavan disease) thinning of the cortex may be obvious. The deep grey matter structures should be assessed for morphological changes (swelling, atrophy) and signal abnormalities. In the acute phase of organic acidopathies, swelling of the basal ganglia is a typical finding, whereas in the chronic stage atrophy is characteristic. These changes are usually associated with increased signal intensity on the T2-weighted images. Hypointense appearance on the long TR images is suggestive of calcifications

or premature iron depositions, which are also characteristic of neurodegenerative diseases. In metabolic diseases presenting with basal ganglia lesions, the claustra may be spared (L-2-hydroxyglutaric aciduria) or involved (Wilson disease). The thalami are quite frequently spared. The subthalamic nuclei are abnormal in kernicterus but in Leigh disease also. The red nuclei are often spared in metabolic disorders but involvement of the surrounding white matter structures and of the substantia nigra with hypersignal on the T2-weighted images results in the so-called 'giant panda face' appearance. The dentate nuclei are often involved in all kinds of metabolic diseases, probably more frequently than previously thought. In the acute phase, when swelling is associated with hypersignal on the T2-weighted images, the depiction of the abnormalities is easy but in the atrophic stage, however, when volume loss is present with less prominent signal changes, identification of the lesions may be very challenging. The cerebellum as a whole, but the cortex in particular, often shows atrophic changes in metabolic diseases; rarely, signal abnormalities are present along the cortical-subcortical interface.

OTHER IMAGING ABNORMALITIES

The identification of additional abnormalities may also be useful in the process of pattern recognition. Macrocephaly in some leucodystrophies (Van der Knaap disease, Canavan disease, Alexander disease), in type 1 glutaric aciduria, GM2 gangliosidosis and L-2-hydroxyglutaric aciduria is an important pattern element. Bony abnormalities in the spine are typical and very characteristic in some forms of mucopolysaccharidoses.

FURTHER READING

Barkovich AJ. MR of the normal neonatal brain: assessment of deep structures. American Journal of Neuroradiology 1998; 19:1397–1403.

Forstner R, Hoffmann GF, Gassner I et al. Glutaric aciduria type I: ultrasonographic demonstration of early signs. Pediatric Radiology 1999; 29:138–143.

Steinlin M, Blaser S, Boltshauser E. Cerebellar involvement in metabolic disorders: a pattern recognition approach. Neuroradiology 1998; 40:347–354.

van der Knaap MS, Valk J, de Neeling N et al. Pattern recognition in magnetic resonance imaging of white matter disorders in children and young adults. Neuroradiology 1991; 33:478–493.

TYPICAL MR IMAGING FEATURES OF METABOLIC DISORDERS

Metabolic disorders have many common features, the awareness and recognition of which is important for raising the possibility of such a disease in as yet unknown central nervous system pathologies.

ATROPHY

Atrophy of different brain structures is common in metabolic diseases. Atrophy may be diffuse but often it is focal, selectively affecting specific structures, such as the cerebellar vermis, the optic nerves or the basal ganglia, which may be important elements

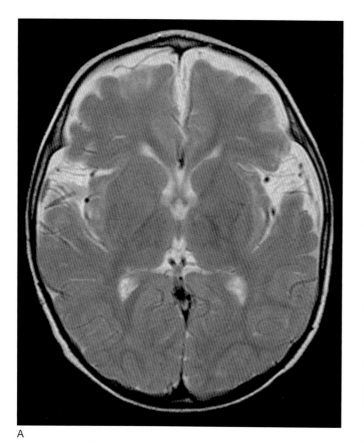
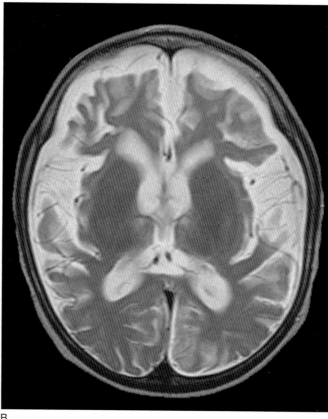

A   B

Figure 12.10.1 Axial T2-weighted fast spin echo images of a patient with biotinidase deficiency at the age of 2 years (A) and 4 years (B) showing progressive diffuse atrophy of the brain.

in pattern recognition. Atrophy is often progressive and may be the sole indicator of an insidious metabolic disorder (Figure 12.10.1). It is, nevertheless, important to note that during an acute metabolic crisis, swelling of grey or white matter structures is typical too.

SYMMETRY

In metabolic disorders, symmetry of the lesions is a characteristic although not a consistent feature. The grey matter structures (basal ganglia, the dentate nuclei) are almost always symmetrically involved. Very rarely asymmetrical involvement of the basal ganglia may be present in metabolic diseases, especially during the early stage of the disease (Figure 12.10.2). The white matter disease in metabolic disorders may be patchy but in extensive disease and in particular in leucodystrophies, the lobar white matter typically shows a fairly symmetrical pattern of involvement. Symmetry is, however, also quite frequent in neurodegenerative processes and even toxic encephalopathies.

MYELINATION ABNORMALITIES

In infants, during the most active period of myelination, delay or hypomyelination is frequently associated with metabolic disorders. These disorders are totally non-specific but important abnor-

malities. In some diseases (Zellweger disease, non-ketotic hyperglycinaemia) it can be very severe; in Pelizaeus–Merzbacher disease, the imaging findings suggest an arrest of the myelination process.

BRAINSTEM AND CEREBELLAR INVOLVEMENT

Cerebral abnormalities in metabolic disorders are much better known and more accurately described in the literature than brainstem and cerebellar changes. Nevertheless, brainstem and cerebellar changes are frequent too. Dentate nucleus lesions are quite frequent in organic acidopathies; the cerebellar white matter may be involved in leucodystrophies (Canavan disease) or in adrenomyeloneuropathy. The pyramidal tracts within the brainstem are always abnormal in X-linked adrenoleucodystrophy. The central tegmental tracts often show signal abnormalities in all kinds of metabolic and neurodegenerative diseases (Figure 12.10.3). As mentioned above cerebellar atrophy may also be associated with metabolic diseases (neuronal ceroid lipofuscinosis, 3-methylglutaconic aciduria, mitochondrial diseases) but prominent brainstem and/or cerebellar atrophy is perhaps more suggestive of neurodegenerative disease (e.g. olivopontocerebellar degeneration). The posterior fossa structures may, however, be totally normal too in metabolic diseases.

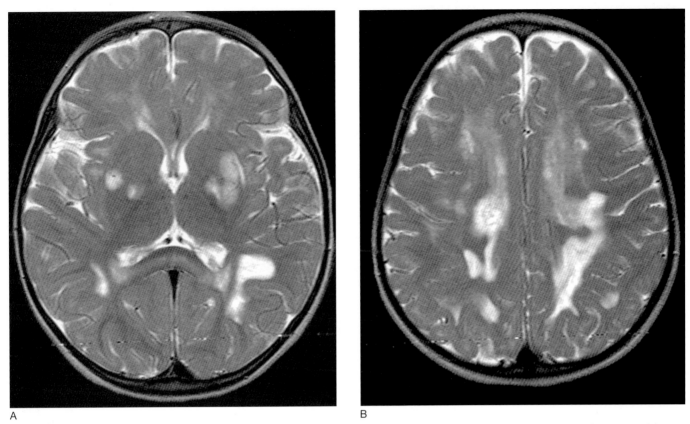

A   B

Figure 12.10.2 Asymmetrical basal ganglia (A) and cerebral white matter (B) lesions on axial T2-weighted fast spin echo images in a 1-year-old female patient with Leigh disease (same patient as in Figure 12.10.22).

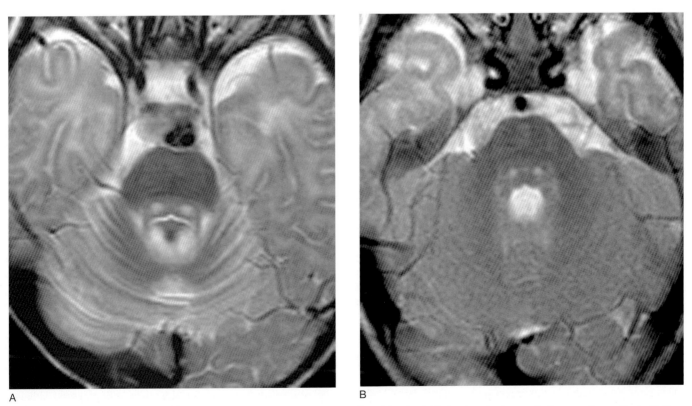

A   B

Figure 12.10.3 Non-specific symmetrical central tegmental tract lesions on T2-weighted axial fast spin echo images in the pons in a patient with 3-methylglutaconic aciduria (A) and in another with type 1 glutaric aciduria (B).

SPINAL CORD INVOLVEMENT

To date, the spinal cord has not been systematically assessed in metabolic diseases, hence literature data is sparse. Evaluation of the spinal cord for possible grey or white matter abnormalities is not easy. It is, however, reasonable to presume that the spinal cord may also be involved in more disease entities than reported so far. Histopathologically, spinal cord involvement has been demonstrated in several metabolic disease entities (Krabbe disease, 5,10 methylene-tetrahydrofolate reductase deficiency, etc.).

CONTRAST ENHANCEMENT

The MR imaging work-up of metabolic disorders rarely requires intravenous contrast injection. In some diseases (e.g. X-linked adrenoleucodystrophy), however, if present, it may be almost pathognomonic.

MALFORMATIONS

The occurrence of brain malformations is surprisingly low in metabolic diseases. It may be explained by the typically postnatal onset of most of the diseases. Callosal abnormalities (hypo- or dysplasia) are always seen in non-ketotic hyperglycinaemia, bilateral cortical dysplasia is a hallmark feature of Zellweger disease and central nervous system malformations have been described in ethylmalonic aciduria also.

FURTHER READING

Nowaczyk MJM, Blaser SI, Clarke JTR. Central nervous system malformations in ethylmalonic encephalopathy. American Journal of Medical Genetics 1998; 75:292–296.

IMAGING PATTERNS IN METABOLIC DISORDERS

Putting together the positive and negative findings during the imaging analysis in metabolic diseases results in various lesion patterns. Unfortunately, many of them are non-specific; nevertheless, they are still important since some of the abnormalities may be useful in raising the possibility of a metabolic disorder among other differential diagnostic considerations. In some diseases, however, the lesion pattern may be suggestive of a specific disease entity or group of diseases, whereas occasionally the imaging pattern is actually pathognomonic.

PATHOGNOMONIC MR IMAGING PATTERNS

This category includes L-2-hydroxyglutaric aciduria, type 1 glutaric aciduria, neonatal maple syrup urine disease, Zellweger disease, X-linked adrenoleucodystrophy, Canavan disease, Alexander disease and Van der Knaap disease.

SUGGESTIVE MR IMAGING PATTERNS

The best known of these metabolic diseases are some forms of methylmalonic, 3-methylglutaconic aciduria, biotin-responsive basal ganglia disease, non-ketotic hyperglycinaemia, Krabbe disease, metachromatic leucodystrophy, Leigh disease, MELAS and mucopolysaccharidoses.

NON-SPECIFIC MR IMAGING PATTERNS

All other metabolic disorders fall into this group. Nevertheless, it is worthwhile mentioning that it comprises many relatively frequent disorders, notably propionic acidaemia, ethylmalonic acidaemia, HMG-coenzyme A lyase deficiency, biotinidase deficiency, phenylketonuria, homocystinaemia and the so-called urea cycle defects.

THE CONCEPT OF DYNAMIC IMAGING PATTERNS

Follow-up studies in inborn errors of metabolism suggest that the imaging patterns may not be stable but are dynamic. This is quite conceivable, since clinically they often present as progressive diseases also. During the early ('subclinical') and late ('burned out') stages of a disease, the imaging patterns may be non-specific or atypical. The 'full-blown' imaging features of a metabolic disease describing a suggestive or pathognomonic pattern may be detected only within a certain period of time during the course of the disease. In the early stage of the disease, the imaging study can even be negative, which makes early diagnosis and more effective treatment difficult or impossible. This means that the imaging patterns during the course of a given metabolic disease may shift from non-specific to suggestive or even pathognomonic and then back to non-specific again.

The most frequently detected interval changes on follow-up imaging studies of metabolic diseases are progressive atrophy, myelination abnormalities and structural lesions.

ATROPHY

The interval enlargement of the extra- or intracerebral CSF spaces on follow-up studies, which is a frequent finding in metabolic disorders, characterizes progressive diffuse brain atrophy. In most cases, simple visual image analysis without volumetric studies is sufficient (see Figure 12.10.1).

MYELINATION ABNORMALITIES

Myelination abnormalities include delayed and/or hypomyelination or progressive demyelination. Interestingly enough, however, the process of brain myelination may still progress, although often at a very slow pace, even in poorly controlled or relentlessly progressive metabolic disorders. Nevertheless, it typically remains delayed or incomplete. The process of demyelination appears to be rather rapid in some diseases, whereas in others it is very slow.

STRUCTURE-SPECIFIC LESIONS

Structure-specific lesions may appear in a given metabolic disorder in a multiphasic fashion. It means that certain structures may be affected early during the disease course and others become abnormal later. This phenomenon may be responsible for significant pattern changes with time. Rarely, structural lesion may improve or totally disappear on follow-up studies.

ADVANCED MRI TECHNIQUES IN THE DIAGNOSTIC WORK-UP OF METABOLIC DISEASES

DIFFUSION-WEIGHTED MR IMAGING

Diffusion-weighted imaging is a true functional imaging modality at the cellular level. This technique was introduced into clinical MRI in the early 1990s and was initially used in the early diagnosis of cerebral ischaemia. More recently, it has been found to be useful in other pathologies, including metabolic disorders.

Water molecules within the cerebrospinal fluid diffuse freely, due to their random Brownian motion. In the brain parenchyma, diffusion of the water molecules is restricted; in the non-myelinated (or demyelinated) brain this is, however, fairly isotropical. As the brain matures and myelinates, water diffusion becomes anisotropically restricted. This means a preferential diffusion of the water molecules along the fibres and a relative restriction of the diffusion across the fibre tracts. This phenomenon is the physiological anisotropy of the white matter in the mature brain.

Oedema is a generic reaction of the brain parenchyma to different insults. Depending on the underlying pathophysiological mechanisms in various pathological processes, different oedema types may develop. Damage to the blood–brain barrier will result in vasogenic oedema, impairment of the Na^+/K^+ pump at the cell membrane level will result in cytotoxic oedema, cerebrospinal fluid (CSF) permeation through the ependymal lining of the ventricles causes interstitial oedema and myelin breakdown may be associated with the so-called myelin oedema, the histopathological substrate of which is vacuolating myelinopathy.

The value of diffusion-weighted imaging lies in its ability to identify precisely different oedema types within the brain. Vasogenic and interstitial oedema are typically associated with isotropically increased water diffusion within the involved brain parenchyma, resulting in decreased signal on the diffusion-weighted images. Conversely, cytotoxic and myelin oedema are characterized by isotropically restricted water diffusion, hence they present with increased signal intensity.

In metabolic disorders, cytotoxic oedema is encountered in acute grey matter disease, whereas active demyelination is often associated with myelin oedema (vacuolating myelinopathy); therefore, an active disease process may be detected easily with diffusion-weighted imaging. The progression of the disease can also be monitored with diffusion-weighted imaging; the disease eventually

leads to necrosis or total demyelination of the involved structures, which will present with hyposignal also. Acute vasogenic oedema may also occur in metabolic disorders. On conventional MR images this may be impossible to differentiate from cytotoxic or myelin oedema but with diffusion-weighted imaging this is usually very straightforward.

PROTON MR SPECTROSCOPY

Magnetic resonance spectroscopy is a technique allowing the *in vivo* detection of the presence of various normal and abnormal metabolites in the brain. For this reason, it has a role in the diagnostic work-up of metabolic diseases. The technique takes advantage of the presence of small but detectable differences in the resonance frequencies of molecules within the brain tissue, which therefore can be identified individually and their relative amounts graphically displayed on so-called spectra. The most commonly used forms of MR spectroscopy are the single voxel and the chemical-shift imaging (CSI) techniques. Single voxel MR spectroscopy is a robust technique, which is capable of producing high-quality spectra within a reasonably short acquisition time of a selected area (volume) of the brain, whereas chemical-shift imaging produces metabolic maps of the brain in a slice-by-slice fashion. Techniques for quantitative analysis of the different metabolites also exist.

The different metabolites have different T2 relaxation properties, therefore their detection may depend on and their appearance may be modified by the applied echo time. Long echo-time (135 and 270 ms) techniques, such as the point-resolved spectroscopy (PRESS), show fewer metabolites but a less noisy background, allowing more accurate peak analysis. Short echo-time (20–30 ms) acquisition techniques, such as the stimulated echo acquisition method (STEAM), demonstrate more metabolites but the background is noisier. The most frequently demonstrated metabolites in the brain and their peak locations on the MR spectra are shown in Table 12.10.2.

NORMAL METABOLITES IN THE BRAIN

In the normal brain, typically three prominent metabolic peaks are invariably detected, notably *N*-acetyl aspartate (a neuronal marker), creatine (an energy metabolism marker) and choline (a myelin marker). Using short echo-time techniques *myo*-inositol is typically seen also. The absolute and relative concentrations of metabolites, however, show age-dependent variations. In the

Table 12.10.2 The most frequently encountered brain metabolites and their peak locations

Metabolite	Peak location (ppm)
Lactate	1.33
N-Acetyl aspartate (methyl)	2.02
Glutamine	2.14–2.46, 3.78
Glutamate	2.11–2.35, 3.76
Creatine (methyl, trimethyl)	3.04, 3.93
Choline (trimethyl)	3.21
Myo-inositol	3.54
Glycine	3.55
Valine (branched chain amino acids)	0.99–1.05

neonate, *N*-acetyl aspartate is a rather small peak, whereas choline is the most prominent. After birth, choline progressively decreases and *N*-acetyl aspartate increases. By the age of 6 months, *N*-acetyl aspartate becomes the most prominent peak on the spectrum.

ABNORMAL METABOLITES IN THE BRAIN

These metabolites are actually present in the normal brain also but in such small quantities that under normal conditions they are undetectable by *in vivo* MR spectroscopy. Their appearance on the spectra therefore may be an indicator of a pathological process. Some of these 'abnormal' metabolites are non-specific (such as lactate, glutamine–glutamate complexes) but in certain settings may be suggestive of metabolic disorders. Other metabolites (e.g. branched chain amino acids, glycine) appear only in specific disease entities; therefore, their detection may be pathognomonic.

QUANTITATIVE ABNORMALITIES

Two rare but specific disease entities constitute a special subset in this group, notably the pathological increase of *N*-acetyl aspartate in Canavan disease and the absence of creatine in guanidinoacetate methyltransferase deficiency.

It is also noteworthy that many metabolic disorders present abnormal MR spectra but the findings are non-specific. This 'generic' pattern is typically characterized by decrease of the

N-acetyl aspartate peak (loss of neuronal integrity) and increase of the choline peak (increased myelin turnover). Occasionally, the *myo*-inositol peak may increase (unknown significance) and various amounts of lactate (impaired energy metabolism) may be present also.

TECHNICAL CONSIDERATION IN MR SPECTROSCOPY

Two important technical aspects of clinical MR spectroscopy need to be discussed here, notably the selection of the acquisition technique (short or long echo-time) and the positioning and size of the sampling voxel.

Acquisition technique

The findings by conventional MR imaging and clinical data influences the strategy of MR spectroscopy. In order to demonstrate *myo*-inositol, glutamine–glutamate complexes and branched chain amino acids, short echo-time (20–30 ms) MR spectroscopy is the technique of choice. *N*-acetyl aspartate, choline and creatine are well assessed on both 135-ms and 270-ms echo-time spectra. Glycine is best identified on the 135-ms spectrum. Lactate has a peculiar presentation on long echo-time MR spectroscopy. With 135-ms echo-time, it presents as a negative peak doublet, whereas with 270-ms echo-time it presents as a positive peak doublet. This is called the J-coupling phenomenon (Figure 12.10.4).

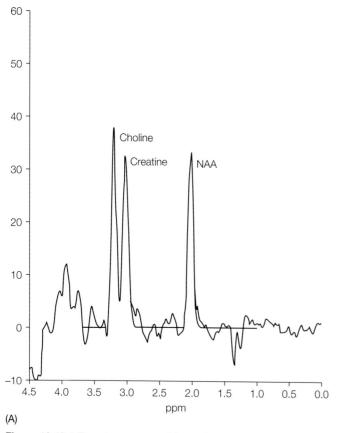

(A)

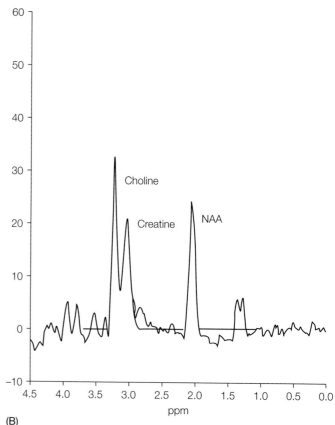

(B)

Figure 12.10.4 The phenomenon of J-coupling in proton MR spectroscopy of the brain in a 3-year-old female patient with metachromatic leucodystrophy (same patient as in Figure 12.10.30). Prominent peak doublets are present at the 1.3 ppm level on both spectra using the PRESS technique. On the spectrum with 135-ms echo time the peak doublet is negative (A); on the spectrum with 270-ms echo time it is positive (B).

Voxel positioning and size

In metabolic disorders, theoretically the sampling voxel may be placed anywhere in the brain, since the abnormal metabolites should be present everywhere within the brain parenchyma. Clear-cut abnormal structures should be avoided whenever possible, since severely damaged (e.g. necrotic) areas are no longer representative of the actual metabolic status of the rest of the brain. Furthermore, in lesion areas, smaller or larger amounts of lactate are almost always present. This should not be misinterpreted as an indicator of 'mitochondrial disease'.

If the voxel size is too small, the background of the spectrum may be rather noisy; hence small peaks may not be identified. Typically, a $2 \times 2 \times 2$ cm or larger voxel provides already interpretable quality spectra.

Occasionally, more than one MR spectroscopy study is performed using the same technique but with voxels positioned on different brain areas in order to demonstrate regional differences in the distribution of metabolites. However, this is more efficiently done by chemical shift imaging, which provides a true metabolic map of the brain.

FURTHER READING

Detre JA, Wang Z, Bogdan AR et al. Regional variation in brain lactate in Leigh syndrome by localized 1H magnetic resonance spectroscopy. Annals of Neurology 1991; 29:218–221.

Rajanayagam V, Balthazor M, Shapiro EG et al. Proton MR spectroscopy and neuropsychological testing in adrenoleukodystrophy. American Journal of Neuroradiology 1997; 18:1909–1914.

Stöckler S, Holzbach U, Hanefeld F et al. Creatine deficiency in the brain: a new, treatable inborn error of metabolism. Pediatric Research 1994; 36:409–413.

Tzika AA, Ball WS Jr, Vigneron DB et al. Clinical proton MR spectroscopy of neurodegenerative disease in childhood. American Journal of Neuroradiology 1993; 14:1267–1264.

Vion-Dury J, Meyerhoff DJ, Cozzone PJ et al. What might be the impact on neurology of the analysis of brain metabolism by in vivo magnetic resonance spectroscopy. Journal of Neurology 1994; 241:354–371.

CLINICAL ASPECTS OF INBORN ERRORS OF METABOLISM

AGE OF ONSET

One of the classifications of metabolic disorders takes into account the age of onset of the disease and is useful clinically. Neonatal, infantile, childhood, juvenile and adult onset diseases are described. The same disease may have different forms (clinical phenotypes) presenting at different ages. As a general rule, the earlier the onset is the more profound the metabolic derangement and the poorer the prognosis.

Devastating metabolic diseases of the newborn is a special category of inborn errors of metabolism, and awareness of this group of diseases and their clinical aspects is important because of the potentially deleterious consequences if not diagnosed and treated early. The infant is typically normal at birth. The prodrome, a few days later, is characterized by the refusal to feed and vomiting. This may occasionally be misinterpreted as pyloric stenosis. This is followed by lethargy and coma, which may mimic central

Table 12.10.3 Devastating metabolic diseases in the newborn

Organic acidopathies	Amino acidopathies	Others
Propionic acidaemia	Urea cycle defects	Zellweger disease
Methylmalonic aciduria	Maple syrup urine disease	Neonatal adrenoleucodystrophy
Isovaleric acidaemia	Non-ketotic hyperglycinaemia	Menkes disease
HMG-CoA lyase deficiency	Nesidioblastosis	
Multiple carboxylase deficiency		
3-methylglutaconic aciduria		
Glutaric aciduria type 2		
Primary lactic acidosis		
5-oxoprolinuria		

nervous system infection, notably meningitis. True meningitis or other infectious complications are not infrequently associated with metabolic diseases. Seizures and changes in muscle tone (hypo- or hypertonia) are often present as well. If the disease is not diagnosed and treated, it then further progresses and leads to irreversible neurological deficit or death. Most of the devastating metabolic diseases of the newborn are organic or amino acidopathies (Table 12.10.3).

SYSTEMIC MANIFESTATIONS OF METABOLIC DISORDERS

As discussed earlier many metabolic disorders have systemic manifestations. They typically include dysmorphic features, organomegaly or skeletal abnormalities. Cardiomegaly is often associated with 'mitochondrial diseases' and hepatosplenomegaly with storage disorders or peroxisomal diseases. Skeletal abnormalities are seen in mucopolysaccharidoses and peroxisomal diseases.

Systemic manifestations such as intercurrent infections, including infections of the central nervous system, notably meningitis or meningo-encephalitis, are frequent. Since devastating metabolic diseases of the newborn may present with meningitis-like signs and an intercurrent infectious disease often triggers symptoms and metabolic crisis situations, the complex association between metabolic diseases and infections may cause challenging differential diagnostic problems. Neutropenia and thrombocytopenia are typically seen in organic acidopathies; haemolytic anaemia is a characteristic complication of 5-oxoprolinuria.

NEUROLOGICAL ABNORMALITIES

SEIZURES

Seizures are frequent but non-specific complications of metabolic disorders. Tonic–clonic seizures occur only after approximately 6 months of age; before that myoclonic seizures may be observed.

PYRAMIDAL SIGNS

Pyramidal signs are typically seen in white matter diseases and are usually progressive. Some metabolic disorders may present with stroke (homocystinuria, Fabry disease, Menkes disease) or stroke-like events (MELAS, urea cycle defects), either due to a true ischaemic complication (occlusive arterial disease, embolism) or metabolic decompensation.

EXTRAPYRAMIDAL SIGNS

Extrapyramidal signs are characteristic in basal ganglia disease. Patients present with dystonia, choreoathetosis or tremor. The onset of these neurological abnormalities may be insidious or sudden, the latter again may mimic stroke.

TONUS ABNORMALITIES

Hypotonia is characteristically seen in propionic acidaemia (ketotic hyperglycinaemia), non-ketotic hyperglycinaemia and urea cycle defects. In propionic acidaemia and non-ketotic hyperglycinaemia this is due to the increased blood glycine levels, since glycine is known to be an inhibitor of the ventral motor neurons in the spinal cord.

Hypertonia is a typical feature of methylmalonic and isovaleric acidaemia. The exact pathomechanism of this is not known.

Alternating hypo- and hypertonia (presenting with opisthotonus) is characteristic to maple syrup urine disease.

ODOUR

Some of the metabolic disorders present with characteristic odour (e.g. 'smelly cheese' in isovaleric acidaemia and 'sweet syrup' in maple syrup urine disease).

FACIAL, EYE AND CUTANEOUS STIGMATA

Patients with organic acidopathies (e.g. propionic acidaemia, methylmalonic aciduria, isovaleric acidaemia, 3-mathylglutaric aciduria) often have a typical organic acidaemia face. This includes a depressed nasal bridge, epicanthic folds and a short or long philtrum. Facial dysmorphia is often present in peroxisomal disorders and characteristic facial changes are seen in mucopolysaccharidoses. Alopecia associated with skin rashes is often seen in biotinidase deficiency. Skin hypopigmentation may be present in phenylketonuria.

Nipple abnormalities (inverted, hypoplastic, supernumerary) may be found in propionic acidaemia patients. Cataracts may occur in 4-hydroxybutyric aciduria galactosemia, isovaleric aciduria, cerebrotendinous xanthomatosis, Cockayne disease and rhizomelic chondrodystrophia punctata; lens dislocations are typical for homocystinuria.

HEAD CIRCUMFERENCE

Head circumference abnormalities, macro- and microcephaly, are frequent in metabolic disorders.

Macrocephalic metabolic diseases include some organic acidopathies (type 1 glutaric aciduria), amino acidopathies (L-2-hydroxyglutaric aciduria), leucodystrophies (Canavan disease, Van der Knaap disease, vanishing white matter disease, Alexander disease) and lysosomal storage disorders (GM2 gangliosidosis, mucopolysaccharidoses). The pathogenesis of macrocephaly, however, differs in these diseases. Early (neonatal or infantile) onset of brain swelling, such as in infantile leucodystrophies or storage disorders, is a common aetiological factor. On the other hand, hydrocephalus (mucopolysaccharidoses) or intracranial arachnoidal cysts (glutaric aciduria type 1) associated with the metabolic disease may also account for the development of macrocephaly.

Microcephaly indicates an abnormal development of the brain. It may be present from birth or develop progressively during the course of the disease. Examples of the latter are the 'microcephalic' leucodystrophies (Cockayne disease, Aicardi–Goutiere disease, Pelizaeus–Merzbacher disease), in which the head circumference is normal at birth but the percentile curve shows progressive downward deviation from the normal afterward path.

FURTHER READING

de Grauw TJ, Smit LM, Brockstedt M et al. Acute hemiparesis as the presenting sign in a heterozygote for ornithine transcarbamylase deficiency. Neuropediatrics 1990; 21:133–135.

Gascon GG, Ozand PT, Brismar J. Movement disorders in childhood organic acidurias. Clinical, neuroimaging, and biochemical correlations. Brain Development 1994; 16 (Suppl):94–103.

Heidenreich R, Natpwicz M, Hainline BE et al. Acute extrapyramidal syndrome in methylmalonic acidemia: "metabolic stroke" involving the globus pallidus. Journal of Pediatrics 1988; 113:1022–1027.

Hsich GE, Robertson RL, Irons M et al. Cerebral infarction in Menkes' disease. Pediatric Neurology 2000; 23:425–428.

MOLECULAR GENETIC ASPECTS OF INBORN ERRORS OF METABOLISM

The molecular genetic basis of the inborn errors of metabolism is being increasingly elucidated. Most metabolic diseases are autosomal recessive; a few of them are autosomal dominant (adult form of Pelizaeus–Merzbacher disease, pigmentary orthochromatic leucodystrophy) or X-linked recessive (X-linked adrenoleucodystrophy, Hunter disease, Fabry disease, Pelizaeus–Merzbacher disease, Löwe syndrome). Some of the so-called 'mitochondrial disorders' have a peculiar inheritance pattern. The genetic abnormality is encoded in the mitochondrial DNA and since the spermatocytes do not contain mitochondria, the diseases show a maternal transmission.

The underlying mutations have been identified in many disease entities. However, there is increasing evidence of genotypic heterogeneity in metabolic disorders. In type 1 glutaric aciduria at least 20 different mutations have been identified, all presenting with the typical biochemical features. The mutations influence the molecular structure and hence the function of the glutaryl coenzyme A dehydrogenase enzyme in different ways, explaining the heterogeneity of the clinical phenotypes. Interestingly enough, some correlation between the clinical (and biochemical) phenotypes and the imaging patterns (radiological phenotype) can also be established (personal unpublished data).

The clinical heterogeneity of metabolic disorders may also be reflected in the age of onset of the disease. Metachromatic leucodystrophy, which has neonatal, infantile, juvenile and adult onset forms, is a good example of this. Metachromatic leukodystrophy is caused by the insufficiency of the arylsulphatase A enzyme. Several different mutations are known: one defining an inactive enzyme (allele I); another an active but unstable enzyme (allele A); and another a so-called pseudodeficient enzyme. Homozygotes or heterozygotes for the pseudodeficient enzyme are clinically normal, whereas homo- or heterozygotes for allele I or A will have clinical disease. This is explained by the fact that homo- or heterozygotes for the pseudodeficient enzyme have some (more than 10%) residual enzyme activity, whereas the disease will manifest only in patients with less than 10% activity. Patients with 2–5% residual enzyme activity have juvenile or adult onset disease and patients with less than 2% present with infantile onset.

Other factors may also play a significant role in the characterization of the clinical phenotype and explain variations even amongst siblings affected by the same disease. They include environmental, alimentary, other metabolic and other as yet unknown factors.

FURTHER READING

Kappler J, Leinekugel P, Conzelmann E et al. Genotype–phenotype relationship in various degrees of arylsulphatase A deficiency. Human Genetics 1991; 86:463–470.

Polten A, Fluharty AL, Fluharty CB et al. Molecular basis of different forms of metachromatic leukodystrophy. New England Journal of Medicine 1991; 324:18–22.

DISEASE ENTITIES AND IMAGING FINDINGS IN METABOLIC DISEASES

ORGANIC ACIDOPATHIES

Many of the organic acidopathies fall into the group of devastating metabolic diseases of the newborn, others have later and an often insidious onset. Typically, grey matter abnormalities dominate the imaging findings; however, white matter involvement may also be present, although this is usually less prominent. Occasionally, organic acidopathies present with a leucodystrophy-like presentation but grey matter lesions are always conspicuous.

PROPIONIC ACIDAEMIA

Propionic acidaemia is a relatively common organic acidopathy. The deficient enzyme is propionyl coenzyme A carboxylase. The inheritance is autosomal recessive.

Patients with propionic acidaemia are encountered in two characteristic situations, notably during metabolic crisis and afterwards in the chronic stage of the disease, with an extrapyramidal syndrome.

IMAGING FINDINGS DURING METABOLIC CRISIS

During metabolic crisis diffuse brain swelling is seen. Signal abnormalities within the basal ganglia, the dentate nuclei are conspicuous on the T2-weighted images. Subtle signal changes may be present within the pulvinar of the thalami. The cerebral and cerebellar cortices are also affected. The involved grey matter structures are swollen at this stage. White matter structures also show signal changes, mainly subcortically, including the subinsular areas (external and extreme capsules). The corpus callosum, the internal capsule and the cortical-spinal tracts appear to be spared (Figure 12.10.5). Diffusion-weighted images usually show moderate signal increase within the involved grey matter structures and the subcortical white matter.

MR spectroscopy demonstrates lactate within the lesion areas, consistent with impairment of the energy metabolism resulting in anaerobic glucolysis. No disease-specific metabolites are identified.

Differential diagnostic possibilities in the acute stage of propionic acidaemia are hypoxic-anoxic brain damage, primary lactic acidosis, Leigh disease or other organic acidopathies (ethylmalonic aciduria, 3-methylmalonic aciduria). In hypoxic-anoxic brain damage, the findings can be quite similar to propionic acidaemia; only the clinical setting and laboratory findings may allow differentiation between the two. Lesions in primary lactic acidosis and ethylmalonic aciduria may be indistinguishable from those in propionic acidaemia from the imaging point of view. In Leigh disease, upper brainstem abnormalities are common; they are absent in propionic acidaemia. In 3-methylglutaric aciduria, the cerebellar vermis is almost always markedly atrophic; this is either absent or less conspicuous in propionic acidaemia.

IMAGING FINDINGS AFTER METABOLIC CRISIS

The brain is usually diffusely atrophic. The basal ganglia and the dentate nuclei are prominently atrophic too and exhibit persistent signal changes, which at the level of the basal ganglia may be conspicuous even on the T1-weighted images. On diffusion-weighted images the basal ganglia lesions are somewhat hypointense. The conventional and diffusion-weighted imaging findings suggest profound tissue damage, probably necrosis. The abnormalities, similar to the findings in the acute stage, are typically symmetrical. The basal ganglia abnormalities constitute the imaging substrate of the extrapyramidal syndrome (choreoathetosis, dystonia).

If the medical treatment was early and adequate the imaging findings may be unremarkable after the metabolic crisis, with almost total normalization of both the grey and white matter changes, perhaps with mild atrophy only.

METHYLMALONIC ACIDURIA

Methylmalonic aciduria is a clinically and biochemically heterogeneous group of diseases. Several clinical phenotypes have been described. Type 3 methylmalonic aciduria is associated with hyperhomocystinaemia.

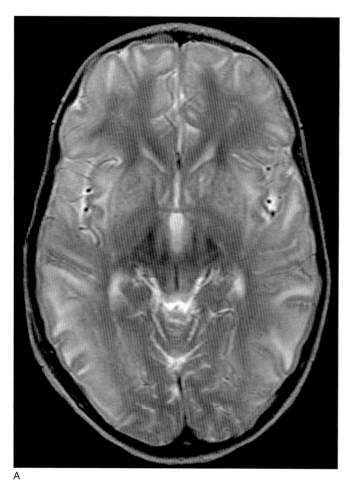
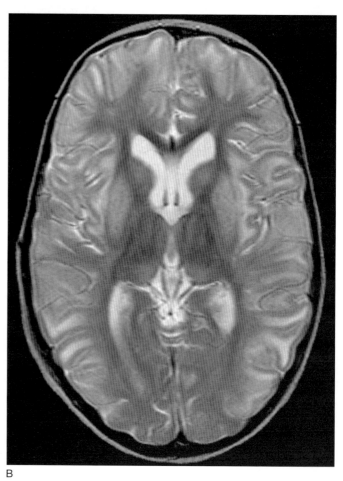

A
B

Figure 12.10.5 (A,B) Axial T2-weighted fast spin echo images in a 6-year-old female patient with propionic acidaemia during metabolic crisis. Diffuse swelling of the brain with abnormal increased signal intensities within the basal ganglia, the cerebral cortex and the subcortical white matter are present. Subtle symmetrical signal changes are also present within the pulvinar of the thalami.

Laboratory findings in methylmalonic acidaemia can be quite similar to those in propionic acidaemia. From the clinical point of view the presentation can also be confusing, with the exception of tonus abnormalities, i.e. in methylmalonic aciduria, hypertonia is found. The imaging findings in methylmalonic aciduria are however quite peculiar and actually quite suggestive. In patients with clinically mild phenotypes, however, the MR imaging findings can be normal.

IMAGING FINDINGS DURING METABOLIC CRISIS

In methylmalonic aciduria, the most typical and often the sole abnormality is the symmetrical signal changes within the globi pallidi, which is associated with swelling (Figure 12.10.6A,B). The caudate nuclei, the putamina and the thalami are spared. The cortex is normal. During the acute metabolic crisis, diffusion-weighted images show hypersignal within the lesion areas. MR spectroscopy may show a small amount of lactate within the lesions. No disease-specific metabolites are demonstrated.

IMAGING FINDINGS AFTER METABOLIC CRISIS

The globus pallidus lesions undergo necrotic changes; they are markedly atrophic and continue to show hypersignal on the T2-weighted images (Figure 12.10.6C,D). Sometimes, mild cerebellar atrophy may be present and subtle signal changes within the dentate nuclei suggest some damage too. In early onset cases, delayed myelination is frequently seen.

Differential diagnoses in bilateral globus pallidus disease without involvement of the other basal ganglia components include methylmalonic aciduria, kernicterus and carbon monoxide intoxication. In kernicterus, lesions to the subthalamic nuclei are associated with the globus pallidus lesions. Carbon monoxide intoxication is usually encountered in suggestive clinical settings.

ETHYLMALONIC ACIDAEMIA

Ethylmalonic aciduria typically presents with basal ganglia disease but patchy white matter lesions may also be present within the

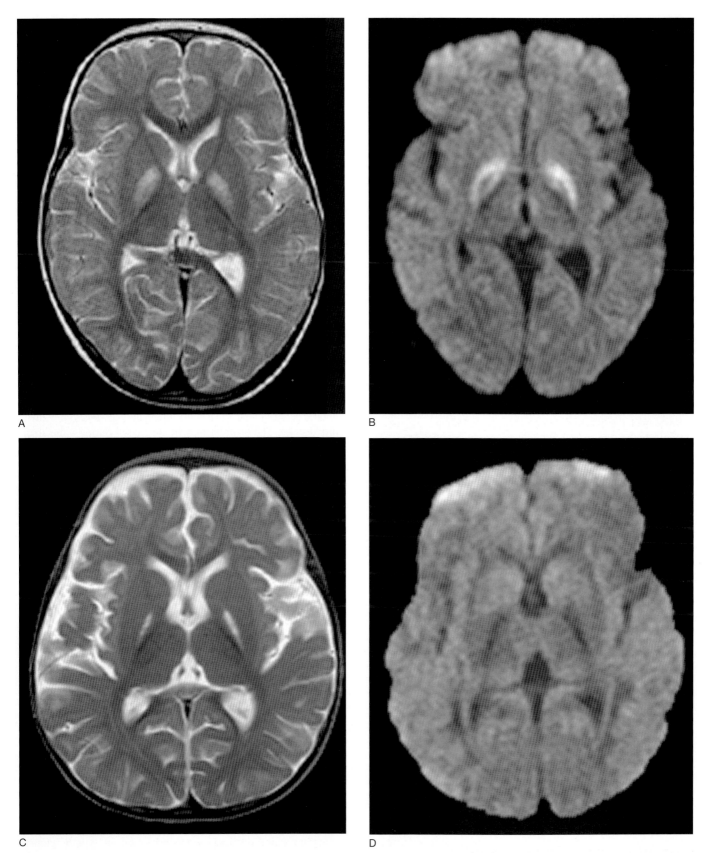

Figure 12.10.6 Axial T2-weighted fast spin echo (A,C) and diffusion-weighted echo planar (B,D) images in patients with methylmalonic aciduria. In a 1-year-old patient during metabolic crisis (A,B), the T2-weighted image shows swelling and abnormal hyperintensity of the globi pallidi. On the diffusion-weighted image in the same patient, hypersignal is seen within the globi pallidi, indicating an active, ongoing disease process. In another 8-month-old female patient examined several months after a metabolic crisis (C,D), the T2-weighted image shows atrophy of the globi pallidi. On the diffusion-weighted image, the globi pallidi exhibit hyposignal, consistent with necrosis.

cerebral hemispheres. The signal changes within the heads of the caudate nuclei and the putamina are somewhat patchy and inhomogeneous. This may help to raise the possibility of the disease and differentiate it from other organic acidopathies. A distinct clinical feature of the disease is the widespread cutaneous petechiae and ecchymoses indicative of vasculopathy.

3-METHYLGLUTACONIC ACIDURIA

The disease has at least four clinical phenotypic presentations. Type 2 has an X-linked inheritance; the others are autosomal recessive. The typical imaging presentation in types 1 and 4 of this metabolic disorder is, as in many other organic acidopathies, also the symmetrical bilateral basal ganglia disease.

IMAGING FINDINGS DURING METABOLIC CRISIS

During the acute stage of the disease the basal ganglia are swollen and exhibit high signal on the diffusion-weighted images, suggestive of cytotoxic oedema. Sometimes, only the globi pallidi, the caudate nuclei and the anterior parts of the putamina are involved; posteriorly they are spared. With the progression of the disease the putaminal abnormalities become complete. In some cases, ill-defined, diffuse cerebral white matter signal changes are also present (Figure 12.10.7A,B). During the metabolic crisis the cerebellar cortex and the dentate nuclei may also show signal abnormalities. Cerebellar atrophy is a very characteristic imaging finding, the vermis usually being more affected than the cerebellar hemispheres. Cerebellar atrophy appears very early during the disease course and may be established during the first metabolic crisis. The association of cerebellar atrophy and basal ganglia disease is a suggestive imaging pattern of 3-methylglutaconic aciduria.

On MR spectroscopy the findings are non-specific. Lactate is present within the lesion areas but no disease-specific metabolite is identified.

IMAGING FINDINGS AFTER METABOLIC CRISIS

In the chronic phase of the disease, the basal ganglia are atrophic and on the diffusion-weighted images they are hypointense. The cerebellar atrophy also progresses and can become very prominent. Diffuse cerebral atrophy also ensues (Figure 12.10.7C,D).

3-HYDROXY-3-METHYLGLUTARYL (HMG)-COENZYME A LYASE DEFICIENCY

This is a relatively rare metabolic disorder on the L-leucine breakdown pathway. The disease may present with metabolic crises with

hypoglycaemia and keto-acidosis. MR imaging usually reveals clear but non-specific abnormalities.

Since the disease usually starts in the early postnatal period or in early infancy, initially the grey matter abnormalities are easier to depict, since the white matter is not myelinated yet. Later, as the brain myelination progresses, the white matter changes, which most probably correspond to demyelination, become more apparent.

The grey matter abnormalities involve the basal ganglia and the dentate nuclei. They are fairly subtle in most cases and do not seem to lead to necrosis if the disease is appropriately treated.

The white matter abnormalities within the cerebral hemispheres are sometimes patchy, but usually confluent. The subcortical U-fibres are often spared (Figure 12.10.8A,B). Diffusion-weighted imaging shows faint hypersignal within the involved white matter structures (Figure 12.10.8C,D).

MR spectroscopy (Figure 12.10.9) invariably demonstrates disease-specific abnormalities with two abnormal peaks at the 1.3 and the 2.4 ppm levels.

GLUTARIC ACIDURIA TYPE 1

Glutaric aciduria type 1 is usually an insidiously developing metabolic disease. The disorder may be diagnosed during a metabolic crisis, which is typically triggered by a febrile illness. In the clinically severe phenotypes of the disease (therapy-resistant and some of the leaky and the non-treated riboflavin-dependent forms), imaging examination shows bilateral basal ganglia disease with sparing of the thalami. The upper brainstem signal changes are reminiscent of the so-called 'giant panda face'. It is characterized by relative hyposignal of the red nuclei and the tectum, and increased signal within the substantia nigra and the tegmentum. The central tegmental tracts along the floor of the fourth ventricle also often show bilateral symmetrical hypersignal. The dentate nuclei may also be abnormal and present with hypersignal on the T2-weighted and FLAIR images. White matter signal abnormalities are also frequent. They are typically seen within the cerebral hemispheres in a subcortical location. These changes are patchy and scattered.

In the clinically mild phenotypes (naturally mild, treated riboflavin-dependent forms), no parenchymal lesions may be seen. Patients with type 1 glutaric aciduria are usually macrocephalic. Another peculiar imaging finding is the bilateral enlargement of the Sylvian fissures. They may correspond to arachnoidal cysts or disturbed and incomplete opercularization. They are usually bilateral but not necessarily symmetrical. Rarely, the abnormality is unilateral. These changes may be detected prenatally or in the early postnatal period by ultrasound. Macrocephaly and Sylvian fissure abnormalities are present in both the clinically benign and malignant phenotypes.

Prominent brain atrophy may also develop. Chronic subdural haematomas are relatively frequently seen in type 1 glutaric aciduria without any evidence of significant head trauma in the patients' clinical history.

The presence of bilateral Sylvian fissure and temporal-polar CSF space enlargement and bilateral basal ganglia lesions in a macrocephalic child are almost pathognomonic of type 1

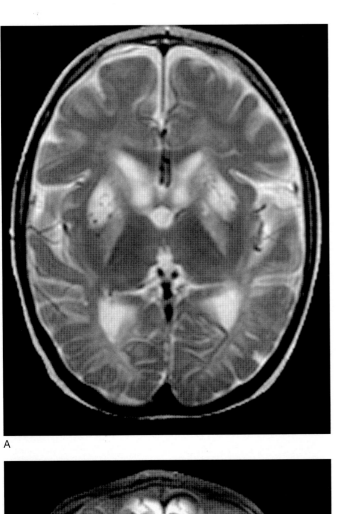
A

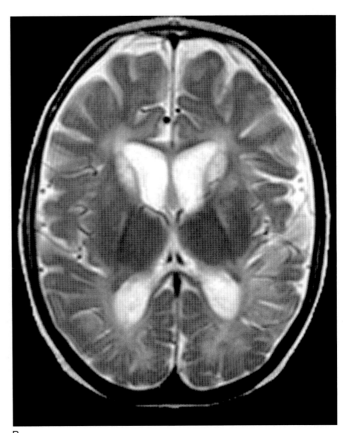
B

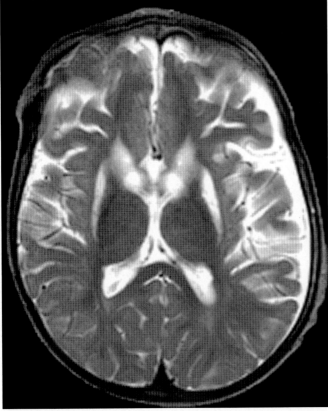
C

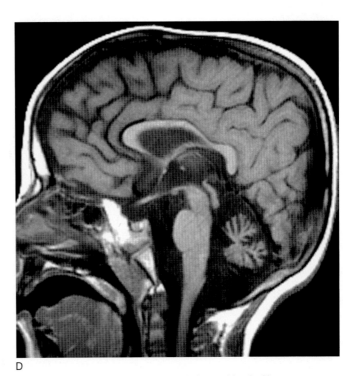
D

Figure 12.10.7 Axial T2-weighted fast spin echo images in a 1-year-old female patient with 3-methylglutaconic aciduria combined with hypermethioninaemia during an acute metabolic crisis (A,B). The heads of the caudate nuclei, the anterior parts of the putamina and the globi pallidi are abnormal. The putamina in the involved areas are swollen, whereas the cerebral hemispheres show mild atrophy and diffuse, dominantly periventricular hyperintensities. In another patient in the chronic phase, the putamina appear to be globally atrophic and the signal abnormalities involve the posterior parts also on the axial T2-weighted fast spin echo image (C). On the sagittal T1-weighted spin echo image (D), the cerebellar vermis is markedly atrophic.

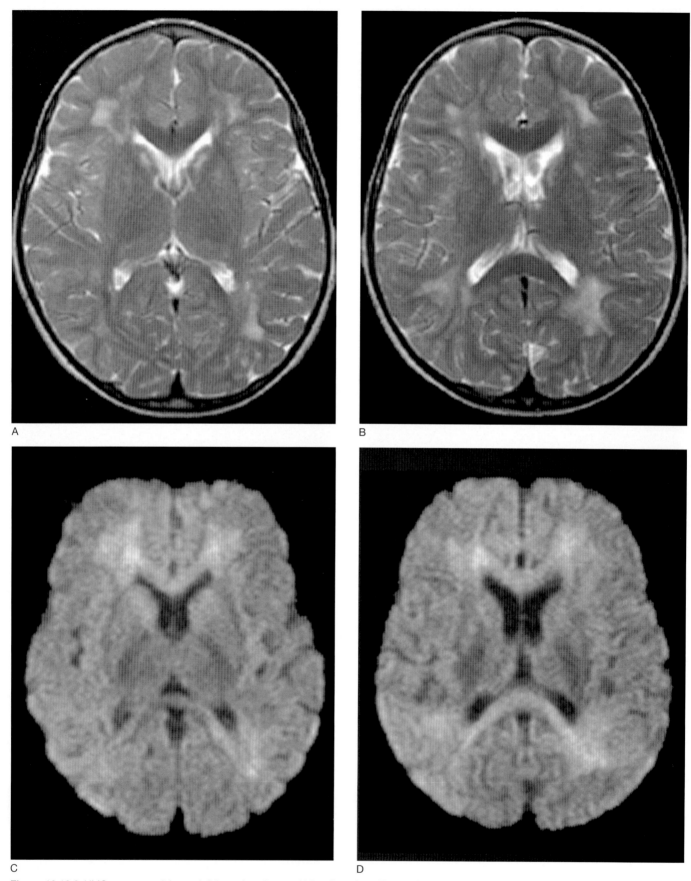

Figure 12.10.8 HMG coenzyme A lyase deficiency in a 3-year-old female patient. The axial T2-weighted fast spin echo images show ill-defined hyperintensities within the heads of the caudate nuclei and perhaps even within the putamina in conjunction with patchy signal changes within the cerebral hemispheric white matter with sparing of the subcortical U-fibres (A,B). On the diffusion-weighted images, increased signal is observed at the level of the white matter lesions with very faint hypersignal within the caudate nucleus lesions (C,D).

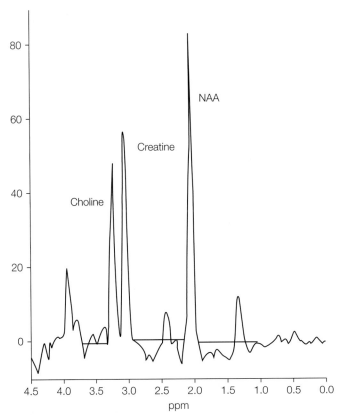

Figure 12.10.9 Single-voxel proton MR spectroscopy in the same patient as Figure 12.10.8. Besides the normal appearance of the NAA, creatine and choline peaks, the study shows two abnormal peaks, at the 1.3 and the 2.45 ppm levels, which are characteristic to HMG coenzyme A lyase deficiency.

glutaric aciduria (Figure 12.10.10). The presence of the aforementioned abnormalities without basal ganglia lesions however should also raise the possibility of the disease and prompt laboratory work-up in order to prevent the devastating consequences of a possible metabolic crisis and the resultant damage to the basal ganglia.

MR spectroscopy may show lactate within the basal ganglia during the acute stage of the disease. Although the possible role of glutamine–glutamate complexes in the pathogenesis of basal ganglia disease has been raised (glutamine 'excitotoxicity' or glutamine 'suicide'), increased glutamine–glutamate levels could not be demonstrated within the basal ganglia by *in vivo* MR spectroscopy.

L-2-HYDROXYGLUTARIC ACIDURIA

L-2-hydroxyglutaric aciduria is a slowly progressive metabolic disorder. The disease is usually discovered in childhood, sometimes later, including young adulthood. The disease however probably starts in early childhood or late infancy. The reason for the relative delay in diagnosis is the rather unremarkable clinical presentation. Patients present with learning difficulties, epilepsy, pyramidal and cerebellar signs. The imaging work-up, which sometimes precedes the laboratory diagnosis, reveals rather promi-

nent brain abnormalities, the overall pattern of which is practically pathognomonic to the disease.

At first glance L-2-hydroxyglutaric aciduria presents with a leucodystrophy-like appearance on MR imaging. The white matter abnormalities exhibit a typical centripetal and slightly anteroposterior gradient, the subcortical U-fibres are most severely affected, and the periventricular white matter and, in particular, the central corticol-spinal tracts and the corpus callosum are spared for quite a long time during the course of the disease. The cerebellar white matter is usually spared. The extreme and the external capsules, as well as the anterior limb and the knee of the internal capsules, are abnormal.

Grey matter structures are, however, also involved. The basal ganglia are always abnormal but this is less prominent than in other organic acidopathies. The thalami are normal. The dentate nuclei are also always abnormal. The involved grey matter structures are often somewhat swollen also (Figure 12.10.11).

With the progression of the disease, atrophic changes develop but much more slowly than in most metabolic disorders and in particular in organic acidopathies. The atrophic changes involve both the cerebral hemispheres and the cerebellum.

Diffusion-weighted images are unremarkable in L-2-hydroxyglutaric aciduria. The most markedly abnormal peripheral hemispheric white matter structures are hypointense. No definite hypersignal is seen elsewhere in the white matter to suggest myelin oedema. This is consistent with a very slowly progressive demyelinating disease, which histologically corresponds to spongiform encephalopathy.

MR spectroscopy shows decreased *N*-acetyl-aspartate and choline peaks. Increase of the *myo*-inositol peak has been described but the significance of this is poorly understood. Typically, no lactate is demonstrated within the brain parenchyma.

PRIMARY LACTIC ACIDOSIS

Primary lactic acidosis represents a complex group of pathologies, some of which belong to the respiratory chain defects, others to the disorders of pyruvate metabolism. They will be discussed in the sections on disorders of mitochondrial energy metabolism (see below).

FURTHER READING

al Aqeel A, Rashed M, Ozand PT et al. 3-methylglutaconic aciduria: ten new cases with a possible new phenotype. Brain and Development 1994; 16 (Suppl):23–32.

Arbelaez A, Castillo M, Stone J. MRI in 3-methylglutaconic aciduria type 1. Neuroradiology 1999; 41:941–942.

Barth PG, Hoffmann GF, Jaeken J et al. L-2-hydroxyglutaric acidemia: a novel inherited neurometabolic disease. Annals of Neurology 1992; 32:66–71.

Bergman AJIW, van der Knaap MS, Smeitnink JAM et al. Magnetic resonance imaging and spectroscopy of the brain in propionic acidemia: clinical and biochemical considerations. Pediatric Research 1996; 40:404–409.

Brismar J, Ozand PT. CT and MR of the brain in glutaric acidemia type I: a review of 59 published cases and a report of 5 new patients. American Journal of Neuroradiology 1995; 16:675–683.

D'Incerti L, Farina L, Moroni I et al. L-2-Hydroxyglutaric aciduria: MRI in seven cases. Neuroradiology 1998; 40:727–733.

Ferris NJ, Tien RD. Cerebral MRI in 3-hydroxy-3-methylglutaryl-coenzyme A lyase deficiency: case report. Neuroradiology 1993; 35:559–560.

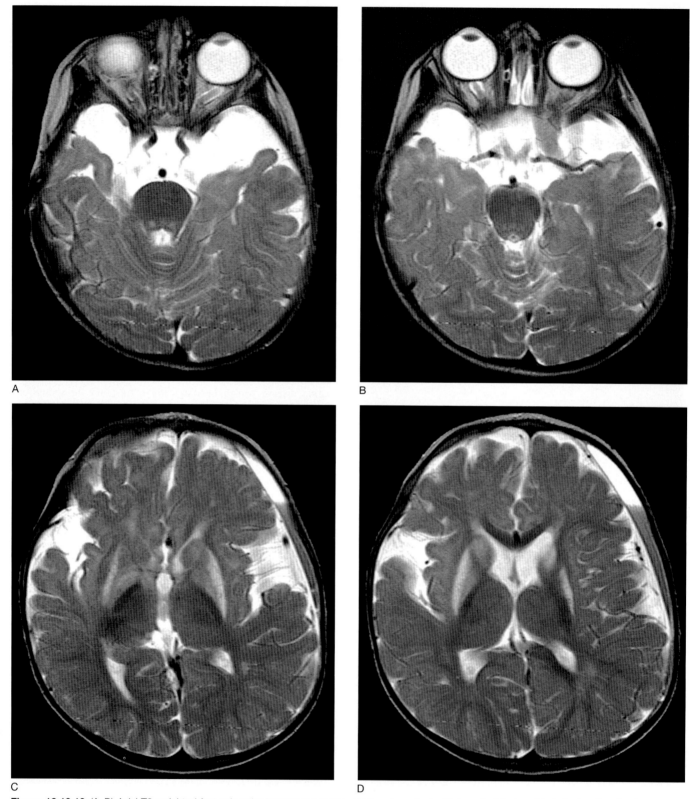

Figure 12.10.10 (A–D) Axial T2-weighted fast spin echo images in a 3-year-old female patient with type 1 glutaric aciduria in the chronic phase of the disease. All the hallmark imaging features of the disease – bilateral temporal-polar arachnoidal cysts, incomplete opercularization, bilateral basal ganglia disease and a chronic subdural haematoma on the left side – are present.

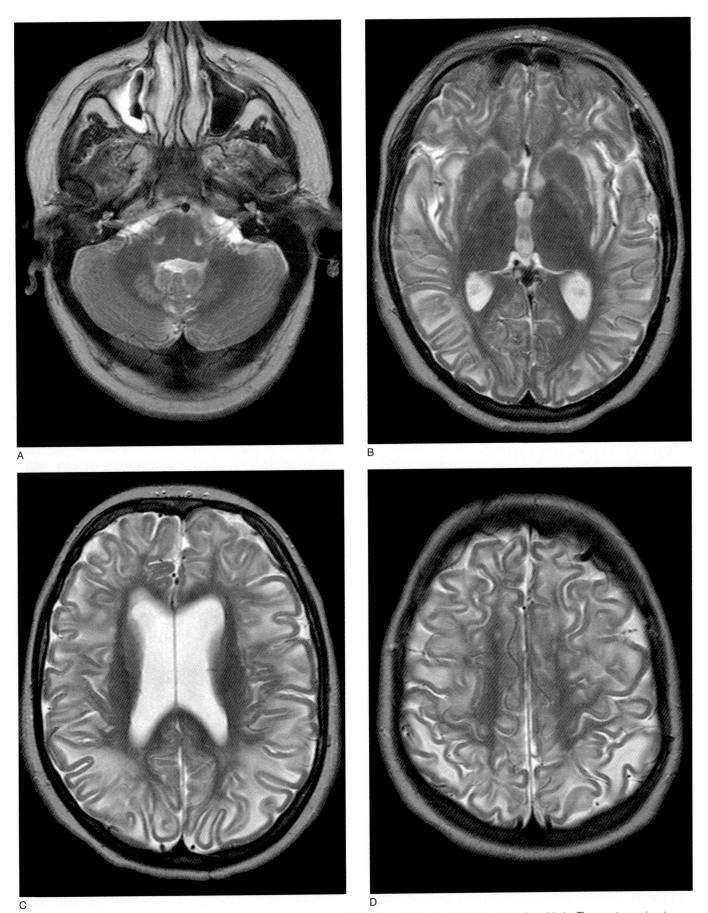

Figure 12.10.11 Axial T2-weighted fast spin echo images in a 21-year-old female patient with L-2-hydroxyglutaric aciduria. The most prominent abnormality in the posterior fossa is the abnormal hyperintense appearance of the dentate nuclei (A). Supratentorially, the images show subtle signal changes within the basal ganglia (B) and the centripetal pattern of the hemispheric white matter disease (C). There is a relative sparing of the white matter in the pre- and postcentral regions (D).

Gordon K, Riding M, Camfield P et al. CT and MR of 3-hydroxy-3-methylglutaryl-coenzyme A lyase deficiency. American Journal of Neuroradiology 1994; 15:1474–1476.

Hanefeld F, Kruse B, Bruhn H et al. In vivo proton magnetic resonance spectroscopy of the brain in a patient with L-2-hydroxyglutaric acidemia. Pediatric Research 1994; 35:614–616.

Iafolla AK, Kahler SG. Megalencephaly in the neonatal period as the initial manifestation of glutaric aciduria type I. Journal of Pediatrics 1989; 114:1004–1006.

Martinez-Lage JF, Casas C, Fernandez MA et al. Macrocephaly, dystonia, and bilateral temporal arachnoid cysts: glutaric aciduria type 1. Childs Nervous System 1994; 10:18–203.

Osaka H, Kimura S, Nezu A et al. Chronic subdural hematoma, as an initial manifestation of glutaric aciduria type-1. Brain and Development 1993; 15:125–127.

Ozand PT, Rashed M, Millington DS et al. Ethylmalonic aciduria: an organic acidemia with CNS involvement and vasculopathy. Brain and Development 1994; 16 (Suppl):12–22.

Pérez Cerdá C, Merinero B, Martí M et al. An unusual late-onset case of propionic acidaemia: biochemical investigations, neuroradiological findings and mutation analysis. European Journal of Pediatrics 1998; 157:50–52.

Topcu M, Erdem G, Saatci I et al. Clinical and magnetic resonance imaging features of L-2-hydroxyglutaric acidemia: report of three cases in comparison with Canavan disease. Journal of Child Neurology 1996; 11:373–377.

van der Knaap MS, Bakker HD, Valk J. MR imaging and proton spectroscopy in 3-hydroxy-3-methylglutaryl coenzyme A lyase deficiency. American Journal of Neuroradiology 1998; 19:378–382.

Yalcinkaya C, Dincer A, Gündüz E et al. MRI and MRS in HMG-CoA lyase deficiency. Pediatric Neurology 1999; 20:375–380.

AMINO ACIDOPATHIES

UREA CYCLE DEFECTS

The urea cycle is a complex metabolic process, the primary role of which is to convert the toxic ammonia into non-toxic urea. Some of the enzymes involved in the urea cycle are located within the mitochondria (carbamyl phosphate synthetase, ornithine transcarbamylase), others in the cytosol (argininosuccinate synthetase, argininosuccinate lyase, arginase). Urea cycle defects are characterized by autosomal recessive inheritance, except ornithine carbamoyl transferase deficiency, which is X-linked. The most common metabolic derangement in each disease entity is hyperammonaemia and impairment of the metabolism of various amino acids (alanine, glutamine, citrulline and arginine).

Some of the urea cycle defects present in neonates as a devastating metabolic disease of almost immediate postnatal onset. If the disease is of later onset (infantile, juvenile or adult), it may manifest with neurological signs and symptoms of acute or chronic encephalopathy.

UREA CYCLE DEFECTS IN THE NEONATE

MR imaging findings in neonates with urea cycle defects are dominated by the prominent brain swelling and white matter signal changes related to vasogenic oedema. The myelinated white matter is less severely affected than the non-myelinated areas (Figure 12.10.12). Diffusion-weighted images show signal inhomogeneities with some prominence of the hypointensities within the lesion areas, consistent with vasogenic oedema. MR spectroscopy with short echo time may show increased glutamine–glutamate peak complexes in the brain parenchyma, indicative of hyperammonaemia. This is a non-specific but, in appropriate clinical setting, highly suggestive finding.

UREA CYCLE DEFECTS OF LATER ONSET

The MR imaging studies during metabolic crises in the later onset forms of urea cycle defects typically show multiple large abnormal signal intensity lesions within the cerebral hemispheres associated with swelling. The lesions, which involve both cortical and subcortical structures, exhibit a stroke-like appearance but they are of metabolic, rather than ischaemic, origin. Occasionally, subtle lesions may be present within the deep grey matter structures as well. In the chronic stage of the disease, ill-defined white matter changes and diffuse brain atrophy are noted (Figure 12.10.13).

MAPLE SYRUP URINE DISEASE

Maple syrup urine disease (MSUD) is an autosomal recessive disorder of the metabolism of amino acids. Four clinical phenotypes are distinguished: the classical, the intermediate, the intermittent and the thiamine responsive. The most severe form is the classical MSUD, characterized by early postnatal onset and rapid progressive neurological deterioration leading to death, if untreated.

The basic metabolic disorder in MSUD is related to the deficiency of the branched-chain alpha-keto acid dehydrogenase enzyme, which is one of the several enzymes on the L-leucine breakdown pathway. As a result, increased concentrations of branched chain amino acids (leucine, valine and isoleucine) and their keto-acid (alpha-ketoisocaproic, alpha-ketoisovaleric, alpha-keto-beta-methylvaleric) and 2-hydroxy derivatives appear in the blood, urine and the CSF.

The neonatal form of the disease typically presents on the seventh day after birth. Conventional MR imaging shows diffuse swelling of the brain. This is mainly due to the vasogenic oedema involving the non-myelinated white matter structures. On the other hand, even more prominent signal changes are also present within the myelinated brain areas (posterior brainstem tracts, central cerebellar white matter, posterior limbs of the internal capsules), representing myelin oedema, secondary to vacuolating myelinopathy.

Identification of the two pathological processes and the resultant distinctly different oedema types is easy when diffusion-weighted images are available. Myelin oedema presents with isotropically restricted water diffusion, hence hypersignal. On the contrary, vasogenic oedema is characterized by isotropically increased water diffusion, which causes hyposignal on the diffusion-weighted images. The sharp contrast between the diffusion-weighted imaging signal properties of these two oedema types and the peculiar distribution of the pathological hypersignal (strictly limited to the myelinated white matter structures) result in a practically pathognomonic imaging pattern (Figure 12.10.14).

MR spectroscopy may also have a role in the diagnostic work-up. Short echo-time MR spectroscopy using the STEAM sequence typically demonstrates prominent peak abnormalities in the 0.9–1.1 ppm range of the spectrum, which corresponds to branched chain amino acids, not detectable in the normal brain. This provides further confirmation of the diagnosis and may warrant specific laboratory tests and adequate treatment.

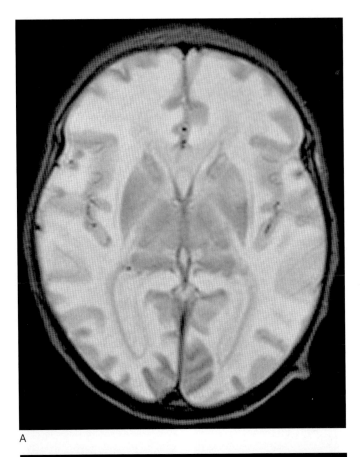

A

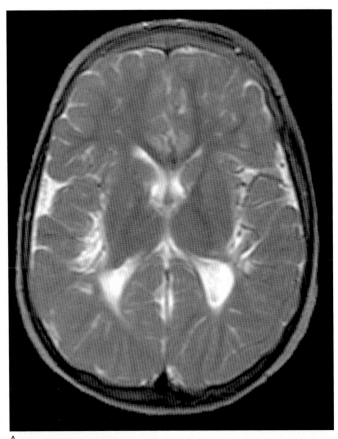

A

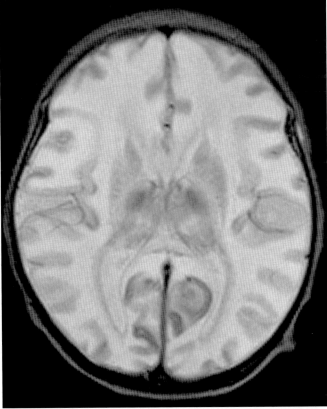

B

Figure 12.10.12 (A,B) Axial T2-weighted fast spin echo images in a 12-day-old male patient with urea cycle defect. The brain is diffusely swollen and the non-myelinated white matter exhibits an abnormal, increased signal intensity appearance. Note the relative sparing of the partially myelinated optic radiations.

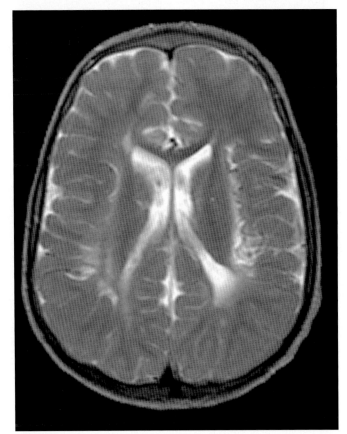

B

Figure 12.10.13 (A,B) Axial T2-weighted fast spin echo images of a 5-year-old male patient with citrullinaemia. Predominantly periventricular white matter changes are seen in conjunction with subcortical atrophy.

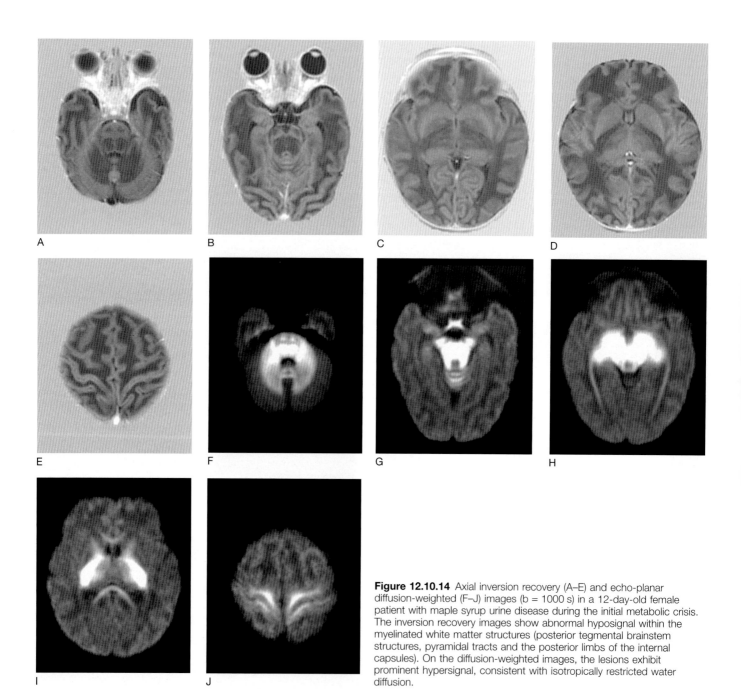

A

B

C

D

E

F

G

H

I

J

Figure 12.10.14 Axial inversion recovery (A–E) and echo-planar diffusion-weighted (F–J) images (b = 1000 s) in a 12-day-old female patient with maple syrup urine disease during the initial metabolic crisis. The inversion recovery images show abnormal hyposignal within the myelinated white matter structures (posterior tegmental brainstem structures, pyramidal tracts and the posterior limbs of the internal capsules). On the diffusion-weighted images, the lesions exhibit prominent hypersignal, consistent with isotropically restricted water diffusion.

The intermittent and intermediate forms of maple syrup urine disease have a more insidious clinical pattern. The first metabolic crisis may appear in late infancy or early childhood. The imaging findings are less characteristic too. Typically, brain atrophy, delayed myelination and pathological signal changes within the upper brainstem structures, the thalami, the globi pallidi and the centrum semiovale are observed. Diffusion-weighted imaging also shows signal abnormalities in the aforementioned areas but they are often rather subtle (Figure 12.10.15). From the imaging point of view, the intermittent form of maple syrup urine disease may therefore be somewhat similar to Canavan disease in the early stage but the clinical context and the laboratory findings allow easy differentiation.

In treated MSUD cases, the conventional MRI and the diffusion-weighted imaging findings rarely return to normal. Typically, variable but prominent residual abnormalities, including diffuse brain atrophy, delayed myelination and structural lesions are noted. The pattern of the structural lesions is very similar to those observed in the intermittent form of maple syrup urine disease; occasionally, however, additional changes are also present, notably in the hypothalamic structures, the dentate nuclei and the cerebellar or the cerebral hemispheric white matter. Subtle residual diffusion-weighted imaging abnormalities may also be noted. In successfully treated cases, MR spectroscopy shows improvement too but total normalization of the branched chain amino acid peak complex is usually not achieved.

PHENYLKETONURIA

Phenylalanine is an essential amino acid. Impairment of the phenylalanine hydroxylating system (i.e. block in the conversion of phenylalanine into tyrosine) results in insufficient breakdown and hence decreased blood concentration of tyrosine and increased blood concentration of phenylalanine (hyperphenylalaninaemia), which leads (through an alternate metabolic pathway) to increased excretion of phenylketones and phenylamines in the urine (phenylketonuria). Two forms of phenylketonuria are known. The more frequent 'classical' phenylketonuria is caused by the deficiency of the phenylalanine hydroxylase enzyme. The other, more 'malignant' and rare form is related to the deficiency of the tetrahydrobiopterin coenzyme, which is also indispensable in the breakdown of phenylalanine into tyrosine.

The clinical and imaging manifestations of the two forms of phenylketonuria are different.

CLASSICAL FORM

In the classical form, the disease usually starts in early infancy. Microcephaly, hypopigmentation, delayed development and infantile spasms are common early clinical features of the disease. Later pyramidal and extrapyramidal signs, generalized tonic–clonic seizures and behavioural changes develop but after childhood further progression is usually very slow.

In the classical type, if dietary restrictions are fully implemented, the MR examination may be totally normal, even on repeated follow-up studies. In non-compliant patients, white matter changes appear, initially in the occipital periventric-ular region, lateral to the optic radiations, later in other regions of the brain. The corpus callosum may also be involved; the internal capsules, the brainstem and cerebellar structures are typically spared.

MALIGNANT FORM

In the malignant form, microcephaly and delayed development are also typical but the disease, if not treated, often leads to death in early childhood. Neurologically, the patients present with prominent extrapyramidal signs (infantile Parkinsonism, choreoathetosis), myoclonic and grand mal seizures. Additionally, progressive pyramidal and bulbar signs develop in conjunction with severe cognitive deterioration.

In the biopterin-dependent form of phenylketonuria, CT examination shows calcifications at the level of the putamina and/or the globi pallidi as well as along the cortical–subcortical junction area in the frontal regions. It is somewhat similar to what may be seen in carbonic anhydrase II deficiency.

The MR imaging study shows signal changes within the calcified areas: hyperintense on the T1- and hypointense on the T2-weighted images. Additionally, white matter lesions are also demonstrated; sometimes they are diffuse, in other cases focal, with cystic degeneration in the parietal-occipital regions.

HYPERHOMOCYSTINAEMIAS

Disorders in this group include cystathionine beta-synthetase enzyme deficiency, folate deficiency, defects of the folate metabolism (5,10-methylene-tetrahydrofolate reductase deficiency), cobalamin (vitamin B_{12}) deficiency and defects of the cobalamin metabolism (isolated methylcobalamin and combined methyl- and adenosylcobalamin deficiencies). Patients with cobalamin and isolated methylcobalamin deficiency, as well as with folate and 5,10-methylene-tetrahydrofolate reductase deficiency present with hyperhomocystinaemia without hypermethioninaemia. Patients with cobalamin and combined methyl- and adenosylcobalamin deficiency present with a dual metabolic disorder, notably hyperhomocystinaemia and methylmalonic aciduria. Patients with cystathionine beta synthetase deficiency present with hyperhomocystinaemia with hypermethioninaemia. Folate and cobalamin deficiencies as well as defects of the cobalamin metabolism are associated with haematological disorders, notably megaloblastic anaemia.

HOMOCYSTINURIA

Homocystinuria is the most common of the hyperhomocystinaemias and is related to a defect of the cystathionine beta-synthetase enzyme. The disease is autosomal recessive and the onset is typically infantile.

The appearance of the patients resembles those with Marfan syndrome. Lens subluxation and vascular complications (premature occlusive arterial disease and thromboembolic strokes) are frequent. Skeletal abnormalities include arachnoclactyly, seniosis, omega epihyses and skeletal osteopenia.

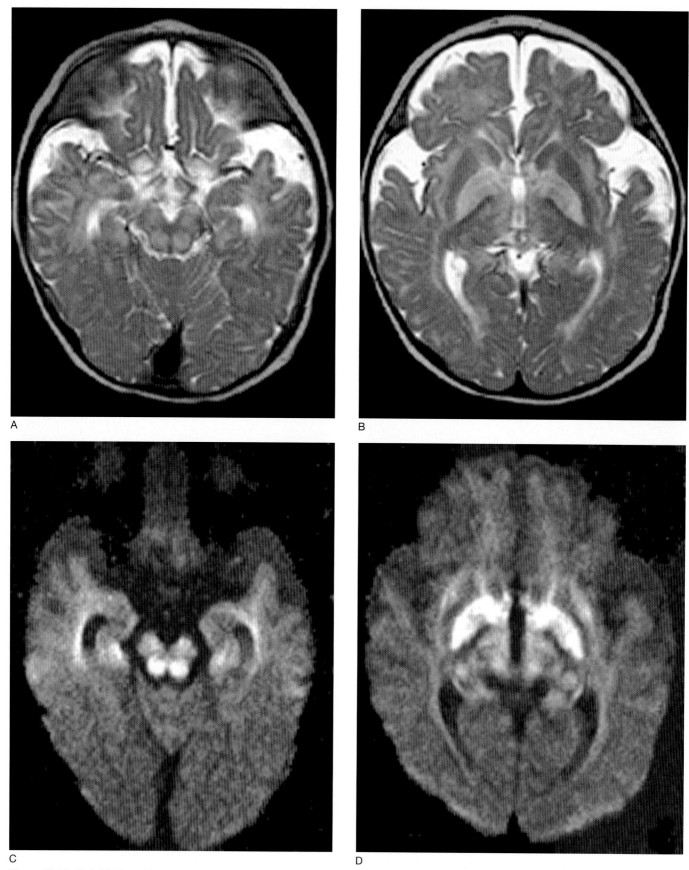

Figure 12.10.15 Axial T2-weighted fast spin echo (A,B) and echo-planar diffusion-weighted (C,D) images (b = strength of diffusion gradient = 1000 s) in a 9-month-old male patient with intermittent maple syrup urine disease. Diffuse brain atrophy. The T2-weighted images show abnormal hypersignal within the upper mesencephalon and the globi pallidi, with corresponding hypersignal on the diffusion-weighted images.

MR imaging in cystathionine beta-reductase deficiency can be very characteristic. Dislocation of the lens, if present, is a highly suggestive feature of the disease (Figure 12.10.16). On the other hand, multiple cortical–subcortical and lacunar infarctions, both within the cerebral and the cerebellar hemispheres may be detected. Nevertheless, the disease may also present with a less specific, diffuse white matter involvement, the pattern of which is suggestive of 'retrograde' demyelination.

5,10-METHYLENE-TETRAHYDROFOLATE REDUCTASE DEFICIENCY

5,10-methylene-tetrahydrofolate reductase deficiency is the best known of the defects of folate metabolism. This form has an autosomal recessive inheritance. The onset of the disease is variable; it is more frequent in infants but later onset cases, including an adult form, are also known. Neurologically, developmental delay is seen in conjunction with signs of spinal cord (combined degeneration of the cord) and peripheral nerve involvement.

MR imaging in 5,10-methylene-tetrahydrofolate reductase deficiency may show rather prominent abnormalities in the brain. The cerebral white matter is diffusely abnormal; the lesions involve the corpus callosum, the external and extreme capsules, the laminae medullares, and the anterior limbs of the internal capsules, with sparing of the posterior limbs. The corticospinal tracts within the centrum semiovale, the subcortical U-fibres in the occipital regions and the optic radiations are also spared. The basal ganglia and the thalami are normal but the globi pallidi show increased signal intensity on the T2-weighted images (Figure 12.10.17). Subtle signal changes may be present within the mesencephalon (hypersignal within the substantia nigra and the periaqueductal regions) and the central tegmental tracts of the pons. The cerebellar white matter is not involved. In some other cases, the MR imaging abnormalities are mild and present with delayed-, hypo- or demyelination.

Diffusion-weighted images show hypersignal within the white matter lesions, suggestive of vacuolating myelinopathy. The diffusion-weighted abnormalities (similar to the conventional MR imaging findings) may remain visible on follow-up studies even after a few years.

NON-KETOTIC HYPERGLYCINAEMIA

Non-ketotic hyperglycinaemia is related to a defect in the glycine cleavage system. Increased plasma urine and CSF concentrations of glycine without ketoacidosis (in contrast to ketotic hyperglycinaemia, notably propionic acidaemia) are the hallmarks of the disease at laboratory work-up. Two clinical phenotypes are known; the more common neonatal type, which is characterized by practically absent glycine cleavage system activity, and the late-onset (infantile and juvenile) form, in which some residual glycine cleavage system activity is present.

The neonatal form presents as a devastating metabolic disorder immediately after birth. The patients are hypotonic (glycine is an inhibitor neurotransmitter at the level of the lower motor neurons), and have frequent myoclonic seizures, hiccups and episodes of apnoea that rapidly progress to lethargy and coma. There is, however, increasing evidence to suggest that glycine is not only an inhibitory but also an excitatory neurotransmitter, the latter seems to be essentially responsible for the devastating effect of the metabolic disorder in the newborn (and most probably in the fetus as well). The late onset form has a milder and rather non-specific clinical presentation.

The imaging hallmarks of non-ketotic hyperglycinaemia are callosal abnormalities and delayed myelination. The spectrum of morphological changes of the corpus callosum ranges from the rare true callosal dysgenesis to the more frequent callosal hypogenesis or hypoplasia but some degree of abnormality is always present (Figure 12.10.18). The delay in myelination is increasingly evident with the ageing of the infant and is probably associated with global hypomyelination. Cortical gyral abnormalities have also been described. Acute hydrocephalus may contribute to the severe clinical picture. In the chronic stage of the disease, progressive atrophy of the brain develops (Figure 12.10.19).

MR spectroscopy is a useful adjunct to the MR work-up of patients with suspected non-ketotic hyperglycinaemia since the concentration of glycine is particularly elevated in the brain. Glycine resonates at the 3.55 ppm level (same as *myo*-inositol) but since it has a much longer T2 relaxation time, in patients with non-ketotic hyperglycinaemia, the abnormal peak on short echo time (20 ms) MR spectrum remains conspicuous on long echo time (135 ms) MR spectra, allowing reliable differentiation between the two metabolites (Figure 12.10.20).

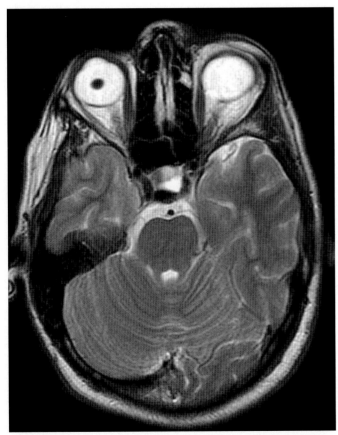

Figure 12.10.16 Axial T2-weighted fast spin echo image in a 19-year-old female patient with homocystinuria showing the characteristic dislocation of the lens within the right eye globe.

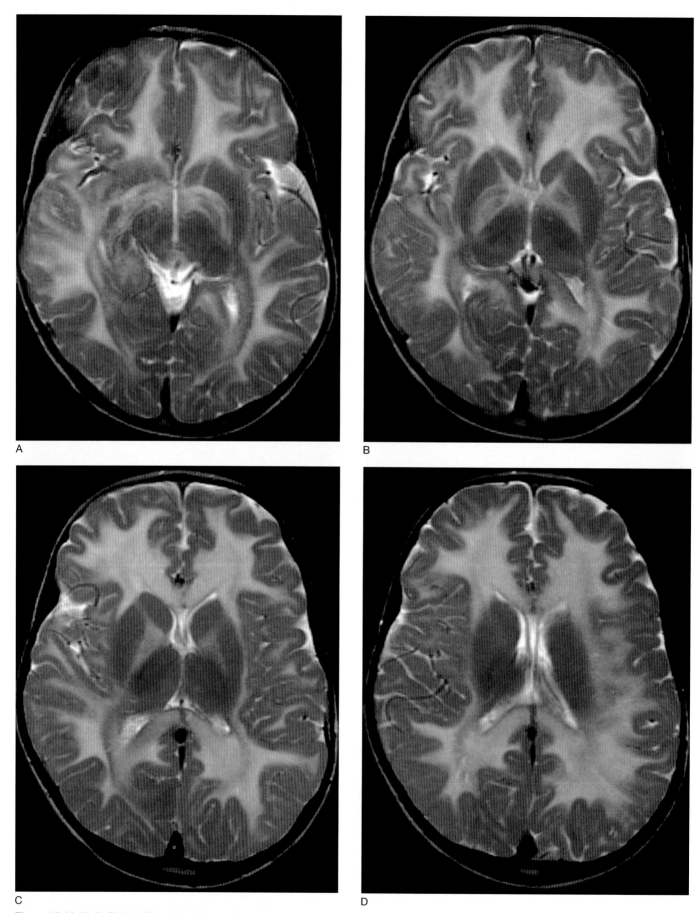

Figure 12.10.17 (A–D) Axial T2-weighted fast spin echo images in a 3-year-old male patient with 5,10-methylene-tetrahydrofolate reductase deficiency. Diffuse white matter changes with some sparing of the posterior limbs of the internal capsules. Note the involvement of the medial and lateral medullary laminae in the globus pallidus regions (A, B).

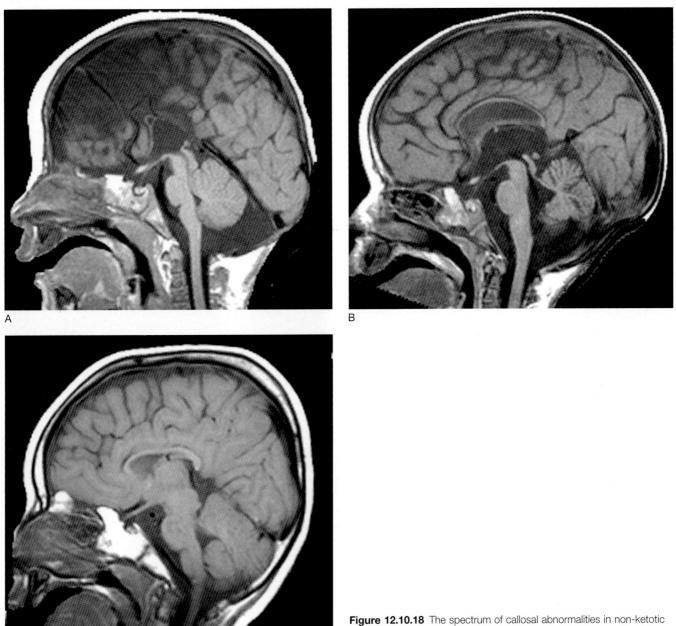

Figure 12.10.18 The spectrum of callosal abnormalities in non-ketotic hyperglycinaemia on sagittal T1-weighted spin echo images. Partial callosal dysgenesis (A), prominent (B) and moderate (C) hypoplasia.

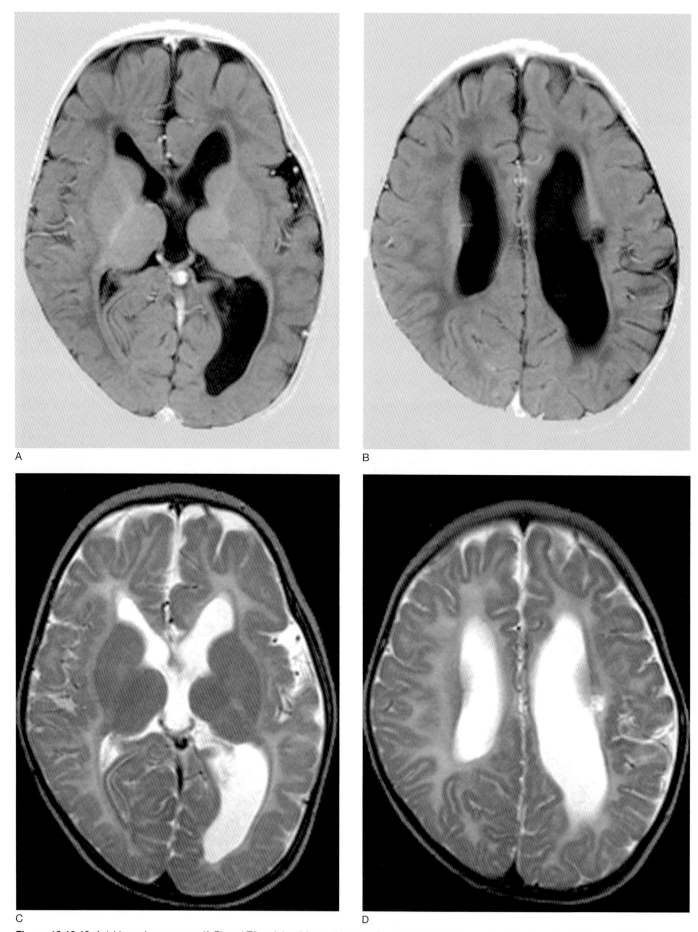

Figure 12.10.19 Axial inversion recovery (A,B) and T2-weighted fast spin echo (C,D) images in a 10-month-old male patient with non-ketotic hyperglycinaemia. Diffuse brain atrophy with prominently delayed myelination. Note that the presence of sparse myelin within the brain (optic radiations, internal capsules) is much better visualized on the T1-weighted than the T2-weighted images. Incidental lacunar subependymal lesion within the left centrum semiovale.

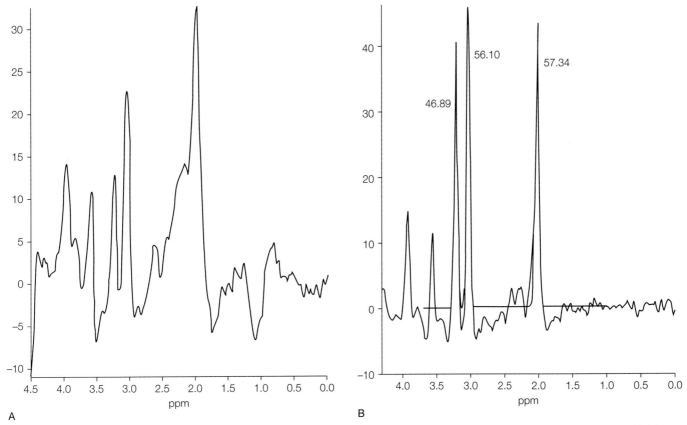

A B

Figure 12.10.20 Single-voxel proton MR spectroscopy in a 10-month-old male patient with non-ketotic hyperglycinaemia. The spectrum with 20 ms echo time (A) shows a prominent peak at the 3.55 ppm level, which remains visible on the spectrum with 135-ms echo time (B), consistent with glycine (see text for explanation).

FURTHER READING

Bick U, Ullrich K, Stöber U et al. White matter abnormalities in patients with treated hyperphenylalaninaemia: magnetic resonance relaxometry and proton spectroscopy findings. European Journal of Paediatrics 1993; 152:1012–1020.

Brismar J, Aqeel A, Brismar G et al. Maple syrup urine disease: findings on CT and MR scans of the brain in 10 infants. American Journal of Neuroradiology 1990; 11:121–128.

Chen YF, Huang YC, Liu HM et al. MRI in a case of adult-onset citrullinemia. Neuroradiology 2001; 43:845–847.

Connelly A, Cross JH, Gadian G et al. Magnetic resonance spectroscopy shows increased brain glutamine in ornithine carbamoyl transferase deficiency. Pediatric Research 1993; 33:77–81.

Engelbrecht V, Rassek M, Huismann J et al. MR and proton MR spectroscopy of the brain in hyperhomocysteinemia caused by methylenetetrahydrofolate reductase deficiency. American Journal of Neuroradiology 1997; 18:536–539.

Felber SR, Sperl W, Chemelli A et al. Maple syrup urine disease: metabolic decompensation monitored by proton magnetic resonance imaging and spectroscopy. Annals of Neurology 1993; 33:396–401.

Heindel W, Kugel H, Roth B. Noninvasive detection of increased glycine content by proton MR spectroscopy in the brains of two infants with non-ketotic hyperglycinemia. American Journal of Neuroradiology 1993; 14:629–635.

Mamourian AC, du Plessis A. Urea cycle defect: a case with MR and CT findings resembling infarct. Pediatric Radiology 1991; 21:594–595.

Press GA, Barshop BA, Haas RH et al. Abnormalities of the brain in nonketotic hyperglycinemia: MR manifestations. American Journal of Neuroradiology 1989; 10:315–321.

Rossi A, Cerone R, Biancheri R et al. Early-onset combined methylmalonic aciduria and homocystinuria: Neuroradiologic findings. American Journal of Neuroradiology 2001; 22:554–563.

Ruano MM, Castillo M, Thompson JE. MR imaging in a patient with homocystinuria. American Journal of Roentgenology 1998; 171:1147–1149.

Uziel G, Savoiardo M, Nardocci N. CT and MRI in maple syrup urine disease. Neurology 1988; 38:486–488.

Van Hove JKL, Kishnani PS, Demaerel P et al. Acute hydrocephalus in non-ketotic hyperglycinemia. Neurology 2000; 54:754–756.

DISORDERS OF METAL METABOLISM

COPPER METABOLISM

Copper is a trace metal and is essential for the appropriate functioning of several enzyme complexes (cytochrome c-oxidase, superoxide dismutase, lysyl oxidase, dopa beta-monooxygenase). Copper is absorbed from the intestines and then transported by plasma albumins to specific organs, notably the liver, brain, kidney and eye. Two specific diseases related to the impairment of copper transport are known to date: Menkes disease and Wilson disease.

MENKES DISEASE

Menkes disease is related to a defect at the level of the membrane copper transport mechanism. One of the consequences of this is the impairment of the normal intestinal absorption of copper, as a result of which a severe copper deficiency develops. On the other hand, transmembrane transport of copper is impaired elsewhere in the organism too, therefore copper cannot be delivered to copper-requiring enzymes, and hence copper is trapped and accumulated in connective tissues, while serum copper and ceruloplasmin levels are low. The most important manifestations of the disease are therefore connective tissue abnormalities and progressive degeneration of the central nervous system, the latter due to global failure of copper-requiring enzymes, in particular cytochrome C-oxidase.

The disease is of X-linked inheritance. The onset of the disease is neonatal but the patients are typically normal during the first 2 or 3 months of life, after which neurological deterioration occurs, with loss of milestones, convulsions, hypotonia followed by spasticity and eventually lethargy. Most affected children die during the first years of life. Menkes disease is often referred to as 'kinky hair' disease because of the peculiar appearance of the hair. Connective tissue abnormalities include bladder diverticula, inguinal hernia, loose skin, hyperflexible joints and vessel wall fragility.

At birth the brain appears normal on MR imaging. During the course of the disease, however, rapidly developing atrophy and prominent delay of the myelination (perhaps with a component of demyelination) become obvious. Shrinking of the brain can be so marked that spontaneous subdural fluid collections (hygroma, subdural haematoma) frequently develop. On the T1-weighted images the basal ganglia exhibit hypersignal, similar to what is seen in chronic hepatic encephalopathies, including Wilson disease. The cerebral vessels are usually tortuous and elongated; this can be seen on conventional images but is better appreciated on MR angiography.

WILSON DISEASE

Wilson disease is of autosomal recessive inheritance. In contrast to Menkes disease, which is essentially intracellular copper transport deficiency, Wilson disease develops due to an extracellular copper transport problem. A deficient transport protein prevents the excretion of copper from the cells, in particular the hepatocytes and incorporation of copper into ceruloplasmin. As a result large amounts of copper are accumulated within the liver and subsequently in other organs (brain, kidney, cornea), leading to degeneration of the involved tissues. This peculiar distribution explains the clinical manifestations of the disease, the hallmarks of which are progressive hepatic insufficiency, neurological deficit (deep cerebral grey matter, brainstem, cerebellar abnormalities) and the so-called Kaiser–Fleischer ring in the cornea.

MR imaging of the brain in clinically symptomatic Wilson disease patients is usually abnormal. The most significant changes are seen at the level of the deep grey matter structures, the brainstem (mesencephalon and pons), the cerebellum and the cerebral hemispheric white matter. At the level of the deep grey matter structures, the T2-weighted images show somewhat ill-defined, bilateral symmetrical hyperintensities involving the caudate nuclei, the putamina, the globi pallidi, the thalami and even the claustra. The latter, if present, is a very characteristic finding and an important differential diagnostic clue in Wilson disease. As in other hepatic encephalopathies, the T1-weighted images may show faint and ill-defined hyperintensities within the basal ganglia and

the thalami even in clinically well-controlled patients who do not have detectable abnormalities on the T2-weighted images. In the brainstem, ill-defined hyperintensities are often found at the level of the pons and the centre of the mesencephalon; nevertheless, the most characteristic (although not pathognomonic) finding is the so-called 'giant panda face' appearance of the upper mesencephalon. This consists of hypersignal within the substantia nigra (mainly in the pars compacta) and the tegmentum of the mesencephalon, in contrast with the normal or hypointense appearance of the red nuclei, the cerebral peduncles and the tectum. In the cerebellum, the dentate nuclei may be involved and patchy lesions are sometimes found in the cerebellar hemispheric white matter also. Smaller or larger white matter lesions within the cerebral hemispheres may also occur; they are usually asymmetrical. T2-weighted gradient echo images often show prominent hyposignal within the putamina, the globi pallidi, the substantia nigra and the red nuclei. The exact nature of the magnetically susceptible substance in these structures is unclear; it may correspond to iron or copper. As the disease progresses diffuse brain atrophy develops (Figure 12.10.21).

Diffusion-weighted images may show hypersignal within some of the lesion areas, including the mesencephalon and the thalami. If paramagnetic substances are present within the deep grey matter structures, they exhibit hyposignal on the diffusion-weighted images.

OTHER METALS

Several rare inherited diseases related to metal metabolism other than copper have been described. They include magnesium (primary hypomagnesaemia, magnesium-losing kidney), zinc (acrodermatitis enteropathica, hyperzincaemia), manganese (prolidase deficiency) and molybdenum (combined deficiency of sulphite oxidase and xanthine oxidase).

FURTHER READING

Barkovich AJ, Good WV, Koch TK et al. Mitochondrial disorders: Analysis of their clinical and imaging characteristics. American Journal of Neuroradiology 1993; 14:1119–1137.

Jacobs DS, Smith AS, Finelli DA et al. Menkes kinky hair disease: Characteristic MR angiographic findings. American Journal of Neuroradiology 1993; 14:1160–1163.

DISORDERS OF THE MITOCHONDRIAL ENERGY METABOLISM

DISORDERS OF THE PYRUVATE METABOLISM

Since the pyruvate metabolism is a pivotal element in energy production and gluconeogenesis, it is obvious that all organs with high energy requirements and, in particular, the central nervous system are vulnerable to any disorder in the process. The two most common abnormalities of the pyruvate metabolism are the

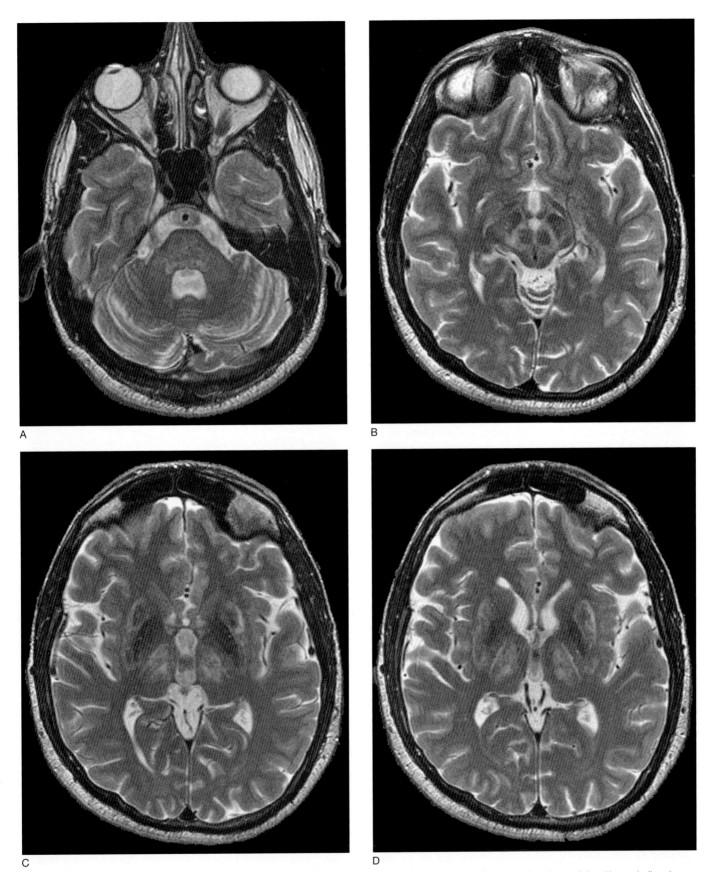

Figure 12.10.21 Axial T2-weighted fast spin echo images in a 28-year-old male patient with Wilson disease, presenting mainly with cerebellar signs. Hypointense lesions are seen within the pons and the middle cerebellar peduncles (A), the pars compacta of the substantia nigra and the tegmental structures in the mesencephalon, characterizing the 'giant panda face' (B), the thalami and the putamina (C,D). Ill-defined hypointensities are shown within the globi pallidi and to a lesser extent within the putamina (C,D), as well as within the pars reticulate of the substantia nigra and the red nuclei (B).

deficiency of the pyruvate dehydrogenase complex and pyruvate carboxylase. Other enzyme defects in the tricarboxylic acid cycle, however, are also known.

PYRUVATE DEHYDROGENASE COMPLEX DEFICIENCY

Most of the genes encoding the different units of the pyruvate dehydrogenase complex are autosomal; one subunit (E1 alpha) is located on the X chromosome. Since this is by far the most frequent site of mutation, most cases of pyruvate dehydrogenase complex deficiency show an X-linked inheritance pattern. In case of deficiency of the pyruvate dehydrogenase enzyme, pyruvate is converted into lactate, which produces significantly less energy than complete oxidation. The disease is therefore characterized by systemic and organ-specific abnormalities related to lactic acidosis and energy failure.

Some degree of involvement of the central nervous system is always present. Affected infants present with delayed development, hypotonia, seizures, ataxia and apnoea, occasionally leading to sudden infantile death. In some cases, the disease may resemble subacute necrotizing encephalopathy (Leigh disease) but only a small fraction of true Leigh disease cases actually are caused by deficiency of the pyruvate dehydrogenase complex.

Imaging studies may show congenital malformations of the brain, in particular, dysgenesis of the corpus callosum. Deep grey matter structures (basal ganglia, upper brainstem) often show abnormalities, although the MR imaging findings may also be quite unremarkable.

PYRUVATE CARBOXYLASE DEFICIENCY

The inheritance of pyruvate carboxylase deficiency is autosomal recessive. The neonatal form of the disease is always very severe and leads to death during the first couple of months of life. It presents with hepatic dysfunction, lactic acidosis, hypoglycaemia, seizures and spasticity. The clinical presentation of patients with the benign form of the disease is quite variable; typically, recurrent episodes of lactic acidosis are encountered with a wide range of associated systemic or central nervous system derangements. Patients with the mild form may live into adulthood without major disability.

DEFECTS OF THE RESPIRATORY CHAIN

The so-called respiratory chain is a complex multi-unit system within the inner membrane of the mitochondria. It consists of five different complexes (complex I–V), each of which has a specific role in the process of the oxidative phosphorylation. The respiratory chain enzymes are genetically encoded by both nuclear and mitochondrial DNA (except complex II, which is entirely encoded by mitochondrial DNA), this gives rise to an often complex inheritance pattern (Mendelian and maternal). Defects of the mitochondrial DNA present with a maternal inheritance.

Multisystem involvement is the rule in the diseases related to defects of the respiratory chain; this can be an important clinical diagnostic clue. In respiratory chain deficiencies, practically any organ or tissue in any combination may be involved; the most frequently affected organs are, however, the central nervous system and the muscles (both skeletal and visceral).

LEIGH DISEASE

This disease is often referred to as subacute necrotizing encephalomyopathy. Besides respiratory chain defects, the disease may be caused by deficiencies of the pyruvate metabolism and the tricarboxylic acid cycle. The inheritance can be both autosomal and maternal. The disease typically appears during infancy and presents with progressive neurological deterioration, including loss of milestones, pyramidal and extrapyramidal signs and symptoms. Respiratory problems and ocular abnormalities (external ophthalmoplegia, nystagmus, strabismus) are also frequently encountered.

The MR imaging findings include abnormalities of the deep cerebral grey matter structures, the brainstem, the deep cerebellar grey matter structures and the cerebral hemispheric white matter. At the level of the upper mesencephalon the pattern of signal changes resembles the 'giant panda face' (hyperintensity within the substantia nigra and the tegmental structures). Prominent signal changes are very often present within the medulla oblongata; this may explain the frequent respiratory problems (episodes of apnoea, sighing) of the patients. Ill-defined, faint hyperintensities may also be present within the centre of the pons. The subthalamic nuclei are almost always involved; the detection of the lesions is however difficult. Basal ganglia changes are typical in Leigh disease; however, their magnitude and extent are quite variable. The thalami are sometimes involved as well. The dentate nuclei frequently, but not always, show abnormalities. White matter lesions in the cerebral hemispheres are usually patchy and predominantly subcortical (Figures 12.10.2 and 12.10.22). The most important differential diagnoses are organic acidopathies but the presence of the peculiar brainstem lesions in Leigh disease usually allows confident differentiation.

Diffusion-weighted images may show hypersignal during the acute metabolic attacks within the lesion areas in the brainstem, the basal ganglia and the dentate nuclei.

MR spectroscopy is helpful by showing the presence of lactate in the brain but obviously this is a non-specific finding (Figure 12.10.23).

MELAS

The acronym MELAS refers to mitochondrial encephalomyopathy with lactic acidosis and stroke-like episodes. This is probably the best known of the so-called 'mitochondrial' diseases. The disease is of maternal inheritance, the mutation occurring on the mitochondrial DNA. In about 80% of cases, the site of the mutation is 3243 (A3243G) but several other rare mutations are also known. As a result, complex I and IV respiratory chain enzymes become deficient.

The clinical phenotypes (tissue involvement, age of onset, severity of the disease) show great variations. The age of onset is typically between 4 and 15 years but early infantile and adult forms have also been reported. The disease is sometimes provoked by a

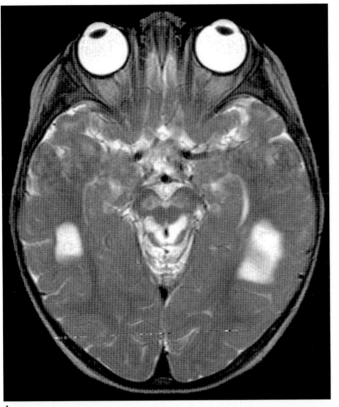

A

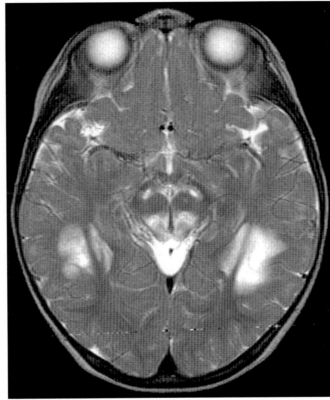

B

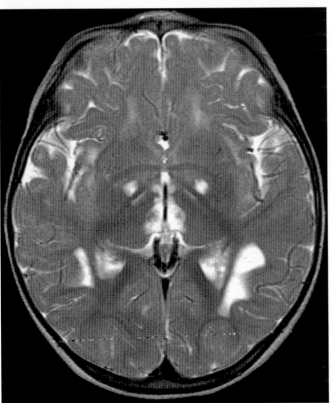

C

Figure 12.10.22 Axial T2-weighted fast spin echo images in a 1-year-old female patient with Leigh disease (same patient as in Figure 12.10.2). The very much characteristic symmetrical lesions within the tectum and tegmentum of the mesencephalon (A), the substantia nigra (B), the thalami, the subthalamic nuclei and the globi pallidi (C) are well demonstrated. Patchy asymmetrical white matter lesions are present within the cerebral white matter in the temporal and occipital lobes.

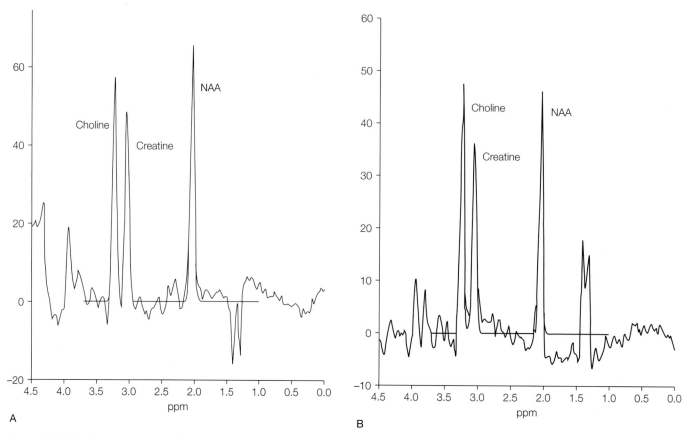

Figure 12.10.23 Single-voxel proton MR spectroscopy in the same patient as in Figure 12.10.22. Both spectra, one with 135-ms (A) and the other with 270-ms (B) echo time, show prominent peak doublets at the 1.3 ppm level, consistent with lactate showing the characteristic J-coupling phenomenon. The sampling voxel was placed on the basal ganglia on the right side.

febrile illness (causing a mismatch between energy requirements and availability); nevertheless, developmental delay and learning disability may be noted before the initial clinical manifestation in some patients. The disease typically presents with sudden onset of headache, vomiting, convulsions and myopathic signs but focal neurological signs soon become obvious as well. Although CSF lactate is sometimes elevated, no systemic lactic acidosis is found. Systemic manifestations of the disease include cardiomyopathy and diabetes (both type 1 and 2).

Imaging studies in MELAS show one or more stroke-like lesions within the brain, typically within the cerebral hemispheres. The most frequently affected areas are the parietal and the occipital lobes, followed by the temporal and frontal regions. The lesions involve both cortical and subcortical structures and in their appearance are quite similar to infarctions. Careful analysis of the lesion areas, however, usually shows a non-territorial pattern, which is the most important differential diagnostic clue (Figure 12.10.24). Another useful sign is the lack of prominent hypersignal in the lesion areas on diffusion-weighted images; this also supports the hypothesis that the lesions are actually not of ischaemic origin but rather secondary to metabolic crash (energetic failure).

MR angiography fails to demonstrate evidence of occlusive arterial disease; in the chronic phase, however, decreased blood supply (due to decreased demand) may result in reduced vascular network in the lesion areas. CT examination in MELAS frequently reveals basal ganglia calcifications.

MR spectroscopy may be a useful complementary test since a small amount of lactate is often detected even in apparently normal brain areas.

In an appropriate clinical setting, the MRI, CT and MR spectroscopic findings provide a highly suggestive pattern and warrant further studies, in particular, muscle biopsy to confirm the diagnosis.

LHON

Leber's hereditary optic neuroretinopathy (LHON) presents with rapidly progressive visual loss, due to degeneration of the optic nerves. The disease typically occurs in young adults. No skeletal muscle involvement has been described in this disease.

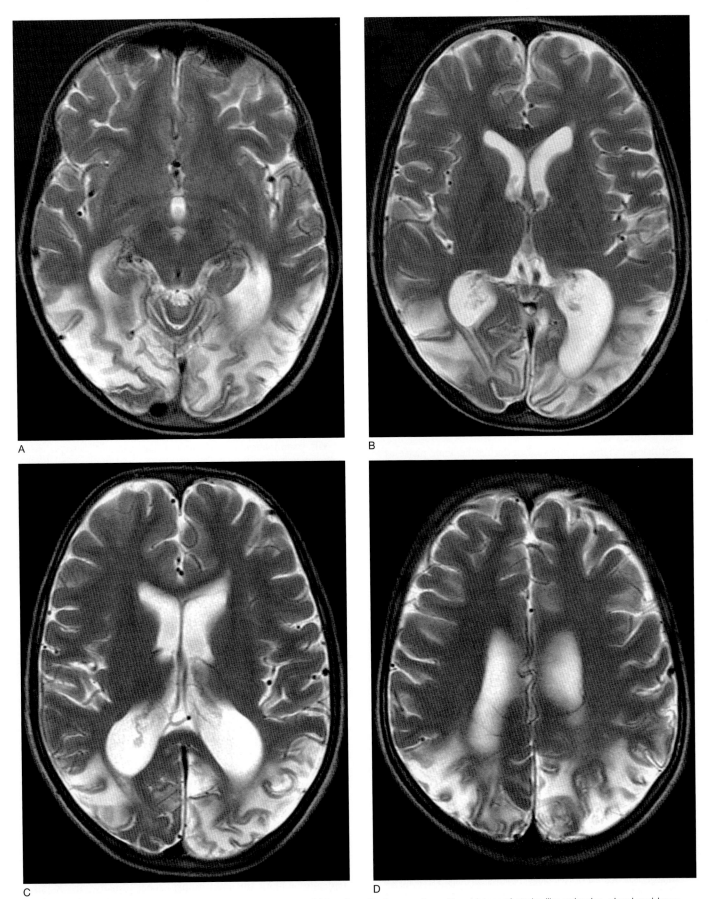

Figure 12.10.24 (A–D) Axial T2-weighted images in a 12-year-old female patient presenting with a history of stroke-like episodes, visual problems and epilepsy. The lesions in the parietal-occiptal regions involve mainly subcortical structures but the cortex is also abnormal in many areas. The lesions do not have a clear vascular territorial pattern (i.e. the lesions extend to both the posterior and middle cerebral artery territories).

MR imaging usually shows signal abnormalities within the distal intraorbital optic nerves. Occasionally, putaminal lesions and scattered white matter lesions within the centrum cerebral hemispheric white matter may be present also.

MR spectroscopy, as in many other 'mitochondrial' diseases, may not show abnormal lactate within the brain parenchyma.

KEARNS–SAYRE DISEASE

Kearns–Sayre disease is a complex syndrome characterized by progressive external ophthalmoplegia and pigmental retinal degeneration associated with either complete heart block, cerebellar ataxia or elevated CSF protein level. The disease is of juvenile onset (by definition, less than 20 years of age).

In Kearns–Sayre disease, CT of the brain may show calcifications within the globi pallidi and the caudate nuclei. On MR examination, extensive involvement of the deep cerebral grey matter structures is seen, with hypersignal of the basal ganglia and the thalami on the T2-weighted images. Within the upper brainstem, the substantia nigra and the tegmental structures are typically abnormal but lesions may also be present within the medulla oblongata. Ill-defined, rather diffuse white matter lesions within the cerebral hemispheres, predominantly in a subcortical location, are frequent also. In the cerebellum, white matter lesions also occur, typically centrally, but may also extend to the middle cerebellar peduncles.

Diffusion-weighted images taken during the acute phase of the disease may show hypersignal within the lesion areas, consistent with isotropically restricted water diffusion.

MR spectroscopy may or may not show abnormal lactate within the brain parenchyma.

FURTHER READING

Arii J, Tanabe Y. Leigh syndrome: Serial MR imaging and clinical follow-up. American Journal of Neuroradiology 2000; 21:1502–1509.

Detre JA, Wang Z, Bogdan AR et al. Regional variation in brain lactate in Leigh syndrome by localized 1H magnetic resonance spectroscopy. Annals of Neurology 1991; 29:218–221.

Medina L, Chi TL, DeVivo DC et al. MR findings in patients with subacute necrotizing encephalomyelopathy (Leigh syndrome): Correlation with biochemical defect. American Journal of Neuroradiology 1990; 11:379–384.

Munoz A, Mateos F, Simon R et al. Mitochondrial diseases in children: neuroradiological and clinical features in 17 patients. Neuroradiology 1999; 41:920–928.

Ohshita T, Oka M, Imon Y et al. Serial diffusion-weighted imaging in MELAS. Neuroradiology 2000; 42:651–656.

Oppenheim C, Galanaud D, Samson Y et al. Can diffusion weighted magnetic resonance imaging help differentiate stroke from stroke-like events in MELAS. Journal of Neurology, Neurosurgery, and Psychiatry 2000; 69:248–250.

Pavlakis SG, Kingsley PB, Kaplan GP et al. Magnetic resonance spectroscopy: use in monitoring MELAS treatment. Archives of Neurology 1998; 55:849–852.

Savoiardo M, Ciceri E, D'Incerti L et al. Symmetric lesions of the subthalamic nuclei in mitochondrial encephalopathies: An almost distinctive mark of Leigh disease with COX deficiency. American Journal of Neuroradiology 1995; 16:1746–1747.

Sue CM, Crimmins DS, Soo YS et al. Neuroradiological features of six kindreds with MELAS tRNA Leu A3243G point mutation: implications for pathogenesis. Journal of Neurology, Neurosurgery, and Psychiatry 1998; 65:233–240.

Valanne L, Ketonen L, Majander A et al. Neuroradiologic findings in children with mitochondrial disorders. American Journal of Neuroradiology 1998; 19:369–377.

LYSOSOMAL DISORDERS

KRABBE DISEASE

The underlying metabolic derangement in Krabbe disease or globoid cell leucodystrophy is the defect of the galactocerebroside beta-galactosidase enzyme, resulting in abnormal accumulation of galactosylsphingosine (psychosine), which is believed to be toxic to oligodendrocytes and Schwann cells, hence the produced myelin becomes unstable and prone to breakdown. Consequently, both the central and the peripheral nervous systems are affected. The disease has an autosomal recessive inheritance.

The disease typically starts in infancy (3–8 months) but later onset forms, including adult onset, may also occur. Initially, the disease presents with irritability, tonic spasms, blindness, deafness and pyramidal signs. As in other demyelinating diseases, CSF protein is elevated. Electrophysiological studies reveal peripheral nerve conduction velocity abnormalities, consistent with peripheral neuropathy. Later, permanent hypertonia, hyperpyrexia and seizures develop, followed by hypotonia, loss of bulbar functions and respiratory failure. The disease is rapidly progressive and death usually occurs between 12 and 18 months of age.

CT studies in Krabbe disease describe hyperdensities within the deep grey matter structures of the brain. This is in keeping with histopathological findings of calcifications in the same areas.

MR examination of the brain often, but not always, shows hypointensities within the basal ganglia and thalami on the T2-weighted images. The most prominent abnormalities in Krabbe disease consist of the widespread white matter changes. Both the cerebral and the cerebellar white matter is involved. In the cerebellum, the most central areas may exhibit a spongy, necrotic appearance. The dentate nuclei are spared. Within the brainstem the pyramidal tracts are usually abnormal. The middle cerebellar peduncles and the lateral parts of the pons also show hypersignal on the T2-weighted images (Figure 12.10.25). Supratentorially, the white matter abnormalities clearly show a centrifugal pattern with an additional posteroanterior gradient. This means that the subcortical U-fibres, especially in the frontal lobes, may show sparing during the early stages of the disease. The posterior limbs of the internal capsules are involved earlier than the anterior limbs. The external and extreme capsules are also relatively spared initially (Figure 12.10.26). With the progression of the disease, practically all white matter structures become abnormal, spongy changes appear in the periventricular regions and diffuse brain atrophy develops (Figure 12.10.27). The supratentorial white matter lesion pattern in the early stage of the disease may be quite similar to that in X-linked adrenoleucodystrophy. Significant differences, however, also exist, both clinically and on imaging. In Krabbe disease, no intermediate zones are seen between the demyelinated and yet 'normal' white matter. Furthermore, although contrast enhancement has been described in Krabbe disease also, it is different from that seen in X-linked adrenoleucodystrophy. In Krabbe disease, it is either along the interface between the deep and the subcortical U-fibres or more frequently in the parietal periventricular zones, whereas in X-linked adrenoleucodystrophy, it is typically within the transitional zone. Finally, in X-linked adrenoleucodystrophy, the cerebellar structures are not involved. In the burned out phase, Krabbe disease may be difficult to differentiate from advanced metachromatic leucodystrophy but

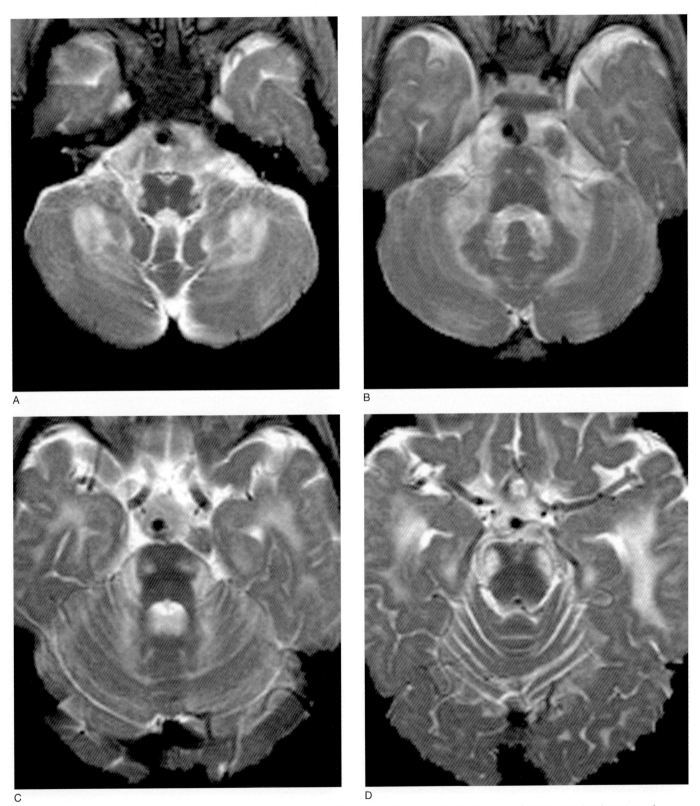

A

B

C

D

Figure 12.10.25 (A–D) Axial T2-weighted fast spin echo images in an 11-month-old female patient with Krabbe disease showing the extent of cerebellar and brainstem involvement.

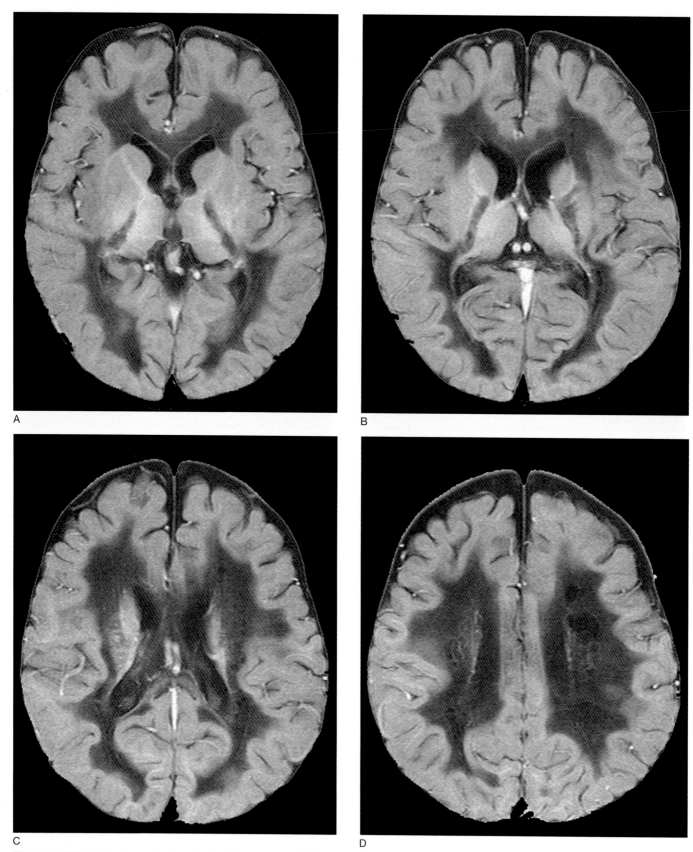

Figure 12.10.26 The rather typical supratentorial lesion pattern in Krabbe disease on axial inversion recovery images (same patient as in Figure 12.10.25). The posterior limbs of the internal capsules are abnormal, whereas the anterior limbs are spared, consistent with the posteroanterior gradient of the white matter disease (A,B). Spongy necrotic changes are seen in the periventricular white matter, consistent with the additional centrifugal progression pattern (D). The corpus callosum and the subcortical U-fibres are involved; the basal ganglia are spared (A–C). The subinsular white matter structures are relatively spared (A,B).

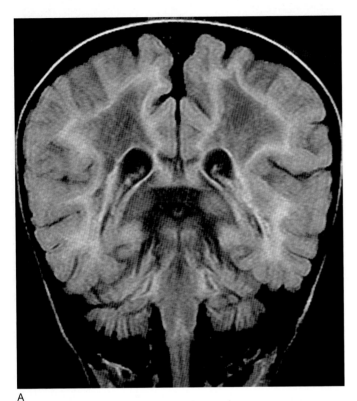
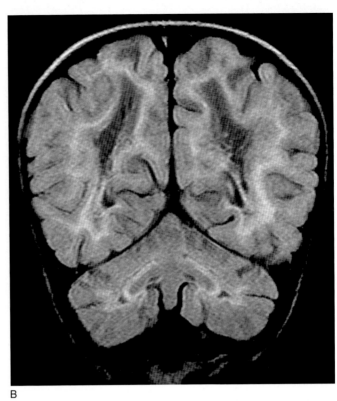

A

B

Figure 12.10.27 (A,B) Coronal FLAIR images in the same patient as in Figures 12.10.25 and 12.10.26. The typical centrifugal gradient of the white matter abnormalities is best demonstrated by this technique, showing the deep spongy white matter lesions and the less severe involvement of the subcortical white matter. Note the same lesion gradient within the cerebellar white matter also.

again cerebellar involvement in the latter is either absent or rather subtle.

It is noteworthy, however, that the imaging findings in the early and late onset forms of Krabbe disease are different. In the late onset forms, the disease predominantly involves the pyramidal tracts and cerebellar and basal ganglia abnormalities are absent.

MR imaging of the spine shows diffuse hypersignal within the spinal cord parenchyma. Nerve root enhancement may also be detected after intravenous contrast injection.

Diffusion-weighted images of the brain show prominent hypersignal along the progression line of the demyelinating process in the early stage of the disease (Figure 12.10.28). However, on follow-up examination these changes may subside quite rapidly and the demyelinated areas turn into hyposignal, indicating fast and complete myelin loss, which is consistent with the usually also rapidly evolving clinical picture.

MR spectroscopy shows significant differences, depending on the positioning of the sampling voxel. In the white matter, a prominent lactate peak is seen in conjunction with decreased N-acetyl aspartate and slightly increased choline peaks. If the sampling voxel is placed on the basal ganglia, the spectrum may be totally normal.

METACHROMATIC LEUCODYSTROPHY

Metachromatic leucodystrophy is related to the deficiency of the cerebroside sulphatase enzyme. The enzyme has two components,

notably the arylsulphatase A enzyme and an activator protein, called saposin B. Clinically, the deficiency of each of the components may lead to metachromatic leucodystrophy but arylsulphatase A deficiency is much more frequent. The impairment of the enzyme leads to accumulation of galactocerebroside sulphate (or sulphatide) within oligodendrocytes and Schwann cells. Thus, as in Krabbe disease, myelin both within the central nervous system and the peripheral nerves becomes unstable and prone to abnormal breakdown.

As discussed above under the heading of the molecular genetic basis of the inborn errors of metabolism, three different abnormal arylsulphatase A enzymes have been identified in metachromatic leucodystrophy. One of them is a truly deficient, inactive enzyme; the other is an unstable but functional enzyme and another is a so-called pseudodeficient enzyme. Homo- or heterozygotes to the pseudodeficient enzyme are clinically asymptomatic; conversely, carriers of the other two mutations develop clinical disease. In case of saposin B deficiency, the patients have normal arylsulphatase A activity, which may be a misleading laboratory finding initially.

Depending on the age of onset, the disease has several clinical phenotypes. The most frequent is the late infantile (onset between 1 and 2 years of age), accounting for 60–70% of cases. Early (3–6 years) and late (6–16 years) juvenile forms are encountered in about 25% and the adult form in about 10% of cases. A neonatal form also exists but is very rare.

As it is typical for leucodystrophies, the disease presents with hypotonia and progressive loss of motor skills, leading to para- and

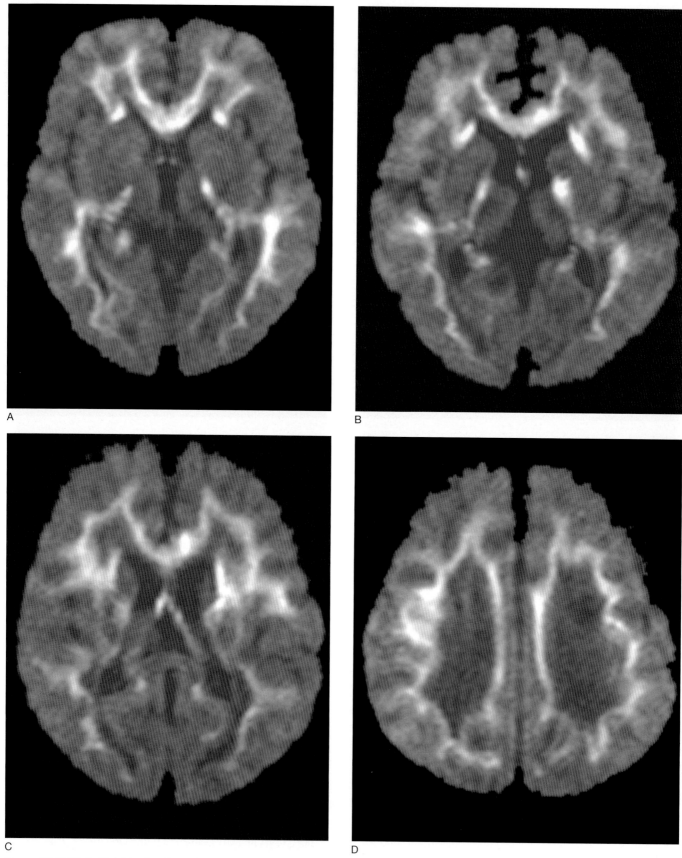

Figure 12.10.28 (A–D) Axial echo-planar diffusion-weighted images in Krabbe disease (same cuts as in Figure 12.10.26). The deep white matter lesions are hypointense (isotropically increased water diffusion), whereas the peripheral, presumably active demyelination zones and the posterior limbs of the internal capsules are hyperintense (restricted water diffusion), consistent with the centrifugal disease progression pattern.

later quadriplegia. Death usually occurs 3–6 years after onset of the disease.

Metachromatic leucodystrophy is a classical leucodystrophy with no apparent involvement of the grey matter structures on MRI. The imaging abnormalities consist of a progressive centrifugal white matter disease but an additional posteroanterior gradient is also present (Figure 12.10.29). The corpus callosum (first the splenium, then the more anterior components), the internal capsules (initially only the posterior limbs, later the anterior limbs too) and the deep hemispheric white matter are always involved. The subcortical U-fibres are typically spared during the initial stages of the disease. The external and extreme capsules are initially spared but are later abnormal. In the early infantile form of the disease, a peculiar 'tigroid' white matter lesion pattern may be seen within the centrum semiovale (Figure 12.10.30). This is most probably due to the initial relative sparing of the perivascular myelin around the transmedullary vessels, the explanation of which is unclear. The 'tigroid' pattern, if present, is a very suggestive pattern element. Signal changes may be present within the upper brainstem and along the cortical-spinal tracts; the latter may be due to Wallerian degeneration. Signal abnormalities within the cerebellar white matter are absent or rather subtle. During the disease course progressive and eventually severe diffuse brain atrophy develops and some degree of cerebellar white matter involvement may become conspicuous. The brain lesions do not show contrast enhancement.

Diffusion-weighted images usually show signal abnormalities. Moderate hypersignal is often seen in the presumed progression zone of the demyelinating process; in the late stage of the disease, diffuse hyposignal is found. The 'tigroid' pattern is also sometimes conspicuous on diffusion-weighted images.

MR spectroscopy shows a decreased N-acetyl aspartate peak, and a normal or increased choline peak. The *myo*-inositol peak may be increased also. Lactate is present during the early stage of the disease within the abnormal white matter areas (Figure 12.10.4).

MUCOPOLYSACCHARIDOSES

Mucopolysaccharidoses are multisystemic diseases with involvement of the skeletal system (dwarfism, bone and joint dysplasias, skull base abnormalities), the eye (corneal opacities), the liver, the spleen (hepatosplenomegaly), the heart (thickening of the valves) and the central nervous system (primary and secondary involvement).

The facial dysmorphias and the skeletal dysplasias (dysostosis multiplex) are often characteristic to the disease and greatly facilitate the diagnosis even on clinical grounds and plain x-ray skeletal survey. In certain conditions, notably when neurological signs and symptoms suggest involvement of the central nervous system, MR imaging of the brain and spine may be indicated for further evaluation of the brain parenchyma, the ventricular system and the craniocervical junction area.

Involvement of the central nervous system in mucopolysaccharidoses may be direct or indirect. The most frequent imaging substrates of direct central nervous system involvement are the enlarged perivascular spaces and white matter lesions, whereas indirect lesions include hydrocephalus and compression of the upper cervical spinal cord due to instability and narrowing in the craniocervical junction area.

Enlargement of the perivascular spaces is believed to be related to abnormal mucopolysaccharide deposition in the leptomeninges,

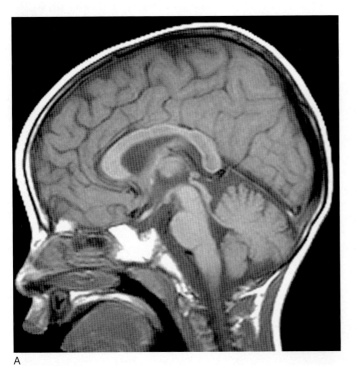
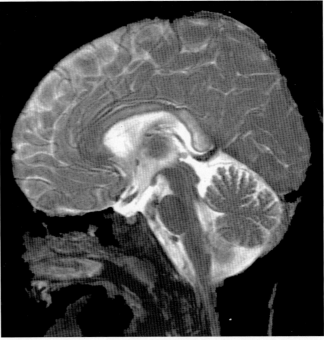

A   B

Figure 12.10.29 (A,B) Sagittal T1- and T2-weighted spin echo and fast spin echo images in a patient with metachromatic leucodystrophy. Although the entire corpus callosum is involved, a posteroanterior gradient is recognizable, especially on the T2 weighted images (B).

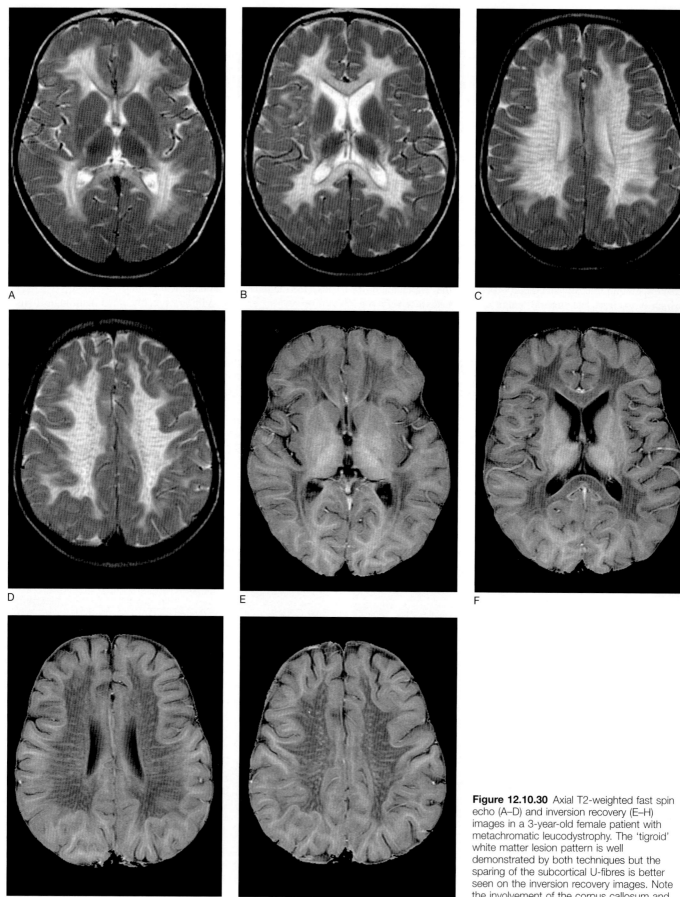

Figure 12.10.30 Axial T2-weighted fast spin echo (A–D) and inversion recovery (E–H) images in a 3-year-old female patient with metachromatic leucodystrophy. The 'tigroid' white matter lesion pattern is well demonstrated by both techniques but the sparing of the subcortical U-fibres is better seen on the inversion recovery images. Note the involvement of the corpus callosum and the posterior limbs of the internal capsules.

A

B

C

D

E

F

G

H

preventing the normal outflow of the interstitial fluid from the parenchyma. Hydrocephalus in mucopolysaccharidoses appears to be non-resorptive, most probably related to dysfunctioning of the Pacchioni granulations, again due to meningeal mucopolysaccharide depositions. Cerebral white matter lesions, which tend to be predominantly periventricular, may be due to delayed myelination and/or demyelination secondary to accumulation of macromolecules within the neurons and oligodendrocytes but transependymal CSF permeation (interstitial oedema), in cases with prominent hydrocephalus, may also play a role. Narrowing of the foramen magnum–upper cervical spinal canal area is due to the combined effects of atlantoaxial instability (odontoid dysplasia in conjunction with ligamental laxity) and mucopolysaccharide depositions within the synovial and dural structures.

In Hurler (MPS-I-H), Hunter (MPS-II) and Sanfilippo (MPS III) disease, the clinical picture is usually dominated by the central nervous system involvement (mental retardation with progressive dementia, gait disturbances). Some degree of intellectual deficit may be present in Scheie (MPS-I-S) and Hurler–Scheie (MPS-I-HS) diseases.

In Morquio (MPS-IV) and Maroteaux–Lamy (MPS-VI) disease, usually no direct involvement of the central nervous system occurs.

The occurrence and magnitude of the characteristic imaging abnormalities is variable in the different forms of mucopolysaccharidoses. Narrowing of the foramen magnum and upper cervical spinal canal is most prominent in Morquio syndrome (Figure 12.10.31) but it is also frequently present in Hunter, Hurler and Maroteaux–Lamy disease. Hydrocephalus is characteristic for Maroteaux–Lamy, Sanfilippo and Hunter disease. White matter changes are typical for Hunter, Hurler–Scheie, Sanfilippo and Maroteaux–Lamy disease. Enlarged perivascular spaces are most frequently encountered in Hurler and Hunter diseases (Figure 12.10.32).

MULTIPLE SULPHATASE DEFICIENCY

This is a rare autosomal recessive but very particular disorder, since it combines the features of mucopolysaccharidoses and metachromatic leucodystrophy from both the clinical and the imaging points of view. As its name indicates, multiple sulphatase enzymes (those involved in metachromatic leucodystrophy and in the various forms of mucopolysaccharidoses) are deficient; however, residual enzyme activities vary considerably. The most frequent form is of early childhood onset; neonatal and juvenile forms also exist but are rare.

Clinically, facial dysmorphia, similar to that seen in mucopolysaccharidoses, hepatosplenomegaly, microcephaly (in the neonatal form macrocephaly), delayed development, progressive spasticity, blindness and deafness are usually found.

Imaging studies of the brain show variable patterns of white matter disease (diffuse or multifocal), ventricular enlargement, occasionally enlarged perivascular spaces and c-c junction abnormalities with stenosis of the upper cervical spinal canal and possible cord compression.

GM GANGLIOSIDOSES

Diseases in this group of lysosomal disorders are characterized by abnormal visceral and neural accumulation of GM1 and GM2

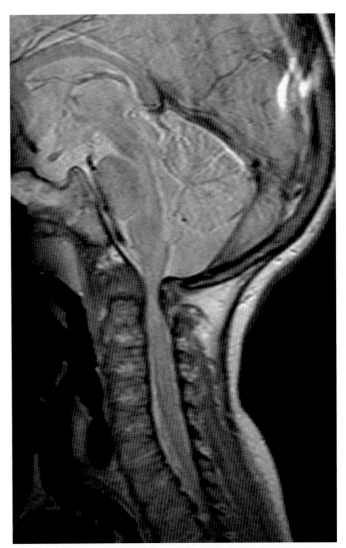

Figure 12.10.31 Sagittal proton density-weighted image of the craniocervical junction area in a 4-year-old female patient with Morquio disease. Severe stenosis of the foramen magnum with compression of the spinal cord. Dysplasia of the odontoid process.

gangliosides. The clinical pictures are therefore dominated by hepatosplenomegaly and encephalopathy.

GM1 GANGLIOSIDOSIS

The deficient enzyme in this group is beta-galactosidase. Three clinical phenotypes of GM1 gangliosidosis, infantile (type 1), juvenile (type 2) and adult (type 3), are known. The infantile type usually leads to death in early infancy; affected patients present with severe developmental delay, progressive spasticity and tonic–clonic seizures as well as hepatosplenomegaly. In type 2 and type 3 GM1 gangliosidoses, a more protracted course is seen; initially gait and speech disturbance and later extrapyramidal signs (choreoathetosis, parkinsonism) dominate the neurological picture.

Data on MR imaging findings in the different forms of GM1 gangliosidosis is very sparse. Type 1 presents with delayed myelination, type 2 with diffuse brain atrophy and extensive white

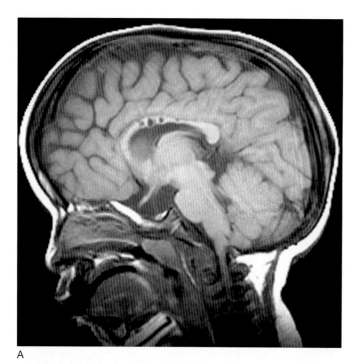

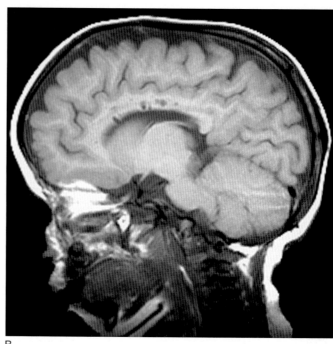

A   B

Figure 12.10.32 (A,B) Sagittal T1-weighted spin echo images in a 2-year-old female patient with Hurler disease. Characteristic enlarged perivascular CSF spaces at the level of the corpus callosum.

matter changes, quite similar to GM2 gangliosidosis, and type 3 shows basal ganglia and white matter abnormalities. The imaging patterns are non-specific.

GM2 GANGLIOSIDOSIS

The deficient enzyme in this group is beta-hexosaminidase. In this group, besides GM2 gangliosides, GA2 gangliosides are also accumulated. According to the proportions between the two substances O, B and AB variants are distinguished. The AB variant only has an infantile form, while the O and B variants have infantile, juvenile and adult forms. The best known disease entities are Tay–Sachs disease (infantile type B) and Sandhoff disease (infantile type O). From the clinical point of view the two diseases are quite similar, except that in Sandhoff disease hepatosplenomegaly may be found, whereas it is absent in Tay–Sachs disease. Patients are macrocephalic and present with a progressive neurological disease, characterized by psychomotor deterioration, pyramidal, later extrapyramidal (choreoathetosis) signs and generalized tonic–clonic seizures.

Imaging findings in Tay–Sachs and Sandhoff disease are quite similar and the pattern is suggestive.

CT examination of the brain shows hyperdensities within the basal ganglia and/or the thalami. This is probably due to calcifications.

The deep grey matter lesions may appear hypointense on T2-weighted and hyperintense on T1-weighted MR images. MR imaging, however, is particularly sensitive in demonstrating the widespread white matter changes within the cerebral hemispheres. Practically all white matter structures are involved, except for the corpus callosum, the anterior commissure and the posterior limbs

of the internal capsules. The external and extreme capsules as well as the laminae medullares between the pars medullaris and lateralis of the globi pallidi and the pars lateralis of the globi pallidi and the putamina are also abnormal. The pattern of the white matter lesions suggests centripetal demyelination. The putamina are always abnormal on the T2-weighted images; subtle hyperintensities may also be suggested at the level of the claustra. The caudate nuclei may be normal but abnormalities similar to the putaminal changes are typically present. Overall, the involved basal ganglia structures appear to be somewhat swollen, at least initially during the disease course. The thalami are spared; in fact, they seem to exhibit hyposignal on the T2-weighted images (Figure 12.10.33). The cerebellar white matter often shows signal abnormalities on the T2-weighted images; the hyperintensities are however less prominent than supratentorially. Typically, no abnormalities are seen within the brainstem and the spinal cord. The overall lesion pattern in a macrocephalic infant can be highly suggestive of the disease

Diffusion-weighted images are usually quite unremarkable, which suggests a relatively slow demyelinating process.

MR spectroscopy shows non-specific alterations of the spectra: the N-acetyl aspartate peak is decreased; the choline peak is slightly increased. No lactate is identified within the brain.

FURTHER READING

Barone R, Nigro F, Triulzi F et al. Clinical and neuroradiological follow-up in mucopolysaccharidosis type III (Sanfilippo syndrome). Neuropediatrics 1999; 30:283–288.

Chen CY, Zimmerman RA, Lee CC et al. Neuroimaging findings in late infantile GM1 gangliosidosis. American Journal of Neuroradiology 1998; 19:1628–1630.

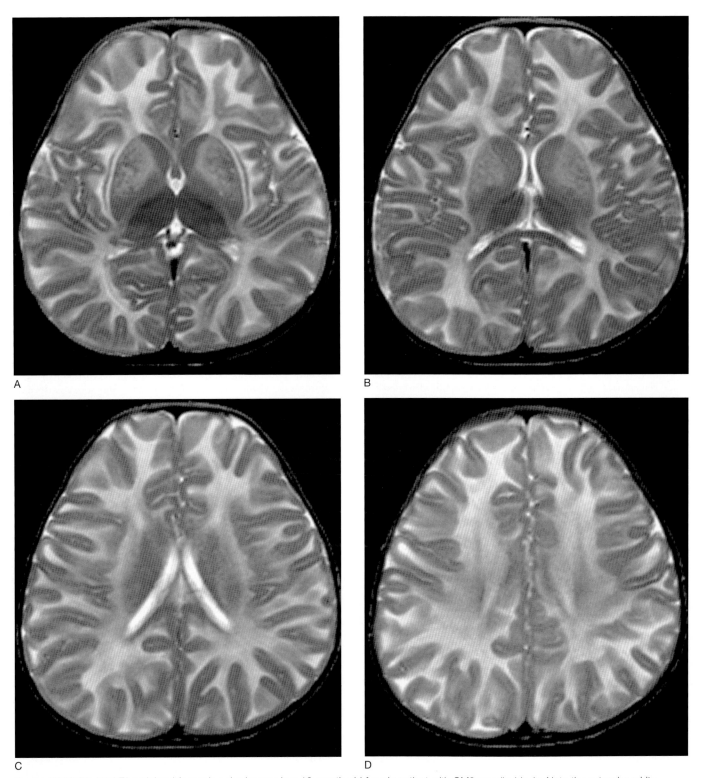

Figure 12.10.33 Axial T2-weighted fast spin echo images in a 16-month-old female patient with GM2 gangliosidosis. Note the extensive white matter involvement (A–D) with relative sparing of the corpus callosum, especially posteriorly (B). The claustra are particularly well delineated because of the prominent signal changes within the external and extreme capsules (A). The putamina exhibit a somewhat swollen and faintly hyperintense appearance; the thalami are hypointense (A,B).

Faerber EN, Melvin JJ, Smergel EM. MRI appearances of metachromatic leukodystrophy. Pediatric Radiology 1999; 29:669–672.

Farina L, Bizzi L, Finocchiaro G et al. MR imaging and proton spectroscopy in adult Krabbe disease. American Journal of Neuroradiology 2000; 21:1478–1482.

Kachur E, Del Maestro R. Mucopolysaccharidoses and spinal cord compression: Case report and review of the literature with implications of bone marrow transplantation. Neurosurgery 2000; 47:223–229.

Kim TS, Kim IO, Kim WS et al. MR of childhood metachromatic leukodystrophy. American Journal of Neuroradiology 1997; 18:733–738.

Kruse B, Hanefeld F, Christen HJ et al. Alterations of brain metabolites in metachromatic leukodystrophy as detected by localized proton magnetic resonance spectroscopy in vivo. Journal of Neurology 1993; 24:68–74.

Loes DJ, Peters C, Krivit W. Globoid cell leukodystrophy: Distinguishing early-onset from late-onset disease using a brain MR imaging scoring method. American Journal of Neuroradiology 1999; 20:316–323.

Uyama E, Terasaki T, Watanabe S. Type 3 GM1 gangliosidosis: characteristic MRI findings correlated with dystonia. Acta Neurologica Scandinavica1992; 86:609–615.

Vasconcellos E, Smith M. MRI nerve root enhancement in Krabbe disease. Pediatric Neurology 1998; 19:151–152.

Yuksel A, Yalcinkaya C, Islak C et al. Neuroimaging findings of four patients with Sandhoff disease. Pediatric Neurology 1999; 21:562–565.

PEROXISOMAL DISORDERS

The remarkable heterogeneity of peroxisomal disorders is explained by the complexity of the underlying biochemical derangements. Schematically, two types of peroxisomal disorders are known. Complex enzymatic deficiencies (so-called peroxisome assembly deficiencies) are caused by the dysfunction of most or all of the peroxisomal enzymes. Disease entities in this group include Zellweger syndrome, Zellweger-like syndrome, infantile Refsum disease, pseudoinfantile Refsum disease, atypical Refsum disease, neonatal adrenoleucodystrophy and some forms of rhizomelic chondrodysplasia punctata. The diseases are typically of early onset and poor prognosis.

The other group of peroxisomal disorders comprises single enzyme deficiencies. The resultant diseases are usually of later onset; the disease course may be more protracted and sometimes more benign, although lethal forms also exist. The best known diseases in this group are X-linked adrenoleucodystrophy, pseudoneonatal adrenoleucodystrophy, classical Refsum disease, pseudoZellweger syndrome, mevalonic aciduria and adrenomyeloneuropathy.

Peroxisomal disorders show great clinical phenotypic heterogeneity but dysmorphic features, neurological abnormalities and hepatointestinal dysfunctions are characteristic for many of them.

ZELLWEGER SYNDROME

Zellweger syndrome is a severe peroxisomal assembly deficiency. The disease is of neonatal onset; affected children present with facial dysmorphia, severe hypotonia, visual and hearing deficit, seizures, hepatomegaly and prolonged jaundice. The disease is also called cerebrohepatorenal syndrome, referring to the typical multiorgan involvement. Indeed, liver and kidney cells are particularly rich in peroxisomes (consistent with their significant metabolic activity); hence their malfunction has serious consequences.

From the MR imaging point of view the hallmarks of the disease are very markedly delayed (sometimes, almost arrested) myelination, brain atrophy, periventricular germinolytic cysts and bilateral, symmetrical perisylvian cortical dysplasia (polymicrogyria) and additional grey matter heterotopias. The combination of the above defines a practically pathognomonic imaging pattern (Figure 12.10.34).

X-LINKED ADRENOLEUCODYSTROPHY

This is the best known and most frequent of the peroxisomal disorders. This entity belongs to the single enzyme (very-long-chain fatty acid-coenzyme A synthetase) deficiencies; the enzyme is either defective or its peroxisomal membrane transport is impaired. The inheritance is X-linked recessive but female carriers are not always entirely asymptomatic. The disease, however, has several clinical phenotypes, the most common being the childhood form. The second most common form is adrenomyeloneuropathy, which is discussed below. Atypical forms have also been described.

The age of onset in the classical clinical phenotype is usually between 4 and 8 years but signs of adrenal insufficiency (pigmentation, frequent intercurrent infections) may appear earlier. The neurological manifestations are slowly progressive. Behavioural disorder, poor concentration (and school performance), gait disturbances, visual and hearing problems, and seizures develop initially, followed by dementia, spastic quadriplegia, blindness and deafness, leading to a decorticate state before death.

The MR imaging findings are very characteristic, in most cases actually pathognomonic. This is a true leucodystrophy, with no involvement of the grey matter structures. The white matter abnormalities typically appear in the occipital region initially. The subcortical U-fibres are spared for quite a long time. The splenium of the corpus callosum, the posterior parts of the posterior limbs of the internal capsules, the geniculate bodies and the pyramidal tracts within the brainstem are involved early in the disease course. The progression pattern is centrifugal and posteroanterior. This results in the most characteristic imaging (and histopathological) feature of the disease. Three distinct zones are identified in the hemispheric white matter lesion areas. The centre of the lesion, which presents with prominent hyposignal on the T1-weighted and hypersignal on the T2-weighted images, corresponds to the fully demyelinated, inactive, burned out zone. Around this area, an intermediate zone is seen, which is best visualized anteriorly. It is only faintly hyperintense on the T2-weighted images and often faintly hyperintense on the T1-weighted images also. After intravenous contrast injection, signal enhancement is frequently seen in this zone; if this is present at the time of the initial MR examination, it may have a predictive value for disease progression. Histopathologically, this corresponds to the inflammatory zone. Anterior to this, another zone is identified; it is only faintly hypointense on the T1-weighted images, while on the T2-weighted images the signal intensity in this zone is between those in the burned out and the inflammatory zones. This is a zone of active inflammation. The separation between this zone and more anteriorly the apparently normal, yet not affected, white matter is ill defined (Figure 12.10.35A–C, F). Rarely, the disease starts in the frontal lobes, in which case the progression pattern is anteroposterior (with involvement of the rostrum of the corpus callosum and the anterior limbs of the internal capsules) but the three zones may also be

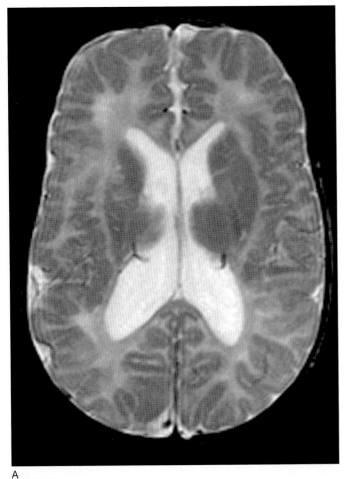
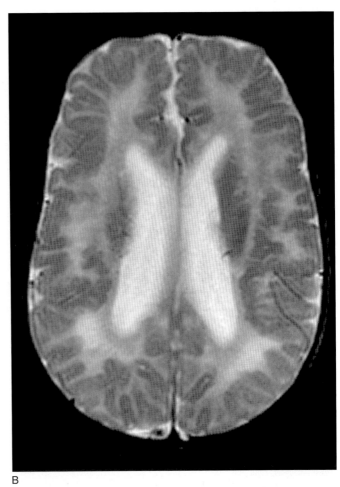

A   B

Figure 12.10.34 (A,B) Axial T2-weighted fast spin echo images in a 3-month-old female patient with Zellweger syndrome, showing bilateral perisylvian cortical abnormalities (polymicrogyria).

recognizable. Exceptionally, the lesions may be asymmetrical. The cerebellar white matter is spared in some cases and is involved in others; perhaps these lesions appear in the more advanced stage of the disease. The middle cerebellar peduncles may show signal abnormalities too. When the cerebellar white matter and the middle cerebellar peduncles are involved at the same time as the occipital white matter, the pattern may be reminiscent of Krabbe disease.

The three distinctly different zones in the cerebral hemispheric white matter lesions are also conspicuous on the diffusion-weighted images. The burned out zone is hypointense, the intermediate inflammatory zone is moderately hyperintense and the most peripheral demyelinating zone is very faintly hyperintense (Figure 12.10.35D,E).

MR spectroscopy shows non-specific abnormalities. In the burnt out zone, all peaks, but in particular the *N*-acetyl aspartate peak, are markedly decreased. Lactate is also present. In the inflammatory and demyelinating zones, the *N*-acetyl aspartate peak is decreased but the choline peak is somewhat increased, consistent with increased myelin breakdown. Lactate is also present in this area, indicative of impaired energy metabolism, as well as a slight increase of *myo*-inositol. In the 'normal' white matter, where conventional and diffusion-weighted images fail to demonstrate

any detectable abnormality, MR spectroscopy still shows a clear increase of the choline peak, which again is suggestive of increased myelin turnover.

ADRENOMYELONEUROPATHY

Adrenomyeloneuropathy is not an independent disease entity; it is actually one of the clinical phenotypes of X-linked adrenoleucodystrophy. The age of onset is usually between 20 and 30 years but since both the clinical and the imaging findings are quite different from those in X-linked adrenoleucodystrophy, it is probably appropriate to discuss the disease separately. Although usually signs and symptoms of cerebellar, spinal cord and peripheral nerve involvement, notably ataxia and paraparesis, as well as peripheral neuropathy, dominate the neurological presentation, mild cognitive disorder is often present as well. Adrenal insufficiency is a frequent associated clinical finding.

The lesion pattern in MR imaging is in keeping with the neurological picture. The lesions are predominantly found within the cerebellum and the brainstem. Both structures are atrophic. The brainstem signal abnormalities can be quite significant but the

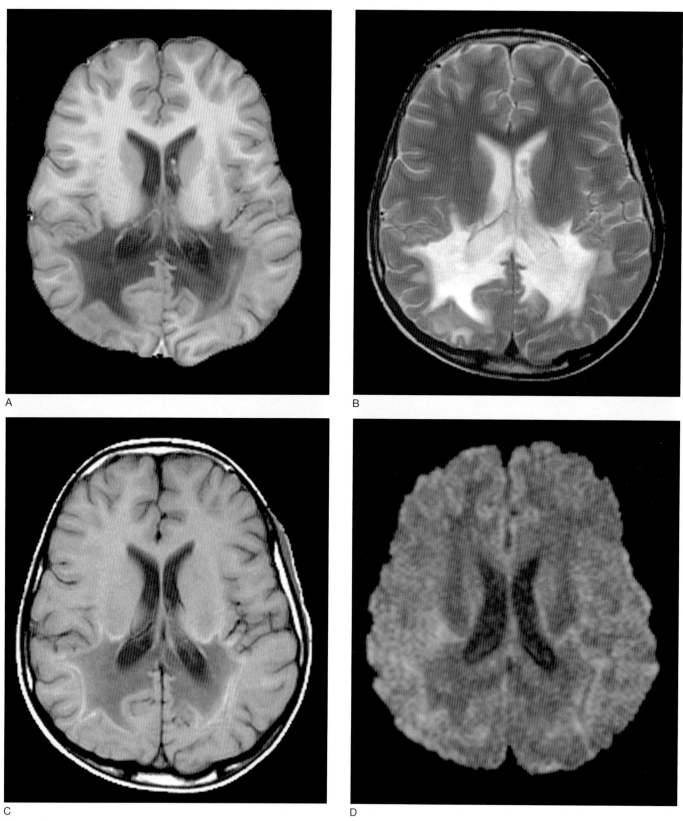

A

B

C

D

Figure 12.10.35 Axial inversion recovery (A), T2-weighted fast spin echo (B), T1-weighted spin echo (C), echo planar diffusion-weighted (D), apparent diffusion coefficient map (E) and contrast-enhanced T1-weighted spin echo (F) images in an 11-year-old male patient with X-linked adrenoleucodystrophy. Typical symmetrical parietal-occipital white matter lesions with sparing of the subcortical U-fibres (A,B), the latter better seen on the inversion recovery images. The intermediate zone of inflammation is spontaneously hyperintense on the T1-weighted (C) and the diffusion-weighted images (D), and after intravenous contrast injection signal enhancement is seen (F). The faint hyposignal on the apparent diffusion coefficient map image (E) suggests isotropically restricted water diffusion within the intermediate zone.

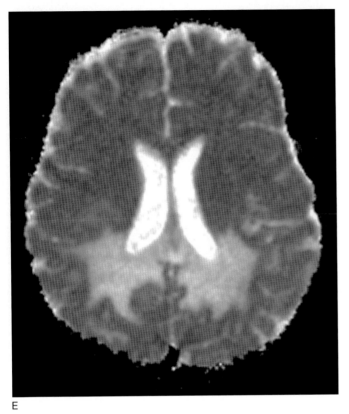

E

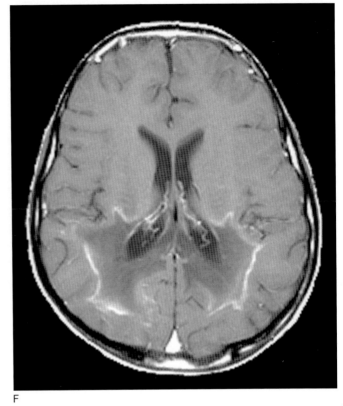

F

Figure 12.10.35 (*Continued*)

tegmental structures are relatively spared. The cerebellar white matter is diffusely abnormal. Involvement of the supratentorial white matter is limited mainly to the posterior limbs of the internal capsules and sometimes the splenium of the corpus callosum (Figure 12.10.36). Occasionally, lesions may be seen within the hemispheric white matter too. Enhancement may also occur within the lesions after intravenous contrast injection.

The diffusion-weighted images show no apparent abnormality.

MR spectroscopy of the cerebellar white matter lesions shows a significantly decreased *N*-acetyl aspartate peak, with grossly normal creatine and choline peaks and a small amount of lactate.

FURTHER READING

Barkovich AJ, Ferriero DM, Bass N et al. Involvement of the pontomedullary corticospinal tracts: A useful finding in the diagnosis of X-linked adrenoleukodystrophy. American Journal of Neuroradiology 1997; 18:95–100.

Barkovich AJ, Peck WW. MR of Zellweger syndrome. American Journal of Neuroradiology 1997; 18:1163–1170.

Confort-Gouny S, Vion-Dury J, Chabrol B et al. Localized proton resonance spectroscopy in X-linked adrenoleukodystrophy. Neuroradiology 1995; 37:568–575.

Melhem ER, Loes DJ, Georgiades CS et al. X-linked adrenoleukodystrophy: The role of contrast-enhanced MR imaging in predicting disease progression. American Journal of Neuroradiology 2000; 21:839–844.

Rajanayagam V, Grad J, Krivit W et al. Proton MR spectroscopy of childhood adrenoleukodystrophy. American Journal of Neuroradiology 1996; 17:1013–1024.

Russel IM, van Sonderen L, van Straaten HLM et al. Subependymal germinolytic cysts in Zellweger syndrome. Pediatric Radiology 1995; 25:254–255.

Tourbah A, Stievenart JL, Iba-Zizen MT et al. Localized proton magnetic resonance spectroscopy in patients with adult adrenoleukodystrophy. Archives of Neurology 1997; 54:586–592.

Tzika AA, Ball WS Jr, Vigneron DB et al. Childhood adrenoleukodystrophy: assessment with proton MR spectroscopy. Radiology 1993; 189:467–480.

van der Knaap MS, Valk J. The MR spectrum of peroxisomal disorders. Neuroradiology 1991; 33:30–37.

Williams GA, Pearl GS, Pollak MA et al. Adrenoleukodystrophy: unusual clinical and radiographic manifestations. Southern Medical Journal 1998; 91:770–774.

UNCLASSIFIED LEUCODYSTROPHIES

A high number of inherited leucodystrophies have been identified in the past few decades and their number is constantly growing. The underlying genetic and metabolic abnormality has been elucidated in some of them and is not yet known in many others. These diseases cannot be classified in any of the previously described categories; however, some of these diseases fall into the category of macrocephalic leucodystrophies, notably Canavan disease, Van der Knaap disease, the vanishing white matter disease and Alexander disease. Other diseases, notably Aicardi–Goutiere disease, Cockayne disease and Pelizaeus–Merzbacher disease, usually present with progressive relative microcephaly.

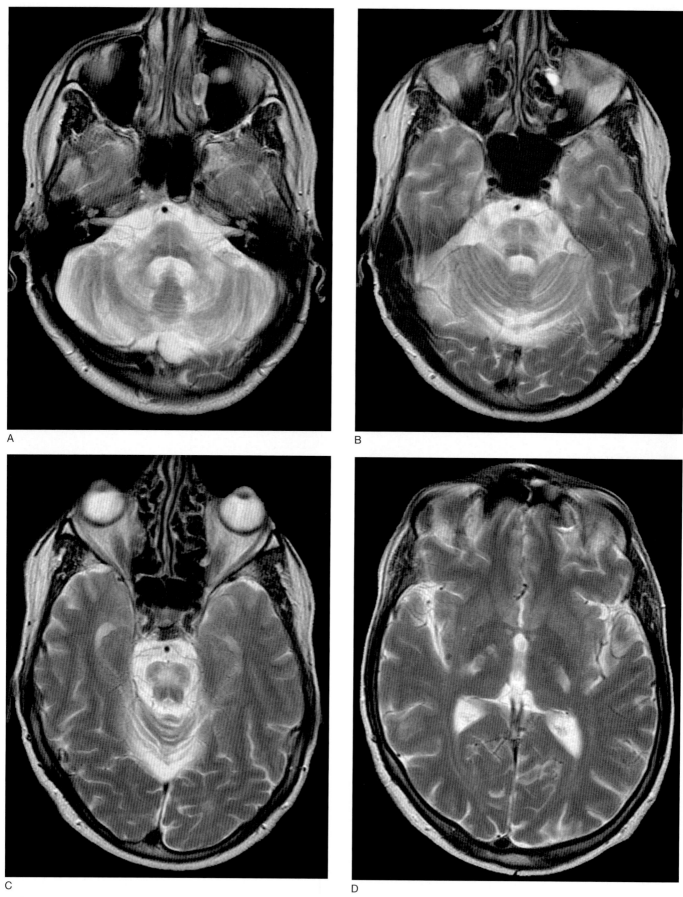

Figure 12.10.36 Axial T2-weighted fast spin echo images in a 30-year-old male patient with adrenomyeloneuropathy. The brainstem and the cerebellum are atrophic. Abnormal, increased signal intensities are present within the pons, the mesencephalon, the cerebellar white matter (A–C) and the posterior limbs of the internal capsules (D).

CANAVAN DISEASE

Canavan disease is related to the derangement of the metabolism of *N*-acetyl aspartate. *N*-acetyl aspartate is a 'brain-specific' substance, the exact role of which is unknown. It is synthesized from acetyl-coenzyme A and aspartate and is metabolized into acetate and aspartate by the aspartoacylase enzyme. Deficiency of the aspartoacylase enzyme causes marked accumulation of *N*-acetyl aspartate in the brain and excretion in the urine. In Canavan disease, histological examination of the brain parenchyma shows spongy degeneration (vacuolating myelinopathy) of the white matter, the exact pathomechanism of the damage, however, is not known. Both direct toxic and indirect mechanisms have been suggested.

The disease has an autosomal recessive inheritance. Although a rare neonatal form is also known, the disease is typically characterized by an early infantile onset. After the first few months of life, patients present with macrocephaly, loss of milestones, hypotonia, irritability and visual loss. Later spasticity of the limbs develops; choreoathetoid movement disorder and seizures may also appear. The disease rapidly leads to severe neurological crippling and a vegetative state. Death occurs after a few years but longer survivals (over 10 years) also exist.

The imaging findings are pathognomonic in the full-blown stage of the disease, in the burned out phase, however, they are non-specific. Practically all white matter structures of the brain are involved but the relative sparing of the internal capsules and the corpus callosum during the early stage of the disease suggests a cen-tripetal progression pattern (Figure 12.10.37). The spongiform changes and hence the imaging abnormalities, however, are not limited to white matter structures only. In keeping with histological observations, MR imaging clearly shows abnormalities within the thalami and the globi pallidi. The caudate nuclei, the putamina and the claustra are spared. In the burned-out phase the brain is atrophic.

Diffusion-weighted imaging shows a rather uniform hypersignal within the abnormal white matter structures, consistent with vacuolating myelinopathy. However, in the burned-out phase of the disease, this significantly decreases and in some areas totally disappears.

Although the diagnosis of Canavan disease is easily made by urine tests, a specific diagnosis may also be made by MR spectroscopy. To date, an increase of the *N*-acetyl aspartate peak has been described only in Canavan disease; therefore, it is considered to be pathognomonic to the disease (Figure 12.10.38).

VAN DER KNAAP DISEASE

This is one of the most recently identified leucodystrophies; it is also called infantile-onset spongiform leucoencephalopathy with a discrepantly mild clinical course or megaloencephalic leucodystrophy with subcortical cysts. The disease has an autosomal recessive inheritance. The onset of the disease is usually during the first year of life but usually it is diagnosed several years later. Patients present with macrocephaly. The initial motor and mental development of the patients is either normal or slightly delayed. The

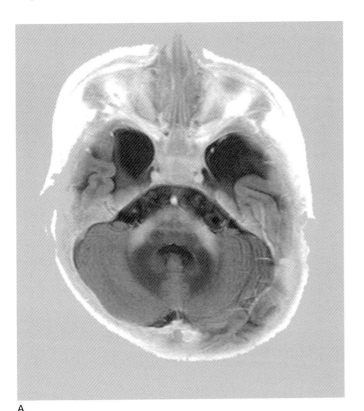
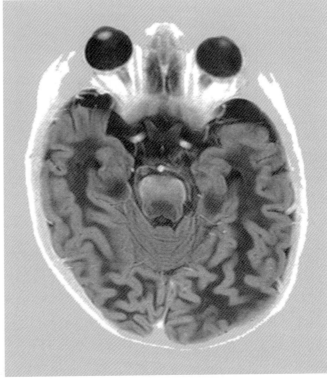

A   B

Figure 12.10.37 Axial inversion recovery images in a 7-month-old male patient with Canavan disease, a very extensive white matter disease involving the brainstem, the cerebellum and the cerebral hemispheres. Some sparing of the middle cerebellar peduncles (A), the ventral brainstem structures (A,B), posterior limbs of the internal capsules (C) and of the corpus callosum (D) is, however, still seen, consistent with the centripetal disease progression pattern.

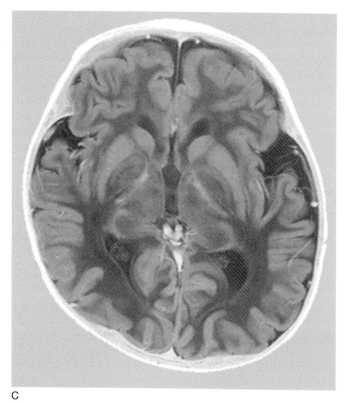

C

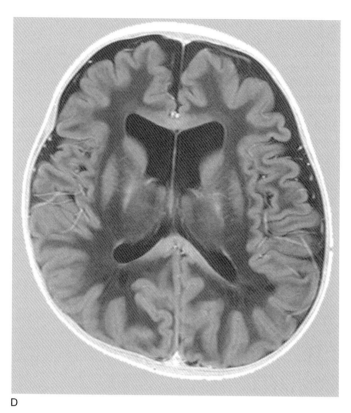

D

Figure 12.10.37 *(Continued)*

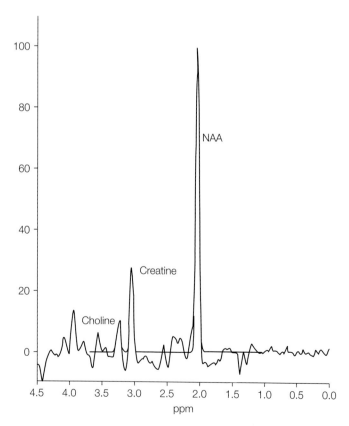

Figure 12.10.38 Single voxel proton MR spectroscopy of the brain in Canavan disease (same patient as in Figure 12.10.37). The prominent increase of the NAA peak is pathognomonic to the disease. The creatine and, in particular, the choline peaks are decreased.

disease is characterized by a slowly progressive course; in particular, ataxia, spasticity, gait disturbances and, in the later stage of the disease, mental deterioration and seizures develop. No peripheral neuropathy is detected. Laboratory tests fail to demonstrate any specific metabolic abnormality. Histologically the findings are consistent with vacuolating myelinopathy.

The MR imaging findings are pathognomonic. The brain is diffusely swollen during the early stage of the disease; later sulcal and ventricular enlargement may be present. The white matter disease is always severe at the time of the initial work-up and it shows a clear centripetal progression pattern (Figure 12.10.39). The peripheral white matter structures of the cerebral hemispheres are the most severely involved, including widespread disappearance of the subcortical U-fibres and the presence of large subcortical cyst formation in the frontoparietal and the temporal regions, best shown by the FLAIR images (Figure 12.10.40). These changes, as well as the initial slight sparing of the periventricular and subcortical white matter in the occipital regions, suggest an additional anteroposterior gradient (Figure 12.10.41). The deep white matter structures, notably the corpus callosum and the internal capsules are spared but the external and extreme capsules are involved. The cerebellar white matter is involved but much less markedly than the supratentorial white matter structures. Subtle signal changes may be present within the brainstem along the pyramidal tracts. The cortical and deep grey matter structures are normal. No abnormal signal enhancement is seen within the brain parenchyma after intravenous contrast injection.

Diffusion-weighted imaging shows prominent hyposignal within the subcortical cysts and somewhat decreased signal within the affected white matter. No definite hypersignal is seen within the non-affected white matter structures or along the interface between the normal and abnormal areas.

The proton spectroscopic findings are non-specific, the N-acetyl aspartate peak is decreased and the choline peak may be increased but no abnormal metabolites are demonstrated.

VANISHING WHITE MATTER DISEASE

This is a recently described, distinct clinical radiological entity. The disease is typically of childhood onset. Initially, the psychomotor development of the patients is normal. Affected patients present with ataxia, spasticity, gait disturbance, but only mildly impaired mental capacities. The clinical manifestation of the disease seems to be preceded by minor head trauma or infections; the same factors are also responsible for episodes of deterioration. During the later stages of the disease optic atrophy and mild epilepsy may develop. The disease is always progressive but the disease course varies. The severe forms lead to death at a relatively young age (2–6 years) but patients with more moderate clinical phenotypes, living into young adulthood, have also been found.

The MR imaging findings are fairly characteristic. The brain appears to be slightly swollen but some of the gyri are somewhat broadened. The lateral ventricles show mild to moderate dilatation. The white matter changes are very prominent; the signal properties of the affected myelin are practically identical to those of the CSF both on the T1- and the T2-weighted images. The posterior limbs of the internal capsules are often involved, whereas the anterior limbs are spared. The corpus callosum is also involved, with

the exception of the outer rim. The cerebellum is usually slightly atrophic; the cerebellar white matter is mildly abnormal. In the brainstem, the posterior tegmental and the pyramidal tracts also show abnormal hypersignal. The grey matter structures, including the basal ganglia, appear to be normal. Diffusion-weighted imaging findings have not been reported as yet.

MR spectroscopy of the affected grey matter shows decreased N-acetyl aspartate, normal or slightly increased choline, rather prominent lactate and glucose (at 3.43, 3.80 ppm) peaks. When the sampling voxel is placed on the affected white matter, very small N-acetyl aspartate, creatine and choline peaks are obtained only. However, small amounts of glucose and lactate are still discernible.

ALEXANDER DISEASE

This is a rare, actually sporadic 'macrocephalic' leucodystrophy without a clear inheritance pattern. The disease has neonatal, juvenile and adult forms. The most frequent form is the neonatal, presenting with macrocephaly, delayed development, spastic quadriparesis and seizures.

The imaging findings are concordant with the histological abnormalities. Extensive, predominantly supratentorial white matter disease is seen, which shows a centripetal progression pattern with an additional anteroposterior gradient. Large cystic lesions are typically seen in the frontal and temporal regions. The cortex is normal but basal ganglia abnormalities are common. The cerebellar white matter is frequently abnormal too. Contrast enhancement may be seen along the ependymal linings of the lateral ventricles, within the basal ganglia or even the dentate nuclei.

AICARDI–GOUTIERE SYNDROME

This rare microcephalic disease is also called leucodystrophy with chronic CSF lymphocytosis and calcifications of the basal ganglia. The disease appears in the neonate or in early infancy. It is a relatively rapidly progressive, devastating disease, characterized by delayed development and spasticity, leading to death in a few months or years.

Computed tomography is an essential diagnostic modality in this disease, since it almost always demonstrates calcifications within the basal ganglia and the periventricular white matter. On MRI, the disease presents with an essentially supratentorial and very extensive white matter disease with possible cystic lesions in the temporal and parietal lobes. The internal capsules are somewhat less affected but are abnormal also. The basal ganglia, the brainstem and the cerebellar structures are spared.

COCKAYNE DISEASE

This is a slowly progressive leucodystrophy, presenting with cachexia, progeric features, delayed development and later with peripheral neuropathy. This disease is also characterized by progressive microcephaly; affected patients are normo-

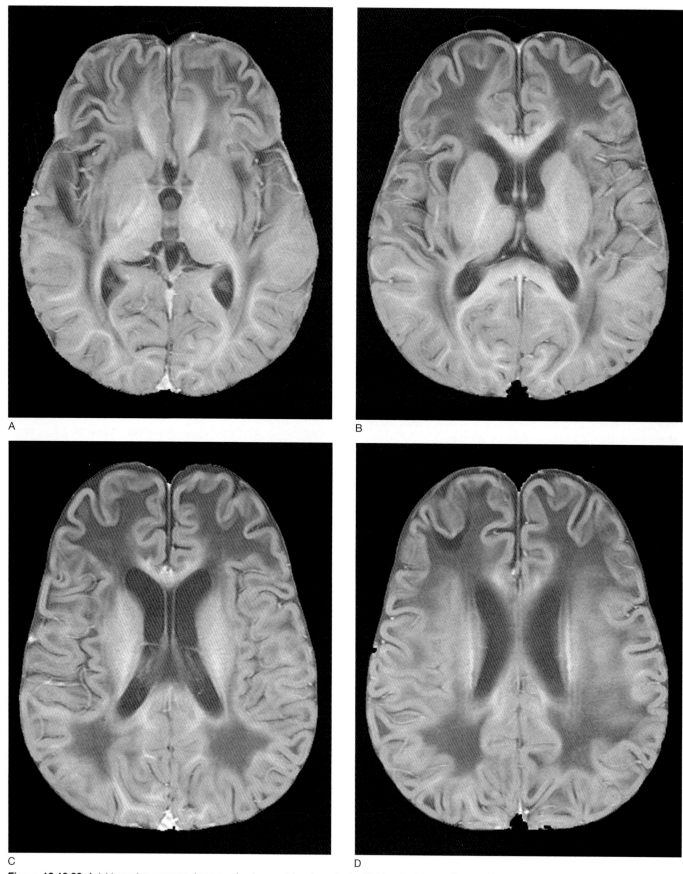

Figure 12.10.39 Axial inversion recovery images of a 4-year-old male patient with Van der Knaap disease. The white matter disease exhibits a centripetal and an additional anteroposterior gradient. The subcortical white matter structures are the most severely involved, especially in the frontal and temporal regions, whereas the subcortical U-fibres are still spared in the occipital lobes (A–C). The deep white matter structures (periventricular white matter, internal capsules, corpus callosum) are relatively spared also (A–D). Note the large subcortical cysts in the right temporal and frontal lobes (A,D).

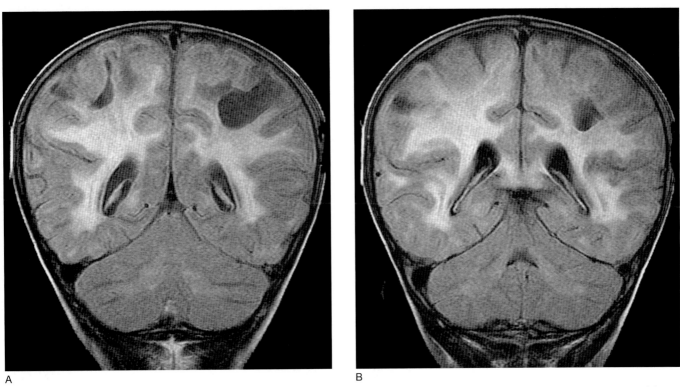

A

B

Figure 12.10.40 Subcortical cysts in Van der Knaap disease (same patient as in Figure 12.10.39) on coronal FLAIR images (A,B). Note the subtle signal changes within the cerebellar white matter.

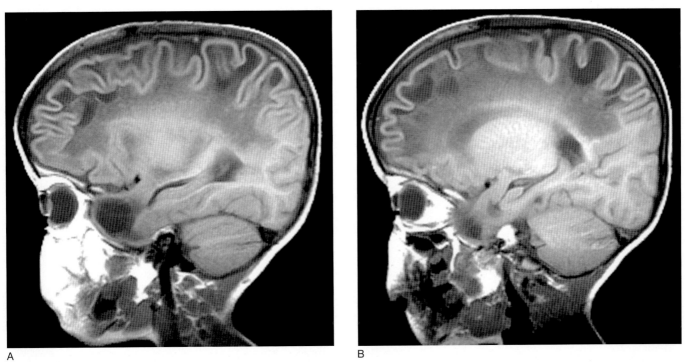

A

B

Figure 12.10.41 (A,B) Sagittal T1-weighted spin echo images in Van der Knaap disease (same patient as in Figures 12.10.39 and 12.10.40). The anteroposterior gradient of the white matter disease (relative sparing of the occipital lobe) and the subcortical cysts in the frontal and parietal regions are well demonstrated.

cephalic at birth, but develop relative microcephaly later during the disease course. One of the hallmark clinical features of the disease is the hypopigmentation of the skin associated with photosensitivity.

Computed tomography is a useful imaging tool. It shows nonspecific calcifications, typically within the basal ganglia and the dentate nuclei. Magnetic resonance examination shows prominent cerebellar and brainstem atrophy. Cerebral atrophy is also present but is usually less severe. Supratentorially, extensive white matter disease is shown. It is less severe than in most other leucodystrophies; it is actually better appreciated on the T2- than the T1-weighted images. The corpus callosum and the deeper white matter structures, including the internal capsules, are somewhat less affected, suggesting a centripetal progression pattern.

PELIZAEUS–MERZBACHER DISEASE

Three forms of this disease are known: the classical infantile type has an X-linked inheritance, the connatal type has both X-linked and autosomal forms, whereas the transitional form is sporadic or autosomal recessive. The disease is most probably due to a defect of the so-called proteolipid protein, which is a major constituent of the normal myelin. Depending on the severity of the defect, it results in impairment of the myelin formation (absence of myelin or dysmyelination with subsequent demyelination).

Clinically, both the connatal and the infantile forms present with severe failure to thrive and developmental delay, nystagmus, extrapyramidal signs and spasticity. Both forms are relentlessly progressive; in the connatal form, death occurs during the first decade of life and in the infantile form, during the second or third decade.

The classical imaging finding in Pelizaeus–Merzbacher disease is almost total absence of myelin within the brain or arrested myelination. In the latter case, the pattern of myelination may be appropriate for a given stage of the myelination process (e.g. birth) but not for the actual age of the patient. This, however, may happen in other pathological conditions, notably after hypoxic-anoxic brain damage or severe central nervous system infections or systemic diseases in infants, which constitute the most important differential diagnoses. Occasionally, a 'tigroid' pattern is also observed; this may indicate some sparing of the perivascular myelin and hence a demyelinating component in the disease process also. The brain is diffusely atrophic.

FURTHER READING

Grodd W, Krageloh-Mann I, Petersen D et al. In vivo assessement of N-acetylaspartate in brain in spongy degeneration (Canavan's disease) by proton spectroscopy. Lancet 1990; 336:437–438.

van der Knaap MS, Barth PG, Gabreels FJM et al. A new leukoencephalopathy with vanishing white matter. Neurology 1997; 48:845–855.

van der Knaap MS, Barth PG, Stroink H et al. Leukoencephalopathy with swelling and a discrepantly mild clinical course in eight children. Annals of Neurology 1995; 37:324–334.

van der Knaap MS, Barth PG, Vrensen GFJM et al. Histopathology of an infantile-onset spongiform leukoencephalopathy with a discrepantly mild clinical course. Acta Neuropathologica 1996; 92:206–212.

Vascular Pathology of the Brain

Francis Brunelle, Valérie Chigot, Hussein Aref

VASCULAR LESIONS OF THE CNS

Vascular diseases affecting the CNS in children are not uncommon. They can be classified under four main aetiologies: vascular malformations, vascular occlusions and associated with ischaemia, venous thromboses and vascular tumours. Atheroma is not a problem in children. When investigating a child for a suspected vascular lesion, imaging will depend on the mode of presentation, local availability of services, the stability of the child and the underlying suspected pathology. In general, acute imaging is by computed tomography (CT) to exclude a lesion that requires urgent surgery but for full assessment, magnetic resonance imaging (MRI) including magnetic resonance angiography (MRA) and possibly MR venography will be required. In a small number of cases, this will need to be supplemented by angiography for further delineation of a lesion and for therapy when appropriate.

VASCULAR MALFORMATIONS

Vascular malformations may affect the brain, meninges and the spinal cord. The arteries, veins and capillaries may be involved. Most occur sporadically and they can present at any age. Syndromes associated with vascular malformations include Sturge–Weber syndrome, hereditary haemorrhagic telangiectasia (Osler–Weber–Rendu disease), rarely ataxia telangiectasia, encephalocraniocutaneous lipomatosis, Cobb's syndrome, Wyburn–Mason syndrome and Klippel–Trenaunay syndrome. In the latter syndrome, the malformations are found in the spinal canal.

Symptoms arise from vascular malformations due to haemorrhage, steal effects and shunt effects, e.g. bruits, visibly enlarged vessels or their effects – pulsating exophthalmos or congestive heart failure.

Clinical presentation of a child with a vascular malformation is usually with an acute bleed and intracranial haemorrhage. Bleeding may occur into the subarachnoid space, intracerebrally, intraventricularly and, if close to the surface, into the subdural space. It may be isolated or occur in a mixture of these locations. Depending on its location and extent it is accompanied by headache, loss of consciousness, fits, cardiac or respiratory arrest or cranial nerve signs. Less acute presentations depend too on the location and include headaches, fits and neurological deficits.

A list of the main vascular malformations is given in Table 12.11.1.

PARENCHYMAL VASCULAR MALFORMATIONS

ARTERIOVENOUS MALFORMATION (AVM)

This is a mass of dilated abnormal vessels, the nidus, which communicates with one or more arterial branches and draining veins without the interposition of capillaries. It is intermingled with the brain parenchyma. Arteriovenous (AV) shunting takes place within the lesion and may divert blood from the surrounding cerebral parenchyma causing hypoperfusion, ischaemia, gliosis and atrophy. High flow within the lesion may result in intralesional aneurysms in the more distal vessels. The lesion itself, if large enough, can cause a mass effect and symptoms before it bleeds. AVMs are said to cause up to 40% of spontaneous intracerebral bleeds. The core of the malformation is called the nidus and describes the centre of the anomaly where most of the fistulas are supposed to be concentrated. The definition of the size and anatomy of the nidus is important for therapeutic purposes. This nidus, however, does not represent a very precise anatomical concept. It may be localized and relatively small or can be very large, involving a large region of the brain or, in some cases, a whole hemisphere.

Several classifications of AVMs are available in the literature but their clinical or therapeutic usefulness have not been clearly established.

Clinically, more than 80% of the malformations present by intraparenchymal (Figure 12.11.1) or intraventricular haemorrhage. The clinical signs of this bleed are sudden headaches with vomiting and depending on the location of the bleed, various neurological deficits such as hemiplegia or hemianopsia. Progressive neurological deteriorating effects of shunting are seen in about 10% of patients but seizures in only 4%. In some patients, there is a history of chronic migraine. Patients who have migraine associated with neurological symptoms should have imaging by CT or MRI to exclude an underlying cause such as a vascular malformation (Figures 12.11.1 and 12.11.2).

Imaging will reveal the intracranial bleed. Contrast enhancement should be performed to identify the diagnosis of brain vascular malformation. The following algorithm is followed in Hôpital des Enfants Malades, Paris.

If the clinical condition is poor, emergency evacuation of the clot is done. In patients with intraventricular haemorrhage, external cerebrospinal fluid (CSF) drainage is performed to reduce the increased intracranial pressure. MRI is performed with MRA to precisely locate the malformation in relation to the adjacent brain structure. MRA provides a road map for the next step, which is an angiogram performed within the next 12–24 h. This provides a precise anatomical location and detailed vascular anatomy. If embolization is appropriate, this is performed during the same session. Indications for embolization include:

- presence of aneurysms of the feeding arteries (rare) in children;
- small nidus;
- few arteries;
- non-eloquent region of the brain; and
- feasibility.

Bleeds occur mainly secondary to rupture of the draining veins.

In most cases of intraventricular haemorrhage, AVMs are drained by subependymal veins that are prone to rupture in the

Table 12.11.1 Vascular malformations

- vein of Galen malformation
- dural arteriovenous malformation
- parenchymal arteriovenous malformation
- isolated venous anomalies
- cavernomatous malformation
- arterial malformation, aneurysms
- syndromes
- spinal arteriovenous malformation
- cavernoma
- vertebral arteriovenous malformation

ventricles (Figure 12.11.3). It goes without saying that treatment of such malformations is better performed in a paediatric neurosurgery/neuroradiology environment.

Other clinical presentations include chronic headaches or migraine, which can be due to AVMs as described earlier. In most cases, with intense migraine major dilatation of the draining veins is seen. External carotid artery injection may reveal the presence of associated dural arteriovenous fistulas (Figure 12.11.4). These complex malformations are difficult to treat, but embolization of the associated dural fistula may improve the headaches. Seizures is another possible presentation. Increased intracranial pressure and chronic papilloedema can be seen. This last presentation is of particular importance as it may lead to sudden blindness. Increased intravenous pressure is probably responsible for the papilloedema. Treatment by embolization should be performed rapidly to avoid blindness (Figure 12.11.5).

TREATMENT

Three treatments are available to take care of brain vascular malformations (BVM): surgery, embolization and stereotactic radiotherapy. The decision is made based on risk/benefit. Surgery is performed if the malformation is small, superficial and in a 'non-eloquent' area. Small temporal lobe BVMs are an example of such 'surgical' lesions. Radiotherapy is performed for small (less than 3 cm) low-flow deep BVMs in dominant hemispheres and in regions with 'eloquent' function. Embolization is performed in other cases.

The use of all three modalities may be required in individual patients. Embolization may be used to reduce the size of the malformation, to make possible radiotherapy, surgery or radiosurgery. Surgery may be performed after embolization. Embolization may be performed after surgery to treat a residual lesion. Similarly, surgery or embolization may be performed after radiotherapy,

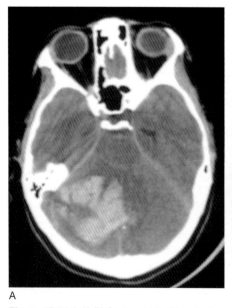
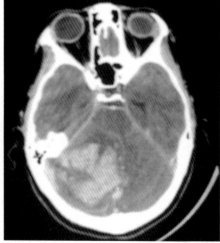
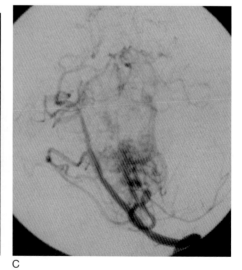

A   B   C

Figure 12.11.1 (A,B) Acute onset of headaches and coma: CT scan with and without contrast shows the presence of a posterior fossa bleed with some abnormal vessels. (C) Angiogram shows the arteriovenous malformation.

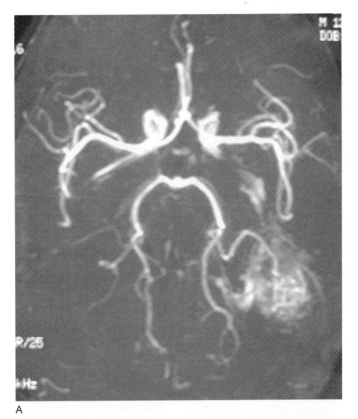

A

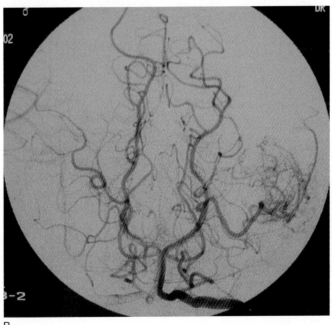

B

Figure 12.11.2 (A) Sudden onset of headaches. The CT revealed the presence of a bleed in the left temporal region. MRA shows the presence of a vascular malformation. (B) The angiogram confirms the vascular malformation. This was embolized during the same session.

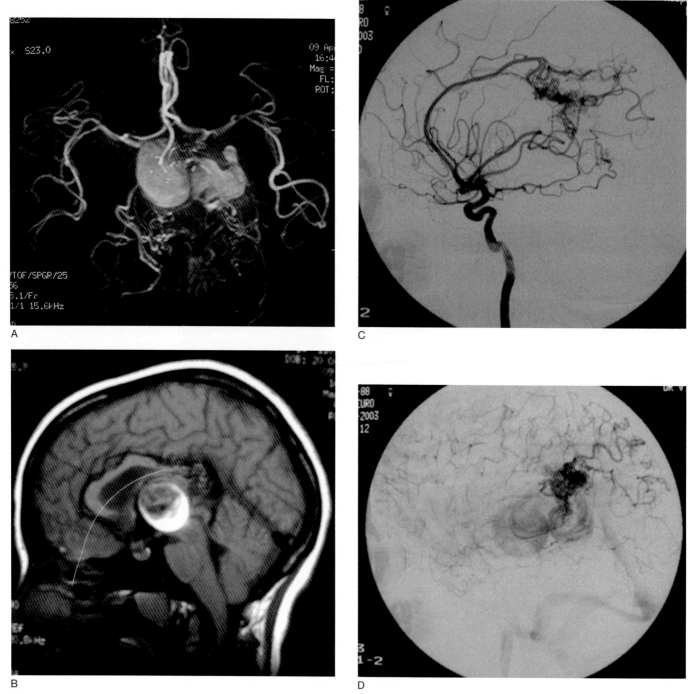

Figure 12.11.3 Sudden onset of headaches, with vomiting and right arm weakness. (A) MRA shows the intraventricular bleed as well as the presence of abnormal vessels. (B) Sagittal MRI shows the presence of a partially thrombosed intraventricular vein. (C) Carotid angiogram, arterial phase. The malformation is fed by the anterior cerebral artery. (D) The venous phase shows the dilated intraventricular vein.

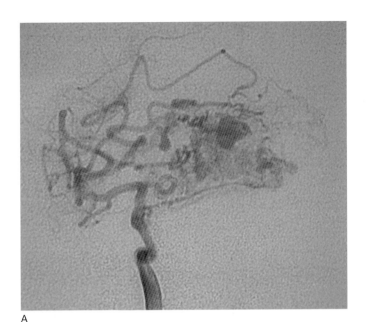

A

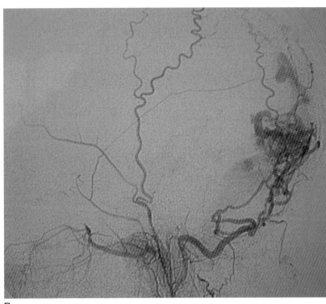

B

Figure 12.11.4 A 12-year-old girl with permanent headaches. The CT scan revealed the presence of a large vascular malformation of the occipital lobe. (A) Lateral view of the internal carotid artery. The complex vascular malformation is seen. Serial embolizations were done. (B) Lateral view of the external carotid artery opacification. Multiple arteriovenous shunts are seen between the meningeal arteries and the lateral sinus. Staged embolization progressively improved the clinical tolerance of the headaches.

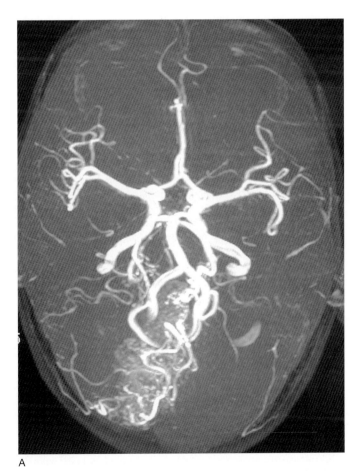

A

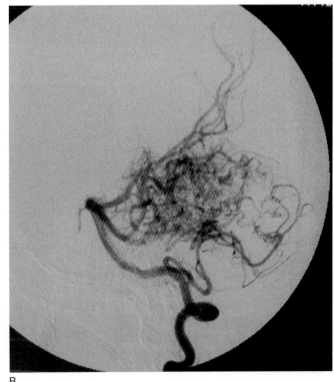

B

Figure 12.11.5 A 10-year-old boy with headaches and papilloedema. MRA revealed the presence of a posterior fossa AVM, responsible for the high pressure in the draining veins of the brain leading to papilloedema. Emergency angiogram and embolization cured the papilloedema.

when a residual lesion is present. In some cases of extensive lesions, no treatment may be feasible because of the risks.

ISOLATED VENOUS MALFORMATIONS

Venous malformations of the brain reflect the persistence of the embryonic venous network of the brain, the so-called medullary veins. They drain centrally towards the internal cerebral veins; this is the opposite of the 'mature' venous network that drains towards the cortical veins. On angiography, they exhibit a very peculiar branching pattern described as a candlestick (Figure 12.11.6). They are usually discovered fortuitously by angiography or MRI. On MRI they are very typical because it can be seen that the vein drains centrally rather than peripherally. They are best seen on T1-weighted scans after injection.

Venous malformations resemble the central veins seen in patients with Sturge–Weber syndrome. They may be seen anywhere on the dorsal neural tube and including the cerebellar hemisphere as well as in the supratentorial hemispheres. They may be

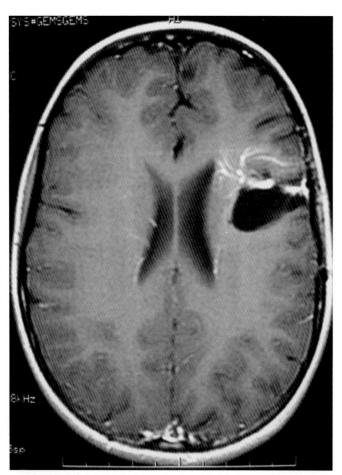

Figure 12.11.6 A 10-year-old girl with a spontaneous intracerebral bleed removed by surgery. Control MRI with gadolinium. The abnormal vein, the so-called venous angioma, is seen in the periphery of the post op porencephaly.

seen during the imaging work-up of patients who present with seizures or intraparenchymal bleed and may be associated with some focal atrophy. Their role in both of these clinical presentations is not established. They are probably thin-walled veins and it is not impossible that sudden increase in venous pressure may induce intracerebral bleed.

SINUS PERICRANII

This describes the finding of a small soft depressible sac under the scalp. This is shown to be a lacuna through the skull through which there is a venous outpouching in connection with the dural sinus.

CAVERNOMATOUS MALFORMATIONS

Cavernomatous malformations of the brain are composed of thin-walled capillaries and venules grouped together to form small to medium lesions. They are also known as cavernomas and cavernous haemangiomas. They are low-flow lesions and as shunting is not present in them the surrounding arteries and veins are not enlarged, but during vascular work-up they are almost invariably associated with venous malformations.

Clinical presentation may be with a bleed or seizures but these lesions may also be found as an incidental finding on neuroimaging performed for another purpose and they should not be mistaken for tumour. They are also incidentally found by pathological examination of resected specimens during surgical removal of intraparenchymal clot. Although not established, the link between venous malformation, cavernoma and sudden bleeding is strong.

When a cavernoma is seen during imaging work-up others should be looked for. There is a 50% incidence in familial cases but this reduces to 12% in sporadic lesions. They are typically iso- or hyperintense on T1-weighted and hypo- or hyperintense on T2-weighted sequences. They may enhance on T1-weighted plus gadolinium sequences. Venous angiomas are seen on those MR sequences.

T2* (GRE sequence) are the most useful sequences to demonstrate brain cavernomas as they contain haemosiderin. Their paramagnetic properties cause them to appear as black (hypointense) lesions in the brain on this sequence and enables their identification. Some cavernomas are only seen on these sequences (Figure 12.11.7).

FAMILIAL CAVERNOMAS AND MULTIPLE CAVERNOMAS

Multiple cavernomas of the brain are seen in some families. Mutation of the KRI gene has been described in these families. The gene locus is on chromosome 7q. When multiple cavernomas are seen in a child, the rest of the family should also be worked-up by MRI. Multiple cavernomas tend to increase in number and size with age in these patients. In addition to clinical presentation with bleeding, they are strongly associated with seizures when located in the

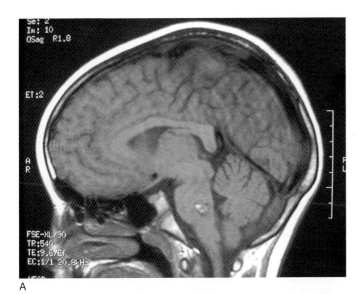

A

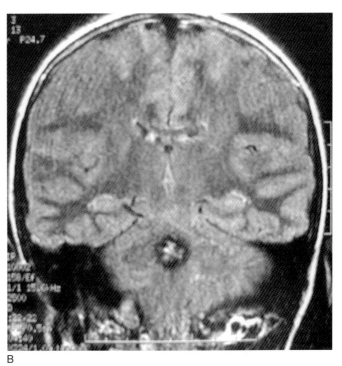

B

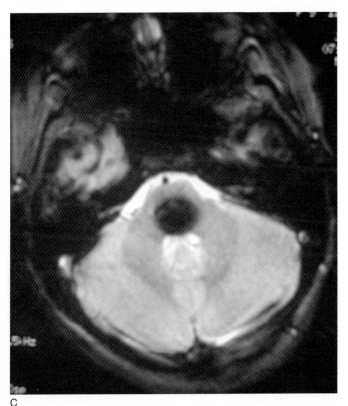

C

Figure 12.11.7 Clinical presentation of sudden brainstem signs, with vomiting. A brainstem tumour was suspected. (A) Sagittal MRI shows the presence of a high signal in the pons. (B) The coronal flair shows the hyposignal characteristic of the presence of haemosiderin in brain cavernomas. (C) The gradient echo (T2*) sequence is even more characteristic on this axial image.

cortex. They may also occur anywhere in the brain and spinal cord (Figure 12.11.8).

ANEURYSMS

Intracranial aneurysms are very rare in children with only one or two cases per year being seen in most specialized centres. They are also associated with brain vascular malformation feeding vessels but this is relatively rare in children. There are several systemic diseases that are associated with cerebral aneurysms (Figure 12.11.9), which are listed in Table 12.11.2.

Other causes of aneurysms in children are also rare but include mycotic aneurysms due to infection and traumatic aneurysms usually due to direct penetrating trauma but they are also recorded from blunt trauma.

Clinical presentation of aneurysms is similar in children and adults. Symptoms are due to meningeal irritation from the subarachnoid blood. The symptoms at the mild end of the spectrum are headache and vomiting but depending on the extent of the bleed may also progress to being obtunded and coma.

Giant aneurysms (greater than 2.5 cm) are more frequent in children and represent about 30% of the total. These may present with focal neurology before they bleed. Aneurysms in children arise most frequently at the internal carotid bifurcation as opposed to the circle of Willis location in adults.

Initial imaging on acute presentation is by CT but this should be followed by MRI and MRA, and where necessary for full delineation angiography during which therapy by embolization may be performed if deemed appropriate for management. The aneurysm is seen as a saccular dilatation arising from a vessel. It may be partially occluded by a clot, especially if large.

MYCOTIC ANEURYSMS

The incidence of these has decreased with the improved treatment of infectious conditions and cyanotic heart disease. They may

Table 12.11.2 Systemic conditions associated with paediatric cerebral aneurysms (reproduced with permission from Barkovich AJ (ed.). Pediatric neuroimaging, 3rd edn. Philadelphia : Lippincott Williams & Wilkins; 796)

Autosomal dominant polycystic kidney disease
Coarctation of the aorta
Tuberous sclerosis
Osler–Weber–Rendu disease
α-Glucosidase deficiency
Klippel–Trenaunay–Weber syndrome
3-M syndrome
α₁-antitrypsin deficiency
Parry–Romberg syndrome

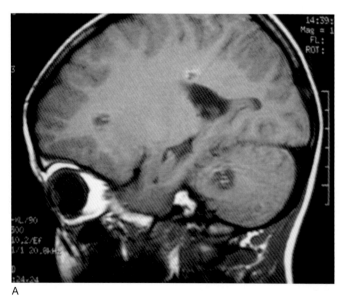

A

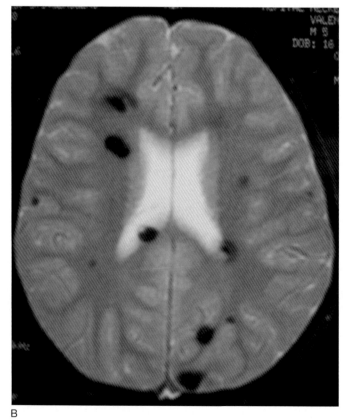

B

Figure 12.11.8 An 8-year-old boy with headaches and seizures. (A) Sagittal T1-W MRI shows the presence of multiple lesions in the brain. (B) The T2* sequence shows the lesions to be multiple cavernomas.

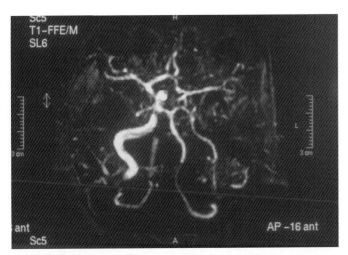

Figure 12.11.9 MRA of the circle of Willis showing a Berry aneurysm on the right. This girl had coarctation of the aorta.

occur from embolization of septic foci in children with bacterial endocarditis or from invasion of the intracranial vessels from adjacent infection of the sinuses or the ear. The underlying pathology is a focal arteritis, which causes degeneration of the arterial lamina and muscularis and thus results in fusiform dilatation. These lesions should be closely searched for in the appropriate clinical circumstances and contrast enhancement is needed with CT and may be helpful with MRI in addition to non-contrast MR angiography. Definitive diagnosis is with contrast angiography. On MRI or CT there may be associated cerebritis, abscess and oedema. Clinical presentation is with a bleed due to rupture, or symptoms associated with the infection.

Children with AIDS may also develop aneurysms and these affect the cavernous portion of the internal carotid artery (Figure 12.11.10). The role of chronic infection of the sinuses by fungus such as *Aspergillus* is suspected but unproven.

TRAUMATIC ANEURYSMS

Traumatic aneurysms may occur from direct penetrating injury, comminuted fractures, and extreme rotatory or flexion and extension movements that cause subintimal tearing of the vessels and disruption of the arterial wall apart from the outside layer or the surrounding tissues, such as may occur in high-velocity accidents, but are also recorded from blunt contusional injury. The aneurysms can be found both intracranially and extracranially. They are often referred to as pseudoaneurysms. Blood flow is preserved through the lesion but may be turbulent. They may enlarge rapidly as their containment is tenuous. Depending on their location they may be initially demonstrated by ultrasound but catheter arteriography is required for full demonstration and therapy by endovascular occlusion of the supplying vessel and the outflow. Therapy may require both an endovascular approach and surgery.

ARTERIAL DYSPLASIA

Rarely, abnormally shaped intracranial arteries are seen on MRA or angiography carried out for other reasons. Segmental dilatation

of the carotid and basilar artery probably represent segmental dysplasias (Figure 12.11.11). Persistence of primitive arteries such as the trigeminal and otic arteries, though occasionally encountered, are not within the scope of this book and are not described here. The reader is referred to specialist texts.

EXTRACEREBRAL VASCULAR MALFORMATIONS

Vascular malformations similar to those that occur elsewhere in the body may also occur in the head and neck. The classification and the approach to their imaging is described in Chapter 8.

CONGENITAL EXTRACEREBRAL ARTERIOVENOUS FISTULAS

Congenital arteriovenous fistulas can occur in the soft tissue. They are rare diseases but may occur in the head and neck region. Several arteriovenous fistulas of the vertebral artery system have been seen in Hôpital des Enfants Malades, Paris. They are discovered either by the mother who finds a palpable mass in the neck or by the paediatrician who hears a murmur while examining the heart. Colour Doppler imaging is used to make the diagnosis by showing the vascular nature of the mass. MRI and MRA easily display the anomaly and provide initial anatomical information about the vascular supply and drainage. Embolization is the treatment of choice. The fistula is catheterized and occluded with coils.

DURAL ARTERIOVENOUS FISTULAS

As elsewhere, dural arteriovenous fistulas represent a direct communication between an artery and a vein. In this situation, the connection is to one of the venous sinuses. These lesions are rare in children and are rarely diagnosed before birth. The clinical signs and symptoms vary and depend on the location of the lesion and the size of the shunt. The cause of the malformation is unknown. Clinical presentation may be with high output cardiac failure, the hearing of a bruit or the palpation of a thrill. Later presentation includes mental retardation or seizures, secondary to chronic brain ischaemia.

Imaging includes both two-dimensional ultrasound, Doppler and colour Doppler, and MRI with MRA and magnetic resonance venography (MRV). Calcification may be seen on CT in areas of chronic brain ischaemia associated with the lesions. For full delineation and for treatment, angiography is required. Multiple arteriovenous fistulas are found between the meningeal arteries and the dural sinuses (Figure 12.11.12); the sinuses are massively enlarged due to the high flow. Embolization is the treatment of choice. Prognosis is poor as these lesions have a tendency to recur. Coil occlusion of the affected sinus or surgical removal is often the only way to treat these patients.

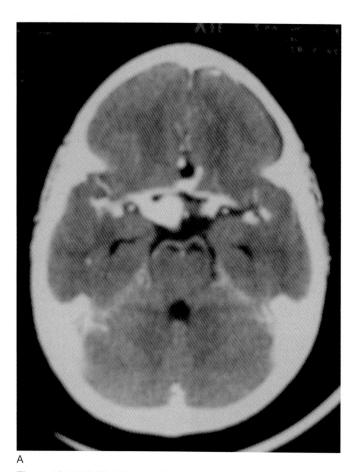

A

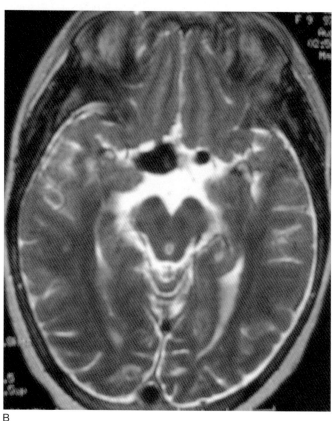

B

Figure 12.11.10 (A) A 7-year-old boy with materno-fetal AIDS who presented with progressive ophthalmoplegia. Axial CT with contrast injection shows the presence of a right sylvian artery aneurysm. (B) Same patient seen on axial T2-W MRI.

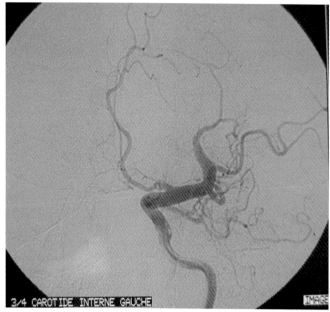

Figure 12.11.11 Incidental discovery on CT of an abnormal vessel. The angiogram shows the presence of a fusiform aneurysm of the left sylvian artery, control angiogram shows stability of the lesion over years.

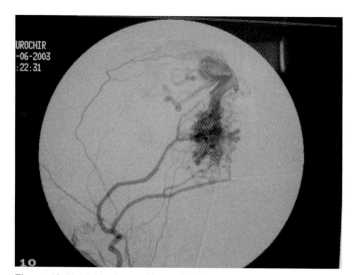

Figure 12.11.12 Newborn with cardiac failure and seizures. External carotid angiogram shows the presence of multiple shunts between the meningeal arteries and the dural sinuses.

CAROTID-CAVERNOUS FISTULA

This condition is due to trauma resulting in a tear in the wall of the carotid artery or one of its branches and a communication is created between this and the cavernous sinus. Because of the pressure differences between the systems, flow is through a fairly high-pressure shunt. Clinical presentation is with headache, proptosis, which may be pulsating, or diplopia. Other symptoms include visual impairment and symptoms of hydrocephalus.

On imaging there is dilatation of the affected cavernous sinus and its entering veins. Proptosis may be demonstrable on the same side.

VEIN OF GALEN ANEURYSM MALFORMATION

Vein of Galen aneurysmal malformations (VGMs) are rare congenital intracranial vascular malformations predominantly diagnosed at the paediatric age (1% of all intracranial and 30% of paediatric vascular malformations). Dependent on the degree of arteriovenous shunting, the condition is often associated with life-threatening congestive heart failure in the neonate. Later in childhood, hydrocephalus may develop either as a result of the direct compression on the aqueduct of Sylvius or because of venous hypertension.

The principal feeding arteries of the malformations are derivatives of those arteries nourishing the prominent choroidal plexus before mature vascularization is fully established. The arteriovenous fistulas occur in early embryogenesis between the choroidal plexus and the forerunner of the galenic vein, the median procencephalic vein, which opens directly into a falcine sinus. The connections between the afferent arteries and the venous aneurysm may consist of either direct fistulas to the venous pouch (type I), indirect arteriovenous fistulas creating an intervening tangle of vessels (nidus) between the arteries and the vein (type II) or a mixture of direct arteriovenous and arteriolovenous fistulas (type III) (Figure 12.11.13).

The neonates presenting with high-flow congestive heart failure have a very high morbidity and mortality rate. The results of neurosurgery are disappointing and the condition is called the Gordian knot of cerebrovascular surgery. Interventional endovascular staged embolization either by the transarterial, transvenous or transtorcular approach has improved the outcome and is regarded as the primary treatment by diminishing the arteriovenous shunting.

Antenatal diagnosis of VGMs is increasing, which is probably due to several factors: sonographers have greater knowledge of its pathology and improvements have been made in techniques and equipment, in particular, colour Doppler imaging. The diagnosis is easily made with colour Doppler imaging. The presence of a cystic structure in the region of the interhemispheric scissure leads automatically to further imaging with colour Doppler, which shows the vascular nature of the structure (Figure 12.11.14).

The main problem is to establish a prognosis to help the family to decide whether the pregnancy should continue or not. Several factors carry a poor prognosis including cardiac insufficiency, fetal

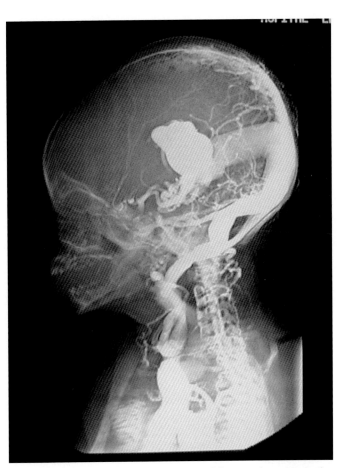

Figure 12.11.13 Postmortem opacification of the vascular network of a fetus with a vein of Galen malformation. Multiple arteries are seen entering the ascending falcine sinus.

growth retardation and brain atrophy identified by the presence of massive ventricular dilatation (Figure 12.11.15). When these signs are not present it is difficult to establish a prognosis.

It is important to differentiate true vascular malformations of the vein of Galen from parenchymal malformations that drain into the vein of Galen and carry an even poorer prognosis (Figure 12.11.16). Treatment strategies should be explained to the family. It is known that cardiac insufficiency can appear suddenly without warning at any moment of the pregnancy or after birth. Overall the prognosis is poor as of over 14 cases diagnosed *in utero* only 4 are alive today without sequelae after treatment.

After birth, the diagnosis can be made because of cardiac insufficiency or progressive hydrocephalus. Treatment is based on serial embolizations. Overall prognosis is still poor as only 30% are cured without sequelae (Figure 12.11.17).

VASCULAR ISCHAEMIA

This chapter will not deal with perinatal ischaemia and anoxia, which are described in Chapter 12.7.

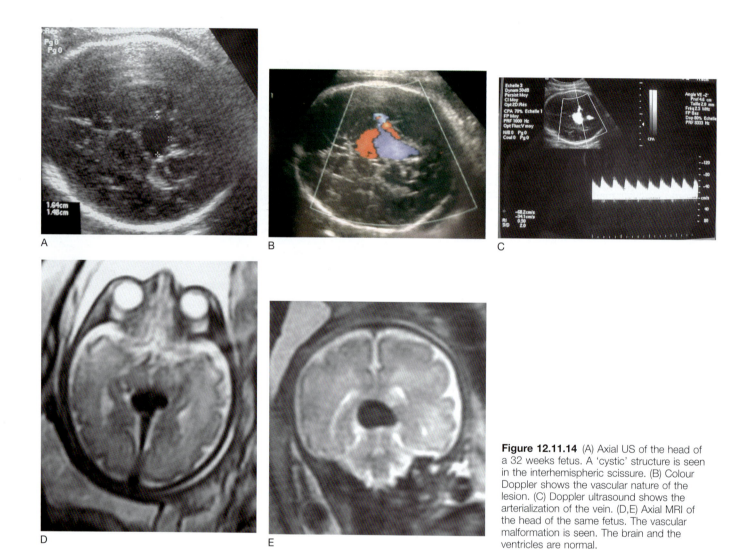

Figure 12.11.14 (A) Axial US of the head of a 32 weeks fetus. A 'cystic' structure is seen in the interhemispheric scissure. (B) Colour Doppler shows the vascular nature of the lesion. (C) Doppler ultrasound shows the arterialization of the vein. (D,E) Axial MRI of the head of the same fetus. The vascular malformation is seen. The brain and the ventricles are normal.

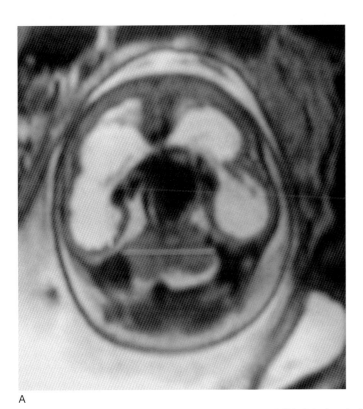

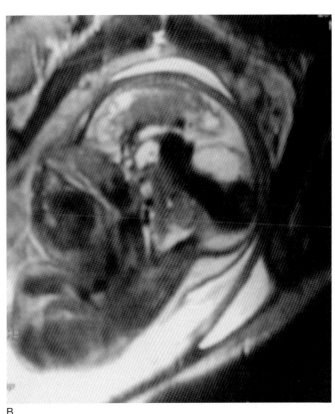

A   B

Figure 12.11.15 (A,B) Axial and sagittal T2-W antenatal MRI of the head of a 33 weeks fetus with a vein of Galen aneurysm. The malformation is well seen as is massive dilatation of the ventricles. The pregnancy was terminated because of the poor prognosis.

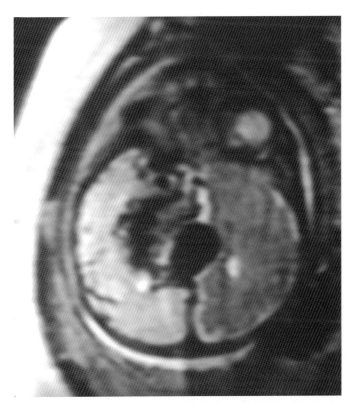

Figure 12.11.16 Axial antenatal head MRI of a 33 weeks fetus with a vascular malformation. The malformation is sited in the temporal lobe but drains into the vein of Galen mimicking a vein of Galen aneurysm.

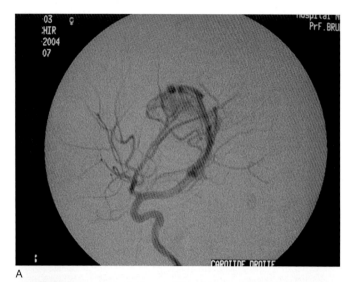

A

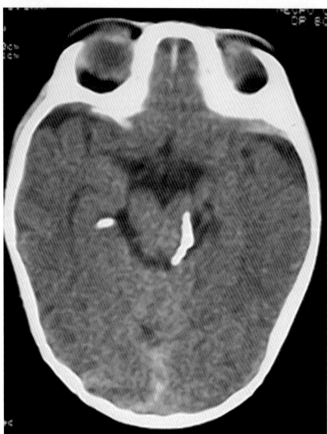

B

Figure 12.11.17 (A) Lateral carotid angiogram showing the multiple fistulas entering the vein. Several were catheterized and embolized with radiopaque glue to diminish the shunt. (B) Axial scan after embolization. The glue is seen in the wall of the dilated vein.

Clinical presentation with symptoms of acute vascular ischaemia, or stroke, though uncommon in children when compared to adults, is still a relatively frequent occurrence. The incidence will be increased in certain geographical regions or ethnic groups who have a high incidence of disease that increases the risk

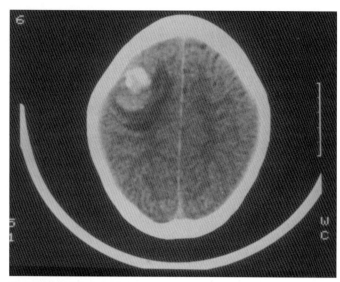

Figure 12.11.18 A 9-year-old girl who presented with an acute onset of headache and loss of power on the left. Unenhanced CT scan showing an acute intracerebral bleed with some surrounding vasogenic oedema.

of stroke, e.g. sickle cell disease. The symptoms include paresis, hemiplegia and aphasia, depending on the location of the ischaemia. The episode may be caused by a cerebrovascular bleed but a variety of other aetiologies may cause similar ischaemic symptoms.

Evaluation of children who present with childhood stroke should include testing for antiphospholipids and factor V Leiden deficiencies in addition to imaging.

IMAGING

All patients presenting with symptoms of vascular ischaemia require imaging. The aim of imaging is to identify the causative lesion, to assess the extent of the insult, and to determine therapeutic options.

Primary imaging is usually by CT to exclude acute haemorrhage as the causative lesion (Figure 12.11.18). This is usually followed by MRI, which should include diffusion weighted imaging, standard T1-weighted (T1-W) and T2-weighted (T2-W) sequences, and MRA and MRV as indicated. As with adults, imaging (apart from diffusion weighted imaging; Fig. 12.11.19) in the acute stage may be normal in the first 6 h or so. Ultrasound with transcranial Doppler is helpful in neonates.

CT APPEARANCES

The earliest change is a loss of contrast between the grey and white matter, due to cytoxic oedema. This progresses over the next hours to days to vasogenic oedema, manifest as an area of low density, which may have mass effect on surrounding structures.

Progression thereafter is resolution of the oedema and the development of an infarct seen as an area of low density (Figure

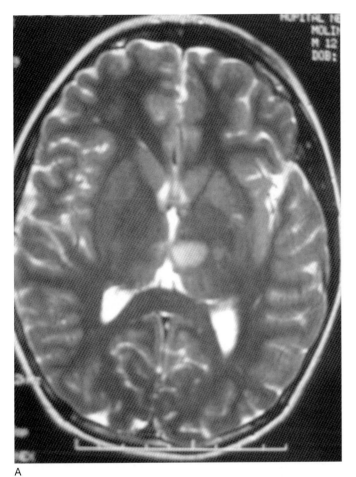
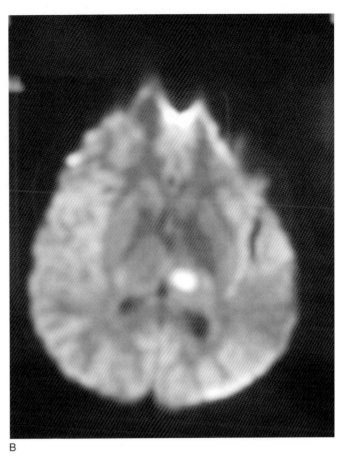

A   B

Figure 12.11.19 Axial T2-W MRI in a 3-year-old boy with sudden onset of a right hemiplegia. (A) A high intensity lesion is seen in the region of the left posterior thalamus and internal capsule. (B) Diffusion study shows a high-intensity lesion characteristic of ischaemia.

12.11.20). The lesions may be in the distribution of a major arterial supply but the lesion may also affect more peripheral end arteries. Haemorrhagic infarction is usually due to thromboembolism. On MRI, the initial changes are best seen on T2-W images as areas of high signal, reflecting the altered water content due to oedema. Subsequent evolution is as for adults, with gliotic scarring and focal atrophy.

HAEMORRHAGIC INFARCTION

This is best seen on CT. On MRI, fresh blood may not be visible on T1-W images in the first few hours. When it is visible, it appears bright on T1-W images. This high signal may persist for weeks in large haemorrhages. On T2-W images, fresh blood deoxyhaemoglobin appears dark and methaemoglobin appears bright. Persistent haemosiderin remains dark. Gliosis and scarring appear bright on T2-W images.

When occlusion takes place, the size of the infarcted area will depend on the location of the occlusion, this obviously being larger with major intracerebral vessels. Collateral flow in children is better than in adults and helps to limit the damage. Cerebral infarction due to a global insult resulting from a drop in cerebral perfu-

sion is most evident at the watershed areas between the arterial territories.

ANGIOGRAPHY

Catheter angiography, which used to be performed routinely, is now replaced by MRA and increasingly MR contrast angiography. Two main groups of patients are identified:

1. Normal MR angiography group. In this group of patients, no arterial anomalies are seen. The sylvian artery is normal. The acute episode will usually be single and regression of the symptoms will occur. The pathophysiology of this disease remains unknown.
2. Abnormal angiography. In this group of patients, stenosis of the sylvian arteries is seen. Non-opacification of the thalamic arteries is present as well. The prognosis is poor and the treatment is difficult. In some cases, this represents the beginning of moyamoya disease.

In patients with Henoch–Schonlein purpura, an unusual pattern is seen. Multiple bilateral cerebral ischaemic lesions are demon-

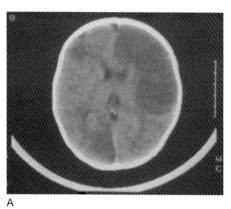 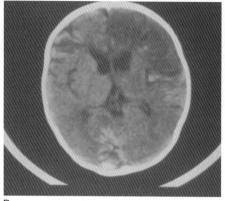 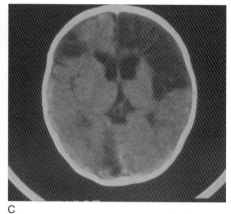

A   B   C

Figure 12.11.20 (A) A child who presented with intractable fits showing multiple areas of developing infarction. (B) Repeat CT scan (without contrast) 2 weeks later showing areas of high attenuation secondary to presumed venous thrombosis and necrosis of the infarcted areas. (C) Follow-up CT scan 6 weeks later showing resorption of most of the haemorrhage and frank residual infarcts. Compared with (A) the ventricles have enlarged indicating diminution in the cerebral oedema.

strated by MRI. These are secondary to involvement of small arterioles of the brain.

ARTERIAL OCCLUSIVE DISEASE

Many of the causes of stroke are listed in Table 12.11.3. The 'stroke' may be the first manifestation of the underlying problem, or the cause may already be obvious and the stroke the complication of the known disease. Imaging reveals the extent of the insult but may not show the causative lesion. This will require other investigations including, as mentioned above, testing for antiphospholipids and factor V Leiden deficiency. All children also require cardiac echo.

Detailed discussions of each of the lesions mentioned in Table 12.11.3 are not given here as they are dealt with elsewhere in this book, e.g. cerebral abscess. A few, however, deserve special mention.

MOYAMOYA DISEASE

Rare in Europe but often seen in Japan, moyamoya disease may be either primary or secondary. The underlying pathology is a progressive vasculopathy. Disorders associated with moyamoya are shown in Table 12.11.4. A genetic basis is also described.

Clinically, patients experience regressive hemiplegias. These are sometimes triggered by other causes of stimulation of the brain metabolism such as classroom activities or mathematics exercises! Seizures and headaches may also be the presenting features. Hemiplegia occurs because of blood diversion towards other sites of the brain. The hemiplegias regress spontaneously in the early stages of the disease but ultimately become established. Progressive stenosis of sylvian arteries leads to the development of multiple collaterals through the basal ganglia. Those collaterals on angiography look like a 'cloud of smoke' (moyamoya) (Figure 12.11.21). Other collaterals can be seen, for example, from the posterior

Table 12.11.3 Aetiology of vascular occlusion in children (modified from Table 10.6.1 1st edn)

Congenital heart disease	Emboli
	Polycythaemia, dehydration
	Congestive heart failure
	Surgery (emboli, hypertension)
Acquired heart disease	Rheumatic disease
	Endocarditis, myocarditis
	Myxoma
	Acute cardiogenic hypotension
Infections: local	Cavernous sinus thrombophlebitis
	Meningitis (purulent, tuberculous, syphilitic)
	Mucormycosis
	Malaria, paragonimiasis (Far East)
	Herpes ophthalmicus
Infections: systemic	Any severe infection that causes hypoxia
Trauma	Direct neck or intraoral trauma
	Closed head trauma
	Strenuous exercise
Arteritis	Moyamoya
	Takayashu
	Collagen diseases (SLE, PAN)
Iatrogenic	Angiography
	Radiotherapy (juxtasellar tumours)
Haematological	Sickle cell disease
	Thrombocytosis
	Polycythaemia
	Intra-ascular coagulopathy
Metabolic disease	Homocystinuria
	Diabetes
	Hyperlipidaemia
	Dehydration
	Fabry's disease
Drug abuse	Arterial spasm (LSD)
	Necrotizing angeitis (amphetamines, cannabis, contaminants)
	Septic emboli (bacterial endocarditis)
Abnormal vessels	Arterial dysplasia, neurocutaneous syndromes
	AVM (with congestive heart failure)
	Fibromuscular dysplasia?
Idiopathic	30–50% of the cases

Table 12.11.4 Disorders associated with moyamoya syndrome (reproduced with permission from Barkovich AJ (ed.). Pediatric neuroimaging, 3rd edn. Philadelphia : Lippincott Williams & Wilkins; 806)

Neurofibromatosis type 1
Down's syndrome
Sickle cell disease
Recurrent thromboembolic events
Radiation therapy
Glycogen storage disease type 1a
Hereditary spherocytosis
Tuberculous meningitis

cerebral artery circulation but this is less often involved in the disease. The hemispheres are then often reperfused through the perforating arteries and other arteries such as the ophthalmic artery in which flow is reversed, and meningeal arteries. Focal areas of frank infarction may be seen on MRI or CT.

Progressive occlusive disease is either primary (moyamoya) or secondary to irradiation of the optic tracts for chiasmatic glioma. In the latter group, irradiation seems to induce a progressive vasculopathy that mimics moyamoya.

Diffusion weighted MRI will differentiate acute infarcts in which there is reduced perfusion from chronic areas of ischaemia in which there is increased diffusion. Contrast administration may show intense enhancement of the basal ganglia.

Although the diagnosis is made by MRI and MRA, angiography (Figure 12.11.21) is usually required for full evaluation of the cerebral and scalp vasculature, to assess the feasibility of surgical anastomoses between the external and internal carotid circulation. Other vascular abnormalities can also be excluded. Following surgery, the external carotid vessels enlarge and collateral circulation develops.

SICKLE CELL DISEASE

Sickle cell disease is a disease that affects patients of African origin. Clinical experience will therefore be influenced by the ethnic mix of the population. Affected patients may be homozygous or heterozygous. The latter are usually less severely affected. The disease, which is a chronic haemolytic anaemia, is caused by a mutation in the β-chain of haemoglobin, which results in the formation of haemoglobin S. This haemoglobin is sensitive to deoxygenation. The red blood cells alter in shape, become rigid and cause thrombosis with resultant damage to the vessel walls. This can cause a sickling crisis, which presents clinically as abdominal or bone pain. Neurological manifestations include altered cognition, stroke, headache and subarachnoid haemorrhage. About 20% of strokes in patients with sickle cell disease are haemorrhagic and result from a ruptured aneurysm.

IMAGING

CT or MR imaging in an acute presentation may show haemorrhage or acute infarction. More chronic presentation may be manifest on imaging as multiple infarcts.

SYNDROMES ASSOCIATED WITH VASCULAR MALFORMATIONS

STURGE–WEBER SYNDROME

This condition, also known as encephalotrigeminal angiomatosis, has the following characteristic components. There is a port wine stain, approximating to the distribution of the trigeminal nerve. It is of variable size and may even be absent, even though the other characteristics are present. Seizures, affecting the contralateral side, occur. These are often progressive. Mental retardation is present in about half of affected individuals. Brain calcification (Figure 12.11.22), ipsilateral to the port wine stain, is present and progressive. Contralateral calcification occurs in about 20% of patients. Ipsilateral congenital glaucoma is present but visual impairment is cortical. Most cases are sporadic.

The underlying pathogenesis is not fully understood but is thought to be due to failure of the primordial vessels to produce normal arterial and venous components and results in inadequate connection between the cortical veins and dural sinuses. There is leptomeningeal telangiectasia covering the affected brain, starting usually in the occipitoparietal cortex. There is abnormal venous drainage of the affected region. Progressive gyriform calcification of the affected region occurs with progressive ischaemia. The calcification may be minimal or absent at birth.

Because of the port wine stain, the diagnosis is usually clinical but may be revealed by imaging of a child presenting with seizures. On CT, the characteristic calcification is seen. This is often initially curvilinear but it may become confluent. This is associated with ipsilateral cerebral atrophy, manifest by enlargement of the ventricle and subarachnoid spaces. The ipsilateral sinuses and choroid plexus may enlarge. Thickening of the skull vault not related to anti-epileptic therapy is frequent. The calcification may be seen on skull x-rays in older children (Figure 12.11.22). On MRI, diffuse high signal is seen on T2-W images.

MANAGEMENT

Control of seizures by anti-epileptic drugs is the first line management but in intractable cases, excision of the affected cerebral hemisphere may be performed.

OSLER–WEBER–RENDU DISEASE

This condition, also known as hereditary haemorrhagic telangiectasia, is an autosomal dominant disease that includes mucocutaneous telangiectatic lesions, which may occur anywhere in the skin or GI tract, arteriovenous shunts in the lung and liver, and vascular malformations of the brain. Primary presentation is usually in adult life but early presentation may also occur. Bleeding may occur from any lesion. A frequent presentation is epistaxis which may be life threatening and require embolization to control the

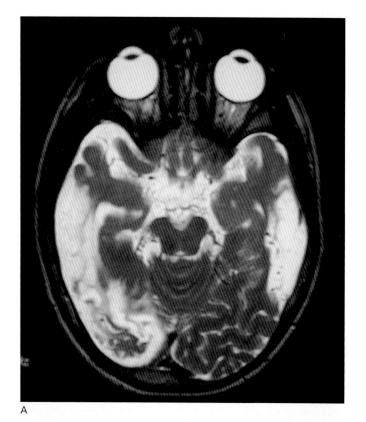

A

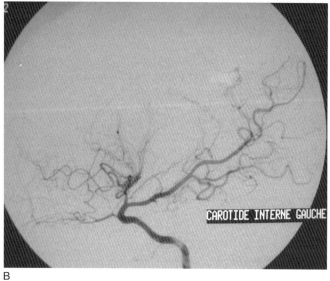

B

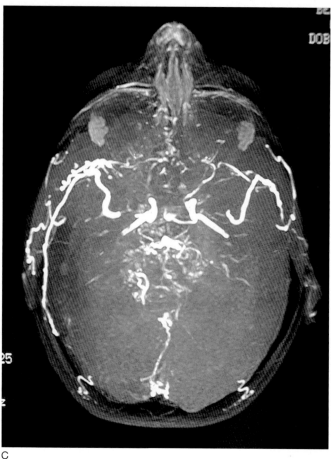

C

Figure 12.11.21 Multiple episodes of neurological deficits. (A) MRI shows multiple infarcts. (B) Carotid angiogram shows sylvian occlusion with multiple collaterals – moyamoya disease. (C) MRA, axial view shows the occlusion of the carotid arteries and the mutiple collaterals.

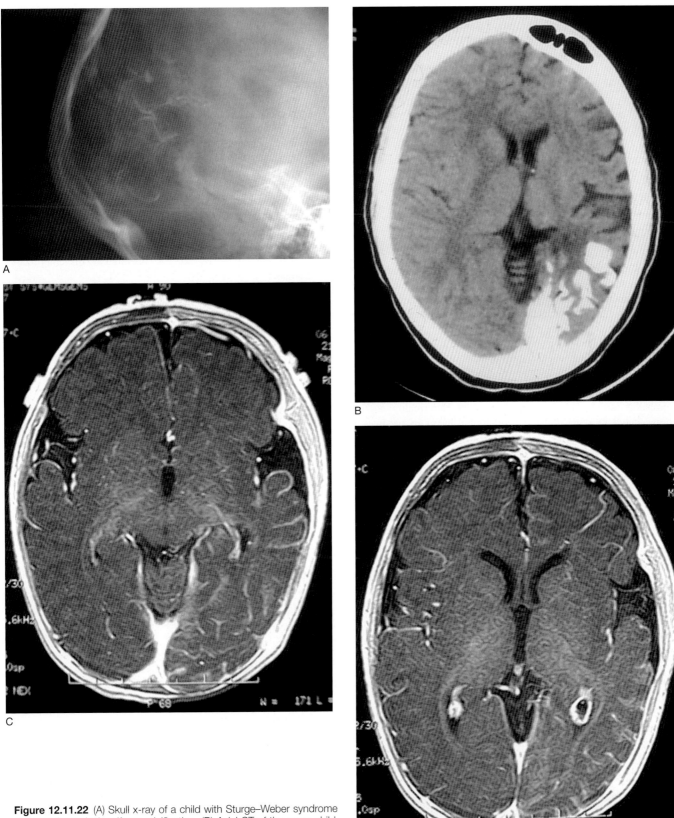

A

B

C

D

Figure 12.11.22 (A) Skull x-ray of a child with Sturge–Weber syndrome showing the typical gyriform calcification. (B) Axial CT of the same child. (C) Axial MRI shows the enhancement of the pial angioma after gadolinium injection on the left side. (D) Same child, lower scan. The hypertrophy of the left choroid plexus is seen.

haemorrhage. Shunting through pulmonary AVMs may cause a cerebral abscess. Polycythaemia may result from AVMs, which in turn cause cerebral vascular thromboses. These complications are more frequent in adults than children.

AVMs and telangiectatic lesions may also occur in the brain or spinal cord. These appear as areas of hypervascularity due to the telangiectasia (Figure 12.11.23). Abnormal vessels may be seen on MRA. Contrast enhancement is marked on both CT and MRI. There is an increased incidence of Berry aneurysm.

ATAXIA TELANGIECTASIA (LOUIS–BARR DISEASE)

CLINICAL DATA

Ataxia telangiectasia is a recessive disorder of DNA synthesis in which cutaneous and scleral telangiectasia, cerebellar ataxia and immunodeficiency occur. There is a high incidence of development of malignant tumours, mainly lymphomas. Hyperglycaemia can be associated.

IMAGING

Cerebellar atrophy is the most prominent abnormality and is shown better by MRI than CT. Intracranial haemorrhage occurs rarely.

Other vascular syndromes with cerebral or spinal cord involvement are very rare. They may be associated with perimedullary AVMs.

ENCEPHALOCRANIOCUTANEOUS LIPOMATOSIS

CLINICAL DATA

Subcutaneous lipomas and ocular choristomas are associated with cranial deformity, seizures and mental retardation.

IMAGING

Unilateral frontotemporal lipomatosis, cervical spinal cord lipoma, leptomeningeal lipogranulomatosis, porencephalic cysts and calcified cryptic cerebral angiomas may be shown using MRI.

COBB'S SYNDROME

CLINICAL DATA

In this cutaneomeningeospinal angiomatosis, a port wine naevus is present at birth and is associated with an angioma of the spinal cord and meninges in the same metameric distribution and often with a high flow AVM in the corresponding vertebrae.

Paraparesis may occur related to the intraspinal angioma. The left-to-right shunting may be sufficient to cause cardiac insufficiency, which may present at birth.

IMAGING

On plain radiography an affected vertebra may be both eroded and sclerotic rather than having the usual honeycomb appearance of a cavernous angioma. The spinal canal is usually enlarged in the region of the angioma.

The abnormality is best assessed using MRI. An enhancing mass is usual in the spinal canal and there may be flow voids outlining enlarged vessels, which may be confirmed by flow-sensitive MR sequences.

Angiography is reserved for presurgical or embolization assessment.

WYBURN–MASON SYNDROME

CLINICAL DATA

1. Facial naevus flammeus or telangectasias.
2. Racemose angioma of the retina.
3. Intracranial AVM(s), which tend to involve any part or the whole of the optic pathway, extending into the basifrontal region or sylvian fissure but may be confined to the brainstem or cerebellum. The AVMs may produce appropriate neurological deficits, seizures or mental retardation.
4. AVM(s) affecting upper or lower jaws, mouth or nasal cavity. These may bleed spontaneously or during dental extraction and are best treated by embolization.

IMAGING

The angiomas are best demonstrated by MRI. Angiography is reserved as a pretherapy measure.

GASS SYNDROME

Gass syndrome associates cavernous angioma of the retina, angiomatous hamartomas of the skin and intracranial cavernous haemangiomas, and is best shown by MRI.

ARTERIAL DISSECTION

Presentation with stroke due to arterial dissection in childhood is very rare (Figure 12.11.24). The two most frequent causes are trauma, and those with syndromes such as Ehlers–Danlos syndrome or fibromuscular hyperplasia. It is also seen with the Klippel–Feil syndrome.

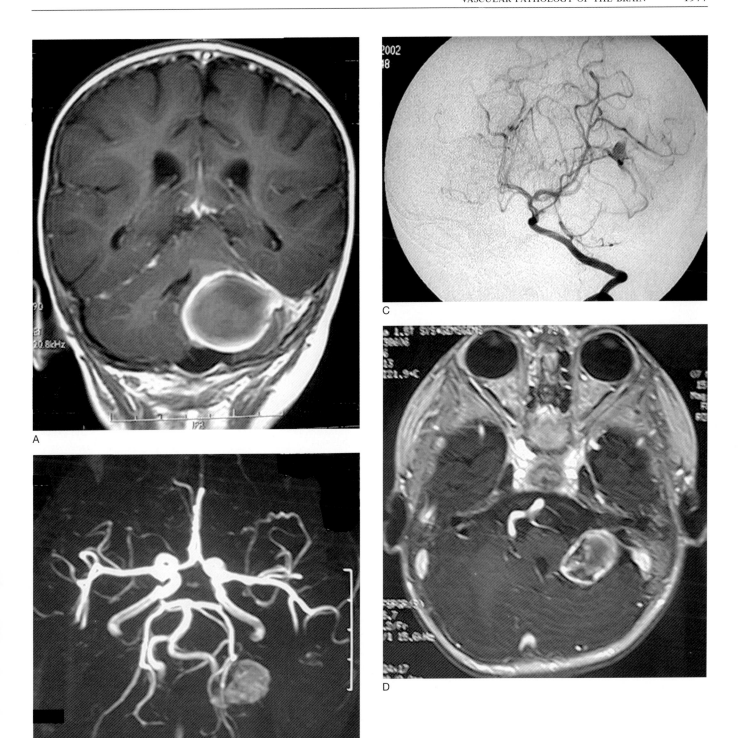

Figure 12.11.23 (A) Sudden onset of headaches, nerve palsies and vomiting. Coronal MRI shows the presence of a hyperacute clot. (B) MRA shows an abnormal vessel feeding the pseudoaneurysm. (C) Angiogram shows the aneurysm that has been embolized with glue. (D) Control MRI 8 weeks later shows the decreased size of the pseudoaneurysm. Genetic and familial study made the diagnosis of Osler–Weber–Rendu disease.

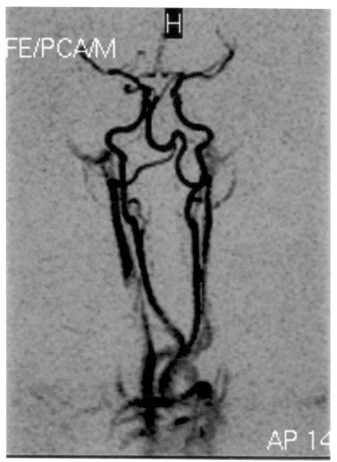

Figure 12.11.24 Angiogram showing occlusion of the right carotid artery, which is due to spontaneous dissection. This child presented with an acute onset hemiplegia following exercise.

Trauma may be obvious, e.g. a penetrating injury, but may be apparently trivial such as occurs following vigorous exercise. The vertebral arteries are most frequently affected by this mechanism. Carotid dissection occurs when a child falls with something in the mouth. The classical clinical setting is falling with a lollipop. The typical location for carotid internal artery dissection is just below the skull base. Vertebral dissections occur mainly between C2 and the occiput.

IMAGING

The initial CT may be normal, demonstrate subarachnoid haemorrhage or an ischaemic brain. There may be haemorrhage in the vessel wall, described as crescentic. This may be visible on CT or MRI. MR angiography usually demonstrates the narrowing in the carotid circulation but has only 20% sensitivity in the vertebral artery. Catheter angiography is required for definitive diagnosis. Findings will include intimal dissection, stenosis, occlusion and false aneurysms.

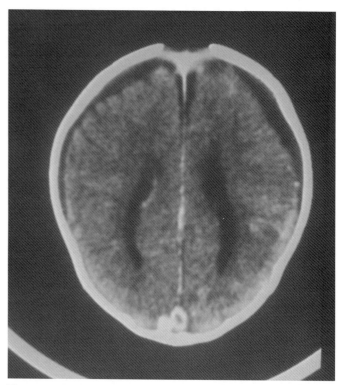

Figure 12.11.25 Contrast-enhanced CT of a boy with sagittal sinus thrombosis. Note the filling defect within the sagittal sinus – the 'empty delta' sign.

DURAL SINUS THROMBOSIS

The incidence of sinus thrombosis has significantly reduced since the advent of antibiotics, earlier recognition of sinus disease and aggressive IV treatment. However, it can still occur and is a potentially catastrophic consequence of sinus disease. Children with thrombophilic conditions may also present with sinus disease. These include nephrotic syndrome, antiphospholipid syndrome and Factor V Leiden deficiency. Symptoms include headache, fluctuating consciousness, cranial nerve paresis and collapse.

Initial imaging is usually with CT. The affected vein may appear hyperdense or the CT may be normal. With contrast enhancement an 'empty delta' sign may be seen due to the thrombus (Figure 12.11.25). On MRI, there is loss of the normal signal void due to flowing blood and collateral enlarged vessels may be seen. The diagnosis may be confirmed by MRV (Figure 12.11.26). Treatment is with anticoagulants and IV antibiotics to treat the sinus disease.

VASCULAR TUMOURS

Haemangioblastomas are rare vascular tumours in children. They occur in patients with Von Hippel–Lindau disease usually during the third decade of life. They usually occur in the cerebellum but

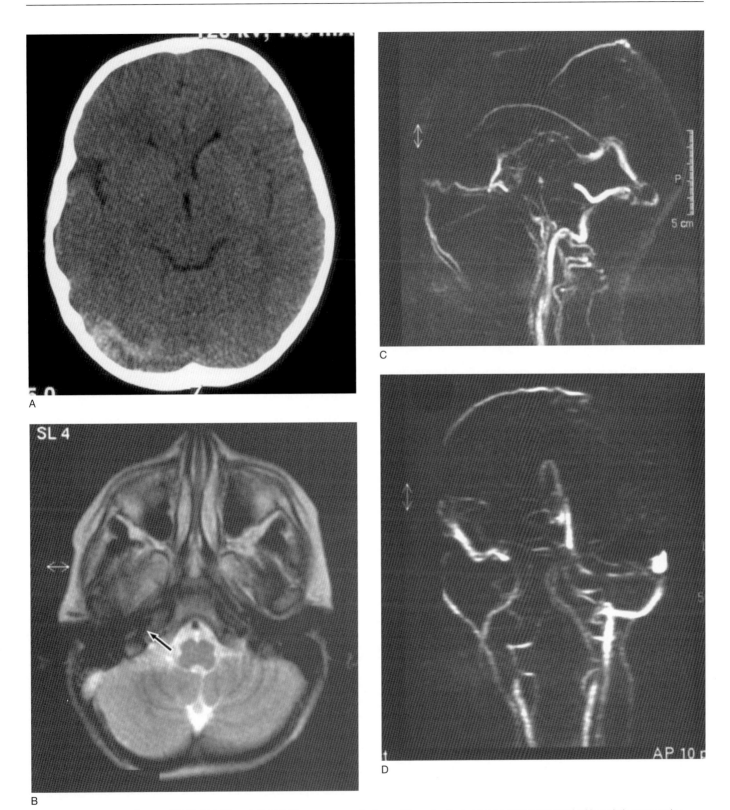

Figure 12.11.26 (A) CT scan, (B) T1-W MRI and (C,D) MR venograms of a boy with nephrotic syndrome who presented with a sixth nerve palsy. Note on the unenhanced CT scan the high attenuation within the thrombosed transverse sinus on the right. On the MRI, there is marked enlargement of the cavernous sinus (arrow). MRV shows thrombosis of both the sagittal and transverse sinus.

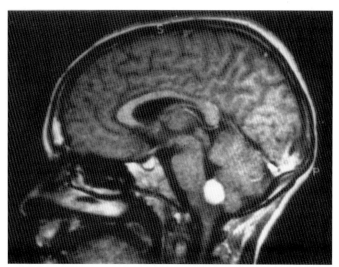

Figure 12.11.27 A 13-year-old boy with polycythaemia and Von Hippel–Lindau disease. Sagittal T1-W MRI with gadolinium injection. The haemangioblastoma is seen in the fourth ventricle.

may occur in the spinal cord. They may be cystic but normally are solid tumours that enhance after gadolinium injection. They are associated with polycythaemia (Figure 12.11.27).

FURTHER READING

Abe M, Hagihara N, Tabuchi K, Uchino A, Miyasaka Y. Histologically classified venous angiomas of the brain: a controversy. Neurol Med Chir (Tokyo) 2003; 43:1–10; discussion, 11.

Ansari I, Crichlow B, Gunton KB et al. A child with venous sinus thrombosis with initial examination findings of pseudotumor syndrome. Archives of Ophthalmology 2002; 120:867–869.

Chevret L, Durand P, Alvarez H et al. Severe cardiac failure in newborns with VGAM. Prognosis significance of hemodynamic parameters in neonates presenting with severe heart failure owing to vein of Galen arteriovenous malformation. Intensive Care Medicine 2002; 28:1126–1130.

Coghlan D, Lynch B, Allcutt D. Hereditary cerebral cavernous angiomas: presentation as idiopathic familial epilepsy. Irish Medical Journal 2002; 95:56–58.

DeVeber G. Stroke and the child's brain: an overview of epidemiology, syndromes and risk factors. Current Opinion in Neurology 2002; 15:133–138.

Fullerton HJ, Chetkovitch DM, Smith WS, Johnston SC. Deaths from stroke in US children, 1979 to 1998. Neurology 2002; 59:34–39.

Hartmann A, Pile-Spellman J, Stapf C et al. Risk of endovascular treatment of brain arteriovenous malformation. Stroke 2002; 33:1816–1820.

Hasan I, Wapnick S, Kutscher ML, Couldwell WT. Vertebral arterial dissection associated with Klippel-Feil syndrome in a child. Childs Nervous System 2002; 18:67–70.

Husson B, Rodesh G, Lasjaunias P, Tardieu M, Sebire G. Magnetic resonance angiography in childhood arterial brain infarcts: a comparative study with contrast angiography. Stroke 2002; 33:1280–1285.

Jones BV, Ball WS, Tomsick TA, Millard J, Crone KR. Vein of Galen aneurysmal malformation: diagnosis and treatment of 13 children with extended clinical follow-up. American Journal of Neuroradiology 2002; 23:1717–1724.

Kehrer-Sawatzki H, Wilda M, Braun WM, Richter HP, Hameister H. Mutation and expression analysis of the KRIT1 gene associated with cerebral cavernous malformations (CCM1). Acta Neuropathology (Berlin) 2002; 104:231–240.

Kincaid PK, Duckwiler GR, Gobin YP, Vinuela F. Dural arteriovenous fistula in children: endovascular treatment and outcomes in seven cases. American Journal of Neuroradiology 2001; 22:1217–1225.

Nagib MG, O'Fallon MT. Intramedullary cavernous angiomas of the spinal cord in the pediatric age group: a pediatric series. Pediatric Neurosurgery 2002; 36:57–63.

Nesdoridi E, Buananno FS, Jones RM et al. Arterial ischaemic stroke in childhood: the role of plasma-phase risk factors. Current Opinion in Neurology 2002; 15:139–144.

Petropoulou F, Mostrou G, Papevangelou V, Theodoridou M. Central nervous system aneurysms in childhood AIDS. AIDS 2003; 17:273–275.

Reich P, Winkler J, Straube A, Steiger HJ, Peraud A. Molecular genetic investigations in the CCM1 gene in sporadic cerebral cavernomas. Neurology 2003; 60:1135–1138.

Sahoo T, Johnson EW, Thomas JW et al. Mutations in the gene encoding KRIT1, a Krev-1/rap1a binding protein, cause malformations (CCM1). Human Molecular Genetics 1999; 8:2325–2333.

Shin DJ, Kim JH, Kang SS. Ophthalmoplegic migraine with reversible thalamic ischemia shown by brain SPECT. Headache 2002; 42:132–135.

Smith ER, Butler WE, Ogilvy CS. Surgical approaches to brain vascular malformation of the child's brain. Current Opinion in Neurology 2002; 15:165–171.

Vorstman EB, Niemann DB, Molyneux AJ, Pike MG. Benign intracranial hypertension associated with arteriovenous malformation. Developmental and Medical Child Neurology 2002; 44:133–135.

Yoon HK, Shin HJ, Chang YW. Ivy sign in childhood moyamoya disease: depiction on FLAIR and contrast-enhanced T1-weighted MR images. Radiology 2002; 223:384–389.

Cerebral and Spinal Infections

Dawn E Saunders, W K 'Kling' Chong

INTRODUCTION

Central nervous system (CNS) infections are much less common than systemic infections in children. This is largely due to the protection of the CNS by the blood–nervous tissue barrier and the contribution by an active immune mechanism. Patients with immunosuppression are particularly susceptible to CNS infections.

Organisms reach the brain via transarterial, transvenous, direct routes and retrograde axonal spread. Transarterial spread usually results from haematogenous dissemination from a distant focus; for example, septic emboli from a lung infection, subacute bacterial endocarditis (SBE) or a systemic infection, particularly in the presence of an arteriovenous shunt, which bypasses the filtering system of the lungs. Transvenous spread occurs in patients with cerebral phlebitis that complicates middle ear infections or sinusitis. Direct spread occurs with penetrating trauma including surgery, congenital cerebrospinal fluid (CSF) leaks including dermal sinuses and middle ear malformations, and epidural sepsis, which may complicate paranasal sinus, mastoid infection or osteomyelitis. Retrograde axonal spread is thought to occur in viruses such as herpes simplex virus.

The timing of the infection in relation to brain development influences the imaging appearances. Infections that occur during the first two trimesters usually result in congenital malformations, whereas those that occur during the third trimester manifest as destructive lesions. The reaction of the CNS to infection differs from that of other organs because neural tissues lack lymphatics. The inflammation often involves arteries and veins, causing stenosis or occlusion and results in vasogenic oedema or parenchymal necrosis. The imaging manifestations of CNS infections are similar in children and adults but the epidemiology and causative organisms tend to be different. These organisms are constantly changing as a result of environmental factors that favour the pathogen, immunization programmes and changes in the virulence of organisms, which results in the emergence of new infections, e.g. Creutzfeldt–Jakob disease, and the submergence of others, e.g. *Haemophilus influenza* and meningococcus C.

Magnetic resonance imaging (MRI) is more sensitive than CT in the detection of both cerebral and spinal pathology and is the imaging modality of choice in CNS infections. Computed tomography (CT) is more sensitive than MRI in the detection of calcification, which is of particular value in the imaging diagnosis of congenital infections. The diagnosis of a specific organism on the basis of imaging alone is limited, and clinical details and serological investigations are usually required. However, certain radiological appearances are characteristic of specific infections, e.g. the temporal lobe involvement of herpes simplex encephalitis and the basal meningeal infection of tuberculosis. In this chapter, the infectious processes that affect both the brain and spine are reviewed with particular emphasis on organisms that more commonly infect the CNS of children. MR spectroscopy has not been discussed as the authors believe it has limited value in the diagnosis of CNS infections. Those readers with interest in the topic should refer to the 'Further Reading' list below.

FURTHER READING

Hunter JV, Wang ZJ. MR spectroscopy in pediatric neuroradiology. Magnetic Resonance Imaging Clinics of North America 2001; 9:165–189.

Pollard AJ, Dobson SR. Emerging infectious disease in the 21st century. Current Opinion in Infectious Disease 2000; 13:265–275.

INTRACRANIAL INFECTIONS

CONGENITAL INFECTION

As mentioned in the introduction, the timing of the fetal insult is more important than the type of insult. Neurons formed at about 8 weeks gestational age migrate to the cerebral cortex by 24 weeks and undergo cortical organization at about 28 weeks' gestation. Therefore, insults in the first 8 weeks result in abnormalities of neuronal production and migration whereas injury after 24 weeks results in abnormalities of cortical organization. The immature brain is not able to mount an astroglial response so it repairs the damage, removes abnormal cells and compensates for missing tissue. The inflammatory response by the immune system, which contributes to the damage produced by infections later on in development, is absent.

The transmission of infectious agents occurs via two main pathways: bacterial infections spread from the cervix to the amniotic fluid while toxoplasmosis, syphilis and viruses spread via the transplacental route. In the developed world, children born with congenital infections have declined in numbers due to a combination of immunization programmes directed at women of child-bearing age and the antenatal diagnosis of intracerebral malformations. However, these infections, including cytomegalovirus (CMV), herpes simplex virus (HSV), toxoplasmosis, syphilis and human immunodeficiency virus (HIV), have not been eliminated. CMV is the most common cause of serious fetal and

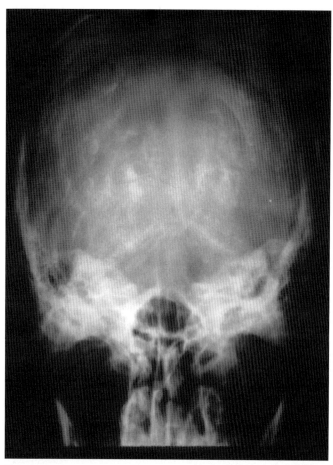

Figure 12.12.1 Skull radiograph of an adult patient with microcephaly demonstrates intracranial calcification compatible with congenital toxoplasmosis, rubella, cytomegalovirus and herpes simplex virus (TORCH) infection.

neonatal encephalitis, affecting 1 in 100 live births in the US. HIV, syphilis and toxoplasmosis are the next most common with rising incidences of syphilis and HIV. HSV and varicella zoster affect 1 in 5000 and 1 in 10 000, respectively, and the incidence of rubella has declined to 1 in a million in the US. Other congenital infections include enterovirus, parvovirus, malaria and tuberculosis. Although the insult is global, one characteristic radiological feature of congenital infection is asymmetry. Calcification is a hallmark of congenital infections and may persist or resolve during the course of the disease (Figure 12.12.1).

FURTHER READING

Ford-Jones EL. An approach to the diagnosis of congenital infections. Paediatrics and Child Health 1999; 4:109–112.

Pollard AJ, Dobson SR. Emerging infectious disease in the 21st century. Current Opinion in Infectious Diseases 2000; 13:265–275.

CONGENITAL AND NEONATAL CYTOMEGALOVIRUS (CMV)

Spread is usually transplacental as a consequence of primary maternal infection and vertical transmission rates are approximately 30–40%. Only 10% of neonates with congenital infection are symptomatic at birth with hepatosplenomegaly, petechiae and thrombocytopenia. Asymptomatic neonates are still at risk of development of sensorineural hearing loss and other neurological deficits in the first 2 years of life. Microcephaly is seen in over half of infected neonates. Mental retardation, deafness, seizures and intracranial calcification are markers of extensive brain damage and are poor prognostic signs.

The mechanism of injury in congenital CMV is thought to be either due to an affinity of the virus to the germinal matrix, resulting in developmental abnormalities, or a primary vascular target leading to ischaemia. An unusual case report of a neonate with CMV from our institution supports the infectious vasculitis theory; both caudate and subarachnoid haemorrhage was thought to result from a small venous haemorrhage. Patients infected with CMV are typically microcephalic with polymicrogyria, reduced white matter bulk, delayed myelination and cerebellar hypoplasia. Isolation of CMV from urine and throat swabs and positive serum CMV-IgM are diagnostic.

Transcranial ultrasound demonstrates branching curvilinear hyperechogenicity in the basal ganglia described as a 'lenticulostriate vasculopathy' (Figure 12.12.2). The appearances are non-specific and similar appearances are seen in anoxic and toxic injury and trisomy 13 and 21. Postmortem studies have shown a mineralizing vasculopathy as the cause. Lissencephaly, hypoplastic cerebellum, delayed myelination, ventriculomegaly and periventricular calcification (Figure 12.12.3) are presumed to result from early second trimester infection whereas later second trimester infection is thought to result in polymicrogyria, less ventricular dilatation and less cerebellar hypoplasia (Figure 12.12.4). Schizencephaly is rarely seen and is also thought to be associated with a second trimester infection prior to the development of cortical gyri, i.e. before 24 weeks (Figure 12.12.5). Infections near the end of gestation or in the early neonatal period have normal gyral patterns, mild ventricular and sulcal prominence, damaged periventricular white matter and scattered periventricular calcification or haemorrhage. Cysts of the temporal pole have been shown to be a feature of CMV.

FURTHER READING

Barkovitch AJ. Infections of the nervous system. In: Barkovitch AJ, ed. Paediatric Neuroimaging. New York: Raven Press; 1995:569–617.

Barkovitch AJ, Linden CL. Congenital cytomegalovirus infection of the brain: imaging analysis and embryologic considerations. American Journal of Neuroradiology 1994; 15:703–715.

Hayward JC, Titelbaum DS, Clancy RR, Zimmerman RA. Lissencephaly-pachygyria associated with congenital cytomegalovirus infection. Journal of Child Neurology 1991; 6:109–114.

Hughes P, Weinberger E, Shaw DW. Linear areas of echogenicity in the thalami and basal ganglia of neonates: an expanded association. Radiology 1991; 179:103–105.

Iannetti P, Nigro G, Spalice A, Faill A, Boncinelli E. Cytomegalovirus infection and schizencephaly: case reports. Annals of Neurology 1998; 43:123–127.

McCraken GH Jr, Shinefield HR, Cobb K et al. Congenital cytomegalic inclusion disease: a longitudinal study of 20 patients. American Journal of Disease in Childhood 1969; 11:522–539.

Melish ME, Hanshaw JB. Congenital cytomegalovirus infection: developmental progress of infants detected by routine screening. American Journal of Disease in Childhood 1973; 126:190–194.

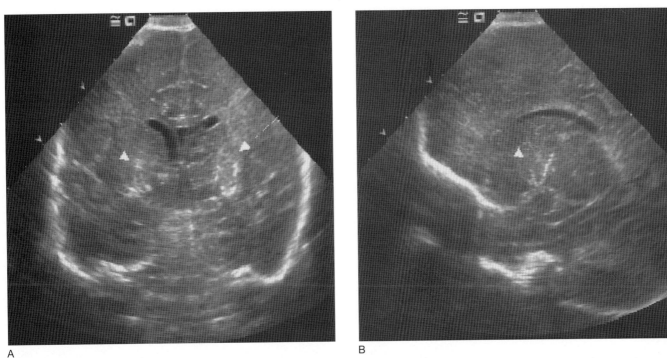

Figure 12.12.2 (A) Coronal and (B) sagittal transcranial ultrasound of a 4-month-old child with a history of a congenital infection demonstrates bilateral branching curvilinear hyperechogenicity in the basal ganglia known as 'lenticulostriate vasculopathy' (arrowheads).

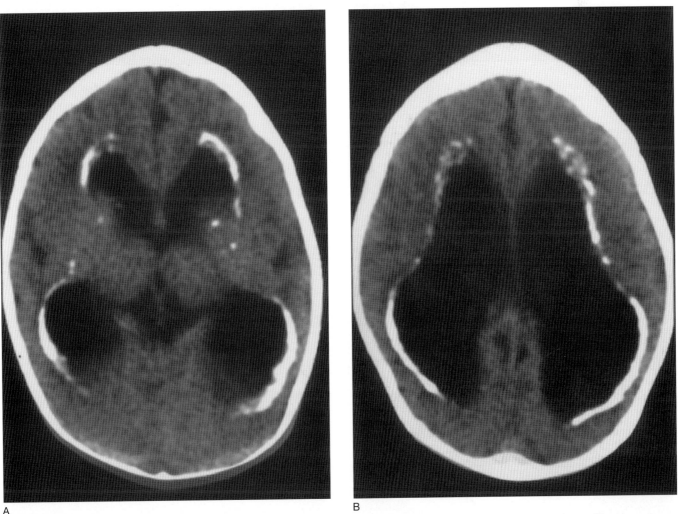

Figure 12.12.3 Congenital CMV. Axial CT scan of a 3-month-old girl demonstrates ventriculomegaly, periventricular calcification and basal ganglia calcification and loss of white matter.

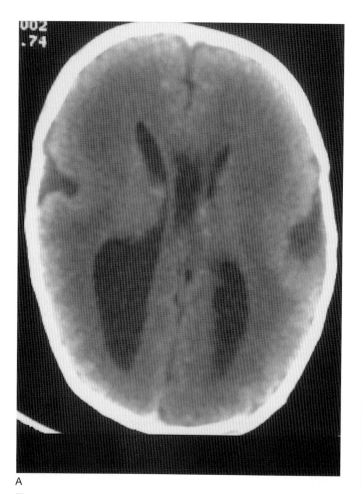

A

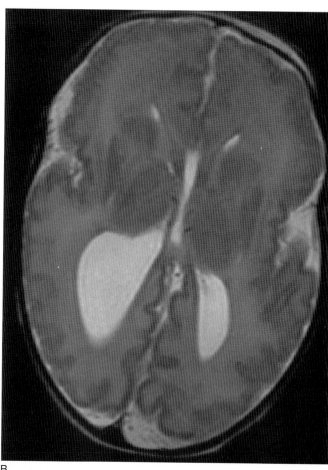

B

Figure 12.12.4 (A) Axial CT and (B) concurrent MRI of a neonate with congenital CMV infection. The thickened cortex seen on the CT scan is shown to be due to polymicrogyria on the MRI scan. These are features of an early infection.

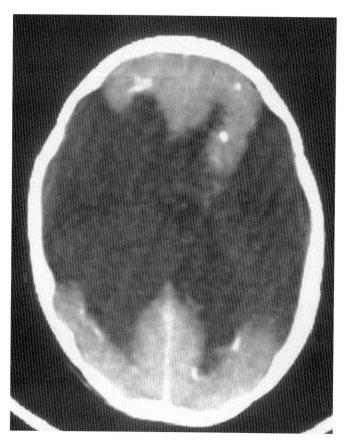

Figure 12.12.5 Axial CT scan of a 3-month-old child requiring intensive therapy support for status epilepticus. There is bilateral symmetrical open lip schizencephaly and subependymal calcification. An organism was not isolated but cytomegalovirus infection is the most likely candidate.

Pass RF, Stagno S, Myers GJ, Alford CA. Outcome of symptomatic congenital cytomegalovirus infection: results of long term follow up. Paediatrics 1980; 66:758–762.

Whitley RJ, Stagno S. Perinatal viral infections. In: Scheld WM, Whitley RJ, Durak DT, eds. Infections of the central nervous system. New York: Raven; 1991:167–200.

CONGENITAL AND NEONATAL HERPES VIRUS

Congenital herpes simplex virus is usually caused by the type II virus (HSV-2) and is most commonly acquired from virus shed in the maternal genital tract at the time of delivery. Less frequently, the virus is acquired through haematogenous spread whilst *in utero*. Neonatal infections caused by HSV type I (HSV-1) are usually acquired postnatally. Congenital infections may lead to death or severe neurological sequelae such as seizures, microcephaly, micropthalmia, ventriculomegaly and multicystic encephalomalacia depending on the timing of the infection. Microcephaly may be seen in association with lissencephaly or polymicrogyria.

Neonatal infection by HSV-2 resulting in multiorgan disseminated infection is likely to be blood-borne and associated with a diffuse encephalitis, resulting in generalized encephalomalacia. Much less frequently in neonates, the disease only affects the CNS and therefore is likely to have been neuronally transmitted to the brain; the appearances are those of herpes encephalitis as seen in older children (see 'Herpes simplex encephalitis'). Babies with HSV-1 infection have a better neurological outcome than HSV-2 and the recent use of high-dose acyclovir in neonatal encephalitis has reduced the mortality to 5% with 40% of children developing normally.

CT and MRI of neonates with herpes encephalitis show patchy, widespread areas of abnormal signal (low attenuation on CT, high signal on T2-weighted images), primarily in white matter. After the first 2 days, there is cortical involvement, which is seen as high attenuation on CT and high signal on T2-weighted images. Enhancement of the meninges may be seen. The cerebellum is involved in about half the patients. Loss of brain substance occurs rapidly, sometimes as early as the second week, which goes on to have the appearance of cystic encephalomalacia. Punctate or gyriform calcification may be seen.

FURTHER READING

Tien RD, Felsberg GJ, Osumi AK. Herpes infection of the CNS: MR findings. American Journal of Roentgenology 1993; 161:167–179.

Whitley RJ. Herpes simplex virus. In: Scheld WM, Whitley RJ, Durack DT, eds. Infections of the central nervous system. Philadelphia: Lippincott-Raven; 1996:73–89.

Whitley RJ, Gnann JW. Viral encephalitis: familiar infections and emerging pathogens. Lancet 2002; 359:507–514.

TOXOPLASMOSIS

Toxoplasmosis is caused by the protozoan *Toxoplasma gondii*, which affects a wide range of birds and mammals. Pregnant women ingest the oocytes in raw or uncooked meat or on vegetables contaminated by cat faeces. The transmission rate during the third trimester of pregnancy increases from 30% at 6 months to nearly 100% during the last weeks of gestation. The incidence of congenital toxoplasmosis is estimated at about 1 in 1000 to 1 in 3400 but may be as high as 1 in 100 when stillbirths are included.

At birth, 80–90% of infants with congenital toxoplasmosis are asymptomatic. Prognosis is poor for both generalized and CNS infection and survivors tend to be educationally subnormal with seizures and spasticity. Amniocentesis or cordocentesis provides the most accurate diagnosis.

Chorioretinitis, hydrocephalus, intracranial calcifications and convulsions are the typical presentation of classic congenital toxoplasmosis. Infection results in an inflammatory infiltration of the meninges with granulomatous lesions or a diffuse infiltration of the brain. The resultant imaging findings are similar to those of congenital CMV infection. Calcifications are common and usually involve the basal ganglia, periventricular region and cerebral cortex and may resolve after antibiotic therapy. Microcephaly, large ventricles and hydrocephalus resulting from ependymitis occluding the aqueduct are commonly seen (Figure 12.12.6).

A spectrum of disease is seen from mild periventricular calcification and mild atrophy to severe disease with total destruction of the cerebral cortex. The severity of brain involvement has been shown to be directly related to the timing of the infection; infection before 20 weeks resulting in more severe brain damage and calcification than after 20 weeks. The radiological appearances are similar to those seen with CMV but the typical brain malformations seen in early CMV infection have not been reported.

FURTHER READING

Bale JF Jr. Viral infections. In: Berg BO, ed. Neurological aspects of pediatrics. Boston: Butterworth-Heinemann; 1992:227–256.

Costa JM, Ernault P, Gautier E, Bretagne S. Prenatal diagnosis of congenital toxoplasmosis by duplex real-time PCR using fluorescence resonance energy transfer by hybridisation probes. Prenatal Diagnosis 2001; 21:85–88.

Diebler C, Dusser A, Dulac O. Congenital toxoplasmosis: clinical and neuro-radiological evaluation of brain lesions. Neuroradiology 1985; 27:125–130.

Dunn D, Wallon W, Peyron F et al. Mother-to-child transmission of toxoplasmosis: risk estimates for clinical counselling. Lancet 1999; 353:1829–1833.

Martin S. Congenital toxoplasmosis. Neonatal Network 2001; 20:23–30.

Patel DV, Holfels EM, Vogel NP et al. Resolution of intracranial calcification in infants with treated congenital toxoplasmosis. Radiology 1996; 199:433–440.

RUBELLA

Since 1988, universal immunization of children in the UK has resulted in a drop in the number of cases of congenital rubella in the UK, from 70 per year to one in 1995. Immigrant populations are still at risk of congenital rubella. Cataracts, glaucoma and cardiac malformations (most commonly persistent ductus and peripheral pulmonary stenosis) occur when the infection occurs in the first 8 weeks of gestation and is almost asymptomatic when infection occurs in the third trimester. Hearing loss and delayed motor development may result from infection in the first trimester. Infants present at birth with seizures, lethargy, hypotonia and a large bulging fontanel but by 4 months of age, affected infants are microcephalic and irritable with vasomotor instability and photophobia.

Infants with congenital rubella are microcephalic with ventriculomegaly secondary to loss of brain tissue. Microphthalmia, cataracts, glaucoma and chorioretinitis are common. A vasculopa-

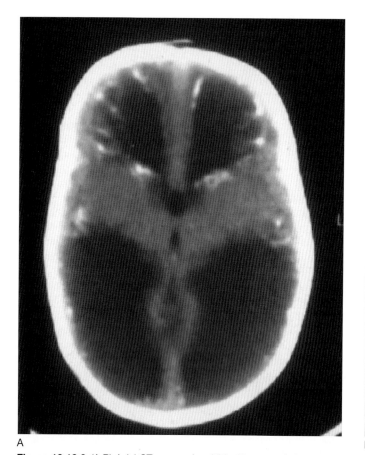
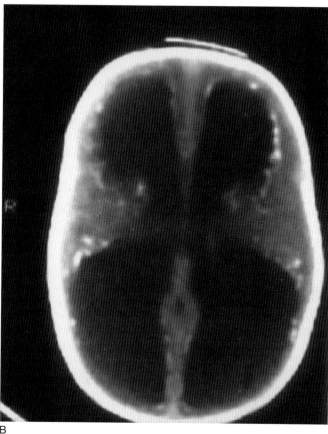

A
B

Figure 12.12.6 (A,B) Axial CT scans of a child with congenital toxoplasmosis with periventricular and cortical calcification. The ventricles are large secondary to extensive parenchymal damage and hydrocephalus at the time of the infection.

thy results in necrosis and gliosis with periventricular white matter, basal ganglia and brainstem calcification. Early infection will result in congenital anomalies, whereas late infections will result in non-specific oedema or loss of brain tissue.

Ultrasound shows a lenticulostriate vasculopathy identical to that in congenital CMV. CT typically shows regions of cerebral white matter hypodensity in association with periventricular calcification and cysts. Less commonly, calcification of the basal ganglia and cortex are seen. In severe cases, brain destruction and microcephaly are present. MR imaging shows delay in the maturation of myelin, in addition to corresponding areas of high signal abnormality on T2-weighted imaging. High-resolution CT of the temporal bone may show malformations of the inner ear structures.

FURTHER READING

Barkovitch AJ. Infections of the nervous system. In: Barkovitch AJ, ed. Paediatric Neuroimaging. New York: Raven Press; 1995:569–617.

Cooper LZ, Ziring PR, Ockerse AB et al. Rubella: clinical manifestation and management. American Journal of Diseases of Childhood 1969; 118:18–23.

Ishikawa A, Murayama T, Sakuma N. Computerised cranial tomography in congenital rubella syndrome. Archives of Neurology 1982; 39:420–422.

Lane B, Sullivan EV, Lim KO et al. White matter hyperintensities in adult patients with congenital rubella. American Journal of Neuroradiology 1996; 17:99–103.

Miller E, Craddock-Watson JE, Pollock TM. Consequences of confirmed maternal rubella at successive stages of pregnancy. Lancet 1982; 2:781–782.

Sheridan E, Aitken C, Jefferies D, Hird M, Thayalasekaran P. Congenital rubella syndrome: a risk in immigrant populations. Lancet 2002; 359:674–675.

Yashimita Y, Matsuishi T, Murakami Y et al. Neuroimaging findings (ultrasonography, CT, MRI) in 3 infants with congenital rubella syndrome. Pediatric Radiology 1991; 21:547–549.

SYPHILIS

In affluent countries, congenital syphilis is very rare but in many poor countries, including the newly independent countries of eastern Europe and the former Soviet Union, the numbers are high and increasing. In much of sub-Saharan Africa, around 10% of pregnant women are affected by syphilis. Congenital infection with *Treponema pallidum* occurs via transplacental spread usually in the second and third trimester. Treatment during pregnancy is effective in preventing transplacental infection in 98% of cases. Most infected neonates are asymptomatic at birth and after the first week of life develop characteristic rashes and mucocutaneous lesions. Metaphyseal abnormalities of the long bones are seen in 20% of clinically asymptomatic newborns.

Neurosyphilis develops in about 60% of infants with congenital syphilis. Neurological signs develop in the first 2 years of life and consist of seizures, cranial nerve palsies and raised intracranial pressure (ICP). Later clinical manifestations include Hutchinson's teeth, optic atrophy, sensorineural hearing loss and spinal cord disease (tabes dorsalis).

The major pathological findings are inflammatory infiltrates of the leptomeninges with mononuclear cells, particularly in the basal meninges surrounding the blood vessels and cranial nerve sheaths. CT and MRI demonstrate leptomeningeal enhancement, which may extend into the cerebral parenchyma through the Virchow-Robin spaces and appear as an enhancing mass. Infarction results from obstruction of the basal meninges by the infected leptomeninges.

FURTHER READING

Alexander JM, Sheffield JS, Sanchez PJ, Mayfield J, Wendel GD Jr. Efficacy of treatment for syphilis in pregnancy. Obstetrics and Gynecology 1999; 93:5–8.

Michelow IC, Wendel GD, Norgard MV et al. Central nervous system infection in congenital syphilis. New England Journal of Medicine 2002; 346:1792–1798.

Walker DG, Walker GJ. Forgotten but not gone: the continuing scourge of congenital syphilis. Lancet Infectious Diseases 2002; 2:432–436.

HUMAN IMMUNODEFICIENCY VIRUS

It has been estimated that more than 60 million people are infected with the human immunodeficiency virus (HIV) and more than a third of these have died. It has been estimated that over the next 20 years 68 million people will die prematurely of AIDS, the largest number being in sub-Saharan Africa. Almost 50% of people infected by HIV are women and this has huge implications in terms of infant health as vertical transmission of HIV accounts for 90% of newly diagnosed cases.

Invasion of the CNS by the virus leads to a subacute encephalitis with an inflammatory reaction and the neuropathological hallmark of HIV encephalitis of multinucleate glial cells and microglial nodules. HIV particles are found in microglial cells and macrophages and both atrophy and impaired brain growth occur as a result. Calcification is seen on pathological specimens in the brain parenchyma and in small and medium-sized blood vessels.

Patients with congenitally acquired AIDS rarely present in the neonatal period. Symptom onset occurs between 2 months and 8 years. Most patients present with non-specific signs such as failure to thrive and hepatosplenomegaly. The major neurological symptoms of HIV in infancy are a progressive and static encephalopathy. In the progressive form, children become demented and spastic, with an increasing head size; the static form consists of a delay in cognitive and motor development.

The commonest imaging abnormalities are global atrophy and bilateral basal ganglia calcification (Figure 12.12.7). Diffuse symmetrical white matter abnormalities with involvement of the periventricular white matter and centrum semiovale are seen in almost half of children with an encephalopathy and are usually associated with mild atrophy. Myelopathy from corticospinal tract degeneration is also seen in children with AIDS encephalitis and therefore imaging of the spine is not usually required.

Opportunistic infection and reactivation of latent infection of the CNS are not often seen in young children, probably because of short exposure times. As a result intracranial neoplasms and infection are rare in children with AIDS. The most commonly reported neoplasm, lymphoma, is seen in only 5% of children. The commonest CNS infection is thought to be progressive multifocal leucoencephalopathy (PML) (Figure 12.12.8);

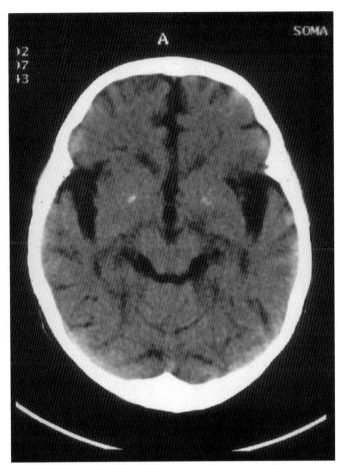

Figure 12.12.7 Axial CT scan of a 5-year-old child with human immunodeficiency virus (HIV) encephalopathy. Basal ganglia calcification and cerebral atrophy are typical features of congenitally acquired HIV.

however, toxoplasmosis, the commonest CNS infection in adulthood, is rarely seen in children. CNS manifestations of HIV infection in children are summarized in Table 12.12.1. In older children, the radiological appearances of AIDS are not very different from adults and are related to a reduction in CD4 levels. Readers are recommended to refer to the adult literature for further information.

Cerebrovascular disease has been documented at autopsy in 24% of children with HIV but stroke occurs in only 1–2%, more commonly in the older child than the infant. The commonest cause of infarction is large vessel vasculopathy and the arteriopathy can be caused by HIV infection itself or superadded infection by viruses such as varicella and CMV. Aneurysmal dilatation of the circle of Willis and moyamoya syndrome have also been described in a child with AIDS.

FURTHER READING

Centres for Disease Control and Prevention: HIV/AIDS surveillance report. 2004 http://www.cdc.gov/hiv/dhap.htm

Fact sheet UNAIDS. The impact of HIV/AIDS; 2002. http://www.unaids.org/barcelona/presskit/factsheet.html

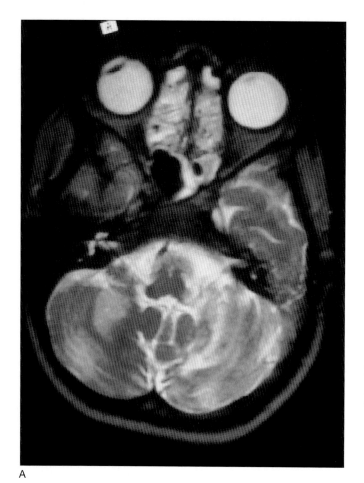

A

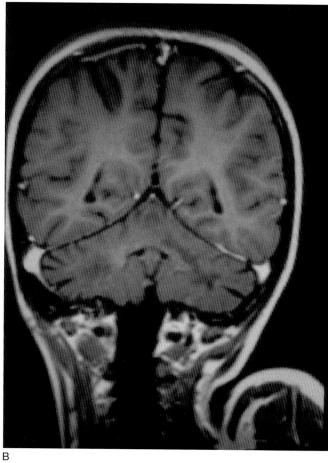

B

Figure 12.12.8 Progressive multifocal leucoencephalopathy. (A) Axial T2-weighted spin echo and (B) postcontrast coronal T1-weighted MR images of a 12-year-old girl with human immunodeficiency virus. The lesions of high signal on T2-weighted and low on T1-weighted images involve the cerebellar white matter bilaterally and there is no mass effect or enhancement.

Table 12.12.1 CNS manifestations of HIV infection in children (modified from States et al. Neuroimaging Clinics of North America 1997; 7:321–339)

Common
HIV encephalitis
Uncommon
Lymphoma
Ischaemic infarction
Haemorrhage
Rare
Toxoplasmosis gondii
Progressive multifocal leucoencephalopathy
Cytomegalovirus
Meningoencephalitis secondary to
    Cryptococcus
    Candidiasis
    Mycobacterium tuberculosis
    Varicella–zoster virus
    Nocardia
    Syphilis
    Staphylococcus aureus, Streptococcus pneumoniae, Haemophilus
      influenzae
Myeloradiculitis
Aneurysmal vasculopathy

Ging-Yuek RH, de Menezes MS. Moyamoya syndrome in a patient with congenital human immunodeficiency virus infection. Journal of Child Neurology 1999; 14:268–270.

Gray F, Scaravilli F, Everall I et al. Neuropathology of early HIV-infection. Brain Pathology 1996; 6:1–15.

Hogg R, Cahn P, Katabira ET et al. Time to act: global apathy towards HIV/AIDS is a crime against humanity. Lancet 2002; 360:1710–1711.

Kieburtz KD, Eskin TA. Opportunistic cerebral vasculopathy in stroke in patients with the acquired immunodeficiency syndrome. Archives of Neurology 1993; 50:430–432.

Morris MC, Ritstein RM, Rudy B, Desrochers C, Hunter JV, Zimmerman RA. Progressive multifocal leukoencephalopathy in an HIV-infected child. Neuroradiology 1997; 39:142–144.

Patsalides AD, Wood LV, Gokce AK et al. Cerebrovascular disease in HIV-infected pediatric patients: neuroimaging findings. American Journal of Roentgenology 2002; 179:999–1003.

Shah S, Zimmerman RA, Rorke LB, Vezina LG. Cerebrovascular complications of HIV in children. American Journal of Neuroradiology 1996; 17:1913–1917.

States LJ, Zimmerman RA, Rustein RM. Imaging of pediatric central nervous system HIV infection. Neuroimaging Clinics of North America 1997; 7:321–339.

Stevens JM, Hall-Craggs M, Chong WK, Murray AD, Lane B. Cranial and intracranial pathology (2): Infections; AIDS; inflammatory; demyelinating and metabolic disease. In: Grainger RG, Allison DJ, Adam A, Dixon AK, eds. Diagnostic radiology. London: Churchill-Livingstone; 2002:2377–2391.

MENINGITIS AND ITS COMPLICATIONS

Meningitis is the most common infection in childhood. Imaging in uncomplicated meningitis is usually normal or may show meningeal enhancement but is not indicated for diagnostic purposes. The diagnosis of meningitis relies on clinical symptoms and signs and lumbar puncture results. Imaging should be reserved for (1) when there is diagnostic uncertainty, (2) the presence of symptoms and signs of raised ICP or focal neurological deficits or (3) when recovery is slow.

PATHOPHYSIOLOGY

Meningitis is relatively uncommon because the subarachnoid space tends to resist infection in normal children but once established causes neurological sequelae by spreading along the adventitia of penetrating cortical vessels in the periventricular spaces. The resultant inflammatory response causes necrosis in the arterial wall and eventually arterial thrombosis. In addition, vessels that traverse the basal exudates result in a vasculitis with inflammation and thrombosis. A similar process in the veins results in venous thrombosis, particularly common when associated with subdural empyemas. Cerebral infarction (venous and arterial) is seen in 30% of neonates with bacterial meningitis and extension of the infection through obstructed vessels into brain parenchyma can result in cerebritis and abscess formation.

Fibropurulent exudates in the basal cisterns, ventricular foramen or over the brain convexity result in hydrocephalus by either obstructing CSF flow or resorption. Ventricular enlargement may persist due to damage to the adjacent periventricular white matter. Ventriculitis occurs in about 30% of children with meningitis and is particularly common in neonates. Ependymal changes are uncommon early on but are seen in severe or prolonged meningitis.

FURTHER READING

Dunn DW, Daum RS, Weisberg L, Vargas R. Ischaemic cerebrovascular complications of haemophilus influenza meningitis. *Archives of Neurology* 1982; 39:650–652.

Friede RL. Cerebral infarcts complicating neonatal leptomeningitis. Acta Neuropathologica 1973; 23:245–251.

Yumashima T, Kashihara K, Ikeda K, Kubota T, Yamamoto S. Three phases of cerebral arteriopathy in meningitis: vasospasm and vasodilation followed by organic stenosis. Neurosurgery 1985; 16:546–553.

EPIDEMIOLOGY

NEONATAL MENINGITIS

The epidemiology of meningitis in the neonatal period is similar to that of neonatal sepsis. Two distinct patterns of disease are identified. Fulminant systemic disease presenting during the first few days of life and associated with complications of labour and late-onset disease, which presents after the first week of life with mild sepsis and usually meningitis. The incidence in the neonatal period is 0.26–1.62 per 1000 live births and mortality is high (between 5% and 75%). Prematurity, maternal colonization by group B streptococcus (GBS), prolonged and premature rupture of membranes, maternal chorioamnionitis, low socioeconomic class, low birth weight and invasive monitoring predispose to meningitis.

The most common organism causing neonatal meningitis is GBS (Figure 12.12.9). Colonization of the neonate occurs during labour or from acquired nosocomial sources. Gram-negative enteric bacteria account for 30–40% of cases of neonatal meningitis. *Escherichia coli* is the most common Gram-negative organism and *Klebsiella* sp. are the second most common while *Enterobacter*, *Citrobacter* and *Serratia* are less commonly isolated. *Listeria monocytogenes* is not often implicated and accounts for between 5% and 20% of cases in some series.

Early diagnosis depends on lumbar puncture being performed on neonates with clinical features of unlocalized sepsis, particularly if seizures occur. Signs of meningeal irritation and raised intracranial pressure appear late in neonatal infection.

The radiological appearances of neonatal meningitis reflect the destructive inflammatory process that occurs throughout the brain. Vasculitis with haemorrhagic necrosis is common (Figure 12.12.10) and complicated by abscess formation. The ventricles tend to become separate from the general CSF circulation by adhesions and aqueduct obstruction. Complications of purulent meningitis in newborns are shown in Table 12.12.2 and discussed further in 'Imaging manifestations' below.

FURTHER READING

Bale JF, Murph JR. Infections of the central nervous system in the newborn. Clinical Perinatology 1997; 4:787–806.

Dawson KG, Emerson JC, Burns JL. Fifteen years of experience with bacterial meningitis. Pediatric Infectious Disease Journal 1999; 18:816–822.

Klein JO. Bacterial sepsis and meningitis. In: Remington JS, Klein JO, eds. Infectious Diseases of the Fetus and Newborn Infant. Philadelphia: W.B. Saunders; 2000:943–998.

Polin RA, Harris MC. Neonatal bacterial meningitis. Seminars in Neonatology 2001; 6:157–172.

Pong A, Bradley JS. Bacterial meningitis and the newborn infant. Infectious Disease Clinics of North America 1999; 13:711–733.

INFANT AND CHILDHOOD MENINGITIS

Acute bacterial meningitis causes a great many deaths and long-term morbidity throughout the world. Mortality is 5% in developed countries and rises to between 12 and 50% in developing

Table 12.12.2 Early and late complications of purulent meningitis in newborns

Early complications
Hydrocephalus
Localized/multifocal abscesses
Empyemas
Ventriculitis
Venous sinus thrombosis resulting in infarction, usually haemorrhagic

Late complications
Subependymal cysts
Multicystic encephalomalacia
Delayed myelination

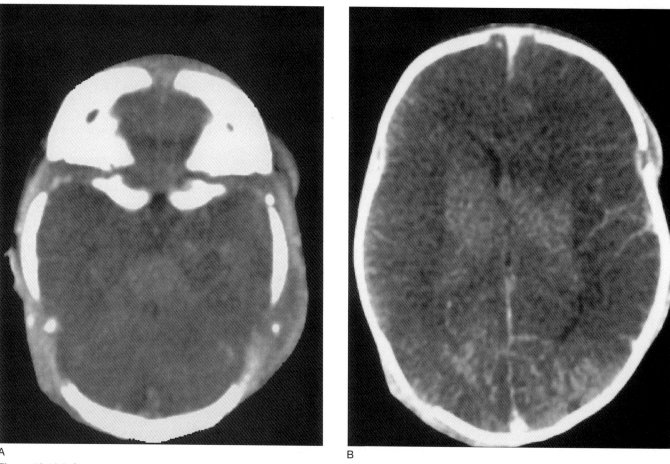

A

B

Figure 12.12.9 β-haemolytic streptococcus in a newborn. (A,B) Axial CT scans show cerebral hypodensity, sulcal effacement and ventricular compression due to widespread cerebral swelling. Involvement of the deep grey structures is also seen. Appearances were suggestive of hypoxic-ischaemic injury but there were clinical signs of meningoencephalitis and β-haemolytic streptococcus was isolated from blood cultures.

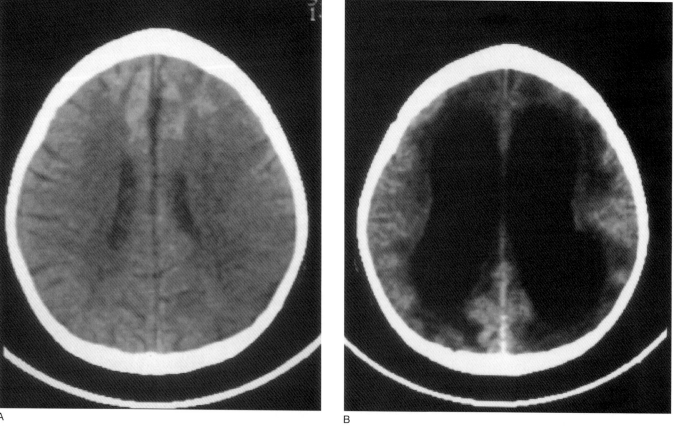

A

B

Figure 12.12.10 (A) Axial unenhanced CT scan of a 1-month-old child with *Streptococcus pneumoniae* sepsis. Haemorrhagic transformation within areas of low density within the grey and white matter of the cerebral hemispheres is indicative of cerebritis. (B) Six months later the CT appearances of encephalomalacia mirror the low-density changes at presentation.

countries. Sequelae are reported in 15–20% of children in developed countries and are probably under-reported in developing countries. The typical presentation is of fever, headache and nuchal rigidity.

Most of the harm caused by bacterial meningitis is through the host defence response to the invading bacteria. The most common meningitis pathogens in childhood are *Streptococcus pneumoniae*, *Haemophilus influenzae* and *Neisseria meningitidis,* which colonize the nasopharynx, enter the bloodstream via the upper respiratory tract and invade the CNS. They cause an intense inflammatory response in the subarachnoid space with resultant hydrocephalus, raised ICP, cerebral oedema and changes in cerebral blood flow.

FURTHER READING

Lebel MH, Hoyt MJ, Wagner DC et al. Magnetic resonance imaging and dexamethasone therapy for bacterial meningitis in children. American Journal of Disease in Childhood 1993; 342:457–461.

Molyneux E, Walsh A, Phiri A, Molyneux M. Acute bacterial meningitis admitted to the Queen Elizabeth Central Hospital, Blantyre, Malawi in 1996–97. Tropical Medicine and International Health 2000; 3:610–618.

Murray JL, Lopez AD. Global burden of disease and injuries series, vol. 2. Global Health Statistics. World Health Organization; 1996:285.

Mustafa MM, Ramilo O, Saez Llorens X et al. Cerebrospinal fluid, prostaglandins, interleukin I beta and tumour necrosis factor in bacterial meningitis: clinical and laboratory correlation in placebo treated and dexamethasone treated patients. American Journal of Disease in Childhood 1990; 144:883–887.

Schuchat A, Robinson K, Wenger JD et al. Bacterial meningitis in the United States in 1995. New England Journal of Medicine 1997; 337:970–976.

IMAGING MANIFESTATIONS

HYDROCEPHALUS

Hydrocephalus is well demonstrated on CT scanning and in the absence of any further complications, MRI is not required. Hydrocephalus results from a combination of factors: (1) impaired CSF resorption due to an increased protein content of the CSF, (2) ependymitis reducing CSF resorption and (3) obstruction at the ventricular foramina and aqueduct resulting in obstruction to CSF flow. CT and MRI may help establish the cause and if the child is symptomatic may guide neurosurgical drainage. In mild cases of meningitis, the hydrocephalus usually resolves with appropriate antibiotic treatment.

EFFUSIONS

Sterile subdural effusions are frequently seen as a complication of meningitis, particularly in neonates (50%) and particularly when the infecting organism is *Streptococcus pneumoniae* or *Haemophilus influenzae* (Figure 12.12.11). Effusions are isointense to CSF on CT and may be slightly hyperintense to CSF on MRI due to the slightly higher protein content and are most commonly situated over the frontal and temporal lobes. The cortical surface of the effusion may enhance, due to the presence of an inflammatory pial membrane or underlying cortical infarction, and differentiation from subdural empyemas is important as the latter require urgent aspiration. Subdural effusions resolve following antibiotic treatment. When a child is imaged for suspected subdural empyemas, contrast enhancement must be used. Subdural empyemas may also occur along the falx as well as over the cerebral convexitus.

VENTRICULITIS

Ventriculitis results from the entry of blood-borne organisms into the ventricles via the choroid plexuses. Both CT and MRI may reveal proteinaceous debris in the occipital horns or trigones of the lateral ventricles and intense ependymal enhancement with contrast. The ventricles dilate as a result of reduced CSF resorption by the inflamed ependyma. A more serious complication is the development of periventricular white matter necrosis, which results from either thrombosis of subependymal or periventricular veins or the release of toxins by the infecting bacteria (Figure 12.12.12).

FURTHER READING

Naidich TP, McLone DG, Yamanouchi Y. Periventricular white matter cysts in a murine model of gram negative ventriculitis. American Journal of Neuroradiology 1983; 4:461–465.

CEREBRITIS AND ABSCESS FORMATION

Cerebritis and abscess develop when the infectious process travels through the thrombosed veins into the cerebral parenchyma (see 'Cerebritis and abscesses' and 'Intracranial dural empyemas' below).

VENOUS THROMBOSIS AND INFARCTION

Thrombosis of deep venous sinuses is an uncommon complication of meningitis and usually occurs in children with dehydration. The symptoms of venous sinus thrombosis (VST) are non-specific (headache, decreased level of consciousness, vomiting, lethargy, anorexia and drowsiness) and cannot be distinguished from the symptoms of the underlying meningitis. Therefore, the diagnosis of VST relies heavily on imaging. Cavernous sinus thrombosis is an uncommon sequela of meningitis, and is more commonly associated with paranasal sinus, dental or ocular infection. In generalized sepsis, the sagittal and lateral sinuses are most commonly involved.

In the acute phase, unenhanced CT scans may detect deep VST as linear densities in the locations of the deep and cortical veins (Figure 12.12.13). As the thrombus becomes less dense, contrast may demonstrate the 'empty delta' sign, a filling defect, in the sinus. However, CT scanning misses the diagnosis of VST in up to 40% of patients. MRI with magnetic resonance venography (MRV) are valuable imaging methods for the diagnosis and follow-up in VST. On MRI, the thrombus is recognizable in the subacute phase as high signal on a T1-weighted scan and further imaging with MRV is usually not required. In the acute phase, the thrombus is isodense on T1-weighted imaging and of low signal on T2-weighted imaging, which can be mistaken for flowing blood but MRV will demonstrate an absence of flow in the thrombosed sinus. Both time-of-flight (TOF) and phase contrast MRV

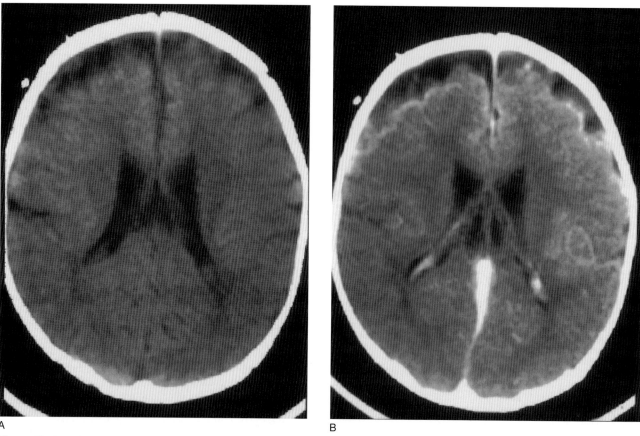

A

B

Figure 12.12.11 (A) Unenhanced and (B) enhanced CT scans of a 4-month-old child with meningococcal meningitis. The CSF overlying the frontal lobes is of normal density and there is pial enhancement reflecting leptomeningeal inflammation. The absence of dural enhancement and presence of low-density extra-axial fluid is against the diagnosis of empyemas.

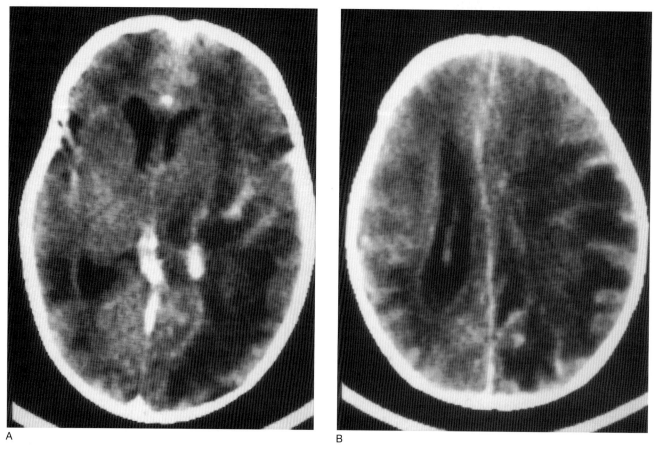

A

B

Figure 12.12.12 Enhanced axial images in a neonate with *E. coli* sepsis. There is evidence of ependymal and choroidal enhancement and ventricular dilatation due to ependymitis and periventricular white matter necrosis in the parietal lobe.

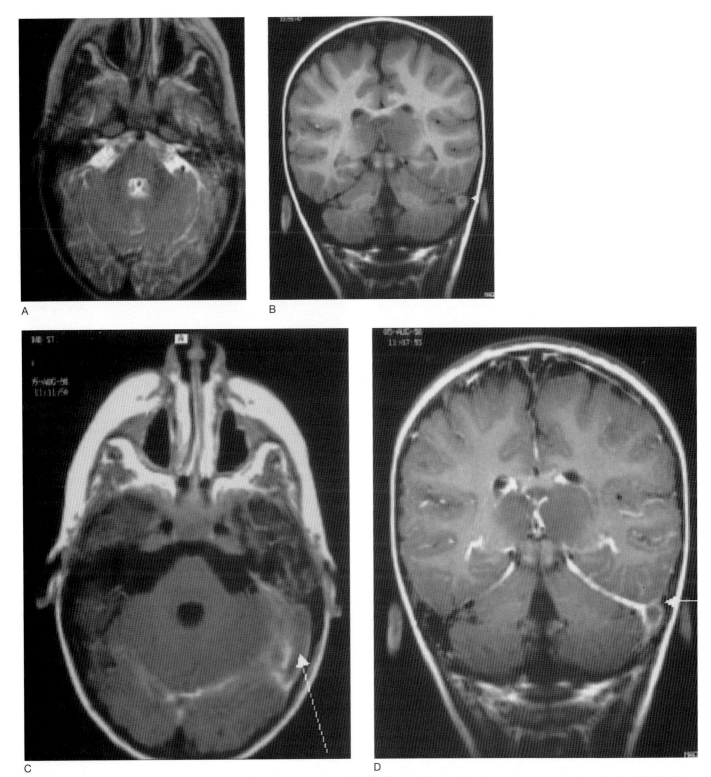

Figure 12.12.13 Venous sinus thrombosis in a child treated for mastoiditis. (A) The axial T2-weighted image reveals pus in the left mastoid air cells. (B) High-signal haematoma can be seen in the adjacent transverse sinus on the precontrast T1-weighted images (arrow). Following the administration of contrast the rim of the haematoma enhances as seen on the (C) axial and (D) coronal postcontrast T1-weighted images (arrows).

methods are available but because TOF techniques are T1-sensitive, a subacute VST will appear as flowing blood using this technique and patients should have phase contrast MRV. In equivocal cases, an endoluminal technique such as high-resolution CT venography or digital subtraction angiography may be required as a final arbiter.

In the largest studies of children with VST from any cause, 40% had associated parenchymal infarcts. Venous infarcts are frequently bilateral, do not conform to an arterial territory but to the territory of venous drainage, and are reported as haemorrhagic in between 25% and 50% of cases.

FURTHER READING

Ball WS. Cerebrovascular occlusive disease in childhood. Neuroimaging Clinics of North America 1994; 4:393–421.

Barkovitch AJ. Infections of the nervous system. In Barkovitch AJ, ed. Paediatric neuroimaging. New York: Raven Press; 1995:569–617.

Barron TF, Gusnard DA, Zimmerman RA, Clancy RR. Cerebral venous thrombosis in neonates and children. Pediatric Neurology 1992; 8:112–116.

Chiras J, Dubs M, Bories J. Venous infarctions. Neuroradiology 1985; 27:593–600.

deVeber G, Andrew M, the Canadian Pediatric Ischemic Stroke Study Group. The epidemiology and outcome of sinovenous thrombosis in pediatric patients. New England Journal of Medicine 2001; 345:417–423.

DiNubile P. Thrombosis of the cavernous sinuses. Archives in Neurology 1988; 45:567–572.

Medlock M, Olivero W, Hanigan W, Wright Rm, Winek SJ. Children with cerebral venous thrombosis diagnosed with magnetic resonance imaging and magnetic resonance angiography. Neurosurgery 1992; 31:870–876.

Pollard AJ, Dobson SR. Emerging infectious disease in the 21st century. Current Opinion in Infectious Disease 2000; 13:265–275.

ARTERIAL INFARCTION

The arteritis complicating meningitis arise from the spread of infection along the perivascular spaces and subsequent involvement of the arterial wall of both large and small vessels. Involvement of the small perforating vessels leads to multiple lacunar infarcts in the distribution of perforating vessels in the brainstem, basal ganglia and white matter. The typical appearance of a subacute infarct is low density on CT and high signal on T2-weighted images on MRI. Petechial, cortical or secondary haemorrhage may be present.

LABYRINTHITIS OSSIFICANS

Meningogenic labyrinthitis is usually associated with bacterial infections and is the commonest cause of acquired deafness in childhood. Infection is thought to spread from the meninges, via the internal auditory meatus, into either the vestibule or through the cochlear nerve foramen into the cochlear apex. In the early phases, faint enhancement of the membranous labyrinth may be seen on postcontrast T1-weighted images. In some children, inflammation persists and labyrinthitis ossificans develops. Prior to the ossifying stage, there is a fibrous stage. High-resolution CT imaging of the temporal bone may reveal hazy increased density within the membranous labyrinth (Figure 12.12.14). High-resolution T2-weighted MRI imaging, which is more sensitive than CT to the changes of labyrinthitis ossificans, at this stage may

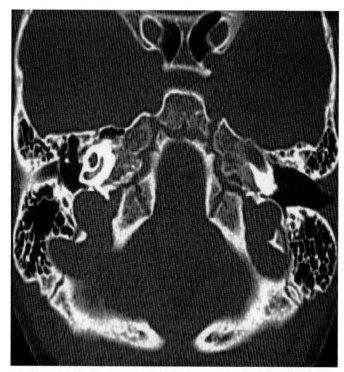

Figure 12.12.14 Labyrinthitis ossificans in a 5-year-old girl presented with bilateral hearing loss following meningitis. High-resolution CT imaging of the temporal bone reveals hazy increased density within the basal turn of the right cochlea. Less marked changes were seen on the left.

Table 12.12.3 Additional features of congenital infections (features in bold are characteristic of the infecting virus)

TORCH infection	Additional features
Toxoplasmosis	Chorioretinitis
	Hydrocephalus
Rubella	Microcephaly
	Micropthalmia
	Deep and subcortical white matter lesions
CMV	**Pachygyria/lissencephaly**
Herpes simplex	Microcephaly
	Hydrocephalus
	Micropthalmia
	Chorioretinitis
	Hyperdense cortex on CT and MRI
HIV	Atrophy

reveal fibrous development of the membranous labyrinth. Early detection is important as children are suitable for cochlear implant at this stage, which may only last a few weeks. Once the typical appearances of diffuse labyrinthitis ossificans develop, a cochlear implant is no longer possible.

FURTHER READING

Casselman JW, Kuhweide R, Ampe N, Meeus L, Steyart L. Pathology of the membranous labyrinth: comparison of T1 and T2 weighted and gadolinium-enhanced spin-echo and 3DFT-CISS imaging. American Journal of Neuroradiology 1993; 14:59–69.

Johnson MH, Hasenstab MS, Seicshnaydre MA, Williams GH. CT of post meningitic deafness: observations and predictive value for cochlear implants in children. American Journal of Neuroradiology 1995; 16:103–109.

Phelps PD, Proops DW. Imaging for cochlear implants. Journal of Laryngology and Otology (Suppl) 1999; 24:21–23.

Swartz JD, Harnsberger HR. The otic capsule and otodystrophies. In: Swartz JD, Harnsberger HR, eds. Imaging of the temporal bone. New York: Thieme; 1998:240–317.

TUBERCULOUS MENINGITIS INCLUDING DURAL-BASED DISEASE

Tuberculous meningitis (TBM) remains a serious paediatric problem, particularly in underdeveloped countries. Although there has been a recent rise in the number of reported cases of tuberculosis in England and Wales (over 6000 cases were reported in the year 2000) this does not appear to have had an effect on the number of cases of tuberculous meningitis in children. This is likely to be due to immunization programmes in neonates of immigrant families. Approximately 260 cases of TB were reported in children under 15 between 1998 and 2000, approximately 15 per year had TBM and numbers have remained static since 1998.

TBM has a significant morbidity and mortality and in a recent long-term follow-up of survivors treated with modern antituberculous agents, only 20% were functionally normal. The clinical presentation can be indolent and the typical signs of meningitis (fever, headache, nuchal rigidity) are often absent. Untreated meningitis results in hydrocephalus and severe brain atrophy due to infarction. Left untreated, tuberculous meningitis rapidly progresses to death, with an average duration of 3 weeks.

FURTHER READING

Rose AMC, Gatto AJ, Watson JM. Recent increase in tuberculosis notifications in England and Wales – real or artefact? Journal of Public Health Medicine 2002; 24:136–137.

Schoeman J, Wait J, Burger M et al. Long-term follow up of childhood tuberculous meningitis. Developmental Medicine and Child Neurology 2002; 44:522–526.

PATHOGENESIS

Tuberculous meningitis is said to almost always accompany miliary tuberculosis but in our experience it is often seen in the absence of involvement of other organs. Inhalation of *Mycobacterium tuberculosis* results in haematogenous infection through the pulmonary alveoli. Once the blood-borne organisms reach the brain, they are distributed throughout the brain and meninges and slowly multiply so that clinical involvement may not be apparent for 6 months. A gelatinous exudate fills the pia-arachnoid along the basal cisterns, particularly the pontine cistern, where it produces an inflammation within the walls of the meningeal blood vessels. As the exudates spreads into the Virchow-Robin spaces, small cortical blood vessels and perforating vessels are involved. The lenticulostriate and thalamo-perforating arteries of the basal ganglia and thalamus are involved in almost half the cases. The thick exudates prevent resorption of CSF and hydrocephalus results. The surrounding membranes of the cranial nerves may become infiltrated resulting in neuropathies, particularly II, VI and VII. Small tubercules may be visible over the convexity of the brain.

IMAGING

The commonest imaging manifestation of TBM is hydrocephalus, which develops in 50% to 77% of affected patients. On non-contrast CT or T1-weighted MR images, the purulent exudates in the basal cisterns may be seen as low density or low signal and may extend into the subarachnoid space. The involved cisterns avidly enhance following the administration of contrast. (Figure 12.12.15).

Meningeal infiltration and the resulting vasculitis cause small infarcts of the basal ganglia and thalamic infarcts. The infarcts appear as low density on CT and high signal on T2-weighted images and once matured appear as low signal on T1-weighted images. Cortical infarcts can result from identical pathology affecting the cortical vessels.

Tuberculomas have a predilection for the grey–white matter junction and are seen as punctate or ring-enhancing foci. Multiple lesions are most common above the tentorium whereas single lesions more commonly occur below the tentorium. On CT, they typically show ring enhancement. On T2-weighted images, the granulomata are hypodense and on T1-weighted images they exhibit a rim of high signal intensity surrounding a complete or partial rim of hypointensity and an isointense centre. Small tuberculomas (< 2 cm) show homogeneous enhancement initially but when they increase in size they exhibit rim enhancement. Tuberculomas may be surrounded by marked vasogenic oedema and when they are large they may be indistinguishable from malignant tumours (Figure 12.12.16). Tuberculomas are usually parenchymal but can be durally based (Figure 12.12.17). Magnetization transfer imaging has been used to differentiate between caseating (hypointense with a hyperintense rim) and non-caseating tuberculomas (hyperintense). Central caseation of tuberculous abscesses results in prolongation of the T2 signal to that close to water and appears as high signal on T2-weighted imaging. Miliary tuberculomas are normally found at the grey–white matter junction and in the basal ganglia and can also be seen disseminated over the pia-arachnoid.

FURTHER READING

Barkovitch AJ. Infections of the nervous system. In: Barkovitch, ed. Paediatric neuroimaging. New York: Raven Press; 1995:569–617.

Gee GT, Bazan C III, Jinkins JR. Miliary tuberculosis involving the brain: MR findings. American Journal of Roentgenology 1992; 159:1075–1076.

Gupta RK, Husain N, Kathuria MK et al. Magnetization transfer MR imaging correlation with histopathology in intracranial tuberculomas. Clinical Radiology 2001; 56:656–663.

Hsieh FY, Chia LG, Shen WC. Locations of cerebral infarctions in tuberculous meningitis. Neuroradiology 1992; 34:197–199.

Kim TK, Chang KH, Kim CJ et al. Intracranial tuberculoma: comparison of MR with pathologic findings. American Journal of Neuroradiology 1995; 16:1903–1908.

Offenbacher H, Fazekas F, Schmidt R et al. MRI in tuberculous meningoencephalitis: report of four cases and review of the neuroimaging literature. Journal of Neurology 1991; 238:340–344.

Wallace RC, Burton EM, Barrett FF et al. Intracranial tuberculosis in children: CT appearance and outcome. Pediatric Radiology 1991; 21:241–246.

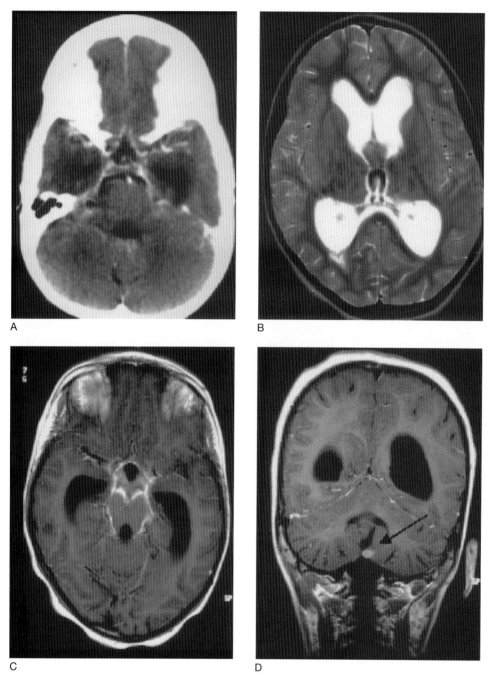

Figure 12.12.15 Tuberculous meningitis in a 15-year-old male. (A) Axial enhanced CT scan demonstrates marked thickening and enhancement of the basal meninges and dilatation of the temporal horns due to the resultant hydrocephalus. In a 5-year-old girl of West African descent, an axial T2-weighted image (B) demonstrates marked hydrocephalus and periventricular oedema, and the (C) axial and (D) coronal postcontrast T1-weighted images shows avid enhancement in the basal cisterns and Sylvian fissures. A meningeal-based nodule is seen overlying the left cerebellar tonsil (white arrow).

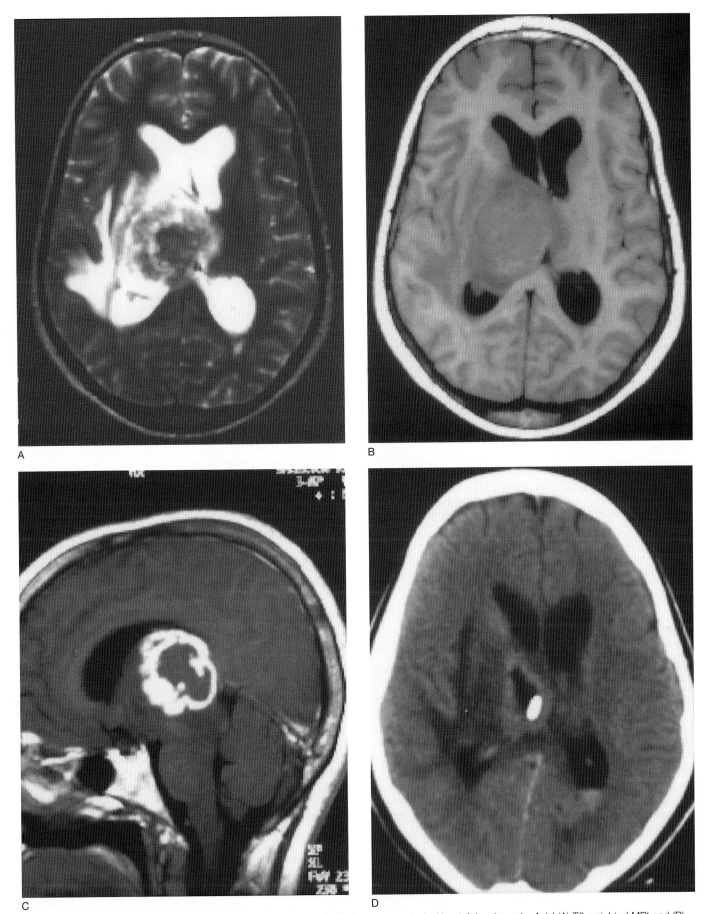

A

B

C

D

Figure 12.12.16 Tuberculoma in an 8-year-old child from the Middle East who presented with a left hemiparesis. Axial (A) T2-weighted MRI and (B) T1-weighted images show a mixed density mass centred in the basal ganglia on the right, with surrounding oedema, mass effect and hydrocephalus. (C) Rim enhancement is seen on the sagittal postcontrast T1-weighted image. The image appearances and site are also compatible with a high-grade glioma. (D) The child responded to surgical drainage and antituberculous treatment leaving an area of residual necrosis.

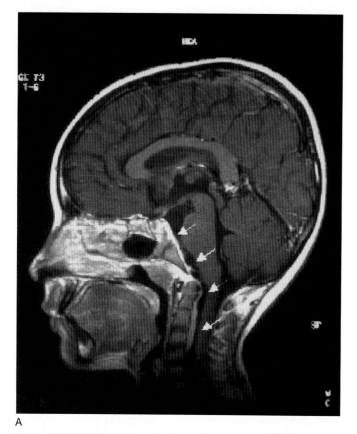
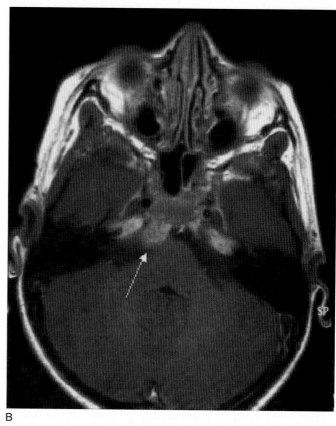

A

B

Figure 12.12.17 Durally based tuberculosis in a 4-year-old girl who presented systemically well with a right 6th nerve palsy. (A) Sagittal and (B) axial postcontrast images reveal marked thickening and enhancement of the dura overlying the dorsal aspect of the clivus (short arrows) and in the region of the proximal right 6th nerve before it enters the cavernous sinus (long arrow).

BACTERIAL, SPIROCHETE AND PARASITE INFECTIONS

CEREBRITIS AND ABSCESSES

Brain abscesses are relatively uncommon in clinical practice, yet remain a serious and life-threatening disease in neonates, infants and children. Predisposing factors to pyogenic infections include: (1) middle ear and paranasal sinus disease; (2) immune deficiency; (3) penetrating injury including neurosurgery; and (4) arteriovenous shunts bypassing the lungs, such as cardiac malformations. The most common cause of intracerebral abscess formation in children is direct or indirect spread from infection in the paranasal sinuses, middle ear and teeth. Frontal, ethmoidal, sphenoid and maxillary sinusitis give rise to frontal and parietal lobe abscess formation whereas mastoiditis results in temporal lobe or cerebellar abscess formation (Figure 12.12.18). The latter can also be associated with dermal sinuses extending into the cerebellum from the occipital region. Abscesses that occur as a result of disease within the cranium tend to be focal whereas those complicating systemic infection, e.g. bacterial endocarditis, tend to be multiple and occur in the parietal and occipital lobes, often in vascular watershed territory. Brainstem and pituitary abscesses are rare but have been reported.

The clinical presentation of brain abscess varies with its size, multiplicity, location and host defence. Symptoms and signs can be categorized into: (1) those arising from systemic infection; (2) those arising from raised ICP; and (3) focal neurology related to the location of the abscess. In most series of brain abscesses, the incidence of *Staphylococcus aureus* has decreased and that of anaerobes has increased. The list of anaerobic organisms causing abscesses is long and includes *Bacteroides*, *Peptostreptococcus* and *Fusobacterium* while aerobic organisms include *Staphylococcus*, *Streptococcus*, *Enterobacteriaceae* and *Haemophilus* species. The organism may give an indication as to the source of the infection; *Staphylococcus aureus* abscess formation occurs most commonly from compound skull fractures, *Bacteroides* and *Haemophilus* are isolated from otogenic abscesses and paranasal sinus infection results in aerobic or anaerobic streptococci abscesses or both. Fungal brain abscesses develop in patients who have impaired host defence and the infecting organisms include *Candida*, *Aspergillus*, *Nocardia* and *Cryptococcus* (see 'Infections in the immunocompromised'). The commonest organisms involved in neonatal abscesses are *Citrobacter* and *Proteus* sp.

Cerebritis is the earliest stage of a bacterial brain infection and untreated can progress to abscess formation, which is characterized by a surrounding impermeable capsule. Brain abscesses in neonates and infants are different from those in older children and adults. They originate in the periventricular white matter, are relatively large and may have poor capsule formation, which allows

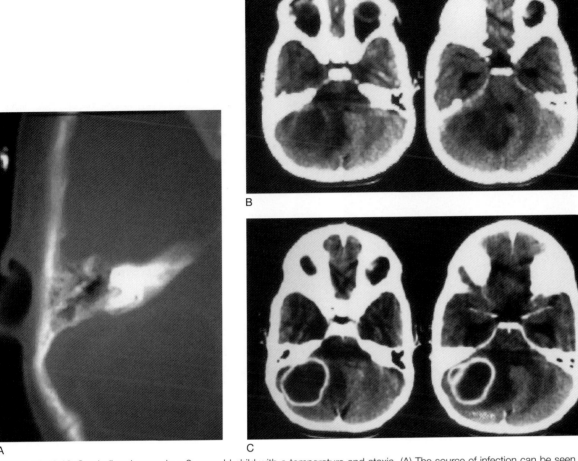

A   C

Figure 12.12.18 Cerebellar abscess in a 2-year-old child with a temperature and ataxia. (A) The source of infection can be seen on the bone windows of the CT as opacification of the right mastoid air cells consistent with mastoiditis. (B) Unenhanced and (C) enhanced axial CT scans show a large right cerebellar hemisphere abscess.

rapid enlargement (Figure 12.12.19). The subcortical white matter and basal nuclei are commoner sites in older children and young adults.

Radiological differentiation between cerebritis and abscess is important because cerebritis responds to antibiotics whereas an abscess usually requires surgical drainage. In the early phase of cerebritis, CT and MRI demonstrate an ill-defined area of oedema (low attenuation and high signal on a T2-weighted and low signal on a T1-weighted scan) with little mass effect, which may undergo haemorrhagic transformation. Poorly defined enhancement of the area may also be seen. Once an abscess has developed, the capsule, which is made up of granulation tissue, becomes visible on CT and MRI. On precontrast T1-weighted imaging, the capsule may appear haemorrhagic (high signal) and usually demonstrates marked enhancement. Typically, there is surrounding oedema and an area of central fluid pus, which demonstrates the non-specific sign of restricted water motion on diffusion-weighted imaging.

Serial imaging by either CT or MRI is used to monitor treatment. A reduction in the degree of enhancement is a useful indicator of resolving cerebritis while a reduction in size and surrounding oedema is used to monitor abscess resolution. In the encapsulated phase, enhancement may continue for some months after the infection has cleared and is not an indication of failure of treatment.

FURTHER READING

Cochrane DD. Brain abscesses: consultation with the specialist. Pediatric Review 1999; 20:209–215.

Fuentes S, Bouillot P, Regis J, Lena G, Choux M. Management of brainstem abscess. British Journal of Neurosurgery 2001; 15:57–62.

Renier D, Flandin C, Hirsch E, Hirsch J-F. Brain abscesses in neonates: a study of 30 cases. Journal of Neurosurgery 1988; 69:877–882.

Shono T, Nishio S, Murantani H et al. Pituitary abscess secondary to isolated sphenoid sinusitis. Minim Invasive Neurosurgery 1999; 42:204–206.

Tung GA, Evangelista P, Rogg JM, Duncan JA 3rd. Diffusion-weighted MR imaging of rim-enhancing brain masses: is markedly decreased water diffusion specific for brain abscesses. American Journal of Roentgenology 2001; 177:709–712.

INTRACRANIAL DURAL EMPYEMAS

Intracranial dural empyemas are relatively uncommon and occur predominantly in children. They most commonly occur as a

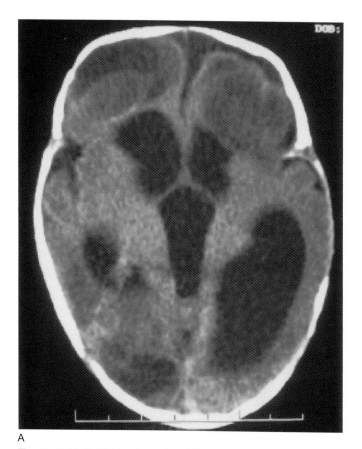
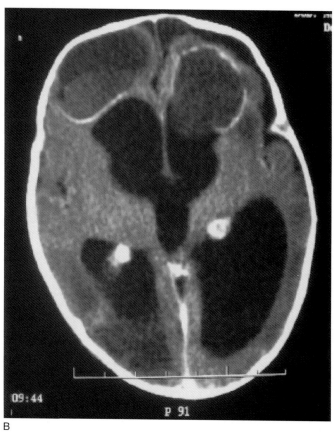

A   B

Figure 12.12.19 (A) Unenhanced and (B) enhanced axial CT scans of a 7-week child with *Serratia* sepsis. There are bilateral frontal lobe abscesses and mild enhancement of the meninges surrounding the Sylvian fissures. There is hydrocephalus and the low density adjacent to the occipital horns is most likely to be due to cerebritis.

complication of paranasal sinusitis (usually frontal and ethmoidal), middle ear sepsis and mastoiditis. Postoperative infection (particularly as a complication of facial or scalp cellulitis), bacterial meningitis, secondary infection of a sterile chronic subdural haematoma, skull fractures involving the paranasal sinuses and osteomyelitis from, e.g. dental sepsis, are less common but recognized causes of intracranial dural empyema. The classical presentation is an acute febrile illness with neurological features such as depressed conscious level, meningism, focal deficits and seizures. Diagnostic difficulties may arise because some children have a more indolent presentation, as is often the case with extradural abscesses.

Subdural empyemas secondary to sinus disease tend to occur anteriorly over the cerebral convexities and in the parafalcine location as well as tracking under the frontal lobes and over the falx cerebri. As a result, the site of the subdural empyema is not always anatomically related to the origin of the infection.

Early diagnosis and neurosurgical intervention are essential to prevent the potentially devastating complications of subdural empyemas, which are (1) venous infarction resulting from thrombosis of major dural venous sinuses or cortical veins, (2) arterial infarction resulting from spasm of the basal arteries and occlusion of small cortical arteries, and (3) cerebral abscess formation. Rarely, pus may collect in the extradural space but these children are more likely to have complications resulting from mass effect as the pus is not as closely related to the brain (Figure 12.12.20).

CT findings are subtle and in the early stages may be missed. Detection requires a high level of clinical suspicion and intravenous contrast should be used (Figure 12.12.21). Typical CT signs are a thin rim of fluid, slightly hyperintense to CSF (because of the presence of protein and cells), overlying a convexity or in the parafalcine space with a thin enhancing margin. Soft tissue swelling over the forehead is a strong indicator that there is a collection and is known as a Pott's 'puffy tumour' (Figure 12.12.22).

Magnetic resonance imaging is more sensitive than CT in the detection of dural empyemas due to the greater contrast between pus collections and the adjacent brain and more marked enhancement of the dura than seen on CT. The multiplanar capability of MRI allows the detection of subfrontal and subtemporal collections, which are often missed on axial CT scanning. Both CT and MRI may provide clues to the underlying aetiology such as paranasal sinus disease, fractures or evidence of neurosurgery. Complications are also more readily demonstrated by MRI. Particularly important is the detection of venous sinus thrombosis (VST), which normally requires anticoagulation (see 'Imaging manifestations' above).

FURTHER READING

Kirkpatrick PJ. Subdural empyema: a continuing threat. British Journal of Hospital Medicine 1992; 48:261–262.

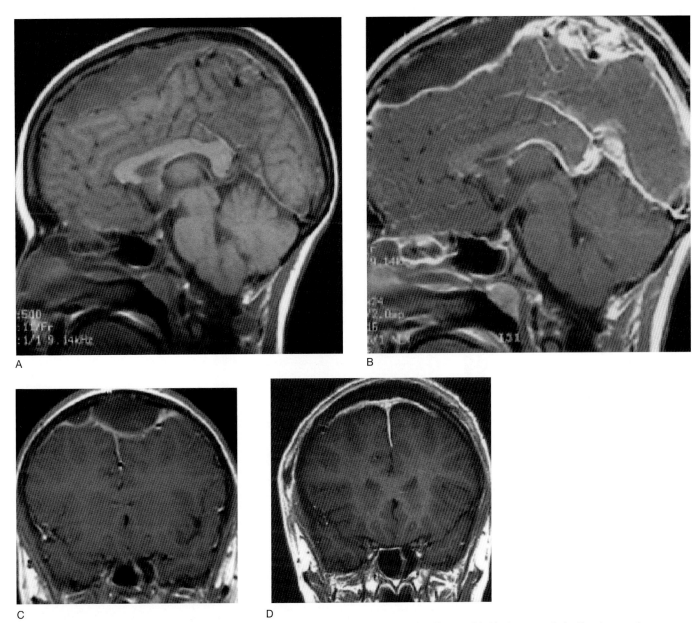

A

B

C

D

Figure 12.12.20 (A,B) Sagittal pre- and postcontrast T1-weighted images of the brain of a 13-year-old girl who presented with a temperature, headache for several days and a reduced level of consciousness. MRI reveals a large enhancing collection crossing the midline that is extra-axial in position. Compare the degree of mass effect to the subdural collection in Figure 12.12.22. (C,D) Pre- and post-treatment enhanced coronal T1-weighted images reveal resolution of the mass effect following surgical drainage.

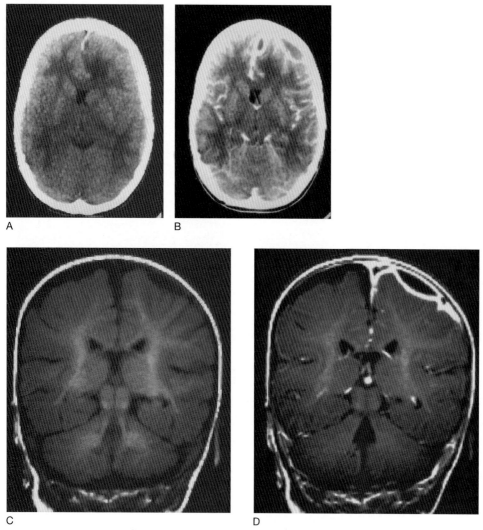

Figure 12.12.21 A 5-month-old child presenting with a temperature and seizures. (A) The unenhanced axial image shows subtle low-density material in the interhemispheric fissure and overlying the left frontal lobe, which become much more conspicuous following the administration of contrast on the corresponding axial image (B). Coronal (C) pre- and (D) post-contrast T1-weighted images also demonstrate the increased conspicuousness following contrast enhancement on MRI.

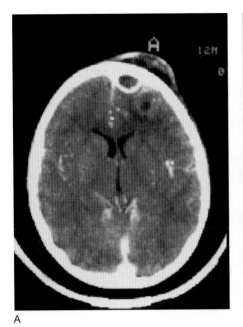
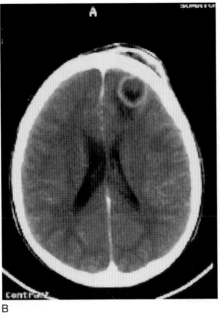
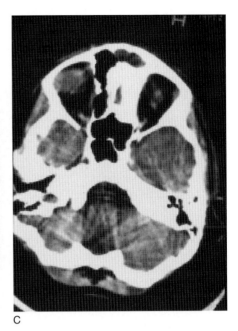

A   B   C

Figure 12.12.22 (A,B) Enhanced CT scans through the cerebral hemispheres of a 7-year-old child showing forehead swelling (Pott's puffy tumour), an underlying subdural empyema and cerebral abscess. (C) Unenhanced CT scan with high-density material in the frontal sinus indicates the source of the infection. *S. milleri* was isolated following surgical drainage.

Krauss WE, McCormick PC. Infections of the subdural spaces. Neurosurgery Clinics of North America 1992; 3:421–433.

Moseley IF, Kendall BE. Radiology of intracranial empyemas, with special reference to computed tomography. Neuroradiology 1984; 26:333–345.

Rich PM, Deasy NP, Jarosz JM. Intracranial dural empyema. British Journal of Radiology 2000;7 3:1329–1336.

Sze G, Zimmerman RD. The magnetic resonance imaging of infections and inflammatory diseases. Radiology Clinics of North America 1988; 26:839–859.

Weisberg L. Subdural empyemas. Archives of Neurology 1986; 43:497–500.

CYSTICERCOSIS

Neurocysticercosis is prevalent wherever pigs are raised in areas of poor sanitation and is the most common cause of new-onset epilepsy in the developing world. As immigration patterns have changed and travel is on the increase, neurocysticercosis is now seen in the UK and US. The infecting organism is almost always the encysted form of *Taenia solium* (tapeworm). Humans are the intermediate host and following ingestion of tapeworm eggs from faecally contaminated food, the eggs hatch and burrow into the small intestine where they penetrate the venules. Mature larvae, or cysticerci, develop after 60–70 days. The most common manifestation of cysticercosis in children is parenchymal cysticercosis, the result of the host response to the dying parasite; children present with seizures but have an excellent prognosis without antihelminthic treatment. The number of lesions or disease activity as determined by CT does not predict seizure control or seizure recurrence rate.

Four forms of the larva are described, which are apparent in the imaging findings (parenchymal cysticerci, leptomeningitis, intraventricular and racemose cysts), but as patients are exposed to the disease on repeated occasions, more than one type may be seen at any one time. Parenchymal cysticercosis occurs most commonly in cerebral grey matter (Figure 12.12.23) but is also seen in the basal ganglia in 25% of patients, brainstem and spinal cord. The lesions are either solid with associated punctate calcification or cystic with calcification within the rim. Completely calcified lesions do not enhance but enhancement is seen when imaging is performed whilst there is an inflammatory reaction associated with the death of the larva.

The radiological appearances of the leptomeningeal form of cysticercosis are those of other granulomatous infections; soft tissue is seen to fill the basal cisterns and there is marked enhancement of the leptomeninges following contrast on both CT and MRI. Calcific granulomata may be seen in the subarachnoid space. Hydrocephalus and vasculitis, most commonly involving the middle cerebral artery are common.

Intraventricular cysticerci result in acute hydrocephalus and are a neurosurgical emergency. MRI may demonstrate the scolex (head) of the parasite within the ventricle as a soft tissue nodule but when situated in the position of a congenital cyst, such as a colloid cyst, the appearances may be indistinguishable.

Racemose cysts are multiple, non-viable cysts located in the subarachnoid space. They may be several centimetres in size, multiple and are commonly situated in the cerebellopontine angle, the suprasellar region, the sylvian fissure and the basal cisterns. They may enhance after contrast administration. Three-dimensional constructive interference in steady-state sequences have been shown to demonstrate intraventricular cysts better than conventional spin echo sequences.

Intraspinal involvement is usually demonstrated on MRI as multiple small intradural extramedullary cysts but intramedullary cysticerci have also been reported. Arachnoiditis may be present in the spinal subarachnoid space. Infestations of the orbit (intra- and extraocular), muscles and soft tissues may support the diagnosis of cysticercosis in a patient with suspected disease.

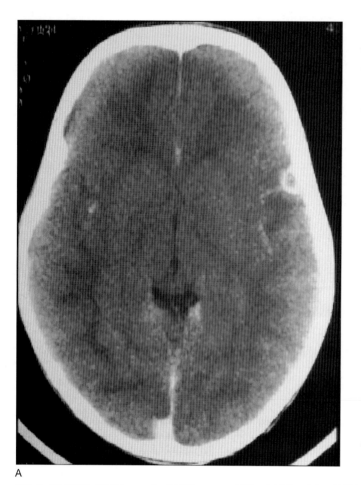

A

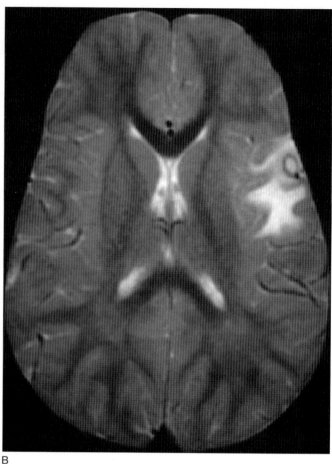

B

Figure 12.12.23 (A) Enhanced axial CT scan and (B) axial T2-weighted MR images of a 3-year-old male with focal seizures. The ring enhancing lesion with surrounding vasogenic oedema in the left frontal cortex is a parenchymal cysticercosis cyst.

FURTHER READING

Barinagarrementeria F, Cantu C. Frequency of cerebral arteritis in subarachnoid cysticercosis: an angiographic study. Stroke 1998; 29:123–125.

Chawla S, Gupta RK, Kumar R et al. Demonstration of scolex in calcified cysticercus lesion using gradient echo with or without corrected phase imaging and its clinical implications. Clinical Radiology 2002; 57:826–834.

Cosentino C, Velez M, Torres L, Garcia HH. Cysticercosis Working Group in Peru. Cysticercosis lesions in basal ganglia are common but clinically silent. Clinical Neurology and Neurosurgery 2002; 104:57–60.

Ferreira LS, Zanardi VA, Scotoni AE, Li LM, Guerreiro MM. Childhood epilepsy due to neurocysticercosis: a comparative study. Epilepsia 2001; 42:1438–1444.

Homans J, Khoo L, Chen T et al. Spinal intramedullary cysticercosis in a five-year-old child: case report and review of the literature. Pediatric Infectious Diseases Journal 2001; 20:904–908.

Mitchell WG. Neurocysticercosis and acquired cerebral toxoplasmosis in children. Seminars in Pediatric Neurology 1999; 6:267–277.

Rahalkar MD, Shetty DD, Kelkar AB et al. The many faces of cysticercosis. Clinical Radiology 2000; 55:668–674.

Suh D, Chang K, Han M, Lee S, Kim C. Unusual manifestations of neurocysticercosis. Neuroradiology 1989; 31:396–402.

Teitelbaum G, Otto R, Lin M et al. MR imaging of neurocysticercosis. American Journal of Neuroradiology 1989; 10:709–718.

LYME DISEASE

Lyme borreliosis is a tick-borne infectious disease transmitted by the spirochete *Borrelia burgdorferi*, which was first identified in 1982. The disease was first described in 1976 in a group of children and adults with arthritis living in Lyme, Connecticut, USA. Lyme disease is the most common vector-borne disease in children in the US but is rarely seen in the UK where it is linked to areas inhabited by deer (e.g. the New Forest), which carry the infected tick. Lyme disease is usually monosymptomatic but can involve multiple organs: the skin (erythema chronicum migrans), the nervous system (neuroborreliosis) and the musculoskeletal system (oligoarthritis).

CNS involvement in children is rare. The most frequent manifestations of patients with neuroborreliosis are peripheral facial nerve palsies (55%), aseptic meningitis (27%) and meningo-radiculoneuritis (3.6%). Cranial nerve palsies, other than of the facial nerves, acute transverse myelitis and large vessel occlusive disease are rare manifestations of the disease. The disease mechanism is unclear and may represent either a direct infection or an autoimmune phenomenon, such as acute disseminated encephalomyelitis.

CT scans are usually normal, although focal low attenuation areas have been reported. Abnormalities on MRI are seen in only

25% of affected patients and show areas of high signal in the white matter on T2-weighted images. In children with cranial nerve palsies, enhancement of the affected cranial nerves may be seen. Primary leptomeningeal enhancement in the absence of parenchymal disease and features of a transverse myelitis have been described in patients with Lyme disease.

FURTHER READING

Belman A. Neurologic complications of Lyme disease in children. International Pediatrics 1992; 7:136–143.

Burgdorferi W, Barbour AG, Hayes SF et al. Lyme disease – a tick-borne spirochetosis? Science 1982; 216:1317–1319.

Christen HJ, Hanefield F, Eiffert H, Thomssen R. Epidemiology and clinical manifestations of Lyme borreliosis in childhood. Acta Paediatrica 1993; 386(Suppl):1–76.

Demaerel P, Wilms G, Van Lierde S, Delanote J, Baert A. Lyme disease in childhood presenting as primary leptomeningeal enhancement without parenchymal findings on MR. American Journal of Neuroradiology 1994; 15:302–304.

Huisman T, Wohlrab G, Nadal D, Boltshauser E, Martin E. Unusual presentation of neuroborreliosis (Lyme disease) in childhood. Journal of Computer Assisted Tomography 1999; 23:39–42.

Klingebiel R, Benndorf G, Schmitt M, von Moers A, Lehmann R. Large cerebral vessel occlusive disease in Lyme neuroborreliosis. Neuropediatrics 2002; 33:37–40.

Shapiro ED. Lyme disease in children. American Journal of Medicine 1995; 98 (Suppl 4A):69–73.

ENCEPHALITIS

GENERAL CONCEPTS

Encephalitis is an unusual manifestation of viral infections. Viruses vary widely in their ability to produce CNS infection. Some viruses, (e.g. mumps virus) commonly infect the CNS but are relatively benign. For other viruses (e.g. Japanese encephalitis), neurological disease is the most significant manifestation of the infection. Other viruses, such as herpes simplex virus (HSV), commonly infect humans but rarely cause encephalitis.

Viruses typically enter the CNS by haematogenous spread but a few pathogens, such as rabies and HSV-1, can spread by ascending along peripheral nerves. In acute viral encephalitis, capillary and endothelial inflammation of cortical vessels occurs primarily in the grey matter or at its junction with white matter. Once the virus enters the CNS, neuronal degeneration and inflammation result. Viruses can also enter the nervous system by intraneuronal routes. Studies in both animals and man have suggested that the olfactory tract is a route of entry of the HSV to the brain. Nucleic acid analysis of brain extract suggests that HSV can exist in a latent state in the brain.

The clinical features of encephalitis are a triad of fever, headache, and altered level of consciousness. Disorientation, behaviour and speech disturbance, and focal and diffuse neurological signs such as hemiparesis or seizures are common neurological signs. In viral encephalitis other than HSV-1, imaging appearances are often not specific for a particular virus. The typical appearances of HSV-1 are thought to result from molecular interactions between proteins expressed on the surface of the virus and receptors on the surface of the host cells.

Examination of the CSF is essential in the diagnosis of encephalitis, unless a lumbar puncture is contraindicated due to the presence of raised ICP. CSF abnormalities include a raised white blood cell count and increased protein levels. New diagnostic assays have simplified the diagnosis of encephalitis. The ELISA assay that detects IgM antibodies in CSF from patients with Japanese encephalitis is both sensitive and specific, and polymerase chain reaction (PCR) applied to the CSF has become the diagnostic method of choice for many CNS infections, especially HSV and enteroviruses. Brain biopsy may be required in cases of diagnostic difficulty.

HSV-1 is the commonest cause of non-epidemic acute focal encephalitis in the US and UK. The frequency of occurrence is 1 in 250 000–500 000 per year and a third of cases are seen in the under 20 age group. Many childhood encephalopathies are attributed to viruses, though viral identification is often not made. Viruses transmitted to humans by the bite of arthropods such as mosquitoes and ticks, i.e. previously known as arboviruses (e.g. Eastern and Western equine virus, Japanese encephalitis virus), are the most important cause of encephalitis worldwide. Rubella, varicella and influenza A are other recognized causes of encephalitis.

MRI is the most sensitive imaging method in the diagnosis of early encephalitis. The initial oedema is seen as areas of high signal on T2-weighted imaging and low signal on T1-weighted imaging. It is not until later on in the disease that regions of low density are seen on CT. A recent study has shown that diffusion-weighted imaging (DWI) is more sensitive than conventional MRI in the detection of encephalitic lesions in the acute period, particularly in the neonatal and infant brain, where the water content is high and the difference between oedematous and normal brain is more difficult to visualize.

The distribution of the abnormalities seen on MRI may aid in identifying a responsible organism. The cingulate gyri and insular cortices are typically involved in herpes encephalitis (see below). Involvement of deep grey structures is characteristic of Japanese encephalitis, while brainstem involvement is more typically seen in encephalitis due to *Mycoplasma pneumoniae* (Figure 12.12.24).

FURTHER READING

Baringer JR, Pasani P. Herpes simplex virus genomes in human nervous system tissue analysed by polymerase chain reaction. Annals of Neurology 1994; 36:823–829.

Domingues RB, Fink MC, Tsanaclis SM et al. Diagnosis of herpes simplex encephalitis by magnetic resonance imaging and polymerase chain reaction assay of cerebrospinal fluid. Journal of Neurological Sciences 1998; 157:148–153.

Gonzalez-Scarano F, Tyler KL. Molecular pathogenesis of the neurotrophic viral infections. Annals of Neurology 1987; 22:564–570.

Johnson RT, Mims CA. Pathogenesis of viral infections of the nervous system. New England Journal of Medicine 1968; 278:54–92.

Teixeira J, Zimmerman RA, Haselgrove JC, Bilaniuk LT, Hunter JV. Diffusion imaging in pediatric central nervous system. Neuroradiology 2001; 43:1031–1039.

Whitley RJ, Gnann JW. Viral encephalitis: familiar infections and emerging pathogens. Lancet 2002; 359:507–514.

HERPES SIMPLEX ENCEPHALITIS

HSV is a ubiquitous organism that commonly infects humans but rarely results in CNS infection. The type 1 virus is associated with

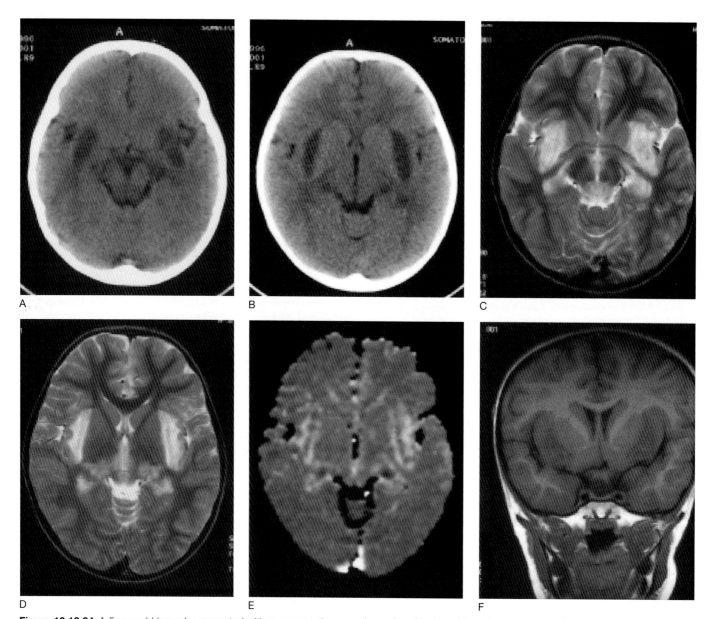

Figure 12.12.24 A 5-year-old boy who presented with recurrent seizures and was found to have *Mycoplasma pneumoniae* encephalitis. (A,B) Axial CT scans show symmetrical involvement of the external and extreme capsules. (C,D) T2-weighted images reveal involvement of the brainstem. (E) A diffusion map acquired on day 2 does not show additional areas of abnormality compared to the corresponding T2-weighted image (C). (F) Coronal T1-weighted images demonstrate symmetrical swelling and low signal of the insular cortex.

orofacial infections and is the commonest cause of herpes simplex encephalitis (HSE) in the majority of children beyond the neonatal period. About one-third of cases are due to primary HSV-1 infection and two-thirds are due to reactivation of the virus. Studies in animals have demonstrated reactivation of the latent virus in the trigeminal ganglion and transmission of the virus along the olfactory tract to infect the brain. HSV-2 is responsible for genital herpes and causes most of the congenitally and perinatally acquired herpes (see 'Neonatal herpes' above).

The radiological picture of HSE is characteristic with asymmetrical involvement of the orbitofrontal and temporal lobes with involvement of the cingulate gyri and insular cortex (Figure 12.12.25). Symmetrical involvement of the hippocampus is seen

in limbic encephalitis (Figure 12.12.26). Meningeal and gyral enhancement after gadolinium diethylenetriaminepentaacetic acid (DTPA) has been reported but is non-specific and does not add to the diagnostic certainty. The MRI and later CT abnormalities are high signal on T2-weighed imaging, low signal on T1-weighted imaging and low attenuation on CT, sometimes with small areas of haemorrhages. Brainstem encephalitis is rare but has been described.

Children present with the clinical triad of encephalitis but more specifically frontal and temporal features of aphasia or mutism, personality change, focal or generalized seizures and, in some cases, coma. In the absence of effective antiviral treatment, the mortality of HSV-1 encephalitis is more than 70%, with only 2.5%

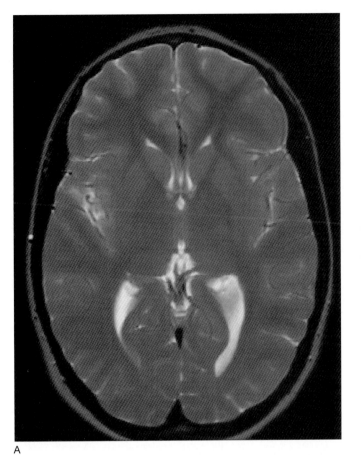

A

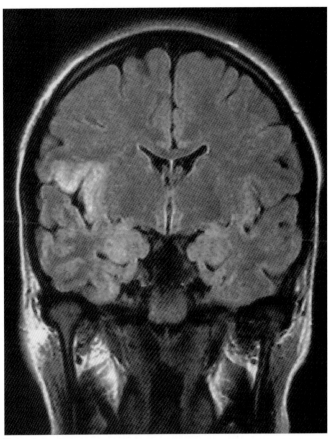

B

Figure 12.12.25 (A) Axial T2-weighted and (B) coronal FLAIR images of a 15-year-old girl who presented with sudden onset of left-sided weakness, dysphasia and an upper motor neurone facial palsy, which resolved quickly but recurred within 24 h. The radiological picture of asymmetrical involvement of the right insular and inferior frontal cortex is characteristic of herpes simplex encephalitis.

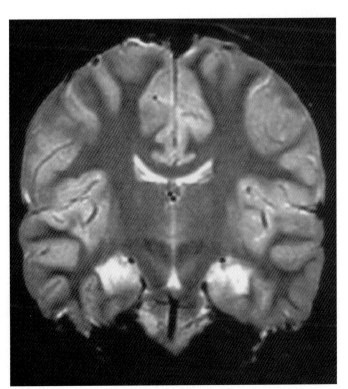

Figure 12.12.26 Coronal T2-weighted image of a 14-year-old girl presenting with features of encephalitis. There is bilateral symmetrical high signal within the hippocampi typical of herpes simplex limbic encephalitis.

of individuals returning to normal function. Despite treatment, mortality (20–30%) and morbidity is still high.

FURTHER READING

Davis LE. Diagnosis and treatment of acute encephalitis. Neurologist 2000; 6:145–159.

Demaerel P, Wilms G, Robberecht W et al. MRI of herpes simplex encephalitis. Neuroradiology 1992; 34:490–493.

Tyler KL, Tedder DG, Yamamoto IJ et al. Recurrent brainstem encephalitis associated with herpes simplex virus type 1 DNA in the cerebrospinal fluid. Neurology 1995; 45:2246–2250.

Whitley RJ. Herpes simplex virus. In: Scheld WM, Whitley RJ, Durack DT, eds. Infections of the central nervous system. Philadelphia: Lippincott-Raven; 1996:73–89.

Whitley RJ, Gnann JW. Viral encephalitis: familiar infections and emerging pathogens. Lancet 2002; 359:507–514.

ARTHROPOD-BORNE VIRUSES

The togavirus (e.g. eastern equine encephalitis), flavivirus (e.g. Japanese encephalitis) and bunyavirus (e.g. LaCrosse encephalitis) families are the commonest arthropod-borne viruses to cause encephalitis. A group related to the flavivirus genus accounts for hundreds of thousands of cases of human encephalitis worldwide: St. Louis encephalitis (North America), Murray valley encephalitis (Australia), Western-Nile virus encephalitis (Africa/Middle East), Far Eastern tick-borne encephalitis (Russia) and Western tick-borne encephalitis (Europe).

Japanese encephalitis virus is transmitted by the mosquito and causes more cases of acute encephalitis than all the other arboviruses combined. Japanese encephalitis has moved from China and southeast Asia, westward to India and Pakistan, northwards to Russia, eastwards to the Philippines and southwards to Australia. In areas where it is common, it is primarily a disease of children. Children present with the typical triad of encephalitis. Characteristic findings are seizures (85%), tremor, dystonia, rigidity and mask-like faces. Recently, a variant that presents like a poliomyelitis acute flaccid paralysis has been described. The MRI features are those of areas of mixed signal intensity in the basal ganglia and midbrain (Figure 12.12.27). Treatment is supportive only. The mortality rate is about 30% and 50% of survivors have neurological sequelae.

In the USA, most cases of arthropod-borne encephalitides in children have been attributed to LaCrosse virus, which causes aseptic meningitis and encephalitis, primarily in school age children. The mortality rate is low but 10–15% of survivors will have neurological deficits. MRI findings are of focal lesions in the basal ganglia, thalami and brainstem.

FURTHER READING

Kalita J, Mista UK. Comparison of CT findings and MR findings in the diagnosis of Japanese encephalitis. Journal of Neurological Sciences 2000; 174:3–8.

McJunkin JE, de los Reyes EC, Irazuzta JE et al. LaCrosse encephalitis in children. New England Journal of Medicine 2001; 344:801–807.

Solomon T, Dung NM, Kneen R, Gainsborough M, Vaughan DW. Japanese encephalitis. Journal of Neurology, Neurosurgery and Psychiatry 2000; 68:405–415.

Solomon T, Dung NM, Kneen R et al. Poliomyelitis-like illness caused by Japanese encephalitis virus. Lancet 1998; 351:1094–1097.

Whitley RJ. Viral encephalitis. New England Journal of Medicine 1990; 323:242–250.

ENTEROVIRUSES

Enteroviruses (including coxsackieviruses and echoviruses) most commonly result in a wide spectrum of disease, most of which are mild and self-limiting. Enteroviruses are frequent causes of aseptic meningitis and meningoencephalitis in young children. Other enteroviruses cause severe neurological disease, the best known being poliomyelitis. Although polio has been eradicated in the western world, it is still seen in underdeveloped countries where the vaccine is not available to all children. The polio virus produces haemorrhagic necrosis of the anterior horns of the spinal cord or brainstem nuclei, progressing to focal atrophy, which may become evident on MRI.

A relatively recent outbreak of enteroviral infection (hand-foot-and-mouth disease and herpangina) in children in Taiwan resulted in an unusually high proportion of neurological complications. Among patients with positive viral cultures enterovirus 71 was isolated from 75% of hospital patients and 92% died. MRI findings were of high-signal lesions throughout the brainstem.

FURTHER READING

Huang CC, Liu CC, Chang YC et al. Neurologic complications in children with enterovirus 71 infection. New England Journal of Medicine 1999; 341:936–942.

Wang SM, Liu CC, Tseng HW et al. Clinical spectrum of enterovirus 71 infection in children in southern Taiwan, with an emphasis on neurological complications. Clinical Infectious Diseases 1999; 29:184–190.

RABIES ENCEPHALITIS

Rabies encephalitis is caused by an RNA virus of the rhabdovirus family; transmission through dog bites and wild animals is rare but well described. The first case for 100 years occurred in an adult in Britain in 2002 as the result of a bite from a bat. The incubation period is from 5 days to over 6 months, the usual period being 20–60 days. Rabies can be prevented by the use of passive and active immunization, even postinfection. After the prodromal period of fever, malaise and anxiety, patients present with predominantly encephalopathic or paralytic CNS findings. Diagnosis is made by the detection of rabies virus RNA in saliva by PCR. The patient progresses to coma, cardiorespiratory failure and ultimately death. As a result, imaging reports are rare but do exist.

CT scanning has demonstrated bilateral and symmetrical low density of the basal ganglia in a child with proven rabies. Symmetrical high signal changes have been reported on MRI in the hippocampus, thalamus, basal ganglia and dorsal aspect of the brainstem, and grey matter of the cord, which correlate with areas of pathological change, in an immunized child with proven rabies. Bilateral symmetrical involvement of the basal ganglia and posterior thalamus have been reported on MRI in an adult with proven rabies but the appearances are non-specific and the differential diagnosis includes toxic encephalopathy (carbon monoxide, methanol, hydrogen sulphide, cyanide), severe hypo-

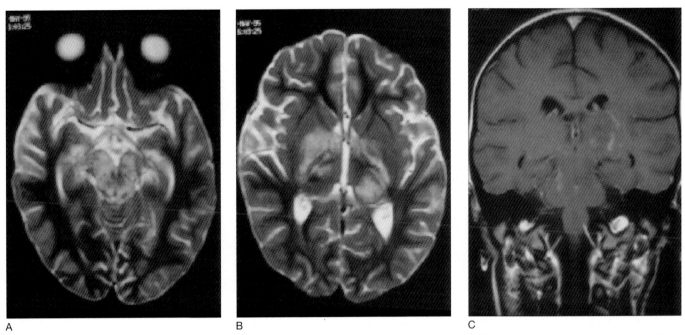

A   B   C

Figure 12.12.27 (A,B) Axial T2-weighted and (C) coronal enhanced T1-weighted scans of a 2-year-old child found to have Japanese B encephalitis. There is mixed signal abnormality seen in the midbrain, mesial temporal lobes, basal ganglia and thalamus on the left. Patchy enhancement is seen within areas of T1 low signal in the thalamus and midbrain.

glycaemia and metabolic disorders such as Wilson's disease and Leigh's disease.

FURTHER READING

Awasthi M, Parmar H, Patankar T, Castillo M. Imaging findings in rabies encephalitis. American Journal of Neuroradiology 2001; 22:677–680.
Desai RV, Jain V, Singh P, Singhi S, Radotra BD. Radiculomyelitic rabies: can MR imaging help? American Journal of Neuroradiology 2002; 23:632–634.
Plontkin SA. Rabies. Clinical Infectious Diseases 2000; 30:4–12.

ACUTE CEREBELLITIS

Acute cerebellitis is an uncommon syndrome characterized by acute onset cerebellar dysfunction. Patients typically present with spontaneous eye movements, myoclonic jerks, truncal ataxia, dysarthria, headaches, tremor and altered mental state. Fever and meningism may be present. Symptoms resolve spontaneously over weeks to months, although permanent disability and even death may ensue. The cause may be infectious, postinfectious as part of acute disseminated encephalomyelitis (ADEM) (see 'ADEM' below) or following vaccination. The infectious agent is usually viral and includes varicella–zoster, Epstein–Barr, measles, pertussis, diphtheria, mumps and coxsackie viruses. Other organisms such as typhoid have been implicated. Non-infectious causes include lead intoxication, cyanide poisoning, demyelination and vasculitis.

Imaging findings in cerebellitis reveal bilateral, symmetrical low attenuation changes on CT, and high signal on T2 and low signal on T1 on MRI in the cerebellar hemispheres; both grey and white matter may be affected (Figure 12.12.28). Localized oedema

can obstruct the fourth ventricle resulting in hydrocephalus, which may require surgical drainage. Contrast enhancement may be seen in the subacute phase.

FURTHER READING

Aylett SE, O'Neill KS, De Sousa C, Britton J. Cerebellitis presenting as acute hydrocephalus. Childs Nervous System 1998; 14:139–141.
Horowitz MB, Pang D, Hirsch W. Acute cerebellitis: case report and review. Pediatric Neurosurgery 1991–2; 17:142–145.
Misra GC, Singh SP, Mohapatra MK et al. Typhoid cerebellitis. Journal of the Indian Medical Association 1985; 83:352–353.
Montenegro MA, Santos SL, Li LM, Cendes F. Neuroimaging of acute cerebellitis. Journal of Neuroimaging 2002; 2:72–74.

ADEM

Postinfectious CNS disease is common in children and is often a single event of inflammation such as the acute cerebellar syndrome that follows infection with the varicella–zoster virus (see above). The symptoms usually appear on day 7–10 following a viral illness.

Acute disseminated encephalomyelitis (ADEM) is a monophasic inflammatory disease that occurs at multiple sites within the CNS. Relapses can occur immediately after ADEM, usually within 6 months, when they are considered to be part of the same acute monophasic process, and are termed 'multiphasic disseminated encephalomyelitis' (MDEM). When relapses occur that are disseminated in time and place, which suggests a chronic immune process, the diagnosis is multiple sclerosis (MS). ADEM and MDEM are considered a monophasic inflammatory disorder and are grouped together in the subsequent paragraphs.

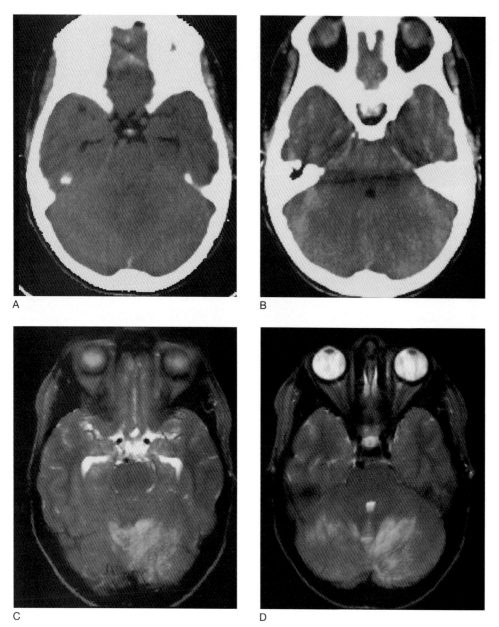

Figure 12.12.28 Acute enterovirus cerebellitis. (A,B) Axial CT images show low density of the cerebellar hemispheres, effacement of the sulci and 4th ventricle and enlargement of the temporal horns, indicating hydrocephalus. (C,D) Corresponding T2-weighted axial images show high signal and swelling of the cerebellar hemispheres and early hydrocephalus.

The clinical and radiological differences between ADEM and MS have been investigated in a group of children followed up for over 5.5 years. Symptoms referable to intracranial pathology, including headache, fever, meningism and seizures, were more common in the ADEM group than the MS group. As a result, two-thirds of the children received initial treatment for infectious meningoencephalomyelitis. A florid, polysymptomatic presentation was common in ADEM, whereas MS patients were more likely to have a monosymptomatic presentation.

MRI of the brain demonstrated asymmetrical white matter abnormalities in both ADEM and MS children, usually following a normal CT scan. ADEM lesions tended to be in the subcortical white matter with relative sparing of the periventricular white matter, whereas MS lesions tended to be in both the periventricular and subcortical white matter. Cortical grey lesions occurred only in the ADEM group and symmetrical involvement of the deep grey structures occurred in both groups, although more frequently in the ADEM group (Figure 12.12.29). The ADEM lesions tended to be poorly marginated, probably due to the presence of oedema, whereas the MS lesions had more discrete margins (Figure 12.12.30). When there is asymmetrical involvement of the cortical grey matter and symmetrical involvement of the deep grey structures, radiological distinction from an acute viral encephalitis may be difficult.

Follow-up MRI has a role in distinguishing between ADEM and MS. Children with ADEM have no new lesions and complete or partial resolution of the majority of old lesions, though residual gliosis and demyelination may occur in some patients. By comparison, follow-up imaging in both children and adults with MS frequently shows new lesions during relapse and asymptomatic lesions during convalescence.

FURTHER READING

Dale RC, de Sousa C, Chong WK et al. Acute disseminated encephalomyelitis, multiple disseminated encephalomyelitis and multiple sclerosis in children. Brain 2000; 123:2407–2422.

Ebner F, Millner MM, Justich E. Multiple sclerosis in children: value of serial MR studies to monitor patients. American Journal of Neuroradiology 1990; 11:1023–1027.

O'Riordan JI, Gomez-Anson B, Moseley IF, Miller DH. Long term follow up of patients with post infectious encephalomyelitis: evidence for a monophasic disease. Journal of Neurological Sciences 1999; 167:132–136.

SUBACUTE SCLEROSING PANENCEPHALITIS

Subacute sclerosing panencephalitis (SSPE) is a disease that predominantly affects children. It is characterized by behavioural changes and mental deterioration followed by ataxia, myoclonia and seizures. Severe dementia, quadriparesis and autonomic failure eventually ensue. The age of onset ranges from 1 to 35 years of age with a mean age of 7; most children are between 5 and 15 at presentation. Half the children have measles infection before the age of 2 and the infection appears to be related to reactivation of the virus many years later. The reason for reactivation of the virus is unclear and is thought to be related to the failure of patients to produce antibodies to the specific virus protein.

Magnetic resonance imaging may be normal in the first few months. Subsequently, lesions start in the cortex and subcortical white matter and spread to the periventricular white matter and corpus callosum (Figure 12.12.31). Basal ganglia changes are seen in about a third of affected patients, usually late on in the disease. In the final stages, T2 abnormalities are seen in the brainstem and

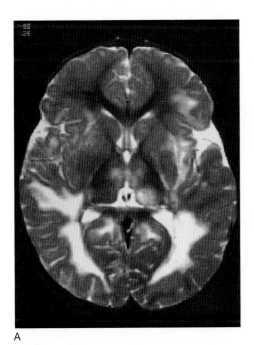
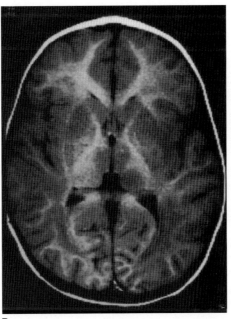

A   B

Figure 12.12.29 (A) Axial T1- and (B) T2-weighted images of a child who presented 2 weeks after an upper respiratory tract infection and was found to have acute disseminated demyelination (ADEM) on the basis of imaging. Confluent asymmetrical T2 high and T1 low signal is seen throughout the cerebral white matter with some sparing of the frontal lobes. Additional asymmetrical poorly marginated lesions are seen in the basal ganglia.

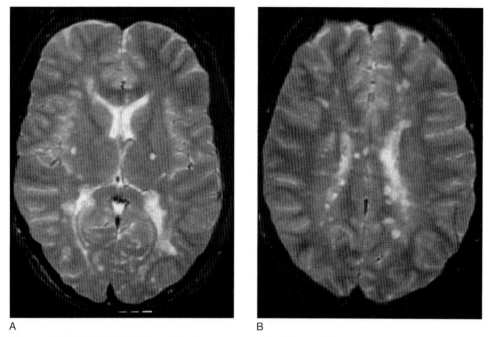

Figure 12.12.30 (A,B) Typical radiological appearances of a 15-year-old male with multiple sclerosis who has multiple well marginated high signal lesions on T$_2$-weighted axial images, concentrated in the periventricular white matter and corpus callosum.

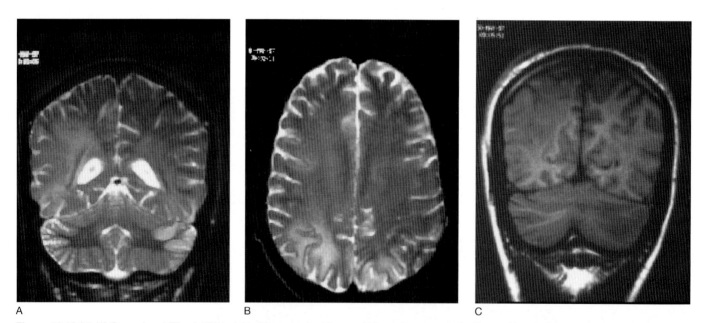

Figure 12.12.31 (A) Coronal and (B) axial T2-weighted images of a 16-year-old boy who presented with cognitive decline and behavioural changes. Subacute sclerosing panencephalitis is characterized by bilateral high-signal lesions in the grey and white matter of the cerebellar and cerebral hemispheres. (C) Pre- and postcontrast coronal T1-weighted images demonstrate the absence of mass effect and enhancement.

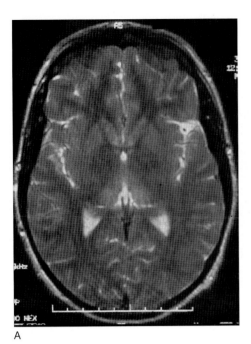 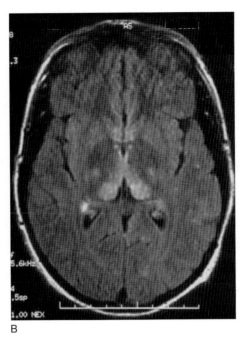

A   B

Figure 12.12.32 Typical MRI appearances of variant Creutzfeldt–Jakob disease. The symmetrical high signal in the posterior thalamus (pulvinar) and the dorsal lateral nuclei result in a 'hockey stick' appearance on both axial (A) T2-weighted and (B) FLAIR images. The changes are more conspicuous on the FLAIR image.

atrophy develops. The extent of the lesions correlate poorly with the clinical state.

FURTHER READING

Akdal G, Baklan B, Cakmakci H, Kovanlikya A. MRI follow up of basal ganglia involvement of subacute sclerosing panencephalitis. Pediatric Neurology 2001; 24:393–395.

Anlar B, Saatci I, Klöse G, Yalaz K. MRI findings in subacute sclerosing panencephalitis. Brain Development 1993; 15:345–355.

Brismar G, Gascon GG, Von Steyen KV, Bohlega S. Subacute sclerosing panencephalitis: evaluation with CT and MR. American Journal of Neuroradiology 1996; 17:761–772.

Cruzado D, Masserey-Spicher V, Roux L et al. Early onset and rapidly progressive subacute sclerosing panencephalitis after congenital measles infection. European Journal of Pediatrics 2002; 161:438–441.

NEW VARIANT CREUTZFELDT–JAKOB DISEASE

New variant Creutzfeldt–Jakob disease (CJD) is one of the subacute spongiform encephalopathies caused by a transmissible protein called a prion and, to date, there have been 147 reported cases in the UK. The combination of a young age at disease onset (mean age of onset 29 years), a prolonged duration of illness, persistent early sensory and psychiatric features, and a non-specific EEG appearance is relatively uniform.

CT scanning is generally normal. The typical MRI features are symmetrical high signal in the posterior thalamus (pulvinar) and the dorsal lateral nuclei, giving a 'hockey stick' appearance (Figure 12.12.32), which are more conspicuous on proton density than T2-weighted imaging. Recent reports have suggested that FLAIR imaging may be more sensitive in the detection of these changes. Appearances correlate with the neuropathology of gliotic change and neuronal loss. The pulvinar changes were found to be 78% sensitive and 95% specific in adults. Wilson's disease and mitochondrial cytopathies may cause similar appearances in children. Other MRI features include increased signal in the caudate head and periaqueductal grey matter.

FURTHER READING

Zeilder M, Collie D, Macleod MA, Sellar RJ, Knight R. FLAIR MRI in sporadic Creutzfeldt-Jakob disease. Neurology 2001; 56:282(letter).

Zeilder M, Sellar RJ, Colllie DA et al. The pulvinar sign on magnetic resonance imaging in variant Creutzfeldt-Jakob disease. Lancet 2000; 335:1412–1418.

Zeilder M, Stewart GE, Barraclough CR et al. New variant Creutzfeldt-Jakob disease; neurological features and diagnostic tests. Lancet 1997; 350:903–907.

RASMUSSEN'S ENCEPHALITIS

Rasmussen's encephalitis is a chronic inflammatory disease of unknown origin that usually affects one hemisphere. In the original description, Rasmussen and coworkers assumed a viral cause but later the disease was linked to circulating autoantibodies. More recently, a cytotoxic T cell reaction against neurones was demonstrated to play a major role but the stimulus for this has not been identified.

The disease is rare and is usually seen in children, although it has been described in adolescents and adults. The typical clinical course is focal onset seizures, characteristically epilepsia partialis continua and a neurological deterioration, most commonly a pro-

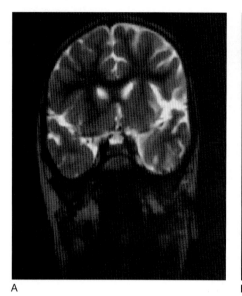
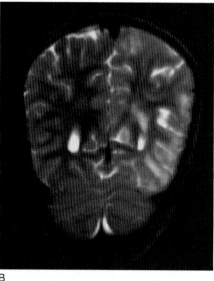
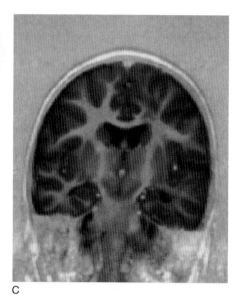

A   B   C

Figure 12.12.33 (A,B) Coronal T2-weighted MR images of a 4-year-old boy who presented with seizures and cognitive decline. The radiological appearances of cortical swelling of the frontotemporal lobes and mild cerebral atrophy are those of Rasmussen's disease. (C) Severe atrophy is seen on the STIR images in the same patient years later. The caudate nucleus and thalamus are atrophic and there is ex vacuo dilatation of the frontal and temporal horns of the lateral ventricle.

gressive hemiparesis. This is followed by a decrease in seizure frequency and stabilization of the hemiparesis.

CT and MRI may be normal in the early course of the disease. Serial MRI reveals a spread of the inflammatory lesion over the affected hemisphere, typically involving the frontal or frontotemporal cortical region. The earliest abnormalities are cortical swelling with high T2/FLAIR signal followed later by atrophy with no cortical signal abnormality evident (Figure 12.12.33). Basal ganglia atrophy has been described in three-quarters of cases in a small series; caudate nucleus involvement was prominent in the majority of cases and putaminal involvement was seen in only 2 of the 21 cases. The clinical course has been correlated to a decreasing number of T cells and reactive astrocytes as assessed by histopathology supporting the theory that the disease is of an active inflammation that burns out later.

FURTHER READING

Bhatjiwale MG, Polkey C, Cox TC, Dean A, Deasy N. Rasmussen's encephalitis: neuroimaging findings in 21 patients with a closer look at the basal ganglia. Pediatric Neurosurgery 1998; 29:142–148.

Bien CG, Bauer J, Deckwerth TL et al. Destruction of neurons by cytotoxic T cells: a new pathogenic mechanism in Rasmussen's encephalitis. Annals of Neurology 2002; 51:311–318.

Bien CG, Urbach H, Deckert M et al. Diagnosis and staging of Rasmussen's encephalitis by serial MRI and histopathology. Neurology 2002; 58:250–257.

Bien CG, Widman G, Urbach H et al. The natural history of Rasmussen's encephalitis. Brain 2002; 125:1751–1759.

He XP, Patel M, Whitney KD et al. Glutamate receptor GluR3 antibodies and death of cortical cells. Neuron 1998; 20:153–163.

Rasmussen T, Olszewski J, Lloyd-Smith D. Focal seizures due to chronic localized encephalitis. Neurology 1958; 8:435–445.

INFECTIONS IN THE IMMUNOCOMPROMISED

In the developed world, children become immunocompromised more commonly from a combination of drug treatment and malignancy than from HIV. Primary causes of immunocompromise such as subacute combined immunodeficiency do occur but are rarely encountered. As vertical transmission accounts for 90% of cases of HIV in children, it is considered in the section on congenital infection (see above). Important causes of immunocompromise in children are diabetes, leukaemia, lymphoma, and prolonged use of antibiotics, corticosteroids, cytotoxic drugs or immunosuppressive treatment. Infections are divided into (1) those that are induced by pathogens and (2) those produced by reactivation of latent infections.

A range of fungal infections, including *Candida*, *Aspergillus* sp. (Figure 12.12.34) and *Mucor* are seen in the immunocompromised. These organisms most commonly cause meningitis (see 'Meningitis and its complications' above), although meningoencephalitis and brain abscesses can also develop (see 'Cerebritis and abscesses' above). In our institution, the Gram-positive bacilli of *Actinomyces* sp., particularly *Actinomyces israelii* and *Nocardia*, and Aspergillosis are recognised causes of intracerebral abscess in the immunocompromised host (Figure 12.12.35). Other infections not specific to the immunocompromised host may be encountered, such as tuberculosis or reactivation of CMV, which can cause encephalitis (see 'Encephalitis'). *Aspergillus* sp. and *Mucor* are associated with sinusitis in immunocompromised children, which may be the source of infection in children who develop meningitis or may cause local aneurysm formation.

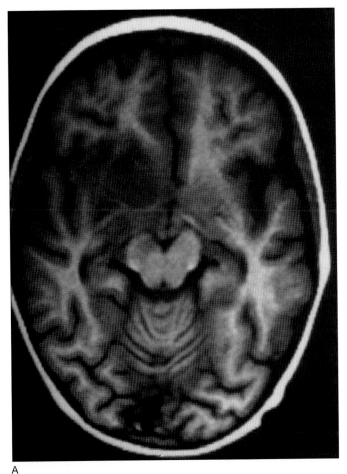 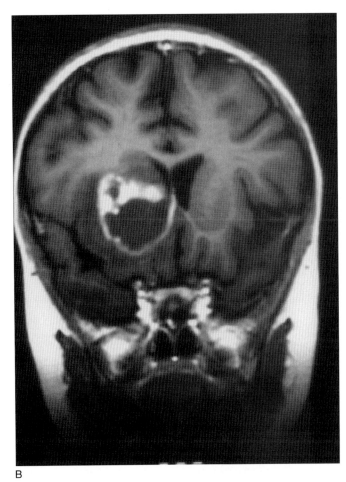

A   B

Figure 12.12.34 (A) Axial pre- and (B) postcontrast T1-weighted images of a 5-year-old child who developed a left hemiparesis whilst receiving chemotherapy for acute lymphoblastic leukaemia. The rim-enhancing low-signal lesion centred on the basal ganglia has a similar appearance to the lesion in Figure 12.12.16. Aspergillosis was diagnosed following surgical drainage.

FURTHER READING

Shrier LA, Schopps JH, Feigin RD. Bacterial and fungal infections of the central nervous system. In: Berg BO, ed. Principles of child neurology. New York: McGraw-Hill; 1996:766–771.

INTRASPINAL INFECTIONS

DISCITIS AND OSTEOMYELITIS

Intervertebral disc infection typically presents in very young children with fever, back pain, irritability and a refusal to walk. The source of the infections is often not identified but it is thought to be due to haematogenous spread. The intervertebral discs of neonates and infants are well vascularized, and the rich supply of vessels to the disc obliterate during development, and from about 13 years of age vessels are not found within the disc on microscopic examination. As a result isolated discitis can occur in childhood but by adulthood, infection starts in the vertebral body and spreads directly to the disc.

Staphylococcus aureus is the most commonly identified organism but in 70% of affected patients an organism is not identified. Other causative organisms include *Streptococcus* sp., Grampositive *Enterococcus*, *Escherichia coli*, *Salmonella* sp., *Pseudomonas aeruginosa* and *Klebsiella* sp. Granulomatous infections can originate from mycobacterium tuberculosis, brucellosis, fungi and parasites including hydatid disease.

MRI is the imaging modality of choice and is more sensitive than plain films and CT, and at least as sensitive as radionucleotide imaging. Plain radiographs are usually normal in the acute phase and after 2–8 weeks may show the typical appearances of disc space narrowing and erosion of the end-plate. Spiral CT scanning has a particular role in CT-guided biopsy for microbiology, and drainage of intradiscal, paraspinal and epidural collections.

The MRI characteristics are severe oedema of the adjacent vertebral marrow (high signal on T2-weighted and low signal on T1-weighted images), disc space narrowing and high signal on T2-weighted images within the disc (Figure 12.12.36). Fat-saturated or short tau inversion recovery (STIR) images improve the conspicuousness of the vertebral body changes. In about 10% of cases, the signal intensity of the disc is low or decreased on the T2-weighted images, especially in the early phase of the disease. L2/3

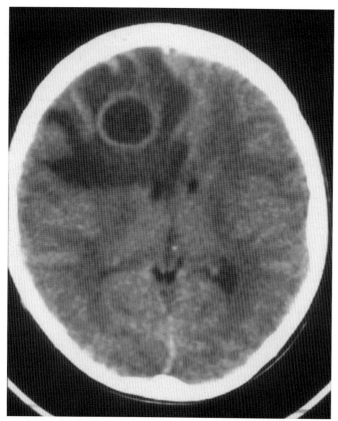

Figure 12.12.35 Enhanced axial CT scan of a 12-year-old immunosuppressed by chemotherapy shows a mass in the right frontal lobe with the typical features of a cerebral abscess and marked surrounding oedema. *Actinomyces* sp. was isolated following surgical drainage.

and L3/4 are the most common disc spaces involved. Because of the well vascularized disc of young children, disc enhancement in this age group can be normal. Chronic infection of the vertebral body may result in collapse and a marked spinal deformity.

The multiplanar capability of MRI allows the demonstration of epidural and paravertebral extension of abscesses, sequestration of bony elements and encroachment of the spinal cord by granulation tissue. Intramedullary abscesses can also result from direct spread from an infected vertebral body or disc, or haematogenous spread. Vascular impairment of the arterial supply to the cord and compression of the epidural veins may result in ischaemia of the cord.

FURTHER READING

Chidambaram B, Balasubramaniam V. Intramedullary abscess of the spinal cord. Paediatric Neurosurgery 2001; 34:43–44.

Crawford A, Kucharczyk W, Rutka J, Smitherman H. Diskitis in children. Clinical Orthopaedics 1991; 266:70–79.

Dagirmanjian A, Schils J, McHenry M, Modic MT. MR imaging of vertebral osteomyelitis revisited. American Journal of Roentgenology 1996; 167:1539–1543.

Onofrio BM. Intervertebral discitis; incidence, diagnosis and management. Clinical Neurosurgery 1980; 27:481–615.

Rubert M, Tillmann B. Lymph node and blood supply of the human intervertebral disc. Acta Orthopaedica Scandinavica 1993; 64:37–40.

Stäbler A, Reiser M. Imaging of spinal infection. Radiology Clinics of North America 2001; 39:115–135.

Sze G, Bravo S, Baierl P et al. Developing spinal column: Gadolinium-enhanced MR imaging. Radiology 1991; 180:497–502.

EPIDURAL EMPYEMA

Spinal epidural empyemas are extremely rare in childhood and associated with osteomyelitis, dermal sinuses (Figure 12.12.37) and direct puncture, e.g. for pain relief and immunosuppression. One third of children do not have a predisposing cause. Spread is usually haematogenous and most commonly caused by *Staphylococcus aureus*. The causative organism in immunocompromised patients is more likely to be unusual, such as *Aspergillus* sp. *Mycobacterium tuberculosis* is a rare cause.

Children classically present with an acute back pain made worse by straining and accompanied by local tenderness 1–2 weeks after an infection. Within a few days, radicular pain develops followed by spinal cord compression. When the infection spreads from an adjacent infected disc, the presentation may be more insidious.

MR imaging is the imaging modality of choice and demonstrates a collection running in the craniocaudal direction in the dorsal epidural space, usually in the lumbar region. The MR signal intensity is variable on precontrast T1-weighted images and usually isodense or hyperintense to CSF on T2-weighted images. The cardinal feature of an epidural empyema is an enhancing epidural collection (Figure 12.12.38). The condition is a neurosurgical emergency as persistent compression of the cord results in thrombosis of the spinal vessels, cord infarction and permanent paralysis.

FURTHER READING

Auletta JJ, John CC. Spinal epidural abscesses in children: a 15-year experience and review of the literature. Clinical Infectious Diseases 2001; 32:9–16.

Barkovitch AJ. Infections of the nervous system. In: Barkovitch, ed. Paediatric neuroimaging. New York: Raven Press; 1995:569–617.

Gupta PK, Mahapatra AK, Gaind R et al. Aspergillus spinal epidural abscess. Paediatric Neurosurgery 2001; 35:18–23.

Numagichi Y, Rigamonti D, Rothman MI et al. Spinal epidural abscess: evaluation with gadolinium-enhanced MR imaging. Radiographics 1993; 13:545–559.

Spears J, Hader W, Drake JM. Spontaneous spinal epidural abscess. Pediatric Neurosurgery 2001; 35:337–338.

MYELITIS AND MYELORADICULITIS

Inflammation of the cord, or myelitis, is more commonly part of ADEM (see above) than due to a direct cord infection. Infective myelitis is usually viral in origin and most commonly caused by enteroviruses. Postinfectious inflammation usually occurs in the presence of cerebral involvement so imaging of the brain in these children is necessary. The radiological appearances of the spinal cord in infectious transverse myelitis and ADEM are similar and

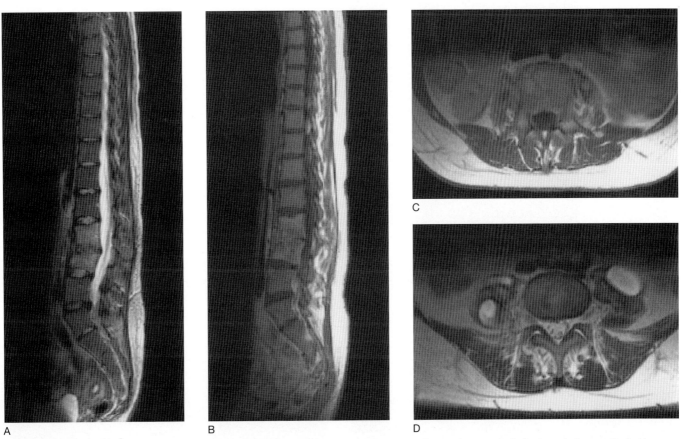

Figure 12.12.36 Images of a 13-year-old child from the Middle East presenting with back pain found to have spinal tuberculosis complicated by psoas abscesses. Sagittal (A) T2-weighted and (B) postcontrast T1-weighted imaging of the lumbar spine demonstrates high signal in the L3 and L4 vertebral bodies and destruction of the L3/4 intervertebral disc. There is enhancement of the vertebral body and intervertebral disc. (C,D) Paravertebral collections at the level of the disc communicate with the psoas muscles abscesses.

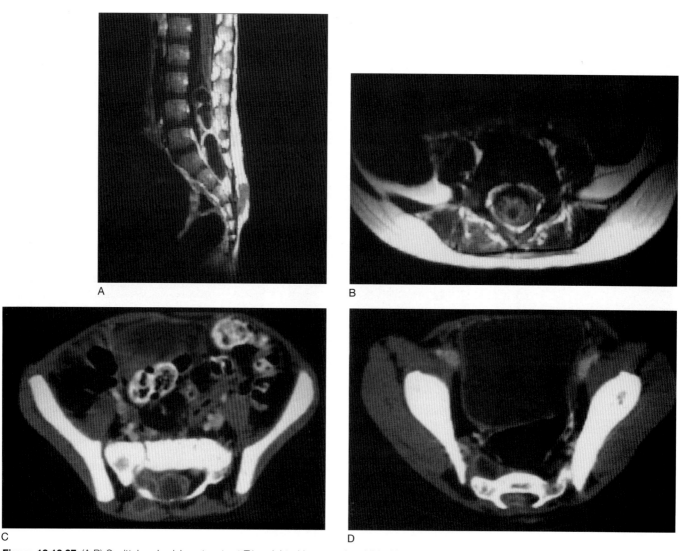

Figure 12.12.37 (A,B) Sagittal and axial postcontrast T1-weighted images of a child with a multiloculated collection surrounding the dura and extending into the overlying soft tissues. *Mycobacterium tuberculosis* was isolated. (C,D) Postcontrast CT scans reveal the deficient posterior arch in addition to the collection. An infected dermoid was resected at surgery.

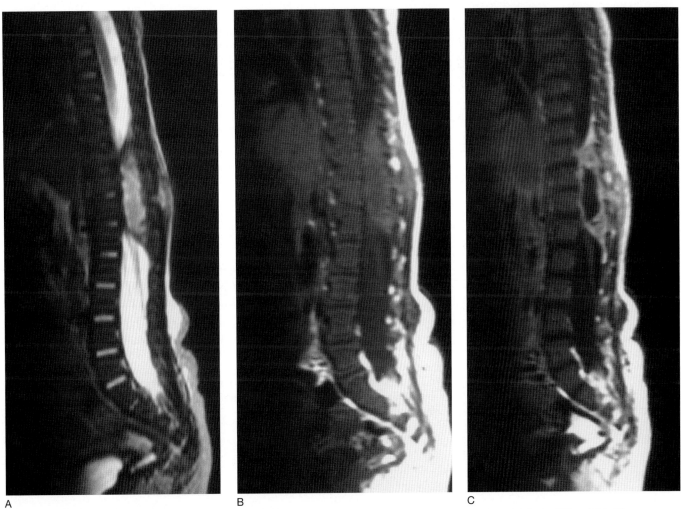

A   B   C

Figure 12.12.38 Epidural empyema in a 2-year-old child following an epidural for pain relief postfundoplication. (A) Sagittal T2-weighted images demonstrate a well-circumscribed collection in the epidural space that is hypodense to CSF. (B,C) Sagittal pre- and postcontrast T1-weighted images reveal marked enhancement of the margins of the collection and a hypointense centre.

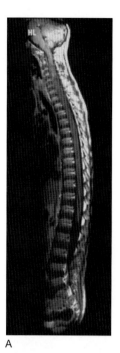
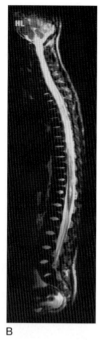

A   B

Figure 12.12.39 Sagittal (A) T1-weighted and (B) T2-weighted images of the spinal cord in a 12-year-old with a renal transplant who presented with a left arm weakness. There is extensive swelling and oedema (low signal on T1-weighted and high signal on T2-weighted images) of the cord. No organism was identified but the symptoms and imaging appearances resolved.

the diagnosis often relies on distinguishing the acute infection from the postinfectious period. Both can cause fusiform swelling of the in the acute phase and the lesions are high signal on T2-weighted and normal or low on T1-weighted images (Figure 12.12.39). The lesions tend to involve most of the diameter of the cord and may be single or multifocal. Cystic necrosis may complicate these conditions. Most of the lesions tend to resolve over a variable period of time but usually within a year. Multiple sclerosis lesions can be differentiated from myelitis when they are peripherally sited within the cord and associated with typical intracranial lesions and progressive disease.

Myeloradiculitis has been reported in middle aged and young adults in association with EBV, HSV and CMV infection; the latter in the context of HIV. Patients present with the clinical features of a myeloradiculopathy and the CSF reflects an inflammatory process. MRI reveals increased signal in the spinal cord and thickening and enhancement of the lumbosacral roots in the cases of EBV and HSV. Enhancement of the leptomeninges over the cord has been reported in a case of proven EBV infection. Although myeloradiculitis has not been reported in children, we have seen cases with similar appearances that resolve spontaneously where an organism has not been identified.

Pyogenic abscesses of the cord are very rare and usually complicate a congenital CSF fistula. Granulomas due to tuberculosis are also rare in children but they can cause intramedullary swelling and arachnoiditis.

FURTHER READING

Kusuhara T, Nakajima M, Inoue H, Takahashi M, Yamada T. Parainfectious encephalomyeloradiculitis associated with herpes simplex virus I DNA in cerebrospinal fluid. Clinical Infectious Diseases 2002; 34:1199–1205.

Majid A, Galetta SL, Sweeny CJ et al. Epstein-Barr virus myeloradiculitis and encephalomyeloradiculitis. Brain 2002; 125:159–165.

Tselis A, Duman R, Storch GA, Lisak RP. Epstien-Barr virus encephalomyelitis diagnosed by polymerase chain reaction: detection of the genome in the CSF. Neurology 1997; 48:1351–1355.

ACKNOWLEDGEMENTS

Some of the images were obtained by Dr W K Chong whilst visiting the Children's Hospital of Philadelphia and The Hospital for Sick Children, Toronto. We thank Dr Robert Zimmerman (CHOP) and Dr Susan Blaser (Toronto) for assisting in their acquisition. Particular thanks goes to Dr Rose de Bruyn, Great Ormond Street Hospital, for providing the ultrasound images of the lenticulostriate vasculopathy.

Intracranial Tumours

*Charles Raybaud, Olivier Levrier,
Nadine Girard*

Cerebral tumours are relatively more frequent in children than in adults. Tumours arising in the nervous system are the second most common type of tumour in this age group with those arising in the haematopoietic system being the most common. Brain cancers in general have a poor prognosis. Cerebral tumours in children are histologically more varied than those in adults; conversely, tumours usually found in adults (glioblastomas, metastases, meningiomas) are very uncommon in children. The tumours in children are located more frequently in the posterior fossa (about 50%), and around the third ventricle, and involve the cerebral hemispheres much less commonly: their clinical expressions therefore include hydrocephalus, visual defects and endocrine disorders. Some are congenital, while others are developmental and are clinically expressed by severe epilepsy. Finally, paediatric brain tumours often disseminate through the cerebrospinal fluid (CSF) along the ependymal surface of the ventricles and within the intracranial and spinal subarachnoid spaces. The preoperative diagnosis depends both on the radiological features of the mass on computed tomography (CT) and magnetic resonance imaging (MRI), and on the topography of the lesion.

CLINICAL PRESENTATION

Paediatric brain tumours are often located along the midline; hydrocephalus is frequent. Involvement of the cortical structures is uncommon and so are seizures.

INTRACRANIAL HYPERTENSION

Signs of increased intracranial pressure – headaches, vomiting, drowsiness, decreased attention, regression – are extremely frequent. In infants, the fontanelle is tense. In older children, macrocephaly is rare, unless the tumour is slow growing. Fundoscopy is useful, by showing papilloedema. If plain radiographs of the skull were made, they might show splayed sutures and digital markings, changes in the morphology of the skull base and local thinning of the vault as well as calcification. However, the value of the investigation is limited; it is not really needed as it can be more usefully replaced by CT or MRI.

NEUROLOGICAL SYMPTOMS AND SIGNS

The neurological examination is more important and the following should be looked for:

- Abnormalities related to the brainstem : (1) long tracts and pyramidal syndromes; (2) vestibular syndrome; and (3) cranial nerve involvement manifesting as oculomotor palsies, incoordinated gaze, nystagmus, Parinaud syndrome, facial palsy, trouble of phonation or swallowing and trigeminal related signs.
- Cerebellar syndromes: dysmetria, instability and incoordination of movement, especially ocular movements.
- Visual impairment: amblyopia, visual field defects and optic atrophy.
- Abnormal tone: torticollis, posterior hypertonicity and decerebrate rigidity.
- Seizures are uncommon, as hemispheric tumours are uncommon, but do occur when the tumour involves the cortex. These may be slow growing tumours and the seizures are one of the presenting symptoms. They may also be developmental tumours and present clinically as a chronic, often refractory epilepsy. In infants, tumour-related epilepsy may present as a West syndrome – infantile spasms and specific EEG abnormalities.

ENDOCRINE STATUS

The endocrine status may be very informative when the tumour is located in the anterior-inferior part of the 3rd ventricle:

- Alterations in the rate of growth or weight: A sudden arrest of growth is a very significant symptom.
- Hypothalamic disorders: Russell's syndrome, hypothalamic obesity.
- Precocious, delayed or absent puberty.

- Diabetes insipidus (DI): a child with DI in whom no explanatory lesion is found should be investigated again in the following months, as germinomas may not be macroscopically apparent for several months or years.

IMAGING METHODS

ULTRASOUND

In the case of infantile tumours, US can be used to rule out other causes of increased intracranial pressure. Modern US equipment yields good images of the parenchyma. It demonstrates hydrocephalus, the mass, its effect on the brain and its location, and may even be sufficient for the diagnosis (e.g. an intraventricular tumour is a choroid plexus papilloma). However, this imaging is limited to young infants as it lacks specificity and the morphological evaluation as a rule needs to be complemented by a more detailed study, usually by MRI.

COMPUTED TOMOGRAPHY

In most cases, this is still the first requested investigation when a physician is faced with a neurological disorder. Except in rare instances, it can diagnose the brain tumour – the lesion, its location, its effects on the parenchyma, its mode of enhancement, its texture, whether it is haemorrhagic and/or necrotic and whether it is well demarcated or infiltrative. Now that MRI is readily available, the role of CT has altered. CT helps to suggest the histological nature of the tumour by showing calcium or fat when performed without contrast injection. It shows the density of the tumour (increased in PNET and germinal tumours mostly) better than MRI and demonstrates subtle calcifications that might not be apparent on MRI. Bone involvement is better depicted by CT. Although no directly related complications as a result of using ionizing radiation have been clinically observed with the use of CT, it is probably better to avoid it as much as possible in young patients. For presurgical evaluation, the better views of anatomy (in various adapted planes) and the better definition (to show the limits of the lesion) that modern, high-definition MRI provides is necessary. CT, if not carried out before MRI, may be useful as a complementary investigation.

MAGNETIC RESONANCE IMAGING

Magnetic resonance imaging has become the imaging modality of choice for investigating the central nervous system and especially for its tumours. It not only gives superb information about the anatomy and condition of the brain, but also gives information about diverse structural, functional, and metabolic changes. Modern equipment is fast but sedation (preferably general anaesthesia) is still needed in young or uncooperative patients. The benefits of MRI are related to the absence of any identified harmful effects, the multiplanarity capability and the ability to use different sequences based on different parameters offering detailed information on the texture of the tissues and the status of the blood–brain barrier (BBB). MR angiography is now a reliable method for the study of the main cerebral arteries and veins. Apart from conventional anatomical MR images, MR technology is now also capable of identifying the circulation of the CSF (by CSF flow imaging), the status of the water compartments by diffusion imaging, the local metabolite contents by MR spectroscopy, the functional anatomy of the cortex by functional MRI, the extent of the vascularity in and around the tumour by perfusion imaging and, more prospectively, the structural anatomy of the white matter by diffusion tensor imaging (DTI).

The imaging protocols usually combine conventional and complementary studies. An important point to remember is that in infants, the design of the imaging sequences should be adapted to the degree of maturation of the brain. Although they may be difficult to apply because of the tumour-related distortion of the anatomy, the reference planes of imaging, bi-commissural or bi-hippocampal, should be respected as much as possible. The minimum protocol includes sagittal (usually T1-weighted), axial and coronal (usually T2-weighted and FLAIR) planes, and T1-weighted images after contrast injection in all three planes. These sequences provide the information about the precise location of the tumour in relation to the surrounding structures, its texture, its limited or infiltrative character, the associated necrosis, haemorrhage and oedema, and whether the blood–brain barrier (BBB) is intact or not. The use of magnetization transfer imaging or of fat saturation imaging, especially in younger children, may enhance the contrast in these postgadolinium images. Because many types of tumours encountered in children tend to disseminate in the subarachnoid spaces (drop metastases) a complete cranial and spinal investigation is often necessary preoperatively, as surgery may induce confusing transient enhancing lesions in the meninges, even at a distance from the operative field.

In practice, the MR evaluation of brain tumours often stops there. However, further possible applications are available if required. MR angiography is now good enough to provide useful images of the proximal portion of the brain vessels, and to replace conventional angiography in most of the indications that remain in the assessment of tumours. Perfusion imaging differentiates a high vascularity from an impaired or absent BBB and evaluates the perfusion of the adjacent tissues. Diffusion imaging is useful for differentiating between true cysts and cyst-like lesions. Proton MR spectroscopy allows identification of neural from non-neural tumours, germ-line tumours and possibly the identification of malignant areas in a generally benign-looking mass; it should be performed before gadolinium contrast agent is administered, as contrast reduces the peak of choline by about 15%. When the intraventricular CSF pathway is obliterated, CSF flow imaging helps in deciding between an extracranial (ventriculoperitoneal) or an internal (ventriculocisternal) drainage. Functional MRI and eventually DTI may help in identifying resection margins that will preserve as much functional tissue as possible.

Whereas CT brings quantitative images (made pixel by pixel according to the Hounsfield unit scale), MRI brings only qualitative images. The window setting has to be adapted individually according to what needs to be shown and the end result depends a great deal on the vision of the attending radiologist. Of course, MRI may miss tiny calcifications, which can be useful in assessing the nature of the tumour. Also, the MR signal does not necessarily reflect the cellular density or the nucleo-plasmic ratio. For these reasons, CT, without contrast enhancement, is still useful in the preoperative assessment of brain tumours in children.

ANGIOGRAPHY

Very few indications remain for conventional intra-arterial angiography in the evaluation of brain tumours in children, as most of the differential diagnosis can be made from MR imaging and MR angiography. It may still be useful in certain types of highly vascularized tumours, such as choroid plexus or dural tumours, or the infrequent haemangioblastoma and rhabdoid tumours. Also, its use as a therapeutic medium for embolization or chemotherapeutic agent infusion should not be neglected as a preliminary or a complementary step to traditional surgery or chemotherapy in selected cases.

MYELOGRAPHY

When adequate postcontrast spinal cord MRI studies were not possible, myelography was used to evaluate spinal spread of the tumour. Because a lumbar tap is dangerous whenever there is an increased intracranial pressure, it was only performed after surgery, causing false positive results. The modern approach is to perform MR spinal imaging before surgery and nowadays there is no indication for myelography and myelo-CT in brain tumours. The same is not completely true for the presurgical evaluation of some other pathologies, such as the spinal malformations.

PATHOLOGICAL-RADIOLOGICAL FEATURES OF BRAIN TUMOURS

Many histological types of cerebral tumours are encountered in children. They develop from all cell types present in the brain. To this should be added specific tumour types derived from poorly differentiated neural cells. The evolution and invasiveness of these diverse tumours is extremely variable: some are stable (dysembryoplastic neuroepithelial tumour, DNT); others, in some instances, may double their volume in weeks or even days; and some may sometimes regress spontaneously (optic gliomas). Dissemination to the subarachnoid space is common for medulloblastomas or germinomas, which are malignant tumours, but not exceptional for juvenile pilocytic astrocytomas, which are benign. Imaging identification of the tumour type depends mainly on its appearance on the various MR sequences and on plain CT without contrast agent, on the type of contrast enhancement and on the tumour location, as well as on the evolution of symptoms and age of onset in a clinical context. As a rule, enhancement by contrast media, oedema or infiltration are not always indicative of malignancy. Haemorrhage and necrosis are more significant. The most significant character of malignancy is probably tumour invasion across anatomical barriers such as the leptomeningeal spaces, although seeding has also been observed with benign gliomas. A

classification of the tumours of the CNS has been devised by the World Health Organization (WHO); however, the various types of tumours encountered in children will be considered here according to their clinical incidence and importance.

JUVENILE PILOCYTIC ASTROCYTOMA (JPA)
(Figures 12.13.1 to 12.13.6)

As indicated by its name this tumour is specific to children and is the most common tumour type in this age group. It is a slow-growing benign lesion and usually develops along the midline, cerebellum, cord and medulla, dorsal pons, anterior third ventricle and anterior optic pathways. It should be remembered here that the optic 'nerves' are not real nerves but ocular extensions of the diencephalic white matter. JPA is classified as grade 1 by the WHO. It is usually sporadic but its association with neurofibromatosis type 1 (NF1) is significant: 15% of cases of NF1 present with a pilocytic astrocytoma, usually optic and anterior 3rd ventricle, and 30% of the optic gliomas are observed in a context of NF1 (Figure 12.13.7). The tumour is characterized by elongated, uni- or bipolar astrocytes with hair-like processes, forming pilocytic areas intermingled with microcysts. These microcysts may coalesce to form huge cystic components, especially in the cerebellar location. Although a nuclear pleomorphism and a marked vascular proliferation are observed, there are no signs of malignancy and the mitotic index is very low. There may be invasion of the meninges, particularly with optic nerve gliomas and occasional seeding in the subarachnoid spaces. The tumour may be well circumscribed as in the cord and cerebellum, or more infiltrative, as in the optic pathways. Occasionally, the tumour is multicentric; it may develop as a malignant lesion in exceptional cases, seemingly more often after radiotherapy. It may be histologically associated with ganglion cells, then forming a ganglioglioma (see below).

The imaging features of the juvenile pilocytic astrocytoma reflect its histology:

- Location. JPA are usually found in the cerebellum, the cord, the medulla, the dorsal pons with an exophytic extension towards the 4th ventricle, the hypothalamus and the anterior optic pathways, where it is, rarely, circumscribed to one optic nerve, making surgical removal easy. More commonly, it infiltrates the chiasm together with parts of the optic nerves, the anterior 3rd ventricle, the optic tracts, and the base of the brain. Occasionally, it is found in the cerebral hemispheres but in such cases a ganglioglioma with a largely predominant glial component should be suspected. Multiple locations are uncommon but do occur.
- Appearance. JPAs may be solid, cystic or both. In the cerebellum and the medulla, they are commonly markedly cystic (Figures 12.13.1 and 12.13.2). Cysts may infrequently develop in optic pathway tumours also. The content of the cyst looks different from CSF on MRI sequences and CT. It has a higher signal on T1-weighted (T1-W) and T2-weighted (T2-W) images because of a higher protein content. Multiple cysts may have different appearances. The solid portion has a low signal on T1-W and a high signal on T2-W images, because of its high water content due to microcysts. It has a low density on CT. Occasionally, necrotic and even haemorrhagic areas are observed,

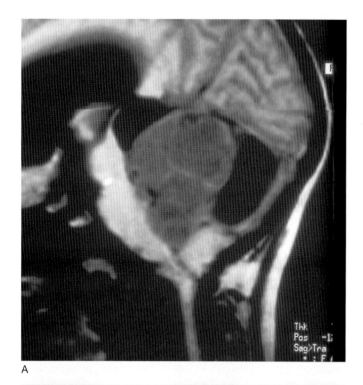

A

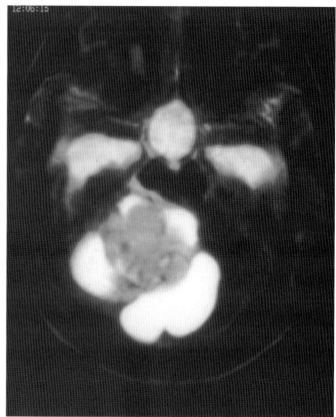

B

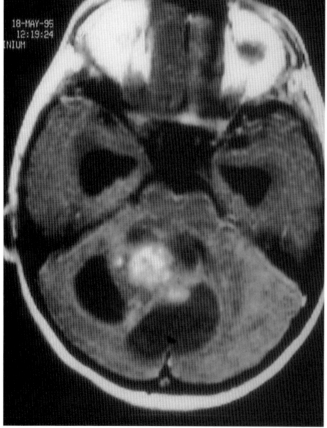

C

Figure 12.13.1 Juvenile pilocytic astrocytoma of the cerebellum, with a low T1-W signal on the sagittal cut (A), a high T2-W signal on the axial cut (B) and clear enhancement of the solid portion (C) surrounded by cysts.

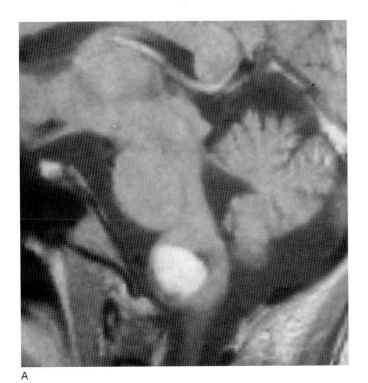

A

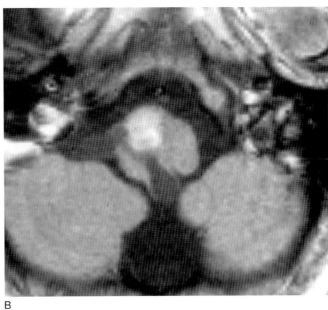

B

Figure 12.13.2 Juvenile pilocytic astrocytoma of the medulla oblongata. Sagittal (A) and axial (B) planes: transmedullary tumour with an anterior enhanced solid portion and a posterior cyst.

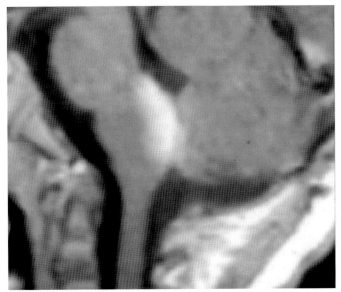

Figure 12.13.3 Juvenile pilocytic astrocytoma of the dorsal pons and medulla, bulging towards the ventricular lumen (T1-W, enhanced).

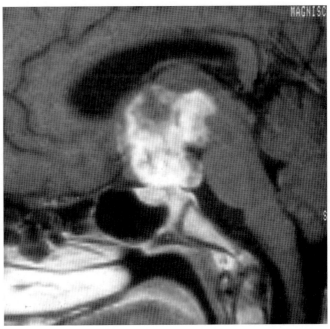

Figure 12.13.4 Juvenile pilocytic astrocytoma of the hypothalamus, extending towards both the ventricular lumen and the interpeduncular cistern, behind the optic chiasm (T1-W, enhanced).

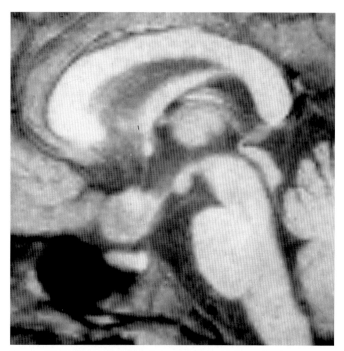

Figure 12.13.5 Juvenile pilocytic astrocytoma of the optic chiasm, sparing the hypothalamus (T1-W without contrast).

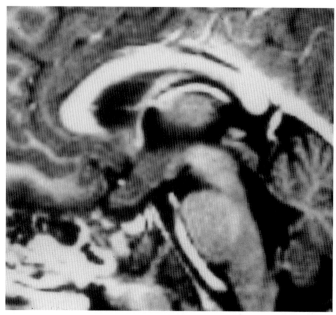

Figure 12.13.7 Juvenile pilocytic astrocytoma in a patient with NF1. The tumour involves the anterior optic pathways as well as the hypothalamus. It is not enhanced by the contrast agent (T1-W with contrast).

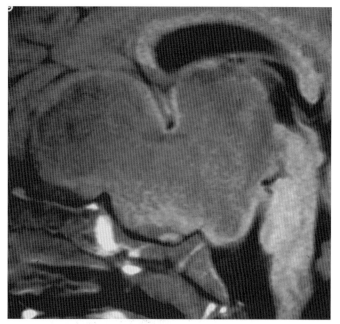

Figure 12.13.6 Juvenile pilocytic astrocytoma with major extension into the 3rd ventricle as well as anteriorly, under the frontal lobes (T1-W without contrast).

which do not indicate malignancy. Drop metastases at a distance from the main tumour into the cisterns and spinal canal may occur. Calcification is uncommon.

• Enhancement. JPAs are highly vascularized tumours with a deficient BBB and therefore typically show marked enhancement (Figures 12.13.1 to 12.13.6). This enhancement obviously does not mean that the lesion is malignant. In the cystic components,

a layering of contrast may be observed at the bottom of the cyst. Infrequently, the wall of the cyst is enhanced also but usually only the solid part of the tumour, the so-called mural nodule, enhances. In the anterior 3rd ventricular and optic gliomas, the enhancement may only affect a portion of the tumour, making the identification of its limits difficult. In NF1-related gliomas, the enhancement, which is often mild, commonly recedes and disappears over time. On rare occasions, histologically typical sporadic JPAs do not enhance at all, even at the time of diagnosis.

• Proton MR spectroscopy is peculiar in the way that it demonstrates a low NAA to choline ratio, similar to the pattern seen in malignant tumours.

DIFFUSE ASTROCYTOMAS

Diffuse astrocytomas are seen mostly in adults, where they are usually located in the cerebral hemispheres. However, they are found also in children, in whom brainstem diffuse astrocytomas (Figure 12.13.8) are the most common form, which are more specifically seen in the pons. These tumours infiltrate the brain tissue but cause little destruction and therefore have relatively mild neurological manifestations, despite appearing large on imaging at the time of the discovery. Infiltration tends to follow the fibre bundles, such as the cerebellar peduncles. Complete surgical removal is as a rule impossible, as major neural structures are included within the mass. Depending on the dominant cell morphology, they are described as fibrillary astrocytomas (the most common), gemistocytic astrocytomas or protoplasmic astrocytomas. The cell density is low, with microcystic cavities that may dominate the histological picture. All diffuse astrocytomas tend to

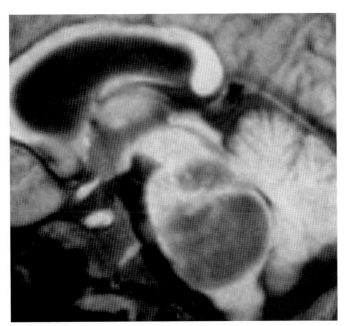

Figure 12.13.8 Infiltrating fibrillary astrocytoma of the brainstem. The neoplasm is located within most of the pons, ill-defined and heterogeneous (T1-W without contrast).

become more malignant with time. According to their malignancy, they are classified as low-grade glioma (grade II), anaplastic glioma (grade III) and glioblastoma (grade IV). The cellular density, the heterogeneity of the tumour, the cellular pleomorphism and the nuclear atypias increase with malignancy.

On imaging, the tumour appears as an ill-defined lesion that is already large at the time of discovery. In the brainstem, it is centred in the pons (Figure 12.13.8), more on its ventral side. The pons is often hugely enlarged, reducing the cisternal spaces and displacing the 4th ventricle posteriorly; but because the pons is enlarged, the ventricle is enlarged also and paradoxically there is no hydrocephalus, or only a mild one. The superficial layer of tissue covering the brainstem usually seems to be preserved, yet the tumour is often exophytic and extends into the cisterns, and characteristically tends to encase the basilar artery. Although there is some diffusion towards the midbrain or medulla, these tend to be compressed rather than invaded. The mass may be symmetrical or more eccentric and commonly invades the middle cerebellar peduncles. The difference between tumour and oedema is difficult to ascertain. The tumour has a low signal on T1-W and a high signal on T2-W images, is occasionally homogeneous and sometimes has areas suggestive of increased cellularity, which may be more malignant, or of necrosis. Coexistence of areas of old and recent haemorrhage can be seen. Typically, there is no enhancement at the first investigation but over time, areas of hypervascularity surrounding areas of necrosis develop, indicating increased malignancy. Distant dissemination of the tumour, especially into the ventricles, may be observed. CT is not particularly helpful for the diagnosis, showing the enlargement of the pons, the displacement of the 4th ventricle and the low density only. The current treatments for these tumours have little effect and the prognosis is generally poor.

Outside the pons, diffuse astrocytomas may be observed in the midbrain, commonly associated with a bilateral extension into the thalami. It may be discovered as a primarily malignant anaplastic glioma (Figure 12.13.9) or, even in children, as a typical glioblastoma: significant mass effect with oedema, central necrosis surrounded by an irregular ring of higher cellular density and irregular peripheral enhancement, usually into the cerebral hemispheres. Diffuse lesions or multicentric lesions indicate a cerebral gliomatosis.

OTHER GLIOMAS

GLIOMATOSIS CEREBRI

The rare condition gliomatosis cerebri is defined by the infiltration of a large part of the brain by a glial tumoral process, affecting large areas of the hemispheres, as well as of the posterior fossa. This extensive involvement contrasts with an often mild clinical picture, with subtle deficits, headaches and changes in mental status. Histologically, it is usually composed of elongated astrocytes. Oligodendrocytic forms may also occur, which infiltrate the myelinated fibre tracts, with a variable mitotic activity but little vascular proliferation. Imaging (Figure 12.13.10) shows abnormal signals or abnormal densities dispersed throughout the parenchyma, with usually little mass effect and no enhancement with contrast agents. In the late stages, a frankly malignant picture may appear with ill-defined heterogeneous enhancement. In typical forms, a biopsy may be needed to ascertain the diagnosis.

OLIGODENDROGLIOMAS

The reported incidence of oligodendrogliomas in childhood varies from centre to centre. They are infrequent in children. These tumours involve the cortex and the adjacent white matter and therefore express themselves by longstanding focal seizures. On imaging, oligodendrogliomas appear as more or less well-demarcated lesions that are hypodense on CT, hypointense on T1-weighted MRI, hyperintense on T2-weighted MRI, usually homogeneous and unenhancing; in fact, they are not essentially different from the diffuse astrocytic glioma, except for a preferential location in the hemispheres. In children, they seem to be less calcified and less typically located in the cerebral poles than in young adults. They may become malignant or a predominantly oligodendroglial malignant tumour may be observed.

PLEOMORPHIC XANTHOASTROCYTOMAS

This is a rare neoplasm predominantly seen in children. It is a well-demarcated cerebral cortical tumour with cystic and solid components, yellowish in colour. The histology is variable, with characteristic multinucleated fat-filled giant cells, together with associated smaller cells with astroglial marking and moderate cellularity. MR imaging demonstrates cortical, heterogeneous tumours that are partly cystic, well demarcated, roughly isointense on T1-W and T2-W sequences and with partial enhancement.

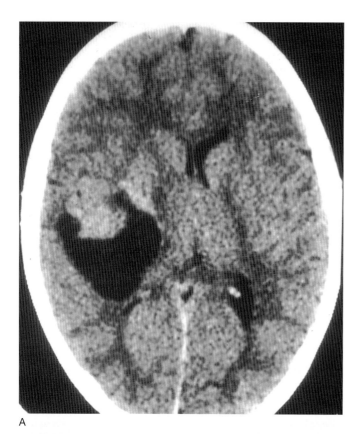

A

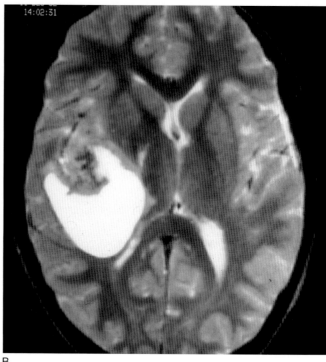

B

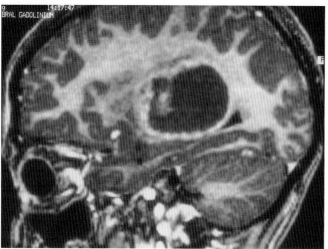

C

Figure 12.13.9 Anaplastic astrocytoma. The tumour is both solid and cystic, the solid nodule being dense on CT (A), heterogeneous and partly haemorrhagic on T2-W images (B). After contrast administration, the rim around the cyst is enhanced (C).

MEDULLOBLASTOMA

After juvenile pilocytic astrocytoma, medulloblastoma of the cerebellum is the second most common brain tumour in children, occurring mostly, but not exclusively, between the ages of 4 and 10 years. Males are more often affected than females. It is characterized by a poorly differentiated neural cell of uncertain origin with a large nucleus and small cytoplasm. Diverse cell types (neuronal, astrocytic and mesenchymal) are observed histologically.

Clinically, the children develop a progressive hydrocephalus, with papilloedema, lethargy and vomiting. Splitting of the cranial sutures is visible on skull x-rays. Acute tumoral haemorrhage or oedema may precipitate the worsening of the clinical condition, because of the sudden increase of the mass effect against the brainstem, or by inferior herniation through the foramen magnum or superiorly, transtentorially, through the tentorium. The tumour typically appears as a well-demarcated compact mass found in the roof of the 4th ventricle, usually to the lower portion of the vermis. It may also develop from the upper portion of the vermis or even

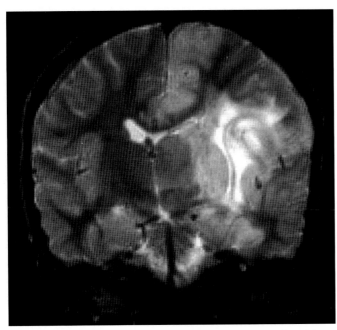

Figure 12.13.10 Gliomatosis cerebri. Diffuse signal abnormality of the left hemisphere, affecting both grey and white matter, contrasting with a minimal clinical deficit in this 9-year-old girl (biopsy proven).

be totally enclosed within the cerebellum with no contact with the CSF spaces. This type of medulloblastoma, which is usually seen in older patients, is called a desmoplastic medulloblastoma and carries a much better prognosis. The expansion is typically within the ventricular lumen, with progressive hydrocephalus. It is a malignant tumour, although amenable to cure in a significant proportion of cases by using a combination of surgery, chemotherapy and radiotherapy. It tends to invade the meninges, either by forming drop metastases into the spinal canal, the intracranial cisterns and the supratentorial subarachnoid spaces, or by infiltrating the pia over the brainstem, the cerebellar folia and the spinal cord.

On neuroimaging (Figure 12.13.11), medulloblastomas appear characteristically as a well-demarcated, compact mass in the centre of the posterior fossa, typically capped by the lumen of the 4th ventricle. On sagittal cuts, it extends upwards from the lower portion of the vermis, compressing and displacing the ventricular lumen, independently from the brainstem, which tends to be pushed forward rather than invaded. Lateral medulloblastomas may extend into the middle cerebellar peduncles; superior ones may extend into the culmen towards the ambient cistern. The mass is finely heterogeneous, has a low T1-W and high T2-W signal on MR images and is sometimes finely haemorrhagic. On unenhanced CT, the tumour appears hyperdense with respect to the cerebellar folia, because of the high nucleo-plasmic ratio. It may be calcified. On CT and MRI, it is usually well enhanced with contrast agent, often with a prominent vessel seen in the centre of the mass. Because of the high metastatic potential of the tumour (Figure 12.13.12), the whole meningeal space should be assessed for dissemination during the preoperative examination.

This typical form of medulloblastoma is observed in roughly half of all cases. Less typical forms include the small principal tumours with diffuse metastatic meningitis (Figure 12.13.13), massive haemorrhagic tumours, and massive oedematous and

necrotic tumours. As a clinical rule, atypical tumours carry a worse prognosis than the typical ones, perhaps because of a higher malignancy, a higher operative complication rate and a higher potential for metastatic diffusion. On rare occasions, histologically typical medulloblastomas may be found in the supratentorial space.

The desmoplastic medulloblastoma presents differently. It occurs in older patients and is located more superficially in the lateral part of the cerebellar hemispheres. It is characterized by an intense network of reticulin isolating the tumour's nodules (Figure 12.13.14). Desmoplastic medulloblastomas do not disseminate and have a much better prognosis. They are about 10 times less frequent than the classical form.

EPENDYMOMAS

This is a group of ependymal neoplasms including not only the classical ependymoma but also the anaplastic ependymomas, the myxopapillary ependymoma and the ependymoblastoma. The two former types are not distinguished by medical imaging. Myxopapillary ependymomas develop in the conus medullaris and the filum terminale. Ependymoblastomas are undifferentiated neuroectodermal tumours, somewhat comparable to the medulloblastoma. Another subvariety of the tumour, the subependymoma, is observed mainly in adults.

The classical ependymoma is observed either in the posterior fossa or in the cerebral hemispheres, the former mostly in younger children. In the posterior fossa, its clinical features include intracranial hypertension with hydrocephalus, vomiting, neck pain and/or torticollis, brainstem-related symptoms and swallowing difficulties. In the supratentorial space, intracranial hypertension, neurological deficit and seizures are more common. The ependymomas are tumours of intermediate cellularity, with relatively 'normal' ependymal cells, often forming rosettes or other cavities, and a heterogeneous fibrillary background. The mitotic activity is low. Necrosis and haemorrhages are not uncommon. In the 4th ventricle, the tumour extends from the ependymal lining of the floor of the cerebellar peduncles and, more rarely, from the roof. Typically, instead of filling the ventricle as a medulloblastoma would do, ependymomas tend to grow outside the ventricular lumen, towards the cisterna magna, the upper cervical spine and the cerebello-pontine angle cistern, where they mingle with the lower cranial nerves. Microcalcifications may develop in the mass. In the supratentorial space, the tumour develops from the walls of the lateral ventricles both into the ventricle and into the parenchyma, forming complex masses with solid and cystic portions, often markedly calcified.

On MR imaging, a posterior fossa ependymoma (Figure 12.13.15) appears as a mass in the inferior part of the 4th ventricle with a low T1-W and high T2-W signal. Characteristically, the tumour extends towards the perimedullary cisterns down to the upper cervical spine, posteriorly and/or laterally, displacing and encasing the brainstem. Assessing this extension is important since much of the surgical difficulties are related to the anatomical relationships of the tumour with the ventricular floor and the lower cranial nerves. On CT, the density of the mass is heterogeneous, iso- and hypodense in respect to the adjacent cerebellum. Hyperdensities may be seen, suggesting calcifications or small haemorrhages. On MRI and CT, the tumour usually enhances clearly, with

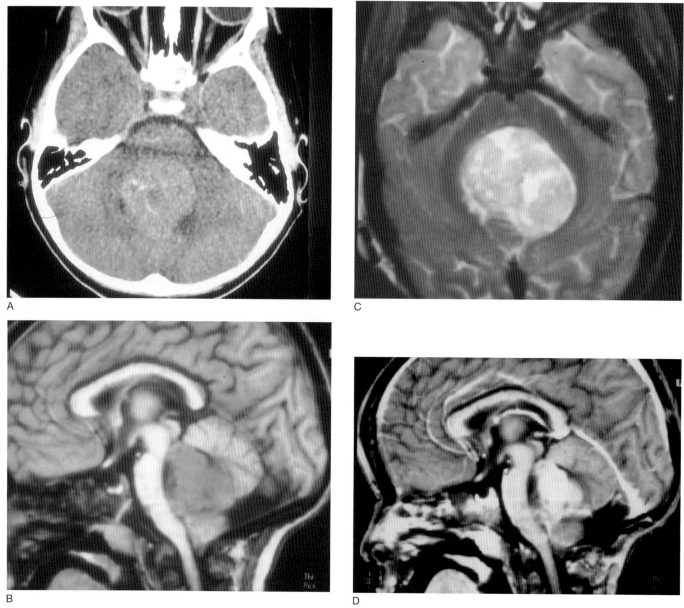

Figure 12.13.11 Medulloblastoma of the 4th ventricle. Central compact, well demarcated, dense mass of the posterior fossa on CT (A). The sagittal cut shows that the neoplasm, slightly hypointense on T1-W images, originates from the lower vermis and extends upwards into the ventricular lumen (B). On T2-W images, the mass again appears well circumscribed, compact, finely heterogeneous (C). It is significantly enhanced by the contrast agent (D).

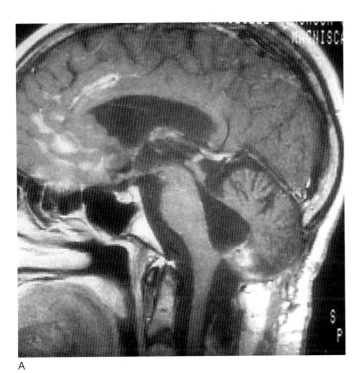

A

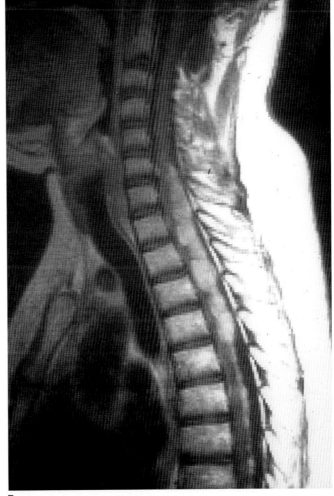

B

Figure 12.13.12 Medulloblastoma of the 4th ventricle. Long-term follow-up. Local recurrence in the wall of the ventricle and distant dissemination into the sulci of the medial aspect of the frontal lobe (A). Disseminated tumour is found also around the cervicothoracic spinal cord (B).

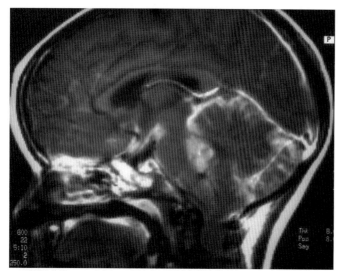

Figure 12.13.13 Medulloblastoma of the 4th ventricle with early dissemination and carcinomatous meningitis in a 14-month-old boy (T1-W with contrast).

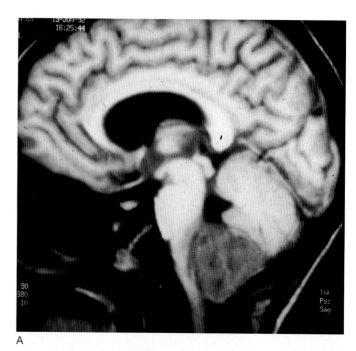

A

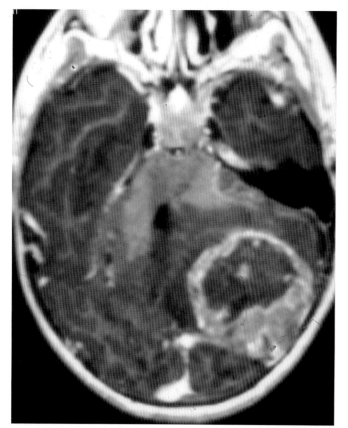

Figure 12.13.14 Desmoplastic medulloblastoma. The tumour has developed in the cerebellar hemisphere and is surrounded by dense fibrous tissue (enhanced).

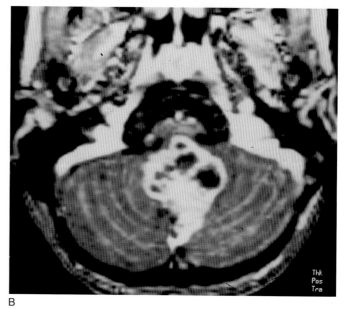

B

Figure 12.13.15 Ependymoma of the 4th ventricle. The mass originates from the ventricular ependyma but extends towards the cisterna magna rather than towards the ventricular lumen (A). Enhancement demonstrates a multiloculated lesion between the cerebellar tonsils (B).

heterogeneity suggesting areas of necrosis. Because of the dissemination potential of the lesion, all of the CSF spaces in the head and the spine should be investigated. The prognosis depends mainly on the quality of the surgical removal. Local recurrences may be reoperated on with good results.

Supratentorial, hemispheric ependymomas (Figure 12.13.16) present differently. They often form huge masses located adjacent to the ventricle into which they may bulge but also extending across the hemispheric white matter towards the cortex. The appearance of the lesion is usually quite characteristic. On CT, it forms a large mass with solid portions isodense to the brain tissue, cystic or pseudocystic portions and marked calcification, with a clear enhancement. The MRI picture discloses the same abnormalities, with an infiltrative mass, iso- or hyposignal on T1-W and hypersignal on T2-W images, a cyst content different from the CSF, calcified masses and marked enhancement. Even with seem-

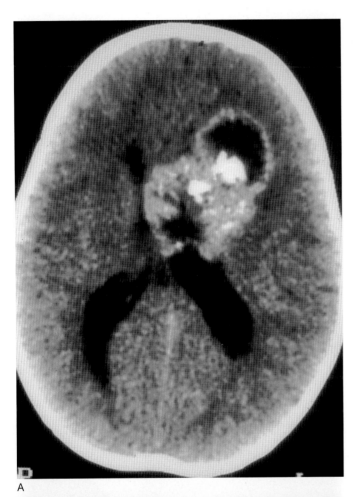

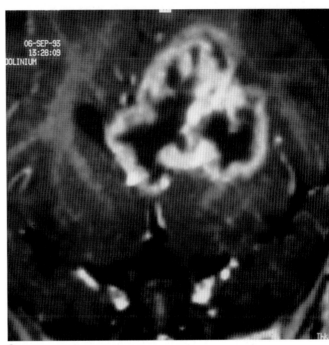

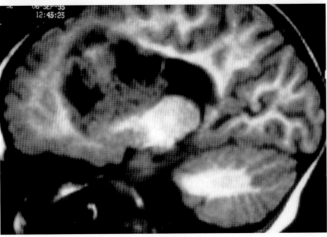

Figure 12.13.16 Ependymoma of the cerebral hemispheres: huge heterogeneous tumour partly solid, partly cystic and partly calcified, mostly dense on CT (A). The lesion develops into the ventricle as well as within the white matter and does not respect the anatomical barriers, which is a sign of malignancy (B). Marked heterogeneous enhancement with the contrast agent (C).

ingly complete transcerebral removal, postoperative recurrences are more common than in the posterior fossa.

More rarely, the tumour develops in the walls of the 3rd ventricle, mostly anteriorly with infiltration of the lamina terminalis. Surgery in this location is not feasible.

CHOROID PLEXUS TUMOURS (PAPILLOMAS AND CARCINOMAS)

These are rare, mainly infantile tumours, which are usually found in infants and young children because of the early hydrocephalus. They are easily diagnosed with CT and/or MRI. They are usually benign (choroid plexus papillomas) and rarely malignant (choroid plexus carcinomas). They develop mostly from the choroid glomus in the atrium of the lateral ventricles, less commonly from the tela choroidea of the 3rd ventricle and, on rare occasions, in the 4th ventricle. In these patients, hydrocephalus raises specific questions as the mass is usually not obstructive. An overproduction of CSF by the tumour was first proposed but the capacity of resorption of CSF is such that this explanation is not really satisfactory. As the mass is generally unilateral, it cannot explain a quadri-ventricular hydrocephalus. Exaggerated pulsatility of the tumoral plexus may modify the normal equilibrium against the pulsating brain mantle and is a further possible explanation. A high level of protein in the CSF has been considered also as a possible factor.

The choroid plexus papilloma is a mass developed from the choroid plexus, usually in the ventricular atrium in children (more often in the 4th ventricle in adults). It is a well-defined compact lesion that is sometimes finely multilobular and usually free in the ventricles but is occasionally incarcerated within the parenchyma without being really invasive. Some tumours may be huge. Haemorrhage may occur within the tumour and CSF-filled cysts may develop. Before the advent of modern imaging techniques, these tumours were usually discovered at an advanced stage and were commonly calcified. With the early diagnosis possible today, it has been shown that calcification is unusual in the first months of life. Histologically, the tumour reproduces the cellular pattern of the normal plexus, with low mitotic activity. As in the normal choroid plexus, the vascularity is abundant.

The discovery of the lesion in a hydrocephalic infant is usually a surprise, as the tumour is rare. On CT as well as on MRI (Figure 12.13.17), the tumour appears as a rather homogeneous intraventricular mass that is isodense with the parenchyma on CT, isointense on MRI on T1-W and T2-W images and markedly enhancing with contrast. Usually, the tumour is of moderate size and contained within the limits of the enlarged atrium. More rarely, it may be incarcerated within the surrounding white matter and, in some instances, the tumour is huge at the time of discovery. Because this tumour is highly vascular, its surgical removal is difficult with a high risk of abundant bleeding in an infant whose blood volume is small. For that reason, presurgical angiography may be useful in assessing the vascularity and allowing for presurgical endovascular embolization through a dilated choroidal artery. Once the surgical difficulties of a complete removal are overcome, sometimes requiring several consecutive operations, the lesion does not recur.

The choroid plexus carcinoma is still less frequent than the papilloma. It is found in young children but usually later than the

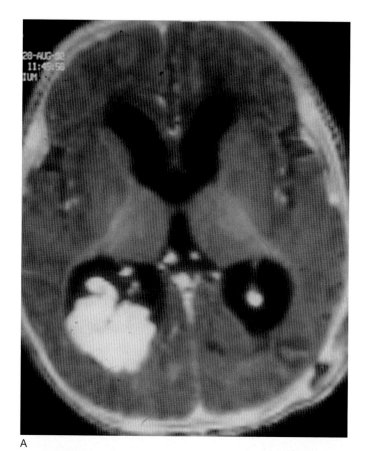

A

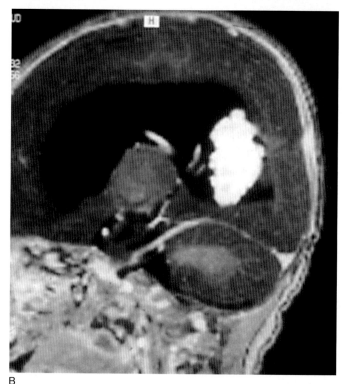

B

Figure 12.13.17 Choroid plexus papilloma in a 4-month-old boy. Compact multiloculated mass, with homogeneous enhancement, located within the ventricular lumen, with bilateral hydrocephalus unexplained by the mass effect. Axial (A) and sagittal (B) slices.

papilloma. It is characterized histologically by its anaplastic features, with an increased mitotic activity, cellular pleomorphism, nuclear atypia, loss of the papillary structure and areas of necrosis. The tumour frequently invades and infiltrates the adjacent parenchyma. Seeding to the other ventricles or into the subarachnoid spaces may occur.

The imaging features of a choroid plexus carcinoma are not very different from those of a papilloma. Characteristically, the tumour invades the walls of the ventricle but this may be difficult to differentiate from a simple incarceration, except when a conventional angiography is performed: it shows the mass to be fed not only by the choroidal arteries but also by the transcerebral perforators from the superficial cortical arteries. Because the tumour invades the parenchyma, complete removal is more difficult to achieve; a combination of adjuvant chemotherapy and/or radiotherapy is needed. The prognosis is then fairly good.

INTRINSIC PINEAL TUMOURS: PINEOBLASTOMA (FIGURES 12.13.18, 12.13.19)

The pineal gland may manifest a variety of tumours, because of the variety of cells it is made up of. This includes gliomas, pineocytomas and pineoblastomas, and germ cells tumours: such gliomas are not different from other gliomas; the pineocytomas afflict mostly adults; and the pineal gland is only one location of the germ cell tumours. In common paediatric clinical practice, the typical intrinsic pineal tumour is the pinealoblastoma. In rare instances, it may be associated with a bilateral retinoblastoma to form the so-called trilateral retinoblastoma.

The intrinsic pineal tumour often presents as a marked enlargement of the pineal gland, developing more towards the ambient cistern than towards the ventricle. It may be well demarcated or it may infiltrate the adjacent structures and, obviously, most commonly the splenium of the corpus callosum. The cellularity is dense, with undifferentiated cells, hyperchromatic nuclei and scanty cytoplasm, a high mitotic activity, necrosis and calcification. On unenhanced CT, the density is therefore high: it has a moderately low signal on T1-W imaging, a high signal on T2-W imaging and it usually enhances. Subarachnoid seeding should be looked for preoperatively.

PINEAL CYST

As indicated later in this chapter, the incidental finding of a small pineal cyst is a relatively frequent finding on MR imaging in adolescents but unusual in infants. It can be regarded as a normal variant. Pineal cysts are recorded as occurring in up to 5% of MR brain scans. They are most easily seen on sagittal images but are also easy to see on T2-W images because of their bright signal. They are isointense with CSF on T1-W images unless they are large, when they can have a higher signal or some heterogeneity because of haemorrhage. Depending on their size, they may cause a slight impression on the superior colliculi or on the third ventricle. They never cause clinical symptoms or hydrocephalus. The wall of the cyst enhances with contrast but not the cyst itself. A

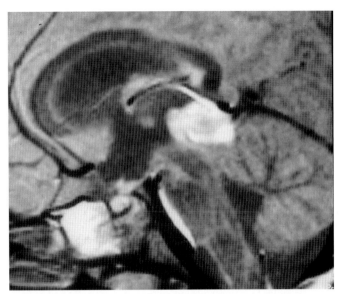

Figure 12.13.18 Pineoblastoma. Well-demarcated mass originating from the pineal gland, expanding towards the ambient cistern, infiltrating the tectal plate and compressing the aqueduct (proton density imaging).

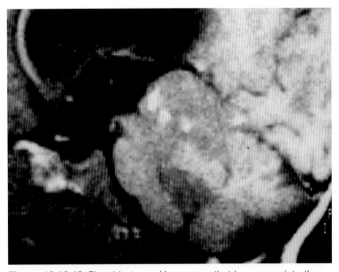

Figure 12.13.19 Pineoblastoma. Huge mass that has grown into the ambient cistern, compressing and invading the posterior 3rd ventricle, the brainstem, the cerebellar vermis and the 4th ventricle (T1-W without contrast).

pitfall is that if the postgadolinium images are significantly delayed there may be some cyst enhancement simulating a tumour.

CRANIOPHARYNGIOMA

A few classical ideas dominate the concept of the craniopharyngioma in children: it is a sellar/suprasellar tumour that is a dysplastic derivative of the remnants of the craniopharyngeal duct or pouch of Rathke (hence its name). It therefore takes its origin somewhere along the pituitary stalk, from where it invades adjacent structures, anteriorly or posteriorly. Depending on the length of the intracranial optic nerves, the expansion is prechiasmatic (postfixed chiasm) or retrochiasmatic (prefixed chiasm). In fact, most of these presumptions are likely to be wrong. It is important to recognize this as it has consequences on the surgical efficacy and can affect considerations in the diagnostic assessment.

The craniopharyngioma is a malformative tumour, which may be found in the sella and in the base of the brain, and also, more rarely, in the pharynx, the sphenoid body and the 3rd ventricle as far posteriorly as the pituitary gland. Surgical removal is difficult and the recurrence rate is quite high for a totally non-malignant lesion. Although it does not disseminate spontaneously, it may recur along the path of surgical resection as well as *in situ*. The cells from which it develops have not been identified but they are known to come from the epiblast. The common assumption is that the tumour is a derivative of the craniopharyngeal duct (Rathke's pouch). This does not correlate with the anatomical organization of the tumour as depicted from MR imaging or with the modern embryological data on the development of the hypophysis and the anterior neural plate. The craniopharyngeal duct is extracerebral, anterior and inferior with respect to the pituitary stalk, and in front of the neurohypophysis; this cannot explain the common occurrence of craniopharyngiomas in the floor of the 3rd ventricle. Furthermore, modern embryological data have shown that the adenohypophysis is a derivative of the outer margin of the anterior neural plate, which induces the diverticulation of the pituitary stalk and neurohypophysis, the interval in between being the pouch of Rathke. Therefore, the tumour develops in different structures that are embryologically clearly separated, such as: the sphenoid body, derived from the facial neural crest; the neurohypophysis, the outer, peripheral aspect of the anterior neural ridge; or the hypothalamus, the lower, central extremity of the floor plate of the neural tube. Craniopharyngiomas are therefore likely to be foci of metaplasia originating in different places, which develop together with the surrounding tissues to which they belong. The feasibility of the resection depends on understanding these complex relationships. In the sella, the tumour is fused with the dura of the cavernous sinuses and with the wall of the carotid syphons. In the infundibulum, it is part of the hypothalamus. The pre- or postchiasmatic extensions of the craniopharyngiomas depend on their site of origin, not on the length of the optic nerves: the natural extension of an intrasellar tumour is upward, under and in front on the optic chiasm. The infundibulo-tuberal tumour is retrochiasmatic from the origin, not by secondary extension.

There are two main histological types: the adamantinomatous craniopharyngioma is the classical type and the one usually observed in children but is also seen in adults; the less common squamous-papillary craniopharyngioma is found mostly in adults. Infrequently, mixed forms are also observed. Craniopharyngioma is a relatively frequent tumour in children and represents 5% to 10% of all intracranial tumours, 12% to 20% of the supratentorial tumours and 50% to 60% of the tumours of the sellar region. Most are discovered between 6 and 16 years of age (80%) but 20% occur before 5 years including neonates and infants. They are histologically benign but due to their location, they are clinically severe and difficult to tackle surgically. The main symptoms and complications are: headaches, either from local sellar-meningeal pressure or from hydrocephalus with increased intracranial pressure; visual defects, as a result of compression of the anterior optic pathways; and endocrine dysfunction, resulting in short stature, diabetes insipidus, delayed puberty and obesity.

Histologically, adamantinomatous craniopharyngiomas are usually both solid and cystic. They consist of a squamous epithelium with a characteristic pattern: nodules of keratin and cysts rich in cholesterol, proteins and blood degradation products. The mass is closely associated with the adjacent tissues in the sella, at the circle of Willis or in the 3rd ventricular floor. In a third of cases, the mass is located within an enlarged sella and the pituitary gland cannot be identified. The extension of the tumour is upward, prechiasmatic (under the optic chiasm, or in front of it between the optic nerves) never towards the interpeduncular cistern. Behind the optic chiasm, the tuber and the infundibulum are always free. In two-thirds of cases, it is located within the tuber cinereum, that is, retro-chiasmatic. The sella is normal or small and the pituitary gland is well identified. The mass then extends into the ventricular lumen, into the interpeduncular cistern, as far as the cisterns of the posterior fossa, the cerebello-pontine angle cisterns and even to the foramen magnum. Giant tumours may extend below and in front of the chiasm but the pituitary gland is always preserved. Rarely, the extension from the tuber is purely inferior behind the stalk into the cistern or purely intraventricular. Exceptionally, the tumour occupies an extended territory including the sella, (the pituitary gland not seen), the stalk, the tuber and the 3rd ventricle almost as far posteriorly as the pineal gland.

On imaging, specific abormalities are observed. Calcification is found in 90% of the paediatric cases; this is described as 'eggshell' when it surrounds the tumour, which may be cystic or solid, or as 'popcorn' when it is nodular or disseminated within the solid tissue (Figure 12.13.20). Cysts are present in most of the adamantinomatous craniopharyngiomas. Commonly both cystic and solid, the tumour may be completely or predominantly cystic. The cyst content is homogeneous. Fluid layering is possible. There are high, varied T2-W signals in different patients or in separate cysts of the same patient. T1-W signal may be high or low and again exhibit diverse degrees of intensity. These signals depend on the amount of protein, cholesterol, desquamated cells, inflammatory reaction and haemorrhagic residue, which looks like 'engine oil' at surgery. The wall of the cyst enhances. Purely cystic craniopharyngiomas have no nodular enhancement. Most, if not all, purely cystic craniopharyngiomas are located in the sella. They affect mostly younger children (Figure 12.13.21). The solid portion is heterogeneous with varying degrees of calcification, which may be eggshell or nodular and diffusely enhancing. It is commonly associated with cystic areas (65%) and is typically located in the 3rd ventricular floor (75%). Completely solid craniopharyngiomas (Figures 12.13.22 and 12.13.23) are less common (9%), and are mostly in the ventricular floor. On occasion, unenhanced portions of the tumour with a relatively homogeneous, hypo T1-W and hyper T2-W signal are observed. They appear 'falsely' cystic. This may represent accumulation of desquamated keratin (Figure 12.13.24).

The intrasellar craniopharyngioma (Figures 12.13.21 and 12.13.22) is found mostly in younger children. The sella is enlarged. The pituitary gland is never identified on the MR images. The extension is mostly superior. The chiasm is pushed upward and backward and visual defects are common. Whether the sphenoidal locations are downward extensions of a sellar tumour or are a primarily sphenoidal tumour is uncertain, but the latter seems more likely. Most, if not all, purely cystic craniopharyngiomas are found in this location, which is of therapeutic significance, but completely solid examples of solid-cystic tumours may be seen

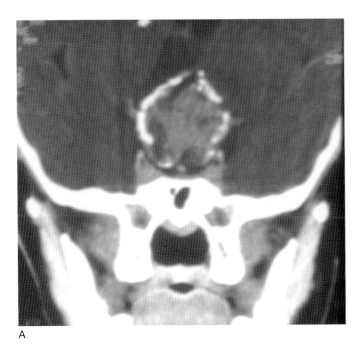

A

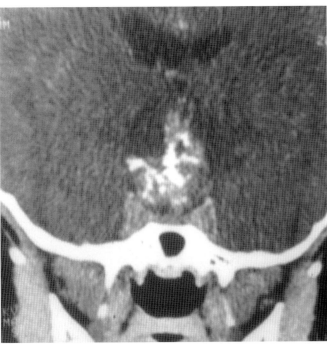

B

Figure 12.13.20 Craniopharyngiomas. Eggshell (A) and popcorn (B) calcifications.

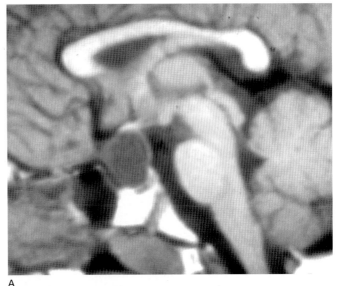

A

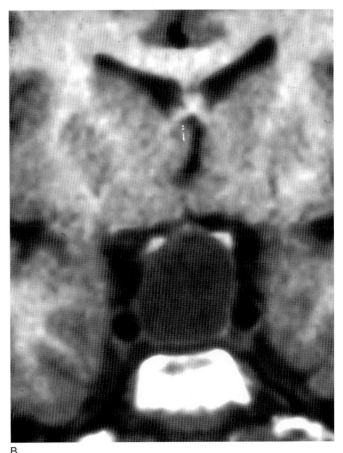

B

Figure 12.13.21 Craniopharyngioma, intrasellar, purely cystic, on sagittal T1-W (A) and coronal T2-W (B) images. The pituitary gland is not seen. The expansion is mainly prechiasmatic. In this 4-year-old boy, the treatment consisted of inserting a shunt into the cyst and injecting bleomycin, with no excision. Excellent clinical status at 12 years follow-up.

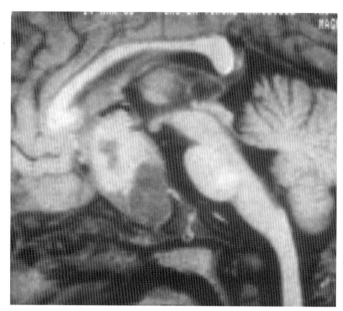

Figure 12.13.22 Craniopharyngioma, intrasellar, solid. The pituitary gland is not seen and the extension is prechiasmatic. Multiple excisions were needed with multiple recurrences.

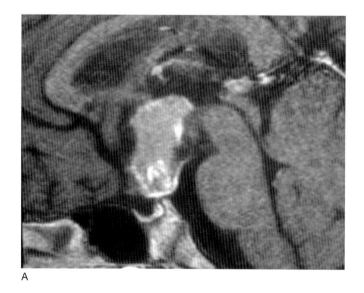

A

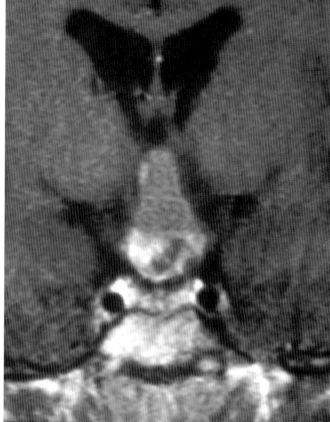

B

Figure 12.13.23 Craniopharyngioma, infundibulotuberal. The mass is retrochiasmatic, mostly solid and enhanced. The pituitary gland is clearly seen on sagittal (A) and coronal (B) cuts. The mass grew into the ventricle as well as towards the interpeduncular cistern.

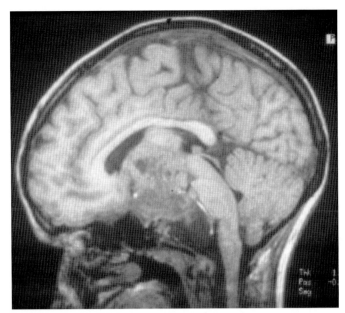

Figure 12.13.24 Craniopharyngioma, infundibulotuberal. A large heterogeneous mass is seen in the floor of the ventricle with a huge extension into the posterior fossa down to the foramen magnum. It is partly solid, partly cystic and partly pseudocystic in its lower portion (T1-W without contrast).

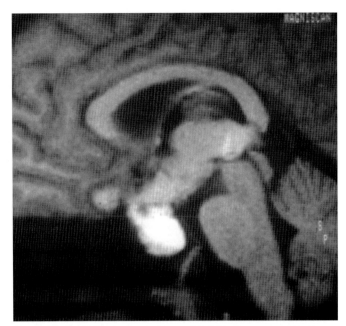

Figure 12.13.25 Craniopharyngioma, global. The mass occupies the whole 3rd ventricle and extends anteriorly along the pituitary stalk towards the (posterior?) pituitary gland. T1-W image: note the heterogeneous signals of the different portions of the mass.

also. The tumour should be resected when it is totally or partially solid. As it is developmentally part of the sella with its related structures, it is commonly not fully resectable safely and the rate of recurrence of solid or solid-cystic intrasellar craniopharyngiomas is high. A fusiform aneurysm of the supraclinoid artery is also a specific and relatively common complication. On the contrary, when the tumour is purely cystic, a drain can be inserted within the cyst for treatment by instillation of a cytostatic agent, without a need for resection, and there is usually no recurrence.

The infundibulotuberal craniopharyngioma (Figures 12.13.23 and 12.13.24) is seen in older children. Hydrocephalus is more common. The tumour is part of the thalamic floor behind the chiasm. The pituitary gland and the sella are normal. It is typically a mixed solid and cystic lesion with extensions towards both the ventricular lumen and the cisterns but purely cisternal or purely intraventricular extensions also occur. The tumour is separate from the brainstem and from the basilar artery system whatever the volume of the extension towards the foramen magnum. This rule has very few exceptions, one being the rare dural insertion in the cerebello-pontine angle cisterns. Other extensions may be lateral and affect the basal ganglia or mesial temporal lobe, or around the chiasm, yet do not affect the pituitary. Surgically, the problem is to dissect the tumour causing as little damage as possible to the surrounding brain, especially to the chiasm, thalami and related structures. As these tumours are typically at least partly solid, instilled cytostatic treatment has no indication in this location. The recurrence rate depends on the ability to achieve a complete removal but has become quite low in recent years.

The uncommon global craniopharyngioma (Figure 12.13.25) extends in both the sella and the ventricular floor; it may be an extension of an infundibulotuberal lesion towards the stalk and the posterior pituitary.

DYSEMBRYOPLASTIC CYSTS

RATHKE'S CLEFT CYSTS

These differ from craniopharyngiomas, as was emphasized above. They are frequently found at autopsy but are usually symptomless. When they display symptoms, they behave like intrasellar, intrapituitary masses with suprasellar expansion and occasional compression of the optic pathways. They occur mainly in adults. In children, a common presentation on MRI is an area of dark T1-W and T2-W signal with no enhancement in the location of the pars intermedia of the pituitary gland (Figure 12.13.26). Repeated studies are recommended at long intervals to check that the lesion does not expand. These lesions are usually found incidentally.

DERMOID CYSTS

Dermoid cysts occur infrequently. They are probably different from the dermal cysts and fistulas that are inclusion defects usually found in the lumbosacral area when the skin remains attached to the otherwise normally closed cord, in the posterior fossa, probably because there was no separation between the skin and the rhombencephalic vesicle, and in the naso-frontal area, when the skin follows the ascent of the dura towards the foramen caecum, in front of the crista galli. All are connected with the surface ectoderm. Dermoid cysts are considered by some to be monotissular benign teratomas. They are also located along the midline, mostly in the sella and the pineal, or within the vault. They contain fat. They have low attenuation at CT, high signal on T1-W imaging, low signal on T2-W imaging with chemical shift artifacts, and at

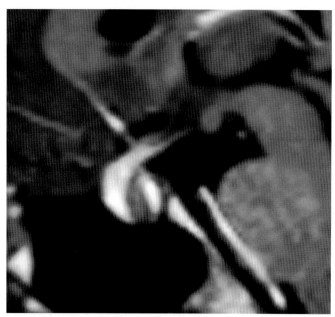

Figure 12.13.26 Rathke's duct residue. Low T1-W signal, with no enhancement, of the pars intermedia of the pituitary gland (T1-W with contrast).

surgical or pathological inspection are found to contain hair. They may leak free fat fluid within the cisterns. They may also have solid portions and may calcify (Figure 12.13.27).

EPIDERMOID CYSTS

Epidermoid cysts (also known as congenital cholesteatoma or pearly tumours) are very rarely discovered in children. They are formed of desquamated epithelium without fatty secretions and are found mostly in the basal cisterns in the cerebello-pontine angle. They also occur in the base of the skull, in the parasellar regions or in the area of the geniculate ganglion of the facial nerve, from where they may destroy the adjacent inner and middle ear structures and expand upwards, epidurally, towards the temporal fossa. They rarely invade the neural axis. Surgery is made difficult by the encasement of the cranial nerves within the mass. They contain keratin, no hair, no fat, and have low T1-W and high T2-W signals (Figure 12.13.28). They may be difficult to differentiate from CSF. If they are suspected because of a local mass effect, diffusion imaging allows for a ready diagnosis, as the motion of the protons in the lesion is more restricted than in CSF.

COLLOID CYSTS

Colloid cysts may be observed in teenagers but less commonly than in adults. They develop from the tela choroidea of the 3rd ventricle in the vicinity of the foramen of Monro and therefore are expressed clinically by episodes of acute headaches caused by acute, transient episodes of intracranial hypertension. They contain hyaline material with varied densities on CT, and varied T1 and T2 signals on MR imaging. The diagnosis is easy as such a cyst

presents as a small rounded mass of the anterior upper 3rd ventricle and usually has an enhancing wall.

GERM CELL TUMOURS

The germ cell tumours form a group of tumours derived from the germ cell lines. They are homologues of the germinal neoplasms found in the gonads. They represent 3% of brain tumours in children and 90% of them present under 20 years of age. There is a marked predominance in boys (about 2 to 1).

The germ cell tumours are classified into six subgroups:

- germinomas (55% in a personal series of 37 cases since the advent of good-quality MRI);
- teratomas, which may be mature, immature or secondarily malignant (22%);
- yolk sac tumours (endodermal sinus tumours);
- embryonal carcinoma;
- choriocarcinoma; and
- mixed cell tumours: instead of arising from a single set of germinal cells, these tumours are composed of a mixture of germ cell-derived tissues. For clinical purposes, these are further subdivided into secreting (13%) and non-secreting (3%) lesions. Also, different types of germ cell tumours may be found in different locations in an individual patient (5%).

Topographically, 80% of the masses are located around the 3rd ventricle, mostly in the pineal region in boys and in the anterior 3rd ventricle in girls. Therefore, the symptomatology is related to these locations: hydrocephalus and Parinaud's syndrome for the pineal masses, diabetes insipidus (DI) and visual alterations for the suprasellar ones. In boys, precocious puberty is a significant feature. A very important fact to remember for radiologists is that even with the best modern imaging techniques, DI may antecede the morphological demonstration of the tumour by several months. This means that in a child with DI, if no explanation is found on imaging, repeated studies are needed every few months to look for the secondary macroscopic appearance of the mass. This mainly occurs with the germinomas.

Owing to the surgical difficulties related to the location of germ cell tumours, especially in the pineal region, and because pure germinomas, the most common germinal tumour, are extremely sensitive to chemotherapy without the need for surgery, it would be ideal to make the diagnosis by non-invasive or minimally invasive techniques. These include imaging, identification of raised tumour markers (alpha fetoprotein, AFP; beta-human chorionic gonadotrophin, β-HCG), stereotaxic needle biopsy and response to chemotherapy. Yet, no non-invasive approach is totally reliable: images may not be specific; tumour markers may be absent; and the needle biopsy may miss a significant cellular component. Therefore, open surgery with total removal of the lesion, complemented by adjuvant therapies may be the safest approach.

As far as MRI is concerned, the goals of the examination are to recognize the presence of the mass, if possible to identify it on its appearance, to evaluate its local effect and, as all members of this group of neoplasms tend to disseminate in the subarachnoid spaces, to look for distant seeding in the skull and in the spine.

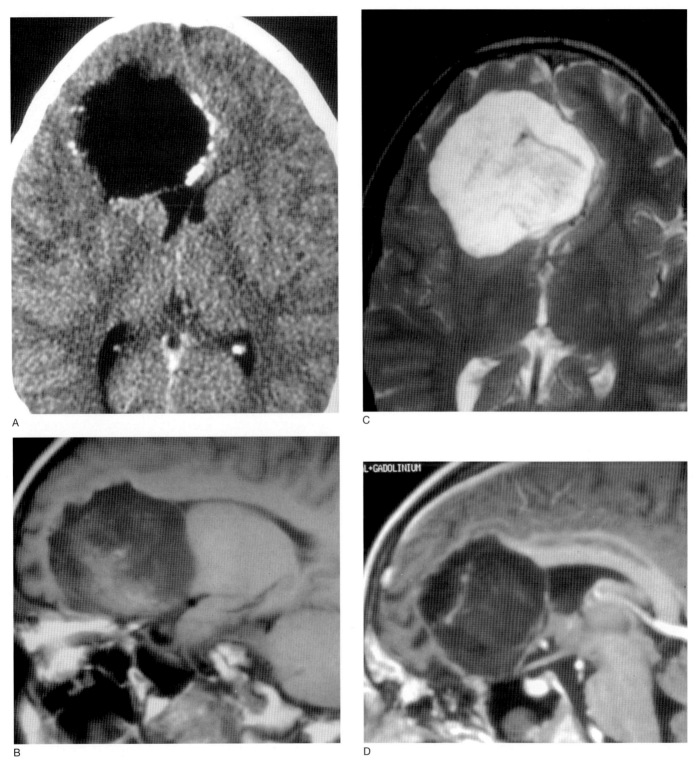

A

B

C

D

Figure 12.13.27 Dermoid cyst. Low-density mass with a calcified rim on CT (A); paradoxically of intermediate signal on T1-W imaging (B). High signal on T2-W imaging (C), heterogeneous. Only minimal partial enhancement after contrast administration (D).

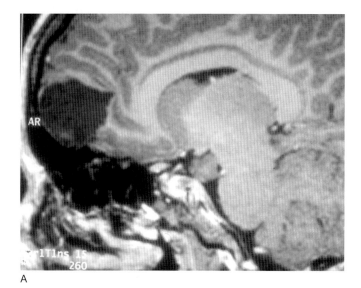

A

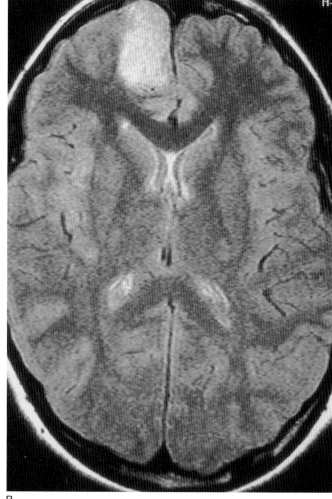

Figure 12.13.28 Epidermoid cyst. Mass with low T1-W signal (A) and high proton density signal (B) incarcerated in the frontal lobe.

B

A germinoma (Figures 12.13.29 to 12.13.34) presents as a well-demarcated mass, occupying the tissue from which it develops rather than displacing it. It is commonly surrounded by a thin rim of oedema (Figure 12.13.29). The main sites are the anterior and the posterior portion of the 3rd ventricle. In the pineal region (Figure 12.13.29), the tumour develops more into the posterior ventricular lumen than towards the ambient cistern but it usually absorbs the pineal gland and the anterior collicular plate. Laterally, it occupies the adjacent portions of the thalami (Figure 12.13.29). An interesting finding is that the pineal gland, usually not yet calcified in young children, is commonly calcified in association with pineal region germ cell tumours (Figure 12.13.31). The other most frequent location is the anterior 3rd ventricle, usually the infundibulum, the chiasm and the pituitary stalk (Figure 12.13.30). Here again, the tumour absorbs the structure in which it sits with practically no mass effect. A typical feature is the presence of a double mass (bipolar germinoma) at both ends of the 3rd ventricle.

On CT, the germinoma appears hyperdense (Figure 12.13.31), sometimes calcified, sometimes haemorrhagic. On MRI, it is iso- or hypointense on T1-W images, slightly hyperintense on T2-W images, finely heterogeneous with microcavities, and sometimes with signs of acute or chronic haemorrhage (Figures 12.13.29 to

12.13.31). As the germinoma is not a neural tissue, it has no blood–brain barrier and it enhances markedly, sometimes with unenhanced areas possibly due to old haemorrhages. Enhancement is helpful in showing ependymal and pial dissemination. After chemotherapy, pineal germinomas often leave a residual cavity (Figure 12.13.29). On the contrary, infundibular germinomas often leave an enhancing, presumably fibrous residue on the floor of the ventricle, which raises the problem of a persisting tumour (Figure 12.13.31).

In the thalami, germinomas are peculiar in that the lesion may be diffusely microcalcified (Figure 12.13.32) or cystic (Figure 12.13.33). They may induce not an expansion but a reduction of the volume of the hemisphere, by diminution of the number of fibres in the corona radiata. Primary germinomas may also be found in the sella, the septum pellucidum, the cord, the cauda equina and the sacrum.

The teratoma is the second most common germ cell tumour of the CNS. In 50% of cases, it is found in the pineal region but it may be seen in any location along the midline, the suprasellar region, 4th ventricle, cisterna magna, spine and cord. It is usually well demarcated and very heterogeneous with bone, fat, cysts (which are sometimes very large) and tissues of varied density and

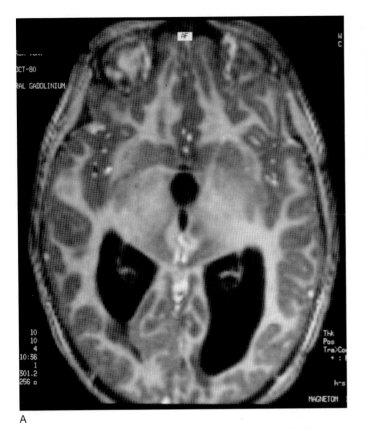

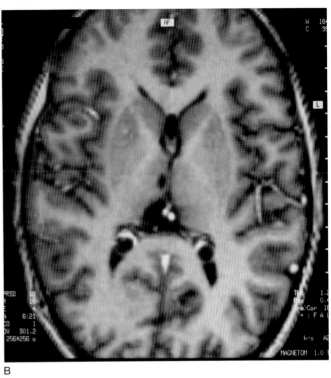

A   B

Figure 12.13.29 Germinoma of the posterior 3rd ventricle. (A) The neoplasm, which has developed towards the ventricle and the adjacent thalami with little mass effect, is surrounded by a rim of oedema (T1-W with contrast). It has disappeared after chemotherapy leaving behind a cavitation (B).

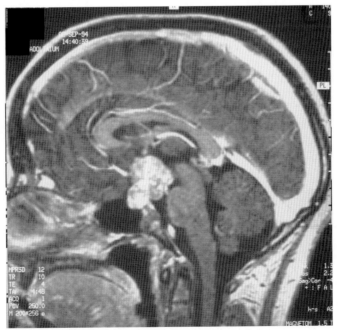

Figure 12.13.30 Germinoma of the anterior 3rd ventricle. The mass occupies the anterior structures of the ventricle, including the optic chiasm, the pituitary stalk and the pituitary gland (T1-W with contrast).

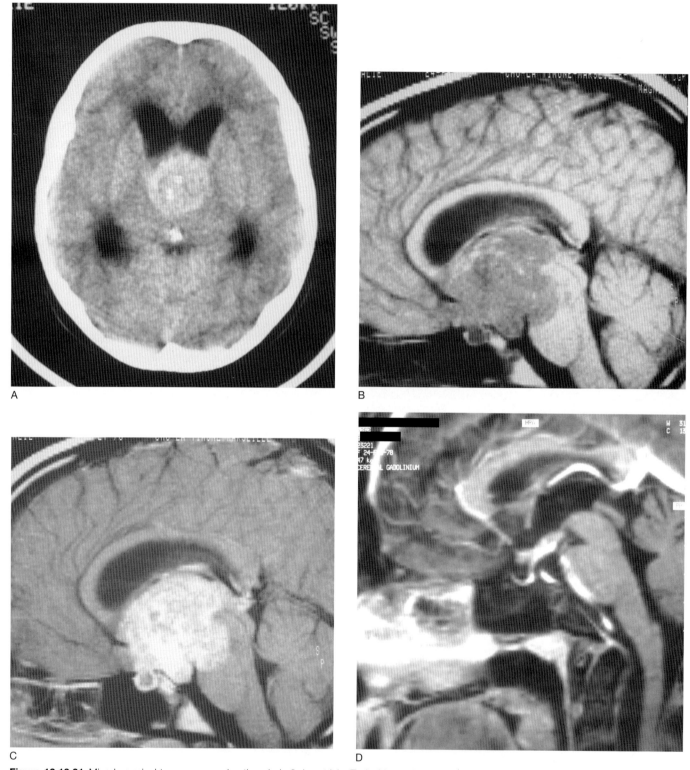

Figure 12.13.31 Mixed germinal tumour occupying the whole 3rd ventricle. Typical hyperdensity on CT (A) with hydrocephalus. The pineal in this 11-year-old girl is calcified. The lesion is moderately hypointense on T1-W imaging (B) and markedly enhanced by the contrast agent (C). After chemotherapy, an enhancing fibrous tissue remains in the floor of the ventricle (D), which is not a residue of the tumour.

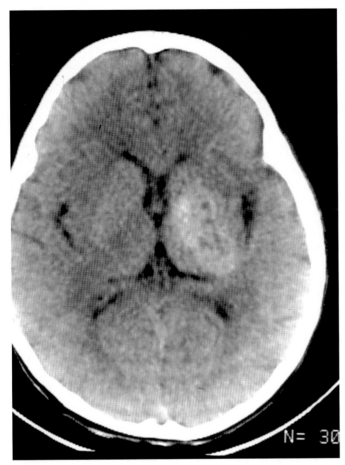

Figure 12.13.32 Calcified germinoma of the thalamus and basal ganglia: finely calcified lesion without mass effect.

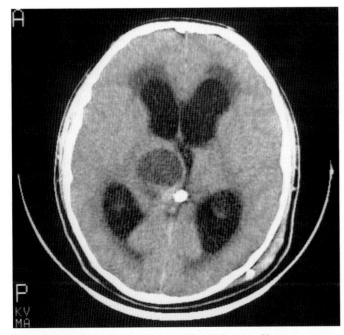

Figure 12.13.33 Cystic germinoma of the thalamus, with hydrocephalus. Note the calcified pineal in this 15-year-old boy.

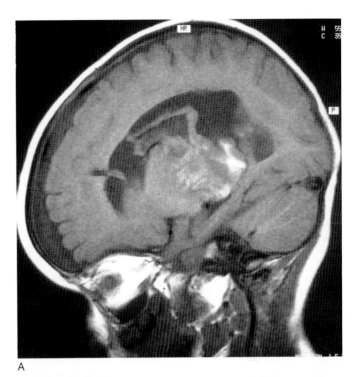

A

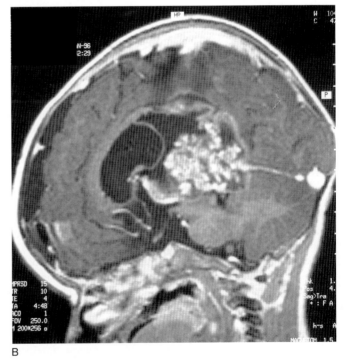

B

Figure 12.13.34 Teratoma of the posterior 3rd ventricle. Heterogeneous mass with a collapsed cyst (surgically punctured) on T1-W imaging (A), irregularly enhanced by the contrast agent (B) in a 7-month-old girl.

variable enhancement, representing diverse tissue differentiation (Figure 12.13.34). The more compact the mass and the more it enhances, the more likely it is to be malignant; it is then also not so well demarcated and may be associated with surrounding oedema.

The other histological types of germ cell tumour, the yolk sac tumour, the embryonal teratoma and the choriocarcinoma, do not have specific features. Yolk sac tumours and embryonal teratomas form heterogeneous masses. Choriocarcinomas are often haemorrhagic but simple germinomas are haemorrhagic also. They are commonly secreting (AFP, β-HCG, PLAP). They are rare and may develop together to constitute the mixed germ-cell tumours with particular dominant tissue types (Figure 12.13.31). These are malignant and disseminate but long-term remission does at least occur. The precise histological identification of the components can be made only by histopathology.

EMBRYONAL NEURAL TUMOURS

Apart from the main types of tumours listed above, the pathology of brain tumours in children is characterized by a multiplicity of poorly differentiated cellular types. The most common and typical of these is the medulloblastoma, which, because of its frequency and its main location in the cerebellar vermis, is described separately. Many other cellular types occur occasionally. The diagnosis is most often made by the pathologist after the tumour has been removed. Most embryonal neoplasms have a predilection for the very young child.

The medulloepithelioma is the most primitive tumour originating from the CNS. Its cellularity reproduces the primitive neural tube. It affects the young child and may even be congenital. It develops more commonly deep in the cerebral hemispheres but may be found anywhere along the neural tube. It is highly malignant and disseminates easily. It appears as a well-demarcated mass on imaging, hypo- or hyperdense on CT, iso- or hypointense on T1-W images, and may be haemorrhagic. It shows little enhancement.

The ependymoblastoma is an embryonal tumour with differentiation potential towards the ependymocyte, containing ependymoblastic rosettes within a globally undifferentiated tumour. The mitotic activity is high. It usually develops close to the ependyma, supra- or infratentorially. Similar to other embryonal tumours, it is well demarcated, often with conspicuous oedema. It enhances with contrast agents.

The central neuroblastomas present in a similar way but with a differentiation more towards the neuroblast. They tend to disseminate. The aesthesioneuroblastoma is a similar tumour developed from the olfactory structures in the roof of the nasal cavity; it is much rarer in children than in adults.

Extracerebellar primitive neuroectodermal tumour (PNET) is the name given to the medulloblastoma when it affects a structure other than the cerebellum. Though uncommon, it is sometimes observed in the cerebral hemispheres (Figure 12.13.35).

The atypical rhabdoid-teratoid tumour is less uncommon. It presents as a solid and cystic or necrotic mass, close to the surface of the brain, irregularly enhanced by contrast agents. It may become large and may disseminate early.

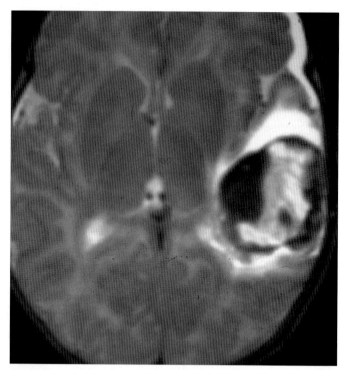

Figure 12.13.35 Primitive neuroepithelial tumour (PNET) of the cerebral hemisphere in a 4-month-old boy. Note the intratumoral haemorrhage.

DYSPLASTIC TUMOURS (EPILEPTOGENIC TUMOURS)

The dysplastic tumours are those intermediate between cortical dysplasia and the real tumours. As they involve both the neuronal (ganglionic) and the glial cellular lineages, they are also identified as neuroglial tumours. They include the dysembryoplastic neuroepithelial tumour (DNT), the ganglioglioma and the desmoplastic infantile ganglioglioma. The three of them primarily affect the cortex and therefore are highly epileptogenic lesions. As developmental lesions, they are characteristically associated with dysplasia of the adjacent cortex. They are essentially dormant neoplasms, although the glial component, in gangliogliomas, may give rise to diverse types of gliomas. Except for the desmoplastic infantile ganglioglioma, which is discovered early because of macrocephaly, the affected patients commonly have a long history of refractory epilepsy at the time of diagnosis, usually with a normal development and intelligence. Because of the sensitivity of modern imaging modalities and the routine investigation of partial onset epilepsies, earlier diagnosis has become the rule.

The dysembryoplastic neuroepithelial tumour (Figures 12.13.36, 12.13.37) was identified by Daumas-Duport from its clinical, imaging and histological features. This tumour typically does not grow and affected patients present with a longstanding (mean duration 9–10 years, between the ages of 2 and 23 years), early onset (the first two decades, mean 9–10 years) partial epilepsy, with no deficit or only a stable, congenital neurological deficit. MRI shows a tumour located in the cortex with deformity

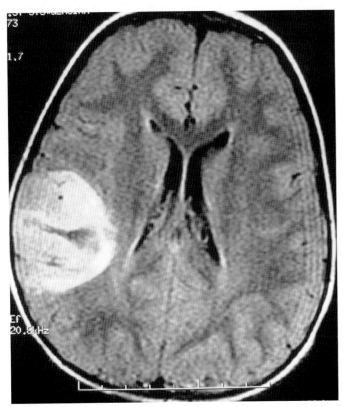

Figure 12.13.36 Dysembryoplastic neuroepithelial tumour (DNT). Well-demarcated cortical-subcortical lesion, slightly heterogeneous, discovered during investigation of longstanding refractory epilepsy.

of the adjacent calvarium. It remains static over time on repeated examinations. However, clinical experience reveals that on occasion some change in the mass may occur with time (Figure 12.13.37). These changes are presumed to result from intratumoral haemorrhages with resulting neoangiogenesis. But whereas the lesion itself may increase in volume, it does not infiltrate into the adjoining tissues in the same way as classical tumours do. There are three histological types of DNT:

- The complex form is a multinodular intracortical mass, with nodules resembling astrocytomas, oligodendrogliomas or oligoastrocytomas, and a peculiar columnar structure perpendicular to the cortical surface. This columnar structure, called the 'specific glioneuronal element', is made up of multiple axonal bundles, surrounded by small oligodendrocytes, and of neurons that appear to be 'floating' in a myxoid interstitial matrix. The surrounding cortex appears dysplastic with abnormal organization. Radiologically, the tumour always affects the cortex. It has clear-cut limits, like a scar, but without atrophy and it does not fit any vascular territory. It is hypodense on CT, sometimes multinodular and occasionally calcified. It may affect the outer portion of the brain only but it may also extend from the ventricle to the cortex. It is hypointense on T1, hyperintense on T2, moderately heterogeneous, without any surrounding oedema, and typically without mass effect, although some deformity of the adjacent structures may be seen on occasions. The overlying inner table of the calvarium, when

the tumour is on the convexity, is slightly expanded, reflecting the developmental nature of the mass. Contrast enhancement is noted in a third of cases.

- The simple form is more uniform and exhibits the specific glioneuronal element only. Radiologically, it appears on CT as a well-delineated pseudocystic hypodensity with a bulging calvarium and occasional calcification. MRI shows cortical location and broad gyri, hyperintensity on T2-W images, and hypointensity on T1-W images; no enhancement is seen in this form.

- The form lacking specific morphological features, conversely, may resemble common astrocytomas, oligodendrogliomas or any other glioma, and does not exhibit the specific glioneuronal elements. The tumour is cortical with broad gyri. It is hypodense on CT and often calcified. On MRI, it is hypointense on T1-W images, hyperintense on T2-W images and enhances in about half the cases.

Classically, all forms are stable on sequential studies. They are more often located in the temporal lobe but may be present anywhere in the cerebral cortex.

The ganglioglioma (Figures 12.13.38 to 12.13.40) is probably the most frequently identified tumour in pharmacoresistant epilepsy in children. It may be found along the whole neural axis (including the spinal cord). It represents 30–40% of the epileptogenic tumours. Histologically, it is located in the cortex and is composed of abnormal, often binucleated ganglion cells mixed with neoplastic astrocytes. The neuronal elements may predominate or may be hard to find distributed within the glial tumour. An extreme variety of neuronal size and density, of degree of lymphocytic infiltrates, of pilocytic elements, or of Rosenthal fibres is found. The ganglionic component of the tumour seems to be purely dysplastic and stable while the glial component accounts for the neoplastic aspects of the lesion. The surrounding cortex is disorganized. Most gangliogliomas are classified as low-grade tumours and may develop as fibrillary or, more rarely, pilocytic astrocytomas but in some the glial component may become anaplastic. Oligodendrocytes are rare. Radiologically, the tumour is well circumscribed, often cystic or pseudocystic and of variable size, sometimes huge. It is found more frequently in the temporal lobe but may be encountered anywhere in the brain. On CT, it is usually hypodense or isodense and is calcified in a third of cases. On MRI, it is heterogeneous, hypointense on T1-W and hyperintense on T2-W images, and partly cystic with a possible mural nodule that usually enhances. When the lesion is solid, there may not be any or only partial enhancement. In many cases, it is impossible to differentiate a ganglioglioma from a typical, conventional glioma. Long-standing epilepsy, however, is unusual in the conventional gliomas and should make one suspicious of the correct diagnosis. Atypical locations for a cystic pilocytic astrocytoma may be suggestive of a ganglioglioma (Figure 12.13.40). Also, the recurrence rate seems higher in large gangliogliomas than it is in common gliomas. Outside the cerebral hemispheres, gangliogliomas are observed in the brainstem, especially the medulla and in the spinal cord. They may be observed also in the cerebellum and rare cases of cerebellar ganglioglioma presenting with epilepsy have been reported, the epilepsy disappearing after removal of the lesion. This, together with the hypothalamic hamartoma, is the only instance of epilepsy originating outside the cerebral hemispheres.

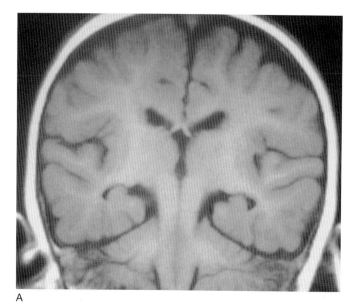

A

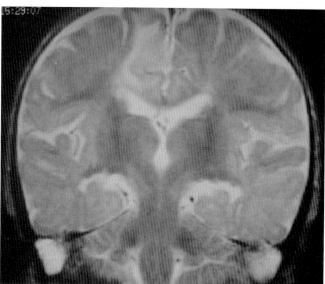

B

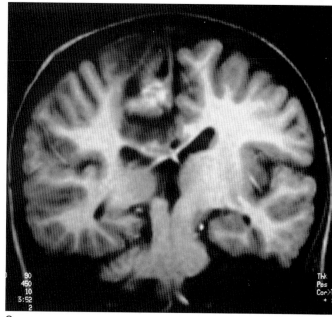

C

Figure 12.13.37 Dysembryoplastic neuroepithelial tumour (DNT). Modification with time. At 9 months, T1-W (A) and T2-W (B) images demonstrate a seemingly dysplastic lesion on the medial aspect of the right hemisphere (blurring of the cortical junction on T1-W, high signal on T2-W). At 4 years, the lesion is markedly modified with pronounced heterogeneity and a moderate mass effect. The diagnosis of DNT was confirmed after surgical excision.

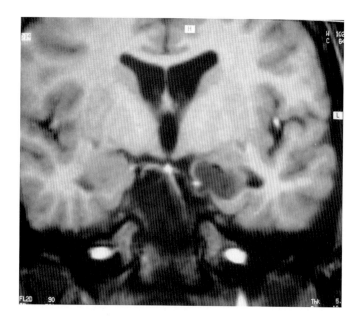

Figure 12.13.38 Ganglioglioma of the mesial temporal lobe. Hypointense T1-W mass in the left amygdaloid nucleus (T1-W without contrast).

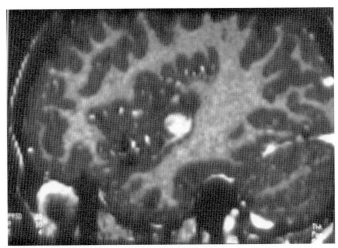

Figure 12.13.39 Ganglioglioma of the posterior planum temporale. Small cortical mass with marked enhancement.

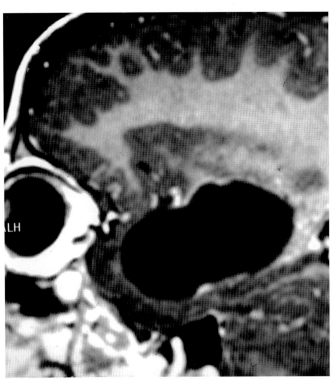

Figure 12.13.40 Ganglioglioma of the temporal lobe with a huge cystic gliomatous component (T1-W with contrast).

The gangliocytoma is a purely neuronal form of ganglioglioma.

The desmoplastic infantile ganglioglioma is considerably more rare than the DNT or the ganglioglioma. It was not identified until 1989. It presents with early seizures, usually before the age of 2 years, sometimes at birth. It represents 15% of the infantile tumours. Affected patients may be developmentally normal or delayed. The epilepsy, partial with frequent generalization, is severe. The tumour may be found anywhere in the brain but occurs predominantly in the frontoparietal area. Pathologically, it is a firm, discoloured region of the cortex, which is focally widened, and of the subjacent white matter, but with attachment to the dura. The cyto-architecture in the lesion is disorganized and the vascularity is increased. Large clusters of dysplastic, embryonal-looking ganglion and glial cells are found within a scant glial background, either scattered or divided into lobules by fibrovascular septa. The abnormal neurons are markedly enlarged, sometimes binucleated and oriented randomly. The mitotic activity is very low. The abnormalities extend into the white matter, where astrocytic gliosis, perivascular chronic inflammation and microcalcification may be associated. The lesion extends into the subarachnoid space. Radiologically, it appears on CT as an iso- or hyperdense, multinodular cortical lesion, which may or may not be calcified, usually with huge cysts. On MRI, the relative signal depends on the maturational stage of the brain and on the degree of calcification. It is typically isointense on T1-W images, and moderately hyperintense and heterogeneous on T2-W images. The nodular portions usually enhance. In fact, clinical experience with these tumours is poor and the reported data are often contradictory.

LHERMITTE–DUCLOS DISEASE (DYSPLASTIC GANGLIOCYTOMA OF THE CEREBELLUM)

Lhermitte–Duclos disease is of uncertain aetiology; it usually affects middle-aged adults but is occasionally discovered in children as well. There is no agreement as to whether it is hamar-tomatous, a malformation or a neoplastic disorder. Histologically, it shows no proliferative activity but regrowth after excision may occur. It is characterized by a thickening of the cerebellar folia, respecting the folial pattern. The external granule cell layer and, in part, the Purkinje cell layer are replaced by a disorganized layer made up of well-differentiated neurons, some large and polygonal, others small with hyperchromatic nuclei. The folial white matter is markedly reduced. Spongy changes and microcalcification are associated. The vermis may be affected like the hemispheres, asymmetrically. The usual clinical features at the time of discovery are hydrocephalus, and cerebellar and brainstem signs and symptoms. On imaging, the lesion appears as a posterior fossa mass. It is hypodense on CT, hypointense on T1-W and hyperintense on T2-W images. The most striking finding is the perfect preservation of the folial pattern. No enhancement with contrast agents is observed.

EXTRACEREBRAL TUMOURS

Meningiomas in children do not differ from those in adults – masses appended to the dural sheaths, usually well demarcated from the brain, isodense on precontrast CT, isointense on precontrast T1-W and T2-W MRI, well enhanced by contrast media, occasionally calcified, rarely intraventricular. They may require diagnostic angiography, which can be used also for a presurgical embolization. Isolated, they are rare in children and when they are found, specific features of NF2 should be looked for. Radiation-induced meningiomas are rarely observed in patients previously treated with cranial radiotherapy for a cerebral or cranial malignancy.

Meningeal sarcomas are rare also. They present like meningiomas but on angiography they demonstrate a more irregular vascularity. Presurgical embolization is useful. Recurrence is unfortunately the rule.

Intracranial schwannomas are also practically non-existent outside the context of neurofibromatosis type 2 (NF2). They appear as extra-axial rounded masses that are isodense on CT, isointense to the adjacent brain on T1-W and T2-W on MR imaging and are usually enhanced 'en masse' by the contrast agents.

Dysembryoplastic (inclusion) cysts are uncommon: epidermoids mainly, in the posterior fossa cisterns (see above). Extracerebral neuroglial (neuroepithelial) cysts are not tumours.

BRAIN TUMOURS RELATED TO HAEMATOLOGICAL MALIGNANCY, GENERAL CANCER OR RADIOTHERAPY

Any tumour developing into the bone adjacent to the brain, especially the blood-forming calvarium, may break the dural protection and invade the brain (Figure 12.13.41), especially when it is of an aggressive type and is developing in a young patient.

Langerhans' cell histiocytosis is the most common of the lesions that affect the brain or its coverings in children. Most often located in the diploe, the disease may also present as epidural plaques of abnormal cellularity. Intracerebral locations are uncommon but where they do occur, the pituitary stalk is the most common location, expressing itself clinically as diabetes insipidus. MRI shows the loss of the high signal of the posterior lobe of the pituitary gland and a thickening of the stalk indicating infiltration by the disease. Another location is in the white matter of the cerebellum, presenting as a high T2 signal corresponding to the infiltration by foamy cells. It should not be mistaken for a metabolic disease.

Leukaemic infiltration of the brain is remarkably rare, at least macroscopically, considering the high frequency of leukaemia in children. When it occurs, the location of the mass is either epidural or both epidural and intradiploic. More rarely, a leukaemic leptomeningeal diffusion with leptomeningeal enhancement is observed. Still more rarely, infiltration of the brain itself by the abnormal blood cells is observed, either in the cortex or deeper into the white matter. An association of several locations may be observed. These lesions should not be confused with the lesions related to the drugs used in this clinical context, especially when injected intrathecally.

Similar observations apply to intracranial lymphoma. While meningeal lymphoma deposits do occur, both in association with bone disease and without it, such lesions are rare and unless there are signs or symptoms relating to their presence, imaging is not indicated. Meningeal lymphoma lesions appear as soft tissue masses in the meninges, mildly hypointense to brain on T1-W and slightly hyperintense on T2-W images. They show diffuse enhancement with contrast. Images should be checked for associated bone involvement. These deposits may extend into the orbits.

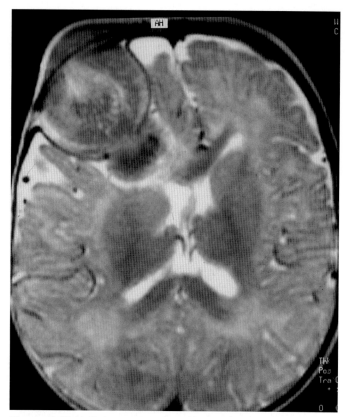

Figure 12.13.41 Ewing sarcoma from the right frontal calvarium in a 7-month-old boy, with intracranial extension, rupture of the dura mater and cerebral invasion to the ventricle.

Intracerebral lesions appear as masses but are rare. A difficult diagnostic problem is the child with known lymphoma, who then presents with acute neurology and is found to have an intracerebral bleed with mass effect. The question is, is this a bleed due to treatment or is this haemorrhage into a lesion? It is often impossible to answer without a biopsy or can only be answered once the lesion has evolved further.

Neuroblastoma metastases may involve the meninges by direct extension through the cranial vault or may involve the meninges and diploic spaces by blood-borne metastases in disseminated stage 4 disease. The lesions, like lymphoma, appear as soft tissue masses in the meninges and may compress the underlying brain. The overlying bone is shown to be involved in most cases and appears as spicules on CT. The cranial sutures are often widened due to sutural deposits. Both the soft tissue masses and the involved periosteum enhance with contrast.

Cerebral metastases of extraneural cancers are remarkably rare and are more often found in the bone than in the brain tissue.

Radiation-induced tumours of the brain usually appear many years after the irradiation and they are more common in children who were young at the time of irradiation. The most common, although infrequent, is the meningioma. Malignant gliomas may be observed. Sarcomas have been described more specifically in the context of radiation treatment of retinoblastomas.

BRAIN TUMOURS RELATED TO NEUROCUTANEOUS AND OTHER INHERITED SYNDROMES

Neuroectodermal syndromes, or phakomatoses, are specific, general systemic disorders that are often genetically determined and usually affect the CNS and the skin, as well as other organs. Our aim here is not to present a description of their clinical-radiological features, which are described elsewhere in this book, but to describe which CNS tumours are likely to develop over the years during the course of these disorders.

Neurofibromatosis type 1 is related to the *NF1* gene on 17q11, coding for neurofibromin. It is the most common genetic disease (1 in 3000–4000 individuals). The clinical features include a multitude of abnormalities of the skin (e.g. café-au-lait spots), the mesenchyme, the peripheral nerves and the CNS. Neurofibromas develop in the nerves distal to the sensory ganglions, often to form plexiform neurofibromas; besides the Schwann cells, they are made up of fibroblasts and may develop into malignant neurofibrosarcomas. The CNS lesions may be purely dysplastic or tumoral lesions. Dysplastic lesions include unilateral or bilateral megalencephaly, areas of abnormal signal in the white matter and the hippocampi, and, very specifically, 'bright spots' in the basal ganglia, the posterior thalami, the brainstem and the deep cerebellar white matter.

Among the tumours, the most common is the pilocytic astrocytoma of the anterior optic pathways and/or of the hypothalamus (Figure 12.13.7). When it develops, it appears in the young child. In NF1, the tumour is somewhat different from that in isolated forms: the meningeal sheaths of the optic nerves are dysplastic and the tumour usually is not as large as in isolated forms. It is more indolent, is often ill enhanced by the contrast agents and commonly stabilizes itself or even regresses at the end of adolescence. Much less commonly, astrocytomas may develop in other areas such as the basal ganglia, the midbrain or the brainstem. It has traditionally been accepted that tumours have a mass effect and enhance with contrast agents, while the 'bright spots' do not; but common clinical experience demonstrates that enhancing masses may disappear spontaneously as well and the general trend now is to follow them using MRI alone. In exceptional cases, however, true high-grade gliomas may develop with their typical poor prognosis. Because of the extreme variety of clinical and morphological features, as well as the unpredictable but generally indolent character of most of the NF1 CNS tumours, there is a trend nowadays not to investigate the patients unless clinical features are present. If a seemingly expanding lesion is uncovered, simple follow-up MR imaging (annual?) is recommended, unless essential functions are compromised.

Neurofibromatosis type 2 can be one of the most devastating diseases of the second and third decades of life (Wishart phenotype), in contrast with the milder form observed in middle-aged individuals (Gardner phenotype). It is related to the NF2 gene on 22q12, coding for the protein merlin. It is characterized by the development of multiple schwannomas, meningiomas (Figure 12.13.42) and ependymomas of the cervical cord and medulla.

The schwannomas are multiple. Typically (but not always) they affect both acoustic nerves, proximal to the geniculate ganglia

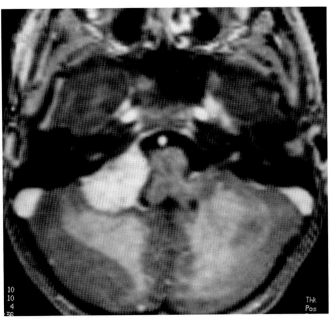

Figure 12.13.42 Bilateral acoustic schwannomas (small discrete areas of enhancement into both internal auditory canals) with a large meningioma of the cerebello-pontine angle cistern in a 7-year-old boy with NF2.

(where they are sometimes hard to separate from the associated meningiomas), the trigeminal nerves, proximal to the Gasserian ganglia, and/or any cranial or spinal nerves, always proximal to the sensory ganglia, on the posterior sensory roots.

The meningiomas are also commonly multiple, nodular on the convexity, or 'en plaque' extensively developed along the base, and able to extend extracranially through the exit foramina of the skull. They are commonly associated with other meningiomas in the spinal canal, and with cranial and spinal schwannomas. When surgery is performed because of their mass effect it produces only transient relief and recurrences as well as emergence of new tumours is the rule.

Ependymomas develop in the cervical cord in the late teens and usually appear on MRI as a mild enlargement with oedema with ill-defined multiple foci of enhancement. They are slow growing. Children suffer more from cord compression by the spinal meningiomas and schwannomas than from the ependymoma itself but, with time, an ependymoma may evolve into a full size, infiltrating mass of the medulla and the cervical cord.

Tuberous sclerosis is another neurocutaneous syndrome, for which two genes have been identified: *TSC1* on 9q34 codes for a protein named hamartin; and *TSC2* on 16p codes for the protein tuberin. The patients have similar phenotypes for both gene mutations. The expression patterns of both proteins seem to overlap, both proteins binding together to form a complex. As well as affecting the CNS, tuberous sclerosis affects the eyes, skin, heart, kidneys, lungs and pancreas. In the brain, it forms cortical tubers, which are considered as focal cortical dysplasias, sometimes with transmantle abnormalities, as well as ependymal small, enhancing nodules. These are commonly calcified on CT; they are usually more or less isointense to the brain in mature children but hyperintense on T1-W and hypointense on T2-W images in infants with unmyelinated brains. All these abnormalities are characterized by the presence of the so-called 'giant astrocyte', which in reality is an ill-differentiated glioneuronal cell. Infrequently (10% of cases), the ependymal nodules, especially those located in the vicinity of the foramina of Monro (Figure 12.13.43), may expand and constitute intraventricular slow-growing, uni- or bilateral (then asymmetrical) subependymal giant cell astrocytomas, which bulge into the ventricles and induce a progressive hydrocephalus. They enhance markedly with contrast agents. Occasionally, they develop acutely as seemingly malignant tumours. The surgical removal of these lesions is controversial.

Other rare inherited syndromes may have brain tumours as part of their expression in children. The Cowden syndrome (*PTEN/MMAC-1* on 10q22-23 coding for PTEN) may be associated with Lhermitte–Duclos disease. The Gorlin syndrome (*PTCH* on 9q31 coding for Patched) may induce the development of medulloblastomas. The Li–Fraumeni syndrome (*TP53* located on 17p13 coding for p53) produces PNETs and astrocytic gliomas. Children with neurocutaneous melanosis develop melanotic

tumours in the leptomeninges, especially in the posterior fossa, that may invade the brain, presumably through the Virchow–Robin spaces. Children with Turcot syndrome (*APC* on 5q21 coding for APC) carry a 100-fold increased risk of developing medulloblastoma; in a subgroup of affected patients, there is a defect in the DNA mismatch/replication error resulting in the development of glioblastomas instead. Von Hippel–Lindau syndrome (*VHL* located on 3q25 encoding pVHL) tends to produce haemangioblastomas in older children and young adults. This is a highly vascular tumour that is often associated with a large cyst in the cerebellum but multiple tumours may also be found in the forebrain and the cord; other extraneural tumours, especially of the adrenal glands, are common.

THE DIAGNOSTIC STEPS

The approach to the diagnosis of a brain tumour in a child can be described as a succession of consecutive steps, starting with the initial symptoms and clinical signs that bring the patient to imaging.

STEP 1: IS THERE A LESION?

This question is now relatively easy to answer, due to the high sensitivity of modern MR imaging techniques, provided the examination has been performed properly. Yet in some strategic areas of the brain, there may be marked clinical signs or symptoms with little detectable abnormality. This particularly applies to the medulla and pituitary stalk. Repeated studies are therefore needed. The main difficulties arise from differentiating an unusual anatomical variant, e.g. a cystic or intensely enhancing pineal gland, or an imaging artifact from a real lesion.

STEP 2: IS THE LESION A TUMOUR?

This is the problem of the differential diagnosis, sometimes the most difficult step of the diagnostic process, when unusual images are found, sometimes incidentally. Some mass lesions are easy to identify as either developmental, e.g. arachnoid cysts, or acquired, e.g. subdural haematomas. Other images are more difficult to characterize and, if there is doubt, repeated studies should be performed after a few months or earlier, depending on the clinical evolution.

A difficult diagnosis may be that of an abscess, when there are no other signs to suggest infection: oedema, ring enhancement and central necrosis are common features. However, the ring enhancement of an abscess is usually thinner, more regularly delineated, and thinner on the cortical side, or on the ventricular side in neonates. Diffusion imaging helps by showing the lack of restriction of proton mobility in cystic tumours, while the mobility is restricted in abscesses.

A hamartoma of the floor of the 3rd ventricle, extra- or intraventricular, is commonly mistaken for a tumour. Although there are specific clinical features (precocious puberty or gelastic

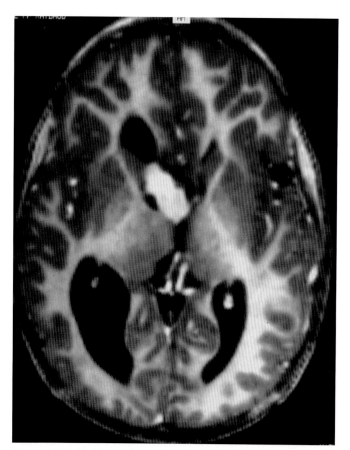

Figure 12.13.43 Giant cell astrocytoma originating in the vicinity of the right foramen of Monro in a 5-year-old boy with tuberous sclerosis. Note the marked enhancement of the neoplasm and the unilateral hydrocephalus. The 'giant astrocyte' in reality is a poorly differentiated glioneuronal cell, somewhat related to the typical cells of Taylor's focal cortical dysplasia.

seizures), the harmartomas appear as normal brain tissue developed from the tuber cinereum, in the interpeduncular cistern or within the ventricular lumen.

Distinguishing an area of focal cortical dysplasia from a dysplastic tumour may prove very difficult, especially as they share the same clinical expression. The treatment, however, is the same and the pathologist ultimately makes the diagnosis. In the same way, subcortical or paraventricular heterotopias may not be correctly identified, as they present as 'masses', often with partial epilepsy of late onset; but they are not space occupying, the ventricle is often locally enlarged instead of compressed and their appearance is that of normal grey matter.

Triventricular hydrocephalus is too often qualified as 'aqueductal stenosis', which is a rare disease, especially in children (3% of non-tumoral hydrocephalus compared with 13% in adults). Therefore, triventricular hydrocephalus should make one suspicious of a midbrain intrinsic mass or a pineal region tumour. Diagnosis can be difficult with CT alone. Good-quality MRI should display the lesion and the correct diagnosis.

The general use of MR imaging has revealed the relative frequency of cystic pineal glands as an incidental finding. These should not be mistaken for tumours and should not even be identified as pathological lesions. They should be considered as anatomical variants, unless they are large enough to compress the aqueduct. Also, the normal pineal may vary in size between individuals and it may also enhance differently. Whenever there is doubt about the size and the enhancement, a control study should be performed after a few months.

Pseudotumour cerebri is a difficult diagnosis to make if no cause, e.g. dural sinus thrombosis, is found. Diffuse, ill-defined brain lesions, with heterogeneous high signal on T2-W imaging may indicate oedema or encephalitis, as well as diffuse tumours.

Intracerebral bleeding in children should never be considered as spontaneous. If no trauma has occurred, no coagulopathy found and there is no vascular occlusion, vascular malformation or hamartoma (cavernoma), a tumoral bleed always remains a possibility. The demonstration of tumour tissue and/or of the enhancement pattern or a history of previous cranial irradiation helps to resolve many difficult cases but surgery with pathological examination of the specimen may be required for the diagnosis.

Focal gliosis is usually associated with atrophy, e.g. enlarged sulci, and enlarged ventricular lumen, while gliomas compress the sulci and distort the ventricles.

Finally, any mass may be confusing, whether enhancing or not: acute inflammatory demyelinating disease, toxic oedema, oedematous ischaemia even. Conversely, in a highly strategic area such as the medulla, a small lesion looking like a small plaque, for example, may prove with time to be a low-grade glioma.

STEP 3: IS THE TUMOUR BENIGN OR MALIGNANT?

The features commonly used in neuroradiology to distinguish malignant from benign cerebral tumours do not always apply to the variety of tumours observed in young patients:

- Is the tumour infiltrative or well demarcated? Benign juvenile pilocytic astrocytoma (JPA) of the anterior optic pathways is typically infiltrative but benign. A malignant atypical rhabdoid-teratoid tumour (well demarcated) is malignant.
- The status of the blood–brain barrier is not always indicative either: a fibrillary astrocytoma enhances when becoming more malignant but the JPA, always benign, nearly always enhances.
- Peritumoral oedema can be seen in nearly every tumour when they are large enough but may be absent around malignant ones. Intratumoral oedema is almost invariable, whatever the tumour type. Necrosis can be observed in any type of tumour of significant volume. Haemorrhage can be seen in JPA and is even a feature of a non-evolving tumour such as the dysplastic DNT.
- Dissemination through the subarachnoid spaces is usually a sign of malignancy and is found in germinomas and other malignant germ cell tumours and medulloblastomas but the anaplastic astrocytomas or the glioblastomas almost never disseminate, whereas again the JPA, although benign, may on occasion disseminate as well.
- In fact, the best indicators for malignancy are the changes in the appearance of the mass over time. A hypodense low-grade fibrillary astrocytoma that presents with higher densities or focal necrosis and with enhancement is likely to have become malignant. Invasiveness across anatomical limits is also a sign of malignancy, e.g. a well demarcated pinealoblastoma invading the nearby splenium.

STEP 4: WHERE IS THE TUMOUR LOCATED?

As will be emphasized later, the topography of a tumour of the CNS in a child is one of the major elements for identifying its nature, as the principal brain neoplasms have a predilection for given areas of the brain. For example, fibrillary astrocytomas occur in the ventral pons, whilst JPA occurs in the dorsal pons. This is helpful as evidence but with invasive lesions, the starting area may not be obvious, especially when the tumour is large and distorts the anatomy. Surgery as a rule is the single most efficient treatment of CNS tumours in children. Therefore, a careful anatomical assessment is a prerequisite for surgical planning. This is required to decide on the feasibility of resection as balanced against the functional risks for the patient; also, to decide on the surgical approach. For example, a 'pineal region' neoplasm developing mostly towards the ventricle may be approached through the corpus callosum and the ventricle, while a mass located mostly in the ambient cistern will be approached through an interoccipital route. Finally, depending on the anatomy and the location of the lesion, the surgical approach through or around the mass can be decided.

STEP 5: WHAT ARE THE EFFECTS OF THE TUMOUR ON THE BRAIN?

Tumours usually are relatively slow-growing processes to which the brain adapts for weeks and months, until the child commonly decompensates rapidly. This may present as a sudden loss of function, for example vision, but is more often related to the complications of increased intracranial pressure with alteration of consciousness and coma. This may occur with massive hydrocephalus with periventricular oedema, transtentorial herniation either upwards or downwards, or transoccipital herniation. It is also important to identify focal compression of, for example, the brainstem or optic chiasm. A supratentorial mass effect may compress the posterior part of the hemisphere between the vault, the tentorium and the posterior falx, resulting in ischaemia. Herniation under the falx may stretch the anterior cerebral artery, which is another cause for ischaemia. All these complications may cause modification of the surgical strategy.

STEP 6: WHICH TUMOUR IS IT?

The identification of the pathology of the most common types of brain tumours during the first two decades of life rests upon two points: the appearance of the lesion, as described above, and the topography, as the most frequently encountered brain neoplasms tend to originate in relatively specific areas of the brain. As these tumours have already been described above, only the topographic distribution is presented below.

POSTERIOR FOSSA

Posterior fossa tumours are frequent in children and represent about 50% of all intracranial tumours. They usually produce hydrocephalus but not always. The mass may be small and away from the ventricular lumen. Even when huge, most brainstem gliomas produce little, if any, hydrocephalus as they enlarge, rather than compress, the 4th ventricle.

BRAINSTEM

Infiltrative tumours of the ventral pons are always fibrillary astrocytomas (Figure 12.13.8). They are rarely nodular, usually diffusely infiltrative, often exophytic within the peritruncal cisterns, encasing the basilar artery, but not in the 4th ventricle; they may or may not be enhanced, haemorrhagic, necrotic or symmetrical. These tumours may infiltrate towards the midbrain or the pons but they more commonly displace and compress them. They may also be centred on the middle cerebellar peduncle.

Tumours of the floor of the 4th ventricle, often exophytic in the ventricular lumen, are usually juvenile pilocytic astrocytomas; they diffusely enhance with contrast agents (Figure 12.13.3). In the same way, tumours of the medulla are typically JPAs. They may be partly cystic. They usually enhance. They may develop anteriorly as well as posteriorly (Figure 12.13.2). They may represent the upper part of a JPA of the cervical cord.

FOURTH VENTRICLE

Besides the exophytic JPA of the dorsal brainstem, only two tumours commonly develop within the 4th ventricle: the medulloblastoma and the ependymoma. The medulloblastoma typically develops from the roof of the ventricle, usually in the inferior vermis, and from there it expands upwards into the ventricular lumen, which usually caps it (Figure 12.13.11). It may compress the floor of the ventricle but usually does not infiltrate it. Hydrocephalus is common, often massive. Although well demarcated, it is a malignant lesion that tends to disseminate (Figure 12.13.12), sometimes being present as early as at the first examination (Figure 12.13.13). It may also be necrotic and/or haemorrhagic. Less commonly, medulloblastoma may develop from the upper or the central vermis, pushing the 4th ventricle forwards rather than invading it.

An ependymoma also develops from the lower part of the 4th ventricle but more from the floor or the lateral recesses. Therefore, it tends to expand below the cerebellar vermis (Figure 12.13.15), towards the foramen magnum and the cervical spine, or, more laterally, towards the cerebello-pontine angle cisterns. It tends to mould the cisterns. It disseminates in the subarachnoid spaces, less commonly than the medulloblastoma.

Rarely, other tumours may be found in this region, e.g. choroid plexus papillomas, carcinomas or dermoids.

CEREBELLUM

The most usual and most characteristic tumour of the cerebellum is the cystic juvenile pilocytic astrocytoma (Figure 12.13.1). It is located in the vermis or lateral to it, is either solid or cystic, and is usually a large mass. Desmoplastic medulloblastomas may grow away from the ventricle, within the cerebellar hemispheres; because of the anatomical arrangement of the cerebellum, they develop in close contact with the arachnoid and develop a strong characteristic fibrotic reaction (Figure 12.13.14). Rarely, cystic haemangioblastomas may be found in older children as part of the von Hippel–Lindau syndrome.

MIDBRAIN

Most of the tumours that develop in the midbrain are astrocytomas, either fibrillary or pilocytic. Fibrillary astrocytomas may infiltrate the ventral midbrain and from there expand towards the thalami. Other less aggressive masses may develop in the collicular plate or around the aqueduct. Many of the so-called 'aqueductal stenoses' are actually dormant astrocytomas of the aqueductal region or postinflammatory stenoses. The primary tectal tumours may be difficult to differentiate from the infiltration of the collicular plate by tumours originating from the pineal region.

THIRD VENTRICLE

ANTERIOR 3RD VENTRICLE: SUPRASELLAR TUMOURS

These have common clinical features: hydrocephalus, visual defects and hormonal disorders. The most common neoplasm expanding from, or in the vicinity of, the anterior 3rd ventricle is the juvenile pilocytic astrocytoma. It may develop either along the anterior optic pathways or from the ventricular floor and is not usually surgically accessible in either location (Figures 12.13.4 to 12.13.7). Optic gliomas (Figure 12.13.5) are usually, but not always, centred at the chiasm, extending more or less into the intracranial portion of the optic nerves (usually asymmetrically), or along the optic tracts. They may preserve the general morphology of the optic pathways or, conversely, be so large as to appear primarily as a giant subfrontal mass (Figure 12.13.6), which is often partly cystic. They may also expand into the 3rd ventricle and obstruct the foramina of Monro, and presumably from the optic tract into the basal ganglia. Exceptionally, an optic glioma develops in the orbit on one optic nerve, away from the chiasm, and can then be removed. The other variety of JPA develops in the tuber cinereum (hypothalamic glioma), behind the chiasm but in front of the mamillary bodies (Figure 12.13.4). In this location, they may be huge, expanding into the lumen of the ventricle as well as into the cisterns. When they are large enough, it is impossible, radiologically or surgically, to identify their site of origin (Figures 12.13.6 to 12.13.7). Both optic and hypothalamic gliomas should be specifically looked for in the assessment of NF1. In general, they tend to be less aggressive in this context and may regress spontaneously. Often, they enhance less in the context of NF1 (Figure 12.13.7) than in the sporadic form. It is usually considered that sporadic suprasellar gliomas have a poorer prognosis than those linked to NF1 but the comparative series are necessarily biased by the fact that in NF1 they are systematically looked for even when they are asymptomatic.

The craniopharyngiomas typically arise either in the sella (Figures 12.13.21 and 12.13.22) or the hypothalamus (Figures 12.13.23 and 12.13.24). The former is within an enlarged sella, the pituitary gland is not seen and extension occurs towards the subfrontal region in front of the chiasm and extracerebrally. The hypothalamic lesions are behind the chiasm and extend towards the ventricular lumen and the posterior fossa cisterns. Both topographic varieties may be solid, cystic or both, the purely cystic forms being found in the sella. The main topographic features of these have been previously described.

Other uncommon tumours of the anterior 3rd ventricle include germ cell tumours, especially germinomas (Figure 12.13.30), ependymomas, congenital lesions like Rathke's cleft cysts (Figure 12.13.26) or dermoids. Tumours limited to the pituitary stalk are either germinomas, histiocytosis or gliomas, and all are rare. Solid hamartomas and neuroglial cysts of the floor of the ventricle are not tumours, although neuroglial cysts may need opening to prevent compression of the third ventricle and the brainstem.

POSTERIOR 3RD VENTRICLE: PINEAL REGION TUMOURS

These also share common clinical features, such as hydrocephalus and Parinaud's syndrome. They are situated in a region of the brain that is surgically difficult to access, deep between the hemispheres and below the splenium of the corpus callosum, where the deep venous system collects to form the great vein of Galen. It is also the region of the brain where the differential diagnosis between the various types of tumours is the most uncertain.

The pineal region is a preferential site for germ cell tumours. The most common are germinomas (Figure 12.13.29), followed by teratomas (Figure 12.13.34), the other histological types being less

common. These tumours tend to develop more towards the posterior 3rd ventricle but they may also expand into the ambient cistern towards the posterior fossa. The presence of multiple cystic components is highly suggestive of a teratoma. A finding common to this class of tumours is early calcification of the pineal gland (Figure 12.13.31).

The second type of tumour in this region is the pineoblastoma (Figures 12.13.18 and 12.13.19). This appears as a sometimes hugely enlarged pineal mass, which lies in the cistern rather than in the ventricle, infiltrating the adjacent structures such as the collicular plate and the splenium, pushing the posterior wall of the 3rd ventricle rather than invading its lumen. Pilocytic astrocytomas may develop here also. The pineal is a classical site for the development of the exceedingly rare dermoid.

TELA CHOROIDEA

The choroidal roof of the 3rd ventricle may also be the site of specific tumours, all uncommon. Choroid plexus papillomas may grow there. Meningiomas are sometimes observed in a context of NF2. In older children, colloid cysts may be observed.

LATERAL VENTRICLES

- At the level of the choroid plexus, papillomas in infants (Figure 12.13.17) and carcinomas in older children may be found. Meningiomas are very rare.
- In patients with tuberous sclerosis, a peculiar type of giant cell astrocytoma may arise, usually at the level of the foramina of Monro (Figure 12.13.43), uni- or bilaterally, infiltrating the adjacent structures, especially the pillars of the fornix, while growing. These giant cell astrocytomas are specific for the disease. Monitoring their development is one of the aims of regular follow-up studies in tuberous sclerosis patients, as the complication of hydrocephalus might induce, or add to, the mental deterioration.
- Rare intraventricular ependymomas may be radiologically confused with choroid plexus carcinomas.

CEREBRAL HEMISPHERES

BASAL GANGLIA

Tumours developing in the basal ganglia are mainly of two types. The thalami are a classical site for germinomas (Figures 12.13.32 and 12.13.33), which in this site are often calcified or cystic. Because of the de-afferentation and the rarefaction of the corona radiata on the affected side, the hemisphere may appear paradoxically smaller on the side of the tumour than on the normal side. The other relatively common type of tumour developing in both the thalami and the basal ganglia are the gliomas, which are most often malignant. Bilateral involvement of the thalami together with the midbrain can be observed in cases of infiltrative fibrillary astrocytomas; it should not be confused with the so-called 'bilateral striatal necrosis', a deadly postinfectious inflammatory disorder that affects the thalami and the midbrain tegmentum also.

WHITE MATTER

All kinds of tumours may be found in the cerebral white matter but the most usual are low- and high-grade gliomas (Figure 12.13.9), the rare gliomatosis cerebri (Figure 12.13.10) and, more commonly, the supratentorial ependymoma (Figure 12.13.16).

CORTEX

The cortex is the elective site for the development of the dysplastic, epileptogenic glioneuronal tumours, especially in the temporal lobe. The most common is the ganglioglioma: it may be restricted to the cortex (Figures 12.13.38 and 12.13.39) or may present with a massive gliomatous component, benign or malignant, extending into the white matter (Figure 12.13.40). The second most common cortical tumour is the dysembryoplastic epithelial tumour (Figures 12.13.36 and 12.13.37). This perfectly static tumour may sometimes become somewhat more space occupying because of intratumoral haemorrhages and neoangiogenesis (Figure 12.13.37). Although cortical in origin, the abnormalities may involve the corresponding subjacent segment of white matter, sometimes as far as the ventricle. In infants, the rare desmoplastic infantile ganglioglioma also is essentially cortical at the beginning.

CEREBRAL TUMOURS IN INFANTS

Cerebral tumours are uncommon in infants but all tumours of the brain have been observed in this age group, sometimes as congenital lesions. A few tumour types are more characteristic of that age: the choroid plexus papilloma (Figure 12.13.17), midline teratomas (Figure 12.13.34), which are sometimes huge, the atypical rhabdoid-teratoid tumours, optic gliomas, ependymomas, the extracerebellar PNET (Figure 12.13.37), metastases of neuroblastomas and extraneural tumours such as the sarcomas (Figure 12.13.41). Epilepsy and intracranial hypertension with macrocrania are common presenting symptoms. The infantile desmoplastic ganglioglioma is quite specific of that age but it is exceedingly rare.

FOLLOW-UP OF BRAIN TUMOURS IN CHILDREN

The follow-up of brain tumours depends on several aspects of their natural history. For tumours that have been operated upon, immediate routine postoperative control with MRI or, more simply and as efficiently, with CT, with and without contrast injection discloses whether any significant amount of the tumour mass has been left behind. As the examination is made before the scarring processes have begun, any enhancement means that some neoplastic tissue is present, provided the tumour was an enhancing one. It is also done to identify any surgical complication. In the first weeks after surgery, CT or MRI may be useful to understand a poor clinical evolution or a secondary deterioration. Later on, MRI is necessary for follow-up of the patient and to observe tumour response to chemotherapeutic or radiotherapeutic agents,

and to detect recurrence. This follow-up is usually conducted according to specific rules related to specific therapeutic protocols. It should concern the site of the primary tumour and if this is of a disseminating kind, the whole craniospinal axis (Figure 12.13.12).

For tumours that have not been operated upon, usually because the risks for the patients outweigh the expected benefits, the follow-up studies are aimed at checking the response to the chemotherapy and/or radiotherapy, according to the same rules as after surgery. Specific evolution of the neoplasm, such as the change from a low-grade to a high-grade tumour, should be looked for, in order to adapt the treatment. The use of MR spectroscopy may be helpful in this respect.

In every case, the occurrence of long-term complications should be monitored; for example hydrocephalus requiring draining. A special problem is that of radionecrosis, which may be difficult to distinguish from a recurrence or from a malignant change, the more so as these are commonly associated. Special imaging techniques such as MR spectroscopy or perfusion may occasionally be helpful.

CONCLUSION

Brain tumours are a common and severe condition in children. Today, diagnosis is mainly made by MR imaging, often complemented by CT – together they are remarkably efficient. Most tumours need a surgical approach, either for tentative complete excision, or for debulking or biopsy. Therefore, neuroradiology should not only recognize the tumour, it should also provide information relevant to the surgical procedure. Recognizing the exact histological nature of the lesion is not so important, except in the particular instance of germinomas, which can be completely cured by medical treatment alone. It is more important to:

- locate the lesion, not only for the anatomy but also because histological probabilities depend on location;
- to study its relationship to adjacent structures, not only in order to evaluate the surgical risks but also the risks of tumour growth;
- to analyze the general effects of the mass on the brain (oedema, hydrocephalus, herniation, vascular compression or stretching); and
- to assess features in favour of benignity or malignancy (infiltration across the natural anatomical barriers, necrosis, haemorrhages), bearing in mind that contrast enhancement, oedema and cyst formation are frequent in benign tumours and that some malignant tumours, e.g. germinomas, have a better prognosis than some perfectly benign ones, e.g. a large infiltrative, non-resectable low-grade glioma.

FURTHER READING

Alvord EC, Lofton S. Gliomas of the optic nerve and chiasm. Journal of Neurosurgery 1988; 69:171–176.

Aoki S, Barkovich AJ, Nishimura K et al. Neurofibromatosis type 1 and 2 cranial MR findings. Radiology 1991; 172:527–534.

Armington WG, Osborn AG, Cubberly DA. Supratentorial ependymomas: CT appearance. Radiology 1985; 157:367–372.

Brunel H, Raybaud C, Peretti-Viton P et al. Les craniopharyngiomes de l'enfant. Etude en IRM d'une série de 43 cas. Neurochirurgie 2002; 48:309–318.

Cha S, Knopp EA, Johnson G et al. Intracranial Mass Lesions: Dynamic contrast-enhanced susceptibility-weighted echo-planar perfusion MR imaging. Radiology 2002; 223:11–29.

Chang T, Teng MMH, Guo WY, Sheng WC. CT of pineal tumors and intracranial germ cell tumors. American Journal of Neuroradiology 1989; 10:1039–1044.

Coates TL, Hinshaw DB, Peckman N et al. Pediatric choroid plexus neoplasms: MR, CT and pathologic correlations. Radiology 1989; 173:81–88.

Jelinek J, Smirniotopaulos JG, Parisi JE, Kanzer M. Lateral ventricular neoplasms of the brain: differential diagnosis based on clinical, CT and MR findings. American Journal of Neuroradiology 1990; 11:567–574.

Kwak R, Sano S, Suzuki S. Ipsilateral cerebral atrophy with thalamic tumor of childhood. Journal of Neurosurgery 1978; 48:443–449.

Lantos PL, Louis DN, Rosenblum MK, Kleihus P. Tumours of the nervous system. In: Graham DI, Lantos PL, eds. Greenfield's neuropathology, 7th edn, vol. 2; 2002: 768–1052.

Lee Y, Vantassel P, Bruner JM, Moser RI, Share JC. Juvenile pilocytic astrocytomas: CT and MR characteristics. American Journal of Neuroradiology 1989; 10:363–370.

Muller-Forell W, Schroth G, Egan PJ. MR imaging in tumors of the pineal region. Neuroradiologie 1988; 30:224–231.

Mutoh K, Okuno T, Ito M et al. Ipsilateral atrophy in children with hemispheric cerebral tumors: CT findings. Journal of Computer Assisted Tomography 1988; 12:740–742.

Peretti-Viton P, Perez-Castillo AM, Raybaud CK et al. MRI in gangliogliomas and gangliocytomas of the nervous system. Journal of Neuroradiology 1991; 18:189.

Rout D, Das L, Rao VRK, Radhakrishnan VV. Symptomatic Rathke's cleft cysts. Surgical Neurology 1983; 19:42–45.

Soejima T, Takeshita I, Yamamoto H. Computed tomography of germinomas of the basal ganglia and thalamus. Neuroradiology 1987; 29:366–370.

Spagnoli MV, Grossman RI, Packer RJ et al. Magnetic resonance imaging determination of gliomatosis cerebri. Neuroradiology 1987; 29:15–18.

Spoto GP, Press GA, Hesselink JR et al. Intracranial ependymomas and subependymomas: MR manifestations. American Journal of Neuroradiology 1990; 11:83–91.

Tamburrini G, Colosimo C, Giangaspero F et al. Desmoplastic infantile ganglioglioma 2003; 19:292–297.

Teo C, Nakaji P, Symons P et al. Ependymoma. Childs Nervous System 2003; 19:270–285.

Tortori-Donati P, Fondelli MP, Cama A et al. Ependymomas of the posterior cranial fossa: CT and MRI findings. Neuroradiology 1995; 37:238–243.

Tortori-Donati P, Fondelli MP, Rossi A et al. Medulloblastoma in children: CT and MRI findings. Neuroradiology 1996; 38:352–359.

Tseng JH, Tseng MY, Kuo MF et al. Chronological changes on magnetic resonance images in a case of desmoplastic infantile ganglioglioma. Pediatric Neurosurgery 2002; 36:29–32.

Yousem DM, Patrone PM, Grossman RI. Leptomeningeal metastases: MR evaluation. Journal of Computer Assisted Tomography 1990; 14:255–261.

Zee CH, Segall H, Apuzzo M et al. MR imaging of pineal region neoplasms. Journal of Computer Assisted Tomography 1991; 15:56–63.

Spinal Cord Neoplasms

Helen Carty

Spinal cord tumours are rare compared with brain tumours in paediatrics. They represent about 10% of all central nervous system tumours in children and can occur at all ages. In general, they are slow-growing lesions. The clinical presentation is often one of subtle symptoms with an insidious onset. The symptoms are usually those of pain and gait disturbance with bowel and bladder sphincter disturbance symptoms occurring relatively late. The pain is dull and aching but may be radicular if there is involvement of a nerve root. Scoliosis is a recognized presentation. Painful scoliosis may be due to a bony vertebral lesion or a spinal cord tumour. Cervicomedullary and cervical cord tumours may present with torticollis.

IMAGING

Once a spinal cord lesion is suspected, magnetic resonance imaging (MRI) is indicated. This should include the whole of the spinal cord with T1-weighted (T1-W) and T2-weighted (T2-W) images in the sagittal plane with axial slices across the whole of the lesion. Gadolinium-enhanced images should be performed in both planes. These views should be supplemented by coronal and oblique views as indicated in individual cases.

Plain radiographs are often initially done in a search for the cause of back pain but have a very low yield in spinal neoplasms. One may see widening of the interpedicular distance with flattening of the medial aspect of the pedicles in slow-growing tumours. Occasionally, a lesion such as an aneurysmal bone cyst with extradural extension may be identified as the cause of the presenting symptom.

When analyzing the MRI, lesions should be classified as intramedullary or extramedullary. Intramedullary lesions expand the cord over the length of the tumour. There is obliteration of the subarachnoid space. They mostly affect the whole width of the cord but they may lie eccentrically and give an apparent extramedullary appearance. Extramedullary lesions displace the cord to one side. These may be intra- or extradural. They usually have sharp outlines and, depending on size, there may be cerebrospinal fluid (CSF) between them and the cord. If large, this space will become obliterated. The administration of contrast may help to separate an extradural mass from the cord.

INTRAMEDULLARY TUMOURS

Intramedullary tumours comprise about 30% of all spinal cord tumours in children. The peak incidence is between about 8 and 12 years but they may occur at all ages in childhood. The clinical presentation is often indolent, with pain being a major symptom. The pain is usually located to the spinal segments surrounding the tumour. Burning pain and paraesthesia located to segments just below the tumour is also described. Weakness of the extremities is frequent.

ASTROCYTOMA

About 60% of intramedullary tumours in children are low-grade astrocytomas. The remainder are ependymomas. Astrocytomas are more frequent in the cervical and upper thoracic cord. Ependymomas tend to be more caudal in location. Other reported intramedullary tumours in children are gangliocytomas and gangliogliomas, and primitive neuroectodermal tumours.

On MR imaging, astrocytomas produce fusiform cord enlargement over the length of the tumour (Figure 12.14.1). The adjacent subarachnoid spaces are obliterated. Though fusiform cord swelling is the norm, sometimes intramedullary lesions may lie eccentrically within the cord to produce an appearance more similar to an extramedullary lesion. Though astrocytomas are basically solid lesions they may be associated with cystic components, which may extend beyond the margins of the tumour.

Within the tumour margins the cystic components may represent necrosis but cysts are also found above and below the more solid component of tumour. Astrocytomas tend to be slightly darker than the cord on T1-W images, often with some heterogeneity. On T2-W images, they have a higher signal than the normal cord. The cysts usually are of low signal on T1-W images and high on T2-W images but high protein content within the cyst may cause them to be of higher signal. Contrast enhancement is seen in astrocytomas and may be homogeneous or heterogeneous. Contrast enhancement may also help to distinguish between cysts and necrosis. Demarcation of tumour margins is poorer with astrocytomas than with ependymomas. With astrocytomas, histologically the tumour margin tends to extend beyond the area of enhancement.

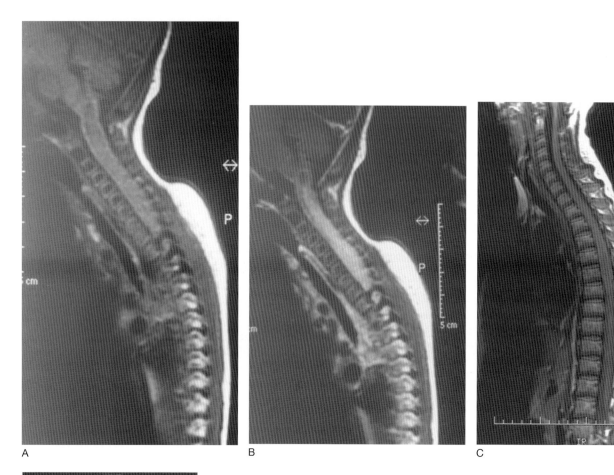

A

B

C

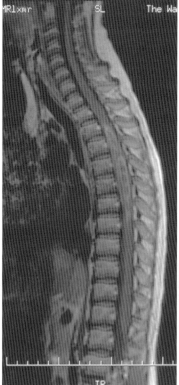

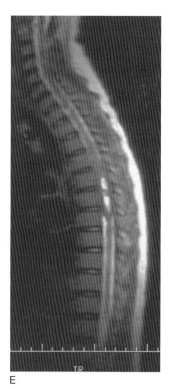

D

E

Figure 12.14.1 (A) T1-W image showing fusiform cord enlargement obliterating the subarachnoid space around the cord. This is the typical appearance of an astrocytoma of the cord. (B) T1-W image with gadolinium showing enhancement of the tumour. (C)–(E) A different child. (C) Sagittal T1-W image without gadolinium, (D) T1-W image with gadolinium and (E) T2-W image of a child with an astrocytoma of the cord, with a cystic component. Note the enhancement with gadolinium.

The prognosis for children with cord astrocytomas depends on the ability to resect the lesion and on the cell type, with pilocytic astrocytomas having the best prognosis.

EPENDYMOMAS

Cord ependymomas tend to occur more caudally than astrocytomas but otherwise present similarly (Figure 12.14.2). Cysts are present above or below the tumour in up to 80% of ependymomas. The precise cause is not known but is probably related to obstruction to CSF flow. Tumour enhancement is concordant with the limits of the tumour margins. Tumour haemorrhage is seen in about 20% of ependymomas, which may be old. If acute, it is of high signal on both T1-W and T2-W images. If old, it is of low signal on T2-W images.

HAEMANGIOBLASTOMA

Haemangioblastoma nodules may affect the cord and appear as an intramedullary lesion. They show marked contrast enhancement due to the vascular nature of the tumour. This too is usually shown by the presence of flow voids from vessels. Cysts are found in 70% of cases. Haemangioblastomas are one component of Von Hippel–Lindau disease.

CAVERNOMA AND ANGIOMATOUS MALFORMATIONS

Spinal cord cavernomas are vascular tumours that often have an acute clinical presentation because of the sudden increase in size caused by haemorrhage (Figure 12.14.3). They represent about 3% of all intramedullary tumours. During an acute presentation with bleeding, there is high signal on both T1-W and T2-W images. A mixed signal intensity is also described. The cord is expanded by the haemorrhage (Figure 12.14.4). Contrast enhancement may occur depending on how much of the lesion is affected by haemorrhage. As the acute haemorrhage resolves, the signal alters and there is then sometimes low signal due to deoxyhaemoglobin or haemosiderin deposits. The lesions may be multiple.

Other angiomatous cord malformations that may present in childhood because of pain or an acute bleed include fistulas and vascular malformations. The appearance on MRI depends on the presence and age of the intramedullary haematoma. The angioma itself has enlarged tortuous vessels with flow voids. For full demonstration of the lesion, spinal angiography is required to identify the vascular anatomy of the feeding vessels, any arteriovenous shunting and the relationship of these to the cord blood supply (Figure 12.14.5).

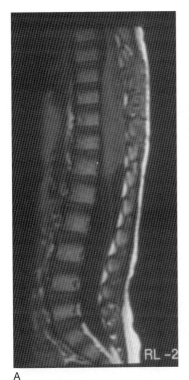
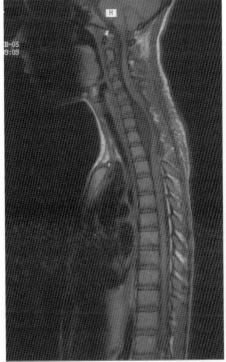
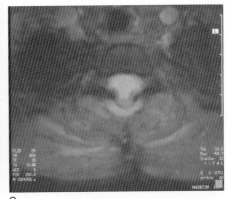

A B C

Figure 12.14.2 (A) Sagittal T1-weighted image of a 3-year-old boy with an ependymoma of the distal cord. (B,C) Images of a different child with a cystic ependymoma arising on the ventral cord and causing very significant attenuation of the residual cord, not involved by the cystic tumour.

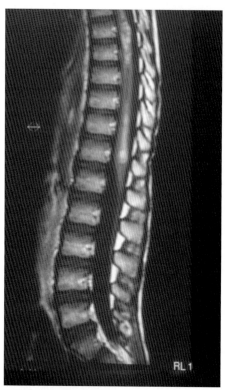

Figure 12.14.3 Sagittal T1-weighted sequence of the lower cord in a boy with two foci of a haemangioma of the cord.

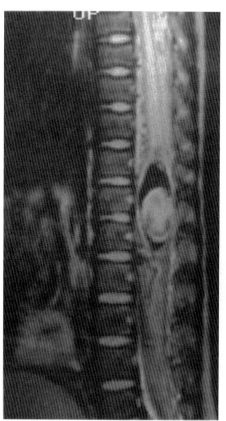

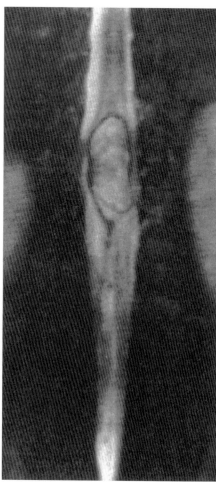

Figure 12.14.4 Angiomatous malformation of the spinal cord with intramedullary haemorrhage. A 5-year-old child who presented with a sudden paraplegia. Sagittal (A) and coronal (B) T2-weighted sequences. The central part of the haematoma is bright due to methaemoglobin and the periphery dark due to haemosiderin plus flow in blood vessels. Note also flow void due to the vessels.

A

B

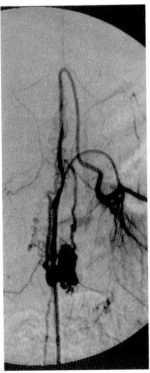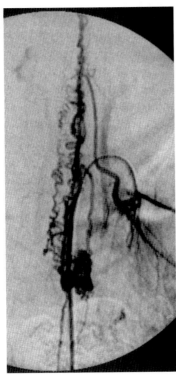

Figure 12.14.5 Intramedullary arteriovenous malformation (AVM). Spinal angiogram shows an enlarged arteria radicularis magna. The anterior spinal artery also is large and is the main feeding vessel of an intramedullary AVM, which drains to the perimedullary venous plexus.

CONGENITAL TUMOURS OF THE SPINAL CORD

Congenital intramedullary spinal cord tumours include lipomas, hamartomas, dermoids and epidermoids.

INTRAMEDULLARY LIPOMA

Most spinal cord lipomas are associated with dysraphism but intramedullary lipomas are rarely reported in children. As with all other intramedullary tumours, presenting symptoms are back pain, gait disturbance, altered sensation and limb weakness. As the lesions are benign, symptoms may be present for a long time. The lesions show as fat signal on T1-W and T2-W images and the signal is suppressed with fat suppression sequences. There is no gadolinium enhancement.

DERMOIDS

Spinal cord dermoids, as elsewhere, are tumours that are lined with squamous epithelium and contain varying tissues such as skin, hair, teeth and sebaceous glands. They are well demarcated round or ovoid tumours, which may be uni- or multilocular. There is an equal sex incidence and they usually present clinically in childhood or before 20 years of age. They are found in association with dermal sinuses in about one-fifth of patients, which brings them to medical attention (Figure 12.14.6A,B). Iatrogenic lesions caused by implantation during procedures has been described. Eighty per cent of spinal dermoids occur in the lumbosacral region. On MR imaging, the most frequent appearance is of low to intermediate signal on T1-W and high signal on T2-W images, but there may be a fatty signal on T1-W images if there is sufficient fat content. They do not enhance with contrast unless infected. This mainly occurs when they are associated with a dermal sinus track. Ascending infection may cause meningitis. They may be discovered on rare occasions by serendipity when a tooth or similar structure is seen in an abdominal x-ray done for some other purpose (Figure 12.14.6C,D).

EPIDERMOIDS

Epidermoid tumours are lined by the skin epidermal elements. They are distributed throughout the length of the spinal canal. They may also be associated with dermal sinuses. Clinical presentation, which is usually that of a slowly progressive myelopathy, is more common in adult life than in childhood. There is a male predominance. About 40% of lesions are intramedullary. On imaging, they are most frequently isointense to CSF on MRI and may be very difficult to diagnose when they are not intramedullary because of the similar imaging characteristics. Flair sequences will show epidermoids as a mass of increased signal compared with surrounding tissue. The space-occupying effect of displacement of the nerve roots and cord also indicate presence of epidermoids (Figure 12.14.7). They do not enhance with contrast unless infected.

HAMARTOMAS

Hamartomas are tumours composed of mesoderm and may contain bone, skin or cartilage. They are usually located in the midthoracic or thoracolumbar region and present clinically as skin covered masses (Figure 12.14.8). Overlying cutaneous angiomas may be present. They are associated with spina bifida in 60% of patients and widening of the spinal canal in 80%. They have been reported to contain choroid plexus tissue and syringomyelia.

SYRINGOHYDROMYELIA

Syringohydromyelia may be associated with congenital brainstem malformations (e.g. Chiari 1 and 2 lesions), bony narrowing of the foramen magnum, may be post-traumatic or may develop in association with tumour or arachnoiditis. As the clinical presentation may be similar to a spinal cord neoplasm it is discussed here. Clinical presentation includes paraesthesias, limb weakness (particularly upper limbs), scoliosis and gait abnormalities. Loss of sensation is described as dissociated. There is loss of pain and temperature sensation while the sense of touch is preserved. In spite of the loss of focal pain sensitivity when tested with pin prick,

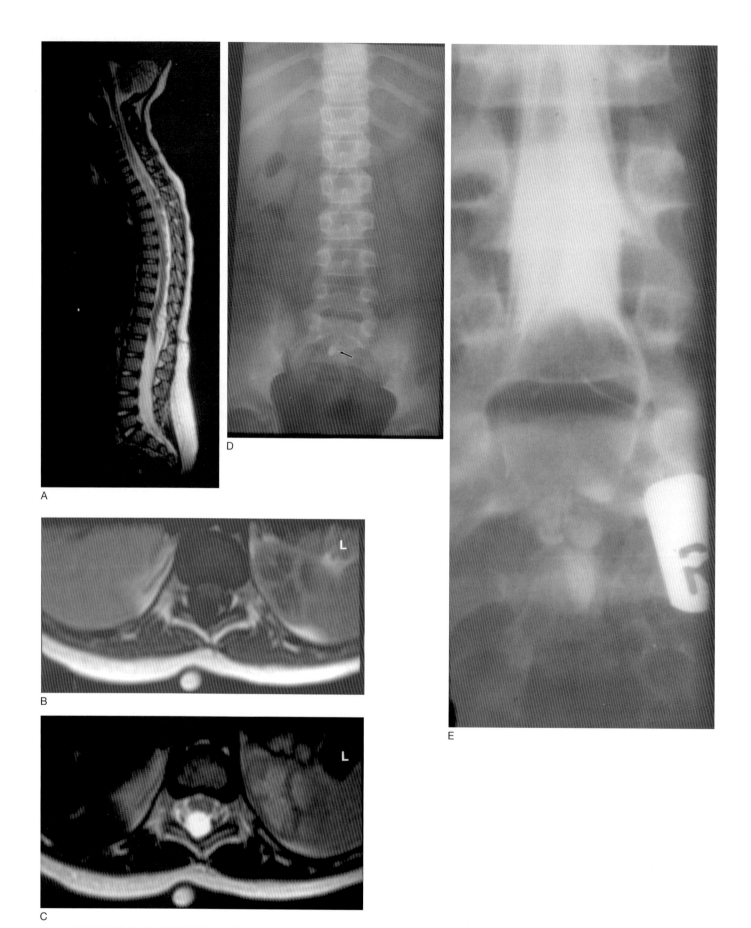

Figure 12.14.6 (A) Sagittal T2-W, (B) axial T1-W and (C) axial T2-W images of a girl with an intradural extramedullary dermoid associated with a dermal sinus track. Note the displacement of the cord by the lesion. (D) Radiograph and (E) myelogram of a different child with an intraspinal dermoid. Note the tooth within the lesion on the x-ray (arrow) and note the displacement of the nerve roots around the tumour on the myelogram (E).

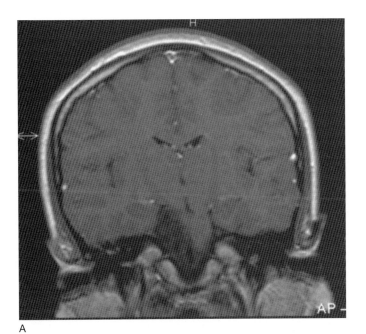
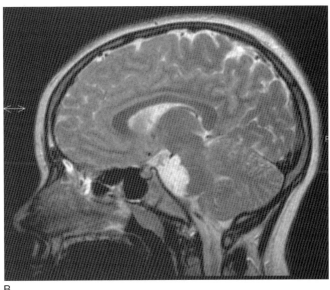

Figure 12.14.7 (A) Coronal T1-W with gadolinium and (B) sagittal T2-W images showing a mass lesion displacing the brainstem away from the epidermoid. Note that the lesion is almost isointense with the CSF on T1-W image and does not enhance.

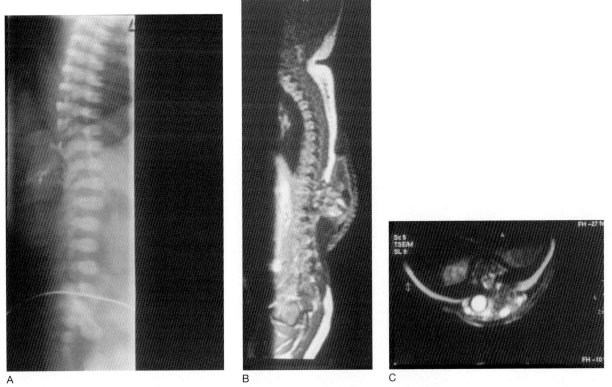

Figure 12.14.8 (A) Radiograph, (B) sagittal and (C) axial MR images of a child with a midthoracic hamartoma. Note, on the x-ray the bony elements within the soft tissue mass and, on MRI, the mixed signal reflecting the underlying mixed tissue. On the axial MR image, the lesion is shown to extend centrally into the spinal canal.

there is often intense pain in the limbs. Symptoms may fluctuate depending on the compressive effect of the cyst. Patients may be asymptomatic and the lesion may be discovered during imaging for another reason. When symptoms occur they most frequently appear in adolescence.

The definition of syringohydromyelia is that there are longitudinal cystic cavities within the cord that pathologically are associated with gliosis. Technically, hydromyelia describes dilatation of the central canal of the spinal cord and syringomyelia describes cysts that extend beyond the canal laterally or do not involve the central canal. The terms are very loosely used in practice and are often used interchangeably. In high lesions, the syrinx may extend proximally to the brainstem and cause an associated syringobulbia. There are several theories as to the causation of syringomyelia and several classifications are described in the neuroradiological literature (see Further Reading). MRI is the imaging technique of choice to demonstrate the lesions. The syrinx cavity has the imaging characteristics of CSF unless it is complicated by haemorrhage (Figure 12.14.9). The examination should include the whole cord, the brain and, in particular, the craniocervical junction, the latter to assess any associated hydrocephalus or malformation such as a Dandy–Walker lesion. Syrinx cavities may be single or multiple. Incomplete septations within a cavity gives the cord a beaded appearance. The cord is usually expanded at the site of the cavities (Figure 12.14.10). Local widening of the arachnoid space with displacement of the cord suggests arachnoiditis as the

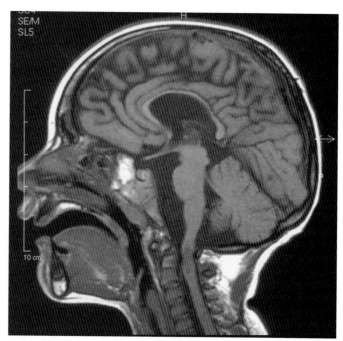

Figure 12.14.9 Sagittal T1-weighted image of a child with a small syrinx cavity in the upper cervical cord, which has intermediate signal within it due to old haemorrhage. This child is also microcephalic.

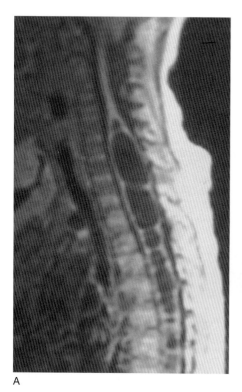

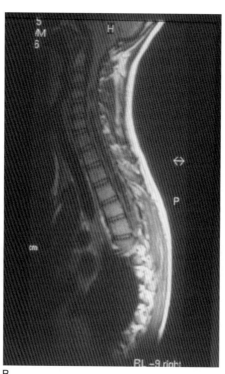

A   B

Figure 12.14.10 (A,B) Two children with septated syrinx cavities within the cord. Note the expansion of the cord (B).

cause of the lesion. Sagittal images of the whole cord using T1-W and T2-W sequences should be followed by axial projections across the whole of the syrinx cavity or cavities.

In children in whom the cause of the syringomyelia is not obvious, e.g. trauma, the first examination should also be performed with contrast enhancement to exclude the presence of a cystic tumour. This also applies to children who have an apparent obvious cause such as a Chiari 1 malformation as some of these children are shown to harbour spinal cord neoplasms as well. CSF flow studies may give further information about the dynamics of the cystic cavities and disturbances to CSF flow. The central canal of the spinal cord is sometimes prominent in children and should not be confused with a syrinx cavity. Slight widening of the canal does not cause cord expansion. If there is doubt, clinical assessment together with follow-up imaging will provide reassurance. Follow-up imaging is dictated by clinical circumstances. Surgical treatment of syringomyelia includes posterior fossa decompression and cyst drainage by shunting into the spinal canal.

DIFFERENTIAL DIAGNOSIS

Cystic cord tumours may be difficult to differentiate from syringo-hydromyelia in the absence of an obvious cause for the syrinx such as an associated Chiari malformation. Contrast enhancement is therefore indicated in all children on discovery of a syrinx on imaging. Cystic tumours usually show peripheral enhancement or enhancement in the adjacent cord whereas a non-neoplastic lesion will not.

Other intramedullary cord tumours will also show contrast enhancement and it is impossible to determine the histology without biopsy.

Not many lesions will mimic an intramedullary spinal neoplasm. One exception is demyelinating plaques from acute disseminated encephalomyelitis or multiple sclerosis, which may cause focal enlargement of the cord and increased signal on T2-W images. If there are associated brain lesions the differentiation is usually straightforward. When the disease is confined to the cord the diagnosis of a plaque is suggested as it is usually wedge- or flame-shaped and does not enlarge the cord to the same extent as a tumour. Plaques may however exhibit contrast enhancement.

EXTRAMEDULLARY SPINAL NEOPLASMS

These are divided into intradural extramedullary tumours and extradural lesions. In children, about two-thirds of all spinal cord tumours are extramedullary. Fifty per cent of these are extradural and up to 15% intradural. The clinical presentation is similar to that with intramedullary lesions. Limb weakness, back pain, torticollis in upper cord lesions and bladder and bowel disturbance are the main presenting complaints. Hydrocephalus is an occasional presentation and is thought to be due to interference with CSF flow.

INTRADURAL EXTRAMEDULLARY LESIONS

METASTASES

Subarachnoid metastases due to drop seedlings from intracranial tumours are the most frequent cause of these lesions. The presence of these carries a poorer prognosis. Medulloblastoma, pineoblastomas and pineocytomas, and ependymoma, particularly ventricular lesions, are the most common brain tumours that cause drop metastases. Ependymoma deposits are more frequent with recurrent tumour. Imaging of these brain tumours should always include spinal cord imaging both on diagnosis and on follow-up. Tumour imaging protocols must include contrast-enhanced sagittal T1-W spinal imaging for these children. Metastases from all these tumours have a similar appearance. They have a signal similar to the cord on T1-W images, high signal on T2-W images and enhance with gadolinium, which is necessary for their demonstration. They are most frequently found in the lumbar region (Figure 12.14.11).

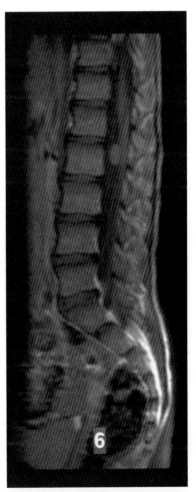

Figure 12.14.11 Subarachnoid metastasis lying anterior to the cord in a child with a medulloblastoma.

MENINGIOMA

Only about 2% of spinal meningiomas occur in children. Meningiomas arise from the meninges. The clinical presentation, histology and management are the same as for older patients. The tumours when found are mainly intradural, extramedullary but may extend into the extradural space. Clinical presentation as one might expect is with symptoms of nerve root pain and spinal cord compression. On MRI, the masses are smooth, sharply demarcated lesions that are nearly isointense with the cord on T1-W and T2-W images but show marked homogeneous enhancement with contrast. The ultimate diagnosis requires histology. They rarely have a signal void due to calcification.

MENINGEAL CYSTS

These are mentioned here as they may compress and displace the cord in a similar fashion to solid meningeal lesions. They may be congenital or acquired. Congenital cysts are arachnoid cysts. On imaging they are smooth, of fluid density on T1-W and T2-W images and do not enhance with contrast (Figure 12.14.12). Meningeal cysts displace the cord and sac away from the lesion. They are most frequently found in the thoracic region and are located behind the cord. Symptoms include pain and weakness, which may be postural. It is postulated that this reflects alteration in the cyst size with filling of the cyst and thus compression of the cord in the erect position.

Acquired meningeal cysts may be inflammatory and secondary to arachnoiditis from infection or haemorrhage, or traumatic and due to avulsion of a nerve root such as is typically described in motor bikers or a tear of the dura. The cysts may be intradural or extradural. They are located mostly dorsal to the cord but may extend into the intervertebral foramina. MRI shows them to be well demarcated fluid-filled lesions that, if large, may displace the cord.

Tarlov cysts are a form of meningeal cyst. These are perineural cysts found most often in the sacral canal and are typically located on the posterior roots (Figure 12.14.13). They are not always symptomatic and careful history taking and assessment is required to determine the relationship of the finding to clinical symptoms. The main reported symptoms are back pain and paraesthesia. On MRI, these cysts are seen as well-defined cystic lesions in the sacral canal.

EXTRADURAL EXTRAMEDULLARY LESIONS

Extradural masses may arise from the meninges, the nerve roots and their surrounding sheaths, the vertebral column and outside the spinal column but extend through the intervertebral foramina or

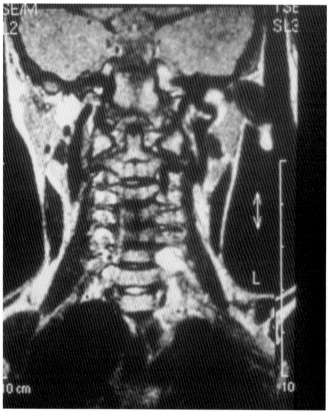

A

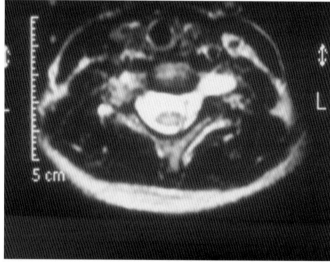

B

Figure 12.14.12 (A) Coronal and (B) axial T2-weighted sequences of a traumatic meningocele secondary to a hyperextension injury, which occurred in a child of eleven who was riding a motor bike.

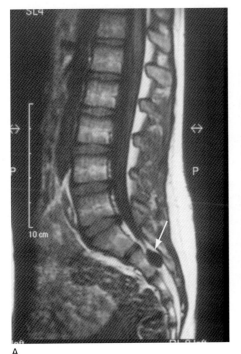
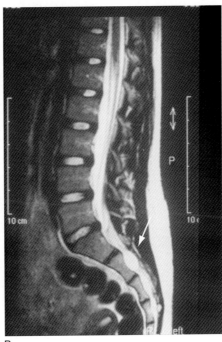

A

B

Figure 12.14.13 (A) T1- and (B) T2-weighted images showing typical appearances of a Tarlov cyst in the sacral canal.

extend into the canal by direct invasion. Clinical symptoms may be dominated by the primary lesion, e.g. neuroblastoma, rather than signs and symptoms directly related to the cord or nerve root compression.

Extradural masses displace the cord and thecal sac away from the surrounding vertebral column and may also surround or displace the emerging nerve roots to cause radicular pain.

PRIMARY MENINGEAL NERVE ROOT TUMOURS

Primary nerve root tumours in children are rare except in patients with neurofibromatosis.

Neurofibromas are also rare as isolated lesions and when seen are almost always found in children with neurofibromatosis 1 (NF 1). They appear as well-defined extradural, extramedullary masses with similar or slightly less signal intensity to skeletal muscle. They frequently extend extradurally into the neural foramina and into the paravertebral space – the 'dumb-bell tumour' (Figure 12.14.14). The expansion of the intervertebral foramen if large enough is seen on radiographs. There is no bone destruction unless there is malignant degeneration. Contrast enhancement of these lesions is variable but most show some enhancement. Malignant degeneration to a neurosarcoma is possible but is more frequent with plexiform neurofibromas (Figure 12.14.15). Paravertebral

tumours arising in the sympathetic chain may also extend through the foramina into the spinal canal and form an extradural tumour (Figure 12.14.16). These lesions include all three neural crest tumours – neuroblastoma, ganglioneuroma and ganglion neuroblastoma (Figure 12.14.17). Primitive neuroectodermal tumours (PNETs) may behave similarly. Both PNETs and neuroblastoma may also invade the bone and cause cord symptoms due to vertebral compression. These tumours usually present because of the extraspinal manifestations or, in the case of benign lesions, their incidental discovery on x-ray. Imaging of all these tumours, which are described elsewhere in this book, should include a careful search for extension through the foramina into the spinal canal and may require thin axial cuts, with contrast for assessment. The thecal sac and cord are displaced away from the lesion.

SCHWANNOMAS

Multiple schwannomas, occasionally seen in older children with NF 2, may also cause intradural extramedullary lesions similar to drop metastases. In children, these are most frequent in the cervical and lumbar regions. About 20% of patients will have an extradural component to the lesion (Figure 12.14.18).

Evidence of NF elsewhere suggests the diagnosis. If the lesions are multiple in the absence of a concomitant brain tumour, the diagnosis of metastases is unlikely.

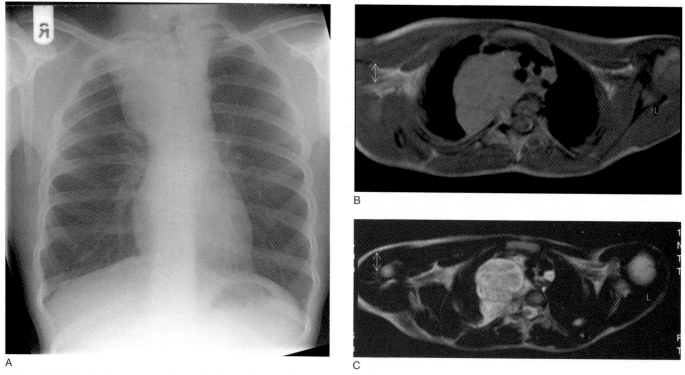

Figure 12.14.14 (A) Chest radiograph and (B,C) axial T1- and T2-weighted sequences of a boy with a large paravertebral neurofibroma that extends through the neural foramen into the spinal canal. Note, on the x-ray, the widening of the posterior rib spaces due to external pressure and displacement of the trachea.

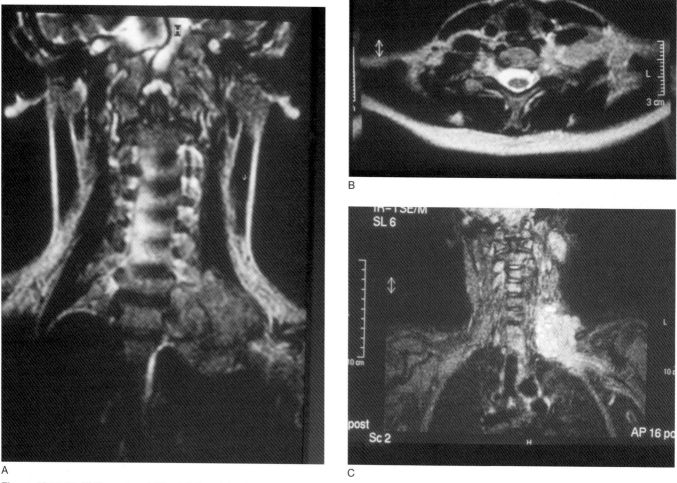

Figure 12.14.15 (A) Coronal and (B) axial T2-weighted sequences and (C) coronal stir in a teenage girl with a malignant neurosarcoma that is mainly in the soft tissues but extends through the neural foramen. This was infiltrating the brachial plexus and caused intense pain.

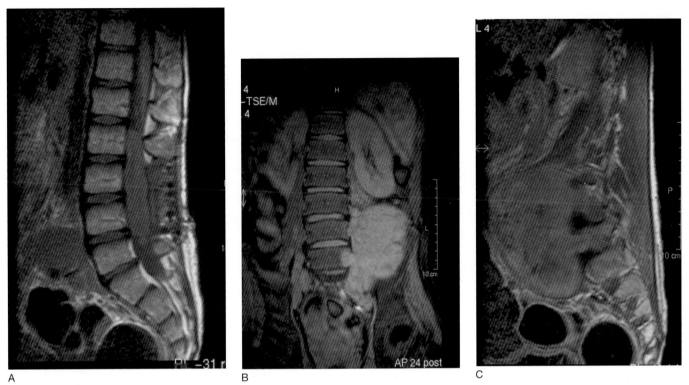

A   B   C

Figure 12.14.16 (A) Sagittal T1, (B) coronal T2- and (C) sagittal T1-weighted images showing a child with a large paravertebral neurofibroma with intraforaminal extension.

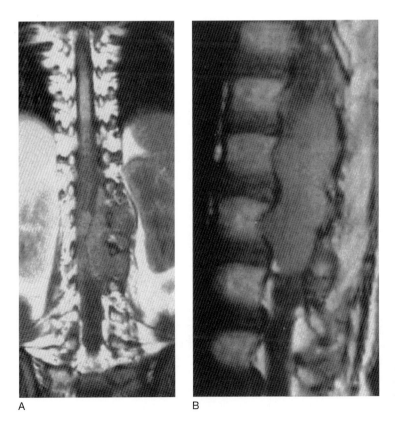

A   B

Figure 12.14.17 (A) Coronal and (B) sagittal images in a girl aged 4 years who has a large paraspinal mass on the left invading the spinal canal and forming a large extradural mass due to a neuroblastoma.

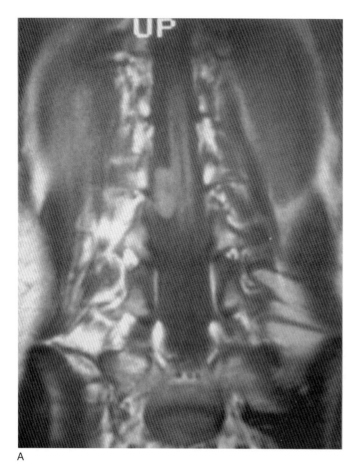

A

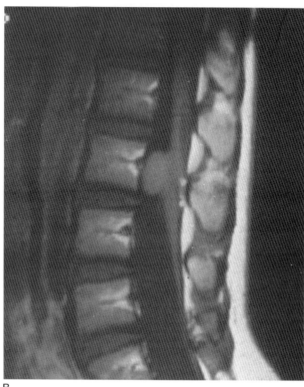

B

Figure 12.14.18 Child aged 9 years with a schwannoma. Coronal (A) and sagittal (B) MRI showing an intradural extramedullary mass on the right. The subarachnoid space is widened around the tumour. The tumour displaces the spinal cord to the left.

SPINAL VERTEBRAL MALIGNANT TUMOURS

These are tumours that may cause cord compression either because of vertebral compression but more frequently as a result of extradural extension of the primary bone lesion.

METASTASES

In adults, the most frequent lesions to cause secondary cord compression are metastases. In children, this is less frequent and unlike in adults, the primary lesion is usually obvious. The most frequent metastatic lesions to cause vertebral destruction and collapse are neuroblastoma, leukaemia or lymphoma. Metastases may affect the vertebral body and appendages. Vertebral collapse and destruction is visible on x-ray.

OSTEOSARCOMA/EWING'S SARCOMA

Primary vertebral osteosarcoma is rare but metastatic osteosarcoma may produce osteoblastic metastases that may affect the cord by extradural compression. Ewing's sarcoma of the spine is more frequent; this mainly affects the vertebral bodies and may involve contiguous segments. Skip segments are due to metastatic lesions. Cord symptoms occur from direct compression or compression by the soft tissue component of the lesion (Figure 12.14.19), both of which may produce bone sclerosis on x-ray. Vertebral compression is more frequent with Ewing's sarcoma than osteosarcoma.

LYMPHOMA/LEUKAEMIA

Bone lymphoma in childhood is rare compared with the adult population. It may rarely be a primary lesion but more frequently it represents Stage 4 disease. It primarily affects the vertebral

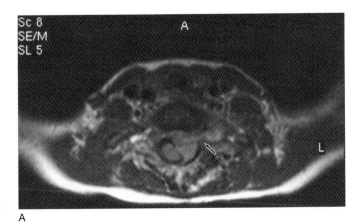

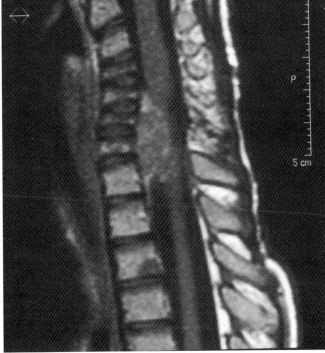

Figure 12.14.19 (A) Axial and (B) sagittal T1-weighted images of a boy with a Ewing's sarcoma of the cervical spine, with a large extradural soft tissue extension. Note the compressed vertebral bodies secondary to the tumour. The tumour lies on the left and extends through the intervertebral foramen. Note also the metastatic lesion in T3.

bodies but a soft tissue component may extend into the extradural space. On MRI, the lesion is of low signal on T1-W and T2-W images with replacement of the normal fatty marrow signal. Leukaemia may cause cord compression due to intrathecal deposits, or due to compression fracture of a vertebral body secondary to malignant infiltration of the marrow. On x-ray, leukaemia produces osteoporosis with vertebral compression fractures. Lymphoma may be sclerotic or destructive.

BENIGN TUMOURS

LANGERHANS' CELL HISTIOCYTOSIS

Most benign tumours affect the vertebral appendages and may produce either cord or nerve root signs. The main exception to this is Langerhans' cell histiocytosis, which typically affects the vertebral bodies to cause a vertebra plana but seldom cord signs. The soft tissue component is small but shows enhancement with gadolinium. The intervertebral discs are preserved. The x-ray appearances of a vertebra plana are characteristic. Usually only one vertebral body is involved but there are reports of more than one with skip lesions. A differential diagnosis in these circumstances is a spondylitis presentation of SAPHO syndrome. This

should be considered as the bone pain responds to pamidronate. Though most patients with SAPHO have peripheral lesions, in addition to the spinal lesions, a primary spinal presentation is described.

Spinal involvement by histiocytosis may also occur in more widespread disease but is rare compared with lesions in the ribs, pelvis, skull or appendicular skeleton.

ANEURYSMAL BONE CYST

This lesion is described in Chapter 2.4. Briefly, a spinal aneurysmal bone cyst affects the vertebral appendages. It may extend into the vertebral body, and into the extradural space, displacing the cord away from the lesion. The bony lesion is a lytic expansile lesion. On MRI, lesions have high signal on T2-W images, fluid signal on T1-W images and may show fluid–fluid levels.

OSTEOBLASTOMA

These lesions typically occur in boys in the second and third decades of life and cause pain by nerve root compression. They are slow-growing lesions that arise in the vertebral appendages or in the posterior sacrum. They are mainly lytic but may cause reactive bone sclerosis. On computed tomography (CT), the lesion is often shown to have calcification in its centre, similar to the nidus of an osteoid osteoma. A soft tissue component may be present. The appearance is characteristic. If MRI is done, the lesion is low signal on T1-W and increased signal on T2-W images, and with extensive surrounding bone oedema. This can cause confusion and lead to a mistaken diagnosis of malignancy.

GIANT CELL TUMOUR

This benign bone tumour also affects the vertebral body or appendages and when found in the spine affects the sacrum most frequently. There is an expansile destructive lesion but usually with intact cortical margins. Spinal cord and nerve root symptoms occur because of encroachment on the canal or foramina. The imaging characteristics are intermediate signal on T1-W and high signal on T2-W sequences. The lesion is well demarcated.

OSTEOCHONDROMA

Osteochondromas may also arise in the spine. If they encroach on a nerve root or the thecal sac they may present with neural symptoms, in addition to pain. They are often only detected on cross-sectional imaging, done to investigate pain. Like osteochondromata elsewhere, they are formed of bone with a cartilaginous cap. Their nature is best appreciated on CT.

CHORDOMA

Chordomas are very rare in children and are found mainly in the clivus and sacrum but may affect vertebral bodies. A chordoma is a slow-growing tumour arising from the notochord. It is technically benign but locally aggressive. It may affect the intervertebral disc and invade the vertebral body and appendages. The soft tissue component extends inwards to form an extradural mass. The lesion is best demonstrated by MRI, its signal characteristics being non-specific with intermediate signal on T1-W and high signal on T2-W sequences (Figure 12.14.20). The lesion is usually well demarcated. Contrast enhancement is variable. On x-ray, a chordoma, though mainly destructive, may be found to cause sclerosis.

EXTRAMEDULLARY HAEMATOPOIESIS

Children who have refractive marrow with failure of formation of haemoglobin produce haemoglobin from sites other than the bone marrow. Typically, this occurs in the liver and spleen, but may also occur in the paravertebral tissues. On x-ray, these appear as paravertebral masses and on rare occasions, these may cause nerve root compression at the foramina and the tissue may even extend through the foramina to form an extradural mass. Affected children usually suffer from thalassaemia or myelofibrosis. In the latter, the bones are sclerotic. In the former, there is usually increased trabecular markings and some osteopenia.

SACRAL AND PRESACRAL MASS LESIONS

Though not strictly spinal cord tumours, these lesions are described in this chapter. Specific masses arising in this region include sacrococcygeal teratoma, presacral PNETs and anterior meningoceles.

SACROCOCCYGEAL TERATOMA

These tumours may be diagnosed on antenatal ultrasound, at birth or in infancy. Though all have attachment to the coccyx, their location varies from being predominantly external extending into the perineum and buttocks, predominantly intrapelvic, or a mixture (Figure 12.14.21). They also vary in consistency from being almost completely solid to mainly cystic, or can be a mixture of both types. Common to all teratomas they may contain calcification, fat, teeth, bony structures and mixed solid mesenchymal elements. There is a 4:1 female:male incidence. Though initially benign, they have a potential to be malignant and need complete excision together with the coccygeal elements. Malignancy is more frequent in tumours that are predominantly intrapelvic as diagnosis is delayed. Metastases occur mainly to the lungs.

Symptoms of lesions that are intrapelvic are mainly pain and constipation, the latter caused by displacement of the rectum. The lesions and their consistency are easily diagnosed by ultrasound but MRI is required for accurate mapping. MR sequences should include T1-W and T2-W images and fat suppression in sagittal and axial planes. Gadolinium enhancement is required and CT of the lungs is necessary at staging to exclude metastases. At diagnosis, the lesions are variable in size and consistency and are usually well defined. The location and imaging are characteristic and therefore primary excision without prior biopsy is the usual management. The tumour marker is alpha fetoprotein (AFP), the levels of which are monitored following treatment to exclude recurrence.

The triad of anorectal atresia, sacral defects and sacrococcygeal teratomas or anterior meningoceles constitute the Currarino triad.

PRESACRAL PNETS

The concavity of the sacrum is a characteristic location for PNETs. These occur in slightly older children aged 2 years or more. Neuroblastoma and ganglioneuroblastoma can also occur here and carry a good prognosis as compared with intra-abdominal neuroblastoma. Clinical symptoms are pain and constipation. The tumours may contain calcification and are mainly solid but may contain areas of necrosis. They enhance with gadolinium. The rectum is displaced anteriorly by the tumour. The tumour may infiltrate through the sacral foramina into the sacral canal. MRI is required for full delineation.

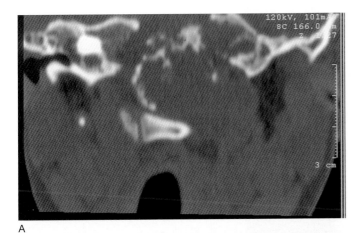

A

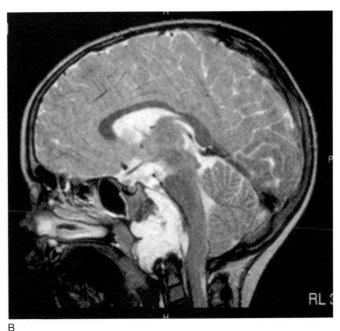

B

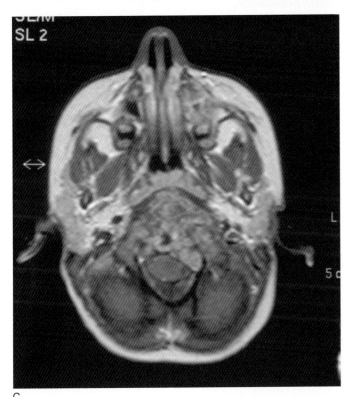

C

Figure 12.14.20 Images of a child with a chordoma of the clivus. (A) CT scan. Note bone destruction and large soft tissue mass. (B) Sagittal T2-weighted and (C) axial T1-weighted MR images with gadolinium, showing the tumour mass, which enhances and displaces the brainstem posteriorly but has not invaded it.

ANTERIOR SACRAL MENINGOCELE

Anterior sacral meningoceles are described in Chapter 12.1 but they are described here also as they may be mistaken for a cystic sacrococcygeal teratoma. Anterior sacral meningoceles are almost invariably associated with sacral abnormalities – most frequently a smooth crescentic defect in the sacrum, which may be eccentric (Figure 12.14.22). By definition they are connected to the spinal canal. They are cystic lesions and MRI, required for diagnosis,

shows their connection to the spinal canal. They may be associated with a tethered cord. They are variable in size and are usually diagnosed either because of the sacral abnormality identified incidentally on radiographs, or because of a cystic mass seen on ultrasound. They are frequently asymptomatic. The differential diagnoses include sacrococcygeal teratoma and ovarian cysts. MRI provides the definitive diagnosis. If these lesions become infected, meningitis is a serious consequence.

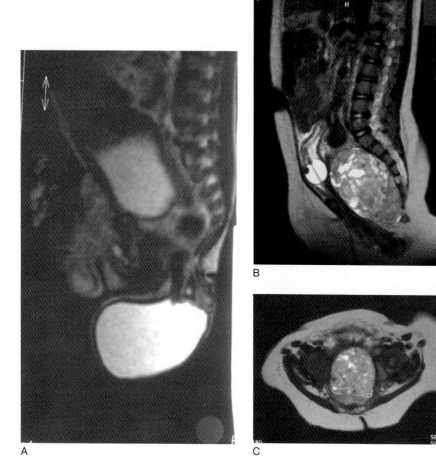

Figure 12.14.21 Two children with sacrococcygeal teratomas. (A) Sagittal T2-weighted image of first child. (B) Sagittal and (C) axial T2-weighted sequences in the second child. In (A), the lesion is predominantly external and is cystic. In (B) and (C), the lesion is predominantly solid and internal. Note in both children the connection of the lesion to the coccyx. Note on (B) the alteration in signal in the lowest sacral segment due to the tumour attachment.

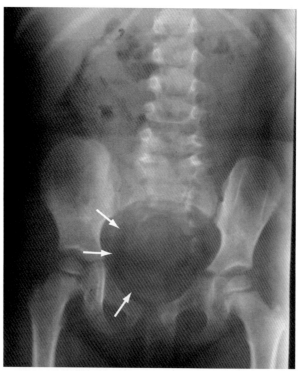

Figure 12.14.22 Abdomen x-ray of a child with an anterior sacral meningocele. Note the displacement of the sacrum to the left by the meningocele.

FURTHER READING

Albright AL. Pediatric intramedullary spinal cord tumors. Childs Nervous System 1999; 15:436–438.

Andersson T, van-Dijk J, Willinsky R. Venous manifestations of spinal arteriovenous fistulas. Neuroimaging Clinics of North America 2003; 13:73–93.

Asazuma T, Toyama Y, Suzuki N, Fujimura Y, Hirabayshi K. Ependymomas of the spinal cord and cauda equina: An analysis of 26 cases and a review of the literature. Spinal Cord 1999; 37:753–759.

Baleriaux DL. Spinal cord tumors. European Radiology 1999; 9:1252–1258.

Barkovich AJ. Neoplasms of the spine. In: Pediatric neuroimaging. Philadelphia: Lippincott Williams & Wilkins; 2000.

Chamberlain MC. Ependymomas. Current Neurology and Neuroscience Reports 2003; 3:193–199.

Constantini S, Houten J, Miller DC et al. Intramedullary spinal cord tumors in children under the age of 3 years. Journal of Neurosurgery 1996; 85:1036–1043.

Deme S, Ang L-C, Skaf G, Rowed DW. Primary intramedullary primitive neuroectodermal tumor of the spinal cord: case review and review of the literature. Neurosurgery 1997; 41:1417–1420.

Deutsch H, Shrivistava R, Epstein F, Jallo G. Pediatric intramedullary spinal cavernous malformations. Spine 2001; 26:427–431.

Fernandez-C, Figarella-Branger D, Girard N et al. Pilocytic astrocytomas in children: prognostic factors – a retrospective study of 80 cases. Neurosurgery 2003; 53:544–553.

Fine MJ, Kricheff II, Freed D, Epstein FJ. Spinal cord ependymomas: MR imaging features. Radiology 1995; 197:655–658.

Furuya K, Sasaki T, Suzuki I, Kim P, Saito N, Kirino T. Intramedullary angiographically occult vascular malformations of the spinal cord. Neurosurgery 1996; 39:1123–1130.

Grattan-Smith P, Ryan M, Procopis PG. Persistent or severe back pain and stiffness are ominous symptoms requiring prompt attention. Journal of Paediatrics and Child Health 2000; 36:208–212.

Greenlee J, Donovan K, Hasan D, Menezes A. Chiari I malformation in the very young child: the spectrum of presentations and experience in 31 children under age 6 years. Pediatrics 2002; 110:1212–1219.

Gupta R, Sharma R, Vashisht S et al. Magnetic resonance evaluation of idiopathic scoliosis: a prospective study. Australasian Radiology 1999; 43:461–465.

Houten JK, Weiner HL. Pediatric intramedullary spinal cord tumors: special considerations. Journal of Neurooncology 2000; 47:225–230.

Innocenzi G, Raco A, Cantore G, Raimondi AJ. Intramedullary astrocytomas and ependymomas in the pediatric age group: a retrospective study. Childs Nervous System 1996; 12:776–780.

Kane PJ, el-Mahdy W, Singh A, Powell MP, Crockard HA. Spinal intradural tumours: Part II – Intramedullary. British Journal of Neurosurgery 1999; 13:558–563.

Kulkarni AV, Armstrong DC, Drake JM. MR characteristics of malignant spinal cord astrocytoma in children. Canadian Journal of Neurological Science 1999; 26:290–293.

Lee M, Epstein FJ , Rezai AR, Zagzag D. Nonneoplastic intramedullary spinal cord lesions mimicking tumors. Neurosurgery 1998; 43:788–794.

Lee M, Rezai AR, Abbott R, Coelho D, Epstein FJ. Intramedullary spinal cord lipomas. Journal of Neurosurgery 1995; 82:394–400.

Lefton DR, Pinto RS, Martin SW. MRI features of intracranial and spinal ependymomas. Pediatric Neurosurgery 1998; 28:97–105.

Mehlman CT, Crawford AH, McMath JA. Pediatric vertebral and spinal cord tumors: a retrospective study of musculoskeletal aspects of presentation, treatment, and complications. Orthopedics 1999; 22:49–55.

Merchant TE, Kiehna EN, Thompson SJ et al. Pediatric low-grade and ependymal spinal cord tumors. Pediatric Neurosurgery 2000; 32:30–36.

Merchant TE, Nguyen D, Thompson SJ et al. High-grade pediatric spinal cord tumors. Pediatric Neurosurgery 1999; 30:1–5.

Mottolese C, Hermier M, Stan H et al. Central nervous system cavernomas in the pediatric age group. Neurosurgical Review 2001; 24:55–71.

Nabors MW, Pait TG, Byrd EB et al. Updated assessment and current classification of spinal meningeal cysts. Journal of Neurosurgery 1988; 68:366–377.

Nadkarni TD, Rekate HL. Pediatric intramedullary spinal cord tumors. Critical review of the literature. Childs Nervous System 1999; 15:17–28.

Patel U, Pinto RS, Miller DC et al. MR of spinal cord ganglioglioma. American Journal of Neuroradiology 1998; 19:879–887.

Prestigiacomo C, Niimi Y, Setton A, Berenstein A. Three-dimensional rotational spinal angiography in the evaluation and treatment of vascular malformations. American Journal of Neuroradiology 2003; 24:1429–1435.

Rodriguez-Casero M, Shield LK, Coleman LT, Kornberg AJ. Childhood chronic inflammatory demyelinating polyneuropathy with central nervous system demyelination resembling multiple sclerosis. Neuromuscular Disorders 2003; 13:158–161.

Schick U, Marquardt G. Pediatric spinal tumors. Pediatric Neurosurgery 2001; 35:120–127.

Schick U, Marquardt G. Pediatric spinal tumors. Pediatric Neurosurgery 2001; 35:120–127.

Seppala MT, Sainio MA, Haltia MJ et al. Multiple schwannomas: schwannomatosis or neurofibromatosis type 2? Journal of Neurosurgery 1998; 89:36–41.

Sevick RJ, Wallace CJ. MR imaging of neoplasms of the lumbar spine. Magnetic Resonance Imaging Clinics of North America 1999; 7:539–553.

Taylor FR, Larkins MV. Headache and Chiari I malformation: clinical presentation, diagnosis, and controversies in management. Current Pain and Headache Reports 2002; 6:331–337.

Thabet F, Mrad S, Abroug S, Hattab N, Harbi A. Medullary arteriovenous malformations in children. Archives of Pediatrics 2001; 8:508–511.

Van-Heesewijk J, Casparie J. Acute spontaneous spinal epidural haematoma in a child. European Radiology 2000; 10:1874–1876.

Zimmermann RA, Haughton VM. Imaging of the tumours of the spinal canal and cord. Radiologic Clinics of North America 1988; 26:965–1007.

Facial Trauma

Benoît Michel

INTRODUCTION

Facial fractures in the paediatric population are infrequent occurrences. They are less common in children than in adults (incidence ranges from 1.5% to 15% of all facial fractures and less than 1% in children under 6 years). Boys are slightly more frequently injured than girls.

Some of the anatomical and physiological aspects of the face in children explain the distinctive features of fractures in this population:

- The cranium/facial ratio is higher in children than in adults (8:1 in infancy and 2.5:1 in adulthood) (Figure 12.15.1).
- There is a lack of pneumatization of the paranasal and frontal sinuses.
- Children's bones have a high proportion of cancellous component, a thin cortex and elastic properties.
- The larger fat pads in children cushion the trauma and lessen the kinetic energy transmitted.

Aside from alveolar fractures, these facts explain why a strong force is necessary to produce a fracture and why fractures are usually either comminuted or greenstick fractures.

Associated injuries are often present: head and cranial injuries (from 42% to 55% of children), extremities (15–24%), thorax or abdomen. They are more commonly found in younger paediatric patients.

AGE AND CAUSES OF ACCIDENTS

The mean age for facial fractures is 10.3 years and half of all cases are aged between 13 and 15 years. Common causes are a fall (30–43%), play and sport (22–23%) and motor vehicle accidents (17–50%). There is a higher percentage of motor vehicle–pedestrian injuries in children compared with adults (20% and 1%, respectively). A fall is the main cause of facial trauma in children under 6 years, where the fractures are usually alveolar or condylar (dental or chin trauma).

FRACTURE TYPE

The most frequent fractures are nasal (60%), mandibular (21%) or maxillary (6%) with alveolar fractures being the most frequent dental injury. The incidence of multiple fractures within the mandible itself is lower than in the adult population but must be looked for. Condylar fractures account for 31% of paediatric mandibular fractures as compared with 24% in the adult group (Figure 12.15.2). Midface fractures comprise 17% of children's facial fractures and are usually seen in older children.

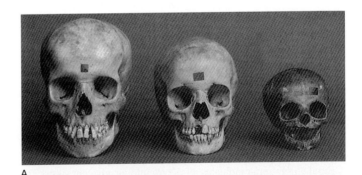

A

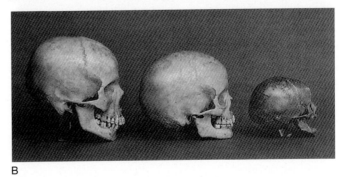

B

Figure 12.15.1 Infant, teenager and adult skulls showing change in cranium/facial ratio with increasing age. (Reproduced with permission from Moos KF, El-Attar A. Plastic surgery in infancy and childhood, 3rd edn. Edinburgh: Churchill Livingstone; 1988:345–364.)

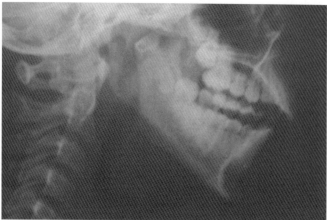

A

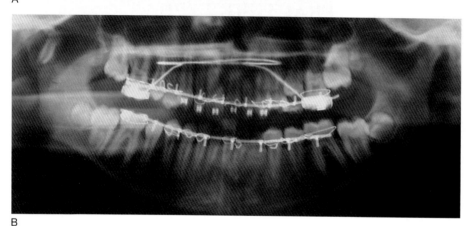

B

Figure 12.15.2 (A) Lateral x-ray of mandible showing a condylar fracture and (B) orthopantomogram of a different child showing a fracture of the right condylar neck.

DIAGNOSTIC METHODS

Clinical examination leads to pertinent complementary radiological examinations. Exploration by palpation of facial bones is essential despite swelling and pain. Deviation of the mandible in occlusion, crepitus and hypoaesthesia occur with facial fractures. Orbital emphysema indicates a fracture into an adjacent sinus. The main clinical signs related to each type of fracture are summarized in Table 12.15.1.

With the exception of orbital fractures and some condylar fractures, diagnosis of displaced fracture is made by inspection or palpation. Non-displaced fractures are nevertheless often seen in children (greenstick fractures). Radiographic diagnosis is always necessary and is based on standard radiographic techniques, panoramic tomography or computed tomographic scanning, the choice of which depends on the type of fracture sustained.

IMAGING METHODS

STANDARD RADIOGRAPHIC TECHNIQUES

Many types of projections have been described but few are now used routinely. A limited number of views is usually sufficient for diagnosis. A computed tomography (CT) scan is presently the most useful examination for complex fractures of the face and renders the multiplication of radiographic projections unnecessary.

Most views are centred on orbitomeatal (OM) and midsagittal planes (S). Towne's view (OM = +25, S = 0°) and the posteroanterior view (OM = +15–20, S = 0) are good views for condylar and mandibular midline fracture visualization. Right and left lateral oblique views are used for mandibular fractures, delineation of the ramus, condylar neck or body when panoramic tomography cannot be done. Waters' view (OM = −45°, S = 0°), an occipitomental projection, is useful for the zygoma and maxilla. In the context of trauma, opacification of or a fluid level of the maxillary sinuses indicates a fracture (Figure 12.15.3): fracture of maxilla (Le Fort I or II), fracture of the zygoma or orbital floor fracture. An interruption of Campbell lines signifies a fracture. A submental vertex view (OM = +75°

Table 12.15.1 Choice of radiographic exploration depending on clinical signs

Fracture type	Main clinical signs	Radiographic explorations
Nasal fracture	Bilateral palpebral haematoma Epistaxis Nasal deformity Nasal mobility	Lateral nasal bones and occipitomental view
Zygomatic fracture	Conjunctival haemorrhage Soft tissue swelling or cheekbone depression External canthal dystopia Paraesthesia in the distribution of the infraorbital nerve Bone assymetry at palpation of the orbital rim +/- signs of orbital floor fracture	Waters' view Submental vertex view +/– CT
Isolated fracture of the zygomatic arch	Depression of the zygomatic area Trismus	Submental vertex view
Le Fort I, II, III fractures	Mobility of the tooth-bearing part of the maxilla	CT
Nasoethmoidal fracture	External canthal dystopia Signs of nasal fracture	CT
Orbital floor fracture	Paraesthesia in the distribution of the infraorbital nerve Palpebral haematoma Vertical diplopia Enophthalmus Crepitus	Waters' view CT (coronal or reconstruction)
Isolated fracture of the orbital medial wall	Same signs as in orbital floor fracture Without paraesthesia in the distribution of the infraorbital nerve With horizontal diplopia instead of vertical diplopia	Waters' view CT
Mandibular fracture	Deviation of the mandible on occlusion Interdental diastasis Fracture mobility (tooth-bearing part of the mandible) Paraesthesia in the distribution of the inferior alveolar nerve	Panoramic x-ray Towne's view
Dental and alveolar fractures	Pathological tooth mobility Abnormal tooth position Tooth fractured or not present at the examination	Intraoral films

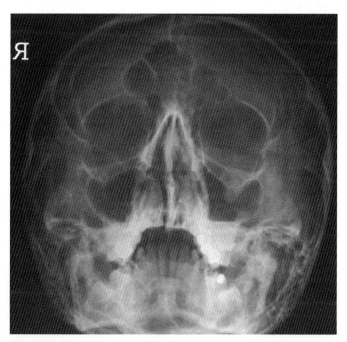

Figure 12.15.3 Blow-out fracture of the orbital floor on the left with trapped orbital content seen superiorly and a fluid level inferiorly.

or –105°, S = 0°) is a good projection for demonstration of the zygomatic arches but it needs a head tilt, which is contraindicated if there is associated cervical trauma. Fortunately, associated cervical injury is seldom seen in the child population. There are two projections that are used to see nasal fractures: lateral nasal bones (OM = 0, S = 90°) and an occipitomental projection (OM = –70°, S = 0°).

Intraoral or occlusal films are the best radiographs for locating alveolar or dental fractures (Figure 12.15.4).

PANORAMIC X-RAY

This rotational tomography is a technique employed to produce tomograms of curved surfaces. It is a helpful examination for mandibular fractures when children have the ability to sit in an upright position and remain still. Care is required in the interpretation of tomograms because of the presence of many artifacts created by, for example, the sinus air.

COMPUTED TOMOGRAPHY

Computed tomography is the most accurate method of imaging paediatric facial trauma. It provides sections of the face with the facility for three-plane and three-dimensional reconstruction

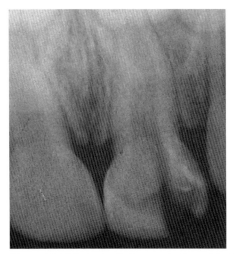

Figure 12.15.4 Anatomical crown fracture of tooth in a 3-year-old child.

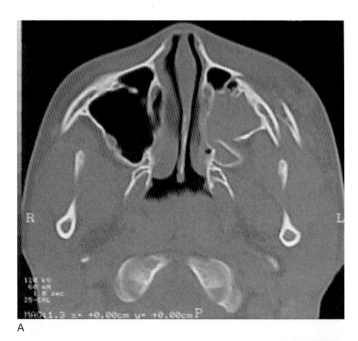

A

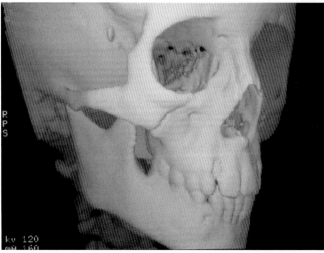

B

Figure 12.15.5 (A) Axial CT showing complex malar fracture on the left and (B) a different child showing undisplaced zygoma fracture with 3D reconstruction.

(Figure 12.15.5). It is required for the full demonstration of facial fractures with orbital involvement (orbital floor, medial wall, zygoma, Lefort fractures) and condylar fractures.

A CT scan is very helpful and can replace orthopantomography in patients who are unable to cooperate or are in pain. It is frequently used initially in patients with head injury requiring imaging of the brain and the facial injury can be imaged at the same time. In orbital trauma, CT is required to assess entrapment of rectus or oblique muscles, the presence of intraorbital haematoma and entrapment of orbital fat.

MAIN TYPES OF FRACTURES

MANDIBULAR FRACTURES

Mandibular fractures in children are less often bilateral or multiple as compared with adults but condylar involvement is more frequent. Fractures of the mandible are classified according to the site of fracture. Most fractures occur at the condyle, angle and body. Other possible sites are the ramus, midline or in the coronoid process. A fracture through the mandible entering a tooth root is a compound fracture and carries the risk of infection (Figure 12.15.6).

Panoramic tomography is the most useful radiograph in evaluation of mandible fractures but it may need to be supplemented by Towne's and lateral oblique projections. However, in younger children (under 6 years) or in children unable to sit in an upright position, standard radiographs (Towne's view and lateral oblique views) may be used. Excellent demonstration of mandibular fractures is achieved with CT, especially for condylar fractures, but panoramic tomography is the initial investigation in older children because of availability.

DENTAL AND ALVEOLAR FRACTURES

These fractures, when they involve the mandible or the maxilla, are not always seen on intraoral radiographs. For these types of fracture clinical evaluation is most important. In most cases, only the incisors are involved (Figure 12.15.7). Dental and alveolar fractures are discussed further in Chapter 15.

NASAL FRACTURE

Nasal fractures along with the alveolar fractures are probably the most common fractures of the face in children but many of them are not reported in clinical studies. This type of fracture is nevertheless not as common as in the adult population because of the immature development of the nasal bones and the greater cartilage component.

Fracture diagnosis is essentially clinical. There is nasal deformation and mobility of the nasal bones. Confirmation of fracture will be given by nasal views. Fractures of the bridge are seen on lateral views and septal deviation on anteroposterior (AP) views (Figure 12.15.8).

ZYGOMATIC FRACTURE

Zygomatic fractures are usually caused by a direct impact on the cheekbone. The bone fractures at four points and may be displaced posteriorly. Pneumatization of the maxillary sinus is necessary to allow bone displacement, which explains why this type of fracture is rare in younger children.

In most cases of isolated trauma, standard radiographs (Waters' view and submental vertex view) are usually sufficient for diagnosis. When there is displacement, a CT scan is required to visualize the bone displacement and to allow planning for repair and reconstruction (Figure 12.15.9). The fracture line runs from the inferior orbital rim through the orbital floor, the lateral orbital rim and through the maxillary sinus. The zygomatic arch is fractured at one point. Bleeding into the maxillary sinus accompanies the fracture. CT is always required in children with diplopia or enophthalmus.

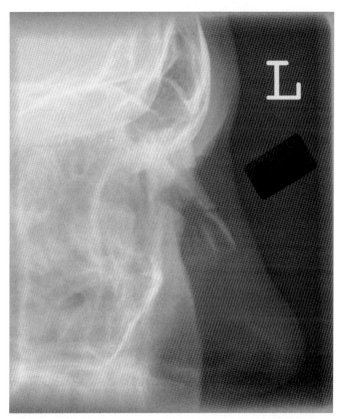

Figure 12.15.8 Lateral view of nasal bones showing undisplaced fracture.

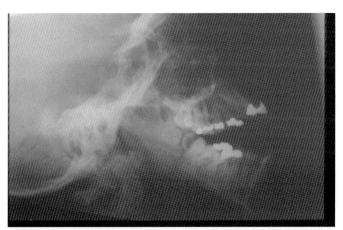

Figure 12.15.6 Bilateral fractures through the angle of the mandible extending into the root sockets.

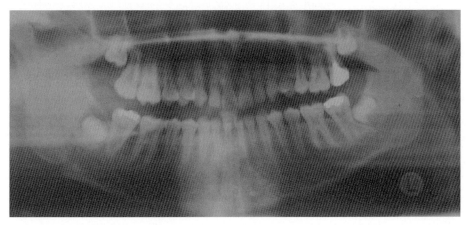

Figure 12.15.7 Orthopantomogram showing displaced fracture of the angle of the mandible in a 14-year-old boy.

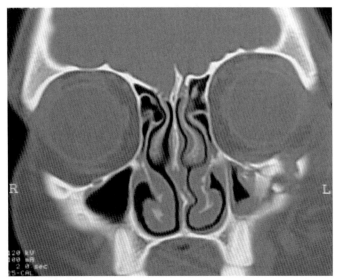

Figure 12.15.9 Comminuted zygomatic fracture in a 14-year-old boy.

ISOLATED ZYGOMATIC ARCH FRACTURE

When there is a lateral facial impact, the zygomatic arch, if fractured, is fractured at three points with medial displacement of the two fragments. The initial diagnosis is made on the submento-vertex projection but will often be supplemented by CT.

ORBITAL FLOOR FRACTURE

Only older children (8 years or more) who have sufficient development of the paranasal sinuses are affected by this type of fracture. Under 7 years old, the orbital roof is far more likely to be injured. This fracture is usually the result of a direct impact on the eye and is called a blow-out fracture (Figure 12.15.3 and Figure 12.15.10). It can also be the result of a direct trauma of the infra-orbital rim. In the first situation, the rise of intraorbital pressure causes depression of the orbital soft tissues into the maxillary sinus. The rectus and oblique muscles may be incarcerated in the fracture resulting in limitation of ocular motility. Standard radiographs (Waters' view) show the opaque sinus due to bleeding or a soft tissue shadow in the upper part of the maxillary sinus and the absence of zygomatic fracture. CT is necessary to determine the extent of the floor defect, the relationship between the fracture and the oculomotor muscles and to evaluate the volume of herniated soft tissues into the sinus. Coronal and sagittal reconstruction must be done in addition to the transverse sections.

MEDIAL ORBITAL WALL FRACTURE

As for the orbital floor fractures, direct impact on the eye may be responsible for medial wall fractures (Figure 12.15.11). Younger children may be affected because of the early development of the

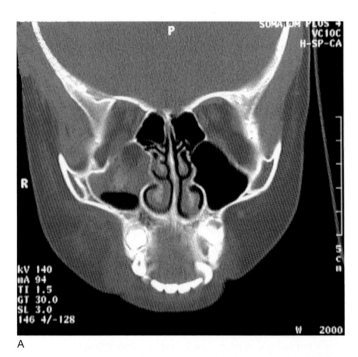

A

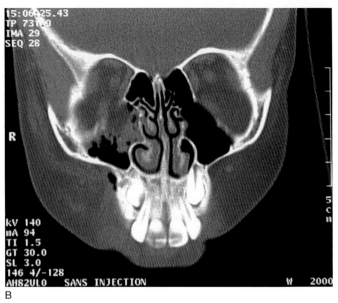

B

Figure 12.15.10 Blow-out fracture of the orbital floor with herniation of orbital contents into maxilla.

ethmoidal sinuses. Soft tissue emphysema without maxillary opacification is highly suggestive of such a fracture. The diagnosis is confirmed by CT.

MISSILE INJURY

In any foreign body injury, such as a missile injury, CT is essential to identify the extent of the soft tissue injury and the location and trajectory of the foreign body (Figure 12.15.12).

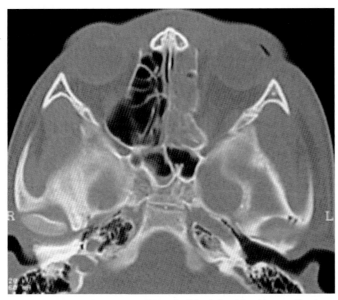

Figure 12.15.11 Fracture medial wall of the left orbit with opacification of the ethmoid sinuses following a direct blow to the face.

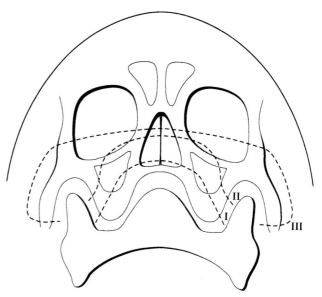

Figure 12.15.13 Fracture lines of the Le Fort classification of facial fractures.

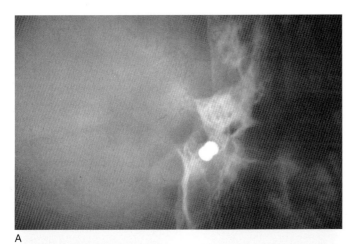

A

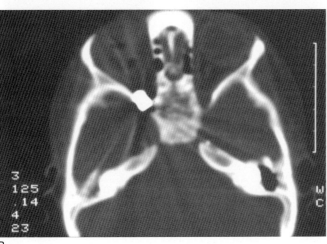

B

Figure 12.15.12 (A) Lateral x-ray of facial bones and (B) CT scan showing an airgun pellet embedded in the posterior wall of the sinuses.

LE FORT FRACTURES

These fractures have varying symptoms and degree of seriousness but have in common a high impact energy of the causative trauma and the relative mobility of the tooth-bearing part of the maxilla from the skull base. Le Fort has described three types of fractures (Figure 12.15.13):

Le Fort I fracture is the result of an impact on the inferior part of the maxilla. Maxillary sinuses are fractured transversely. There are no orbital or nasal fractures. The pterygoid apophysis and vomer are fractured in their inferior part.

Le Fort II fracture is more extensive and is the consequence of a violent impact on the maxilla or the nasal bones in an up-down direction. The fracture line runs inferiorly and laterally through the medial and inferior walls of the orbits and then through the lateral walls of the maxillary sinuses. The pterygoid apophysis is fractured on its median third.

Le Fort III fracture is a complete craniofacial disjunction resulting from a high-energy trauma of the nasal bones. The fracture line runs through the nasal bones, the lateral orbital wall and the zygomatic arch. The nasal septum and pterygoid apophysis are fractured superiorly. Fracture extension to the skull base is possible.

This classification allows the description of complex facial fractures in just a few words. Different Le Fort fracture types may affect both sides of the face simultaneously. CT is required for assessment of the degree of displacement. Three dimensional reconstruction is helpful for planning of reconstruction.

NASOETHMOIDAL AND FRONTAL FRACTURES

A violent impact between the eyes may lead to a comminuted fracture of the higher part of the maxilla, ethmoid, nasal, lacrimal or frontal bones. There is often cerebral involvement. The main clinical sign is telecanthus. CT is the best way of imaging these fractures.

EVOLUTION

In children, bone healing occurs within a shorter period than in adults and most fractures are firmly healed 2–3 weeks after the injury. Radiological signs of fracture will disappear within 3 months. Non-union of children's fractures is exceptional.

Facial fractures need appropriate management to avoid functional or aesthetic sequels. In children, continual growth allows anatomical bone adaptation, especially in the case of a condylar fracture. Fractures may also be responsible for major aesthetic deformity because of mandibular growth inhibition (temporomandibular ankylosis) or increased depression or deviation from nasal fractures.

CONCLUSION

Excluding alveolar fractures, facial fractures in children are usually the result of a violent facial trauma. Associated injuries are thus usual. A multidisciplinary management is often necessary and maxillofacial management takes place once other serious injuries are attended to. The diagnosis of facial fractures is essentially clinical. When suspected, plain radiographs are usually necessary and should include, as required, a Waters' view, a Towne's view, panoramic tomography and intraoral films. CT is still the most precise method of investigation, especially in younger children, and will be required for the assessment of all serious facial trauma at all ages.

FURTHER READING

Bansagi ZC, Meyer DR. Internal orbital fractures in the pediatric age group: characterization and management. Ophthalmology 2000; 107:829–836.

Gussack GS, Luterman A, Rodgers K, Powell RW, Ramenofsky ML. Pediatric maxillofacial trauma: unique features in diagnosis and treatment. Laryngoscope 1987; 97:925–930.

Hall RK. Injuries of the face and jaws in children. International Journal of Oral Surgery 1972; 1:65–75.

Holland AJ, Broome C, Steinberg A, Cass DT. Facial fractures in children. Pediatric Emergency Care 2001; 17:2001.

Hunter JG. Pediatric maxillofacial trauma. Pediatric Clinics of North America 1992; 39:1127–1143.

Kaban LB. Diagnosis and treatment of fractures of the facial bones in children 1943–1993. Journal of Oral Maxillofacial Surgery 1993; 51:722–729.

Koltai PJ, Amjad I, Meyer D, Feustel PJ. Orbital fractures in children. Archives of Otolaryngology and Head and Neck Surgery 1995; 121:1375–1379.

Lizuka T, Thoren H, Annino DJ, Hallikainen D, Lindqvist C. Midfacial fractures in pediatric patients. Archives of Otolaryngology and Head and Neck Surgery 1995; 121:1366–1371.

Mac Coy FJ, Chandler RA, Crow ML. Facial fractures in children. Plastic Reconstructive Surgery 1966; 37:209–212.

Mac Graw B, Cole RR. Pediatric maxillofacial trauma. Otolaryngology and Head and Neck Surgery 1990; 116:41–45.

Mac Ivor J. Maxillofacial radiology. In: Grainger RG, Allison DJ, eds. Diagnostic radiology: an anglo-american textbook of imaging, 2nd edn. Edinburgh: Churchill Livingstone; 1992:2165–2170.

Reil B, Kranz S. Traumatology of the maxillo-facial region in childhood: (statistical evaluation of 210 cases in the last 13 years). Journal of Maxillofacial Surgery 1976; 4:197–200.

Rowe NL. Fracture of the facial skeleton in children. Journal of Oral Surgery 1967; 26:505–515.

Spring PM, Cote DN. Pediatric maxillofacial fractures. Journal of the Louisiana State Medical Society 148:199–203.

Head Trauma

Francis Brunelle, Valérie Chigot,
Hussein Aref

In western society, head trauma is the commonest cause of death and disablement in persons under the age of 20 years. Overall, most severe head injuries are due to road traffic accidents and falls from heights, and these account for 50% of the deaths. However, non-accidental injury (NAI) is involved in 25% of head injuries in children and is the most frequent cause of severe head injury in infants, accounting for over 80% of the deaths.

The management of the acute stage of head injury may considerably modify the outcome. Potentially preventable causes of death and disability include hypoxia, brain swelling and some intracranial haemorrhages. Management is based to a large extent on clinical and biological observation but imaging is essential in the detection of intracranial bleeding and lesions with significant mass effect. In infants, extra-axial bleeding may present as insidious anaemia without signs of raised intracranial pressure.

The necessity for and timing of imaging is determined clinically. Most head injuries in young children are relatively mild and when recovery from concussion is rapid without residual impairment of consciousness or focal neurological deficit, imaging is generally unnecessary. It should not be used for documentation for medicolegal purposes, except in suspected NAI in which both cranial imaging and a skeletal survey may be in the interest of the child. Brain death is a clinical diagnosis, documented if necessary by electrophysiological tests.

In severe head trauma, brain death is suspected on EEG but imaging still has a legal role to play and is used in some societies. The role of imaging is to prove the absence of brain perfusion. Traditionally, angiography was the imaging technique of choice but this has been replaced by angio computed tomography (CT).

An upper cervical fracture should be suspected clinically if respiratory insufficiency or difficulty in maintaining blood pressure occurs. In severe head injuries, a lateral radiograph of the cervical spine is an absolute prerequisite prior to other imaging, since movement of the head and neck may be required, which in the presence of an unstable fracture or subluxation of the spine could potentially damage the spinal cord. However, the incidence of such fractures is low in children; when present they may result from high-momentum accidents. The lateral radiograph can be obtained during the acquisition of the scout view during the CT scan of the head (Figure 12.16.1). Increasingly in adult practice, CT of the cervical spine is used in trauma patients. It should be used selectively in children and not routinely to avoid unnecessary thyroid irradiation.

SKULL FRACTURES

A fracture of the skull can be shown overall in about 27% of children with head injury, in 75% of severe head injuries, but in under 10% of more minor injuries admitted for hospital inpatient observation. The incidence varies between studies and reflects the cohort and the severity of the injury on which the study was based and, as such, quoting such figures is not very meaningful. Other studies document a skull fracture in less than 2% of minor head injury. The majority of fractures are parietal and linear, with an overlying cephalhaematoma and they heal spontaneously. Fractures are not excluded by a normal skull x-ray and the mere demonstration of a simple vault fracture gives inadequate information about intracranial damage and should not modify management. Only 40% of children with extradural and 15% with subdural haematoma have a fracture, so that significant treatable pathology, including extra-axial haematoma in children, is not infrequent in the absence of any fracture. Potentially significant fractures are evident on CT and the presence of any embedded bone fragments and mass lesions requiring surgery, as well as an indication of the amount of damage to the brain or meninges, will be given. It is also well documented that fractures may be missed on CT because of the incident plane of the scan. This is of little importance in most patients as it is the presence of brain injury that matters but in NAI the demonstration of the fracture is important even in the absence of brain injury, and skull x-rays are still indicated in this group.

The most frequent type of skull fracture in children of all ages is a simple linear fracture of the parietal bones (Figure 12.16.2). It may be horizontal or vertical. Short vertical fractures (Figure 12.16.3) can be difficult to distinguish from accessory fissures or strip sutures in young children as these, unlike normal sutures, have straight edges. Scalp swelling over the lesion helps to distinguish them. Frontal and occipital fractures tend to occur from direct impact trauma over them. The accessory sutures that may mimic fractures are the metopic and cerebellar sutures. Both of these are in the midline. The presence of scalp swelling over a fracture indicates it is recent, i.e. within 1 week of x-ray. Delayed presentation of scalp swelling over a fracture is a rare but well-recorded occurrence. This is thought to be due to slow leakage of CSF into the scalp. The detection of scalp swelling is also influenced by the amount of hair on the head and its type. Indian children have thick black hair, which may cover a visible swelling, although it will be palpable.

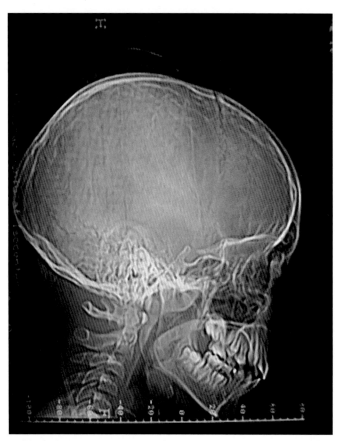

Figure 12.16.1 Lateral view of the upper cervical spine obtained during head CT for trauma.

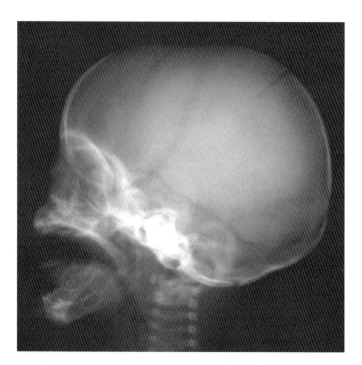

Figure 12.16.3 Short vertical fracture of the upper part of the parietal bone. This film is oblique and thus appears to widen the fracture. This type of injury is very difficult to distinguish from a strip suture, which is a normal variant. The presence of overlying soft tissue swelling helps.

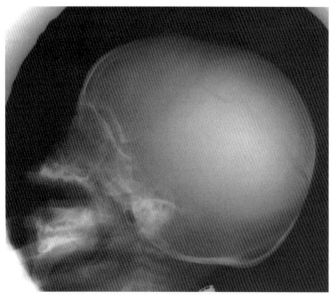

Figure 12.16.2 Linear parietal fracture sustained during a fall.

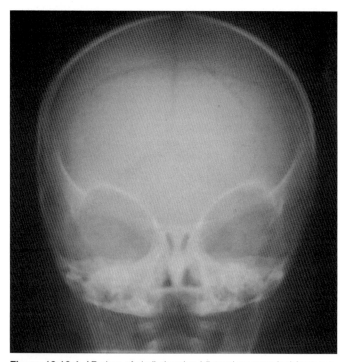

Figure 12.16.4 AP view of skull showing bilateral symmetrical fractures of the parietal bone.

Vertical or horizontal biparietal fractures may occur from a single impact in a young child. The fractures occur at the point of maximum deformity of the skull and spread backwards to meet in the midline (Figure 12.16.4). This is easily appreciated on CT with vertical fractures, provided high enough slices are taken. On x-ray, obliquity of the film may apparently separate the fracture lines.

The plasticity of the infant skull allowing deformities is the cause of biparietal fractures.

Skull bones are membranous bones and repair does not excite much periosteal reaction. Some thickening may be evident on CT. It is impossible to age skull fractures reliably. The presence of scalp swelling indicates that fractures are recent and fresh fractures on x-ray have crisp edges. After about 2 weeks the edges lose their sharpness. The length of time for a fracture to disappear is variable but most have healed by 3 months. Some fracture lines may persist for months. Wide fractures (greater than 3 mm) are said to be more frequent in non-accidental than accidental injury and this is in general true, but caution should be exercised before using this attribute to declare a fracture non-accidental as oblique projections can give the false impression of a wide fracture because of magnification.

Depressed fractures can occur from forceful focal impaction, such as being hit with a golf club, or falling onto a stone or rock. A palpable deficit may be detected clinically. Radiographically, a depressed fracture may appear as a lucency or a sclerotic line depending on the projection (Figure 12.16.5). It will appear sclerotic if it lies in the plane of the incident beam. A tangential view was traditionally done to identify depression but CT is indicated to correctly assess the extent of the depression and any underlying brain injury. Surgical decisions about fracture elevation are based on CT.

PING PONG FRACTURES

Ping pong fractures may occur as a result of forceps delivery or an overlay injury. The latter occurs when the pliable infant skull is depressed. It appears on radiographs as a large smooth depression (Figure 12.16.6).

GROWING FRACTURE

When the dura underlying a fracture has been torn, intracranial contents may impinge on the fracture. The transmitted intracranial pulse erodes the margins of the fracture and a pulsating swelling is clinically evident on the scalp (Figure 12.16.7).

The condition usually occurs in children under 1 year of age and 90% of all cases are under 3 years of age. The fracture may be caused by forceps delivery or by postnatal violent trauma or by surgery. It usually involves a parietal bone, though the occipital, mastoid or frontal bones may be affected. In the latter two sites, herniating soft tissue may encroach into the middle ear cleft, frontal sinus or orbit causing a post-traumatic encephalocele and/or CSF leak.

The interval between trauma and diagnosis may be weeks to years but is usually 4–6 months and, in addition to the pulsatile mass, there may be focal neurological deficits relating to the damaged underlying brain.

The enlarging bone defect may be documented on radiographs. It is usually tapering with bevelled edges and sclerotic margins. The fracture is almost always associated with underlying brain damage apparently initiated and/or perpetuated by trauma to the cortical vessels where they pass through the cranial defect unprotected by dura. The damage should always be elucidated by CT and/or MRI. There is usually focal encephalomalacia with dilatation of the ventricle and cerebral herniation. A leptomeningeal cyst or segment of the subarachnoid space walled off by adhesions is the cause of the erosion in only a minority of cases. Rarely, erosion

is caused by a false aneurysm. Effective treatment requires repair of the dural tear.

BASE OF SKULL FRACTURES

These may present clinically with bruising around the eyes or ears, bleeding from the nose or ear, fluid discharge due to CSF leakage from the nose or ear, cranial nerve abnormalities, or deafness. Once suspected, CT is indicated (Figure 12.16.8). High-resolution, thin-slice images viewed on a variety of windows may be required for their demonstration. Fluid levels in the sinuses, fluid in the mastoid air cells or middle ear cleft and abnormal locations of air around the sinuses or in the intracranial cavity are all imaging features. CT will also distinguish fractures through the otic capsule from ossicular disruption as a cause of deafness.

Most base of skull fractures are managed conservatively with antibiotics and do not require surgery. It is important that they are diagnosed, as failure to treat with antibiotics may result in meningitis. A base of skull fracture into a sinus or into the mastoids is a compound fracture.

PENETRATING INJURY

Penetrating intracranial injury is fortunately a relatively rare occurrence in children, most occurring during 'play'. Most occur through the orbit or face but high-velocity injury, such as airgun pellets fired at close range, may penetrate the skull vault. The aim of imaging is to identify the depth of the intracranial extension of the wound, the structures injured, the extent of the damage and the presence and location of residual foreign bodies, e.g. bullet fragments. Initial imaging should be by CT as many such injuries are with ferromagnetic substances. Once these have been excluded as being present, magnetic resonance imaging (MRI) may then also be required.

RECURRENT MENINGITIS OR INTRACRANIAL ABSCESS AND/OR CSF RHINORRHOEA OR OTORRHOEA

These may result from trauma involving the air sinuses, middle ear or cribriform plate. Most fractures involving the sinuses, mastoids or middle ears spontaneously seal off from the cranial contents in the acute phase of head injury. A small proportion continue to communicate and constitute a potential route of infection. Meningitis and extracerebral or intracerebral abscesses may result. The fracture line itself may be visible on CT or a small amount of air may be present within the cranial cavity adjacent to the fracture, or fluid or cerebral substance may herniate through it and may be identified on CT or MRI. This is particularly true of fractures involving the middle ear or mastoid antrum or occasionally the posterior wall of a frontal sinus. If none of these features are visible at a time when the leak is still clinically manifest the site may be identified with MR cysternography.

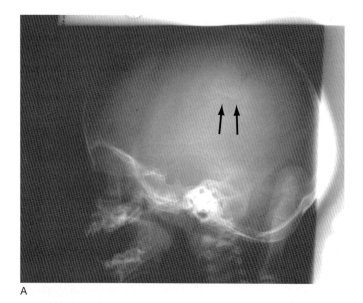

A

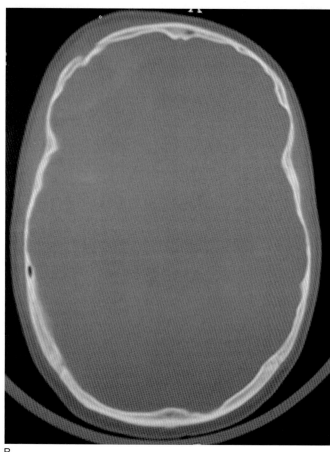

B

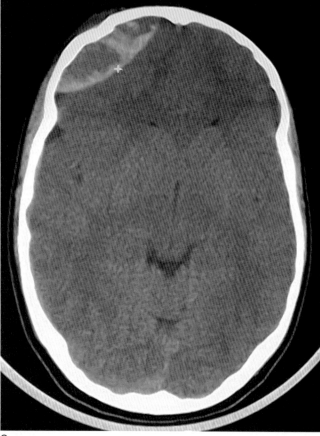

C

Figure 12.16.5 (A) Lateral radiograph of a child with a depressed fracture. Note the sclerotic line on the radiograph. (B) Another child who was in a motor vehicle accident. Direct trauma in the frontal region. (C) CT scan, bone window shows the presence of a depressed fracture. Soft tissue window shows an extradural haematoma as well as hypodensity of both frontal lobes due to contusion and oedema.

The leakage may be increased during the study by jugular compression or a Valsalva manoeuvre after elective positioning of the patient.

Coronal thin scans on T2-weighted sequences with fat saturation show the CSF spaces and outline the fistula when present (Figure 12.16.9).

Nuclear medicine studies with intrathecal injection of DTPA via a lumbar puncture have recently been abandoned.

BIRTH TRAUMA

Skull fractures in the neonatal period are a recognized though rare consequence of instrumental delivery, mainly forceps. These fractures may be linear or depressed fractures and there is usually a significant cephalohaematoma associated with them. There are three forms of extracranial bleeding that may occur secondary to birth trauma:

1. Subgaleal bleeding. This term describes haemorrhage under the scalp aponeurosis and may be very extensive with blood loss severe enough to cause symptoms, require transfusion and even lead to death (Figure 12.16.10).

2. Cephalohaematoma. This may occur without a fracture or without instrumental delivery. A cephalohaematoma is due to encapsulated bleeding between the pericranium and a skull vault bone. Thus, it does not cross a suture. The parietal bone is most often affected with the occipital bone being the next most frequently involved. Periosteal new bone is laid down on the outer edge of the haematoma, which then gradually fills in. It may calcify initially and is seen on x-ray as a calcific opacity projected over the skull vault (Figure 12.16.11). It may remould completely but there may be some residual thickening. There may be some underlying subdural bleeding both under a cephalohaematoma and under subgaleal bleeding.

3. Caput succedaneum. This is not confined by sutures and is due to diffuse bleeding and oedema under the scalp. It is a common problem following vaginal delivery, especially if prolonged. It does not require imaging.

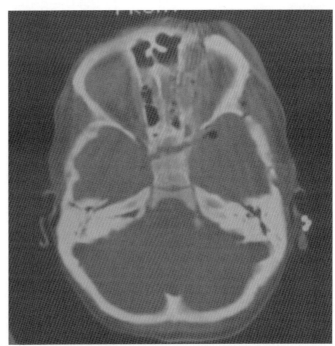

Figure 12.16.8 CT scan of a child who has a fracture of the right frontal bone just above the right orbit but in addition has a fracture of the sphenoidal bone. Note air in the right temporal region.

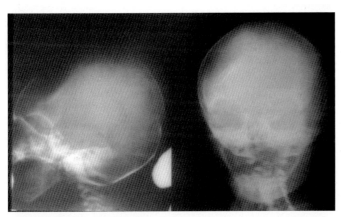

Figure 12.16.6 Anteroposterior (AP) and lateral view of skull of a child with a depressed fracture of the right frontal bone and a haematoma, secondary to a forceps delivery.

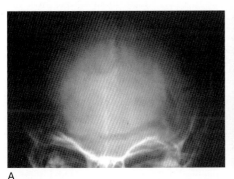

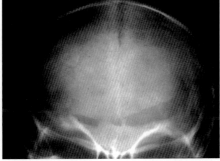

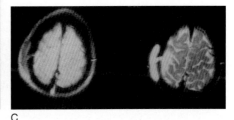

A   B   C

Figure 12.16.7 Growing fracture. (A) Initial x-rays: a fracture extending into the posterior fossa is visible. (B) A year later the fracture has grown. (C) Axial T1- and T2-weighted MRI shows the presence of a dural tear and a post-traumatic meningocele communicating with the CSF spaces.

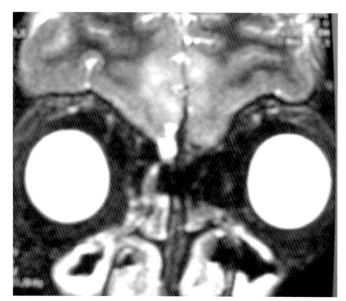

Figure 12.16.9 Post-traumatic CSF leak secondary to ethmoidal fracture. Coronal T2-weighted MRI shows the right-sided CSF fistula through the fractured ethmoidal cribriform plate.

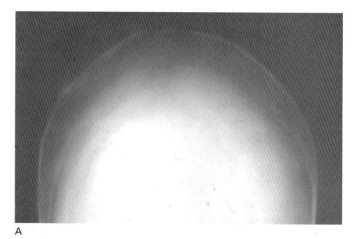

A

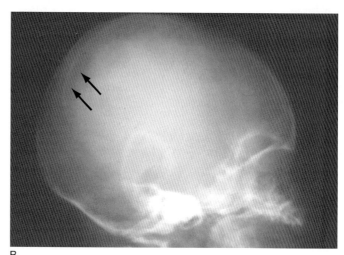

B

Figure 12.16.11 (A) Towne's view of skull with calcified cephalohaematoma on the right. (B) Different infant showing large, calcified cephalohaematoma projected over the parietal bone.

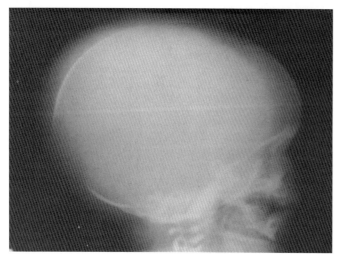

Figure 12.16.10 Lateral skull radiograph of an infant showing a large soft tissue swelling on the top of the head, secondary to subgaleal haemorrhage from birth injury.

difficult to identify in the infant brain, as it is normally more hypodense than normal due to a high water content. Delayed tentorial tears have been described, with the infant presenting in the first few days after birth. More recent work with MRI in asymptomatic children has shown that small silent subdurals are more frequent than previously appreciated. These resolve without sequelae.

IN UTERO INJURY

In utero skull fractures due to direct abdominal trauma have been reported. Most *in utero* injury to the infant brain is due to ischaemia or disruption of fetal circulation and is not discussed here. Scalp and other injury to the fetus as a result of amniocentesis is also recorded, though rare. This must be distinguished from aplasia cutis, a rare congenital defect of the scalp, which may be associated with underlying skull table defects.

Most infants imaged for signs of intracranial injury following birth have symptoms, e.g. irritability, fits, abnormal posturing, or respiratory or feeding difficulties. This can occur even without instrumental delivery. Brain injury and its imaging in the premature infant is described elsewhere in this book. The main intracranial traumatic lesions encountered in the symptomatic term infant are subdural haematomas, both convexity and infratentorial, subarachnoid bleeding and evidence of asphyxia. The latter can be

CRANIOTABES

There is compression of the skull vault *in utero* against the maternal sacrum or by the infant fist. This is often associated with oligohydramnios (Figure 12.16.12). The infant is born with the depression but there is no overlying scalp swelling. Gradual remodelling of the skull vault is the natural history.

CLOSED HEAD INJURY

This term defines intracranial injury without external evidence of trauma or a skull fracture. The raised intracranial pressure is confined to the cranium, without decompression, which may occur with a complex fracture. It is therefore potentially very serious. It may occur with both accidental and non-accidental trauma. Clinically, it presents with neurological signs – headache, irritability, loss of consciousness and fits. The underlying lesions may be focal or diffuse. Focal lesions include epidural and subdural haematomas. Diffuse lesions are mainly those of brain swelling. Death occurs from coning if the pressure is not relieved.

IMAGING

In the acute situation, skull radiographs may waste valuable time: if imaging is required, it is best to proceed without delay to CT. Other indications for skull radiography include:

1. A history of a CSF shunting procedure. Plain radiographs are the best way to show disconnection of shunt catheters.
2. In NAI as part of the skeletal survey.
3. When CT is not easily available, skull radiography may be helpful in the selection of patients for further imaging. The detection of a skull fracture is often one such criterion.

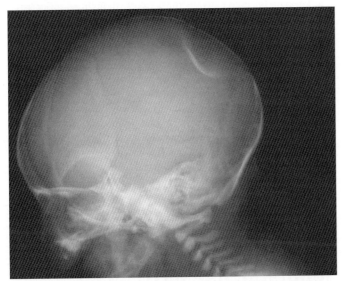

Figure 12.16.12 Lateral view of skull of an infant born with depression of the skull vault secondary to *in utero* compression. There had been maternal oligohydramnios.

The standard radiographs should include a posteroanterior (PA) and lateral view with the addition of a Towne's view for occipital injury. They should be exposed to see the scalp as well as the bone. Today, base of skull and mastoid views are not indicated and have been replaced by CT.

Guidelines are now published that broaden the indications for CT scanning in order to avoid missing a clinically significant head injury. Many of these are based on the evidence of the 'Canadian Rules'. If these guidelines are not used locally, the following indications should apply:

1. Disturbance of consciousness, especially if there is delay in onset after the trauma or deterioration or even lack of improvement within 1 h of the trauma. In practice, some temporary deterioration of conscious level during the hours following a head injury is not uncommon in the absence of any abnormality on CT and is thought to be due to delayed convulsive activity.
2. Increasing or unexplained focal neurological signs. Early treatment of brain compression improves the prognosis, so that imaging should be repeated to elucidate any potentially significant deterioration in the clinical status of the patient. Indeed, in about 50% of severe head injury cases, early CT scans are normal; some of these cases show intracranial haemorrhage requiring evacuation, or oedema or infarction on a later study. Hyperacute haemorrhage is isointense on CT scan. Persisting neurological signs and seizures occuring after 24 h are usual indications. Imaging is frequently normal in such cases and is of good prognostic significance.
3. The presence of a skull fracture on x-ray if done, even in the absence of clinical signs, is now regarded as an indication for CT in most hospitals.
4. Suspected intracranial or intraorbital foreign body after penetrating injuries. Ferromagnetic foreign bodies should be excluded by a skull film or CT prior to study by MRI.
5. History of a previous craniotomy or shunt procedure.

CT is generally freely available in most Western societies. It is relatively inexpensive and other parts of the body can then be scanned should this prove necessary in polytrauma patients. The head scan should be done before administration of intravenous (IV) contrast. CT is the initial imaging technique of choice in acute trauma and identifies conditions requiring surgical intervention. Acute intracranial haematomas and haemorrhagic mass lesions amenable to surgical correction as well as intraventricular and subarachnoid haemorrhage are revealed using CT. Enhancement is rarely necessary in the acute phase but may be useful to confirm:

1. isodense extracerebral effusions considered equivocal on plain CT;
2. the size of a resolving haematoma by ring enhancement;
3. vascular and inflammatory complications; and
4. the presence of a vascular malformation.

This is not contraindicated since the advent of isomolar nonionic agents.

CT is better than MRI for the clear demonstration of some types of foreign body, potentially disfiguring depressed fractures, pneumocephalus and the majority of fractures. Surgical repair of torn dura will prevent additional brain damage and growth of fractures, and early evaluation of depressed fractures in older children improves cosmetic results. This is unnecessary in young children since remodelling occurs and there is no good evidence that the incidence of post-traumatic epilepsy is reduced.

The correlation between CT appearances and both focal neurological deficits and the clinical indicators of severe global brain injury is often poor. Even with repeated studies and using high-resolution CT, many lesions shown at autopsy are not revealed by imaging. This is not surprising because CT is inefficient for the detection of lesions particularly in the posterior fossa, with absorption coefficients approaching those of the surrounding brain and which cause little anatomical distortion.

Microhaemorrhagic and non-haemorrhagic shear strain injuries including diffuse axonal and subcortical grey matter injury, which are over twice as common as frankly haemorrhagic lesions and particularly brainstem and hypothalamic contusions and infarcts and which are important causes of prolonged alteration of consciousness and disability, are often not visible on CT but at least are partly revealed as so-called marker lesions by MRI. The multiplanar facility of MRI is excellent for precise localization of these lesions and from this the pathology can generally be deduced.

MRI is useful in selected cases during the subacute phase of trauma, particularly for assessment of prognosis. Examples are:

1. major clinical abnormalities without a correlating lesion on CT;
2. minor head injuries with persisting unexplained disability; and
3. suspected non-accidental injury when repeated trauma may have occurred; MRI may show evidence of both recent haematoma and haemoglobin degradation products, in particular on gradient echo T2-weighted sequences, and thus suggests that bleeding has occurred on more than one occasion.

MRI is the indicated imaging technique for the follow-up of head injury patients.

CT is the initial imaging technique and is the preferred technique for monitoring acute complications. In severe trauma, the scan should be performed as soon as the child is stable enough to move to the scan room. Scanning in children who do not present with acute major trauma but are being imaged because of protocols should be done according to these, modified locally if necessary to avoid unnecessary disturbance to staff or child. In a small number of children, in particular those with cerebral oedema, small subdurals and epidurals, early scanning may be normal or only subtly abnormal, if insufficient time has elapsed for imaging signs to become apparent. Repeat scanning after a few hours, if required clinically, may show the development of lesions.

Follow-up scanning for prognosis, once the acute injury is managed, should be performed by MRI. This is particularly valuable for demonstrating gliosis in shear injuries, which though volumetrically small, may have serious neurological consequences. These may be found anywhere but are characteristically seen in the corpus callosum, the temporal lobes and the inferior surface of the frontal lobes. T1-weighted (T1-W), T2-weighted (T2-W) and FLAIR sequences are required in the axial and coronal plane, together with sagittal T1-W and T2-W sequences, and a gradient echo T2-W sequence in the coronal and sagittal planes.

Though CT remains the initial imaging technique because of its high yield and accessibility, the advent of diffusion and perfusion weighted MR imaging is increasing the importance of early MR imaging as abnormalities seen by these techniques are of prognostic importance.

TYPES OF LESIONS

Intracranial lesions can be divided into those caused directly by the trauma and reactive changes initiated by the trauma, the effects of which may be delayed. The latter include loss of autoregulation of cerebral vessels, vasogenic oedema and loss of cerebral perfusion with ischaemia or infarction, related to the compressive effects of brain swelling.

PRIMARY TRAUMATIC HAEMORRHAGES

These may be due to tearing of arteries or veins or of smaller vessels. They are far less frequent in children than adults but are an important cause of compression and displacement of brain substance, which may result in irreversible and sometimes fatal brain damage, and it is therefore important to diagnose them early for surgical consideration. They may be extra-axial, in the extra or subdural space, or intra-axial. All extra-axial fluid collections displace the brain surface and grey–white matter interface away from the skull.

EXTRADURAL HAEMATOMAS

These are also known as epidural haematomas. They are relatively uncommon in children and are usually of venous origin: a dural or meningeal vein may be torn in the absence of any fracture, especially in the very young. The traumatic incident may be relatively minor. Compared with adults the haematomas tend to be less acute. In young children with compressive lesions, a lucid-free interval is less common. The haematoma is situated over the temporal or temporoparietal convexity in most cases, though posterior fossa extradural haemorrhage is relatively common in young children. An acute haematoma is of high density on CT and isointense to brain substance on MRI if performed. In arterial haemorrhage, there may be flowing blood within the haematoma adjacent to the torn vessel. This part is of lower density on CT (Figure 12.16.5C and Figure 12.16.13) and hypointense on MRI; it enhances markedly after intravenous contrast medium. The medial border of the haematoma is convex towards the brain, with a well-defined inner margin formed by the displaced dura. The dura itself is not visible as a separate structure on CT but shows as a hypointense band on MRI. Extradural haematomas due to venous bleeding are often adjacent to a large sinus, which may be displaced away from the vault by a haematoma extending across the midline or across the tentorial attachment. Epidural haematomas with mass effect are a neurosurgical emergency.

SUBDURAL HAEMATOMAS

Minor subdural haematomas may be seen after trauma in infants and young children and are believed to be caused by shearing

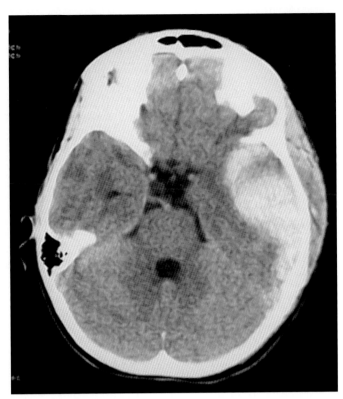

Figure 12.16.13 Direct trauma on the left temporal region. A large extradural haematoma is seen as well as mild temporal herniation.

injuries, which commonly induce simultaneous brain damage and tear the transdural segment of cortical veins. The haematomas are more common over the supratentorial convexities but are not infrequent over the cerebellar convexities in the newborn, particularly following breech or difficult deliveries and along the falx and tentorium. Delayed presentation of a supratentorial tear and a consequent subdural haematoma is described in newborns days after delivery. MRI has shown that small subdural haematomas are frequent in the posterior fossa even after normal deliveries. They are without any clinical significance. They may extend over the occipital cortex into the falx cerebri. This distribution is also seen in shaking non-accidental injury but usually not in acute accidental trauma.

Traumatic subdural haematomas may be unilateral or bilateral. When associated with a fracture, they are often unilateral. An associated mass effect depends on the size of the collection and brain swelling. If there is major brain swelling, a small contralateral subdural may be compressed against the bony skull, only to become evident on follow-up.

The juxtacerebral surface of the haematoma conforms to the shape of the brain, which is displaced away from the dura. An acute clot is generally of high density on CT, though the density may be less in anaemic patients or due to dilution with CSF if the arachnoid is torn. On MRI, the appearance of the bleed varies considerably with the age of the clot. It is generally hyperintense on

T1-weighted sequences. Its intensity depends on dilution of the blood with CSF.

As the blood ages, the CT density of a haematoma is reduced and eventually becomes lower than the adjacent brain. In general, the high density of fresh haemorrhage disappears by 1 week but may persist longer in neonates and young children. For a short time, the density may be close to that of the brain substance and the extracerebral effusions may not be directly visible, though their presence can usually be recognized by displacement of the hemisphere (Figure 12.16.14). Intravenous contrast medium may outline cortical vessels or an enhancing inner membrane, the latter in particular with chronic subdurals (Figure 12.16.15). Such haematomas contain methaemoglobin, which is bright on both T1- and T2-weighted MR sequences and thus easily distinguished both from brain substance and CSF. MRI is particularly useful for showing thin layers of subdural blood which, even in the acute phase, despite being of high density, may be difficult to recognize on CT against the high density of the bone of the vault due to beam-hardening effects. Transversely orientated high cerebral convexity, juxtatentorial and basal subdural effusions are optimally demonstrated in the coronal plane on MRI (Figure 12.16.16).

In the context of acute trauma, the finding of a fresh subdural haematoma and its natural evolution until resorbed presents no diagnostic difficulty. The discovery of a subdural haematoma without a history of trauma must raise concerns about a non-accidental causation. Rare causes of an acute subdural haematoma without an accidental aetiology include haemorrhagic meningitis, for which there is an obvious history, rupture into the subdural space of a subdural or peripheral cerebral vascular malformation. MR imaging will usually show the underlying pathology.

Chronic subdural collections may be the result of bleeding or more rarely meningitis, for which there should be an appropriate history. Glutaric acidurea type 2 and coagulopathies may also result in chronic subdural haematomas but are both identifiable by appropriate investigations.

AGEING OF SUBDURAL HAEMATOMAS

Guidelines and tables as to the appearance of a subdural haematoma on CT and MRI are published and serve as a useful guide. In most instances, the ageing of a subdural is of no clinical relevance as the incident that caused the bleed is well documented. The problem arises in children with suspected non-accidental injury, in which ageing may be important, as is the presence of lesions of more than one age.

The age of a subdural in infants is more reliably assessed by CT than MRI, especially in the acute situation. The persistence of high-attenuation blood indicating fresh haemorrhage lasts for a longer time in young infants than adults. In adults, it is accepted that fresh haemorrhage loses its high attenuation by 7 days. In very young infants, this may persist for up to 2 weeks, and for longer on MRI, especially if the blood is compartmentalized by a membrane. The presence of a membrane does indicate an older lesion. Table 12.16.1 shows the signal intensity of haemorrhage at different ages. This should only be used as a guide as it may take longer for acute blood to disappear in young infants.

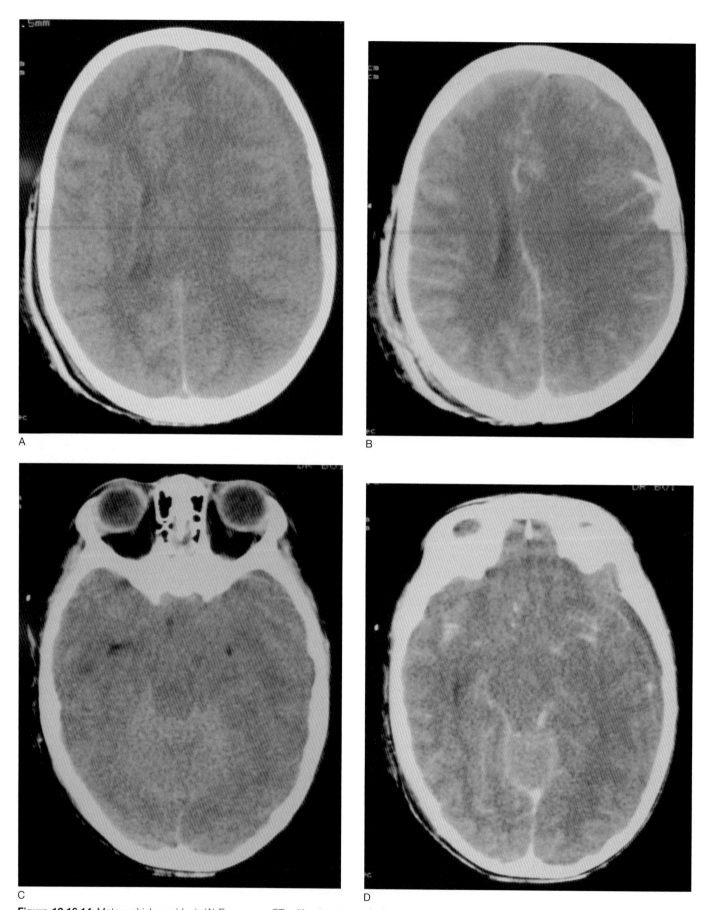

Figure 12.16.14 Motor vehicle accident. (A) Emergency CT, without contrast. An isodense subdural haematoma is seen. (B) After contrast injection an acute bleed is visible in the subdural effusion. (C,D) Same patient, axial scan at the level of the tentorial incissura. Oedema of the brain is visible as well as left tentorial temporal lobe herniation.

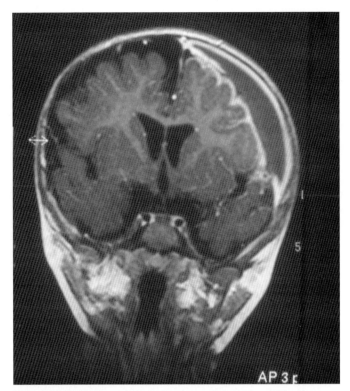

Figure 12.16.15 Coronal contrast-enhanced scan of a child with an enhancing membrane around a subdural haematoma.

PRIMARY POST-TRAUMATIC INTRACEREBRAL HAEMATOMAS

These most frequently occur in the frontal, temporal and basal ganglion regions (Figure 12.16.17). Extensive damage around a haemorrhage suggests that is has occurred as a secondary event into ischaemic or contused brain substance. Acute haemorrhage with normal surrounding brain is seen without contusion. The possibility of a delayed onset intracerebral haematoma should be considered if acute deterioration occurs in a previously stable head injury patient. Intracerebral haematomas are evident in the acute phase on CT as high-density circumscribed masses (Figure 12.16.18). When examined after 2–3 weeks they may become isodense with brain substance on T1-weighted images. They are hyperintense on T2-weighted images. On echo gradient echo T2-weighted images (T2*) the haemosiderin deposition is visible as a dark rim around the haematoma.

SUBPIAL HAEMORRHAGE

During deceleration in traffic accidents or in shaken baby syndrome small haemorrhages occur at the root of torn small cortical veins. Such small bleeds are best seen on coronal scans on T1-weighted images. When CT imaging is performed, the scan should cover the vertex in order not to overlook such lesions.

INTRAVENTRICULAR AND SUBARACHNOID HAEMORRHAGES

These may be due to extension of intracerebral haematomas but are more commonly the result of shearing injuries tearing surface vessels (Figures 12.16.19 and 12.16.20). Acute subarachnoid haemorrhage is best seen on CT and may be missed on routine T1- and T2-weighted MR sequences, although it may be visible on FLAIR sequences. The blood remains high signal on FLAIR, whereas CSF is of low signal.

Callosal, septal and/or forniceal injury should be suspected in intraventricular haemorrhage. These imply a poor prognosis. Parafalcine subarachnoid haemorrhage, especially posteriorly in infants, should suggest non-accidental injury. The parafalcine collection is evident on CT. It is distinguished from the normal high-density falx seen, especially if there is an oedematous brain, by noting the thicker irregular outline of the haemorrhage in the falx. Associated shearing injuries are best revealed by MRI. They may also be seen in the frontal lobes on transfontanellar ultrasound. The presence of large quantities of blood in the CSF may be followed by hydrocephalus requiring external drainage.

Table 12.16.1 MRI (1.5T) signal intensity of haemorrhage on different pulse sequences

T1 – weighted Haemorrhage/ appearance	Time frame	T2-weighted Haemoglobin state/ appearance
Hyperacute (intracellular)/ isointense or hypointense	4–6 h	Oxyhaemoglobin/hyperintense
Acute (intracellular)/ isointense or hypointense	6 h to 3 days	Deoxyhaemoglobin/hypointense
Early subacute (intracellular)/ hyperintense	First week (>3 days)	Methaemoglobin/hypointense
Late subacute (extracellular)/ Hyperintense	Second week to 3 months (>7 days)	Methaemoglobin/hyperintense
Chronic (within isointense or hypointense phagocytes)	2 weeks to months (>14 days)	Ferritin and haemosiderin/ hypointense or hyperintense with a hypointense rim

Reproduced from Fitz CR, Byrd SE. Trauma. In: Caffey's pediatric diagnostic imaging, 10th edn. Elsevier; 2004:548.

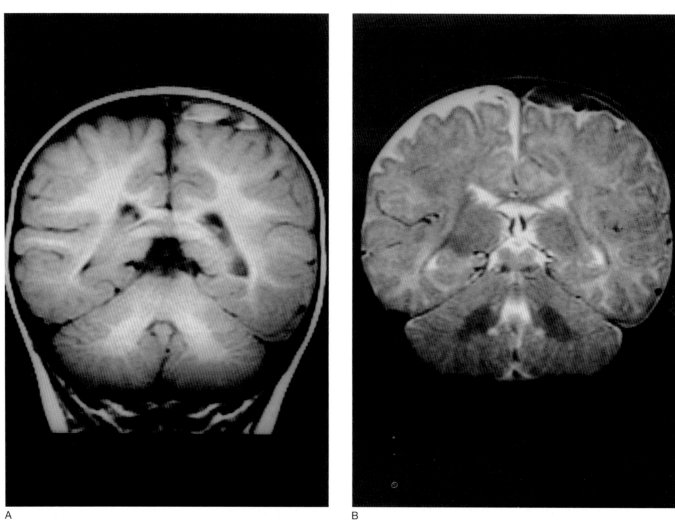

A   B

Figure 12.16.16 Coronal T1-weighted (A) and T2-weighted (B) images taken after trauma in a child with chronic subdural. On the left the haematoma is hyperintense on T1-weighted and hypointense on T2-weighted images. The CSF subdural on the right exhibits a reverse signal.

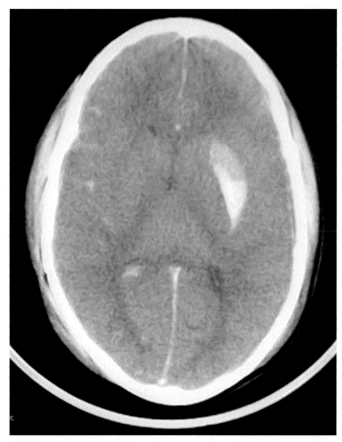

Figure 12.16.17 Major trauma after a fall from a building. Haematoma is seen in the left basal ganglia as well as intraventricular haemorrhage. Brain oedema is present with obliteration of the ventricle lumen. The patient died the next day.

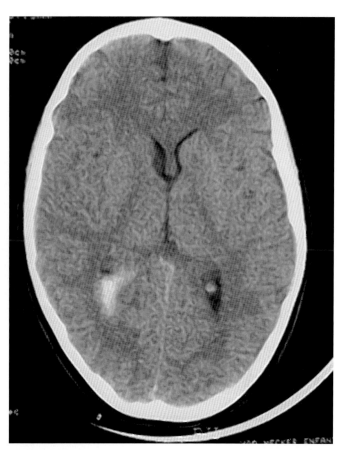

Figure 12.16.19 Intraventricular haemorrhage. Left intraventricular haemorrhage; the left hemisphere is swollen.

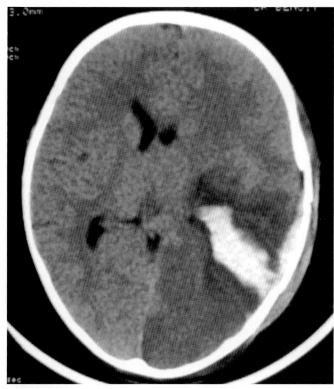

Figure 12.16.18 Fall from the fourth floor. An acute hyperdense haematoma is seen in the left posterior parietal region. Oedema of the affected brain is seen as well.

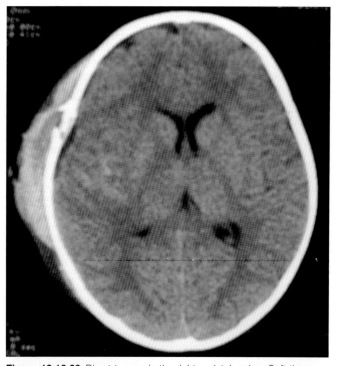

Figure 12.16.20 Direct trauma in the right parietal region. Soft tissue oedema is seen as well as small haematomas in the brain substance in the right cerebral hemisphere.

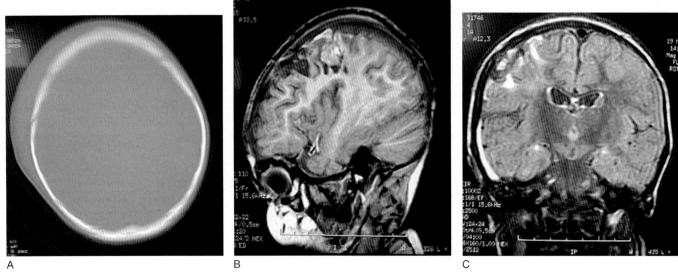

Figure 12.16.21 Direct trauma after a fall. (A) CT shows presence of a right parietal fracture. (B) Sagittal T1-weighted MRI demonstrates brain contusion and haemorrhage. (C) Coronal FLAIR shows the extent of brain contusion.

PRIMARY INJURIES TO BRAIN SUBSTANCE

CEREBRAL LACERATION

This is caused either by a penetrating injury or by a direct blow causing a depressed fracture or transient depression of the bone. Localized brain damage simulating haemorrhagic infarction is evident on both CT and MRI (Figure 12.16.21). Penetrating injuries carry a high risk of infection as a complication. Small fragments of the object may be deposited in the track in the brain. The causation of penetrating injuries depends in part on the play activities of children. Mock duelling may cause transorbital penetrating brain injuries, destroying the orbit in the process. The velocity of air rifle pellets is fortunately seldom sufficient to penetrate the skull vault but they too may enter the brain by the transorbital route. The outcome of such injuries depends on the amount of brain damage and what structures are involved. Initial imaging should be by CT. A fine, penetrating injury, particularly when accidentally self inflicted, may not be detected until late and may present with an intracranial abscess, meningitis or CSF leak (Figure 12.16.22).

SHEAR STRESS INJURY

This is a common cause of damage following head trauma. Strain occurs at points of relative fixation and at interfaces of differing density at times of rapid deceleration. The commonest such lesion following severe head injury is diffuse axonal damage. Tearing of the axons is most frequent in the cerebral hemispheres near the junction of grey and white matter, particularly in the frontal lobes,

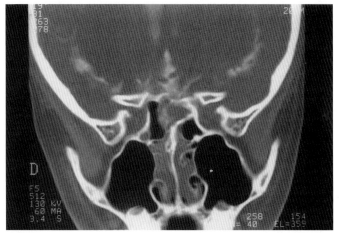

Figure 12.16.22 Post-traumatic CSF rhinorrhoea. Coronal CT after lumbar injection of contrast media. The fistula is well seen in the right part of the sphenoid sinus.

in the parasagittal regions and in the temporal lobes. Other parts of the cerebral white matter and the cerebellum are involved less frequently.

A more severe strain associated with axial rotation tends to cause tearing in the splenium and posterior part of the body of the corpus callosum. The depth of the falx posteriorly causes the posterior parts of the hemispheres, including the splenium of the corpus callosum, to be relatively fixed, compared to the shallower anterior parts of the hemispheres and corpus callosum. Stress develops in the posterior parts of the body and in the splenium, which tend to be damaged, usually unilaterally, but with increasing severity of injury, the entire body of the corpus callosum and the septum pellucidum, usually at the site of attachment to the corpus callosum, and/or the fornices may be involvedl.

With even more severe injuries, axonal tearing may occur in the peripheral parts of the midbrain and rostral pons, resulting in decerebration and/or cranial nerve palsies. The superior cerebellar peduncles and medial lemnisci and, less commonly, the cerebral peduncles are particularly affected.

The immediate effects of diffuse axonal shearing are generally non-haemorrhagic lesions, confined to white matter orientated in the long axis of white matter tracts; the lesions vary from a few millimetres up to 2 cm in length. The lesions are usually multiple and are often poorly shown by CT when clearly visible on MRI (Figure 12.16.23). However, release of vasoactive substances and slowing of blood flow tends to cause some secondary oedema and haemorrhage occurs into about 20% of lesions. Sometimes confluence of lesions occurs and they may thereby become apparent on delayed CT studies made 24–48 h after trauma. Even acute MR imaging does not reflect the full extent of the damage, which may be followed within 3–4 weeks by atrophy and demyelination.

Cortical contusions are usually caused by shear stress of the brain substance at its junction with the dura and skull (Figure 12.16.24); they may also arise from direct trauma or contre coup injury. Clinical accompaniments include coma, focal neurological deficits, seizures and raised intracranial pressure. These contusions are less frequent than diffuse axonal tearing but they tend to be larger; over 50% develop haemorrhagic foci, which tend to increase in extent over several hours and may become confluent, and are then conspicuous on CT. They may burst through the cortex and cause an acute subdural haematoma. Smaller lesions with lesser amounts of extravasated blood may be shown only by MRI. The non-haemorrhagic components are best appreciated as bright lesions on T2-weighted MRI. Haemorrhage varies in appearance with the state of the blood products, but often contributes a mottled pattern.

Cortical contusions particularly involve the lateral and anterior aspects of the temporal lobes and the lateral and inferior frontal

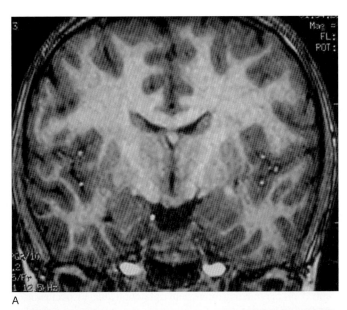

A

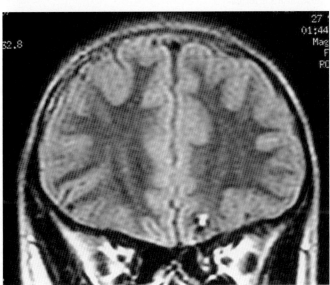

B

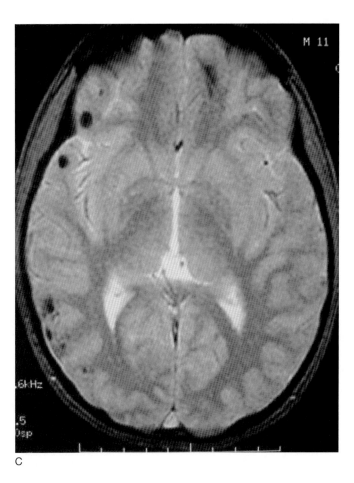

C

Figure 12.16.23 Unexplained coma after a motor vehicle accident. (A) Coronal T1-weighted MRI show very little. (B) Coronal FLAIR shows a small subfrontal haemorrhagic lesion. (C) Axial T2* shows the multiple hypointense lesions corresponding to diffuse axonal lesions.

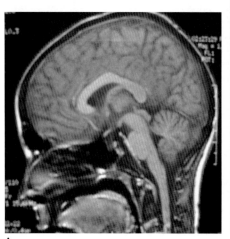
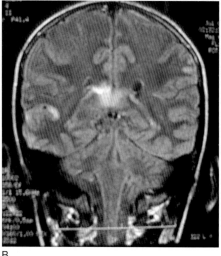
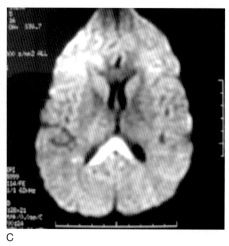

A   B   C

Figure 12.16.24 Deceleration injury. (A) Sagittal T1-weighted MRI. The posterior part of the corpus callosum is hypointense. (B) Coronal FLAIR shows the hyperintensity of the corpus callosum lesion. (C) Axial diffusion image shows the high diffusion coefficient of the injured corpus callosum.

regions. Less often, contusions involve the parietal and occipital lobes and the peripheral parts of the cerebellar hemispheres and vermis. This peripheral distribution adjacent to a rigid structure involving the cortex and sometimes subadjacent white matter, which may be oedematous, followed by focal atrophy constitutes an appearance so typical as to be virtually diagnostic of previous trauma in the absence of any history.

Severe trauma can also cause damage to the peripheral segments of small perforating arteries resulting in small regions of brain damage, often haemorrhagic, in the thalami (Figure 12.16.25) and rostral brainstem, and less frequently in the basal ganglia. Because of their location these lesions are frequently symptomatic.

Lesions of the basal ganglia are very difficult to diagnose by CT. MRI is the modality of choice for imaging the brainstem. In some rare cases, trauma will result in avulsion of a cranial nerve resulting in cranial nerve palsy (Figure 12.16.26).

NON-TRAUMATIC ENCEPHALOPATHY

It must also be remembered that the brain substance may undergo severe injury from encephalopathy from any cause. Ischaemic brain injury in the neonate is described elsewhere. Causes of encephalopathy include infection, substance abuse, status epilepticus, drowning, asphyxiation and inhalation. All may result in hypoxic encephalopathy. The earliest sign as seen on CT is loss of the grey/white matter differentiation, followed by loss of sulcal and cisternal fluid and ventricular compression. Progressive swelling causes tentorial herniation and coning. On MR, the initial signs may be very subtle, with increased signal seen on T2. Depending on the degree of injury and the timing of scans, one may see haemorrhagic infarction occur in the affected areas of brain, with high attenuation of the cerebral cortex on CT, which may have a gyriform pattern. If the child survives, and depending on the age, this may proceed to encephalomalacia.

Diffusion weighted imaging is more sensitive than standard MR sequences in showing early changes of injury.

SECONDARY AND/OR REACTIVE CHANGES

Mass effects from head injury may involve the supratentorial compartment on one or both sides and may cause subfalcine and/or transtentorial herniation. Trapping of an anterior cerebral artery against the free edge of the falx may cause infarction of parafalcine brain substance. Entrapment of the posterior cerebral artery against the tentorium may cause temporal and/or occipital lobe, or central or paramedian brainstem infarction due to occlusion of perforating arteries.

Unilateral lesions with midline shift and compression of the third ventricle cause contralateral hydrocephalus. These appearances on imaging correlate with clinical signs of raised intracranial pressure.

Acute generalized cerebral swelling occurring usually shortly after but sometimes up to 5 days after severe coma-producing head trauma is a frequent condition apparently confined to young children. It is poorly understood but appears to be related to loss of ability of the cerebral vessels to autoregulate, resulting in cerebral vasodilatation and increased blood flow; it is likely that hypoxia and hypotension play a significant role. The swelling is accompanied by compression of the intracranial CSF spaces and may cause transtentorial herniation. Secondary obstruction of the superior sagittal sinus may add to congestion and elevation of intracranial pressure, which may be further exacerbated by resistance to CSF absorption due to blockage of pacchionian granulations by blood products following trauma-induced subarachnoid haemorrhage. A slight increase in CT brain density has been described but the brain substance generally appears normal initially on imaging; cerebral oedema may supervene and cause diffuse low density with loss of

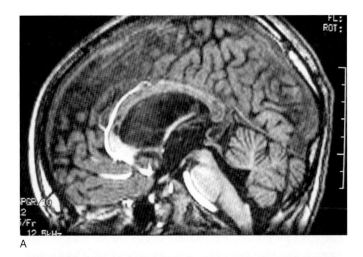

A

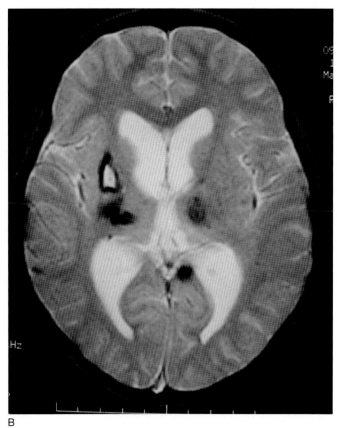

B

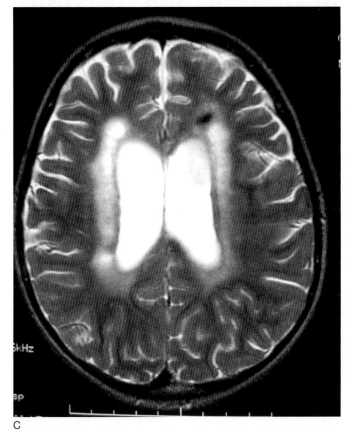

C

Figure 12.16.25 Severe head trauma. (A) Sagittal T2-weighted MRI shows multiple injuries of the corpus callosum. (B) Axial T2-weighted MRI shows multiple haemorrhagic lesions of the deep grey matter. (C) Transependymal resorption is seen on the axial T2-weighted MRI secondary to acute posthaemorrhagic hydrocephalus.

the normal grey/white matter differentiation. The supratentorial ventricles often appear relatively small but there is no lower limit to normal ventricular size, so that brain swelling cannot be recognized at the time of an initial scan on the basis of relatively small ventricles alone unless a baseline study is available confirming an otherwise inexplicable diminution in size. Complete obliteration of the basal cisterns is a much more reliable sign of high intracranial pressure.

Acute generalized cerebral swelling has a poor prognosis with a mortality rate of over 50%. In the survivors, the swelling usually resolves with conservative measures within a few days. Manage-

ment includes insertion of intracranial pressure monitoring and medical measures to decrease intracranial pressures.

Secondary hypoxia or hypoxic ischaemia due to respiratory and/or cardiac insufficiency or severe hypotension most commonly causes border zone ischaemia, which may be superimposed on the primary lesions of head trauma.

Large vessels may be injured by both penetrating and blunt trauma. Laceration of the walls of a major artery may result in intramural haematoma or dissection with narrowing or occlusion of the lumen and compromised flow. Clinical evidence of ischaemia in the distribution of the vessel may be immediate or

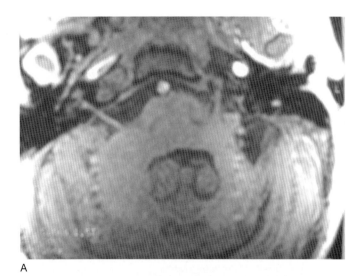

A

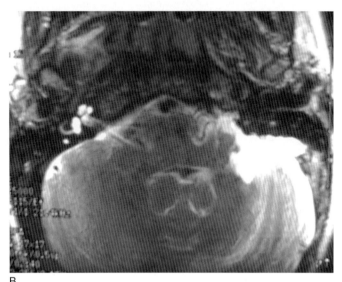

B

Figure 12.16.26 Motor vehicle accident with deceleration. Seventh nerve palsy, left ear deafness. (A) Axial T1-weighted MRI. The left facial and acoustic nerves are not visible. (B) A large CSF sac is seen on T2-weighted image.

delayed by up to 2 weeks. Intramural haematoma is best shown by MRI. The clot is hyperintense on T1-weighted images and the narrowed lumen of the affected vessel may be shown by flow void or by MR angiography.

A fracture crossing the superior sagittal or a dominant transverse sinus even when there is no depression may precipitate occlusion of the sinus. This may cause cerebral oedema or haemorrhagic infarction, which may be suspected clinically by recurrent seizures and/or a pseudotumour cerebri type syndrome; it may be confirmed by MRI. MR venography will confirm the diagnosis of sinus occlusion.

FISTULAS

Damage to the arterial wall, by direct injury or by deceleration, may cause it to rupture. Other consequences are intimal dissection

and fistula formation. Dissection may lead to clinical presentation with a stroke. Though both are rare, the two most frequent fistulas are corticocavernous and vertebrovertebral fistulas. The veins become distended because of the high blood flow. The typical clinical presentation of a carticocavernous fistula is a pulsatile proptosis, an audible bruit, enlargement of the facial and conjunctival veins, loss of vision and ophthalmoplegia. Fistulas may be evident immediately following trauma and may spontaneously regress. However, onset is frequently delayed by days to weeks, and in such cases spontaneous regression is rare. When clinical signs are typical, selective angiography is indicated to show the anatomy of the fistula as a prelude to treatment by interventional angiography.

LONG-TERM SEQUELAE OF HEAD INJURY AND FOLLOW-UP NEUROIMAGING

Dependent on the severity of the initial insult, the patient may recover completely or be left with varying degrees of emotional, mental and physical retardation or a mixture of all three. Severe impairment is obvious. Minor degrees may not be overtly evident but the consequences for education and employment are significant. Active programmes for rehabilitation of head injury victims and increased educational support have been shown to be effective in limiting the sequelae.

Post-traumatic epilepsy complicates 6.5–10% of childhood head injuries. It occurs in about 5% of blunt head injuries and is relatively more frequent (about 15%) when the injury is accompanied by seizures in the acute phase that continue for more than 24 h. Epilepsy follows 30% of penetrating injuries, usually associated with a meningocerebral cicatrix; fibrosis and gliosis may be accompanied by focal ventricular dilatation and arachnoid cyst formation.

Damage to the infundibulum may cause pituitary dysfunction with panhypopituitarism or isolated growth hormone deficiency; diabetes insipidus, which is usually transient, is common in the acute phase.

Most post-traumatic epilepsy is secondary to a structural lesion; this is evident on MRI but occasionally single photon emission computed tomography (SPECT) imaging will be required to confirm that the locus is the focus if surgery is being considered.

During the immediate recovery phase from a significant head injury it is important to ensure that the patient's swallowing mechanism is intact and it is safe to feed him/her. Functional barium swallow studies using liquids of varying thickness are indications for this. Orthopaedic management and appropriate imaging may be required for resultant postural problems.

Follow-up neuroimaging should be by MRI, which is by far the most sensitive modality for identifying brain damage. As experience with diffusion tensor imaging and other functional imaging grows, it is likely that these techniques will play an increasing role in both the prognosis of head injury and the identification of structural lesions causing neurological sequelae. Brain injury may appear as:

1. Haemosiderin residues, indicating previous haemorrhagic lesions, causing dark foci on T2-weighted sequences, especially

on high field units. When the blood–brain barrier is intact these residues persist for a long time and sometimes indefinitely. If there is no history of trauma, the possibility of previous non-accidental injury should be considered.

2. Gliosis, necrosis or encephalomalacia, causing low density on CT, dark regions on T1- and bright on T2-weighted MRI sequences. Multiple sclerosis and/or small vessel disease causing white matter infarction, which are important considerations in adults, are too uncommon in children to be considered in differential diagnosis in the clinical context.

3. Focal and/or generalized atrophy causing ventricular and sulcal dilatation, which may be evident within 4 months of head injury and may progress. This may be accompanied by wallerian degeneration affecting descending tracts, which become bright on T2-weighted sequences and there may be loss of volume in the corresponding pyramidal tract.

Treatable complications may also be shown. These include:

1. chronic extracerebral effusions; and
2. hydrocephalus.

SUBDURAL HYGROMA

This usually accumulates within 2 weeks of trauma, presumably as a result of a tear in the arachnoid membrane. CT density and MR brightness is similar to that of CSF at all times from the onset. Hygromas frequently absorb spontaneously within 3 months and generally do not require surgery. Like subdural haematomas, they may be complications of arachnoid cysts.

POST-TRAUMATIC HYDROCEPHALUS

Post-traumatic hydrocephalus usually presents within a month of the injury, but occasionally occurs as late as 3 months postinjury. It should be suspected if there is failure to improve to the degree expected after head injury. This hydrocephalus is usually communicating with generalized distension of the ventricular system, due to bleeding into the CSF so that blood breakdown products cause obstruction of pacchionian granulations; adhesions in the subarachnoid spaces or ventricles may contribute to the block.

Hydrocephalus, due to clot obstruction, usually at the posterior part of the third ventricle or aqueduct, is a less frequent and generally more acute and early complication.

Distinction between communicating hydrocephalus and atrophy can be difficult in the absence of macrocrania or progessive cranial enlargement. It is facilitated by prominent distension of the temporal horns, reduction of the angle between the roofs of the lateral ventricles and distension of the recesses of the third and roof of the fourth ventricle, best shown by MRI. MRI may also show increase in the water content of the periventricular white matter with a sensitivity greater than that of CT.

The hydrocephalus may resolve spontaneously or become balanced to a state of normal pressure hydrocephalus. Prolonged monitoring of the pressure may show periodic abnormal elevations, which increase the likelihood of response to shunting procedures.

Recurrent or chronic headache following head injury may accompany subdural effusion or hydrocephalus but in many cases computed imaging remains normal. If there is evidence of raised intracranial pressure, such cases are usually called benign intracranial hypertension. In most, there are no abnormal physical signs and the headache is often classified as being due to tension or migraine.

INFANTILE CHRONIC SUBDURAL HAEMATOMA

When a child who presents with a large head and previous history of accidental trauma and is discovered on imaging to have bilateral chronic subdural collections, the aetiology of the subdurals is not in doubt. A child presenting similarly without an antecedent history of trauma presents a clinical dilemma, as the question of a previous non-accidental aetiology has to be considered.

In addition, these children must not be confused with children who have macrocrania, often familial, in whom there is excess fluid in the extracerebral fluid spaces. This fluid lies in the subarachnoid space; thus, it is easily identifiable on MRI and has the same imaging characteristics as CSF (Figure 12.16.27). The fluid is around the convexities and extends into the interhemispheric fissure. The ventricles are normal in size. When imaged, these children are often diagnosed erroneously as having 'cerebral atrophy' because of the excess fluid. This is a normal finding in these children and reimaging at about 2–3 years of age will show the fluid to be reabsorbed and the brain returned to normal. The children's heads are big and do not show any sudden jump on head circumference charts. The children are physically and mentally normal. This condition is perhaps best described as benign macrocrania of infancy.

This condition is also sometimes called benign external hydrocephalus, communicating hydrocephalus or extraventricular hydrocephalus (Figure 12.16.28). It cannot be distinguished on imaging grounds from communicating hydrocephalus. Progressive head circumference growth and raised pressure at lumbar puncture or the presence of symptoms will distinguish the conditions.

The question arises as to whether infants with benign macrocrania of infancy may develop subdural bleeds silently or from minor trauma, as a small number of these children may be discovered to have a subdural collection on imaging without any other signs of NAI, e.g. a normal skeletal survey, no retinal haemorrhages and generally no neurological problems. Opinions vary as to the aetiology of the subdural bleeds in these children (Figure 12.16.29).

The MR intensities of acute and subacute subdural haematomas are similar to those of intraparenchymal haematomas but it appears that methaemoglobin is absorbed from or diluted in subdural haematoma, so that T1 shortening is less pronounced in chronic subdural haematoma than in intraparenchymal lesions. Chronic subdural haematomas are usually hypointense to grey matter on T1-weighted images. On T2-weighted images the collections are hyperintense without dark components indicative of haemosiderin deposition unless there has been recurrent haemorrhage, when haemosiderin is often present in the thickened membranes.

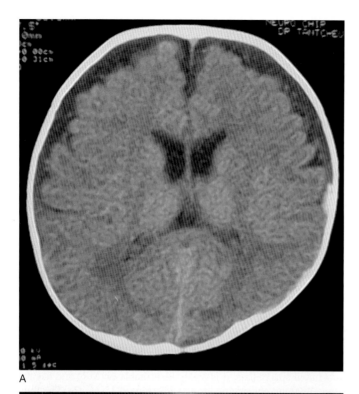

A

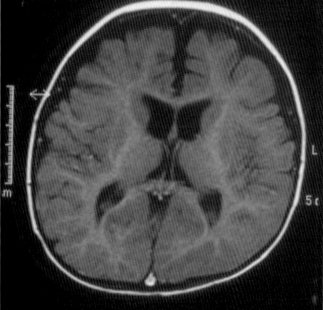

B

Figure 12.16.27 (A) Enlarging head, no history of trauma. Extracerebral collections are seen. The ventricles are not dilated. The diagnosis is benign external hydrocephalus. (B) MRI of a different child showing similar collections, which have the same signal intensity as the CSF in the ventricles.

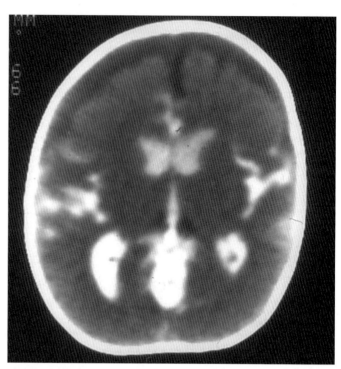

Figure 12.16.28 Benign external hydrocephalus. CT scan performed after lumbar injection of contrast media; the subdural effusion does not communicate with the CSF spaces.

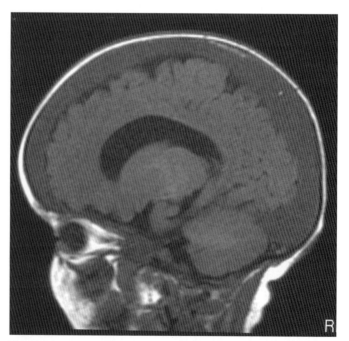

Figure 12.16.29 Sagittal T1-weighted MRI of a child who presented with a large head without history of injury and with no other features of concern in the family. The diagnosis was presumed to be chronic subdurals arising in a child with extraventricular hydrocephalus/macrocrania of infancy.

Childhood chronic subdural haematoma is uncommon, except as a complication of ventricular shunt procedures, and usually follows significant trauma. It forms a lentiform collection similar to that found in adults. It usually has an enhancing peripheral membrane. Calcification may develop.

Subdural hygroma is more common. It usually accumulates within 2 weeks of trauma, presumably resulting from a tear in the arachnoid membrane. CT density and MR brightness is similar to that of CSF at all times. Hygromas frequently resorb spontaneously and generally do not require surgery. Like subdural haematomas, they may be complications of arachnoid cysts.

FURTHER READING

Arnholz D, Hymel KP, Hay TC, Jenny C. Bilateral pediatric skull fractures: accident or abuse? Journal of Trauma: Injury, Infection, and Critical Care 1998; 45:172–174.

Cohen MD, McGuire W, Cory DA et al. MR appearance of blood and blood products: an in vitro study. American Journal of Roentgenology 1986; 146:1293–1297.

Gruen P. Surgical management of head trauma. Neuroimaging Clinics of North America 2002; 12:339–343.

Dubowitz DJ, Bluml S, Arcinue E, Dietrich RB. MR of hypoxic encephalopathy in children after near drowning: correlation with quantitative proton MR spectroscopy and clinical outcome. American Journal of Neuroradiology 1998; 19:1617–1627.

Eidlitz-Markus T, Shuper A, Constantini S. Short term subarachnoid space drainage: a potential treatment for extraventricular hydrocephalus. Childs Nervous System 2003; 19:367–370.

Han BK, Towbin RB, De Courten-Myers G, McLaurin RL, Ball WS Jr. Reversal sign on CT: effect of anoxic/ischaemic cerebral injury in children. American Journal of Neuroradiology 1989; 10:1191–1198.

Hawley CA, Ward AB, Long J, Owen DW, Magnay AR. Prevalence of traumatic brain injury amongst children admitted to hospital in one health district: a population-based study. Injury 2003; 34:256–260.

Hayman LA, Taber KH, Ford JJ, Bryan RN. Mechanisms of MR signal alteration by acute intracerebral blood: old concepts and new theories. American Journal of Neuroradiology 1991; 12:899–907.

Herskovits EH, Gerring JP, Davatzikos C, Bryan RN. Is the spatial distribution of brain lesions associated with closed-head injury in children predictive of subsequent development of posttraumatic stress disorder? Radiology 2002; 224:345–351.

Hilmani S, Bertal A, El Malki M et al. Acute subdural hematoma of the posterior fossa in the child. Case report. Neurochirurgie 2003; 49:44–46.

Hirsch W, Schobess A, Eichler G et al. Severe head trauma in children: cranial computer tomography and clinical consequences. Paediatric Anaesthesia 2002; 12:337–344.

Kieslich M, Fiedler A, Heller C, Kreuz W, Jacobi G. Minor head injury as cause and co-factor in the aetiology of stroke in childhood: a report of eight cases. Journal of Neurology, Neurosurgery and Psychiatry 2002; 73:13–16.

Lloyd DA, Carty H, Patterson M, Butcher CK, Roe D. Predictive value of skull radiography for intracranial injury in children with blunt head injury. Lancet 1997; 349:821–824.

Loh JK, Lin CL, Kwan AL, Howng SL. Acute subdural hematoma in infancy. Surgical Neurology 2002; 58:218–224.

Noguchi K, Ogawa T, Seto H et al. Subacute and chronic subarachnoid hemorrhage: diagnosis with fluid-attenuated inversion recovery MR imaging. Radiology 1997; 203:257–262.

Perrin RG, Rutka JT, Drake JM et al. Management and outcomes of posterior fossa subdural hematomas in neonates. Neurosurgery 1997; 40:1190–1200.

Poussaint TY, Moeller KK. Imaging of pediatric head trauma. Neuroimaging Clinics of North America 2002; 12:271–294.

Rugg-Gunn FJ, Symms MR, Barker GJ et al. Diffusion imaging shows abnormalities after blunt head trauma when conventional magnetic resonance imaging is normal. Journal of Neurology and Psychiatry 2001; 70:530–533.

Rupprecht H, Mechlin A, Ditteich D, Carbon R, Bar K. Prognostic risk factors in children and adolescents with craniocerebral injuries with multiple trauma. Kongressbd Dtsch Ges Chir Kong 2002; 119:683–688.

Rutherford M. MRI of the neonatal brain. London: W.B. Saunders; 2002.

Takaoka M, Tabuse H, Kumura E et al. Semiquantitative analysis of corpus callosum injury using magnetic resonance imaging indicates clinical severity in patients with diffuse axonal injury. Journal of Neurology, Neurosurgery and Psychiatry 2003; 73:289–293.

Tong KA, Ashwal S, Holshouser BA et al. Hemorrhagic shearing lesions in children and adolescents with posttraumatic diffuse axonal injury: improved detection and initial results. Radiology 2003; 227:332–339.

Woodstock RJ, Davis PC, Hopkins KL. Imaging of head trauma in infancy and childhood. Seminars in Ultrasound, CT and MR 2001; 22:126–182.

Young RJ, Destian S. Imaging of traumatic intracranial hemorrhage. Neuroimaging Clinics of North America 2002; 12:189–204.

Zapalac JS, Marple BF, Schwade ND. Skull base cerebrospinal fluid fistulas: a comprehensive diagnostic algorithm. Otolaryngology – Head and Neck Surgery 2002; 126:669–676.

Epilepsy

Helen Carty

This section on the role of imaging in epilepsy is included in the neuro section as it is a frequent clinical indication for a request for MR imaging.

Epilepsy is present when the child suffers from recurrent fits due to repeated primary cerebral dysrhythmias. Not all fits and seizures equal epilepsy. The fits may involve the motor system, e.g. tonic–clonic, or may be non-convulsive such as occur in absence seizures or complex partial seizures. Gelastic seizures are characterized by sudden outbursts of laughter, usually occurring at the onset of a seizure. These are associated with hypothalamic hamartomas (Figure 12.17.1), which may range in size from tiny lesions in the tuber cinereum to large tumours. Because of the location, the children may also suffer from precocious puberty.

CLASSIFICATION OF EPILEPSY

The classification of epilepsy is complex but it is mostly classified by seizure type, i.e. partial or generalized, then further subdivided by the type of fit, e.g. tonic, clonic or myoclonic, or absence, and whether there is loss of consciousness, complex, if there is, and simple, if not. In addition to the above, there are the numerous epilepsy syndromes.

All types of epilepsy, whatever the classification, may be associated with a structural cerebral abnormality, but in most cases imaging is normal. Epilepsy associated with lesions (Table 12.17.1) does not necessarily present as focal epilepsy and, conversely, fits caused by metabolic disease may present with a focal fit.

The incidence of epilepsy in adults is variously quoted in texts. One figure from a large population study quotes a lifetime incidence of 3%. Fifty out of a thousand children will suffer one fit during childhood but this includes conditions such as febrile convulsions and breath-holding attacks. Approximately one-third of all childhood epilepsy patients will undergo spontaneous remission by puberty and not recur in adult life. Death due to epilepsy is comparatively rare but may occur in status epilepticus, or as a complication of a seizure, e.g. aspiration or suffocation. Death may also be due to the underlying disease that caused the epilepsy, e.g. tuberous sclerosis, neurodegenerative disease or cerebral palsy. It may also be due to one of the epilepsy syndromes.

AETIOLOGY

In between 70% and 75% of children, no structural underlying aetiology is identifiable but in up to one-third of these, there may be a genetic basis for the epilepsy. In the 25% of children in whom a cause is found, a genetic basis may also coexist for their disease, e.g. neurofibromatosis 1 and tuberous sclerosis (Figure 12.17.2). A list of those currently known is given in Table 12.17.1. In addition to the conditions given in this list, epilepsy is a frequent and prominent feature of children with trisomy 21, 12 and ring chromosome 14, fragile X syndrome, MELAS (mitochondrial encephalopathy, lactic acidosis and stroke episodes) and MERRF (myoclonic epilepsy and ragged red fibres on muscle biopsy). These latter two conditions are linked to DNA point mutations. Other aetiological causes for epilepsy demonstrable by imaging are listed in Tables 12.17.2 and 12.17.3.

The role of imaging is to try to define an underlying structural cause for the epilepsy which, in a small number, if it is concordant with clinical and EEG evidence as the focus for the epilepsy might be amenable to surgery if satisfactory control of the seizures cannot be achieved by anti-epileptic drugs. The other role of imaging is to identify a cause for the epilepsy for genetic counselling, prognosis and to provide an explanation to the parent and child for the condition.

A detailed description of most of the structural lesions is included in the relevant chapters in this book and the reader is referred to these. It cannot be overstressed that the imaging must be correlated with clinical and EEG features before ascribing an imaging finding as the causative lesion that might be amenable to surgical excision.

EPILEPSY SYNDROMES AND SPECIFIC LESIONS

Some of the more frequent and important lesions are briefly discussed here. The reader is referred to specialized texts for a more detailed description.

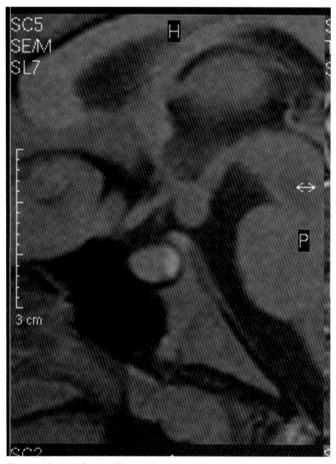

Figure 12.17.1 Sagittal T1-weighted image of a child who presented with gelastic seizures. There is a moderate-sized hypothalamic hamartoma.

Table 12.17.1 Genetics of epilepsy – chromosomal localization

Epilepsy/epilepsy syndrome/disease	Chromosome location
Benign familial neonatal convulsions	8q and 20q
Hyperekeplexia	5q
Tuberous sclerosis complex 1	9q 3.4
Tuberous sclerosis complex 2	16p 13.3
Early infantile neuronal ceroid lipofuscinosis (Batten's disease)	1q
Late infantile neuronal ceroid lipofuscinosis	11p15
Neurofibromatosis type 1	17q 11.2
Miller–Dieker syndrome (characterized by lissencephaly)	17p
Autosomal dominant nocturnal frontal lobe epilepsy	20q
Huntington's disease	4p
Partial epilepsies (including partial epilepsy with rolandic spikes)	10q 2.3
Juvenile myoclonic epilepsy	6p and 15q
Progressive myoclonic epilepsy (Mediterranean and Baltic myoclonus and Unverricht–Lundborg disease)	21q

Reproduced with permission from Appleton R, Gibbs J, eds. Epilepsy in childhood and adolescence, 2nd edn. London: Martin Dunitz; 1998:56.

Table 12.17.2 Causes of epilepsy that may be demonstrated by imaging

Consequences of perinatal asphyxia
Cerebral malformations, e.g. both focal and generalized cortical dysplasia, megalencephaly, etc.
Neurocutaneous syndromes
Cerebral infarction and porencephaly
Tumours – hamartomas and malignant lesions
Vascular malformations
Congenital and acquired infection, e.g. toxoplasmosis, tuberculosis, cysticercosis
Post head injury traumatic lesions
Neurodegenerative disease
Mesial temporal sclerosis
Rasmussen's encephalitis

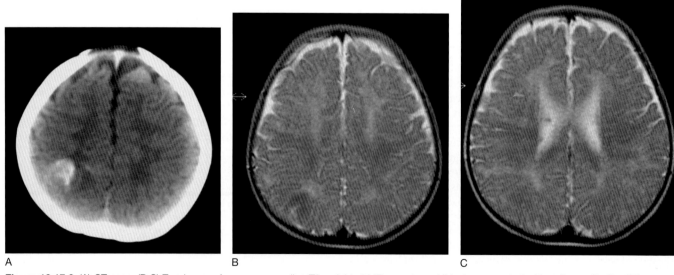

A   B   C

Figure 12.17.2 (A) CT scan. (B,C) Two images from corresponding T2-weighted MR scan in a child who presented with epilepsy. On the CT scan, a calcified hamartoma is present posteriorly on the right. Due to the calcification, this shows as low signal on MRI. Note the subependymal nodules in the ventricles in (C). These are the typical imaging features of tuberous sclerosis.

Table 12.17.3 Neurocutaneous syndromes associated with cortical dysplasia and epilepsy

NFI
Tuberous sclerosis
Sturge–Weber syndrome
Linear sebaceous naevus syndrome
Miller–Dieker syndrome
Aicardi's syndrome
Angelman's syndrome
Opercular dysplasia

MESIAL TEMPORAL SCLEROSIS

Mesial temporal sclerosis is an important cause of complex partial epilepsy, often refractory to medical treatment. There is disruption of the normal architectural structure of the hippocampus with loss of neural tissue and astrogliosis. This is seen on magnetic resonance imaging (MRI) as varying degrees of hippocampal atrophy and increased signal on T2-weighted (T2-W) and FLAIR sequences (Figure 12.17.3). The appearances may be subtle and are particularly difficult to appreciate if bilateral. Coronal thin-section volume gradient echo T1-weighted (T1-W) sequences and also thin-section coronal T2-W sequences are required for demonstration of this pathology. Contrast enhancement is indicated to exclude a small tumour that may mimic mesial temporal sclerosis.

Other lesions located in the medial temporal lobe that cause complex partial seizures, or temporal lobe epilepsy include small slow-growing tumours, cortical dysplasia and hamartomas (Figure 12.17.4). Clinically, children with lesions here may present with varied and odd symptoms in addition to fits. These symptoms include automatism, auras, hallucinations, behavioural changes and memory disturbances. They may also have learning difficulties.

RASMUSSEN'S ENCEPHALITIS

This condition is a chronic progressive focal encephalitis associated with intractable epilepsy, hemiparesis and a slowly progressive, regressive neuronal development and dementia. MR imaging shows progressive atrophy of the affected hemisphere. If demonstrated, and the major epileptogenic focus is shown to be in that hemisphere, hemisphrectomy is considered as a treatment option.

EPILEPSY SYNDROMES

These syndromes are characterized by high seizure frequency resistant to medical management. They are associated with cognitive impairment and have a high incidence of neurodevelopmental delay and regression with progressive dementia. They are sometimes known as malignant epileptic syndromes. The most frequent are given below.

OHTHARA SYNDROME

In this condition, there is early infant epileptic encephalopathy with an age of onset before 3 months. Imaging may show cortical dysplasia or histopathological evidence of dysgenesis at autopsy. The prognosis is poor.

WEST'S SYNDROME

This syndrome is also known as infantile spasms. The age of onset is under 1 year with peak presentation at 3–6 months. About 75% of cases have a demonstrable cause such as tuberous sclerosis, hypoxic ischaemic change, congenital infection, structural brain malformation or biochemical metabolic abnormality. The prognosis depends on the cause. If no cause is found, the prognosis is good.

LENNOX GASTAUT SYNDROME

In this syndrome, the age of onset is between 1 and 8 years. About 20% of cases have preceding West's syndrome. The same cerebral abnormalities may be demonstrated. The prognosis is poor.

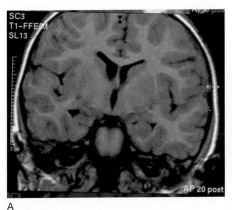
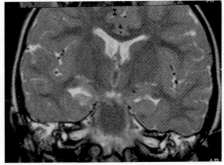
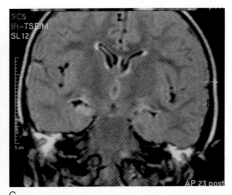

A   B   C

Figure 12.17.3 (A) T1-weighted (B) T2-weighted and (C) FLAIR sequences of a child with right-sided mesial temporal sclerosis. Note the slightly small hippocampus on the right with the enlarged temporal horn. The high signal seen on T2-W image and FLAIR represents gliosis.

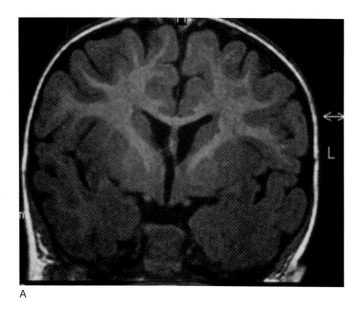

A

B

Figure 12.17.4 (A) T1- and (B) T2-weighted MR images of a child with extensive cortical dysplasia of the left temporal lobe. On the T2-weighted sequence there is also high signal in the right temporal lobe, which suggests that there is a further area of dysplasia here.

PROGRESSIVE MYOCLONIC EPILEPSY SYNDROME

In this syndrome, the age of onset is variable and in part is dependent on the causative lesion. It is associated with Batten's diseases (neuronal ceroid lipofuscinosis) and mitochondrial cytopathies, e.g. MELAS, MERRF. There are many other associations without imaging abnormalities.

LANDAU–KLEFFNER SYNDROME

The age of onset in this syndrome is between 2 and 10 years. These children have acquired aphasia with loss of language and autistic behaviour. The aetiology is unknown but it may be associated with a vasculitis. Imaging is usually normal.

KOJEWNIKOV'S SYNDROME

In this syndrome, there is progressive continuous partial epilepsy. The age of onset is under 10 years. It may be associated with Rasmussen's encephalitis and the mitochondrial cytopathies.

SELECTION OF PATIENTS FOR IMAGING

It will be seen from the brief discussion above that selection of patients for imaging is not always easy. Furthermore, expectations in different societies vary so that the threshold for imaging varies considerably. Most would agree that the indications outlined in Tables 12.17.4 and 12.17.5 are reasonable guidelines.

IMAGING

Imaging of epilepsy is initially structural but functional imaging both with MRI and nuclear imaging play an increasing role. The procedure of choice for imaging of children with epilepsy should be MRI. Imaging is primarily structural but techniques such as T2 mapping or relaxometry, spectroscopy and functional MRI are increasingly valuable in selected patients. It is of paramount importance that good-quality images are obtained. Arrangements should be in place so that, where required, sedation or general

Table 12.17.4 Imaging not indicated

Childhood primary idiopathic generalized epilepsy
Typical absence epilepsy (petit mal)
Juvenile myoclonic epilepsy
Febrile convulsion
Benign partial epilepsy with centrotemporal or occipital spikes on EEC

Adapted from Wright NB. Review article: imaging in epilepsy. British Journal of Radiology 2001; 74:575–589.

Table 12.17.5 Imaging indicated

Epilepsy commencing in first year, excluding febrile fit
Focal neurological signs
Asymmetrical fits
Evidence of a neurocutaneous syndrome
Evidence of a developmental regression
Simple or complex partial seizures
Suspected genetic cause
Infantile spasms or myoclonic fits
Suspected epilepsy syndrome
Refractory epilepsy
Gelastic seizures
Intractable seizures
Alteration in seizure pattern when previously controlled

anaesthesia is available. Information about any EEG focus should be available.

Routine structural imaging sequences in a child with epilepsy should include sagittal T1-W, axial T1-W and T2-W, coronal FLAIR and inversion recovery sequences. In addition to these, thin-section volume coronal T1-W and thin-section T2-W sequences are required if there is an EEG focus that suggests a structural cause such as cortical dysplasia or a temporal lobe lesion. Contrast enhancement is used if a tumour is suspected. Three-dimensional reconstruction may be helpful in demonstrating cortical dysplasia.

T2-W RELAXOMETRY

Measurement of the T2-W relaxation time of each pixel provides an objective grey scale map of the area chosen, as opposed to subjective viewing of the cortex to identify attenuation differences and this allows subtle changes that might indicate pathology (Figure 12.17.5). The normal T2-W relaxation time is generally less than 115 ms but there is some variation between scanners. The T2-W relaxation time is increased in pathological cortex, such as mesial temporal sclerosis. It should be performed when there is clinical or EEG evidence to suggest a focus and nothing is seen on conventional imaging. One of the problems with this technique in young children is that the immature brain with areas of non-

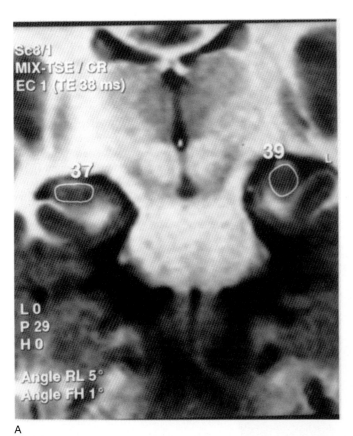

A

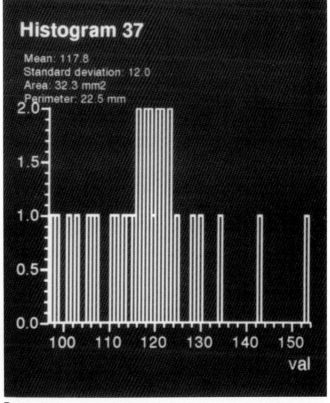

B

Figure 12.17.5 Sample of T2 mapping. (Courtesy of Dr N. Wright, Manchester Children's Hospital, Pendlebury)

myelination will result in high T2-W relaxation times. The results, therefore, should be interpreted with caution below the age of complete myelination, i.e. about 3 years of age.

SPECTROSCOPY

Magnetic resonance spectroscopy (MRS) is used to evaluate brain metabolism *in vivo*. Measurement of *N*-acetylaspartate (NAA), choline (Cho) and creatinine (Cr) can be made by ('H) proton spectroscopy. Neuronal loss results in reduced NAA levels. Astrocytosis and gliosis result in increased levels of Cho and Cr. The intensity ratio of NAA/Cho and Cr signal is accepted as a useful index of metabolic abnormality in the underlying brain. Data can be acquired from any area of brain suspected as being the epileptogenic focus. MRS is useful in lateralizing a lesion and in particular in bilateral pathology when absolute values are abnormal. There is good correlation of ('H)MRS with interictal single photon emission computed tomography (SPECT).

^{31}P MRS measures energy metabolism by measuring phosphorylation potential and phospholipid metabolism. An abnormal ratio of these has been demonstrated in the temporal lobes in epileptic children.

FUNCTIONAL MRI (fMRI)

Blood oxygen level dependent fMRI or BOLD fMRI can create a functional map of an area of brain that can then be image fused with anatomical data. An increased BOLD signal has been shown in sites of electrical discharge activity on EEG in interictal states, this localizing a focus. It can also be used to localize functional motor cortex preoperatively in children with tumours. It is being investigated as a tool for lateralizing memory and correlates with the WADA test in children in whom surgery is being contemplated for temporal lobe epilepsy.

NUCLEAR IMAGING

Functional nuclear medicine imaging is a useful imaging tool in epilepsy if used selectively. It is a useful tool in children in whom

MRI is either normal or shows a lesion that does not correlate with clinical or EEG assessments. Two nuclear medicine techniques are used. SPECT imaging is most frequently performed with technetium 99m hexamethylpropylenamine oxime (HMPAO). Newer radiopharmaceuticals such as iomazenil I[123] are now available.

SPECT imaging with HMPAO reflects the regional cerebral blood flow distribution. This differs in the ictal and interictal states (Figure 12.17.6). Epileptogenic foci usually show increased activity during ictus and decreased activity interictally. For an ictal study, the radiopharmaceutical must be injected during the fit, with imaging done subsequently when control of the seizure is achieved. The logistics of this are obvious and therefore, in general, ictal studies are only feasible in specialized units. High-quality images are essential and sedation or anaesthesia is often required for imaging. Interictal SPECT can be performed at any time.

PET (positron emission tomography) imaging using F18 fluorodeoxyglucose FDG reflects brain glucose metabolic activity, but as it takes 45 min for PET uptake, it is used only interictally. FDG uptake is reduced in areas of hypometabolism. It is of most value in the temporal lobes but is not a routine investigation. Access to PET scanning is limited in much of the world. The main uses currently of PET are to lateralize a focus when other techniques have failed, for research purposes and for correlating differing imaging techniques.

With increasing sophistication of image fusion techniques it is becoming possible to merge functional with anatomical data, thus improving localization of pathology and opening up surgical possibilities.

THE WADA TEST

In this test, a catheter is placed in the internal carotid artery via a standard cerebral arteriographic technique and a barbiturate, usually sodium amytal, is directly injected, this anaesthetizing the ipsilateral cerebral hemisphere for a short time. The child, who has been previously rehearsed, is then given the same neuropsychological tests to assess memory. The procedure is repeated in the contralateral carotid. Thus, memory is localized. This is of utmost importance, prior to surgery. The test is only feasible in children who are cooperative.

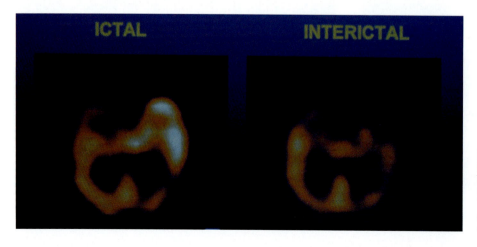

Figure 12.17.6 HMPAO SPECT brain imaging. On the ictal image, there is increased activity in the left temporal region which, on the interictal image, shows decreased activity. These are the typical imaging findings of an epileptic focus. This still needs to be correlated with the EEG and MR images.

COMUTED TOMOGRAPHY (CT)

CT has no primary role to play in imaging epilepsy since the advent of MRI. It is more sensitive than MRI in the detection of calcification and provides confirmatory evidence of suspected lesions but does not alter management. CT is, however, helpful in status epilepticus in those children in whom hypoxic ischaemic encephalopathy is suspected secondary to the status.

FURTHER READING

Appleton RE. Mortality in paediatric epilepsy. Archives of Disease in Childhood 2003; 88:1091–1094.

Appleton R, Gibbs J. Epilepsy in childhood and adolescence, 2nd edn. London: Martin Dunitz; 1998.

Baldwin GN, Tsuruda JS, Maravilla KR, Hamill GS, Hayes CE. The fornix in patients with seizures caused by unilateral hippocampal sclerosis: detection of unilateral volume loss on MR images. American Journal of Roentgenology 1994; 162:1185–1189.

Bookheimer SY, Dapretto M, Karmarkar U. Functional MRI in children with epilepsy. Developmental Neuroscience 1999; 21:191–199.

Cakirer S, Basak M, Mutlu A, Galip GM. MR imaging in epilepsy that is refractory to medical therapy. European Radiology 2002; 12:549–558.

Cendes F, Andermann F, Gloor P et al. MRI volumetric measurement of amygdala and hippocampus in temporal lobe epilepsy. Neurology 1993; 3:719–725.

Chan S, Erickson JK, Yoon SS. Limbic system abnormalities associated with mesial temporal sclerosis: a model of chronic cerebral changes due to seizures. Radiographics 1997; 17:1095–1110.

Chen C-Y, Zimmerman RA, Faro S et al. MR of the operculum: abnormal opercular formation in infants and children. American Journal of Neuroradiology 1996; 17:1303–1311.

Commission on Classification and Terminology of the International League Against Epilepsy. Proposal for revised clinical and electroencephalographic classification of epileptic seizures. Epilepsia 1981; 22:489–501.

Commission on Neuroimaging of the International League against Epilepsy. Recommendations for neuroimaging of patients with epilepsy. Epilepsia 1997; 38:1255–1256.

Cross JH, Gordon I, Connelly A et al. Interictal 99Tc(m) HMPAO SPECT and 1H MRS in children with temporal lobe epilepsy. Epilepsia 1997; 38:338–345.

Devous MD Sr, Thisted RA, Morgan GF, Leroy RF, Rowe CC. SPECT brain imaging in epilepsy: a meta-analysis. Journal of Nuclear Medicine 1998; 39:285–293.

El-Koussy M, Mathis J, Loveblad KO et al. Focal status epilepticus: follow-up by perfusion and diffusion MR. European Radiology 2002; 12:568–574.

Grant PE, Barkovich AJ, Wald LL et al. High-resolution surface-coil MR of cortical lesions in medically refractory epilepsy: a prospective study. American Journal Neuroradiology 1997; 18:291–301.

Guerrini R, Carrozzo R. Epilepsy and genetic malformations of the cerebral cortex. American Journal of Medical Genetics 2001; 106:160–173.

Hanefeld F, Kruse B, Holzbach U et al. Hemimegalencephaly: localized proton magnetic resonance spectroscopy in vivo. Epilepsia 1995; 36:1215–1122.

Iannetti P, Spalice A, Atzei G et al. Neuronal migrational disorders in children with epilepsy: MRI, interictal SPECT and EEG comparisons. Brain Development 1996; 18:269–279.

Killgore WD, Glosser G, Casasanto DJ et al. Functional MRI and the Wada test provide complementary information for predicting post-operative seizure control. Seizure 1999; 8:450–455.

Kodama F, Ogawa T, Sugihara S et al. Transneuronal degeneration in patients with temporal lobe epilepsy: evaluation by MR imaging. European Radiology 2003; 13:2180–2185.

Kuzniecky RI, Jackson GD. Magnetic resonance spectroscopy. In: Magnetic resonance in epilepsy, 1st edn. New York: Raven Press; 1995:289–314.

Li LM, Cendes F, Antel SB et al. Prognostic value of proton magnetic resonance spectroscopic imaging for surgical outcome in patients with intractable temporal lobe epilepsy and bilateral hippocampal atrophy. Annals of Neurology 2000; 47:195–200.

Meiners LC. Role of MR imaging in epilepsy. European Journal of Radiology 2002; 12:499–501.

Meiners LC, Gils A, Jansen GH et al. Temporal lobe epilepsy: the various MR appearances of histologically proven mesial temporal sclerosis. American Journal of Neuroradiology 1994; 15:1547–1555.

Montenegro MA, Guerreiro MM, Lopes-Cendes I et al. Bilateral posterior parietal polymicrogyria: a mild form of congenital bilateral perisylvian syndrome? Epilepsia 2001; 42:845–849.

O'Brien TJ, Zupanc ML, Mullan BP et al. The practical utility of performing peri-ictal SPECT in the evaluation of children with partial epilepsy. Pediatric Neurology 1998; 19:15–22.

Ohtsuka Y, Tanaka A, Kobayashi K et al. Childhood-onset epilepsy associated with polymicrogyria. Brain and Development 2002; 24:758–765.

Otsubo H, Hwang PA, Gilday DL, Hoffman HJ. Location of epileptic foci on interictal and immediate postictal single photon emission tomography in children with localization-related epilepsy. Journal of Child Neurology 1995; 10:37–81.

Pauli E, Eberhardt KW, Schafer I et al. Chemical shift imaging spectroscopy and memory function in temporal lobe epilepsy. Epilepsia 2000; 41:282–289.

Robinson RO, Ferrie CD, Capra M, Maisey MN. Positron emission tomography and the central nervous system. Archives of Disease in Childhood 1999; 81:263–270.

Sato N, Hatakeyama S, Shimizu N et al. MR evaluation of the hippocampus in patients with congenital malformations of the brain. American Journal of Neuroradiology 2001; 22:389–393.

Sisodiya SM. Surgery for malformations of cortical development causing epilepsy. Brain 2000; 123:1075–1091.

Sitoh YY, Tien RD. Neuroimaging in epilepsy. Journal of Magnetic Resonance Imaging 1998; 8:277–288.

Spencer DC, Morrell MJ, Risinger MW. The role of the intracarotid amobarbital procedure in evaluation of patients for epilepsy surgery. Epilepsia 2000; 41:320–325.

Tasch E, Cendes F, Li LM et al. Hypothalamic hamartomas and gelastic epilepsy: a spectroscopic study. Neurology 1998; 51:1046–1050.

Wang ZJ, Zimmerman RA. Proton MR spectroscopy of pediatric brain metabolic disorders. Neuroimaging Clinics of North America 1998; 8:781–807.

Watson C, Jack CR, Cendes F. Volumetric magnetic resonance imaging. Archives of Neurology 1997; 54:1521–1531.

Won HJ, Chang KH, Cheon JE et al. Comparison of MR imaging with PET and ictal SPECT in 118 patients with intractable epilepsy. American Journal of Neuroradiology 1999; 20:593–599.

Wright NB. Review article: imaging in epilepsy. British Journal of Radiology 2001; 74:575–589.

Yune MJ, Lee JD, Ryu RH et al. Ipsilateral thalamic hypoperfusion on interictal SPECT in temporal lobe epilepsy. Journal of Nuclear Medicine 1998; 39:281–285.

SECTION | 13

THE EYE AND ORBIT

The Eye and Orbit

Laurence J Abernethy

IMAGING MODALITIES FOR EVALUATION OF THE EYE AND ORBIT

PROJECTIONAL RADIOGRAPHY

Conventional projectional radiography of the orbit remains the first line of investigation for orbital trauma and suspected intraorbital foreign bodies. The main advantages of projectional radiography are that it is fast, non-invasive and widely accessible. It may also be valuable in the assessment of other diseases affecting the bony orbit but gives little information about the orbital soft tissues, and so in most cases some form of cross-sectional imaging is usually more appropriate.

ULTRASOUND AND COLOUR FLOW IMAGING

Ultrasound of the eye and orbit is a valuable imaging technique, particularly when cataract or opaque media makes fundoscopy impossible. In children, eye ultrasound is usually performed with a high frequency, small footprint transducer placed over the closed eyelid, using a non-irritating sterile aqueous gel for acoustic contact. With patience, useful images can be obtained even with a restless child; careful explanation and demonstration of the technique are important. Ultrasound is unique in providing real-time imaging, which enables kinetic evaluation of mobile intraocular abnormalities such as retinal detachment. Colour flow imaging allows immediate assessment of the vascularity of an ocular or orbital lesion.

MAGNETIC RESONANCE IMAGING

Magnetic resonance imaging (MRI) is particularly well suited to imaging the eye and orbit because of its high intrinsic contrast and multiplanar capability. Fat saturation sequences are useful to make pathological lesions more conspicuous by reducing the signal from normal orbital fat. Calcification and cortical bone are poorly seen on MRI, which limits its value in the evaluation of some tumours such as retinoblastoma. Long imaging times present practical dif-

ficulties in imaging infants and young children, who may need sedation or general anaesthesia.

COMPUTED TOMOGRAPHY

Computed tomography (CT) of the orbit produces high-resolution images with short scan times and is excellent for demonstration of calcification and lesions involving the bony orbit. However, the benefits of CT must be balanced against the risks of exposure to ionizing radiation. The lens of the eye is particularly sensitive and large exposures carry a long-term risk of cataract. Scan parameters should be optimized to reduce the dose to the lens as much as possible and repeated CT scans of the orbits should be avoided.

VENOGRAPHY AND ARTERIOGRAPHY

Orbital venography (phlebography), with direct injection of contrast into the orbital veins, is used in the assessment of orbital vascular malformations and is an essential precursor to sclerotherapy of these lesions. It is still occasionally used in the evaluation of lesions in the region of the cavernous sinus but non-invasive cross-sectional imaging obviates the need for conventional venography in most cases. Cavernous sinus thrombosis can readily be demonstrated by contrast-enhanced CT or MR venography.

Catheter arteriography is also mainly used for the detailed assessment of vascular malformations and post-traumatic caroticocavernous fistula; it is now rarely required in the investigation of orbital masses. The orbit is supplied by branches of both the internal carotid artery (ophthalmic artery) and the external carotid artery (middle meningeal artery, lacrimal artery and deep temporal artery), and so selective catheterization of both arteries is necessary.

DACROCYSTOGRAPHY (CONVENTIONAL, RADIOISOTOPE AND MRI)

Obstructed lacrimal drainage may be investigated by conventional dacrocystography, in which a fine catheter is introduced into a

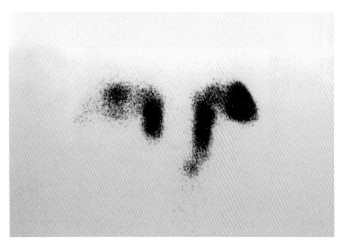

Figure 13.1 Radioisotope lacrimal drainage study showing bilateral obstruction of the lacrimal ducts.

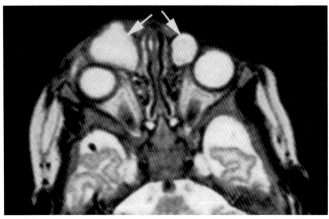

Figure 13.2 Congenital lacrimal duct obstruction: heavily T2-weighted axial MRI scan shows bilateral dacrocystoceles (arrows) on the medial sides of the orbits.

canaliculus (usually the superior canaliculus), and a small amount of water-soluble contrast is injected, after which projectional radiographs, tomograms or a CT scan is obtained. Radioisotope lacrimal drainage scans are non-invasive and provide better functional information but less anatomical detail; a drop containing Tc-99m pertechnetate is placed in the eye with the child in front of the gamma camera and a sequence of images is obtained to provide a physiological demonstration of lacrimal drainage (Figure 13.1). Normally, drainage of activity into the nose is visible within a few minutes. Obstructed nasolacrimal ducts may also be demonstrated by heavily T2-weighted MRI scans (MR dacrocystography) without the use of catheters or contrast media (Figure 13.2).

FURTHER READING

Byrne SF, Green RL. Ultrasound of the eye and orbit. 2nd edn. St Louis: Mosby; 2002.

Enriquez G, Gil–Gibernau JJ, Garriga V, Ribes I, Lucaya J. Sonography of the eye in children: imaging findings. American Journal of Roentgenology 1995; 165:935–939.

Hopper KD, Sherman JL, Boal DKB. Abnormalities of the orbit and its contents in children: CT and MR findings. American Journal of Roentgenology 1991; 156:1219–1224.

DEVELOPMENTAL ABNORMALITIES OF THE EYE

ANOPHTHALMIA AND MICROPHTHALMIA

Anophthalmia is a rare congenital condition in which there is complete absence of one or both eyes. MRI is helpful to confirm the diagnosis of true anophthalmia by showing absence of the optic nerve (and, in bilateral anophthalmia, the optic chiasm and optic tracts), and to identify associated structural brain abnormalities.

Microphthalmia refers to a small eye, which may be congenital or acquired. Congenital microphthalmia is associated with a number of multisystemic syndromes, including Fanconi syndrome and Diamond–Blackfan syndrome, and with several chromosomal anomalies. Acquired microphthalmos may be a sequel to trauma or infection, particularly during the first year of life, when most growth of the eye occurs. Imaging will typically show a small remnant of the eye with an intact optic nerve (Figure 13.3).

CONGENITAL CATARACT

Congenital cataract may cause complete lens opacification, making opthalmoscopic examination impossible. Ultrasound is then very valuable to exclude a posterior segment abnormality such as a retinoblastoma or persistent hyperplastic primary vitreous (PHPV). In simple congenital cataract, ultrasound shows increased echogenicity within the lens, with thickening of its posterior wall. In many cases, the lens has an abnormal spherical shape.

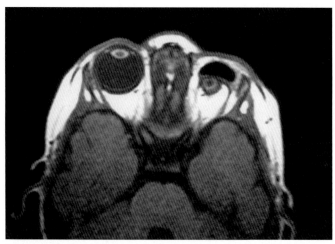

Figure 13.3 Microphthalmos: axial T1-weighted MRI scans demonstrate a normal right eye. A tiny, dysplastic left eye is present. A tissue expander is in place in the anterior part of the left orbit.

OPTIC NERVE DRUSEN

Optic nerve drusen are benign calcifications, which may simulate papilloedema on ophthalmoscopy. They are usually bilateral and are recognized on ultrasound as focal areas of intense echogenicity within the optic nerve heads, which cast dense acoustic shadows (Figure 13.4). It is important to show that the appearances remain consistent as the transducer is moved to different positions, particularly in oblique projections, as the normal optic nerve head may appear echogenic when it is at right angles to the incident ultrasound beam.

PERSISTENT HYPERPLASTIC PRIMARY VITREOUS (PHPV)

PHPV results from incomplete regression of the embryonic hyaloid artery and hyperplasia of adjacent connective tissue. Clinically, the diagnosis is suggested by a small cornea and prominent ciliary processes. Ultrasound shows microphthalmia; the lens is abnormally thin and the posterior capsule is irregular. The persistent hyaloid vessel is visible as an echogenic band extending across the vitreous from the posterior lens capsule to the optic disc (Figure 13.5).

Sporadic PHPV is usually unilateral but bilateral PHPV occurs in Norrie's disease, an X-linked recessive syndrome, and is also associated with trisomy 13, 15, 18 and 21.

COATS' DISEASE

Coats' disease (congenital retinal telangiectasia) is a congenital vascular malformation that affects the retina; it is characterized by leaking telangiectatic vessels, which cause a lipid exudate within the retina. It occurs most commonly in boys. The disease is usually unilateral; it is present from birth but does not become symptomatic until retinal detachment occurs. It may present with impaired visual acuity, leukokoria (white eye) or squint, usually between 6 and 8 years of age. Imaging is helpful to confirm the diagnosis. Ultrasound typically shows a retinal detachment with echogenic subretinal fluid. CT may be helpful to confirm the absence of a calcified mass and so effectively exclude the possibility of a retinoblastoma (non-calcified retinoblastomas may occur but are very rare). MRI shows subretinal fluid, which is hyperintense on both T1-weighted and T2-weighted images.

RETINOPATHY OF PREMATURITY

Retinopathy of prematurity is typically a bilateral condition, affecting the peripheral retina and vitreous. In severe cases, ultrasound may show dense retrolental membranes and extensive retinal detachment with retinal hoops. Haemorrhage or cholesterol debris may be visible within the subretinal space.

COLOBOMA

Colobomas arise from a defect in the closure of the embryonic optic fissure. Most cases are inherited as an autosomal dominant trait; some are associated with cerebral malformations such as Aicardi syndrome or multisystemic syndromes such as the CHARGE association (coloboma, heart defects, choanal atresia, genital and ear anomalies). There is microphthalmia with a focal cystic outpouching of the vitreous, which is anechoic on ultrasound and isointense with normal vitreous on MRI (Figure 13.6).

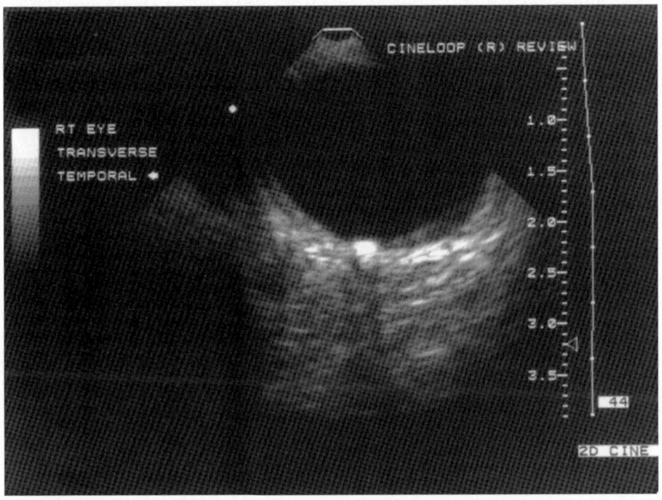

Figure 13.4 Optic nerve drusen. Ultrasound shows a densely echogenic focus within the optic nerve head, casting distal acoustic shadows.

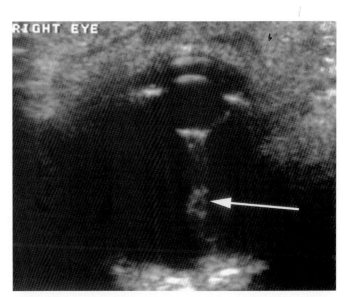

Figure 13.5 Persistent hyperplastic primary vitreous (PHPV). Ultrasound shows a band of echogenic tissue (arrow) extending across the vitreous from the posterior surface of the lens to the optic nerve head.

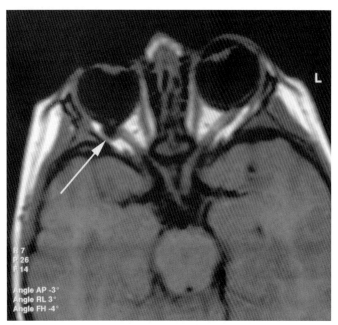

Figure 13.6 Coloboma: axial T1-weighted MRI scan shows a focal cystic outpouching of the vitreous (arrow).

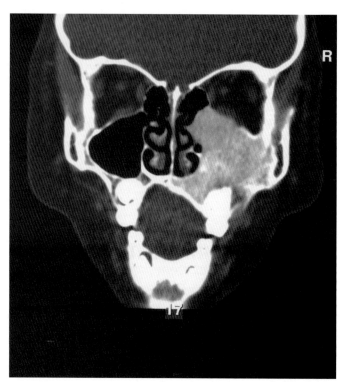

Figure 13.7 Fibrous dysplasia of the maxilla: direct coronal CT shows thickened, sclerotic bone with an amorphous 'ground glass' appearance, completely replacing the maxillary antrum and involving the floor of the orbit.

DEVELOPMENTAL ABNORMALITIES OF THE ORBIT

CRANIOSTENOSIS

The shape of the orbit is often affected by premature fusion of cranial sutures. Premature fusion of the coronal sutures results in hypertelorism (widely spaced eyes), shallow orbits and exophthalmos. Premature fusion of the metopic suture causes hypotelorism and trigonocephaly. Syndromes that are associated with premature fusion of multiple sutures, such as Crouzon syndrome and Apert's syndrome, are often associated with midface hypoplasia and orbital hypoplasia, and marked exophthalmos.

ORBITAL ENCEPHALOCELE

Orbital encephaloceles typically present with pulsatile exophthalmos. Encephaloceles may extend into the orbit anteriorly, through the frontoethmoidal suture, or posteriorly, through the sphenoid bone.

FIBROUS DYSPLASIA

Fibrous dysplasia is a benign skeletal disorder in which the affected bone is replaced by dense fibrous tissue, leading to pro-gressive enlargement, hyperostosis and deformity, which usually occurs between 5 and 15 years of age. Stabilization usually occurs after puberty. Fibrous dysplasia affecting the orbit and maxilla may present with progressive exophthalmos. Skull base lesions may cause cranial nerve compression, resulting in impaired vision or ophthalmoplegia. Projectional radiography and CT show characteristic appearances of thickened, sclerotic bone with an amorphous 'ground glass' appearance (Figure 13.7). Rarely, fibrous dysplasia may be complicated by benign or malignant degeneration. Benign degeneration is due to cystic change or haemorrhage. Malignant transformation to osteosarcoma, chondrosarcoma or fibrosarcoma occurs in less than 1% of cases but should be considered if there are signs of rapid enlargement, particularly after puberty.

NEUROFIBROMATOSIS TYPE 1 (NF-1)

NF-1 may present with congenital glaucoma (buphthalmos). Hypoplasia or complete absence of the greater wing of the sphenoid allows protrusion of the temporal lobe into the orbit and typically causes pulsatile exophthalmos (Figure 13.8). Plexiform neurofibromas may occur within the orbit along the course of the cranial nerves.

Optic gliomas occur in up to 20% of children with NF-1 (see below). However, these tumours remain stable or are very slowly progressive in most cases and only a minority have progressive symptoms. MRI screening for optic gliomas in children with NF-1 is therefore recommended only if there are clinical signs of visual impairment, raised intracranial pressure or precocious puberty.

FURTHER READING

Bilaniuk LT, Farber M. Imaging of developmental abnormalities of the eye and orbit. American Journal of Neuroradiology 1992; 13:793–803.

INFECTION AND INFLAMMATION

ORBITAL CELLULITIS

In children, orbital infection usually arises from paranasal sinus infection, facilitated by the presence of open sutures and large communicating veins. In particular, infection can readily spread from the ethmoid air cells through the thin and incomplete medial wall of the orbit. Periorbital cellulitis is the first stage of this process, in which inflammation is limited to the preseptal tissues (eyelids and anterior orbits). Extension of infection results in post-septal orbital cellulitis, in which there is subperiosteal oedema along the medial orbital wall. In the early stages, antibiotic therapy may produce rapid improvement but without effective antibiotic therapy, an inflammatory mass or phlegmon may develop in the subperiosteal space, progressing to form a subperiosteal abscess. Severe infection may extend into the extrinsic ocular muscles and retrobulbar fat, leading to proptosis and visual impairment, and may be complicated by thrombosis of the superior ophthalmic vein and cavernous sinus.

The primary role of imaging in orbital infection is to identify subperiosteal or orbital abscesses that require surgical drainage. Urgent imaging is not necessary in uncomplicated acute periorbital cellulitis but is indicated if there is no response to antibiotic therapy, and if there are signs of proptosis or visual impairment. The imaging modalities of choice are contrast-enhanced CT, with direct coronal scans, or MRI, as subperiosteal abscesses are diffi-cult to demonstrate with ultrasound, and axial CT scans may miss superomedial collections. Both CT and MRI will show fluid within infected ethmoid air cells and inflammatory changes in the orbit. When an inflammatory mass or phlegmon has developed, there is displacement of the medial rectus and proptosis (Figure 13.9). Abscess formation results in an enhancing wall surrounding a central fluid collection (Figure 13.10). Thrombosis of the superior ophthalmic vein and cavernous sinus produces a filling defect within the vessels on contrast enhanced CT or MRI (Figure 13.11). MR venography is helpful to assess the full extent of intracranial sinus thrombosis.

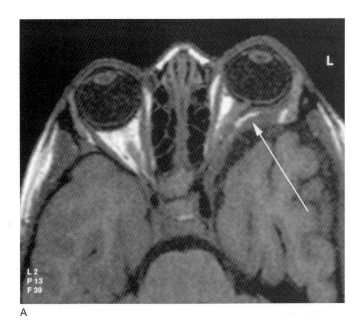

A

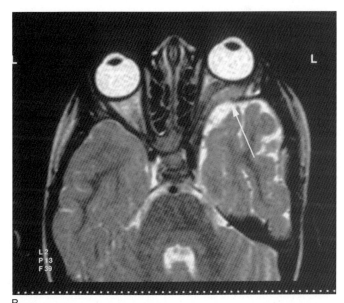

B

Figure 13.8 Neurofibromatosis type 1. Axial T1-weighted (A) and T2-weighted (B) MRI scans show absence of the greater wing of the sphenoid on the left side (arrows), with protrusion of the temporal lobe into the orbit and exophthalmos.

TOXOCARIASIS

Toxocara infection (larval granulomatosis) causes a peripheral granuloma, which may be associated with retinal folds and a pos-terior retinal detachment. It is usually unilateral and the size of the eye remains normal. Imaging may be helpful if the condition is difficult to distinguish clinically from retinoblastoma; absence of calcification is usual but not invariable.

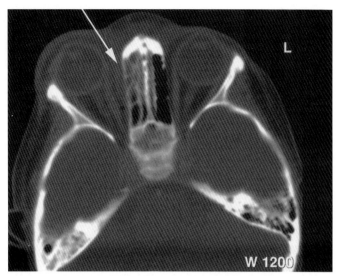

Figure 13.9 Orbital cellulitis. Axial CT scan shows fluid within infected ethmoid air cells and signs of an inflammatory mass (arrow) causing displacement of the medial rectus.

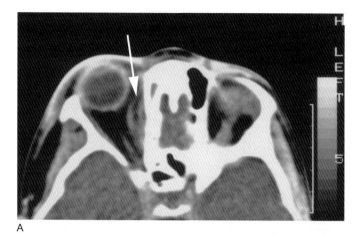

A

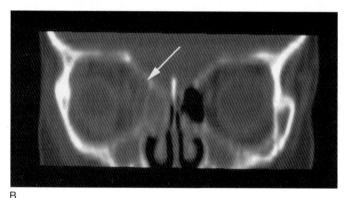

B

Figure 13.10 Orbital cellulitis with subperiosteal abscess. (A) Axial and (B) coronal CT scans following intravenous contrast show a subperiosteal fluid collection on the medial wall of the orbit, with an enhancing rim.

IDIOPATHIC ORBITAL INFLAMMATION (INFLAMMATORY PSEUDOTUMOUR)

Infiltration of orbital structures by lymphocytes and plasma cells may occur in the absence of any specific local infection or systemic cause, causing painful proptosis and ophthalmoplegia. The condition is usually unilateral and may affect the lacrimal gland, extrinsic ocular muscles, sclera, optic nerve and orbital fat. CT typically shows diffuse swelling of the affected structures, with intense enhancement following intravenous contrast. On MRI scans, the lesions are usually isointense with muscle on T1-weighted images and hyperintense on T2-weighted images (Figure 13.12). The diagnosis is confirmed by a rapid and sustained resolution with steroid therapy. Residual or recurrent lesions following steroid therapy require biopsy to exclude an underlying disorder such as lymphoma.

FURTHER READING

Castillo M, Mukherji SK. Orbital complications of sinusitis. In: Imaging of the paediatric head, neck, and spine. Philadelphia: Lippincott-Raven; 1996.

ORBITAL TUMOURS

PROLIFERATIVE HAEMANGIOMA

Proliferative haemangiomas are benign vascular tumours, which usually appear shortly after birth. They undergo a proliferative phase of rapid growth, becoming raised, bulky, compressible lesions with a characteristic strawberry-red colour. Following a few weeks of proliferation and growth, they typically enter a phase of stabilization lasting for several months, followed by a phase of involution. In some cases, proliferation is biphasic. The rate of regression is variable; 50% enter the phase of involution by 5 years of age and 90% by the age of 9 years. The prognosis for cosmetic outcome is not universally favourable; even after involution, some residual abnormality is present in 20–40% of cases, ranging from mild telangiectasia, hyperpigmentation or hypopigmentation to persisting fibrofatty masses.

Proliferative haemangiomas occur more frequently in girls than in boys; there is a significant association with prematurity. Although eventual stabilization and involution can be expected, proliferative haemangiomas may cause significant symptoms. There is a special category of lesions at dangerous sites, including

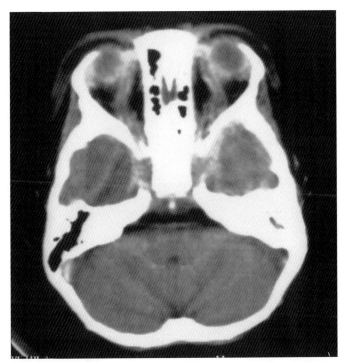

Figure 13.11 Thrombosis of superior ophthalmic veins and cavernous sinuses. Axial, contrast-enhanced CT scan shows filling defects within the superior ophthalmic veins and cavernous sinuses on both sides.

those close to the eye, where rapid proliferation may have disastrous consequences. In the young infant, permanent visual impairment may occur if the eye is occluded for longer than 1 week; a large proliferative haemangioma on the eyelid therefore requires urgent investigation and treatment. Medical management of symptomatic or dangerous proliferative haemangiomas involves the use of high doses of steroids. If steroid therapy is ineffective, alfa-interferon or chemotherapy with vincristine may be used. Direct steroid injection is used for rapid control of orbital lesions. If none of these is effective, surgical excision may be necessary, although surgery is avoided wherever possible because of the risks of haemorrhage and long-term scarring.

Imaging is not usually necessary for typical cutaneous proliferative haemangiomas but it can be very valuable in determining the extent of large periorbital lesions, particularly to determine whether there is retrobulbar extension. The differential diagnosis of a superficial soft tissue mass in an infant includes infantile fibrosarcoma, rhabdomyosarcoma, neurofibroma, nasal glioma and vascular malformation. If the nature of the lesion is not clinically certain, ultrasound and colour flow imaging may be helpful in showing a typical appearance of a well-defined, solid, echogenic mass, which is intensely hypervascular. In difficult cases, high vessel density and high-peak arterial Doppler shift can help to distinguish haemangiomas from other vascular soft tissue masses such as arteriovenous malformations and vascular malignant tumours. Vessel density in excess of five per square centimetre, and peak arterial Doppler shift greater than 2 kHz, taken together are highly specific and give a positive predictive value of 97% for the diagnosis of proliferative haemangioma.

MRI of haemangiomas in the proliferative phase typically shows a lobulated, solid mass with intermediate signal on

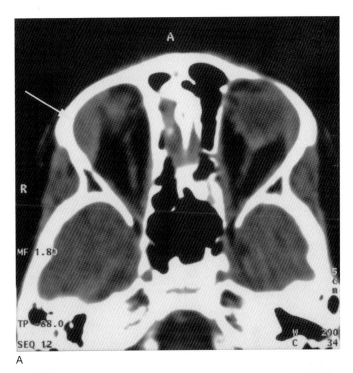

A

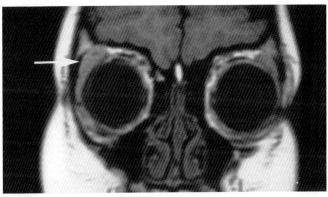

B

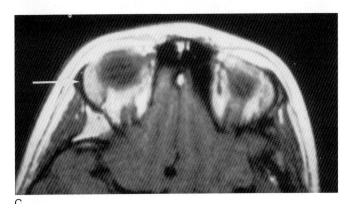

C

Figure 13.12 Idiopathic orbital inflammation. (A) Axial CT and (B) coronal T1-weighted MRI scans show diffuse swelling of the right lacrimal gland (arrow). (C) Axial T1-weighted MRI , following intravenous gadolinium, shows intense enhancement of the swollen lacrimal gland (arrow).

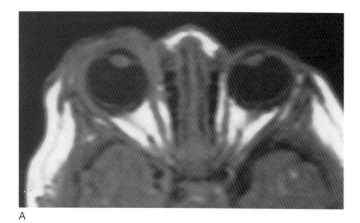

A

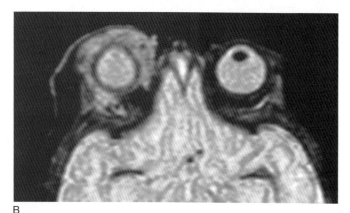

B

Figure 13.13 Proliferative haemangioma. (A) T1-weighted and (B) T2-weighted axial MRI scans show that the right eye is surrounded by a mass of solid tissue, within which flow voids are visible.

T1-weighted images and high signal intensity on T2-weighted images (Figure 13.13). Flow voids may be visible within feeding arteries and draining veins. There is intense, uniform enhancement following intravenous gadolinium. In the involuting phase, appearances are more varied and heterogeneous, as the lesions contain varying amounts of fibrous tissue, fat, blood breakdown products and calcification.

LYMPHATIC MALFORMATIONS

Orbital lymphatic malformations are benign developmental lesions but they may grow progressively, causing proptosis and orbital deformity. They may also bleed spontaneously, causing acute or recurrent proptosis. They tend to present at a later age than proliferative haemangiomas. Like lymphatic malformations elsewhere in the body, they may be capillary (consisting of a mass of normal-sized lymphatic vessels), microcystic or macrocystic (cystic hygroma). The lesions do not communicate with the normal lymphatic system and are filled with serous fluid. They are usually non-encapsulated, diffusely infiltrating lesions. Ultrasound of the microcystic form typically shows a densely echogenic mass, within which tiny cysts may sometimes be visible. In the macrocystic form, thin-walled cysts of varying size predominate within an echogenic, solid matrix. Colour Doppler may show some intrinsic blood flow but the lesion is usually much less vascular than a

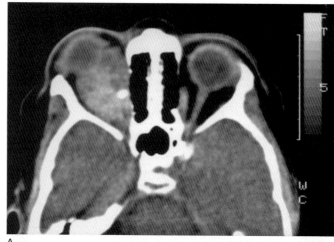

A

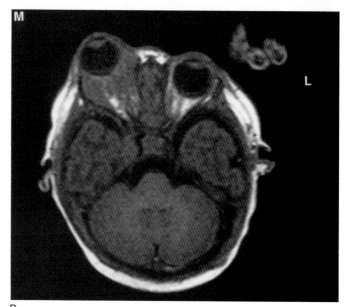

B

Figure 13.14 Lymphatic malformation. (A) CT and (B) T1-weighted MRI scans show a large, solid mass in the posterior part of the right orbit, infiltrating both extraconal and intraconal spaces, with marked proptosis. The CT scan shows focal calcification in the medial part of the mass.

proliferative haemangioma or vascular malformation. On CT and MRI scans, the lesions show mixed characteristics; the cystic elements may contain fluid–fluid levels, particularly when haemorrhage has occurred. Focal calcification may be present (Figure 13.14). Following intravenous contrast, there is often ring enhancement around the cystic components.

DERMOID CYST

Dermoid cysts are developmental tumours, which arise from failure of the ectoderm to separate from the underlying structures along embryonic lines of closure. It follows that, in the orbit, dermoid cysts occur at the site of sutures, most commonly the zygomaticofrontal, at the lateral canthus of the eye. Dermoid cysts have characteristic appearances on CT; they usually have a well-

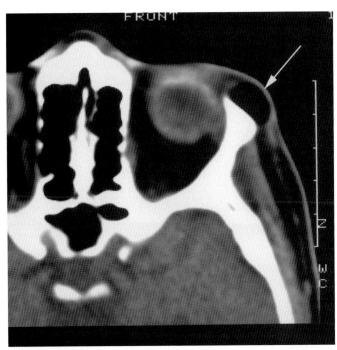

Figure 13.15 Orbital dermoid. Axial CT scan shows a well-defined, thin-walled lesion with low attenuation contents closely applied to the bone at the lateral canthus of the left eye (arrow).

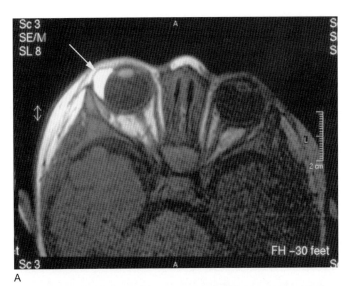

A

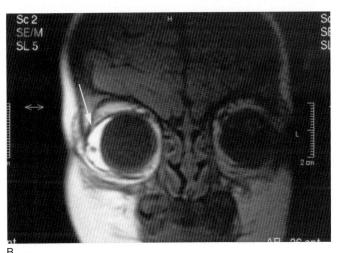

B

Figure 13.16 Orbital dermoid. (A) Axial and (B) coronal T1-weighted MRI scans shows a well-defined crescentic mass with high-signal intensity in the anterolateral part of the right orbit (arrow).

defined, thin capsule surrounding contents, which show uniform low attenuation (equal to or lower than orbital fat) and there is frequently flattening or scalloping of the adjacent bone, to which the lesion may be closely adherent (Figure 13.15). On MRI scans, the cyst contents show high-signal intensity on T1-weighted images (Figure 13.16).

RETINOBLASTOMA

Retinoblastoma is the most common intraocular tumour in childhood. It is a highly malignant tumour, which is bilateral in 30% of affected children. The average age at diagnosis is 13 months. Most cases are sporadic but there is an hereditary form, which is associated with a high frequency of other malignancies, particularly osteogenic and soft tissue sarcoma. Retinoblastoma may present with leukokoria (white eye), reduced visual acuity, eye pain or strabismus. The tumour arises in the retina and usually grows anteriorly into the vitreous, but there may be posterior growth into the subretinal space and sclera. Extraocular extension of the tumour, involvement of the optic nerve and intracranial extension may occur with advanced tumours and are poor prognostic factors.

Ultrasound usually shows an irregular retinal mass with evidence of calcification, sometimes extending into the vitreous (Figures 13.17 and 13.18). The eye is usually normal in size or enlarged, which helps to distinguish retinoblastoma from other causes of leukokoria. In some cases, retinoblastomas form diffuse infiltrating lesions within the retina, which may be difficult to identify with ultrasound. The differential diagnosis of calcified retinal lesions includes benign calcifications such as optic nerve drusen but, in practice, a calcified ocular mass lesion in a child below the age of 3 years is highly likely to be a retinoblastoma.

CT without contrast enhancement detects calcification in over 95% of retinoblastomas. CT is more sensitive for extraocular extension of the tumour than ultrasound; up to 50% of patients may have extraocular spread of tumour at diagnosis. The noncalcified parts of the tumour typically show intense enhancement following intravenous contrast.

MRI is less sensitive for the presence of calcification but its high intrinsic contrast and multiplanar capability makes it the optimal modality for the demonstration of tumour extension into the optic nerve and metastatic disease in the CSF spaces. The tumour is usually hyperintense to vitreous on T1-weighted images and hypointense on T2-weighted images. MRI is particularly helpful in follow-up surveillance after treatment.

RHABDOMYOSARCOMA

Rhabdomyosarcoma is the most common primary orbital malignancy in childhood. The tumour occurs more commonly in boys

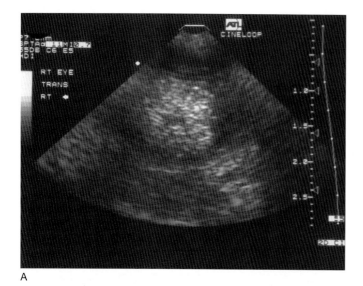

A

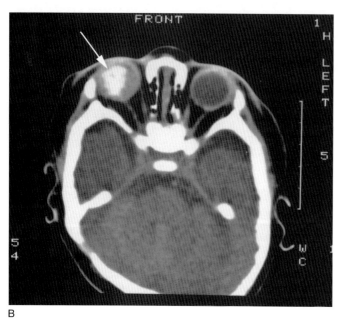

B

Figure 13.17 Retinoblastoma. (A) Ultrasound shows an echogenic retinal mass extending into the vitreous. (B) CT confirms the presence of a densely calcified intraocular tumour (arrow) with no evidence of extraocular extension.

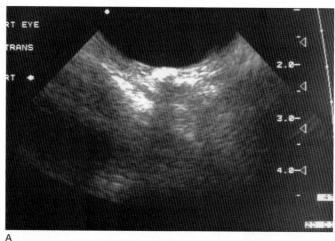

A

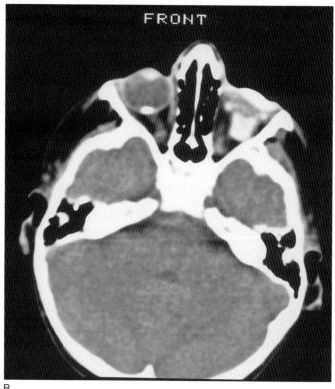

B

Figure 13.18 Retinoblastoma. (A) Ultrasound and (B) CT scans of a child previously treated for retinoblastoma in the left eye. A small, calcified tumour, confined to the retina, has developed within the right eye.

and the age distribution is bimodal, with peak incidences at 2–6 and 14–18 years. The typical presentation is rapidly developing exophthalmos. Acute pain, redness and swelling may initially suggest periorbital cellulitis.

The tumour may occur anywhere in the orbit but usually arises from rests of embryonal muscle cells within mesenchymal tissue rather than the extrinsic ocular muscles; the tumour may therefore be intraconal or extraconal and sometimes appears to arise from the lacrimal gland.

Ultrasound appearances are non-specific, typically demonstrating a solid mass with low or intermediate echogenicity. Colour Doppler may show blood flow within the tumour but it is usually much less vascular than a proliferative haemangioma. CT and MRI

may both be used for local staging (Figure 13.19). Invasion of the bony orbit is best appreciated with CT, which shows an irregular, infiltrating mass with similar attenuation to muscle. Necrotic tumours may show mixed patterns of attenuation. CT scans following intravenous contrast show patchy enhancement. MRI typically shows a solid mass, which is isointense to muscle on T1-weighted images and hyperintense on T2-weighted images. Fat saturation techniques to reduce the signal from orbital fat are helpful for precise delineation of the tumour. MRI is most sensitive for soft tissue and intracranial extension of tumour but is less

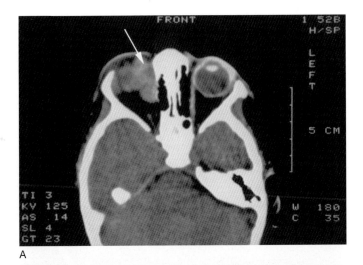

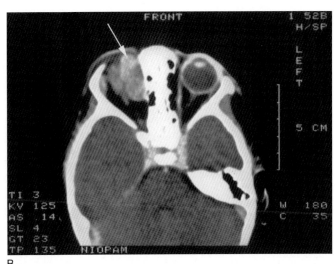

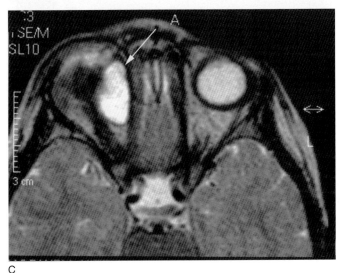

Figure 13.19 Rhabdomyosarcoma. (A) Axial CT scan shows a solid mass in the upper, medial quadrant of the right orbit (arrow). (B) Axial CT scan following intravenous contrast: the tumour shows patchy enhancement. (C) Axial T2-weighted MRI scan: the tumour is visible as a well-defined, hyperintense mass (arrow).

sensitive than CT for bone destruction. Lymphatic metastasis to the cervical lymph nodes and distant metastasis to lung and bone may occur. CT of the neck and chest and a radioisotope bone scan are recommended for complete staging.

OPTIC NERVE GLIOMA

Optic glioma is a slowly progressive neoplasm, which can occur anywhere within the optic pathways; histologically, the tumours are usually pilocytic astrocytomas. Optic gliomas often diffusely involve the intracranial optic pathways but may occasionally be localized to the intraorbital portion of the optic nerve, presenting with proptosis and impaired visual acuity. About 50% of cases occur in children affected by neurofibromatosis type 1. CT and MRI scans typically show a fusiform mass involving the optic nerve. MRI is more sensitive than CT for small lesions and is particularly helpful in the assessment of diffuse intracranial disease involving the optic tracts and optic radiations (Figure 13.20). Optic

gliomas show similar signal intensity to grey matter on T1-weighted images, with variable enhancement following intravenous gadolinium, and usually show high signal intensity on T2-weighted images. Large lesions may have both solid and cystic components.

METASTATIC NEUROBLASTOMA

The orbit is a common site for neuroblastoma metastases, usually from an abdominal primary. Proptosis and bruising of the eyelids may be the presenting features in a child with neuroblastoma and so investigation of a suspected orbital mass should include abdominal ultrasound. Orbital metastases from neuroblastoma are usually bilateral and often involve the roof and lateral walls of the orbit. CT typically shows bone destruction with a soft tissue mass, which shows inhomogeneous contrast following intravenous contrast. Intense uptake of activity on scintigraphy with I-131 metaiodobenzylguanidine (MIBG) is highly specific (Figure 13.21).

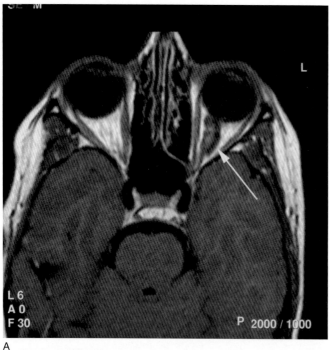

A

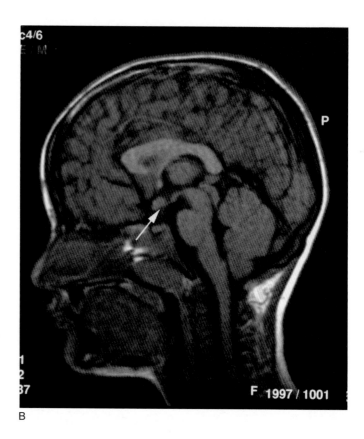

B

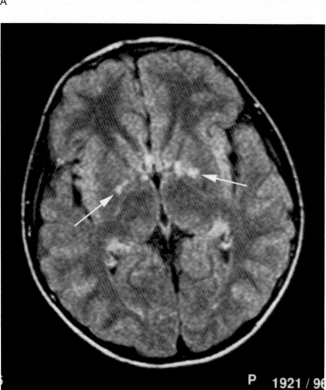

C

Figure 13.20 Optic pathway glioma. (A) Axial T1-weighted MRI scan of the orbits shows diffuse enlargement of the intraorbital portion of the left optic nerve (arrow). (B) Sagittal T1-weighted image shows a tumour mass involving the optic chiasm (arrow). (C) Axial FLAIR image shows multiple nodules of high signal intensity in the optic radiations in both cerebral hemispheres (arrows).

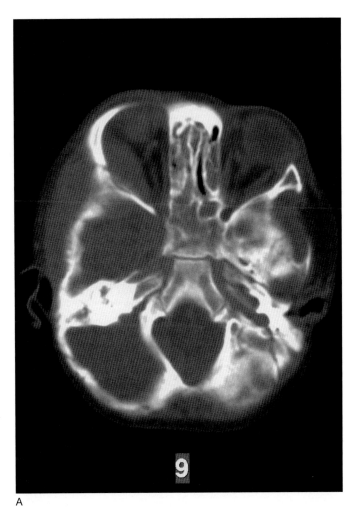

A

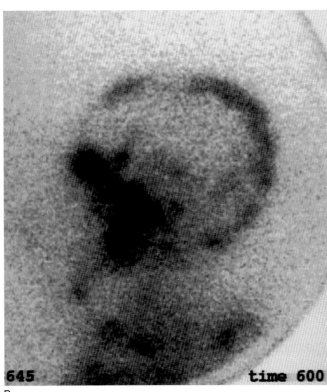

B

Figure 13.21 Metastatic neuroblastoma. (A) Axial CT scan shows bone destruction with a soft tissue mass involving the lateral wall of the right orbit and the adjacent temporal bone. (B) Scintigraphy with I-131 metaiodobenzylguanidine (MIBG) shows intense uptake of activity in the orbits and skull base.

LYMPHOMA AND LEUKAEMIA

Non-Hodgkin lymphoma may occur in the orbit. Acute leukaemia may occasionally present with similar appearances to metastatic neuroblastoma, due to solid leukaemic deposits (granulocytic sarcoma or chloroma). Meningeal infiltration and cranial nerve involvement may present with ophthalmoplegia, which is a frequent sign of CNS relapse. CT and MRI scans may show abnormal meningeal enhancement, particularly around the base of the brain, but in many cases a definite diagnosis is made only by CSF cytology.

LANGERHANS' CELL HISTIOCYTOSIS (LCH)

LCH frequently causes lytic skull lesions, which may be single or multiple. Lesions which involve the bony orbit may present with proptosis. Projectional radiography and CT show a characteristic appearance of well-defined, geographic lytic lesions (Figure 13.22) associated with soft tissue masses, which show uniform enhancement on scans following intravenous contrast. LCH involving the orbit is usually present in children with widespread disease.

FURTHER READING

Bilaniuk LT. Orbital vascular lesions. Role of imaging. Radiologic Clinics of North America 1999; 37:169–183.

Chawda SJ, Moseley IF. Computed tomography of orbital dermoids: a 20 year review. Clinical Radiology 1999; 54:821–825.

Graeb DA, Rootman J, Robertson WD et al. Orbital lymphangiomas: clinical, radiologic, and pathologic characteristics. Radiology 1990; 175:417–421.

McHugh K, Boothroyd AE. The role of radiology in childhood rhabdomyosarcoma. Clinical Radiology 1999; 54:2–10.

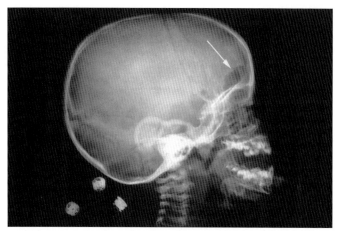

Figure 13.22 Langerhans' cell histiocytosis. Lateral skull radiograph shows a well-defined lytic lesion involving the roof of the orbit and frontal bone (arrow).

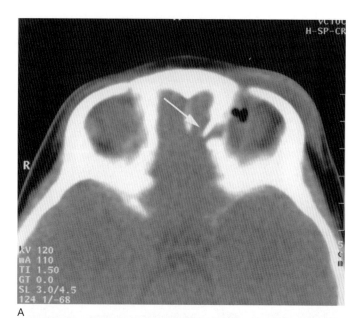

A

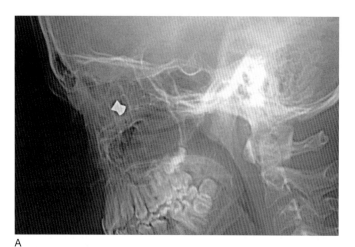

A

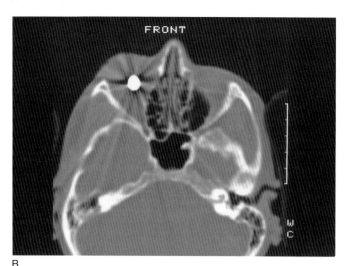

B

Figure 13.23 Intraorbital foreign body (air gun pellet). (A) Lateral radiograph and (B) axial CT scan demonstrate the position of the foreign body within the orbit.

B

Figure 13.24 Penetrating eye injury. Axial CT scans on (A) soft tissue and (B) bone windows show air within the orbit and a depressed fracture of the superomedial wall of the orbit (arrow).

ORBITAL TRAUMA

PENETRATING EYE INJURY

Projectional radiography is usually employed as the first line of investigation for a suspected intraorbital foreign body. Standard occipitofrontal and lateral projections will localize most radio-opaque foreign bodies but may be supplemented with tangential craniocaudal and lateral projections using small dental films. Occipitofrontal projections with the eyes in different directions of gaze have been used to localize intraorbital foreign bodies but where CT is available this can be achieved much more precisely (Figure 13.23). CT can also demonstrate foreign bodies, which are not sufficiently dense to be visible on conventional radiographs.

Ultrasound can be used very effectively, particularly for foreign bodies, which are not radio-opaque. Ultrasound can also demonstrate injury to the lens and ciliary apparatus, vitreous haemorrhage and retinal detachment. However, local pain and tenderness may make it difficult to obtain a satisfactory examination in an injured child without general anaesthesia. One major problem with ultrasound is the possibility that air bubbles introduced by a penetrating injury may simulate foreign bodies. Examining the eye in different directions of gaze is often helpful as air bubbles are usually mobile.

MRI is contraindicated if there is any suspicion of a ferromagnetic foreign body within the eye; such foreign bodies may move under the influence of the intense magnetic field and cause irreversible damage.

ORBITAL FRACTURES

Orbital fractures may occur as part of major maxillofacial trauma or may result from a deep penetrating injury. Orbital injuries

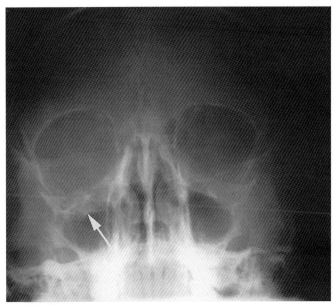

Figure 13.25 Fracture of the floor of the right orbit. Occipitomental radiographs show a soft tissue mass in the upper part of the right maxillary antrum (arrow).

require thorough investigation as there may be unrecognized intracranial injury (Figure 13.24). A direct blow to the eye may result in a 'blow-out' fracture of the floor of the orbit. The inferior rectus muscle may prolapse through the fracture and become entrapped. This may be recognized clinically by loss of eye movement in the vertical plane, associated with infraorbital loss of sensation. The cardinal radiological sign is a soft tissue mass in the upper part of the maxillary antrum (Figure 13.25). The orbital floor fracture itself may be difficult to identify on projectional radiographs but can be demonstrated optimally with direct coronal CT.

SECTION | 14

THE EAR, THE NOSE AND THE THROAT

The Ear, the Nose and the Throat

Neville B Wright

INTRODUCTION

Imaging of the ear, nose and throat (ENT) in children is a challenging area for the radiologist. The complexities of middle and inner ear structure, the various convolutions of the turbinates and sinuses, and the detailed assessment of the swallowing mechanism reflect on the varied nature of paediatric ENT radiology. Many of the techniques used are similar to those used in adult practice but the spectrum and types of disease encountered may be entirely different. Plain radiography has to a large extent been replaced by computed tomography (CT), especially in respect to imaging the ear and sinuses. However, it is important to minimize radiation exposure in children. Magnetic resonance imaging (MRI) has an expanding role and bronchography is being used increasingly for dynamic assessment of the upper airway.

EAR

EMBRYOLOGY

The inner ear forms from the otic capsule at about the third week of gestational life. The middle ear, external auditory meatus and pinna arise from the first and second branchial arches around 8 weeks of gestation. The malleus, short process and head of the incus and tensor tympani muscle arise from the first arch (Meckel's cartilage), the other parts of the ossicular chain and stapedius muscle from the second arch (Reichart's cartilage). Thus, abnormalities of the middle and external ear are commonly associated, whereas the inner ear abnormalities tend to be found in isolation. By the time of birth, the inner and middle ear is the size and shape of that of an adult, although the mastoid region and temporomandibular joint are still developing. With further development there is growth and pneumatization of the mastoid process.

IMAGING TECHNIQUES

PLAIN FILMS

Although there are a number of radiographic projections that can be used to assess the petrous bone and mastoid, detailed assessment is now performed using CT. There is still a role for obtain-ing mastoid views to assess the degree of pneumatization of the air cells but this should be limited to requests from ENT specialists. For historical purposes the following views can be performed:

- lateral oblique – to assess mastoid pneumatization;
- oblique posteroanterior (PA) view (Stenver's projection);
- 30 degree half-axial (Towne's) view;
- axial or submentovertical view; and
- per orbital view.

Previously, x-ray tomography was frequently used to image the petrous bone but this has been replaced by CT.

COMPUTED TOMOGRAPHY

With the development of faster scan times and improved resolution, CT now provides excellent images of the middle and inner ears. Generally, high-resolution 1-mm scans should be obtained in the transverse and coronal planes. With some of the more modern scanners, transverse images can be obtained and then the coronal images reconstructed from the scan dataset without loss of detail. This helps to reduce the radiation exposure to the child. The cross-sectional anatomy is the same as that in an adult (Figure 14.1). The images should all be postprocessed using a sharp filter.

MAGNETIC RESONANCE IMAGING (MRI)

There is increasing use of MRI, not just to assess the cerebellopontine angle and other intracranial structures but also inner ear abnormalities. Transverse and coronal T2-weighted sequences provide the best information about the inner ear, clarifying the presence of fluid-filled structures, such as the cochlea, vestibule and semicircular canals, but occasionally T1-weighted and post-contrast images may be helpful. When intracranial extension of disease occurs there may be involvement of the venous sinuses and then MR venography provides a non-invasive method of assessing vessel patency. Further advances in MR technology now permit exquisitely detailed three-dimensional reconstructions of the inner ear.

CONGENITAL EAR DEFORMITIES

Many congenital abnormalities of hearing do not result in structural changes of either the bone or soft tissue. Despite this, it is

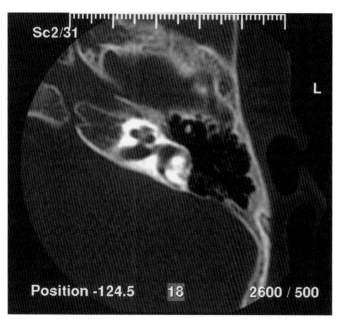

Figure 14.1 Transverse section through the left petrous temporal bone, demonstrating the internal auditory meatus, cochlea, vestibule and lateral semicircular canal.

clear that CT has a role in demonstrating some of the bony deformities that do occur, and that MRI is also able to define soft tissue abnormalities and problems related to the labyrinth of the inner ear and the cerebellopontine angle. Unfortunately, many of the young children requiring assessment will need general anaesthesia or sedation to obtain appropriate images.

There are a number of clinical features that may alert the paediatrician to the possibility of hearing impairment but most often this is identified as a result of a screening programme. Clinical pointers include a family history of deafness or neonatal jaundice, external ear deformity, a history of maternal rubella during pregnancy, or the presence of syndromes such as Treacher–Collins or Pendred syndrome.

Radiology has a complementary role to other electrophysiological techniques which can be used to assess the child with suspected hearing impairment, such as auditory brainstem response, electrocochleography and impedance audiometry.

TYPES OF DEAFNESS AND RADIOLOGICAL ASSESSMENT

The causes of deafness can be divided into those that are congenital, or acquired in the neonatal period, and those that are acquired in the older child. In addition, the type of hearing loss can be divided into that which is conductive and that which is sensorineural. When considering the auditory pathway, conductive deafness suggests an abnormality somewhere between the external auditory meatus and the middle ear cavity, possibly affecting the ossicular chain. Sensorineural deafness suggests either a central neurological cause or an abnormality somewhere in the

inner ear. Sensorineural deafness should be investigated with a combination of MRI and CT, and conductive deafness by CT. Clearly this is a generalization but it is helpful to consider deafness in these terms.

Radiological assessment of deafness requires evaluation of the state of the brainstem, inner ear and middle ear. Features to note are as follows:

Brainstem and inner ear:

1. Appearances of the brainstem and vestibulocochlear nerves.
2. Assessment of the state of the cochlea, vestibule and semicircular canals.
3. Assessment of the presence of a wide vestibular aqueduct
4. Exclusion of a cerebrospinal fluid fistula.

Middle ear:

1. Identification of a normal ossicular chain.
2. Assessment of adequate pneumatization of the middle ear cavity and mastoid region.
3. Identification of potential surgical hazards.
4. Assessment for feasibility for improved sound conduction (BAHA – bone anchored hearing aids).

The age of the child gives some indication of the type of problem that may be encountered. Identification of hearing problems up to the age of 3 months is difficult and most often suspected when the child has external signs of ear deformity or other syndromic abnormalities. These would include conditions such as Treacher–Collins syndrome, hemifacial microsomia and Klippel–Feil syndrome. Assessment of both ears is crucial in these children since bilateral lesions that are clinically occult are common.

Between 6 months and 4 years, there may also be reasonably obvious clinical features to point to the cause of hearing loss, such as otitis media or glue ear. These do not require imaging unless there is reason to perform exploratory surgery. Deafness associated with cerebrospinal fluid (CSF) otorrhoea, rhinorrhoea or meningitis needs careful evaluation of the temporal bones. Patients with significant deafness and language abnormalities may have severe inner ear abnormalities and should be assessed with CT and MRI. These children may need sedation and/or general anaesthesia to obtain adequate images.

RADIOLOGICAL TECHNIQUE

High-resolution CT scanning in the transverse and coronal planes provides exquisite detail of the inner and middle ear structure and should be obtained at 1-mm intervals. Where there is sensorineural hearing loss, it is also prudent to obtain an MR scan through the posterior fossa to assess the brainstem and vestibulocochlear nerves. The latter are not clearly demonstrated on CT, but should be identified prior to surgery for cochlear implantation. In general, T2-weighted sequences provide the best information with most of the normal structures in the ear showing as high signal. Plain films are generally unhelpful and should not be performed.

PREOPERATIVE ASSESSMENT

The important features to look for in assessing a child prior to ear surgery for deafness are as follows:

1. presence, shape and size of the middle ear cavity;
2. presence of the oval and round windows;
3. the course of the facial nerve; and
4. the state of the ossicles.

In general, these features are best assessed by CT although further tissue characterization of any soft tissue density seen within the middle ear cavity is not possible.

INNER EAR DEFORMITIES

The most recent classification divides these into five types:

1. Complete absence of the labyrinth of the inner ear that occurs at 3 weeks' gestation constitutes the Michel deformity and is very rare. The inner ear is replaced by cystic cavities.
2. The primitive otocyst (Figure 14.2) constitutes a much more common cause of deafness but importantly neither abnormality has a risk of CSF fistula, although there is complete anacusis.
3. Cessation of development at a slightly later stage (about 4 weeks' gestation) gives rise to the 'common cavity' abnormality first described by Cock and the importance of this lesion is its high risk of spontaneous CSF fistula and or meningitis. The cochlea and vestibule form a common cavity.
4. The Mondini deformity represents an abnormality of the distal cochlea turns towards the apex. There is a normal basal cochlea turn and because of this there is some hearing preserved in the true Mondini deformity. There may be associated abnormalities of the vestibular aqueduct (Figure 14.3).
5. In cochlear aplasia, the vestibule and semicircular canals may be normal or malformed. In cochlea hypoplasia, there is a small cochlear with a normal shape and number of turns but this is often associated with a normal or malformed vestibule and semicircular canals. These abnormalities may occur in the branchio-oto-renal syndrome.

Syndromes associated with the Mondini defect include di George, Waanderberg's, Alagille, Klippel–Feil and Pendred's syndromes.

A complete absence of the semicircular canals is seen in CHARGE (coloboma of the iris or retina, heart defects, atresia of the choanae, retarded growth and development, genital abnormalities and ear abnormalities) syndrome and in the majority of cases this is associated with complete anacusis. Otherwise, the semicircular canals may be absent or dilated to varying degrees. The commonest labyrinthine abnormality is a solitary dilated dysplastic lateral semicircular canal.

Abnormalities of the internal auditory meatus include abnormalities of the direction, commonly the result of abnormalities of the skull base, a very narrow (Figure 14.4) or double internal auditory meatus which is often associated with severe or total deafness, and dilatation of the internal auditory meatus producing a bulbous appearance. This latter feature may be associated with one type of X-linked deafness.

VESTIBULAR AQUEDUCT SYNDROME

Enlargement of the vestibular aqueduct may give rise to progressive and fluctuant hearing loss as part of the wide vestibular aqueduct syndrome. The aqueduct is deemed enlarged when it measures more than 1.5 mm in diameter. This can be demonstrated on CT or MRI (Figure 14.5). Classically, there is stepwise sensorineural hearing loss often following relatively minor head trauma. Most cases are sporadic. Syndromes associated with this include CHARGE syndrome and branchio-oto-renal syndrome.

A large endolymphatic sac is a very suggestive feature of Pendred's syndrome, a condition where there is a combination of congenital deafness and thyroid dysfunction.

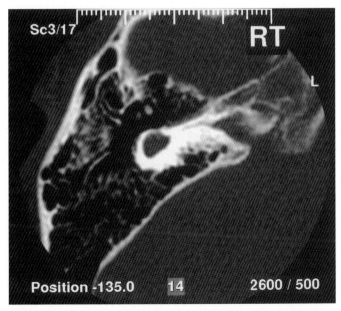

Figure 14.2 Transverse CT section shows a single cavity consistent with a primitive otocyst.

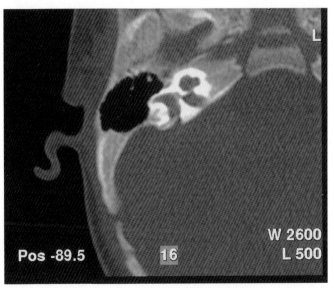

Figure 14.3 Transverse CT section showing a Mondini abnormality of the cochlea, with failure of partition of the cochlea.

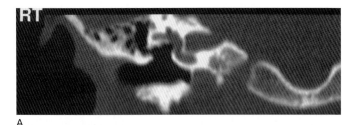

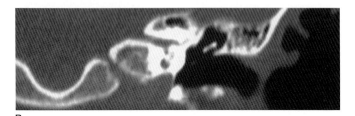

Figure 14.4 Coronal CT image shows (A) a normal internal auditory meatus and (B) an abnormally narrowed left internal auditory meatus.

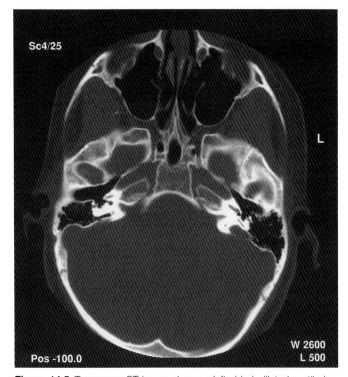

Figure 14.5 Transverse CT image shows a left-sided, dilated vestibular aqueduct. Normal right side.

INNER EAR LESIONS ASSOCIATED WITH CSF FISTULAS

Congenital CSF fistulas into the middle ear cavity are potentially fatal; they are often misdiagnosed but are rare. Clinical suspicion usually arises from one of three clinical settings:

1. CSF rhinorrhoea if the ear drum is intact; there is a nasal discharge related to CSF passing down the eustachian tube into the nasal airway;

2. CSF otorrhoea if there is perforation of the ear drum or if there has been surgery for suspected serous otitis media; and
3. recurrent attacks of meningitis.

The deafness associated with these conditions is usually severe or complete. It frequently goes unrecognized if it is unilateral, and is difficult to diagnose and assess in the young child. Spontaneous CSF fistulas from the subarachnoid space into the middle ear cavity can be classified into either perilabyrinthine or translabyrinthine:

*   Perilabyrinthine fistulas are usually associated with normal hearing and are extremely rare. Bone defects may be very subtle and may require contrast administration or radionuclide studies to define them further. High-resolution CT may be helpful.
*   Translabyrinthine fistulas are frequently associated with anacusis, severe labyrinthine dysplasias and communication via the internal auditory meatus. The labyrinthine deformity is typically described as being more severe than that classically described by Mondini. The cochlea lacks a modiolus or central bony spiral. There is no appropriate basal turn and there is wide communication between the cochlea sac and the vestibule, which is often abnormal and enlarged. The lateral semicircular canal is particularly dilated, but all of them may be abnormal to varying degrees. The labyrinthine malformation is often associated with a defective stapes, with the exit route for CSF being via the oval or less commonly the round window. The fistula is usually spontaneous or precipitated by relatively minor head trauma. CSF fistula detection requires a high clinical suspicion.

MIDDLE EAR DEFORMITIES AND THE EXTERNAL AUDITORY MEATUS (Figure 14.6)

Most unilateral atresias of the external auditory meatus have a deformed pinna but no other congenital abnormality. The mastoid is usually normally formed in these cases, with good pneumatization and a relatively normal middle ear cavity. In bilateral atresia, however, the situation is usually more severe. Often the middle ear cavity contains undifferentiated mesenchyma, which radiologically mimics other soft tissues or retained mucus. Rarely, there is complete absence of the middle ear, there usually being at least a small hypotympanum lateral to the basal turn of the cochlea. The middle ear cavity itself may be reduced in size by the atretic plate laterally, descent of the tegmen, or a high jugular bulb. In hemifacial microsomia and mandibular facial dysostosis, the attic and antrum are typically absent or slit-like, being replaced by inferior descent of the tegmen or simple solid bone. When the middle ear cavity contains air, its shape and contents are relatively easy to assess but when the undifferentiated mesenchyme is present evaluation is more difficult. Preauricular pits or cysts result from abnormalities of the first brachial cleft and are often asymptomatic unless they become infected. Ultrasound or MRI can be used to assess the extent of the lesions and occasionally sinography can be helpful. Care must be exercised in excising the lesions since they are intimately related to the facial nerve.

FACIAL NERVE ABNORMALITIES

Although the facial nerve may be hypoplastic, it is very rare to find it completely absent. The main problems are related to variation

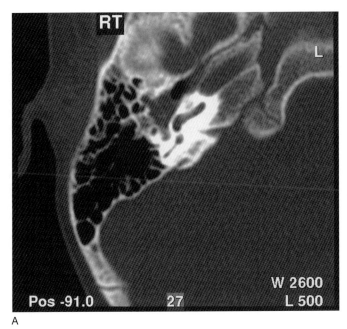
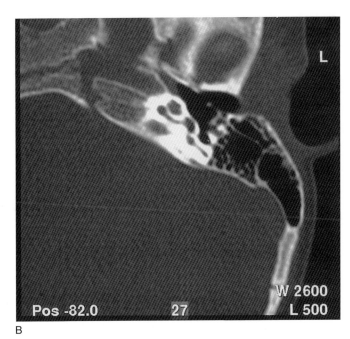

A   B

Figure 14.6 Transverse CT images show an absent external auditory meatus on the right (A), with soft tissue density material in the middle ear cleft and poorly discernible ossicles. The left side (B), shown for comparison, is normal.

in its course. The first part of the facial nerve is rarely affected unless a primitive otic sac is present, in which case the facial nerve lies anterior to the otocyst. The course of the second and third parts depends on normal development of the branchial arches, in particular the second arch. In general terms, the greater the deformity, the more marked is the likelihood for the facial nerve to follow a direct course into the soft tissues of the face. Minor abnormalities of the first branchial arch leads to maldevelopment of the tympanic ring and no change to the course of the second and third parts of the facial canal, but more severe problems lead to increasing deformity. An exposed facial nerve in the middle ear cavity is a common finding at surgery for congenital malformation. Absence of the second genu of the facial nerve is a usual finding in Treacher–Collins syndrome resulting in difficult access to the oval window. Preoperative assessment of the facial canal requires both coronal and sagittal CT sections, with transverse images showing the descending canal to the stylomastoid foramen in profile.

OSSICLES

When there is atresia of the external ear, a normal ossicular chain is rare, although complete absence of the ossicles is unusual. The vestigial ossicles are often thicker and heavier than normal and may be fixed to the walls of the middle ear cavity. A common finding is fusion of the bodies of the malleous and incus, which may be bony or fibrous. The identification of the individual ossicles is not of great importance, although the handle of the malleous is often the most abnormal and most easily recognized. The handle of the malleous is usually angled towards the atretic plate to which

it may be fixed, giving a typical 'L'-shaped appearance to the ossicular mass.

EXTERNAL AUDITORY MEATUS

The external auditory meatus may be narrow, short, completely or partly atretic, or it may be orientated in an abnormal direction. Obstruction may be due to bone or soft tissue, although in the majority of cases both are involved. The tympanic bone may rarely be hypoplastic, deformed or absent. The atretic plate may be composed of a number of surrounding bones, a deformed tympanic bone or portion of the squamous temporal bone or mastoid.

SYNDROMES ASSOCIATED WITH HEREDITARY DEAFNESS

There are numerous syndromes associated with hereditary deafness and more exhaustive accounts are given in the Further Reading section with concentration here on some of the more common and important syndromes. Most can be adequately assessed with high-resolution CT, supplemented with MRI where appropriate to assess associated intracranial abnormalities.

OCULO-AURICULO-VERTEBRAL SPECTRUM (HEMIFACIAL MICROSOMIA)

This is primarily a unilateral malformation of the structures originating from the first and second branchial arches. The ear is small, often with preauricular tags along the line between the front of the

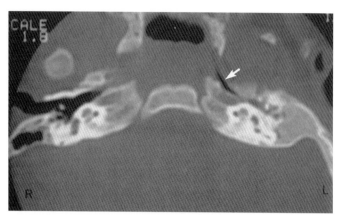

Figure 14.7 Hemifacial microsomia. Transverse CT section shows greatly reduced middle cavity with an absent external meatus. The ossicles are left and there is a dilated eustachian tube (arrow).

ear and the side of the mouth. There is microstomia and failure of formation of the mandibular ramus and condyle. If there is an epibulbar dermoid present, this constitutes Goldenhar syndrome. Cervical vertebral anomalies and cardiac defects are common. More than 50% have both conductive and less often sensorineural hearing loss. This may be associated with anomalies of the middle and external ears, hypoplasia or agenesis of the ossicles, aberrant nerves, a wide open eustachian tube and abnormalities of the skull base with descent of the tegmen (Figure 14.7). There are often associated anomalies of the inner ear. Most cases are sporadic and hemifacial microsomia represents the most common of the otocraniofacial syndromes. However, there are a few families where the disorder is autosomal dominant.

TREACHER–COLLINS SYNDROME

Treacher–Collins syndrome contrasts with hemifacial microsomia by being a symmetrical, bilateral condition and having

characteristic middle ear abnormalities. The incidence is approximately 1 in 50 000 and the typical features are abnormalities of the pinnae, atresia of the external auditory canals and anomalies of the middle ear ossicles, hypoplasia of the facial bones, antimongoloid slanting of the palpable fissures, with colobomata of the lower eyelids with a lack of eyelashes medial to the abnormality, and a cleft palate. A spectrum of abnormalities may be present, although the inner ear is usually normal. CT demonstrates symmetrical lesions with a slit-like appearance of the attic and the antrum on coronal CT (Figure 14.8). In general, the external auditory canal is atretic, although it may be normal. The atresia may be cartilaginous or bony. In most cases, the middle ear cavity is hypoplastic or occasionally absent. Abnormalities of the ossicles are common and the facial nerve follows a more direct route. The ossicles may be hypoplastic or even absent. Ankylosis to the lateral or medial wall of the tympanic recess is common. In general, increasing degrees of outer canal malformation are reflected by increasingly abnormal ossicle and cavity formation. Although the patients largely have conductive deafness, some have a sensorineural component, though the reasons for this is not clear. The general hypoplasia of the structures makes treatment extremely difficult.

OSSEOUS DYSPLASIAS

There is a wide spectrum of differing bone dysplasias that commonly may lead to deafness, some of which produce reduced bone density, some sclerosis. Most of them are very rare. Osteogenesis imperfecta tarda is a cause of conductive, sensoneural or mixed hearing loss. There is generalized demineralization of the labyrinthine capsule and a large proportion of the petrous bone. Hearing loss in osteogenesis imperfecta is unusual before the age of 10 years but may be related to fractures through the stapes. Osteopetrosis, craniometaphyseal dysplasia, craniodiaphyseal dysplasia, frontometaphyseal dysplasia and Camurati–Engelmann syndrome may all be associated with hyperostosis and sclerosis of the skull bones. This may result in mixed hearing loss, which is slowly progressive.

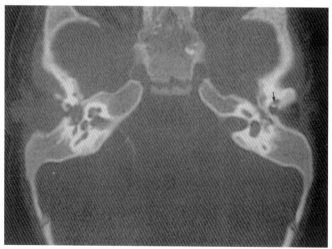

A

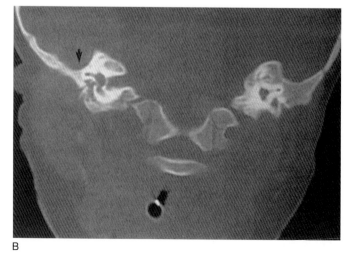

B

Figure 14.8 Treacher–Collins syndrome. Normal inner ears. The small middle ear cavities are opaque, and only one small hypoplastic ossicle (small arrow) can be seen on the transverse section (A). The coronal section (B) shows depression of the floor of the middle cranial fossa to the level of the lateral semicircular canal (large arrow).

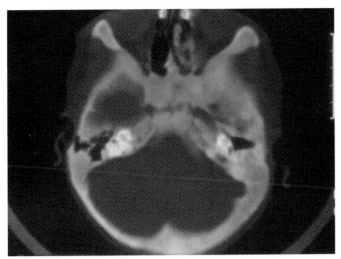

Figure 14.9 CT scan of a child with fibrous dysplasia affecting the sphenoidal bones and left temporal bone. Note the expansion of the diploic spaces.

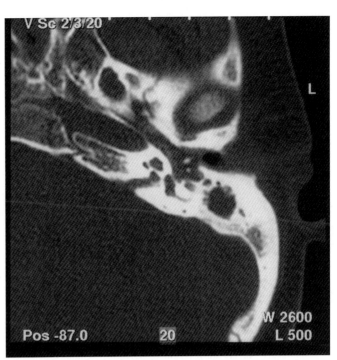

Figure 14.10 Otitis media. Transverse CT image shows soft tissue density material filling the middle ear and surrounding the ossicles.

Some of this may be related to bony encroachment on the cranial foramena, but in general, cross-sectional imaging shows an increased sclerosis of the petrous temporal bone and narrowing of the internal auditory meatus (IAMs). Bony encroachment into the middle ear cavity may also contribute to conductive hearing loss. Fibrous dysplasia may also affect the cranial foramina. It involves the temporal bone most frequently when polyostotic. Deafness is conductive. Fibrous dysplasia causes expansion of the diploic space and extends along the temporal bone towards the petrous apex (Figure 14.9).

CHARGE SYNDROME

CHARGE is an acronym for Coloboma of the iris or retina, Heart defects, Atresia of the choanae, Retarded growth and development, Genital abnormalities and Ear abnormalities. There is a spectrum of ear abnormalities including:

* protrusion of external ears;
* deformed or absent semicircular canals;
* Mondini dysplasia;
* absence of the utricle;
* absent incus or stapes;
* absent oval windows; and
* absent stapes.

OTITIS MEDIA

Acute otitis media is very common in infants and young children and refers to inflammation of the middle ear and its associated air spaces in the petrous temporal bone. It is a clinical diagnosis and imaging is not usually required, although CT will show non-specific soft-tissue density material within the middle ear surrounding the ossicles (Figure 14.10). Persistence of the inflammatory process leads to chronic otitis media with mastoiditis and

breakdown of the air cells. Although the infection is usually viral, the most common bacterial organisms implicated are *Streptococcus pneumoniae* and *Haemophilus influenzae*. Imaging by contrast-enhanced CT is generally required to delineate the complications of acute otitis media, which are rare. These include:

* Acute mastoiditis. Today, this is usually contained by antibiotic treatment. Extension of infection to cause serious complications may occur from direct erosion of the bone, haematogenous spread or thrombophlebitis.
* Petrous apicitis. Clinically, this presents classically as Gradenigo syndrome with otitis media, abducens nerve palsy and pain in the distribution of the trigeminal nerve.
* Subperiosteal and Bezold abscess formation. The former occurs by direct extension of infection and may occur in any direction. The latter results from osteolysis at the mastoid tip with extension of inflammation into the neck and deposition of infected debris (Figure 14.11).
* Subdural and epidural abscess formation.
* Meningitis.
* Dural venous sinus thrombosis.
* Cerebral/cerebellar abscess formation.

The intracranial complications may be life threatening and are described elsewhere in this book. They are best demonstrated by MRI.

Mastoiditis may be seen on radiographs but high-resolution CT is required for the demonstration of any suspected complication or prior to surgery. In acute mastoiditis, there is clouding of the mastoid air cells. In chronic disease, there is poor pneumatization and sclerosis of these.

The complications of chronic otitis media differ and include:

- deafness – following labyrinthitis ossificans and osteoneogenesis (Figure 14.12);
- formation of giant cholesterol cysts and granulation tissue;
- cholesteatoma formation;
- labyrinthine fistula;
- facial nerve palsy;
- ossicle fixation and erosion;
- tympanic membrane retraction; and
- chronic secretory otitis media.

CHOLESTEATOMA

Cholesteatomas (epidermoids) have traditionally been divided into congenital and acquired forms, the majority being considered acquired in nature with a small number (2–5%) congenital. Cholesteatomas can arise at any site in the intracranial cavity but are more common in the middle ear (Figure 14.13). Congenital cholesteatomas develop behind an intact ear drum with no history of otitis media or obvious connection with external auditory meatus. Acquired cholesteatoma are seen in children with a history of otitis media. In both acquired and congenital forms, the hearing loss is generally of a conductive type unless complications occur, when a sensorineural element may develop. The acquired lesions can be further divided into those seen in the region of the pars flaccida (attic cholesteatomas) and those associated with the pars tensa. The role of imaging in cholesteatoma is to define the extent of disease and identify any particular complications. CT is the imaging modality of choice and features that suggest the presence of a cholesteatoma in the middle ear are:

1. a homogeneous soft tissue density mass within the middle ear cavity possibly extending into the mastoid region;
2. bone destruction – this is the cardinal feature and in particular the scutum should be carefully assessed as this is the earliest site of destruction;
3. remodelling of the middle ear cavity;
4. ossicular displacement – attic cholesteatomas tend to produce medial displacement and pars tensa (sinus) cholesteatomas lateral displacement of the ossicles.

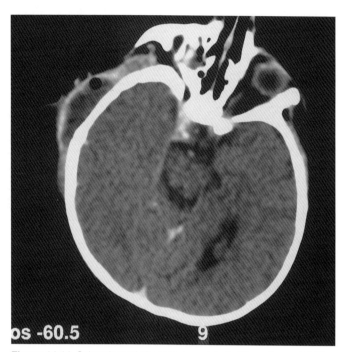

Figure 14.11 Subperiosteal abscess associated with acute mastoiditis and otitis media. Transverse CT image shows an abscess containing gas over the right temporal region.

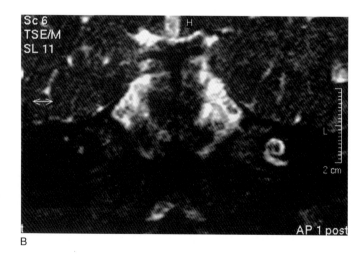

Figure 14.12 Labyrinthine ossification. (A) Transverse CT examination shows ossification of the right cochlea. (B) Coronal T2-weighted MRI clearly shows the cochlea 'whorl' on the left but no cochlea fluid on the right.

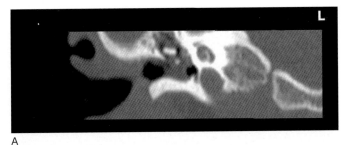
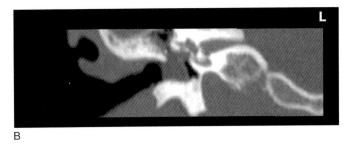

Figure 14.13 (A,B) Two CT images of a child with a cholesteatoma in the middle ear.

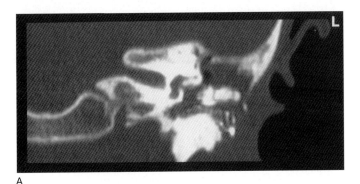

Figure 14.14 CSF fistula. (A) Coronal CT image showing appearances following cholesteatoma surgery. A breach in the tegmen is shown with soft tissue density material in the mastoid and middle ear. (B) Coronal MR scan shows high signal adjacent to the temporal lobe and within the mastoid and middle ear on the left.

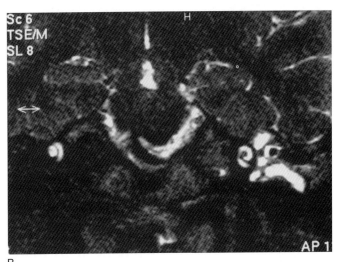

Unfortunately, CT is a poor discriminator for the determination of the differing types of soft tissue present in the middle ear cavity but the combination of the clinical and imaging features usually suggests the diagnosis. On MRI, cholesteatomas are of intermediate signal on T1-weighted and high signal on T2-weighted sequences. The complications of cholesteatoma formation are as follows:

1. ossicular damage;
2. inner ear or intracranial fistulas (Figure 14.14);
3. facial nerve involvement;
4. extension into the petrous apex – to produce apicitis;
5. complete hearing loss;
6. automastoidectomy; and
7. intracranial extension with possible venous sinus thrombosis.

Congenital cholesteatomas arise from aberrant embryonic epithelial rests and are identical to epidermoids. They usually develop within the middle ear cavity although they can be in the external canal or at other sites in the petrous temporal bone. When encountered early in development they can be removed easily. CT is the best imaging modality to demonstrate the localized soft tissue density lesion, usually adjacent to the tympanic membrane.

NEOPLASMS

In general, temporal bone tumours can be divided into three main groups by site; the squamous temporal bone and the external ear, the middle ear and mastoid, and the cerebellopontine angle. The reader is referred to the Tables 14.1 to 14.3 for a more exhaustive list, but the following conditions merit special mention. Clinical presentation depends on the location of the lesion and includes a soft tissue mass, pain, tinnitus, deafness and facial nerve palsy (Figure 14.15).

The most common neoplasm to be encountered in the petrous temporal bone of a child is a rhabdomyosarcoma. A facial nerve palsy with acute otitis media suggests an underlying tumour may be present. Occasionally, a tumour polyp may perforate through the ear drum. Cross-sectional imaging with MRI and CT is essential to define the extent of disease, with CT defining the limits of bony destruction. The reader is referred to other sections within the text on rhabdomyosarcoma for staging and evaluation. There are no specific imaging features to enable one to make a tissue diagnosis. This will require biopsy.

Other less common tumours encountered around the petrous bone and cerebellopontine angle include schwannomas and, rarely, acoustic neuroma. Acoustic neuromas in childhood are usually associated with neurofibromatosis type 2 (NF 2). These lesions are well defined.

Table 14.1 Tumours of the squamous temporal bone and external ear

Soft tissue neoplasms	Bony neoplasms
Lymphangioma	Exostosis
Haemangioma	Osteoblastoma
Haemangioendothelioma	Chondroblastoma
Langerhans' cell histiocytosis	Aneurysmal bone cyst
Rhabdomyosarcoma	Ewing's sarcoma
Adenoid cystic carcinoma	
Myofibromatosis	
Fibrosarcoma	
Neurofibroma	
Meningioma	
Yolk sac tumour	
PNET	

Table 14.2 Tumours of the middle ear and mastoid

1. Rhabdomyosarcoma
2. Langerhans' cell histiocytosis
3. Endolymphatic sac tumour
4. Ewing's and osteogenic sarcoma
5. Lymphoma and leukaemia
6. Chondro- and fibrosarcoma
7. Germ cell tumour
8. Malignant neuroectodermal tumour

Table 14.3 Tumours of the cerebellopontine angle

1. Epidermoid and dermoid
2. Arachnoid cyst
3. Lipoma
4. Acoustic and trigeminal schwannoma
5. Meningioma
6. Neurofibrosarcoma
7. Choroid plexus papilloma
8. Craniopharyngioma
9. Teratoma
10. Fibrosarcoma
11. Granulocystic sarcoma

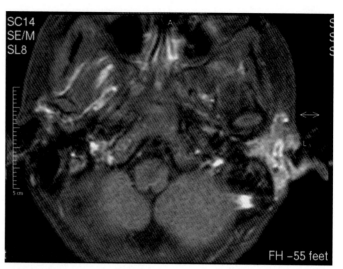

Figure 14.15 Axial T1-weighted image with fat suppression and gadolinium of a girl who presented with a small mass lesion in the preauricular region on the left which, on biopsy, was proven to be a PNET. Note the soft tissue mass, which shows some enhancement with gadolinium.

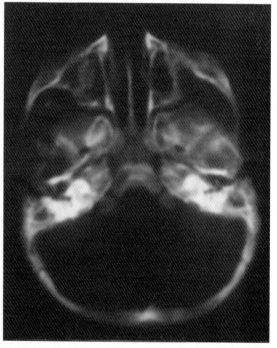

Figure 14.16 CT scan, presented on bone window settings, of a boy with histiocytosis causing destruction of the right temporal bone. This boy presented with a discharging ear.

Langerhans' cell histiocytosis is a condition producing widespread bone destruction associated with massive infiltration of histiocytes. The precise pathogenesis is unknown but children will present with a soft tissue mass around the external auditory meatus with persistent discharge (Figure 14.16). There may be other focal areas of bone destruction seen elsewhere in the skeleton and skeletal survey is indicated for full assessment. There may also be associated pituitary abnormalities with the child presenting with diabetes insipidus. In general, CT evaluation produces excellent demonstration of any bony involvement of the inner ear with MRI showing the soft tissue component.

ACOUSTIC SCHWANNOMA

Most children presenting with deafness secondary to an acoustic neuroma have NF 2. The neuromas are usually bilateral but may be asymmetrical in size. The tumours affect the vestibular division of the acoustic nerve more frequently than the cochlear division.

The tumours are located in the internal auditory canal and expand it towards the meatus. They may occasionally arise in the labyrinth and extend towards the middle ear. Clinical presentation is with tinnitus, sensineuronal hearing loss and sometimes vertigo. On imaging, the IAM is enlarged. A well-defined, enhancing soft tissue mass is seen with MRI, which is required for their demonstration. Prior to contrast, the neuroma has a slightly higher signal than brain on T1-weighted images.

TEMPORAL BONE TRAUMA

Temporal bone fractures are rare. They are bilateral in approximately 40% of patients. Direct impact trauma to the temporal or parietal bone is the cause. They should be suspected when there are clinical features of a base of skull fracture, such as conductive deafness, discharge of CSF, bleeding from the ear or facial nerve paralysis. High-resolution CT is the investigation of choice and has high sensitivity (Figure 14.17) in their detection. In the acute setting, children are usually referred for head CT to identify the intracranial complications of trauma. If there are clinical features suggesting a base of skull fracture, high-resolution scans can be obtained at this stage but more often this is deferred until any potential life-threatening, neurological complication has been treated and the child stabilized.

Ideally, both transverse and coronal images should be obtained to assess the extent of the fracture and the status of the ossicular chain. MRI may also be helpful to identify any fistulas but this is usually not practical in the acute stage. In general, temporal bone fractures lie obliquely, although classical description defines them as longitudinal or transverse with respect to the long axis of the petrous bone. Usually the fracture extends into the squamous temporal bone and petrous apex and overall the fractures are best assessed on the transverse image. Longitudinal fractures are more commonly associated with fractures of the external auditory canal, particularly its posterior-superior aspects. Fractures of the anterior tympanic plate may also occur from direct blows to the mandible with force transmitted to the temperomandibular joint into the external auditory canal.

The complications of temporal bone trauma are primarily related to four areas:

- CSF fistula formation;
- deafness;
- facial nerve injury; and
- intracranial injury.

When CSF fistula is suspected, MRI may be useful in distinguishing between CSF and blood within the middle ear cavity, although this is by no means easy. CSF fluid leaks usually resolve spontaneously and only require conservative management. Deafness is a common feature of the acute stages of temporal bone fracture but only a minority persist with hearing problems after a month or two. Conductive hearing loss is the most common problem, either caused by haemorrhage within the middle ear or disruption of the ossicular chain. Those with persisting deafness usually have ossicular damage. Sensorineural hearing loss is less common and occurs in approximately one in six of children with temporal bone fractures. Again, this is more likely to persist than conductive deafness.

Facial nerve injury is seen in about 3% of children with temporal bone fractures. CT and MRI may be useful to define the site of abnormality and guide surgical decompression. The spectrum of intracranial injury following temporal bone fracture includes temporal lobe contusion and extra-axial haematomas. Clearly, these

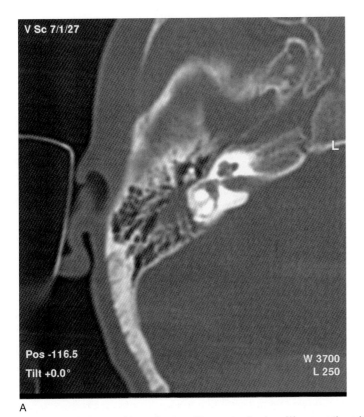
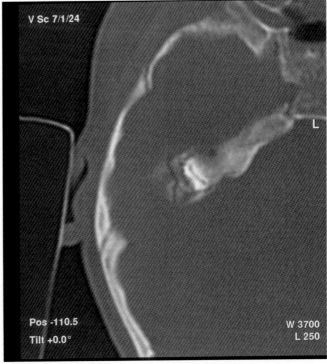

Figure 14.17 Temporal bone fracture. Transverse fracture (A) across the middle ear cavity associated with some blood around the ossicles and extending into the mastoid region, and (B) passing lateral to the superior semicircular canal.

require neuroradiological and surgical evaluation. In general, in the acute phase, CT should still be performed, with a low threshold to proceeding to MRI for more detailed evaluation.

IMAGING RELATED TO EAR SURGERY

In general this relates to three areas:

1. Recognition of the presence of grommets inserted for treatment of glue ear and postsurgical packing. Clearly, there should be a history of grommet insertion but it is often all too easy for the clinician to forget this relevant piece of information when requesting scans. Grommets usually appear on CT scans as short parallel linear structures at the level of the tympanic membrane. They are easy to miss on brief reviews of images, especially when the middle ear cavity is fluid filled. Bismuth packing is sometimes used following surgery and may produce unusual densities mimicking other foreign bodies (Figure 14.18).
2. Recognition of previous mastoid surgery. Imaging of the postoperative middle ear cavity and mastoid region is difficult to interpret as the CT and MR changes are non-specific. Generally, a well-pneumatized postoperative cavity is an encouraging feature, whereas residual soft tissue material may mimic residual disease or simply postoperative fluid.

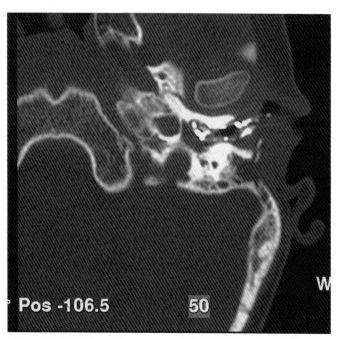

Figure 14.18 Postoperative packing. High-density opacities within the left external meatus and middle ear represent bismuth packing following recent surgery.

3. Awareness of the appearances of cochlear implants. Imaging related to cochlear implants is beyond the scope of this text but in general terms there will be external and internal components and intracochlear and extracochlear electrodes. A combination of plain films and CT are required to assess the postoperative appearances.

BELL'S PALSY

Clinical presentation with Bell's palsy is rare in childhood compared with adults. The aetiology is thought to be viral in the absence of an underlying tumour. The natural history is for resolution in about 8 weeks but steroids are now used to hasten resolution. Imaging is not usually performed or required in a typical case but anxiety about sinister underlying pathology may lead to it being done. This should be performed with MRI. This may be normal but subtle enlargement of the inflamed nerve in the bony canal may be seen. There is enhancement with contrast. Bell's palsy may rarely be due to destructive base of skull lesions such as Langerhans' cell histiocytosis or rhabdomyosarcoma. The diagnosis is easily demonstrated by imaging.

FACE AND SINUSES

DEVELOPMENT

The development of the sinuses is as follows:

- Maxillary sinus – present at birth in a rudimentary form, the maxillary sinus enlarges to lie below the level of the medial orbital wall by 1 year and the hard palate by 9 years of age, although there is much variation.
- Ethmoid sinus – develops from anterior to posterior, expanding rapidly in the first 2 years of life and again just before puberty.
- Sphenoid sinus – initially filled with red marrow which then becomes fatty, the sphenoid sinus can show pneumatization as soon as 2 years of age but is very varied. It is generally adult-like by puberty.
- Frontal sinus – begins pneumatization from the anterior ethmoid air cells at about 2 years but is visible in the anterior vertical part of the frontal bone by 10 years.

IMAGING TECHNIQUES

Evaluation of the plain radiographs of the paranasal sinuses in the young child is difficult as opacification is not necessarily pathological. Plain films should generally be deferred until the child is about 5 years of age. A single occipitomental (OM) view and/or a lateral film will be sufficent in most circumstances. In the younger child, less angulation is required to obtain adequate films of the maxillary antra. Sinus radiographs should only be requested by ENT surgeons and the indications are as follows:

- a single OM or lateral film to identify a foreign body;
- a single OM film to confirm a maxillary empyema prior to surgery; and

- a lateral view of the posterior nasopharynx to confirm adenoidal hypertrophy in a child with suspected sleep apnoea who cannot be adequately examined.

CT provides better assessment of the sinuses and will allow three-dimensional reconstructions to be performed in complex cranio-facial malformations but it is important to utilize a low-dose technique to minimize the radiation burden to the child. For sinus disease, CT images are best obtained in the coronal plane, which shows the ostiomeatal complex to advantage (Figure 14.19) but transverse images are also useful, particularly for evaluating the sphenoethmoid recess. In complex craniofacial abnormalities, transverse images are generally used to reconstruct the face in three dimensions. When assessing tumours in the nasopharyngeal area, MR should be used, with fat-suppressed sequences being especially helpful in assessing lymphadenopathy. Coronal, transverse and contrast-enhanced images should be obtained routinely.

CONGENITAL ABNORMALITIES

CHOANAL ATRESIA

The most frequently encountered bony atresia or stenosis of the nasal cavity is posterior choanal stenosis/atresia. They may be unilateral or bilateral and are due to abnormal development of the oronasal membrane. Fifty per cent of children have associated anomalies or syndromes, with the incidence being higher in those with bilateral abnormalities. Common associations are CHARGE, Treacher–Collins and Pierre Robin anomalad syndromes. Infants with bilateral obstruction present at birth or during their first feed with respiratory distress, which may be improved with crying. Children with unilateral obstruction tend to present later. Transverse and coronal CT images should be obtained and vasoconstrictive drops may be instilled into the nasal airway to help to reduce the quantity of mucous.

The classical features include:

- thickening or deviation of the vomer;
- medial deviation of the medial walls of the maxillary wall; and
- presence of a bony, fibrous or membranous bar across the posterior choanae (Figure 14.20).

There may also be elevation of the hard palate, an air–fluid level within the obstructed airway and hypoplasia of the inferior turbinates.

CONGENITAL NASAL MASSES

These include nasal encephaloceles (Figure 14.21), nasal dermoids and nasal gliomas. They result from the failure of regression of dura which crosses the prenasal space during the second month of gestation. Herniation of grey matter into the defect results in an encephalocele, sequestration of glial tissue results in a nasal glioma, and persistence of a tract of dura, which communicates with the skin, results in a dermoid/epidermoid. The latter may partly seal off but there is a potential for intracranial communication leading to recurrent meningitis and CSF leakage. These lesions may present clinically in a variety of ways. They may be an incidental finding on inspection, associated with facial malformation or present with feeding difficulties because of obstruction of the nasopharyngeal airway.

CT and MRI are the imaging modalities that best demonstrate the extent and connections of these lesions. High-resolution targeted CT of the floor of the anterior cranial fossa, especially around the crista galli, can be very informative, but MRI with direct sagittal and coronal images often more fully evaluates the lesions. Basal encephaloceles, which can be transethmoidal, sphenoethmoidal and nasoethmoidal, can herniate into the nasal cavity and MRI shows the intracranial communication. The con-

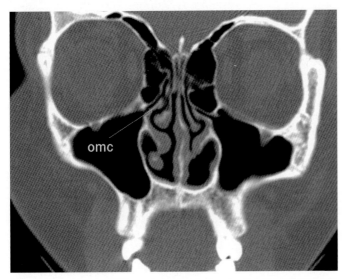

Figure 14.19 Coronal CT scan of sinuses showing the normal anatomy and ostiomeatal complex (arrowed omc).

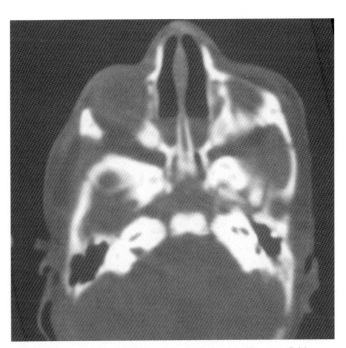

Figure 14.20 A child with bilateral choanal atresia with some fluid retention in the nares. There is a complete bony bar on the right and an incomplete one on the left.

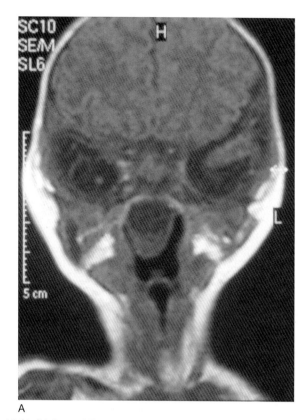

A

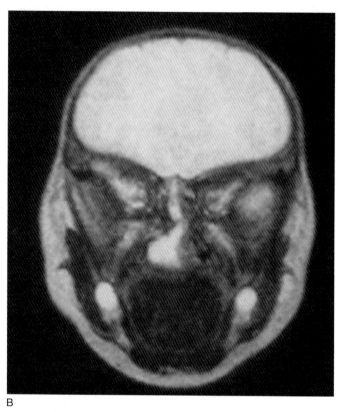

B

Figure 14.21 (A) Coronal T1- and (B) T2-weighted images, in slightly different planes, of a child with a nasal encephalocele. Note the cystic lesion projecting into the pharynx and the connection through to the brain, as shown by the high signal track on T2.

tents may be dysplastic brain tissue, gliotic tissue or brain tissue of normal appearance. As a point for differentiation, nasal encephaloceles tend to lie just off centre, whereas nasal dermoids tend to lie in the midline, possibly splitting the crista galli. Large midline defects may require vascular assessment to define the course of the anterior cranial vessels and status of the hypothalamic-pituitary axis.

NASAL DERMOIDS

These are midline lesions, presenting as a mass of variable size anywhere along the midline of the nose but most typically at the tip or at the junction of the nose and forehead (Figure 14.22). Like all dermoids the mass is basically solid and contains fatty and cholesterol components. The reason for imaging is to exclude deep connections, particularly intracranially before excision.

SINUS DISEASE

There is considerable variation in the appearance of the sinuses with age, which makes their assessment difficult. Thirty to fifty per

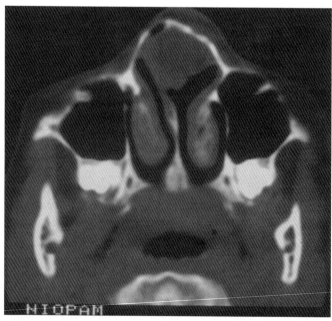

Figure 14.22 CT scan showing typical features of a large nasal dermoid, distorting and expanding the nasal bones.

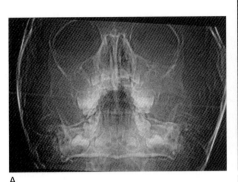
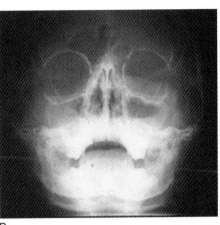
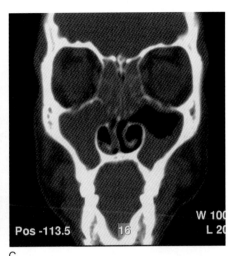

A   B   C

Figure 14.23 Sinusitis. (A) OM view showing opacity of both antra in a child with acute sinusitis. (B) A slightly older child with an air–fluid level in the left antrum due to sinusitis. Note also, almost complete opacification of the right antrum. (C) Coronal CT image of another child shows diffuse mucosal thickening with soft tissue density material filling the ethmoid sinuses, the right maxillary antrum and a large proportion of the left maxillary antrum. Note, there has been previous surgery on the left with removal of the osteomeatal complex.

cent of x-rays will show abnormalities in asymptomatic children confirming their poor sensitivity and specificity for sinusitis. CT suffers from similar problems, although the anatomical definition of the extent of any disease is superior. Both techniques can demonstrate mucosal thickening and fluid levels (Figure 14.23). Anatomical features that predispose to sinus disease as they block the ostia and thus drainage of the sinuses include a deviated nasal septum or middle turbinate and large concha. Retention cysts may develop in the sinuses (Figure 14.24).

Diffuse symmetrical changes are suggestive of allergic rhinosinusitis. Accurate definition of the extent of disease is important especially when infection extends out of the sinus into the surrounding tissues. This is particularly relevant in orbital cellulitis, where there is a risk of visual loss and cavernous sinus thrombosis in unrecognized cases. A child with acute sinus infection and proptosis requires urgent evaluation with contrast-enhanced CT. Complications of sinusitis include:

- Orbital cellulitis – usually associated with acute sinusitis, especially in the ethmoid sinuses where the lamina papyracea forms a very thin boundary between the sinus and the orbit (Figure 14.25).
- Intracranial abscess formation – especially frontal extradural empyema with frontal sinus disease (Figure 14.26).
- Cavernous and superior sagittal sinus thrombosis.
- Osteomyelitis.
- Mucocele formation – most commonly with chronic sinusitis and secondary to chronic obstruction. They may become infected or present because of mass effect. Most (60%) are frontal, with ethmoidal and maxillary being much less common (30% and 10%, respectively). Sphenoidal mucoceles are rare. Typically, CT shows an expanded, fluid-filled sinus (Figure 14.27), with a thick-enhancing rim suggesting the lesion is

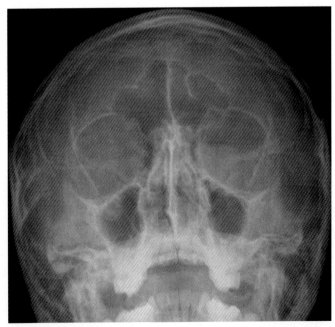

Figure 14.24 OM view of a child with a retention cyst in the superior wall of the right antrum.

infected (mucopyocele). Clearly, the lesions may have mass effect on adjacent structures producing proptosis or neurological symptoms.

- Pott's puffy tumour. This condition, which is an osteomyelitis of the frontal bone secondary to sinus infection, is rare today. Clinically, the child presents with pain over the forehead and swelling. On imaging, the destructive osteomyelitis with the associated abscess is seen. This extends intracranially to form an epidural collection.

OSTEOMAS

Osteomas may arise in the sinuses, especially the frontal sinus. They may occur in isolation but may also be part of syndromes

such as Gardner's syndrome. The bony masses may obstruct the ostia, leading to pain, sinusitis, mucocele or intracranial complications (Figure 14.28).

POLYPS

Nasal polyps are unusual in children but when they occur are most commonly associated with cystic fibrosis. In addition to the polyposis, there may be generalized thickening of the mucosal lining of the sinuses. Antrochoanal polyps also occur in the slightly older child (5–15 years) and may mimic other causes for nasopharyngeal masses such as juvenile angiofibromas, encephaloceles, intranasal dermoids and nasal gliomas. One distinguishing feature is their lack of bone erosion, a particular feature of angiofibromas.

TUMOURS OF THE SINUSES AND NASOPHARYNX

JUVENILE ANGIOFIBROMA

This is the most common benign nasopharyngeal tumour but even so is rare. It is a vascular tumour of developmental origin. It typically occurs in adolescence. The median age is 15 years and it almost exclusively affects males. Severe epistaxis, a blood-stained nasal discharge, obstruction or a mass are common clinical features. Extensive local invasion may produce cranial nerve abnormalities, proptosis or deafness. Biopsy of this very vascular lesion may produce significant bleeding.

Although a benign condition, it does have locally invasive, aggressive properties with a tendency to infiltrate and displace surrounding soft tissues. Bone destruction or bowing of the base of the pterygoid plates, especially the medial plate, is also a

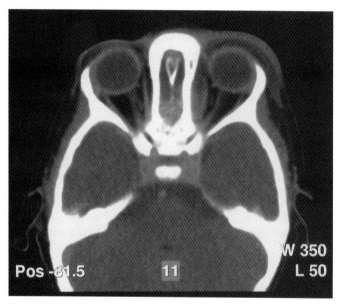

Figure 14.25 Orbital cellulitis. Transverse contrast-enhanced CT image shows left-sided orbital cellulitis with a subperiosteal abscess along the medial wall (lamina papyracea).

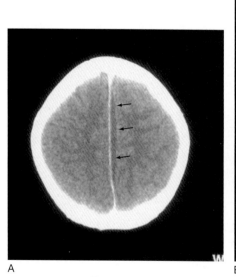

A

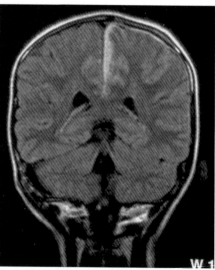

B

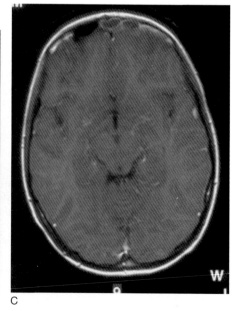

C

Figure 14.26 (A) Contrast-enhanced CT, (B) T2-weighted flair MRI and (C) T1-weighted MRI with contrast of a child with a parafalcine subdural empyema secondary to left frontal sinusitis.

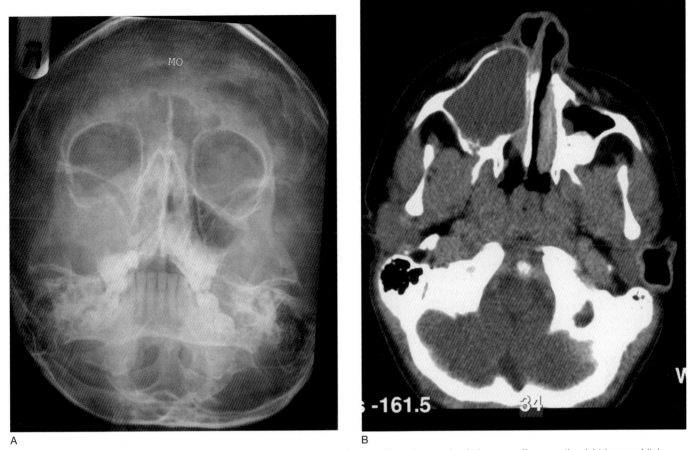

A

B

Figure 14.27 Maxillary mucocele. (A) Plain radiograph shows an opaque right maxillary sinus and soft tissue swelling over the right lower orbital margin; (B) transverse CT image shows an expanded, fluid-filled maxillary antrum.

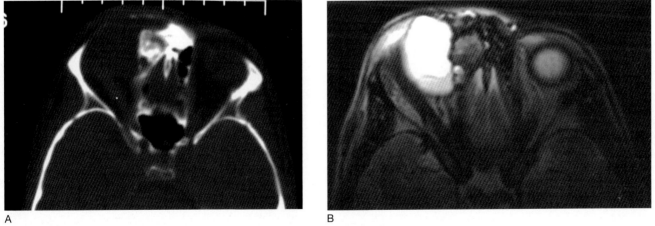

A

B

Figure 14.28 (A) Axial CT and (B) axial T2-weighted MRI of a teenager with an osteoma in the right frontal sinus causing a mucocele.

characteristic, frequently identified and an almost pathognomic finding. The lesion originates from the pterygopalatine fossa, enlarging the sphenopalatine foramen and destroying adjacent bone including the floor of the sphenoid sinus and posterior wall of the maxillary antrum.

Transverse and coronal CT gives excellent bony definition and this should be supplemented with multiplane soft tissue assessment with MRI (Figure 14.29). The tumour typically shows intense contrast enhancement, reflecting its very vascular nature. With MRI, it may also show serpiginous signal voids typical of high-flowing vascular lesions. Fat suppression should also be used and may be helpful in follow-up for disease recurrence. The sphenoid sinus should be carefully assessed, as its involvement often leads to recurrence. In some centres, formal angiography is performed routinely with preoperative embolization. Most tumours receive their vascular supply from the external carotid artery, although there may be some cross-supply from the internal carotid or, rarely, the entire lesion is fed via internal carotid branches. Thus, both internal and external carotid assessment is required.

NEOPLASMS

Other soft tissue neoplasms involving the nasopharynx and sinuses include lymphoma (Figure 14.30), rhabdomyosarcoma, neuroblastoma and nasopharyngeal carcinoma. These are discussed later in this chapter. Although not strictly a neoplasm, Langerhans' cell histiocytosis also causes marked bony destruction mimicking some of the 'true' neoplasms.

The clinical features are generally similar regardless of the underlying cause with nasal obstruction, epistaxis, proptosis and pain being typical features. The tumours may be part of a systemic, multifocal process, such as lymphoma, or may be localized to the nasopharynx, such as nasopharyngeal carcinoma. In either event,

the role of the radiologist is to define the extent of the disease process for staging purposes, and perhaps aid in localization for biopsy. CT is useful in assessing bony involvement (Figure 14.31) but generally MRI, supplemented with contrast-enhanced images, provides a better overall assessment of disease. Staging of disease may also require chest CT and isotope imaging, perhaps with positron emission tomography (PET). Careful evaluation as part of clinical trials has had a significant impact on some childhood malignancies. In rhabdomyosarcoma the overall survival has improved from 25% in 1970 to 75% in 1990. One of the consequences of treatment is growth failure of the facial structures, if radiotherapy is part of the treatment.

Bone and cartilage tumours such as chordoma, Ewing's and osteogenic sarcoma, chondromas and chondrosarcoma may also occur and generally the principles of imaging are similar to those above, although bony lesions require CT evaluation (Figure 14.32). Chordomas arise from notochordal remnants in the basisphenoid bone and may extend anteriorly into the nasopharynx and posteriorly to abut the pons and brainstem (Figure 14.33). The lesions are generally heterogeneous in appearance and are best demonstrated with MRI. Ewing's tumour and osteogenic sarcoma are rare and have imaging features similar to those seen elsewhere in the body. Dense plaques of calcification within a soft tissue mass typify chondroma and chondrosarcoma, and are best demonstrated by CT. These may occur in the nasal cavity or sinuses. Fibrous dysplasia produces typical appearances of ground glass enlargement of the facial bones (Figure 14.34) but may clinically mimic a more aggressive lesion.

FACIAL TRAUMA

Imaging of facial trauma is dealt with in depth in Chapter 12.15.

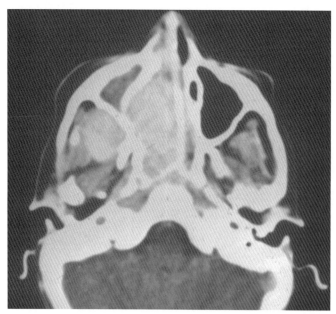

Figure 14.29 Juvenile angiofibroma. Transverse contrast-enhanced CT scan shows a large enhancing mass in the nasopharynx extending into the infratemporal fossa and right nasal airway.

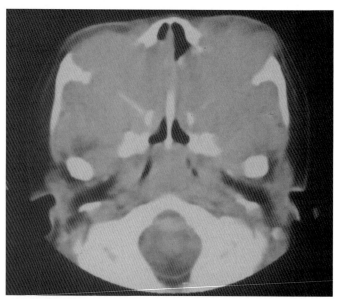

Figure 14.30 Child of 4 years of age who presented with epistaxis. Note total infiltration of sinuses and nasal cavity with soft tissue masses. On biopsy, this was found to be B-cell lymphoma.

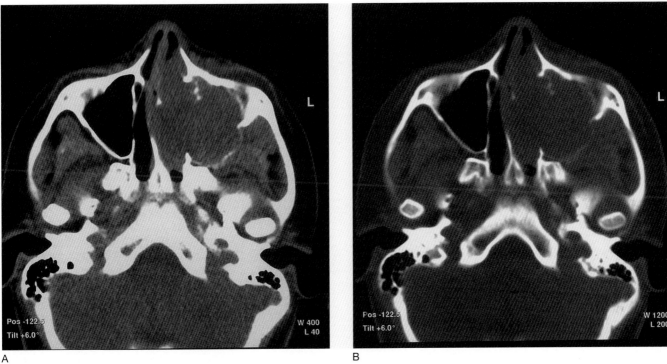

A   B

Figure 14.31 Paranasal rhabdomyosarcoma. Transverse CT images on (A) soft tissue and (B) bony setting show an expansile mass involving the left maxillary sinus with destruction and distortion of the medial and lateral walls of the antrum.

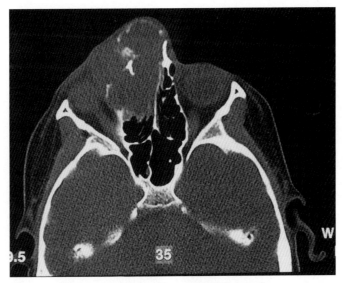

Figure 14.32 Ewing's sarcoma. Transverse CT image shows a destructive, expansile soft tissue mass involving the right anterior ethmoid region and extending into the orbital roof.

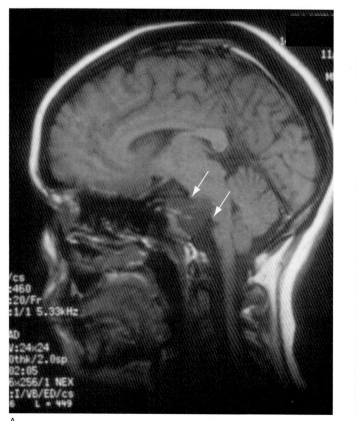

A

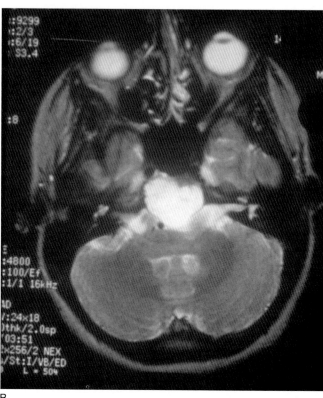

B

Figure 14.33 (A) Sagittal T1- and (B) axial T2-weighted images of a child with a clivus chordoma that extends posteriorly towards the brain-stem. The location is typical.

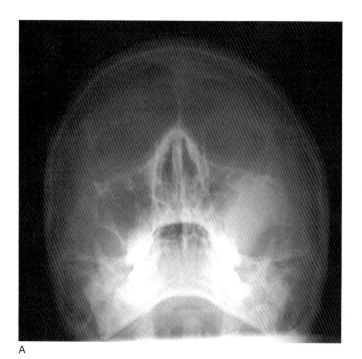

A

Figure 14.34 Fibrous dysplasia. (A) Plain film shows typical appearances with a ground glass density and expansion of the lateral wall of the left maxillary antrum. (B) Transverse CT image confirms the extent of the abnormality, almost filling the antrum on this single slice.

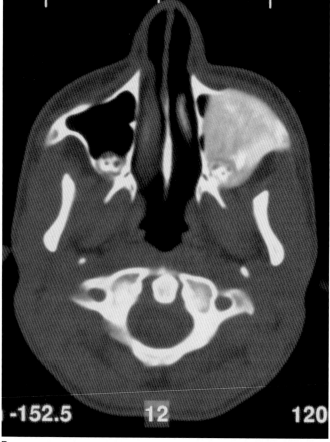

B

THROAT AND UPPER AIRWAY

PATHOPHYSIOLOGY

From an ENT perspective, the airway can be divided into five main regions:

1. nasal airway;
2. pharyngeal airway;
3. larynx;
4. trachea; and
5. bronchial airway.

The airway above the larynx is easily distended and its patency is determined by muscle tone. The part of the airway with most tendency to close is the upper oropharynx at the level of the soft palate. Also, the tonsils and adenoids can have considerable influence on the calibre of the nasopharynx and oropharynx in the young child. The airway below the larynx may initially be quite soft and collapse in the first few years of life until cartilaginous development forms a more rigid, supportive structure.

IMAGING TECHNIQUES

RADIOGRAPHY

Plain radiography of the airway is generally restricted to a lateral film, where air acts as a negative contrast medium to outline the structures. The film should be obtained during inspiration and the neck slightly extended if possible, as there is considerable variation in appearances with posture in the young child. This is particularly so when the neck is flexed and the child is breathing out, to the extent where soft tissue swelling can mimic a pharyngeal mass. High kilovoltage radiography with added tube filtration used to be recommended for airway assessment but this is no longer required since the advent of digitally enhanced computed radiography (Figure 14.35), multislice CT and MRI, all of which give much better detail.

FLUOROSCOPY

Assessment of swallowing and phonation requires fluoroscopy of the upper airway and most importantly the assistance of a speech therapist. For swallowing, sequential analysis of the swallowing cycle requires recording of data on videotape or other media storage device for careful assessment. In general, lateral screening only will suffice and the following features should be noted:

- tongue movement;
- presence of nasopharyngeal reflux;
- time of initiation of the swallow;
- presence of pooling in the hypopharynx before or after swallowing;
- presence of laryngeal penetration of contrast; and
- presence of aspiration and whether it induces a cough reflex.

Most children require assessment with at least three types of food consistency. Yoghurt mixed with barium, thickened barium

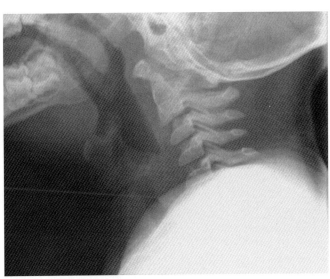

Figure 14.35 Lateral view of the soft tissues of the neck. Normal computed radiography image.

and liquid barium should all be assessed, with other foodstuffs used as appropriate. In the very young child, the yoghurt should be omitted. For phonation studies, ideally a small quantity of barium is administered to each nostril, then sniffed so as to coat the soft palate. Clearly very young children find this distressing and barium may have to be omitted. Fluoroscopy is performed with the child in a modified Towne's view (chin-tuck) to obtain a tangential view of the velopharyngeal portal and then subsequently in the lateral projection. When no barium has been administered only the lateral projection is performed. Again the examination is recorded on videotape.

Velopalatine movement can also be successfully performed with MRI, using short T1-weighted sequences during phonation of different sounds and replaying them in cine mode. In cooperative children, this is a satisfactory alternative to fluoroscopy.

CT AND MRI

CT and MRI are also useful tools in assessing the larynx and upper airway, although more specialized MRI is required to allow snapshot images that are free from movement artifact. Volume acquired CT information can be used to assess the upper airway and may be used to generate virtual bronchoscopic images.

BRONCHOSCOPY

Some children benefit from careful evaluation of the airway using dynamic bronchography, where a small quantity of non-ionic water-soluble contrast is injected into the trachea and bronchi (Figure 14.36). This is limited to children requiring full ventilatory support and should only be done with full resuscitation facilities available. Clearly its use is restricted to specialized paediatric centres. It is mainly used for confirmation of suspected anatomical abnormalities or to confirm the extent of tracheobronchomalacia.

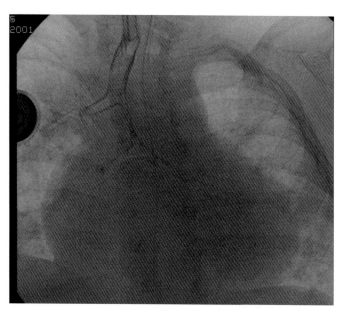

Figure 14.36 Tracheobronchogram. Single frontal image from a dynamic study shows a bronchus suis and diffuse narrowing of the distal trachea.

ULTRASOUND

Ultrasound is a valuable and important method of assessing the neck and thoracic inlet, and combined with Doppler studies and colour flow provides essential information about neck masses. More recently, ultrasound has been used to assess the unossified, cartilaginous structures of the larynx with some success. It has the advantages of providing real-time images under physiological conditions and is generally performed in the transverse plane. It is particularly useful in assessing vocal cord movement (Figure 14.37) and subglottic lesions such as haemangiomas. High-resolution linear array probes with a small footplate are used. The examination should be video recorded.

Ultrasound is the initial imaging technique for neck masses.

AIRWAY OBSTRUCTION

Airway obstruction often results in abnormal upper airway sounds, stertor or stridor. Stertor results from sounds arising in the nasopharyngeal region and is typically associated with obstructive sleep apnoea. Stridor arises from further down the airway at a laryngeal or tracheal level.

OBSTRUCTIVE SLEEP APNOEA SYNDROME

This condition is characterized by intermittent partial or complete obstruction of the upper airway during sleep. Snoring is a characteristic clinical feature, with day-time features being irritability, mouth-breathing, behaviour disturbance, cognitive dysfunction and hyperactivity. The causes can be divided into four main areas:

1. Oropharyngeal – tonsillar enlargement, macroglossia, retrognathia.
2. Nasal/nasopharyngeal – adenoidal enlargement, allergic rhinitis, deviation of the nasal septum.
3. Systemic disease – cerebral palsy, reticuloses, sickle cell disease, Prader–Willi syndrome, achondroplasia, glycogen storage disease;
4. Craniofacial syndromes – Down's, Apert's, Treacher–Collins and Crouzon's syndromes.

Imaging should include a lateral neck x-ray with the mouth closed and the neck in a neutral position to assess the patency of the nasopharyngeal airway. Fluoroscopy and cross-sectional imaging may also be helpful.

Adenoidal enlargement is frequent in young children, especially in geographical areas with damp climates and pollution (Figure 14.38). Tonsillar enlargement is not dependent on similar factors and is due to infection.

Central causes of sleep apnoea include damage to the respiratory centres in the brainstem following trauma or infection such as encephalitis. This is known as Ondine's curse. The Pickwickian syndrome describes children who are pathologically obese, with poor respiratory drive who become chronically hypoxic and

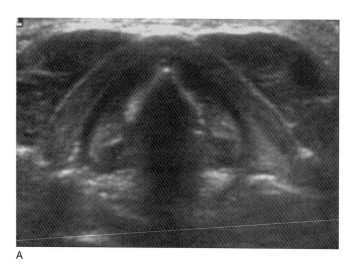

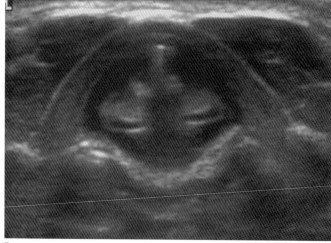

Figure 14.37 Ultrasound of the larynx showing transverse images (A) relaxed and (B) during phonation.

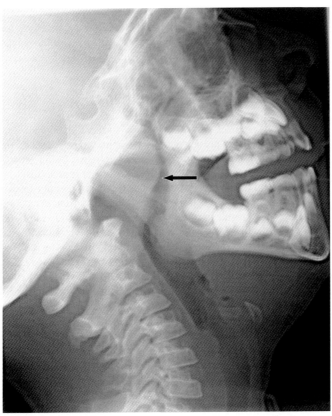

Figure 14.38 Lateral radiograph of upper airway demonstrating extensive adenoidal enlargement (arrow), narrowing the nasopharynx.

develop respiratory failure. These children may also suffer sleep apnoea.

STRIDOR

Stridor is a high-pitched musical noise resulting from obstruction in the larynx or upper trachea. The causes can be divided into supraglottic, glottic and subglottic:

Supraglottic causes:

1. Laryngomalacia – a clinical and endoscopic diagnosis.
2. Epiglottitis – a clinical diagnosis (see below).
3. Extrinsic compression – from masses, vascular lesions and cysts. These generally require ultrasound and subsequent cross-sectional imaging for further assessment.
4. Laryngeal cyst – intrinsic cyst may be shown endoscopically or on imaging.
5. Foreign body.

Glottic causes:

1. Laryngeal web or cleft – an endoscopic diagnosis, occasionally requiring contrast studies for confirmation of communication between oesophagus and trachea.
2. Recurrent respiratory papillomata – an endoscopic diagnosis, with human papilloma virus, types 6 and 11 implicated, and transmitted via the birth canal from maternal condylomata (Figure 14.39).
3. Vocal cord palsy – endoscopic or ultrasound diagnosis but the underlying cause will need defining with neck and chest

imaging using CT or MRI. Assessment of the brainstem and craniocervical junction may also be warranted.
4. Foreign body.

Subglottic causes:

1. Laryngotracheobronchitis (Croup) – see below.
2. Subglottic stenosis – congenital or acquired. A history of previous intubation suggests an acquired cause (Figure 14.40). Endoscopy may be supplemented with plain films or CT with multiplanar reconstruction. It is important to define the length of the stenosis prior to any surgery. MRI may be indicated to delineate any vascular compression.

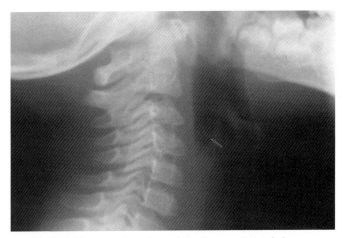

Figure 14.39 Pharyngeal papilloma. Note the rounded soft tissue mass lying in the pyriform fossa behind the epiglottis (arrow).

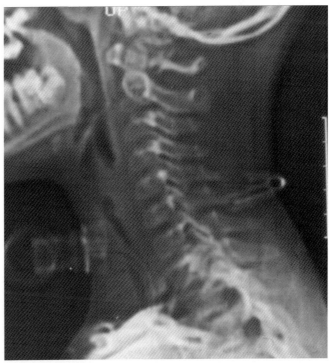

Figure 14.40 Lateral scout CT image of a boy with a tracheostomy tube *in situ*. Note subglottic narrowing of the airway. This was due to prolonged intubation required to manage a severe head injury.

3. Tracheomalacia – generally a diagnosis confirmed by endoscopy. In selected cases dynamic bronchography may be very informative in ventilated patients, especially when combined with airway pressure evaluation. Electron beam CT may also be useful. It may occur as a primary condition, be associated with vascular rings, and to some degree is invariable with tracheoesophageal fistulas. Tracheobronchomalacia is frequent in children with Down's syndrome in early life.

4. Haemangioma – usually presents at 1–2 months of age and is confirmed endoscopically but can also be demonstrated with ultrasound. As with other haemangiomata in infants, it tends to increase in size initially and then involute. The clinical challenge is managing the airway during the growth period. Assessment with CT and MRI may be useful to monitor the progress and assess the extent of the lesion outside direct endoscopic visualization.

5. Abnormal vessels – when endoscopy suggests an extrinsic pulsatile lesion, MRI or contrast CT should be used to define vascular anatomy. The commonest abnormal finding is a distal origin of the right subclavian artery, resulting in the vessel crossing anterior to the trachea. Other vascular causes may include, for example, a double aortic arch (Figure 14.41).

6. Complete tracheal ring – a variant of complete tracheal stenosis. Plain films and CT may help to make the diagnosis.

7. Foreign body.

INFLAMMATORY LESIONS

TONSILLITIS

This is a common paediatric condition that generally does not require imaging, unless there is failure to respond to treatment and extratonsillar spread or abscess formation is suspected. In these cases, contrast-enhanced CT provides excellent detail on disease extent. Ultrasound may also be helpful in localizing collections for aspiration. On a lateral radiograph, tonsil, at the back of the palate, is seen projecting into the pharynx (Figure 14.42).

RETROPHARYNGEAL ABSCESS

Fever, dysphagia, neck stiffness, drooling and swelling are all clinical pointers to the presence of a retropharyngeal abscess. In general, if an inflammatory tonsillar or pharyngeal lesion fails to respond adequately to treatment, with a persistent leucocytosis, an abscess should be excluded. Pharyngeal perforation either from a foreign body, iatrogenic (Figure 14.43) cause or non-accidental injury may also result in a retropharyngeal abscess. On radiography, there is widening of the soft tissues in the retropharyngeal area. An air–fluid level may be present and there is loss of the normal cervical lordosis (Figure 14.44). Contrast-enhanced CT is the modality of choice, with an abscess shown as a focal ring-enhancing, low attenuation lesion within an area of soft tissue swelling (Figure 14.45). The abscess may be multilocular. The relationship to adjacent vessels will also be useful information to the surgeon contemplating drainage. Unrecognized pharyngeal perforation may cause a diverticulum with or without associated mediastinitis.

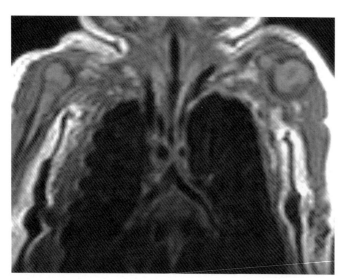

Figure 14.41 Double aortic arch producing tracheal compression; coronal T1-weighted MR image.

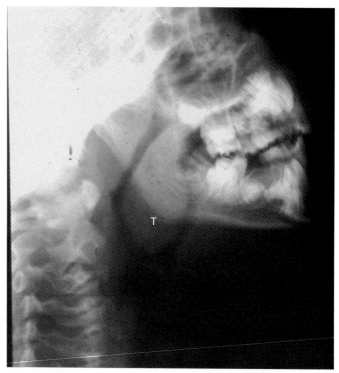

Figure 14.42 Lateral radiograph of the nasopharynx showing massive tonsillar enlargement in addition to adenoidal enlargement, causing marked airway narrowing.

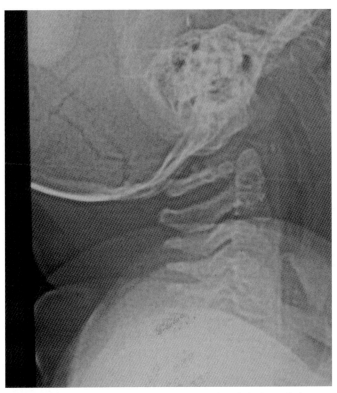

Figure 14.43 Lateral radiograph of neck showing air in the soft tissues surrounding the pharynx and extending in the precervical region behind the trachea. This was due to a pharyngeal perforation caused by incorrect nasogastric intubation.

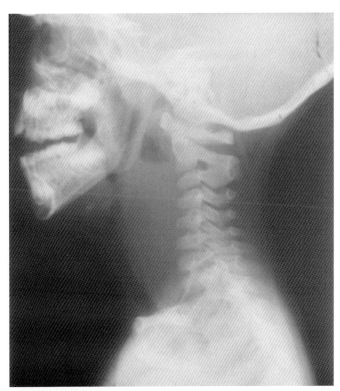

Figure 14.44 Lateral radiograph of neck showing marked widening of the prevertebral soft tissues with an air–fluid level. These are the appearances of a retropharyngeal abscess. Note also loss of cervical lordosis.

CERVICAL ADENITIS

Cervical lymphadenopathy is a common finding in children, the majority of cases being due to infection. This is usually bacterial but with persistent non-responsive adenopathy, atypical mycobacterium or tuberculosis should be considered. Sinus formation is more common in the latter conditions. Rarely, non-infective lymphadenopathy is encountered due to, for example, histiocytosis or systemic lupus.

The lymph nodes in the neck of children are generally larger and more numerous than in adults. They also tend to be bilaterally symmetrical. The oropharynx is constantly exposed to new organisms during childhood and this probably accounts for the increased size and reactivity of the surrounding lymph nodes. Ultrasound should be used and is generally the only modality required to confirm the diagnosis. There is considerable variation in the size of normal lymph nodes but important ultrasound features of normal lymph nodes are (Figure 14.46):

1. hypoechoic hypertrophied germinal cortex;
2. hyperechoic central medullary lymphoid; and
3. active vascular pattern.

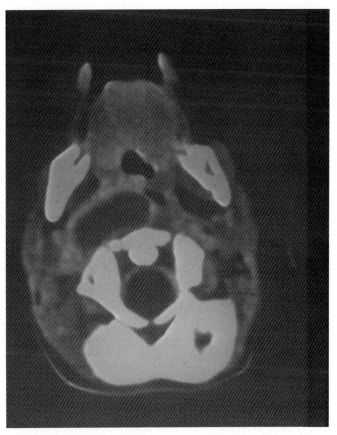

Figure 14.45 Transverse contrast-enhanced CT image of the neck shows a retropharyngeal abscess on the right.

Abnormal lymph nodes are typified by (Figure 14.47):

1. rounded appearance;
2. generalized hypoechogenicity;
3. increased vascularity (relative to other nodes); and
4. increased echogenicity of perinodal fat.

With further progression of inflammation, necrosis and abscess formation can occur, resulting in hypovascular areas, a hyperechoic 'snow-storm' echopattern and eventually a hypoechoic collection. The presence of a 'collar stud' rupture appearance and calcification is highly suggestive of tuberculous infection. Assessment of other anatomical sites for lymphadenopathy, may give support to a diagnosis of viral infection, such as cytomegalovirus, glandular fever or varicella-zoster. Rarely, assessment with CT or MRI is required, especially to assess more deeply placed nodes. Fat suppressed MR sequences should be used routinely.

Lymphoma or leukaemia may occasionally cause some confusion, although clinically they are usually easy to distinguish from infective causes.

ATYPICAL MYCOBACTERIUM

There are numerous types of mycobacteria in the environment that do not normally cause disease. Infection with atypical mycobacteria that becomes clinically manifest usually presents in children as cervical adenopathy. Unlike inflammatory adenopathy from other organisms, this does not respond well to antimicrobial treatment. Surgical excision is the treatment of choice if it is resistant. As previously stated, atypical mycobacterial nodes are particularly prone to forming a sinus track (Figure 14.48). This may lie in close proximity to the salivary glands. Radiographically, atypical mycobacterial glands and tuberculous glands cannot be distinguished unless there is calcification or concomitant chest disease. On ultrasound the glands are matted together and may have necrotic centres.

ACUTE EPIGLOTTITIS

This is a life-threatening condition, usually occurring between 2 and 4 years of age. In those countries where *Haemophilus influenzae* vaccination is routine, there has been a dramatic reduction in

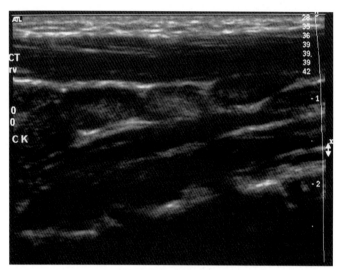

Figure 14.46 Normal ultrasound cervical lymph nodes. Ovoid shape with typical echopattern demonstrated.

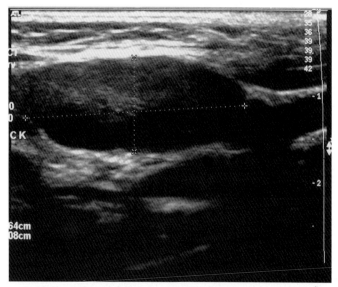

Figure 14.47 Abnormal ultrasound of cervical lymph node. Enlarged node with prominent hypoechoic area typifies pathological adenopathy.

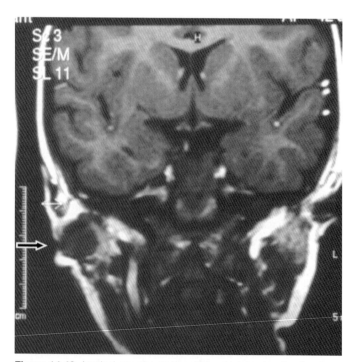

Figure 14.48 Atypical mycobacterium. Note sinus track extending from the parotid region to the neck.

the incidence of acute epiglottitis. The diagnosis is a clinical one, with the typical child being feverish, drooling and sitting upright to maintain the airway. There is inspiratory stridor. The epiglottis is swollen and cherry-red in appearance. Children are prone to acute laryngospasm and therefore distress should be minimized. Radiography is not indicated unless the condition of the child is so stable as to question the diagnosis. In practical terms, it is far safer to obtain appropriate ENT or anaesthetic support than obtain any radiographs. If a radiograph is taken, the epiglottis is swollen (Figure 14.49).

LARYNGOTRACHEOBRONCHITIS (CROUP)

Croup is a common condition caused by parainfluenza and influenza viruses. It is more common in the winter months and usually affects children between 1 and 3 years old. Children have a barking cough and stridor. There is subglottic oedema resulting in a tapered appearance to the upper trachea, sometimes termed a 'steeple-shaped' or 'wine-bottle' appearance. Radiographs of the trachea are not usually indicated but chest x-rays may be performed. These may show lung changes associated with infection, such as atelectasis but also may demonstrate the upper tracheal tapering. More severe bacterial tracheobronchitis may present similarly but there is associated high fever.

GRISEL'S SYNDROME

Grisel's syndrome, or non-traumatic subluxation of the atlantoaxial joint, is a rare condition resulting from inflammatory liga-

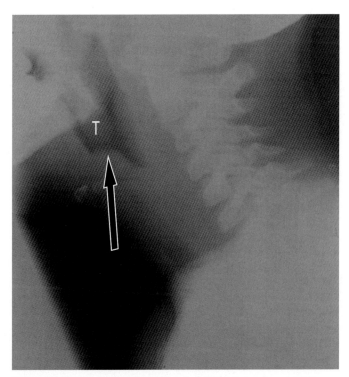

Figure 14.49 The lateral radiograph of a child with acute epiglottitis. Note the swollen epiglottis (arrow). T, tonsil.

mentous laxity secondary to pharyngeal infection tracking back to the C1/2 articulation. The child presents with torticollis, which if it does not resolve, results in atlantoaxial rotatory fixation requiring halo traction. Persistence of torticollis for more than 1 week is an indication for orthopaedic referral. Most inflammatory neck infections have been associated with the condition. Evaluation requires plain films and cross-sectional imaging.

THYROIDITIS

Imaging of this condition is described in Chapter 6.4.

MASSES OF THE NECK AND AIRWAYS

CONGENITAL NON-VASCULAR NECK MASSES

THORNWALDT'S CYST

This is an embryological remnant that is usually of no clinical significance unless it becomes infected. It lies in the posterior-superior pharyngeal wall and is usually an incidental finding. Typically, it appears as a fluid-filled cyst and is most obvious on MRI. When infected it can form a large inflammatory mass.

PYRIFORM SINUS FISTULA (ABSCESS)

This rare branchial pouch abnormality connects the apex of the pyriform sinus with the thyroid gland. They are frequently left-sided, occasionally right-sided or bilateral. They usually present with a neck abscess, rarely a sinus or suppurative thyroiditis. CT or MRI is useful in the acute phase but a contrast study may show the sinus track if performed after the acute inflammatory changes have resolved.

PLUNGING RANULA

These are acquired inflammatory retention cysts of the sublingual glands that subsequently rupture into the submental region to form a pseudocyst. US will confirm a cystic lesion but MRI delineates the presence of submandibular fluid connecting to the floor of the mouth (Figure 14.50).

BRANCHIAL CLEFT ANOMALIES

During embryological development, a membrane separates the branchial clefts, which arise from the ectoderm, from the pharyngeal pouches, which arise from the endoderm. There are six branchial arches in all but the first and second are the most important pathologically (Figure 14.51). The first arch abnormalities give rise to submandibular and preauricular lesions and cause cleft defects in the palate and lips and mandibular hypoplasia. Abnormalities of the third and fourth arches are extremely rare and occa-

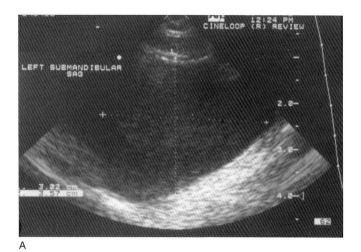

A

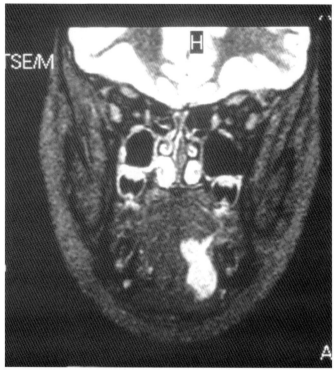

B

Figure 14.50 (A) Ultrasound and (B) coronal MR scan in two children with a plunging ranula. Note on the ultrasound, the slightly echogenic fluid. On the MRI, the track from the ranula to the floor of the mouth is elegantly demonstrated.

sionally produce deep cysts. The fifth and sixth are rudimentary. Developmental anomalies of the second arch result mainly from overgrowth of this arch in a caudal distribution and are more common than anomalies of the other five arches. These include cysts, sinuses, fistulas and cartilaginous remnants with skin tags. The clinical presentation of anomalies of the branchial clefts depends on which portions remain patent. If a branchial cleft remains patent then there is a sinus draining to the skin surface (Figure 14.52). Cysts have no communication with the pharynx or skin but lie along the tract of the branchial cleft or pouch. Sinuses

are blind-ended and either communicate with the skin, an external sinus, or the pharynx, an internal sinus. Fistulas are duct-like structures connecting the skin to the pharynx. A branchial sinus is situated laterally on the neck at the anterior border of the sternomastoid muscle. This distinguishes it from a thyroglossal fistula, which is in the midline. Children with branchial sinuses present with recurrent discharge. Secondary infection can occur but is more frequently found in blind cysts. Though the lesion can be shown by MRI, a sinogram may be needed to outline the anatomy prior to surgery.

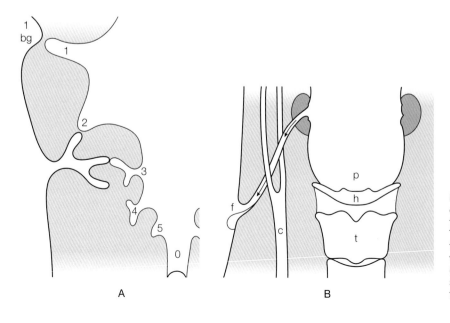

A   B

Figure 14.51 (A) Schematic drawing of the development of branchial arches and grooves. The first becomes the external acoustic meatus by term. The other grooves, which lie opposite, the second, third and fourth arches, form the cervical sinus, which is obliterated by term as the neck develops. (B) Schematic drawing of the position of a branchial sinus fistula. p = pharynx, h = hypoid bone, t = trachea, c = common carotid artery, f = fistula.

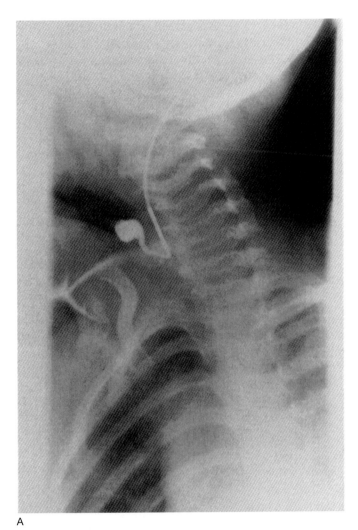

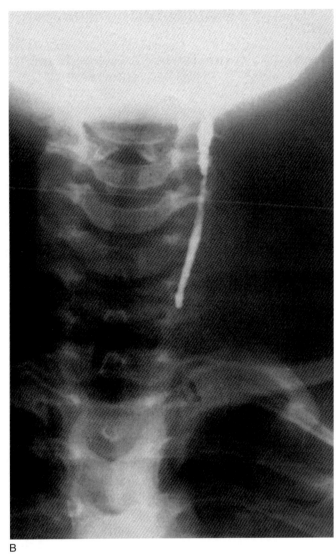

A

B

Figure 14.52 (A) Sinogram of a branchial sinus. A sialographic cannula, inserted into the orifice, fills a fluid sac. (B) Sinogram of a branchial sinus showing the characteristic location of the track anterior to the sternomastoid muscle.

Generally, cysts can be assessed with ultrasound initially to confirm their nature, although they can be rather echogenic if they contain keratin and cholesterol crystals. Contrast-enhanced CT demonstrates a thin-walled uni- or multilocular cyst, with wall enhancement suggesting infection. Fluid is usually of water density unless infected. MR imaging can demonstrate a characteristic beak extending between the internal and external carotid arteries, which is pathognomonic for a second branchial cleft cyst. Depending on the contents, T1-weighted images may show high signal if there are blood products, protein or cholesterol crystals present.

STERNOMASTOID 'TUMOUR'

This condition is also known as fibromatosis colli or congenital muscular torticollis. Birth trauma is thought to be the primary underlying pathology, although intrauterine posture has also been suggested as a possible cause, since fibrotic changes can be well established. Fibrosis and shortening of the sternomastoid muscle results in head and neck rotation. The mass is usually seen between 2 and 8 weeks of age. Ultrasound is used to demonstrate increased echogenicity and typically fusiform thickening of the sternomastoid, although occasionally the entire muscle is involved. The distal third is most commonly affected, with no predilection to either side of the neck. Most cases respond to physiotherapy, although a small number will require surgery to prevent development of facial hemihyperplasia.

THYROGLOSSAL DUCTS

For a description of thyroglossal ducts please refer to Chapter 6.4.

MALIGNANT TUMOURS OF THE NECK AND AIRWAYS

Malignant tumours arising in the neck include the following:

1. lymphoma;
2. rhabdomyosarcoma;
3. nasopharyngeal carcinoma;
4. neuroblastoma;
5. thyroid carcinoma (see Chapter 6.4);
6. sarcomas – osteogenic sarcoma, Ewing's sarcoma, neurofibrosarcoma; and
7. germ cell tumours.

Malignant tumours of the head and neck may represent part of a more generalized disease, e.g. lymphoma, or they may represent local disease such as occurs with neck nodes in Hodgkin's disease with disease confined to the neck. They may also be the location of a primary tumour that may occur anywhere in the body, e.g. rhabdomyosarcoma or primitive neurectodermal tumours. A primary head and neck tumour is a nasopharyngeal carcinoma. Clinical presentation of head and neck tumours may be the presence of a neck mass or lymph nodes, a blocked nose, pain and in the case of a cervical neuroblastoma, Horner's syndrome.

IMAGING

The role of imaging is to define the extent of disease for staging purposes and possibly to guide biopsy. Initial imaging for a focal mass is usually ultrasound. The appearances are usually non-specific. Calcification may be present in neuroblastoma but is not specific to it. Nodes other than the mass may be seen. Cross-sectional imaging will be required for full assessment, accurate staging and follow-up, combined with bone scintigraphy and, increasingly, PET studies.

The decision to use MRI or contrast-enhanced CT will depend on their availability and the child's cooperation. Even though chest CT will be performed to assess for metastases, a baseline chest film will be necessary for comparison during follow-up. Particular note should be made of any tracheal compression or deviation so that the anaesthetists can be alerted to the problem prior to intubation. MRI should include T1-weighted, T2-weighted and fat suppressed sequences in axial and coronal planes. Particular note should be made of any extension into the infratemporal fossa.

Initial staging and follow-up should be performed in concordance with the tumour protocols in use in that country. The role of PET in the management of children's head and neck tumours has yet to be established. At present in the UK it is used sporadically and mainly to try and resolve the significance of any persisting nodal enlargement after treatment.

LYMPHOMA

Head and neck lymphoma may affect the retropharyngeal tissues, the sinuses, the orbits and the neck nodes. B-cell lymphoma is the more usual in the retropharynx, orbits and sinuses. Burkitt's lymphoma, seen in particular in African children, has an association with Epstein–Barr virus. This produces massive swelling of the mandible and neck nodes. Hodgkin's disease is more frequent in older children than in those younger than 10 years of age. T-cell lymphoma may affect children of all ages and is usually associated with extensive mediastinal disease.

The imaging appearances are non-specific. There is nodal enlargement, which is usually extensive. It may be unilateral or bilateral. Soft tissue masses are seen in the sinuses, retropharynx and orbits when disease is present here. In general, bone destruction is less extensive with lymphoma than with rhabdomyosarcoma. Contrast enhancement with gadolinium occurs but this is moderate.

RHABDOMYOSARCOMA AND PRIMITIVE NEUROECTODERMAL TUMOURS (PNETS)

Both of these can have similar appearances on imaging (Figures 14.53 and 14.54). They are soft tissue masses with, in general, poorly defined margins. PNETs tend to be confined to the soft tissues at presentation while rhabdomyosarcomas frequently involve bone destruction especially in the region of the sinuses, orbits and retropharynx. They both enhance with gadolinium. Both CT and MRI are required for the demonstration of the full extent of the disease. Unlike lymphoma, the disease is usually unilateral. Both tumours have a high likelihood of local recurrence. Distant metastases are to nodes, soft tissues and the lung.

NASOPHARYNGEAL CARCINOMA

This tumour is less frequent than lymphoma, rhabdomyosarcoma and PNET as a head and neck tumour in childhood. Its clinical presentation and imaging appearances are similar to a rhabdomyosarcoma or PNET (Figure 14.55). Recurrent disease is mainly local. The prognosis for nasopharyngeal carcinoma in children is better than for rhabdomyosarcoma and PNET.

NEUROBLASTOMA

The imaging characteristics and the staging of neuroblastomas are described in Chapter 6.7. The presentation is variable and includes stridor, pain, a palpable mass and, as described above, Horner's syndrome. The prognosis for cervical neuroblastoma is better than for abdominal lesions.

SARCOMAS

The imaging appearance of sarcomas of the neck and airways is similar to sarcomas found elsewhere in the body. Confusion arises because of the unusual location.

SECOND MALIGNANCIES

The development of second malignancies is one of the rare but tragic occurrences in children who survive treatment for childhood cancer. The reasons for this are probably multifactorial and include genetic predisposition, chemotherapy and radiation treatment. The most frequent primary neoplasms associated with second malignancies are lymphoma, leukaemia, retinoblastoma, medulloblastoma and neuroblastoma. The most frequent second malignancies

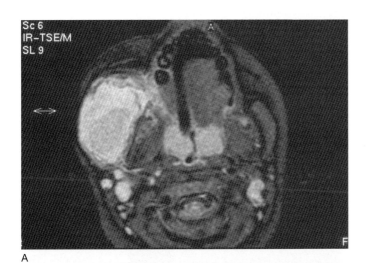

A

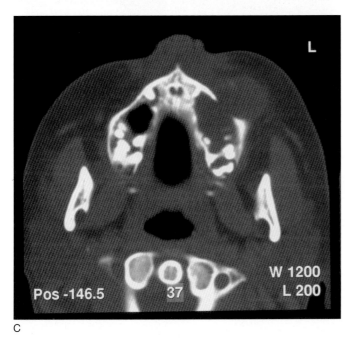

C

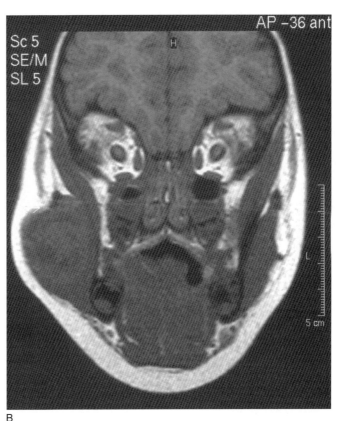

B

Figure 14.53 (A) Axial fat suppressed and (B) coronal T1-weighted image of a child with a facial rhabdomyosarcoma. The MRI features are non-specific but indicate a solid tumour. (C) CT scan of a different child showing a rhabdomyosarcoma eroding the left maxilla.

are those in the CNS, sarcomas, thyroid and parotid gland tumours and acute myelogenous leukaemia. The imaging appearances of the second tumour are those that one would expect for the tumour. There are no specific features to mark it as a second malignancy.

VASCULAR LESIONS OF THE HEAD AND NECK

Vascular lesions of the head and neck are common in children. Their terminology and classification has caused considerable confusion in the past. They are discussed more fully in Chapter 8.

Two of these lesions are a glomus jugulare tumour and jugular venous ectasia. The latter may present as a soft cystic swelling in the lateral aspects of the neck. The diagnosis is easily made, both by duplex and colour Doppler. A glomus jugulare tumour, also known as a chemodectoma, is a solid vascular tumour arising in the region of the jugular vein, and may even lie within it. On ultrasound, it is shown to be a solid mass but is not necessarily very vascular.

The following conditions are described in Chapter 8:

- Vascular tumours
  - Haemangioma
  - Kaposiform haemangioendothelioma
- Vascular malformations
  - Capillary malformation
  - Venous malformation
  - Lymphatic malformation – formally cystic hygroma, lymphangioma
  - Arteriovenous malformation
  - Combined vascular malformation.

FOREIGN BODIES

For the purposes of this section, comments are restricted to the postnasal space and upper airway, although children may also put objects up their nose. When unobserved and not removed foreign

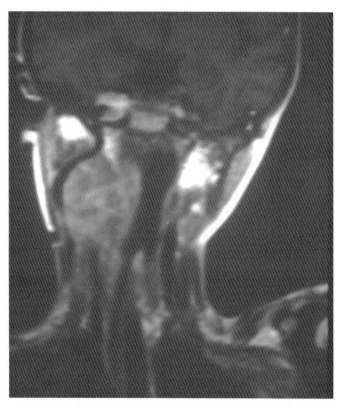

Figure 14.54 Coronal T1-weighted image with gadolinium of a child with a large soft tissue tumour on the right side of the neck that, on biopsy, was a PNET. Note that the appearance of this is very similar to the rhabdomyosarcoma seen in Figure 14.53.

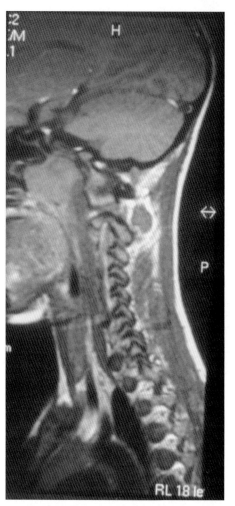

Figure 14.55 Sagittal T1-weighted image with gadolinium showing a retropharyngeal mass extending proximally towards the infratemporal fossa. This, on biopsy, was a nasopharyngeal carcinoma but any soft tissue tumour would have the same appearance.

bodies (FBs) can lead to purulent nasal discharge. While opaque objects will be seen on x-ray, non-opaque ones will not.

It is important to emphasize that not all FBs are radiopaque and children may not give any history of inhalation. Clinical features depend on the site of the FB but include nasal discharge, pain on swallowing, drooling, food refusal and stridor. A lateral film may confirm the presence of a radiopaque FB. It is important to remember that thyroid and cricoid calcification is unusual before the third decade. The tonsils are a typical site for impaction but more important is identification of an FB lying just above the larynx, since these are at risk of completely occluding the airway. Fish or chicken bones (Figure 14.56) are commonly implicated as causes for impacted FBs and visualization depends on the degree of calcification of the 'bone' involved and a good quality lateral radiograph of the pharynx with it well distended with air. They appear as linear opacities projected across the airway. Non-opaque FBs cannot be seen without contrast studies but if located in the pharynx are best identified at endoscopy.

When an FB impacts slightly more distally, the common location is at the level of the thoracic inlet. Opaque FBs, such as a coin,

are visible on x-ray. A lateral radiograph confirms the oesophageal location. Non-opaque FBs will require a contrast study for their demonstration. Children often complain of the FB being stuck even though it has passed, hence it is important to have a radiograph performed if the object is opaque, immediately prior to any planned endoscopy.

TRAUMA

Neck injury is unusual in children. Injuries may be penetrating or blunt.

PENETRATING INJURY

Typical penetrating injuries in children occur when the child falls with an object in the mouth, such as a pencil or 'ice-lolly' stick. Surgical emphysema may be seen on plain lateral radiographs in

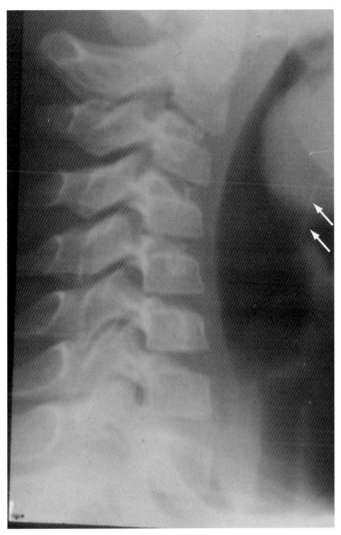

Figure 14.56 Lateral radiograph of neck showing a fish bone projected across the airway and the tonsil.

the prevertebral space and retropharyngeal abscesses can develop. A retained portion of the foreign body is rarely present but may be visible. The injury may penetrate the skull base, pass through the sinuses, and enter the intracranial cavity, damaging the pituitary gland or intracranial vessels. Spinal injury can also occur. Imaging should be guided appropriately. Young children are also prone to attack by dogs, which often bite the neck, damaging soft tissues and inflicting serious injuries. Glass laceration, stabbing and gunshot wounds will all produce potentially life-threatening injury, despite apparently innocuous skin entry wounds. Contrast-enhanced CT may be very informative once the child's condition is stable. With vascular injury formal angiography may be required.

BLUNT TRAUMA

Injuries are commonly due to bicycle or horseriding accidents and falls from trees. It is important to be aware that there may be associated cervical spine injury. The larynx in the young child is relatively protected, as it lies higher and is shielded by the mandible. The cartilaginous nature of the child's larynx also means it has a greater tendency to stretch and bend, producing mucosal damage and avulsion injuries to the vocal cords and arytenoids, rather than fractures. Plain films may show surgical emphysema but indirect laryngoscopy may suffice in assessing the cords. Otherwise CT and MRI may be required.

FURTHER READING

Adams DA, Cinnamond MJ. Paediatric otolaryngology. Scott-Brown's otolaryngology, vol. 6. Oxford: Butterworth Heinemann; 1997.

Ahuja AT, Yuen HY, Wong KT, Yue V, van Hasselt. Computed tomography imaging of the temporal bone – normal anatomy. Clinical Radiology 2003; 58:681–686.

Chong VFH, Khoo JBK, Fan Y-F. Imaging of the nasopharynx and skull base. Head and neck MR imaging II. Magnetic Resonance Clinics of North America. Philadelphia: Saunders; 2002.

Davidson HC. Imaging of the temporal bone. Head and neck MR imaging II. Magnetic Resonance Clinics of North America. Philadelphia: Saunders; 2002.

King SJ, Boothroyd AE. Pediatric ENT radiology. Berlin: Springer; 2002.

Kronbach GA, Schmitz-Rode T, Presher A et al. The petromastoid canal on computed tomography. European Radiology 2002; 12:2770–2775.

McDowell HP. Update on childhood rhabdomyosarcoma. Archives of Disease of Childhood 2003; 88:354–357.

Nakashima K, Morikawa M, Ishimaru H et al. Three-dimensional fast recovery fast spin-echo imaging of the inner ear and the vestibulocochlear nerve. European Radiology 2002; 12:2776–2780.

Swartz JD, Harnsberger HR. Imaging of the temporal bone. New York: Thieme; 1998.

Vasquez E, Castellote A, Piqueras J et al. Imaging of complications of acute mastoiditis in children. RadioGraphics 2003; 23:359–372.

Vasquez E, Castellote A, Piqueras J et al. Second malignancies in pediatric patients: Imaging findings and differential diagnosis. RadioGraphics 2003; 23:1155–1172.

Witte RJ, Lane J, Driscoll C et al. Pediatric and adult cochlear implantation. RadioGraphics 2003; 23:1185–1200.

Yates PD, Flood LM, Banerjee A, Clifford K. CT scanning of middle ear cholesteatoma: what does the surgeon want to know? British Journal of Radiology 2002; 75:847–852.

Yuen HY, Ahuja AT, Wong KT, Yue V van Hasselt. Computed tomography of common congenital lesions of the temporal bone. Clinical Radiology 2003; 58:687–693.

SECTION | 15

DENTAL RADIOLOGY

Dental Radiology

Martin Payne

Before discussing the more common dental and jaw abnormalities that might present to the paediatric radiologist it is helpful to briefly outline normal dental development, dental notation and radiological anatomy. In the primary or deciduous dentition there are 10 teeth in each jaw: 4 incisors, 2 canines and 4 molars. Using the Palmer system of notation, which is widely used in the UK, these teeth are designated by capital letters from the midline (see Table 15.1). The primary teeth are eventually replaced by the secondary or permanent teeth, of which there are 16 in each jaw: 4 incisors, 2 canines, 4 premolars and 6 molars. In Palmer notation, these teeth are designated by numbers from the midline (see Table 15.2).

These eruption dates are approximate. Individual variation exists and sometimes eruption is affected by lack of space, particularly with the upper canine and lower third molars. As a general rule, however, with regard to the secondary dentition, the paediatric radiologist might find it useful to remember that 'the 6's erupt at 6'. Using Palmer notation (Figure 15.1) when referring to a particular tooth one would write, for example, 'the upper left C' (deciduous canine) or 'lower right 7' (permanent second molar).

An alternative and widely used system of notation is the FDI (Federation Dentaire Internationale), which numbers the secondary tooth quadrants:

1 Right Maxilla
2 Left Maxilla
3 Left Mandible
4 Right Mandible.

The deciduous tooth quadrants are numbered:

5 Right Maxilla
6 Left Maxilla
7 Left Mandible
8 Right Mandible.

The number of each particular tooth then follows the quadrant number. For example, the patient's upper left deciduous canine would be numbered 6 (deciduous left maxilla) 3 (canine) – 63, whilst the lower right permanent second molar would be numbered 4 (right mandible) 7 (second molar) – 47.

The crown of each tooth has a very opaque outer layer of enamel beneath which is the slightly less opaque dentine. The dentine surrounds the pulp chamber and its extension, the root canal, down into the root. The pulp and root canal are radiolucent as they contain blood vessels, nerves and lymphatics rather than calcified material. The root dentine is covered in a thin layer of cementum which, via the radiolucent periodontal ligament, attaches the root to the dense lamina dura of the surrounding bone (Figure 15.2).

DEVELOPMENTAL ABNORMALITIES OF THE TEETH AND JAWS

There are many abnormalities that can affect the number, eruption, size, shape and structure of the teeth. Only the most frequent are covered below.

HYPODONTIA

It is extremely rare for a complete dentition to be congenitally absent (anodontia) but it is fairly common for one or two teeth not to develop (hypodontia). The teeth that are most often absent are third molars, second premolars (Figure 15.3) and upper permanent lateral incisors. Hypodontia and even anodontia can be seen in association with systemic defects – typically ectodermal dysplasia. Chemotherapy or radiotherapy in childhood (Figure 15.4) can result in various dental abnormalities including hypodontia.

HYPERDONTIA

The presence of extra teeth is fairly common, particularly in the anterior region of the permanent dentition. These extra teeth can sometimes affect the normal eruption of adjacent teeth (Figure 15.5). Hyperdontia can be associated with cleidocranial dysplasia, Gardner's syndrome and palatal clefts.

DENTINOGENESIS IMPERFECTA

This is a rare autosomal hereditary disease that affects the dentine in both dentitions. It is sometimes associated with osteogenesis imperfecta. Radiologically, the teeth have short roots and the pulp chambers and root canals within are often absent, having been

Table 15.1 The Palmer system of notation for primary teeth

Tooth	Palmer notation	Eruption date (months)
Central incisors	A	6–8
Lateral incisors	B	8–10
Canines	C	16–20
First molars	D	12–16
Second molars	E	20–30

Table 15.2 The Palmer system of notation for secondary teeth

Tooth	Palmer notation	Eruption date (years)
Central incisors	1	6–8
Lateral incisors	2	7–9
Canines	3	9–12
First/second premolars	4 & 5	10–12
First molars	6	6–7
Second molars	7	11–13
Third molars ('wisdom teeth')	8	17–21

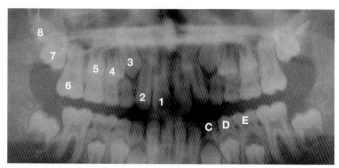

Figure 15.1 Dental panoramic tomograph of a 9-year-old patient showing normal complement of primary (CDE) and secondary (1–8) teeth for this age.

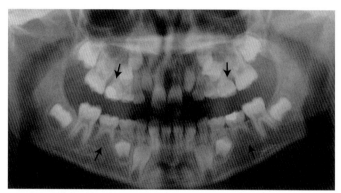

Figure 15.3 Dental panoramic tomograph showing absence of all four second premolar teeth.

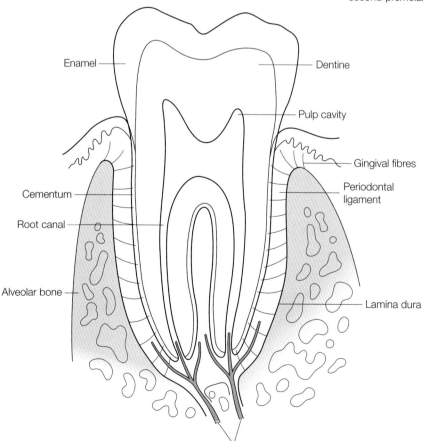

Enamel — Dentine

Pulp cavity

Gingival fibres

Cementum

Periodontal ligament

Root canal

Alveolar bone

Lamina dura

Nutrient vessels

Figure 15.2 Diagram illustrating normal dental anatomy.

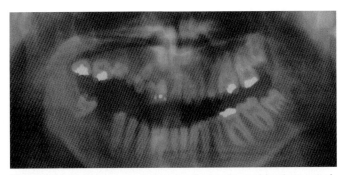

Figure 15.4 Dental panoramic tomograph showing maldevelopment of right-sided teeth in a patient who had received radiotherapy to the right face as an infant for a local malignancy.

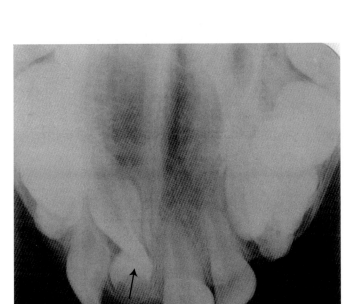

Figure 15.5 Upper anterior occlusal radiograph showing a supernumerary tooth, which has prevented normal eruption of the right central incisor tooth.

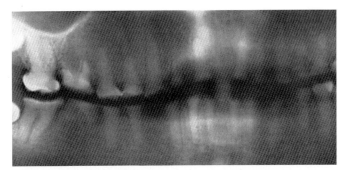

Figure 15.6 Cropped dental panoramic tomograph showing gross occlusal wear, stunted roots and general pulpal obliteration in a case of dentinogenesis imperfecta.

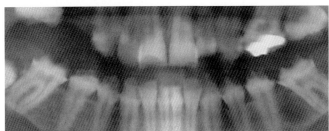

Figure 15.7 Cropped dental panoramic tomograph showing generalized thinning or loss of the enamel layer in amelogenesis imperfecta.

obliterated by dentine (Figure 15.6). The enamel layer is rapidly lost exposing the softer layer of dentine underneath, which quickly becomes worn down.

AMELOGENESIS IMPERFECTA

This rare inherited condition affects the enamel layer of the teeth in both dentitions. There are many variants but the usual radiological findings include a particularly thin enamel layer with an unusual square or rectangular appearance to the crowns (Figure 15.7). As with dentinogenesis imperfecta, there may be pulpal obliteration and the teeth may become worn down.

DENS INVAGINATUS

The alternative name for this is dens in dente or 'tooth within a tooth', which describes the radiological appearance nicely. It results from an invagination of the enamel and dentine towards the pulp or root canal with the result that a carious lesion in the crown can rapidly involve the pulp leading in turn to infection of the bony tissues at the end of the root-periapical infection (Figure 15.8). The upper permanent lateral incisor is most commonly affected.

ODONTOMES

These are hamartomas within the jaw comprising variable amounts of the different dental tissues. When calcification is complete there is no further growth. Radiologically, there is usually a well-defined radiolucent area within which is either an irregular collection of dental tissue (Figure 15.9) or an arrangement of several small tooth-like structures (Figure 15.10). The former type are referred to as 'complex' and these favour the posterior mandible, while the latter are known as 'compound' and are usually found in the anterior maxilla. Odontomes are often detected incidentally although they may affect the normal eruption of adjacent teeth.

CLEFT LIP AND PALATE

Clefts may form in the lip, the palate or in both. Cleft lip (1:600) is more common than cleft palate (1:2500). A cleft palate results

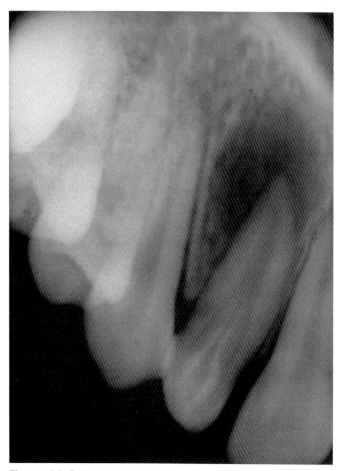

Figure 15.8 Periapical dental radiograph showing an area of apical rarefaction associated with this malformed 'dens in dente' upper right lateral incisor.

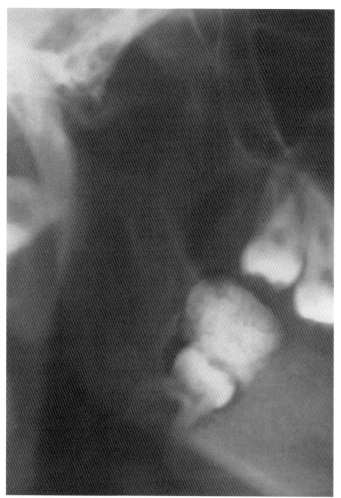

Figure 15.9 Cropped dental panoramic tomograph showing well-defined mass of tissue of similar density to adjacent impacted third molar – complex odontome.

from total or partial failure of fusion of the palatine process. It may be detected by antenatal ultrasound. Cleft deformities are associated with many syndromes and skeletal dysplasias.

In addition to a cleft in the alveolar bone (Figure 15.11), a radiograph may reveal dental anomalies such as the presence of supernumerary teeth or an absent lateral incisor. Maleruption may occur. An increased incidence of hypodontia in both jaws has been noted in patients with cleft palate. Long-term problems associated with repaired clefts include mid-face hypoplasia, nasal speech due to a short deformed palate, with failure of closure of the palatopharyngeal mechanism, and escape of fluid during drinking due to a persistent cleft. Phonetic studies are required to assess movement. These are performed using videofluoroscopy following nasal instillation of barium and repeating sounds. Dynamic magnetic resonance imaging (MRI) of the palate may give further information. Computed tomography (CT) of the facial bones with three-dimensional reconstruction is required before facial reconstructive surgery.

HEMIFACIAL MICROSOMIA

This condition, in which there is underdevelopment of one half of the face, is unilateral in 80% of cases. Even when bilateral, some

asymmetry should be detected between the two sides. CT will demonstrate the soft tissue hypoplasia (Figure 15.12), whilst the affected bones, which will be small in size, and the asymmetry will be nicely demonstrated on a dental panoramic tomograph. There may be fewer teeth than normal on the affected side and those that are present may be unusually small. In addition, the ear canal is often absent and the pinna deformed. There is also underdevelopment of the soft tissues and ipsilateral parotid gland.

MANDIBULOFACIAL DYSOSTOSIS

Mandibulofacial dysostosis, sometimes known as Treacher Collins syndrome, is bilateral. The severity varies. Some patients will present with many anomalies such as underdevelopment of the condyle and ramus of the mandible, and zygomatic bones, as well as ear deformity and cleft palate. The appearance of the mandible can be quite striking (Figure 15.13). The underdevelopment also affects the soft tissues but to a lesser degree than with hemifacial microsomia.

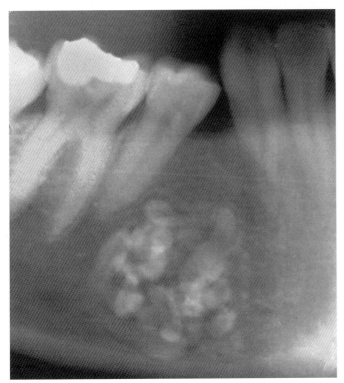

Figure 15.10 Cropped dental panoramic tomograph showing a collection of tooth-like structures in the right body of mandible – a compound odontome.

HEMIFACIAL HYPERPLASIA

This is a condition in which half of the face undergoes excessive growth, sometimes in conjunction with other parts of the body. The affected primary teeth may be prematurely lost and rapidly replaced by secondary teeth, which are larger than normal (Figure 15.14). As would be expected, the bones on the affected side will be enlarged. This condition is associated with various neoplasms such as hepatoblastoma and Wilms' tumour of the kidney as well as mental defects, anomalies of the genitourinary tract and scoliosis.

CONDYLAR HYPERPLASIA

In this developmental condition, there is excessive growth of one of the mandibular condyles, which often leads to either deviation of the chin towards the normal side or a vertically enlarged mandible on the affected side. Aside from facial asymmetry, the patient may present with temporomandibular discomfort and restricted jaw movement. The morphology of the normal and abnormal condyles is nicely demonstrated on a dental panoramic tomograph (Figure 15.15), while radionuclide imaging (Figure 15.16) is used to try and assess whether the abnormal condylar growth has stopped, an important factor with regard to the timing of corrective surgery.

FIBROUS DYSPLASIA AND CHERUBISM

Fibrous dysplasia is a self-limiting fibro-osseous disease that can affect just one bone or several. In the jaws, the maxilla is more commonly affected and the usual clinical finding is one of painless swelling, usually noticed in childhood or adolescence. The radiological appearance is variable and depends upon the stage of lesion development. Early lesions tend to be radiolucent and well defined but with time bone will be laid down producing a mixed-density appearance (Figure 15.17). Eventually, the margins will tend to blend in with the adjacent bone. Aside from the bony expansion, teeth may be displaced and eruption may be severely affected.

Although not identical pathologically, cherubism can be regarded as a familial type of fibrous dysplasia that develops in infancy, initially presenting as a painless bilateral enlargement of the posterior mandible and in time progressing to involve the maxilla, leading to the characteristic cherubic appearance. The radiological appearance is striking (Figure 15.18) with bilateral multilocular radiolucencies starting at the mandibular angle spreading to the ramus and body. Developing teeth are often adversely affected, particularly the lower second and third molars.

FURTHER READING

Acton CH, Savage NW. Odontomes and their behaviour; a review. Australian Dental Journal 1987; 32:430–435.
Kaste SC, Hopkins KP, Jenkins JJ. Abnormal odontogenesis in children treated with radiation and chemotherapy: Imaging Findings. American Journal of Roentgenology 1994; 162:1407–1411.
White SC, Pharoah MJ. Oral radiology, 4th edn. St. Louis: Mosby; 2000.

CARIES (TOOTH DECAY)

Caries is an extremely common disease caused by the action of acid that is produced by bacteria present in plaque on tooth surfaces. The acid causes demineralization of the enamel layer, which can then lead to involvement of the underlying dentine and, ultimately, without intervention, infection of the pulp. Caries tends to develop in those stagnation areas of the tooth that are more likely to retain bacteria-containing plaque such as the proximal surfaces adjacent to other teeth and within the occlusal fissures. The early carious lesion can be very difficult to detect clinically, particularly when it involves the proximal surface of the tooth, and intraoral radiographs are an essential aid to diagnosis. Certain individuals are more at risk from caries than others and as such will benefit from more frequent radiographic examination in order to detect this condition.

Radiologically, caries manifests as a radiolucency in the enamel or dentine (Figure 15.19) and in the early stages this may be quite difficult to detect – ideal film viewing conditions are crucial and even then different dentists may reach different conclusions with regard to the presence or otherwise of caries!

As the carious lesion progresses through the dentine it will become more obvious radiologically and, given sufficient time, it

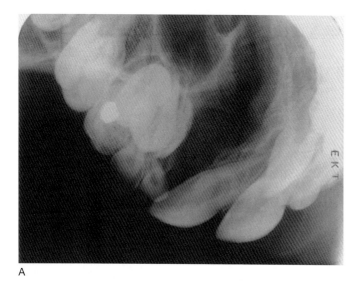

A

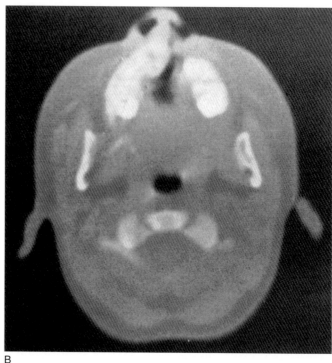

B

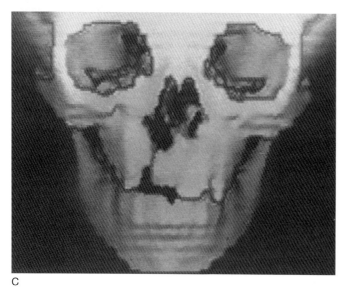

C

Figure 15.11 (A) Oblique upper occlusal radiograph showing a right-sided cleft of the palate. (B) Axial CT scan showing a cleft lip and palate. (C) Three-dimensional CT reconstruction.

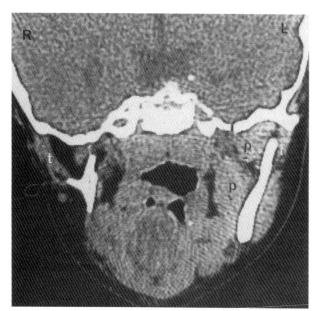

Figure 15.12 Coronal CT section of a severe case of hemifacial microsomia. Note the gross hypoplasia of muscles on the right side as well as the deformity of the mandible. Note also the small tag representing the auricle on the right. p, pterygoid muscles; t, temporalis.

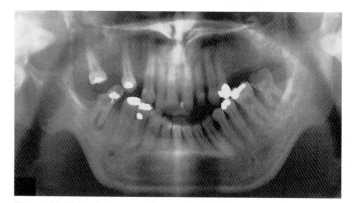

Figure 15.13 Dental panoramic tomograph of a patient with Treacher Collins syndrome.

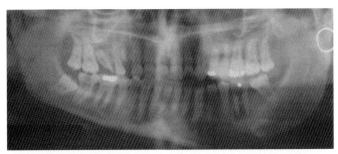

Figure 15.14 Hemifacial hyperplasia. Dental panoramic tomograph showing gross enlargement of the left side of the mandible.

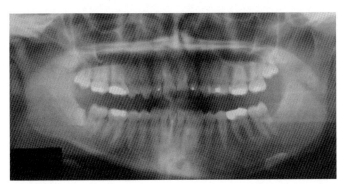

Figure 15.15 Dental panoramic tomograph showing left-sided condylar hyperplasia.

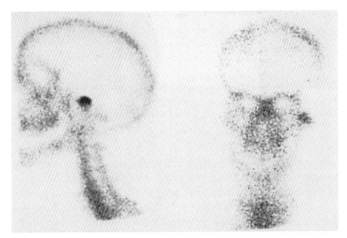

Figure 15.16 Radionuclide scans showing increased uptake in the left condyle.

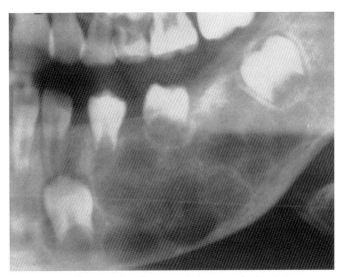

Figure 15.17 Cropped dental panoramic tomograph showing an area of fibrous dysplasia within the left mandible.

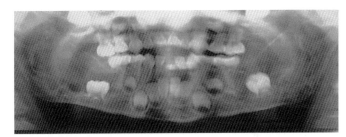

Figure 15.18 Dental panoramic tomograph showing bilateral well-defined multilocular radiolucent lesions affecting both jaws in a 4-year-old boy with cherubism.

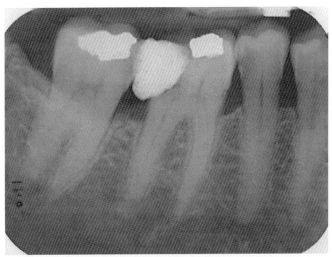

Figure 15.19 Periapical dental radiograph showing distal caries in the lower right second premolar tooth extending into dentine. Also revealed, a huge overhanging restoration in the first molar.

may appear to involve the pulp but one should always remember that because the radiograph is only two-dimensional a radiolucency projected over the pulp does not always mean that the pulp has been breached.

While a carious lesion confined to enamel may remineralize given appropriate conditions, once the dentine becomes involved the dentist must intervene and place a restoration after removing the caries. However, even after such treatment, the tooth may develop recurrent caries, which may manifest as a radiolucent zone adjacent to one of the margins of the restoration (Figure 15.20).

Incidentally, it is not uncommon for bits of dental restorative materials to be swallowed during treatment and these, particularly dental amalgam, may show up as opaque foreign bodies on an abdominal film, which may cause some confusion to the radiologist.

FURTHER READING

Faculty of General Dental Practitioners (UK). Selection criteria for dental radiography. The Royal College of Surgeons of England; 1998:29–41.

JAW INFECTION

Untreated caries can lead to pulpitis, which may in turn cause infection of the tissues at the end of the root(s) – periapical periodontitis. In the early stages of this condition, the periapical tissues may appear quite normal radiologically but, given time, the apical periodontal ligament space will appear widened, the lamina dura will be lost and an area of ill-defined rarefaction in the bone may develop – rarefying osteitis (Figure 15.21). With chronic low-grade infection there may well be a sclerotic bony response called sclerosing osteitis, and in such situations granulomatous and even cystic change may eventually occur. While it is impossible to radiologically differentiate with absolute certainty a granuloma from a cyst, an apical radiolucency greater than 2 cm in diameter is highly suggestive of cystic change.

OSTEOMYELITIS

Although uncommon in children, osteomyelitis may occur in the jaws, particularly if the immunity is impaired in some way. In infancy, haematogenous spread of infection is thought to be the usual cause of this condition, which at this age favours the maxilla reflecting the excellent blood supply to this structure. In contrast,

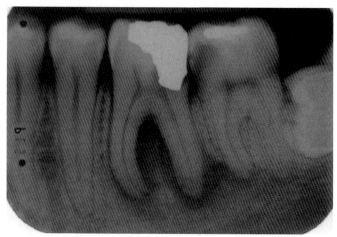

Figure 15.21 Periapical dental radiograph showing an area of apical rarefaction associated with the deeply restored lower left first molar. Also mesial decay in the crown of the adjacent second molar and an impacted lower left third molar.

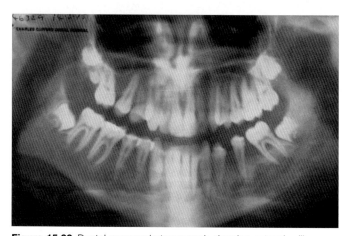

Figure 15.22 Dental panoramic tomograph showing extensive ill-defined areas of rarefaction in the left body of the mandible in a patient with acute osteomyelitis.

osteomyelitis in older children and adults almost always occurs in the posterior aspect of the mandible, with its poorer blood supply, as the result of local uncontrolled spread of infection usually from a tooth that has lost its vitality. In the early stages, the bone will look normal radiologically but once the condition is established one can expect to see areas of ill-defined rarefaction (Figure 15.22), leading to severe bony destruction and ultimately formation of sclerotic 'islands' of sequestrum.

In time, one may detect a layer or several layers of new bone, which is produced by the periosteum as it is lifted from the surface of the mandible by the inflammatory exudate. Radiologically, this will appear as alternating radiolucent and radiopaque lines adjacent to the edge of the mandible. This process is called proliferative periostitis and it can be particularly marked in children (Figure 15.23).

Usually, the clinical picture will make the diagnosis of acute osteomyelitis quite straightforward but sometimes in children other conditions may have to be considered and radiological findings can be very helpful where there is uncertainty. In fibrous dysplasia, for example, bony enlargement occurs as a result of new bone produced inside the outer cortex, while with osteomyelitis,

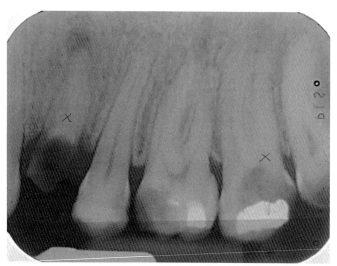

Figure 15.20 Periapical dental radiograph showing gross breakdown of the upper left first premolar tooth with associated apical rarefaction. Also, recurrent gross caries in the upper left second molar tooth.

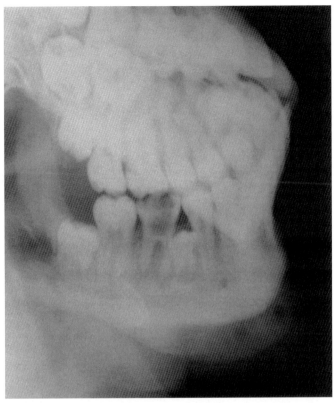

Figure 15.23 Oblique lateral radiograph showing periosteal new bone related to the adjacent osteomyelitis in a 15-year-old patient.

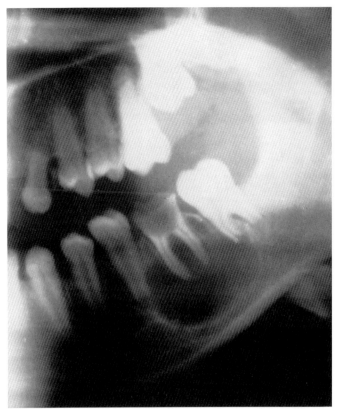

Figure 15.24 Cropped dental panoramic tomograph showing well-defined radiolucent lesion (radicular cyst) associated with the grossly carious lower left first molar tooth.

enlargement results from periosteal new bone being laid down on the outside of the cortical plate.

Another condition to consider is Langerhans' cell histiocytosis, particularly the eosinophilic granuloma form. Eosinophilic granuloma (EG) tends to affect children or young adults and aside from the bony destruction there is a tendency to form periosteal new bone, which can mimic that seen in osteomyelitis, making for diagnostic difficulty when the EG is solitary.

Ewing's sarcoma (see below) may mimic osteomyelitis but this disease is rare in the jaws.

FURTHER READING

White SC, Pharoah MJ. Oral radiology, 4th edn. St. Louis: Mosby; 2000.
Zain RB, Roswati N, Ismail K. Radiographic evaluation of lesion sizes of histologically diagnosed periapical cysts and granulomas. Annals of Dentistry 1989; 48:3–5.

CYSTS

The radicular (dental) cyst is by far the most common that affects the jaws. This originates from a dead tooth and thus can be a long-term complication of untreated caries, although it should also be noted that a tooth can lose its vitality as a result of local trauma, particularly in the upper anterior region, in which case the crown of the tooth may appear sound. Radicular cysts manifest radiologically as a well-defined radiolucent lesion closely associated with the dead root apex (Figure 15.24). If the causative tooth is removed but the radicular cyst is left behind then this cyst is referred to as being 'residual' (Figure 15.25).

The next most common cyst in the jaws is the dentigerous cyst. The characteristic radiological feature here is one of a well-defined radiolucent lesion that envelops all or part of the crown of an unerupted tooth (Figure 15.26). This may well prevent normal eruption and sometimes the tooth will be displaced quite some distance away from its usual position.

The teeth that are more prone to impaction such as the lower third molar and upper canine are usually affected. Many will be detected in adolescents and young adults.

The eruption cyst is a type of dentigerous cyst that arises in the superficial soft tissues overlying a tooth that is about to erupt. They are only seen in children (Figure 15.27).

Odontogenic keratocysts are certainly not as common as those just described but they are very important because of their tendency to recur after surgical removal. Most appear during the second and third decades and the vast majority develop in the third molar and ramus region of the mandible. Radiologically, they present as well-defined radiolucent lesions, sometimes with multilocularity, and occasionally they can involve the whole length of the mandible with minimal expansion. Sometimes, a keratocyst will grow around an unerupted tooth crown thus mimicking the less significant dentigerous cyst.

The tendency for recurrence dictates that affected patients will be followed up and re-radiographed for many years after surgical

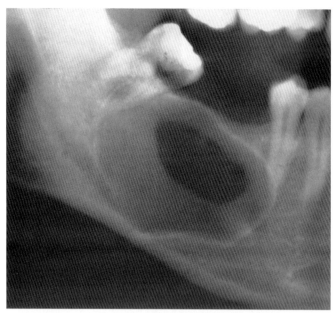

Figure 15.25 Cropped dental panoramic tomograph showing well-defined corticated radiolucent lesion in the right body of the mandible – residual cyst. The area of increased radiolucency within the lesion is a sign of perforation of either the buccal or lingual bony plate.

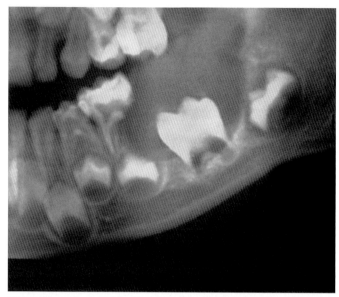

Figure 15.27 Cropped dental panoramic tomograph showing well-defined soft tissue lesion (eruption cyst) overlying the unerupted lower left first permanent molar. Note the resorption of the adjacent distal root of the deciduous molar.

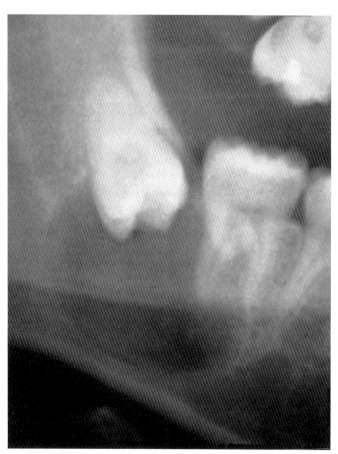

Figure 15.26 Cropped dental panoramic tomograph showing well-defined radiolucent lesion around the crown of the impacted third molar – dentigerous cyst.

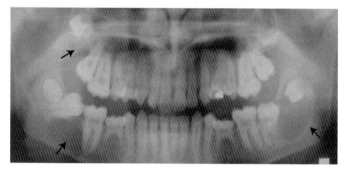

Figure 15.28 Dental panoramic tomograph showing three well-defined radiolucent lesions (keratocysts) in the jaws of this patient with Gorlin–Goltz syndrome. Note also the absence of the lower second premolar teeth.

excision. Multiple keratocysts of the jaws are a feature of Gorlin–Goltz syndrome, which is usually detected in childhood (Figure 15.28).

The nasopalatine cyst is probably about as common as the odontogenic keratocyst and, as its name implies, it occurs in the midline of the anterior maxilla, usually presenting as a swelling just behind the central incisors, although most are asymptomatic.

Radiologically, the lesion presents as a well-defined heart-shaped radiolucency (Figure 15.29) that when small (<6 mm in diameter) may be difficult to differentiate from the incisive foramen.

Although not strictly speaking a true cyst, the simple bone cyst, sometimes known as 'traumatic' or 'haemorrhagic' cyst, is included in this section because it is common and usually presents in the late teens. These often occur in conjunction with fibrous dysplastic lesions and the mandible is invariably affected. Radiologically, the most characteristic feature is one of a radiolucency,

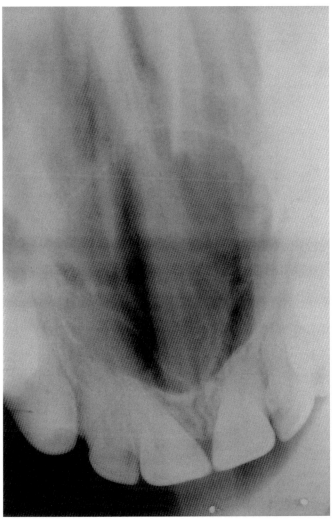

Figure 15.29 Upper anterior occlusal radiograph showing well-defined radiolucent lesion splaying the roots of the central incisor teeth – nasopalatine cyst.

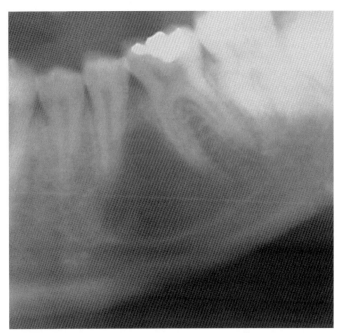

Figure 15.30 Cropped dental panoramic tomograph showing well-defined radiolucent lesion extending up between the roots of the lower left second premolar and first molar teeth – simple bone cyst.

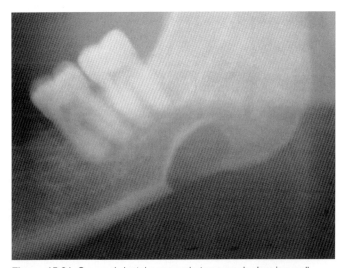

Figure 15.31 Cropped dental panoramic tomograph showing well-defined radiolucency at the left angle of the mandible – Stafne bone cavity.

which has a scalloped upper border between the roots of the adjacent teeth (Figure 15.30). Expansion is unusual and most lesions are detected incidentally.

The Stafne bone cyst is another condition, which is inappropriately named as it is not truly cystic. Basically, this is a developmental well-defined concavity in the lingual aspect of the mandible, which sometimes contains some submandibular salivary gland tissue. These cysts classically present on panoramic dental films as an incidental radiolucency just below the inferior dental canal at the angle of the mandible (Figure 15.31). Although they can appear quite striking, these 'lesions' should be easily recognized for what they are and should be left well alone.

FURTHER READING

Gorlin RJ, Goltz RW. Multiple nevoid basal cell epithelioma, jaw cysts, and bifid rib: a syndrome. New England Journal of Medicine 1960; 262:908–912.

REACTIVE BONE LESIONS

CENTRAL GIANT CELL GRANULOMA

This is a benign lesion of uncertain origin usually treated by enucleation or curettage. Most lesions present in adolescents or young adults and the area anterior to the first permanent molar in the mandible is invariably affected. It usually presents as a painless swelling although sometimes it will be detected incidentally on radiographic examination. Growth is usually slow but can be rapid; involved teeth may be loosened and there is sometimes root displacement and resorption.

Radiographically, early lesions tend to present as small, well-defined, non-corticated radiolucencies but with growth there is a tendency for lesions to appear multilocular often with a wispy pattern of trabeculation within (Figure 15.32). Large lesions may result in significant cortical expansion.

ANEURYSMAL BONE CYST

Another lesion of uncertain origin, possibly related to pre-existing bony pathology such as fibrous dysplasia. Badly named because, although vascular, it does not contain aneurysms nor is it truly a cyst. The vast majority occur in teenagers and the posterior aspect of the mandible is the usual site. It usually presents as a tender swelling, which is sometimes fairly quick to develop. Adjacent teeth may be displaced and there may be root resorption.

Aneurysmal bone cyst is usually treated by curettage or even resection; recurrence is fairly common and so patients will require follow-up. The radiographic appearance depends upon the stage of development: early lesions usually present as a poorly defined area of radiolucency but with further growth the border becomes better defined and there may be faint trabeculation within. Given time there may well be gross expansion, often with a multilocular appearance (Figure 15.33).

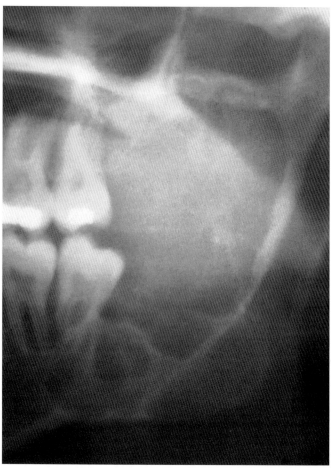

Figure 15.33 Cropped dental panoramic tomograph showing expanded large multilocular radiolucent lesion in the left ramus – aneurysmal bone cyst.

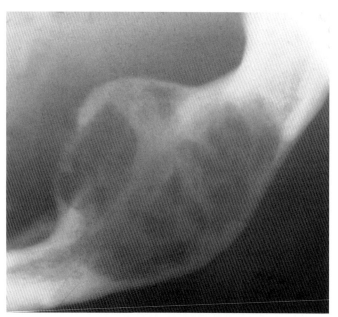

Figure 15.32 Cropped occlusal radiograph showing expanded radiolucent lesion with internal pattern of trabeculation – central giant cell granuloma.

NEOPLASMS

BENIGN ODONTOGENIC NEOPLASMS

The commonest odontogenic neoplasm is the ameloblastoma and although uncommon in children, cases do occur. Radiologically, these present with a well-defined, often multilocular, radiolucent lesion that may cause bony expansion and often causes root resorption (Figure 15.34). If the lesion is intimately related to the crown of an unerupted tooth then it may well be mistaken for a dentigerous cyst. Although they can occur anywhere in the jaws the vast majority are found in the posterior mandible.

The adenomatoid odontogenic tumour (AOT) is an uncommon lesion that is typically found in teenagers, particularly females. The anterior maxilla is almost invariably affected. Radiologically, the AOT presents as a well-defined unilocular radiolucent lesion that usually totally surrounds an unerupted tooth – typically a canine (Figure 15.35). Thus, it may resemble a dentigerous cyst. However, in most cases, there will be multiple radiopacities within the lesion, which would be most unusual for a dentigerous cyst.

Another benign neoplasm that mainly affects the young is the odontogenic myxoma. Females tend to be favoured and the usual

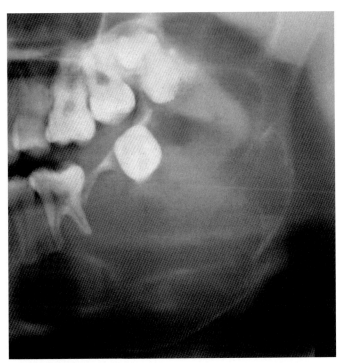

Figure 15.34 Cropped dental panoramic tomograph showing large radiolucent lesion involving the left angle and ramus of the mandible with gross expansion and some root resorption – ameloblastoma.

site is the posterior tooth-bearing area of the mandible. Often a tooth will not have formed or will be unerupted in the area affected. Associated teeth may be displaced and given time there may be gross expansion of the jaw. Radiologically, the myxoma presents as a generally well-defined radiolucency, which is usually but not invariably multilocular. The pattern of bony trabeculation that often occurs within these lesions has been likened to the strings of a tennis racket (Figure 15.36).

The cementoblastoma is a lesion that tends to affect adolescents or young adults and it usually involves the first molar or a pre-molar in the lower jaw. The lesion is often painful and given enough time there may be a localized bony swelling or even displacement of adjacent teeth. The usual radiological finding is of a rounded, well-defined radiopacity attached to the involved root surrounded by a radiolucent zone or 'halo' (Figure 15.37).

Space does not allow inclusion of some of the other benign odontogenic neoplasms but as a general rule they present radiologically as well-defined radiolucent lesions, which may or may not be associated with unerupted teeth. Clinical details are therefore essential in trying to arrive at a meaningful differential diagnosis.

BENIGN NON-ODONTOGENIC NEOPLASMS

Osteomas are fairly common in the jaws, especially in the mandible, but they are usually detected in middle-aged rather than young patients. However, an important condition that might be detected in the second decade is Gardner's syndrome in which multiple osteomas of the jaws (Figure 15.38) and sebaceous cysts

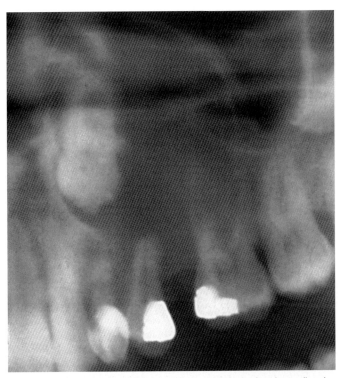

Figure 15.35 Cropped dental panoramic tomograph showing unilocular radiolucent lesion surrounding an unerupted maxillary canine – adenomatoid odontogenic tumour.

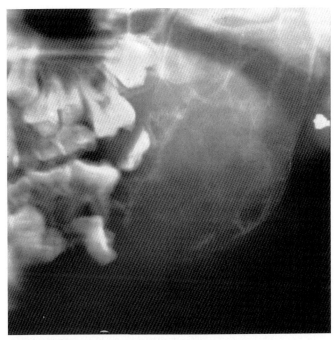

Figure 15.36 Cropped dental panoramic tomograph showing multilocular radiolucent lesion in the left ramus of the mandible of this 9-year-old patient – odontogenic myxoma.

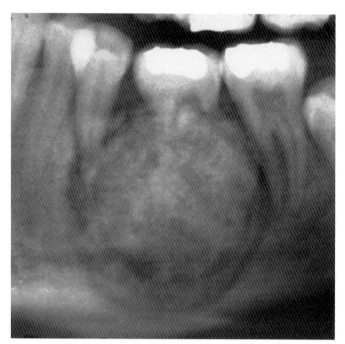

Figure 15.37 Cropped dental panoramic tomograph showing well-defined radiopaque lesion attached to the crown of the lower left first molar – cementoblastoma.

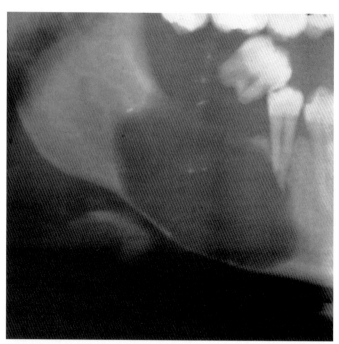

Figure 15.39 Cropped dental panoramic tomograph showing large well-defined radiolucent lesion in the right body of the mandible with extensive root resorption – neurilemoma.

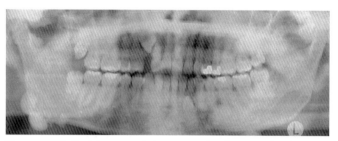

Figure 15.38 Dental panoramic tomogram showing several osteomas of the jaws together with a generalized increase in mandibular bone density – Gardner's syndrome. (Reproduced with kind permission from Payne M et al. British Dental Journal 2002; 193:383–384.)

usually manifest themselves before the development of multiple intestinal polyps, which have a marked tendency to undergo malignant change before the age of 40.

The neurilemoma, sometimes known as a Schwannoma, is the most common neoplasm of nerve tissue that occurs within bone. They usually arise in the second and third decades and the mandible is a common site, often presenting as a painless swelling, although there may be some paraesthesia. Radiologically, there is usually an ovoid expansion of the inferior dental canal (Figure 15.39).

Another benign nerve neoplasm to consider and one that has been known to undergo malignant change is the neurofibroma. This often presents as a firm swelling and there may be some associated pain or paraesthesia. Radiologically, as with neurilemoma, if the inferior dental nerve is affected then there will be an oval or fusiform enlargement of the canal.

In neurofibromatosis, patients develop multiple neurilemomas and neurofibromas in addition to the characteristic areas of skin pigmentation and a variety of other abnormalities. When the jaws are affected the inferior dental canal is usually enlarged and, in addition, the surrounding bone and overall appearance of the mandible may be extremely unusual (Figure 15.40).

MALIGNANT NEOPLASMS

Malignancy involving the jaws is thankfully most uncommon in children but cases do occur and radiologically one of the key features to note, whatever the type of tumour, is diffuse destruction of alveolar bone from around the roots, leading to the appearance of the teeth 'floating in air' (Figures 15.41 to 15.43).

In east central Africa, Burkitt's lymphoma is the most common malignant disease of childhood and the jaw is commonly affected, particularly the molar region. The condition is more prevalent in boys. Clinically, loosening of the primary teeth without obvious cause is a common sign as is gingival swelling and ulceration. Radiologically, expect to see ill-defined radiolucencies in the bone, which will destroy or displace developing teeth as well as sometimes cause gross bony expansion. Maxillary lesions will destroy the normal antral outlines (Figure 15.44).

Another largely childhood malignancy to consider is Ewing's sarcoma. A minority of cases involve the jaws, usually the posterior mandible. Radiologically, there will be a destructive radiolucent lesion, which may mimic osteomyelitis. Given time, the periosteum may produce layers of new bone leading to the so-called 'onion skin' appearance. Many lesions produce a 'sunray' pattern at the cortex but this is not specific to Ewing's sarcoma and may be found in osteosarcoma and other rapidly growing lesions such as neuroblastoma (Figure 15.45).

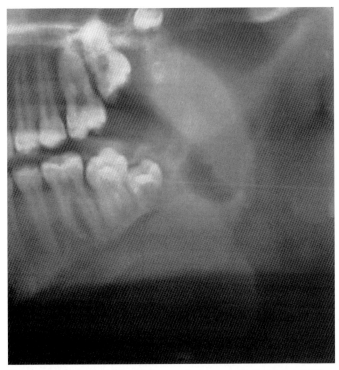

Figure 15.40 Cropped dental panoramic tomograph showing central radiolucent lesion within distorted left ramus of the mandible – neurofibroma.

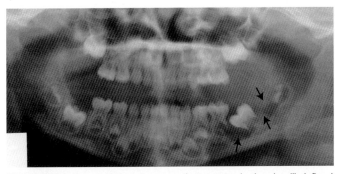

Figure 15.41 Cropped dental panoramic tomograph showing ill-defined alveolar bone destruction around the lower left first and second permanent molars in a 5-year-old girl with Langerhans' cell histiocytosis.

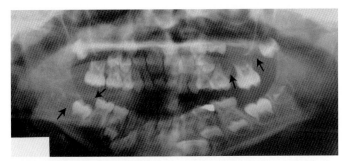

Figure 15.42 Dental panoramic tomograph showing areas of ill-defined alveolar bone destruction around the developing lower right first and second permanent molars and around the erupted upper left first permanent molar in a 6-year-old girl with non-Hodgkin's lymphoma.

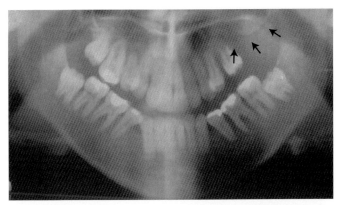

Figure 15.43 Dental panoramic tomograph showing ill-defined loss of alveolar bone and destruction of the antral floor on the left side in a 15-year-old girl with antral carcinoma.

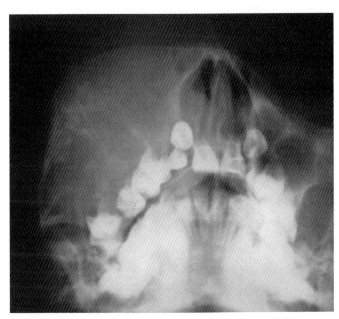

Figure 15.44 Occipitomental radiograph showing gross soft tissue swelling and destruction of the right antral outline in a young boy with Burkitt's lymphoma.

FURTHER READING

Cawson RA et al. Lucas's pathology of tumours of the oral tissues, 5th edn. London: Churchill Livingstone; 1998.

White SC, Pharoah MJ. Oral radiology, 4th edn. St. Louis: Mosby; 2000.

COMMON CHILDHOOD SYSTEMIC CONDITIONS THAT MAY MANIFEST IN THE JAWS

HYPERPITUITARISM

In this condition, there is an excess of circulating growth hormone, which in a child before fusion of the epiphyses, will result in

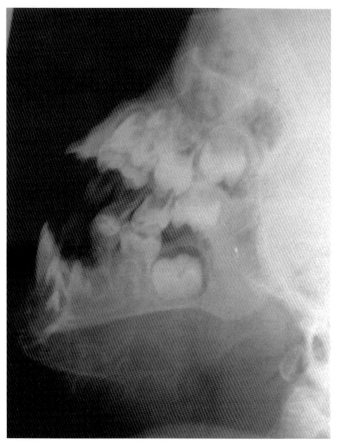

Figure 15.45 Oblique lateral radiograph showing ill-defined bony destruction at the inferior border with 'sunray' pattern of spiculation in an infant with mandibular neuroblastoma.

THALASSAEMIA AND SICKLE-CELL DISEASE

In both conditions, there is hyperplasia of the bone marrow resulting in a generally radiolucent appearance radiologically, which is well demonstrated in the jaws (Figure 15.46). With thalassaemia, in particular, the paranasal sinuses may be obliterated as a result of the hyperplastic marrow and there may be quite marked expansion of the jaws. With both conditions the diploic space in the skull will be wider than normal and the inner and outer tables will be thinned – in a small minority, the outer table will be replaced by a 'hair-on-end' appearance (Figure 15.47). Bony infarcts may occur in sickle-cell disease and these manifest radiologically as areas of osteosclerosis (Figure 15.46).

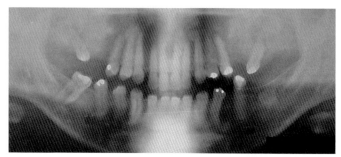

Figure 15.46 Dental panoramic tomograph of a young adult patient with sickle-cell disease. Note the bony infarcts in the maxilla and in the left body of the mandible.

gigantism. More commonly, the excess growth hormone production occurs in adult life and acromegaly ensues but if the excess hormone production starts in adolescence and persists then the two conditions may be combined. Affected children may become extremely tall and the mandible may be quite enlarged. The frontal air sinuses are often huge although this tends to occur more with acromegaly. Dental development may be accelerated and the roots of posterior teeth can be larger than normal as a result of hypercementosis.

HYPOPITUITARISM

When there is a deficiency of growth hormone the jaws will be much smaller than normal. The teeth, however, tend to be of normal size but there may be a delay of several years before the primary dentition is replaced by the secondary.

HYPOTHYROIDISM

In children, a lack of circulating thyroxine will result in abnormally small jaws with teeth that erupt late and which have short roots.

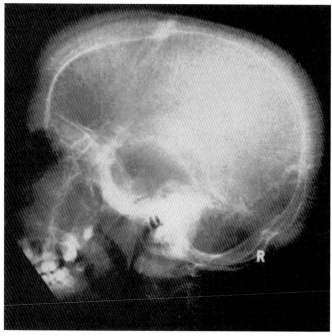

Figure 15.47 Thalassaemia. A gross 'hair-on-end' appearance affects the basiocciput and squamous temple regions.

OSTEOGENESIS IMPERFECTA

In this condition, the bones exhibit cortical thinning and generalized demineralization – this will be evident in the mandible and will be well demonstrated on a panoramic film. In 10–30% of cases, the characteristic dental findings of dentinogenesis imperfecta (see above) will be present.

OSTEOPETROSIS (ALBERS–SCHONBERG DISEASE)

This disease is caused by faulty osteoclasts leading to the production of abnormally dense bone that is fragile and, because of the compromised blood supply, more susceptible to severe infection. In the jaws, the mandible is particularly at risk from osteomyelitis.

Radiologically, the jaws will be abnormally opaque, sometimes so much so that it is difficult to actually see the roots of teeth. A characteristic sign of osteopetrosis that may be present is that the lamina dura around the roots and the inferior dental canal is thickened, although if the jaws are completely opaque it will be impossible to detect this (Figure 15.48). If the bone is very dense then this may cause delayed eruption of the teeth and the teeth themselves may be subject to various abnormalities such as enamel defects and root deformity.

CLEIDOCRANIAL DYSPLASIA

The characteristic dental findings are the excessive retention of the primary teeth and the delayed eruption of their permanent successors. In addition, there may be many supernumerary teeth that remain unerupted in the jaws (Figure 15.49). The maxilla and paranasal sinuses are usually hypoplastic.

FURTHER READING

White SC, Pharoah MJ. Oral radiology, 4th edn. Mosby; 2000.

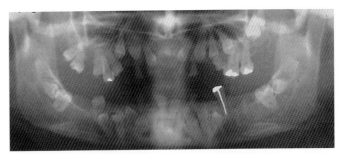

Figure 15.49 Dental panoramic tomograph showing multiple, unerupted, supernumerary teeth in a patient with cleidocranial dysplasia.

TRAUMA

Dental injuries in children are common and, not surprisingly, most involve the upper central incisor teeth, particularly when these are more prominent (proclined). A variety of dental injuries are possible ranging from concussion, in which the tooth is intact but the surrounding structures bruised, to fracture of the crown/root and even complete loss (avulsion) of the tooth. Intraoral periapical or occlusal radiographs are required following significant dental injury in order to reveal the state of root development and to detect any injury to the root and the surrounding tissues.

With dental concussion, radiologically one may initially only detect some widening of the periodontal ligament space but, given time, perhaps months or years later, the pulp chamber and canals may become obliterated and there may be apical rarefaction as a result of chronic infection (Figure 15.50). Traumatized teeth, no matter how innocuous the injury may appear, should therefore be reviewed regularly by the dental practitioner.

Sometimes the trauma results in displacement and mobility (luxation) of the affected tooth. Teeth can be forced upwards (intruded) into the supporting bone or, conversely, they may be displaced some distance out of the socket (extrusion). Intraoral radiographs will demonstrate such displacement relative to the adjacent uninjured teeth and a common finding is widening of the periodontal ligament space as with dental concussion. Again, given time,

Figure 15.48 Osteopetrosis. A 'bone-within-a-bone' appearance may be seen in the mandibular condyles. The mandible as a whole is grossly deformed and bone texture grossly abnormal with overall increase in density. The dentition is abnormal. The teeth are hypoplastic and the enamel poorly formed.

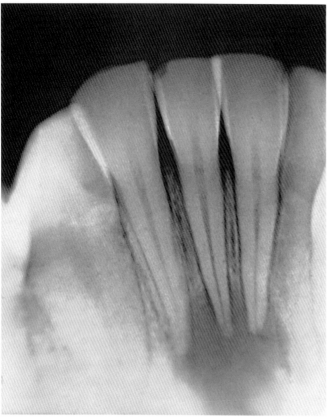

Figure 15.50 Periapical dental radiograph showing an area of apical rarefaction associated with these previously traumatized lower incisors.

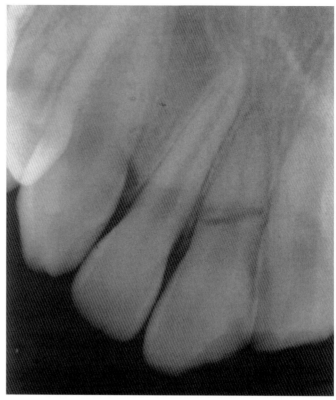

Figure 15.52 Dental radiograph showing root fracture of this chipped, upper central permanent incisor.

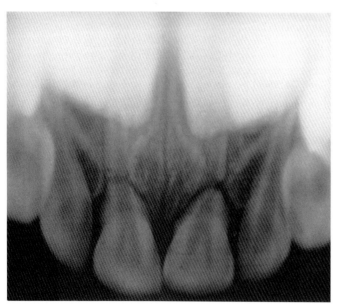

Figure 15.51 Dental radiograph showing fracture of the roots of these primary, central upper incisors.

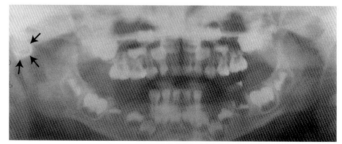

Figure 15.53 Dental panoramic tomograph showing fracture of the right mandibular condyle in a 4-year-old patient.

further radiographs may reveal pulpal obliteration and even signs of apical infection if the tooth loses its vitality.

Fractures of the crown are quite common and radiographic examination in this situation is useful because the stage of root development will be revealed together with some idea regarding the size of the pulp – information that is very helpful to the dentist when considering restorative dental treatment. If there has been partial loss of the crown and laceration of the adjacent soft tissues, particularly the lip, then a soft tissue radiograph is essential in order to ensure that there are no buried fragments that may cause trouble in the future.

Root fractures (Figures 15.51 and 15.52) are less common and the affected tooth will be mobile as with luxation injuries. Intra-oral radiographs are required to diagnose some fractures and sometimes two or even three periapical views, taken using different vertical angulation, are needed to detect these fractures. When assessing periapical radiographs taken for trauma, the radiologist should take care not to confuse superimposed soft tissue shadows such as the lip with root fractures!

Sometimes, trauma results in complete loss of the tooth from the socket – radiographic examination may still be worthwhile in order to confirm that the tooth has actually been lost and not displaced into nearby soft tissues or intruded. If there is uncertainty about whether a displaced tooth might have been inhaled then a chest radiograph is mandatory. Sometimes, these can be very difficult to see and if there is serious concern then the patient should be referred to a paediatrician for possible bronchoscopy.

Fractures of the facial bones in children are infrequent – only about 5% of facial fractures occur in children – the nasal bones and mandible being the usual sites involved. In the mandible, the condyle area (Figure 15.53) is most frequently affected – a dental panoramic tomograph taken in the mouth open position is especially useful for detecting these fractures. Generally, surgical intervention is not required for fractured condyles in children but as a general rule it is advisable for these cases to be assessed by a maxillofacial surgeon.

FURTHER READING

Andreason JO, Andreason FM. Textbook and colour atlas of traumatic injuries to the teeth, 3rd edn. Munksgard, Copenhagen; 1994.

Rowe NL, Williams JL. Maxillofacial injuries, 2nd edn. Edinburgh: Churchill Livingstone; 1994.

White SC, Pharoah MJ. Oral Radiology, 4th edn. St Louis: Mosby; 2000.

Index